LWW PHARMACY TECHNICIAN E

# PRACTICAL PHARMACOLOGY *for the* PHARMACY TECHNICIAN

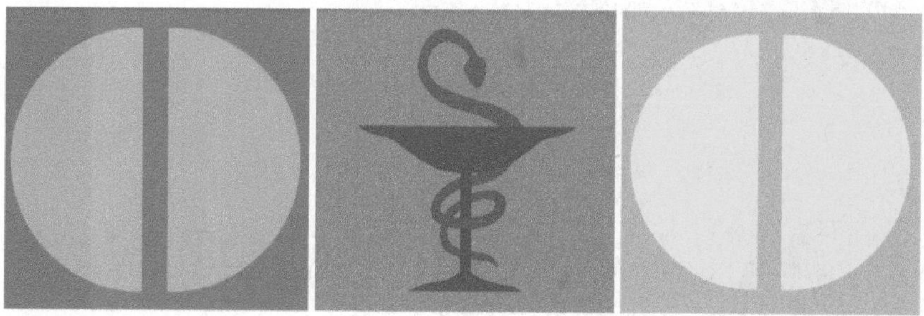

LWW PHARMACY TECHNICIAN EDUCATION SERIES

# PRACTICAL PHARMACOLOGY *for the* PHARMACY TECHNICIAN

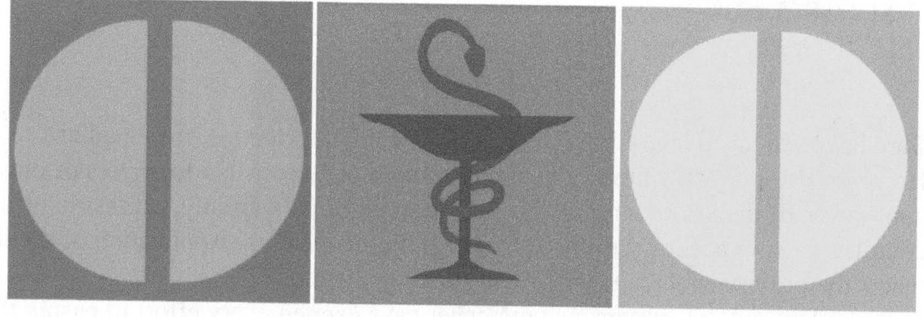

**JOY BELLIS SAKAI,** PHARM D

Instructor, College of the Sequoias
Clinical Pharmacist, Kawea Delta Health Care District
Rx Consultants

Wolters Kluwer Health | Lippincott Williams & Wilkins

Philadelphia • Baltimore • New York • London
Buenos Aires • Hong Kong • Sydney • Tokyo

Executive Editor: John Goucher
Managing Editor: Meredith L. Brittain
Project Editor: Beth Martz
Marketing Manager: Christen D. Murphy
Creative Director: Doug Smock
Production Service: Maryland Composition
Artist: Accurate Art, Inc.


**530 Walnut Street**
**Philadelphia, PA 19106 USA**
**LWW.com**



Library of Congress Cataloging-in-Publication Data

Sakai, Joy Bellis.
Practical pharmacology for the pharmacy technician / Joy Bellis Sakai.—1st ed.
p. ; cm.
Includes bibliographical references and index.
ISBN 978-0-7817-7348-5
1. Pharmacology. 2. Pharmacy technicians. I. Title.
[DNLM: 1. Pharmacists' Aides. 2. Pharmacology—methods. 3. Drug Therapy—methods. 4. Pharmacokinetics.
QV 21.5 S158p 2008]
RM300.S15 1008
615'.1—dc22

2007046068



To purchase additional copies of this book, call our customer service department at (800) 638-3030 or fax orders to (301) 223-2320. International customers should call (301) 223-2300.

Visit Lippincott Williams & Wilkins on the Internet: at LWW.com. Lippincott Williams & Wilkins customer service representatives are available from 8:30 am to 6 pm, EST.

10 9 8 7 6 5 4 3

This book is dedicated to every member of the Bellis-Sakai family tree: the roots that give it strength, the branches that provide shade and shelter, and all the little nuts that give joy and meaning to our lives.

# This Book and the LWW Pharmacy Technician Education Series

*Practical Pharmacology for the Pharmacy Technician* is part of a series of texts that embodies a shift between eras. Previously, on-the-job training of technicians was considered acceptable, but the recent realization of those in the field is that pharmacy technicians must be educated professionals. The changing role of the pharmacist and the emergence of a new definition of pharmaceutical care dictate that competent, well-trained technicians be prepared to assume most of the dispensing functions previously performed by pharmacists. The conceptual organizational approach of the LWW Pharmacy Technician Education Series is to educate the technician as an invaluable member of the pharmacy team and to assist in the development of the decision-making ability required for the technician's practice.

Current texts emphasize the mechanics of performing functions under the direct supervision of a pharmacist. This concept of direct supervision is beginning to change and will continue to evolve as pharmacists assume responsibility for greater numbers of technicians. Technicians need the tools to make important decisions and the confidence to trust their decisions, while retaining the ability to discern when pharmacist consultation is needed. The LWW Pharmacy Technician Education Series is written by premier educators in the field of pharmacy technician education to provide technician students with the confidence-based knowledge required for their practice today and in the future. Each title is accompanied by a strong ancillary package of instructor and student resources.

The following titles will appear in the series:

- *Practical Pharmacology for the Pharmacy Technician,* by Joy Sakai
- *Pharmaceutical Calculations for the Pharmacy Technician,* by Barbara Lacher
- *Standards of Practice for the Pharmacy Technician,* by Mary Mohr
- *Lab Experiences for the Pharmacy Technician,* by Mary Mohr

In *Practical Pharmacology for the Pharmacy Technician*, Joy Sakai, a respected educator with years of experience in pharmacy, nursing, and pharmacy technician education, has presented a complex subject in a format that can be readily understood by the pharmacy technician student. Her experience as a pharmacy practice clinician brings an authenticity to the text, which provides guidance for instructors and facilitates comprehension by the student. This book is an up-to-date, comprehensive pharmacology text that will prepare technician students for their expanded role in pharmacy practice.

Mary E. Mohr

# Preface

Pharmacology is an incredibly complex and rapidly growing field of study. Most pharmacists need reference books of many hundreds of pages to keep up, some of them updated on a monthly basis. New drug approvals continue at a rapid pace, with 22 completely unique prescription drugs added in 2006. The rapid growth in the number of available drug products is accompanied by a rapid increase in information that can impact the practice of both pharmacists and technicians. Partly because of a nationwide shortage of pharmacists, the job of the pharmacy technician is becoming more demanding and is likely to require even more accountability on the part of future technicians.

At present, there is little in the way of regulated structure for pharmacy technician training courses in most states. As instructors of pharmacy technology courses know, students come from a variety of educational backgrounds and most often without experience in a pharmacy practice setting. For pharmacy technician students and their instructors, these factors make learning and teaching pharmacology a challenge. *Practical Pharmacology for the Pharmacy Technician* is designed with these challenges in mind.

The problems encountered over years of teaching pharmacy technician students using other pharmacology texts, which often lack a systematic approach to learning or an application to pharmacy practice, were kept clearly in mind while writing this book. It is written in a narrative style with a natural approach to learning pharmacology and information is tailored to the needs of pharmacy technicians. The highly regarded *Lippincott's Illustrated Review: Pharmacology* originally inspired the organization of this textbook. *Practical Pharmacology for the Pharmacy Technician* is unique among pharmacology books used in technician training programs because of its intuitive approach, with emphasis on drug classes instead of individual drugs. Because technicians can easily integrate information on new drugs into their understanding of a drug class, learning pharmacology in this manner provides technicians with a system that will serve them well into the future.

## Organizational Philosophy

A few fundamental education principles form the foundation for the organization of this textbook. The most profound learning occurs when goals are clearly understood from the beginning, material is organized systematically, and connections are made to past experiences, current knowledge, or to understandable realistic situations. Understanding general principles results in greater retention of related knowledge than does rote memorization of facts without a grasp of fundamental principles. Material that is expressed pictorially as well as verbally will be more accessible to learners with different learning styles. Finally, when students are allowed to pursue in-depth study in areas of their own choosing, they develop interest in the material and will begin to direct their own life-long learning process.

To facilitate learning, units in this book are organized by body systems and drug classes used in diseases of these systems. The most frequently prescribed drugs are emphasized. Each unit begins with a review of foundational knowledge of anatomy and physiology necessary to understand the concepts covered. Drug class discussions include actions and indications, side effects, administration, and specific and practical information useful in the pharmacy workplace. Students are encouraged to learn the most important characteristics of the drug group so that as additional drugs are encountered, educated generalizations can be made. Chapters are sprinkled with real life situations that will connect the material covered with actual experience and emphasize the important role technicians play in the practice of pharmacy. Using the review questions at the end of each chapter will further bolster learning. An open-ended, student-directed opportunity for further inquiry is included with each chapter review to encourage readers to pursue further exploration on the subject of their choosing.

The appendices include answers to the cases in the book, auxiliary prescription drug labels, and a table of error-prone drug names and abbreviations. A glossary of the key terms that are boldfaced in the body of the text is also included. (Answers to the book's review questions are found in the instructor's resources only.)

## Pedagogical Features

Pedagogical features incorporated into this textbook are designed to aid and reinforce student learning. Each chapter includes:

- Chapter objectives: This list of competencies at the beginning of each chapter should be mastered upon the completion of the chapter.
- Drug classes covered: This feature provides an overview of drugs discussed in the chapter, with a brief description of each. Many drugs have multiple uses and are discussed in more than one chapter.
- Key terms: The student must know the basic vocabulary to attain a full understanding of the material. Key terms, which appear at the beginning of the chapter and are highlighted in color throughout the text, are defined in the margins and in the glossary.
- Tips for the technician: This feature provides practical information and application tips geared to the pharmacy technicians' workplace.
- Cases: These real-world situations will stimulate discussion and critical thinking, and encourage students to apply their newly acquired knowledge. Case studies are useful because the reader is asked to take the place of the decision maker to help solve a problem. Although many cases can be answered intuitively by the experienced practitioner, students will, through their reading of the chapter, group discussions, and guiding questions included in the cases, develop decision making processes and the ability to think in terms of the problems that will face them as technicians. Answers to the cases can be found in Appendix A.
- Analogies: These features provide another way of envisioning material.
- Review questions: At the end of each chapter are 20 questions for review, including multiple-choice, true/false, matching, and short answer. Answers to these questions are available to the instructor only.
- For further inquiry: This section gives students the opportunity to extend the depth of their knowledge by exploring a subject related to, but not covered in, the text.

## Illustrations and Tables

To illustrate the textbook, some of the drawings from *Lippincott's Illustrated Review: Pharmacology* have been redesigned for pharmacy technician students' ease in understanding and new illustrations have been added. The illustrations provide pictorial reinforcement of the material covered and are blended with very brief verbal explanations that allow integration of knowledge without constant shifting between text and illustrations. Anatomy and physiology chapters include supporting illustrations of organ structure and function. A table included in each drug class section provides easy access to brand and generic drug names, available formulations, and important additional information for the most frequently used products.

# Student and Instructor Resources

## Student Resources

A Student Resource Center at http://thePoint.lww.com/sakai includes the following materials:

- A Quiz Bank with 370 multiple-choice and true/false questions
- Student worksheets on the topics of abbreviations, conversions, dosage and administration, equations, and prescriptions
- Pharmacology animations
- A Stedman's Audio Glossary of select key terms
- Two supplements to the text on the topics of Topical and Locally Acting Drugs and Complementary and Alternative Medicines
- Suggested additional readings for each of the chapters as well as for the two supplements

## Instructor Resources

We understand the demand on an instructor's time, so to help make your job easier, you will have access to Instructor Resources upon adoption of *Practical Pharmacology for the Pharmacy Technician.* In addition to the student resources just listed, an Instructor's Resource Center at http://thePoint.lww.com/sakai includes the following:

- A Test Generator with 740 multiple-choice questions
- PowerPoint slides for every chapter
- Hands-on activities for most of the chapters and for the two supplements, as well as comments on those activities
- An Image Bank that contains the figures and tables from the textbook and the two supplements
- WebCT/Blackboard-ready cartridge
- Answers to the review questions found in the text and in the two supplements
- Answer key to student worksheets
- Answers to the case studies found in the two supplements

Quiz bank and test generator questions by Cristina Kaiser, CPhT, MA. PowerPoint slides by Betty J. Klein, MS, RN.

# Summary

This textbook is not intended to be a reference for pharmacy practice but rather an organized approach for learning the basic pharmacology required by pharmacy technicians.The dynamic nature of the pharmaceutical industry and pharmacy practice prevents any textbook from being fully inclusive of every drug product or absolutely accurate by the time it is published. Although every conceivable effort has been made to present accurate information, the author makes no warrant, implied or otherwise, as to the accuracy of the information contained herein.

*Practical Pharmacology for the Pharmacy Technician* is designed to assist student learning while providing instructors with a comprehensive approach to teaching basic pharmacology. My experience teaching pharmacology to pharmacy technicians informs the organization and approach to learning presented in this textbook, but it is also the product of 30 years of clinical pharmacy practice and many years of instruction to pharmacy and nursing students. Every effort was made by the publishing team to create a practical and informative tool for learning pharmacology. It is my sincere hope that we have succeeded.

# Acknowledgments

Writing a book is a little bit like climbing a mountain; it requires planning, preparing for the unexpected, plenty of encouragement, hard work, and guides to get you through the rough terrain that is certain to be part of any such journey. In short, it requires teamwork, and I will be forever grateful to everyone who contributed to this project. The entire team at Lippincott Williams and Wilkins deserves a big "thank you!" Among others, David Troy, Barrett Koger, Matt Hauber, and my managing editor for most of the project, Meredith Brittain, are experienced professionals, readily available with answers when I had questions, and capable of handholding when necessary. The editorial reviewers for this text provided ideas and constructive criticism for every chapter. I thank them for their many contributions that ultimately resulted in a better book.

A number of my colleagues came to my aid by reading chapters, reviewing the content when I felt I needed the additional input, and helping in other ways. My thanks go to Ray Vella, Pharm D; Leland Beggs, MD; Celeste Riley, RPh; Bill Koole, Pharm D; Steve Waite, Pharm D; Gale Thomas CPhT; and pharmacy staff members at both Children's Hospital of Central California and Kaweah Delta Health Care District. Thanks go to my sisters-in-spirit, Cathy, Charlene, Char, Mary Ann, and Susan for their unbridled enthusiasm and moral support throughout what sometimes seemed like an endless project.

By the time I was 5 years old, I knew I wanted to become a pharmacist. My father was a pharmacist, and some mornings he would take me to the drug store with him. On busy days I would dust shelves and stay out of the way. When the day was quiet, my dad would set me on the counter and let me count the medicine, although I was always a little insulted to see him rechecking my work. In a family-run business, everyone helps out, and my sisters and brother and I spent many vacations and holidays decorating the drug store, working the register, wrapping gifts, and delivering prescriptions. Just like the family efforts of my past, writing this book was, more than anything else, a family effort. My brother Will and sisters Pam and Diane provided emotional support throughout these many months of work, and graciously excused me for not making appearances when I should have.

I am fortunate to have children and a husband who could and did provide expertise in a variety of ways. Our daughter Rebecca, now a veterinarian, edited many chapters and contributed hundreds of chapter review questions while still in veterinary school. Rachel, a graphic artist, gave up hours of potential "travel time" to create a number of concept designs and completed illustrations for the book, and to contribute editorial advice and parts of the glossary. Our son Russell, while in his third year as a biochemistry major at the University of California, contributed chapter review questions and plenty of computer technical support. Most of all my long-time husband and partner, Richard I. Sakai, Pharm D, put up with my nearly complete abandonment of the house and our social life so that I could write this book. He gave me ideas for cases, read chapters, provided access to knowledgeable staff members, arranged for dinner, and made tea for 2 years running, without complaint. I could not have done this without you—thank you all!

Joy Bellis Sakai, Pharm D

# Reviewers

**Jane Alcorn, DVM, PhD**
Associate Professor of Pharmacy
College of Pharmacy and Nutrition
University of Saskatchewan
Saskatoon, Saskatchewan, Canada

**Eric L. Barker, PhD**
Assistant Dean for Graduate Programs
Associate Professor of Medicinal Chemistry and Molecular Pharmacology
College of Pharmacy, Nursing, and Health Sciences
Purdue University
West Lafayette, Indiana

**Bobbi Chacon**
Everest College at Alhambra
Alhambra, California

**Scott Higgins, MA**
Chair, Pharmacy Department
Technology Education College
Columbus, Ohio

**Joycelyn D. Moore, CPhT, MS**
Health Science Education
Florida Metropolitan University
Tampa, Florida

**Gloria Pring**
Chair, Pharmacy Department
National Institute of Technology
Cross Lanes, West Virginia

**Anne Redmond, BA**
Hospital Technician Instructor
Baker College
Flint, Michigan

**Douglas Scribner, CPhT, BA**
Pharmacy Technician Program Chair
Central New Mexico Community College
Albuquerque, New Mexico

**Cynthia Lynn Speetzen-Thoma, AA, CPhT**
Pharmacy Technician Program Director/Instructor
Silicon Valley College
Walnut Creek, California

# User's Guide

This User's Guide introduces you to the many features of *Practical Pharmacology for the Pharmacy Technician*. Taking full advantage of these features, you'll discover how drugs affect human function. Moreover, they'll help you perform the duties of a pharmacy technician correctly and safely.

Each chapter is loaded with features that help you focus on the key points, quickly develop your knowledge, and put your new knowledge into practice.

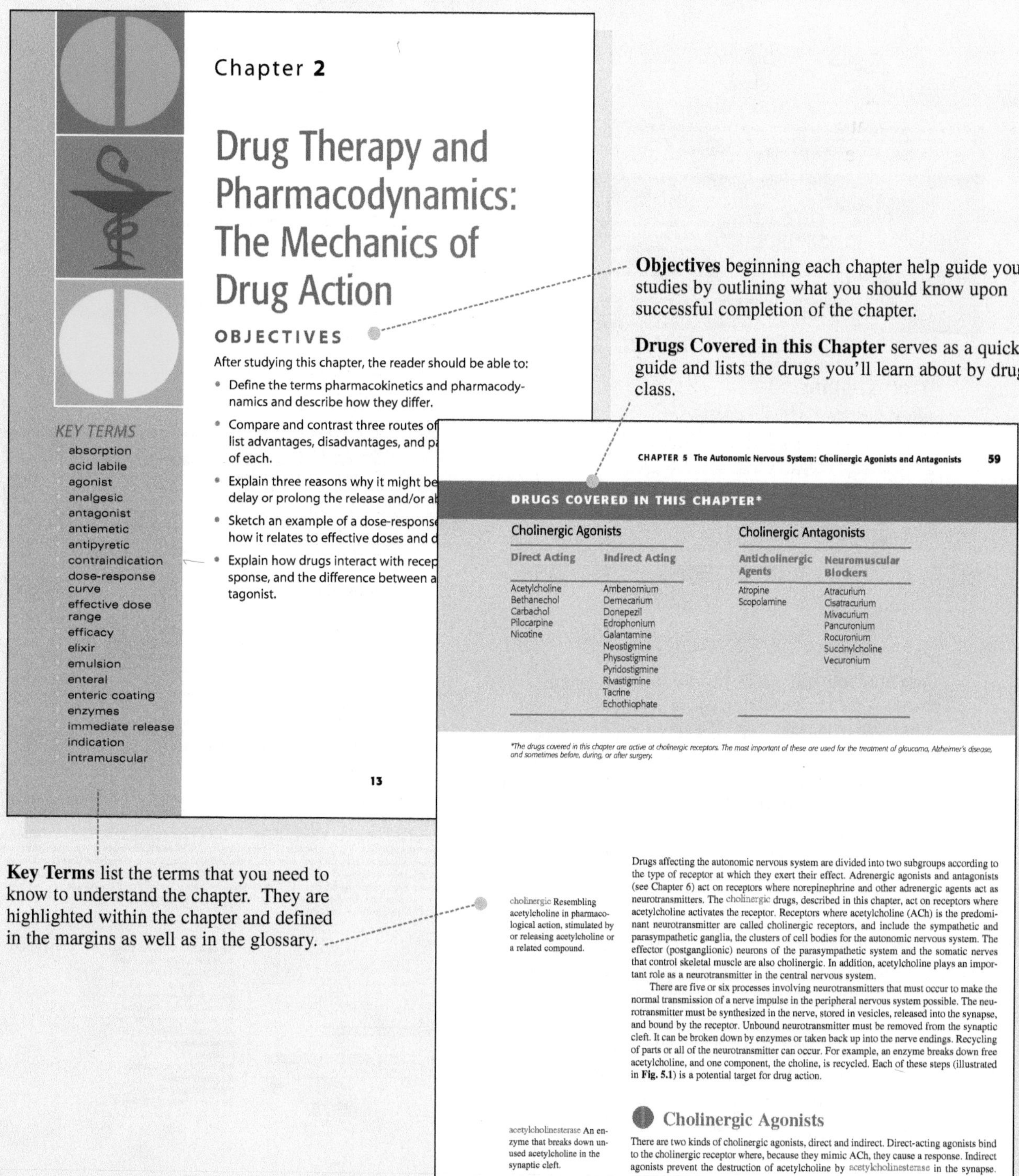

Chapter **2**

Drug Therapy and Pharmacodynamics: The Mechanics of Drug Action

OBJECTIVES

After studying this chapter, the reader should be able to:

- Define the terms pharmacokinetics and pharmacodynamics and describe how they differ.
- Compare and contrast three routes of list advantages, disadvantages, and p of each.
- Explain three reasons why it might be delay or prolong the release and/or a
- Sketch an example of a dose-respons how it relates to effective doses and
- Explain how drugs interact with recep sponse, and the difference between a tagonist.

KEY TERMS

absorption
acid labile
agonist
analgesic
antagonist
antiemetic
antipyretic
contraindication
dose-response curve
effective dose range
efficacy
elixir
emulsion
enteral
enteric coating
enzymes
immediate release
indication
intramuscular

13

CHAPTER 5 The Autonomic Nervous System: Cholinergic Agonists and Antagonists 59

DRUGS COVERED IN THIS CHAPTER*

| Cholinergic Agonists | | Cholinergic Antagonists | |
|---|---|---|---|
| Direct Acting | Indirect Acting | Anticholinergic Agents | Neuromuscular Blockers |
| Acetylcholine<br>Bethanechol<br>Carbachol<br>Pilocarpine<br>Nicotine | Ambenonium<br>Demecarium<br>Donepezil<br>Edrophonium<br>Galantamine<br>Neostigmine<br>Physostigmine<br>Pyridostigmine<br>Rivastigmine<br>Tacrine<br>Echothiophate | Atropine<br>Scopolamine | Atracurium<br>Cisatracurium<br>Mivacurium<br>Pancuronium<br>Rocuronium<br>Succinylcholine<br>Vecuronium |

*The drugs covered in this chapter are active at cholinergic receptors. The most important of these are used for the treatment of glaucoma, Alzheimer's disease, and sometimes before, during, or after surgery.

cholinergic Resembling acetylcholine in pharmacological action, stimulated by or releasing acetylcholine or a related compound.

Drugs affecting the autonomic nervous system are divided into two subgroups according to the type of receptor at which they exert their effect. Adrenergic agonists and antagonists (see Chapter 6) act on receptors where norepinephrine and other adrenergic agents act as neurotransmitters. The cholinergic drugs, described in this chapter, act on receptors where acetylcholine activates the receptor. Receptors where acetylcholine (ACh) is the predominant neurotransmitter are called cholinergic receptors, and include the sympathetic and parasympathetic ganglia, the clusters of cell bodies for the autonomic nervous system. The effector (postganglionic) neurons of the parasympathetic system and the somatic nerves that control skeletal muscle are also cholinergic. In addition, acetylcholine plays an important role as a neurotransmitter in the central nervous system.

There are five or six processes involving neurotransmitters that must occur to make the normal transmission of a nerve impulse in the peripheral nervous system possible. The neurotransmitter must be synthesized in the nerve, stored in vesicles, released into the synapse, and bound by the receptor. Unbound neurotransmitter must be removed from the synaptic cleft. It can be broken down by enzymes or taken back up into the nerve endings. Recycling of parts or all of the neurotransmitter can occur. For example, an enzyme breaks down free acetylcholine, and one component, the choline, is recycled. Each of these steps (illustrated in **Fig. 5.1**) is a potential target for drug action.

acetylcholinesterase An enzyme that breaks down unused acetylcholine in the synaptic cleft.

Cholinergic Agonists

There are two kinds of cholinergic agonists, direct and indirect. Direct-acting agonists bind to the cholinergic receptor where, because they mimic ACh, they cause a response. Indirect agonists prevent the destruction of acetylcholine by acetylcholinesterase in the synapse.

**Objectives** beginning each chapter help guide your studies by outlining what you should know upon successful completion of the chapter.

**Drugs Covered in this Chapter** serves as a quick guide and lists the drugs you'll learn about by drug class.

**Key Terms** list the terms that you need to know to understand the chapter. They are highlighted within the chapter and defined in the margins as well as in the glossary.

CHAPTER 5 The Autonomic Nervous System: Cholinergic Agonists and Antagonists 73

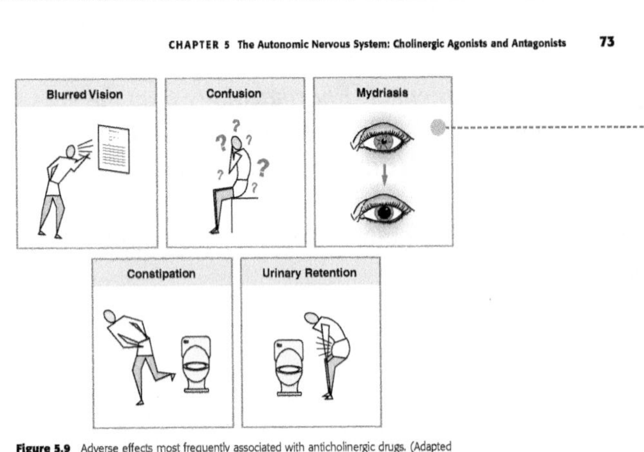


**Figure 5.9** Adverse effects most frequently associated with anticholinergic drugs. (Adapted with permission from Harvey RA, Champe PC, Howland RD, et al. *Lippincott's Illustrated Reviews: Pharmacology*, 3rd ed. Baltimore: Lippincott Williams & Wilkins, 2006.)

**Side Effect Figures** offer simple illustrations of common adverse effects that you need to remember.

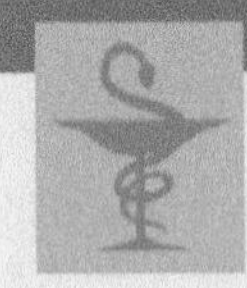

Tips for the Technician

Patient profiles usually contain information about clients' diagnoses. It is important to alert the pharmacist of a diagnosis of glaucoma or benign prostatic hypertrophy (a common condition in men that causes bladder obstruction) on the profile of a patient that brings in a prescription for a product containing belladonna alkaloids, or other anticholinergic agents. These drugs are contraindicated in glaucoma and benign prostatic hypertrophy.

Hospital pharmacy technicians are often responsible for setting up the trays of emergency medications that are kept in "crash carts," the carts equipped with emergency supplies that are wheeled to cardiac and respiratory emergencies. Atropine is always included, but a number of strengths and sizes are available from manufacturers. To avoid errors, use a double-checking process before the pharmacist checks the trays.

**Tips for the Technician** offer you practical application tips specifically written for pharmacy technicians.

Neuromuscular Blocking Agents

Early in the nineteenth century, Sir Walter Raleigh and other European explorers witnessed the use of poisoned arrows and darts for hunting by the native people of South America. The tips of the arrows were dipped in a dark, sticky paste made from the bark of native plants of the loganaceae family. Minutes after the arrows pierced the animals they were dead. Much later, pharmacologists identified the plant alkaloids in arrow poisons as curare and tubocurarine, examples of neuromuscular blocking agents. The arrow poison works by paralyzing skeletal muscles (including the muscles involved in respiration) until the animals die of lack of oxygen.

CHAPTER 8 Central Nervous System Depressants: The Anxiolytic and Hypnotic Drugs 119

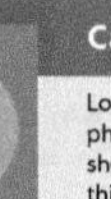

Case 8.1

Long ago and far away, an eager intern pharmacist, excited about practicing clinical pharmacy, took it upon herself to counsel every patient about all new prescriptions she dispensed in the pharmacy where she worked, although the law did not require this at the time. Her employer barely tolerated this practice and the pharmacy clerk routinely smirked during her discussions with patients, until the Valium® incident.

On this occasion, a patient (call him Mr. Sweet) came in with a new prescription for diazepam, which the intern carefully filled and had checked. She reviewed the risks of taking the medication with the patient, including the possibility of drowsiness and the additive effect of taking other CNS depressants, and especially warned him about alcohol. Mr. Sweet appeared unimpressed and only half listened, and claimed he wasn't much of a drinker.

The following Monday Mr. Sweet came back into the pharmacy, looking rather sheepish. He asked to speak to the pharmacist in charge, and thanked him effusively for the intern's warning, which unfortunately, he disregarded. That weekend he had taken his diazepam as directed, but went to visit friends for a barbecue, and consumed a couple of beers. On his way home he made a right turn into his driveway, or so he thought. Actually, he missed the driveway, ran over the curb, and on through his neighbor's living room window. Fortunately, no one was hurt. Nobody in the pharmacy ever snickered about the intern's enthusiasm again either.

What could have been the result in this situation if the patient had not been counseled? Whose responsibility is it to make sure patients are informed about the risks of taking prescription medications?

**Case Studies** place you in the role of a practicing pharmacy technician, asking you to apply your knowledge to manage a specific situation. Answers to case studies are in Appendix A.

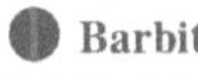

## Barbiturates

The barbiturates were formerly the mainstay of treatment of anxiety and insomnia. Today, they have been largely replaced by the benzodiazepines. This is because the barbiturates induce tolerance, and cause physical dependence associated with severe withdrawal symptoms when the drug is discontinued. Furthermore, they cause coma in toxic doses. For many years they were the agents of choice for people trying to commit suicide. Now, prescribing and dispensing of the most dangerous barbiturates is tightly controlled. Three barbiturates are still widely used in medicine for conditions other than anxiety or as sedatives. Thiopental and methohexital (Brevital®) are used for anesthesia, and phenobarbital is often prescribed for the treatment of seizure disorders.

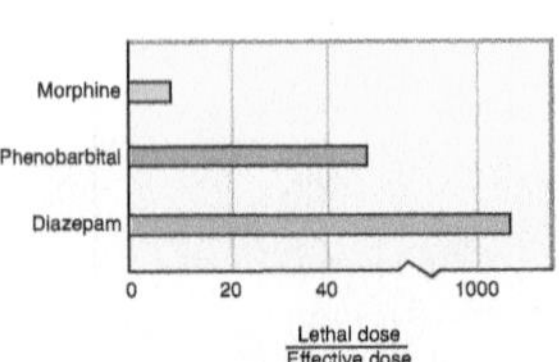


**Figure 8.3** The relative safety of the benzodiazepines as compared to morphine and phenobarbital. The graph shows the relationship between lethal dose and effective dose. The lethal dose of diazepam is more than 1,000 times the effective dose. (Adapted with permission from Harvey RA, Champe PC, Howland RD, et al. *Lippincott's Illustrated Reviews: Pharmacology*, 3rd ed. Baltimore: Lippincott Williams & Wilkins, 2006.)

248 Practical Pharmacology for the Pharmacy Technician

Table 16.2 Summary of Drugs Used for Angina, with Available Formulations and Indications.

| Generic | Brand Name | Available as | Indications | Notes |
|---|---|---|---|---|
| **Nitrates** | | | | |
| Isosorbide dinitrate | Isordil® | Tablets, ER tabs, ER capsules, chewable | Angina prophylaxis | Not for acute angina |
| Isosorbide mononitrate | Imdur®, Monoket® | Tablets, ER tablets | Angina prophylaxis | Not for acute angina |
| Nitroglycerin | Nitrostat®, Nitrodur®, others | Sublingual tabs, ER tabs and caps, ointment, IV transdermal patches, buccal tabs | Acute angina, Angina prophylaxis hypertension | Spray, sublingual for acute attacks, IV for HF |
| **Beta-Blockers** | | | | |
| Acebutolol | Sectral® | Capsules | PVCs, angina | Not 1st choice for angina |
| Atenolol | Tenormin® | Tablets, injection | HTN, angina, atrial arrhythmias | Useful after MI |
| Metoprolol | Lopressor®, Toprol® | Tablets, ER tabs, injection | Angina, post MI, hypertension, | |
| Propranolol | Inderal® | Tablets, oral soln, injection ER capsules | Angina, post MI, hypertension, others | |
| **Calcium Channel Blockers** | | | | |
| Amlodipine | Norvasc® | Tablets | Chronic angina, HTN | |
| Diltiazem | Dilacor®, Cardizem® | Tablets, ER tabs and capsules | Chronic angina, HTN, arrhythmias | Vasospastic and chronic angina |
| Nicardipine | Cardene® | Capsules, ER capsules, injection | Hypertension, chronic angina | Regular release for angina |
| Nifedipine | Procardia®, Adalat® | Capsules, ER tablets | Angina, hypertension | |
| Verapamil | Calan®, Isoptin® | Tablets, ER tabs & capsules, injection | Angina, HTN, arrhythmias | For all variants of angina |

ER, extended release; HF, heart failure; HTN, Hypertension; MI, Myocardial Infarction; PVC, premature ventricular contraction.

erance to this effect. High doses of organic nitrates can also cause postural hypotension, facial flushing, and tachycardia. Patients using sublingual tablets may experience some burning under the tongue with use. Headache and other side effects are a direct result of the vasodilation caused by the nitrates.

Tolerance to the actions of nitrates develops rapidly, and the blood vessels become less responsive to the vasodilating effects. Although a number of drug combinations have been used to try to prevent tolerance, the only sure way tolerance can be avoided is by provid-

**Comparison Tables** in each drug class section provide easy access to brand and generic drug names, available formulations, and additional key information.

**Analogies** offer creative and alternative ways to help you understand key concepts.

## Analogy

When we were young, we played a game called "red light, green light." To play this game, a leader is chosen, who will act as the "light" and the rest of the players line up and follow directions. When the leader turns to face the group, she says "red light" and no one can move. When she turns her back on the group, she says "green light" and players can move forward at will. Now, imagine a cardiac version of this game. All the players (and there are thousands of them) are in a circle, and when the leader says "green light," everyone takes two steps, in unison, towards the center of the circle (contraction of the myocardium). When the leader says "red light" everyone takes two steps out, and rests for a moment before the green light (relaxation of the myocardium). But what if, after about the ten millionth round, a couple of wise-guys in the circle got bored and gave the "green light" signal between the leader's signals? Undoubtedly, some of the players who become confused will step forward at the wrong time and generate disorganization among the players. Perhaps the group nearest the leader would follow her commands, while the people near the troublemakers would follow their signal. Worst of all, mass confusion might ensue, with no one moving on command at all. In this analogy, the players represent myocardial cells and the leader represents the SA node. The players who try to take the leader's role represent cells with abnormal automaticity that can trigger arrhythmias, a form of myocardial confusion and disorganization.

## FOR FURTHER INQUIRY

Go to the American Heart Association web site and investigate the Advanced Cardiac Life Support treatment recommendations for one of the arrhythmias discussed here. What is always the first treatment instituted? If you found someone unconscious would you know what to do? Contact your local hospital, Red Cross, or Heart Association and find out if there are basic life support classes available to the public at no cost. If you do not already have a basic life support card, consider taking a class.

**For Further Inquiry** enables you to extend your knowledge by exploring subjects related to, but not covered in the text.

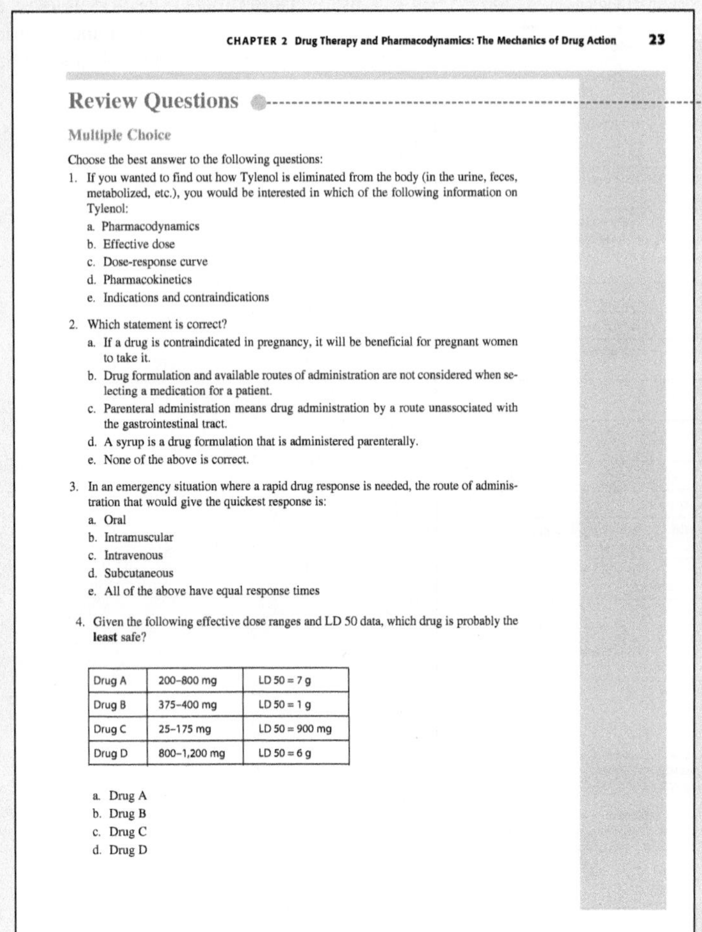

CHAPTER 2 Drug Therapy and Pharmacodynamics: The Mechanics of Drug Action 23

Review Questions

Multiple Choice

Choose the best answer to the following questions:

1. If you wanted to find out how Tylenol is eliminated from the body (in the urine, feces, metabolized, etc.), you would be interested in which of the following information on Tylenol:
   a. Pharmacodynamics
   b. Effective dose
   c. Dose-response curve
   d. Pharmacokinetics
   e. Indications and contraindications
2. Which statement is correct?
   a. If a drug is contraindicated in pregnancy, it will be beneficial for pregnant women to take it.
   b. Drug formulation and available routes of administration are not considered when selecting a medication for a patient.
   c. Parenteral administration means drug administration by a route unassociated with the gastrointestinal tract.
   d. A syrup is a drug formulation that is administered parenterally.
   e. None of the above is correct.
3. In an emergency situation where a rapid drug response is needed, the route of administration that would give the quickest response is:
   a. Oral
   b. Intramuscular
   c. Intravenous
   d. Subcutaneous
   e. All of the above have equal response times
4. Given the following effective dose ranges and LD 50 data, which drug is probably the **least** safe?

| | | |
|---|---|---|
| Drug A | 200–800 mg | LD 50 = 7 g |
| Drug B | 375–400 mg | LD 50 = 1 g |
| Drug C | 25–175 mg | LD 50 = 900 mg |
| Drug D | 800–1,200 mg | LD 50 = 6 g |

   a. Drug A
   b. Drug B
   c. Drug C
   d. Drug D

**Review Questions** at the end of each chapter help you assess your grasp of the material as you advance in the text.

# Additional Learning and Teaching Resources

This textbook features a companion website: http://thepoint.lww.com/sakai

## Student Resource Center

- Chapter quizzes
- Worksheets
- Animations
- Stedman's audio glossary
- Full text online

## Instructor's Resource Center

- Test generator
- Image collection
- PowerPoint presentations
- Answers to questions and worksheets
- Hands-on activities

# Contents

UNIT I

# Introduction to Pharmacology

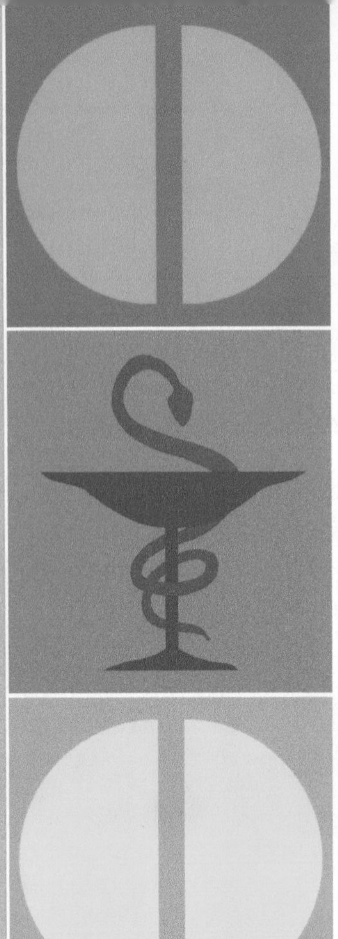

Chapter 1

# Pharmacology and Pharmacy: Past, Present, and Future

## OBJECTIVES

After studying this chapter, the reader should be able to:

- Define the term pharmacology.
- List three significant turning points in the development of Western medicine and discuss why they are important.
- Explain why drug therapy can never be both completely safe and effective.
- Define the terms: chemical name, generic name, and trade name and describe the purpose of each name.
- Compare the role of the pharmacist and the pharmacy technician in the delivery of pharmaceutical care.

## KEY TERMS

- adverse drug event
- adverse effect
- antimicrobial
- cardiac glycoside
- cathartic
- chemical name
- drug
- enantiomer
- generic name
- materia medica
- noncompliance
- pharmaceutical care
- pharmacology
- pharmacopoeia
- stereoisomer
- therapeutic effect

The word pharmacology is derived from the Greek word *pharmakon* meaning remedy, and the suffix *-logy*, meaning the study of. No one knows what motivated the first human to try to treat an illness, but it is easy to imagine that ancient people inhabited a world filled with risks. They would have been familiar with pain, injuries, burns, wounds, infections, and many of the same diseases that plague humankind today. Perhaps some lucky accident or possibly the observation of animal behavior led the first human to apply cool mud to a burn, or a medicinal herb to a cut. Whatever the origin, there is ample evidence to demonstrate that humankind has a long history of treating ailments.

pharmacology The study of drugs, including their origin, composition, actions, uses, and side effects.

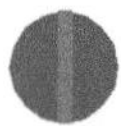

## A Brief History of Pharmacology

In the worldview of prehistoric societies, events and occurrences were linked to spirits. Since disease was thought to be an invasion of evil spirits, spiritual leaders such as shaman or medicine men were responsible for treatment. The healer might perform an incantation or hang a special healing amulet around the patient's neck. Perhaps he would burn an aromatic plant for the patient to inhale in order to drive out the evil spirit. Magic and spiritual beliefs were the most potent treatments available to prehistoric societies.

As human society became more advanced, written language developed, as did our ability to connect an action with a subsequent response. Magic and spiritualism still played a central role in healing, but humans were becoming more dependent on the use of medicinal compounds for treatment of disease. Archeologists have discovered clay tablets from ancient Mesopotamian societies (two to three thousand years before the Common Era) with directions for making medicinal infusions and extracts. Use of cathartics, such as senna or castor oil is documented in both ancient Egypt and Mesopotamia. More than 250 different drugs of plant origin, 120 of mineral origin, and 180 from other sources were identified in written artifacts from these cultures. Materials were boiled, pulverized, filtered or extracted, and mixed in bases of oil, alcohol, wine, fat, honey, milk, or wax for medicinal use.

cathartic A medication used to stimulate the clearing of the intestinal contents.

Similar approaches of treating illness can be found in ancient Chinese and Indian societies of about the same time period as the Mesopotamian culture. These cultures studied plants and other medicinals and collected data on their appropriate applications. They recorded this information in what is referred to as a materia medica, the equivalent of a modern formulary, or listing of available medications.

materia medica Materials used in the composition of remedies, also a general term for all the substances used as curative agents in medicine.

The ancient Greeks fostered and nurtured a rational approach to medicine. They looked for physical causes of disease rather than spiritual. This rational approach to diagnosis and treatment became the basis for Western medicine as it is practiced today. Although it was based on an incomplete and inaccurate understanding of the human body, Hippocrates (probably born in 460 BCE), who founded this rational approach, directed treatment based on a diagnosis of the four "humors," phlegm, blood, black bile, and yellow bile. For example, fever and sweats were thought to be caused by an excess of blood, the humor associated with heat and moisture. The prescription for this condition might be leeches, to remove blood. As a logical outcome of too much of a certain "humor" cathartics, emetics, diuretics, and expectorants were identified and used.

The most significant contribution of all the ancients to pharmacology was made by Dioscorides in 50 to 70 AD (**Fig. 1.1**). Dioscorides, often considered the father of pharmacy, wrote *de Materia Medica*, a compilation of information on more than 600 plants, 35 animal products, and 90 minerals for medicinal use. His work was unique because he included botanical descriptions and information on habitats and harvesting, as well as descriptions of use, side effects, dosages, and directions for preparation and storage of remedies. *De Materia Medica* was the essential medicinal authority for more than 1,500 years.

As scientific inquiry became more knowledge-based, understanding of chemistry, anatomy, and physiology expanded quickly, especially during and after the Renaissance. Tools became more advanced, and discovery of the cause of a disease uncovered opportunities to find specific treatments. Anton van Leeuwenhoek, who is credited with inventing the first truly useful microscope in the 1670s, was the first to see microscopic organisms in pond water. Eventually the "germ theory" of disease was proposed, suggesting that mi-

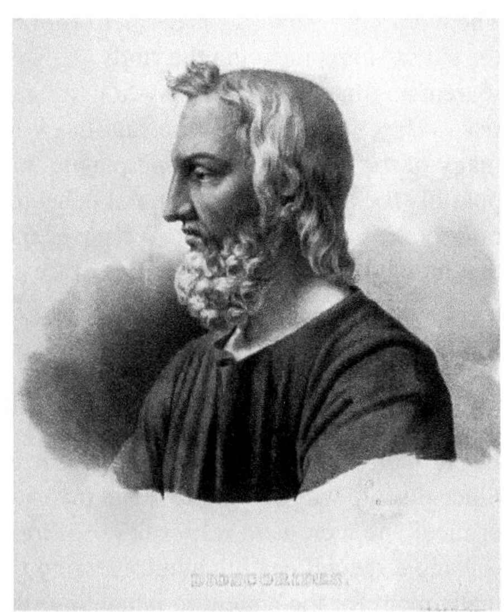

**Figure 1.1** Dioscorides, considered the father of pharmacy, wrote *de Materia Medica*, the most important source of information on medicinals for more than 1,500 years. (Courtesy of the National Library of Medicine, available on-line at http://www.ihm.nlm.nih.gov/.)

crobes cause infectious diseases. This proved to be the most important and revolutionary idea in pharmacology because, once accepted, the germ theory led to the discovery and use of antibiotics, saving millions of lives in the process.

Two centuries after van Leeuwenhoek, Louis Pasteur proved that specific microbes cause infectious diseases and used this research to encourage cleanliness in medical practice. Edward Jenner (1796) and Pasteur (1881) were responsible for developing the earliest vaccines to prevent communicable diseases. In the early 20th century, Paul Ehrlich began the search for chemical compounds designed to kill or inhibit infectious organisms without harming the body. He coined the term "chemotherapy" to describe the idea of using chemistry to design a medication specific to the treatment of a particular illness without causing unwanted effects. In 1908 Ehrlich discovered that the arsenic compound arsphenamine could be effectively used to treat syphilis. Not long after, sulfanilamide, the first sulfa antimicrobial, and penicillin were discovered and put to use.

antimicrobial A drug used to kill, or suppress the growth of, micro-organisms.

pharmacopoeia A book describing the drugs and preparations used in medicine, usually issued by an officially recognized authority, and serving as a standard.

While new drugs were being created, many older remedies were discarded from pharmacopoeias when judicious observation led to the realization that they didn't work or might even do harm. Oliver Wendell Holmes, renowned American physician and poet of the 19th century, wrote "I firmly believe that if the whole materia medica, as now used, could be sunk to the bottom of the sea, it would be all the better for mankind—and all the worse for the fishes" (Massengill SE. *A Sketch of Medicine and Pharmacy*. Bristol, Tennessee: SE Massengill Company, 1943.)

As newer, more specific treatments, like arsphenamine, were put to use, patients who might have died from disease were saved, only to suffer severe toxicity or death due to drug therapy. It became apparent that the ideal of treating disease without ever causing harm to the patient was unrealistic.

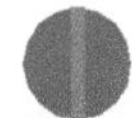

## Risks of Drug Therapy

drug Any compound taken with the intent to alter some form or function of the body or treat a disease.

therapeutic effect The positive, or desirable, effect expected to occur when a drug is administered.

adverse effect An unwanted or dangerous reaction to a drug.

Simply defined, the word drug means any compound taken with the intent to alter some form or function of the body, or treat a disease. It is important to remember that no drug has just one specific effect. Any drug with a therapeutic effect on the body also has potential for adverse effects (undesirable effects). Some compounds studied as potential drugs have no desirable effects, and still have unwanted effects. More often, a compound has desirable effects, but is unacceptably toxic. Some drugs have an acceptable balance of desirable effects with an acceptable rate of undesirable effects, and it is these that are most likely to make it to the consumer. It is important to remember that a drug that is purported to have no side effects undoubtedly has no salutary effects either.

In the early 20th century, remedies could be marketed to the public without any proof that they were either safe or effective. The Food, Drug, and Cosmetic Act, passed in 1938, was the first piece of legislation that required drugs to be proven safe before marketing. It was passed because more than 100 people died from taking the life-saving sulfa antimicrobial drug, sulfanilamide, in a new formulation that had recently been marketed. The S. E. Massengill Company decided to market a liquid formulation of sulfanilamide, and found that it would dissolve in diethylene glycol. Diethylene glycol is familiar to us as antifreeze, a compound we all recognize as highly toxic. Because there was no requirement for testing the safety of drugs, this product was released in 1937, and was withdrawn within 2 months because of the deaths. This event gave Congress the impetus to reinforce the authority of the fledgling Food and Drug Administration (FDA), and to charge it with protecting the public from unsafe and improperly labeled drugs. However, the best efforts of science, pharmaceutical companies, health professionals, and oversight organizations like the FDA cannot make drug therapy risk-free.

Consider the case of thalidomide, introduced to Europe in 1958 for use as a sleep aid and to prevent nausea in pregnancy. It was marketed as a "harmless" sleep inducer that provided a normal night's sleep. Over the next 3 years, European physicians noted a surge of severe limb deformities in newborns, called phocomelia (**Fig. 1.2**). Through the efforts of several European physicians, the connection between these birth defects and the mother's use of thalidomide in the first three months of pregnancy became established. Fortunately for Americans, thalidomide was never approved for use in the United States because of suspicions within the FDA that it was not safe.

The goal of developing perfectly targeted drugs that treat disease without causing side effects (Paul Ehrlich's concept of chemotherapy), the pharmaceutical "magic bullet," has remained elusive. In its efforts to protect the public from dangerous medicines, FDA regulations require drug manufacturers to do extensive clinical testing on animals and large numbers of both healthy and ill patients before drugs are approved for marketing. The studies are designed to explore the actions of the drug in the body, prove their efficacy, and look for potential side effects. Before they can be marketed, the FDA reviews the studies, and decides if the benefit of the drug outweighs its associated risks (**Fig. 1.3**). Because of this process, it can take ten or more years and cost as much as a billion dollars to bring a truly unique compound to consumers.

Increasingly stringent testing to prove drug safety and efficacy does not guarantee that all potentially grave adverse drug effects will be discovered before FDA approval. Vioxx® and Bextra®, two commonly prescribed pain medications, were removed from American

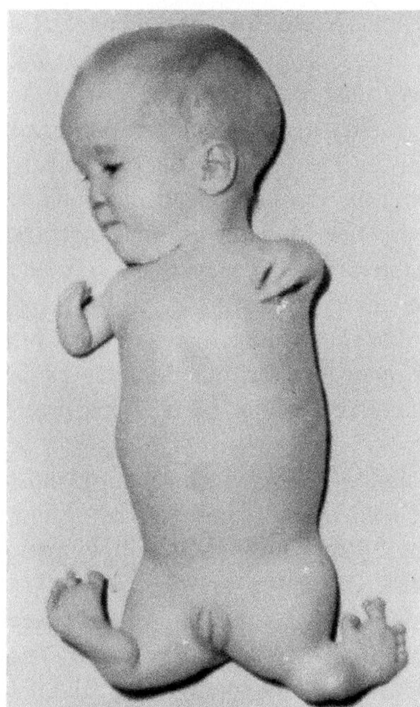

**Figure 1.2** An infant born with phocomelia. (Reprinted with permission from Sadler T. *Langman's Medical Embryology*, 9th ed. Baltimore: Lippincott Williams & Wilkins, 2003.)

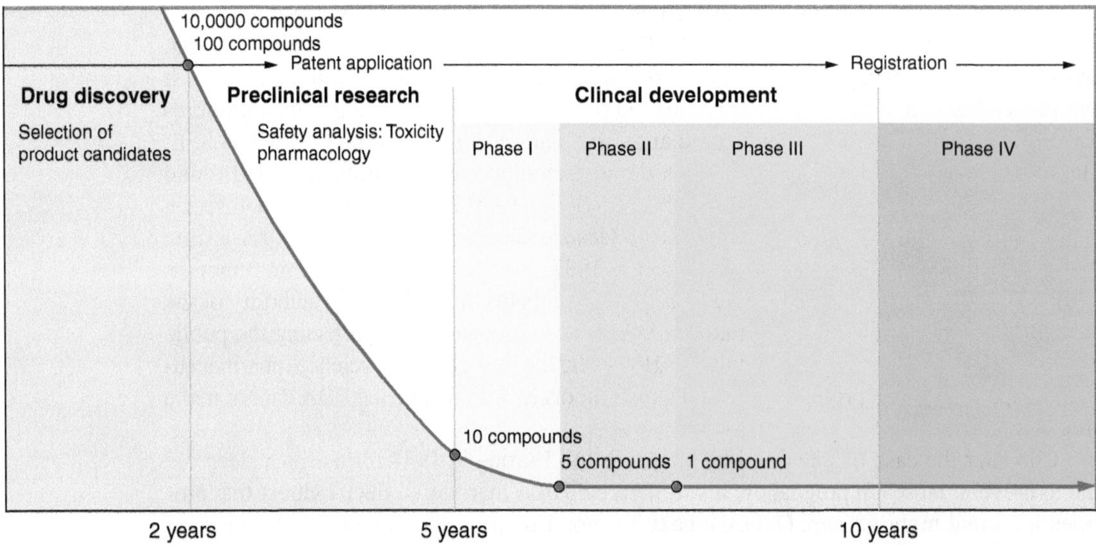


**Figure 1.3** The stages of new drug development with typical time periods required for drug approval. The pharmaceutical industry estimates that they study 10,000 compounds for every one approved drug. (Adapted with permission from F. Hoffmann-LaRoche Ltd.)

pharmacy shelves more than four years after their approval because of unacceptably high risks in certain patients who took the medication. Some side effects go undiscovered in premarketing studies because they are rare. Very serious side effects may only occur once in every 10,000 to 100,000 patients treated, so are difficult to connect to the drug that may be the cause. Because side effects can be rare and difficult to identify, and because drugs have multiple effects, we must accept that there can never be a completely safe and effective drug.

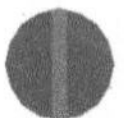

## The Pharmacopoeia Today

chemical name The proper scientific name, based on the chemical structure, for a drug.

generic name Nonproprietary name assigned to a drug or chemical recommended or recognized by an official body.

In order to understand the medications currently available, it is important to understand how they are named. Before a drug is approved for use, it is given at least two names and sometimes three or more different names. The chemical name is derived systematically from the chemical structure of the compound.The chemical name is universally recognized. The generic name is the nonproprietary name recognized in the United States by the United States Pharmacopoeia (USP) and the National Formulary (NF), the official national standard-setting authorities. The generic name usually refers in some way to the pharmaceutical class of the drug. When a manufacturer holds a patent on newer drugs, they assign proprietary, or brand (trademarked), names. These names will be used in advertising and marketing, and are usually created to suit marketing needs. Once the patent on a newer drug expires, the medication can be sold less expensively as a generic (nontrademarked) product. Many pharmacies organize drugs by their generic names, since there may be multiple proprietary names for any one generic drug. To illustrate the naming process, consider the chemical name N-(4-hydroxyphenyl) acetamide, which will probably not sound familiar. The generic name of the same compound, acetaminophen, is easier to pronounce and quite familiar, but the trade name Tylenol®, used in extensive marketing, may be the most familiar of all. In this textbook, drugs will be referred to by their generic names.

cardiac glycoside Drugs derived from the foxglove plant that increase the contractility of the heart muscle.

In spite of tremendous advances in the laboratory sciences, a great majority of the most important drugs used today originated from a natural source, and some from the same sources as those written about by the ancient physicians. Many people grow willow trees, foxglove, and vinca in their gardens. Aspirin, the cardiac glycosides, and the vinca alkaloids (cancer chemotherapy agents), respectively, come from these common plants (see **Figs. 1.4, 1.5, and 1.6**). Other compounds, such as insulin, thyroxin, or other hormones originated from animal sources, and some important nutrients, such as iron and calcium,

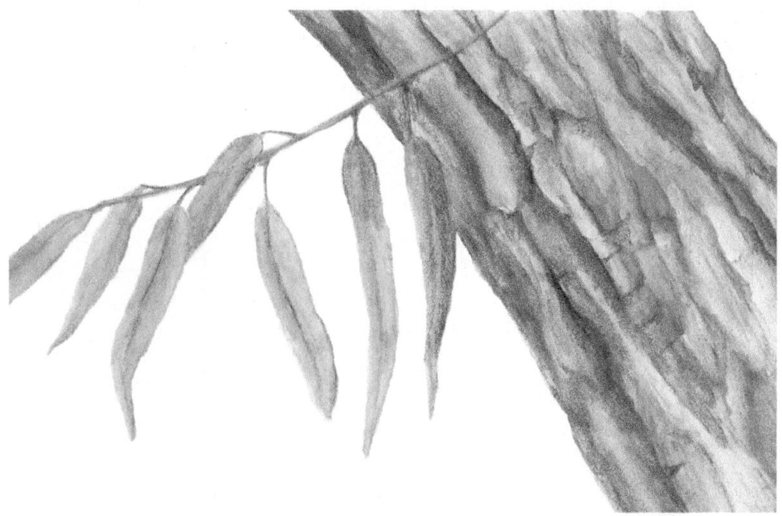

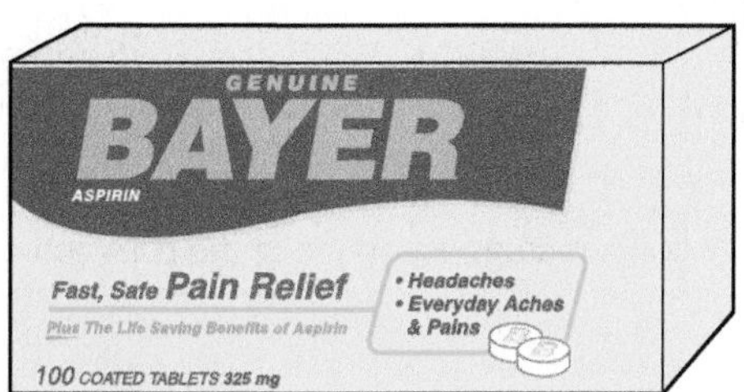


**Figure 1.4** Native Americans used the bark of the willow tree (Salix nigra) to treat pain and fevers.The bark contains salicylates, the family of drugs to which aspirin belongs. (Plant image by Rachel Sakai.)

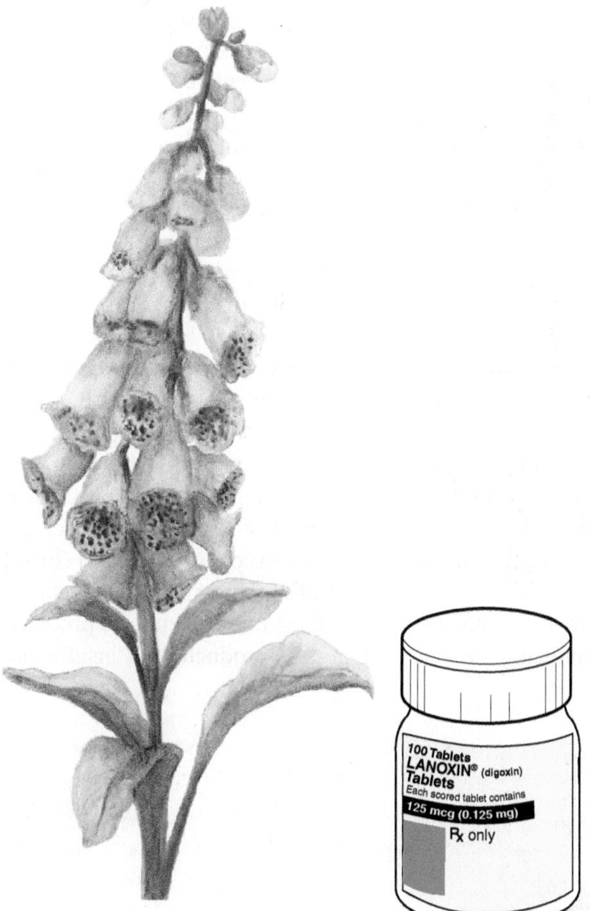


**Figure 1.5** Foxglove plants (Digitalis purpurea) contain the toxic, but effective, cardiac glycosides used in congestive heart failure. (Plant image by Rachel Sakai.)

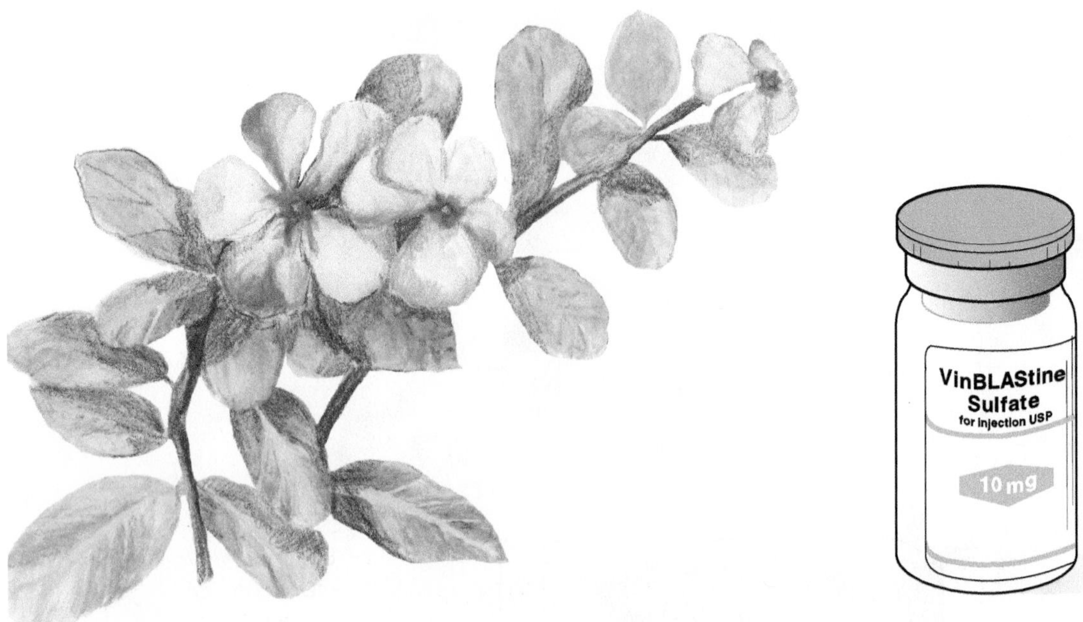


**Figure 1.6** The vinca alkaloids, potent anticancer drugs, are found in the common periwinkle, Vinca minor. (Plant image by Rachel Sakai.)

came from mineral sources. Today, most drugs are synthesized in laboratries because of the requirement for purity and consistency set by the USP and NF.

Many so-called "new" drugs are not new at all, and take relatively little time and effort on behalf of pharmaceutical companies to bring to the market. Pharmaceutical companies may make small adjustments to older drugs for which the patent is expiring, in order to extend the high earnings made from branded drugs. Consider Prilosec® (omeprazole) and Nexium® (esomeprazole) good examples of this practice. At about the time the patent on Prilosec®, one of the best-selling drugs ever marketed, was set to expire, AstraZeneca Pharmaceuticals was also anticipating the approval of omeprazole as a nonprescription drug. In a move calculated to maintain sales, the drug manufacturer introduced Nexium®, a single enantiomer of omeprazole that would only be available by prescription. The original compound was composed of two enantiomers, stereoisomers with the same chemical composition and physical properties, except that they rotate polarized light passing through in opposite directions (see **Fig. 1.7**). Names of enantiomers that rotate light to the left usually begin with the prefix levo-, l-, or s- (in this case esomeprazole), and those that rotate light to the right usually begin with the prefix dextro- or d-. The FDA approved this new prescription version of omeprazole even though it is chemically identical, not proven to be any better, and sells for almost ten times the price of nonprescription, generic omeprazole. Although many authorities have condemned this practice, pharmaceutical companies continue to use it to extend their profits.

enantiomer Either of a pair of chemical compounds whose molecular structures have a mirror-image relationship to each other.

stereoisomer Molecules with the same formula in which atoms are linked in the same order, but differ in their spatial arrangement.

Although pharmaceutical companies are profit oriented in their exploration of new drugs, university and government supported research on diseases and their treatment continues at a rapid pace. Some of the newest additions to the pharmacopoeia were developed because of advances in genetic research that led to the use of recombinant DNA technology. This technology allows nonhuman organisms to produce human hormones, proteins, and antibodies. For example, the human gene that regulates the production of insulin can

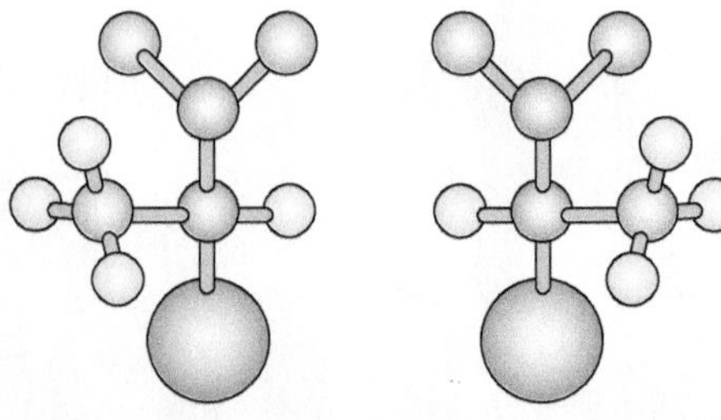

**Figure 1.7** These two chemically identical compounds are mirror images of each other and are not superimposable. They are called stereoisomers and represent the L and R forms of a drug.

be implanted in the bacteria *Escherichia coli*. The gene, once implanted, is replicated in huge numbers of these organisms, and becomes a "manufacturing plant" for human insulin, which is removed and purified for use. While this modern technology has helped create both brand new compounds and older compounds of greater purity, consistency, and specificity, it also forces the costs of drugs higher every year.

As new technologies are developed and knowledge of human proteins, genes, and chemical messengers expands, some drug manufacturers plan to design drugs that are individually tailored to specific patient needs. The desired result of these technological advances is improved drug safety and longer and healthier lives for patients. Clearly, however, the financial cost of progress will be very, very high.

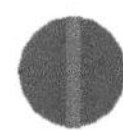

## Pharmacology and the Practice of Pharmacy

We have explored some of the reasons that drug therapy is intrinsically risky. It is important to understand that other, avoidable risk factors, such as inappropriate dosing or selection of medication, interactions with other medications, and inappropriate administration of medications can add to these dangers. The longer a patient takes a drug, the higher the dose that is taken, and the more concurrent therapies that are taken, the greater the risk of adverse effects. It is estimated that each year more than 2 million Americans suffer some kind of adverse drug effect.

In *To Err Is Human*, the Institute of Medicine states that more than 7,000 people died from acknowledged medication errors in 1993 alone. This number increased more than 2.5 fold over the previous decade and does not include deaths from medications used appropriately or deaths from undiscovered side effects, or unreported errors. Overall, medication errors are estimated to occur at a rate of anywhere from 3 to 5 errors per 1,000 medication orders or prescriptions processed. There are many reasons that errors are made; illegible handwriting, names or packaging that look or sound like other drugs, chaotic workplaces, or fatigued employees are all potential causes of errors.

While bad results can occur when patients take medications, they also occur when patients do not take their medication. Noncompliance is the term used to describe the lack of patient adherence to dosing directions. When patients do not take their medications, the results can be disastrous. For example, people who do not take their blood pressure medication have a much higher risk of developing strokes. People who do not comply with directions while taking antibiotics run the risk of developing infections that are more difficult to treat. Patients who are encouraged by pharmacy employees to take their medications may have a better chance of avoiding these bad results.

The most important responsibility of every person working in the field of pharmacy is to do their part to deliver the most appropriate drug therapy to every patient. This concept is called pharmaceutical care, and pharmacy technicians play a key role in this charge.

noncompliance Failure or refusal to comply with instructions for taking prescribed medication.

pharmaceutical care Direct involvement of the pharmacist in the design, implementation, and monitoring of a therapeutic drug plan intended to relieve symptoms, or treat disease.

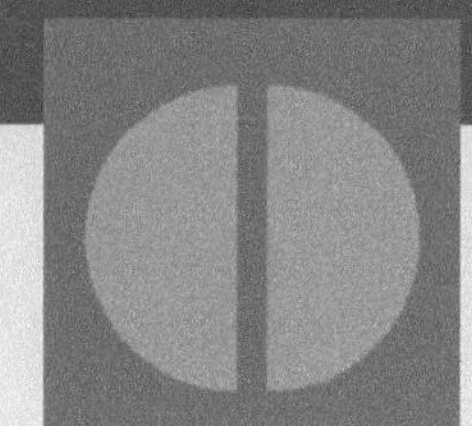

### Case 1.1

Ann, a pharmacy technician who learned and keeps up with the basics of pharmacology, receives the following, partially legible prescription:

Hydr***zine 25 mg, dispense #60, one tablet twice daily for blood pressure.

She checks the pharmacy shelf and finds two products that fit the spelling and strength indicated on the prescription, hydroxyzine 25 mg and hydralazine 25 mg tablets. She says she knows which of the medications is used for blood pressure, but you, the pharmacy technician extern, are not sure. What would you do if you received a prescription like this and were unsure which medication to take from the shelves? Which medication is the one for blood pressure control?

Although pharmacy technicians are not allowed to manage problems that require clinical decision-making, they can alert the pharmacist to potential errors or other problems before they occur. As a technician enters information into the patient profile, receives and enters prescriptions into the pharmacy computer system, carefully selects medications from the shelf, and double-checks medication before it is dispensed, he or she can screen for errors, check for drug allergies, and report any computer generated warnings to the pharmacist. Technicians may have more time to interact with clients and build rapport than pharmacists do. This rapport can lead to a discussion of medication-related problems, or compliance issues that patients might otherwise be inclined to dismiss. The technician can then direct concerned patients to the pharmacist for help.

The alert and informed technician plays a vital role in the delivery of the best possible pharmaceutical care. Pharmacists want to work with a professional and responsible technician who is willing to step into this role, and can assist the pharmacist in preventing adverse drug events. A technician who understands the basic concepts of pharmacology and possesses an array of general drug knowledge, combined with a healthy respect for the risks of drug therapy will be perfectly suited to fulfill the vital role of assistant to the pharmacist.

adverse drug event Any unexpected or unwanted effect caused by the administration of a drug.

# Review Questions

## Multiple Choice

Choose the best answer to the following questions:

1. Dioscorides' *de Materia Medica* was a drug resource used for more than 1,500 years. Which of the following information did it contain?
   a. Descriptions of the properties of remedies
   b. Directions for preparing remedies
   c. Dosages of remedies
   d. Information on the habitat of botanical compounds used in remedies
   e. All of the above

2. The germ theory of disease says that:
   a. An excess of certain "humors" in the body is the cause of infectious disease
   b. Microbes cause infectious disease
   c. Magic and spiritual beliefs will cure infectious diseases
   d. Microbes cause infectious diseases in animals, but not in humans
   e. None of the above

3. What is the name of the government organization that is responsible for ensuring that drug manufacturers provide safe and effective products to consumers?
   a. The Drug Enforcement Administration
   b. The United States Department of Pharmaceuticals
   c. The Food and Drug Administration
   d. The United States Department of Agriculture
   e. The Drug Council of America

4. Which of the following changes would increase the risk of adverse drug effects?
   a. Decreasing the duration of drug therapy
   b. Lowering the drug dosage
   c. Adding additional drugs to a therapeutic regimen
   d. Discontinuing a patient's drug therapy
   e. All of the above

5. Which of the following personnel are responsible for delivering a safe, effective, and accurate pharmaceutical product to the patient?
   a. Pharmacist
   b. Drug Manufacturers
   c. Pharmacy Technician
   d. Only a and b
   e. a, b, and c

## True/False

6. Pharmacology is the study of drugs and remedies.
   a. True
   b. False
7. Vioxx®, Bextra®, and thalidomide are all drugs that were eventually found to cause harmful effects in patients.
   a. True
   b. False
8. Diseases can always be treated without any risk to the patient.
   a. True
   b. False
9. With all of today's advanced technology, medication errors no longer occur.
   a. True
   b. False
10. Pharmacy technicians fill a crucial role in pharmacy by double-checking medications before they are dispensed.
   a. True
   b. False

## Matching

Match the word or phrase with the correct lettered choice from the list below. Choices will not be used more than once and may not be used at all.

11. Chemotherapy
12. Adverse drug effect
13. Pharmacopoeia
14. Vaccine
15. Therapeutic drug effect

a. An undesirable effect produced by a drug
b. An official listing of drugs or remedies
c. Used to prevent contagious disease
d. The use of compounds designed to treat
e. A desired effect produced by a drug
f. An allergic reaction
g. Dioscorides authored this

## Short Answer

16. What is the role of the Food and Drug Administration in pharmacy and why is it so important?
17. You are a pharmacy technician working in a very busy pharmacy. You and your fellow technicians are often tired and overworked. Also, since things get so busy during the workday, the workspace is often disorganized, and drugs sometimes get misplaced on the shelves. What could you do in this situation to prevent the occurrence of drug errors?
18. Is drug therapy risk free? Why or why not?

19. Why was the discovery of the germ theory of disease so important?

20. Why should pharmacy technicians learn pharmacology?

## FOR FURTHER INQUIRY

Research a significant turning point in the history of pharmacy and medicine and explain why it is important. What was gained by humanity at this juncture? In what way did these changes negatively impact health care? Potential topics include the change from a spiritual-based treatment approach to a rational one, the acceptance of the germ theory of disease, or development of recombinant DNA technology.

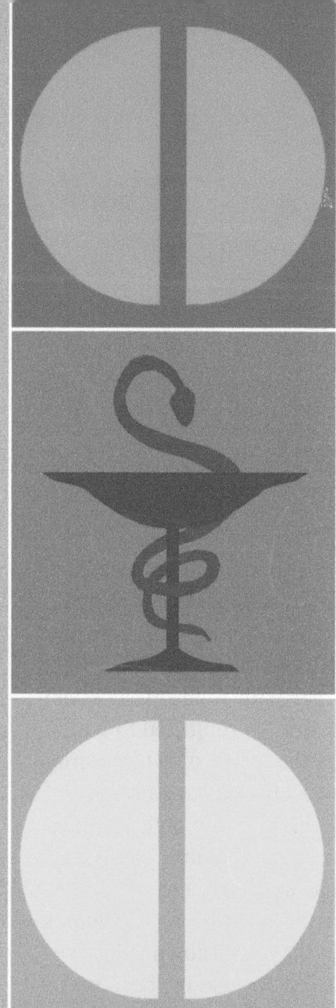

Chapter **2**

# Drug Therapy and Pharmacodynamics: The Mechanics of Drug Action

## OBJECTIVES

After studying this chapter, the reader should be able to:

- Define the terms pharmacokinetics and pharmacodynamics and describe how they differ.
- Compare and contrast three routes of administration and list advantages, disadvantages, and patient acceptability of each.
- Explain three reasons why it might be advantageous to delay or prolong the release and/or absorption of a drug.
- Sketch an example of a dose-response curve and explain how it relates to effective doses and drug safety.
- Explain how drugs interact with receptors to initiate a response, and the difference between an agonist and antagonist.

*KEY TERMS*

- absorption
- acid labile
- agonist
- analgesic
- antagonist
- antiemetic
- antipyretic
- contraindication
- dose-response curve
- effective dose range
- efficacy
- elixir
- emulsion
- enteral
- enteric coating
- enzymes
- immediate release
- indication
- intramuscular

- intravenous
- lozenge
- oral
- otic
- parenteral
- pharmacodynamics
- pharmacokinetics
- potency
- rectal
- structure-activity relationships
- subcutaneous
- sublingual
- suspension
- sustained release
- syrup
- systemic
- therapeutic index
- tincture
- topical
- toxicity
- transdermal
- troche

pharmacodynamics A branch of pharmacology dealing with the reactions between drugs and living systems, including the correlation of effects of drugs with their chemical structure.

pharmacokinetics The study of the characteristic interactions of a drug and the body, including its absorption, distribution, metabolism, and excretion.

indication A disease or symptom that suggests the use of a specific drug treatment or procedure.

contraindication A condition that makes a particular drug or procedure inadvisable.

The aim of drug therapy is to prevent, cure, or control disease without causing unnecessary harm to the patient. Most people take medications with the hope of achieving this aim and never think about how drugs work. Drugs alter biochemical processes within the body in a number of ways, through their interaction with existing physiological processes. Pharmacodynamics is the science that studies how drugs interact with living tissues and pharmacokinetics is the study of the physiologic processes that a drug is subjected to within the body over time. More simply stated, pharmacodynamics is the study of what a drug does to the body, and pharmacokinetics is the study of what the body does to a drug.

To achieve successful treatment of a disease without undue harm to the patient, physical and chemical characteristics of the medication, as well as individual characteristics of the patient need to be considered. Individual differences, such as age, size, race, and conditions, such as illnesses or pregnancy for example, can affect the way the body handles drugs. Drugs are indicated for use in particular conditions when they are known to be useful and are either approved by the Food and Drug Administration for use or, because of thorough investigation and experience, are considered accepted practice for the condition. A drug is contraindicated when a separate condition or disease exists that makes use of the drug inadvisable. When a medication and dosing regimen is selected for use in a patient all of the following features of the drug are considered:

- Drug formulations and available routes of administration
- Effective dose
- Expected response
- Potential unwanted effects, including drug interactions

In addition to the characteristics of the drug, certain individual patient variables must also be considered:

- Age, height, weight
- Drug allergies
- Organ function
- Pertinent health issues
- Contraindications to drug use (pregnancy, for example)
- Any other medications, including supplements and herbal remedies, that the patient is taking

Clearly, because of the many variables, there are many opportunities for errors in the selection and use of medication. To reduce the risk of errors, it is important that pharmacists have access to correct patient information so that they can assess and review prescriptions before dispensing them to patients. Pharmacy technicians can improve the chances of successful use of medications by communicating effectively, and carefully collecting necessary patient information for patient profiles.

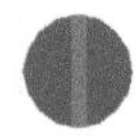

# Drug Formulations and Routes of Administration

Drugs are manufactured in a variety of formulations for enteral administration (any route that utilizes the gastrointestinal tract for absorption), or parenteral administration (any route of administration not associated with the gastrointestinal [GI] tract; see **Fig. 2.1**). The chemical and physical properties of a drug, such as water or fat solubility, the size and ionization state of the molecule, and its stability in the presence of acid, largely determine what formulations are made by pharmaceutical companies. Products for oral administration (administration by mouth) are the least expensive to make and the easiest for patients to take, but are subject to many biological processes in the body before delivery at the site of action (see Chapter 3).

The rectal route of administration, while effective, is generally less accepted by patients. However, it is especially useful when nausea or vomiting prevents patients from keeping oral medications in the GI tract long enough to be absorbed. This route is also useful in very young children who cannot swallow a medication or in older or debilitated patients who have difficulty swallowing. Rectal formulations are available for antipyretic (fever reducing), analgesic (pain relieving), laxative, and antiemetic (treatment of vomiting) medications and for drugs used to treat seizures and diseases of the colon.

Formulations for enteral (oral or rectal) administration include:

- Tablets or capsules, both immediate-release and sustained-release preparations
- Troches, lozenges, and suckers, all designed to slowly dissolve in the mouth
- Syrups

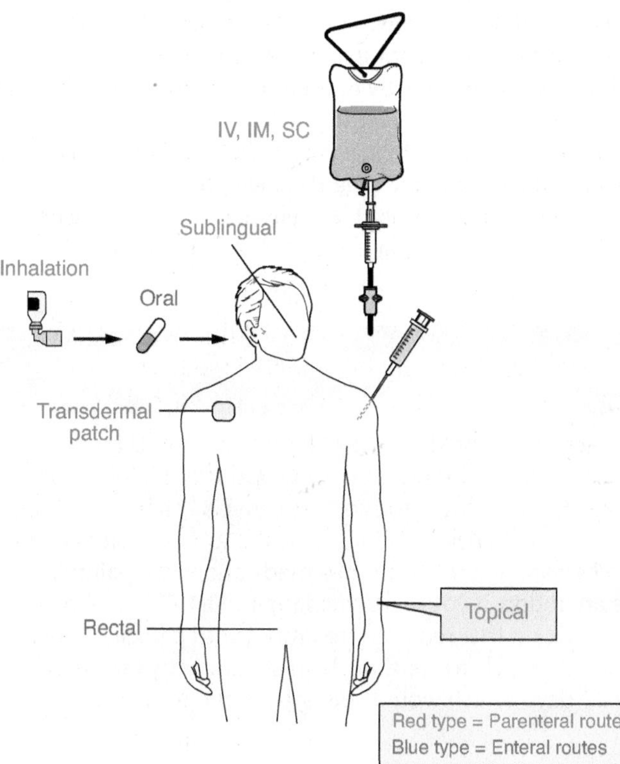


**Figure 2.1** Commonly used routes of drug administration include administration by enteral routes (oral and rectal) as well as parenteral routes (sublingual, transdermal, or by injection for example). (IV, intravenous; IM, intramuscular; SC, subcutaneous.) (Adapted with permission from Howland RD, Mycek MJ, Harvey RA, et al. *Lippincott's Illustrated Reviews: Pharmacology,* 3rd ed. Baltimore: Lippincott Williams & Wilkins, 2006.)

enteral A route of nutrient or drug delivery where delivery is made directly into the gastrointestinal tract.

parenteral Introduced into the body other than by way of the intestines; usually relates to drug administration by injection

oral Pertaining to the mouth; route of administration of medication given or taken by mouth.

rectal Pertaining to the rectum; as in rectal suppository.

antipyretic An agent that relieves or reduces fever.

analgesic An agent that relieves pain without causing loss of consciousness.

antiemetic A drug used to prevent or alleviate nausea or vomiting.

immediate-release Drug formulation with normal dissolution characteristics; not delayed release.

sustained-release A drug formulation designed to slowly release the active ingredient over an extended period of time; also known as delayed or extended release.

troche Lozenge.

lozenge Small, flavored, solid medication formulation designed to be held in the mouth for slow dissolution; also known as a troche.

syrup Concentrated solution of sugar and water; in pharmacy, flavored and used as a vehicle for a medicinal substance.

elixir A drug preparation in which the active ingredients are dissolved in an alcohol-based, sweetened liquid.

tincture A formulation of a drug in an alcoholic solution.

suspension A drug formulation of fine, insoluble particles dispersed evenly throughout a suitable vehicle.

emulsion Pharmaceutical preparation of one liquid dispersed in small globules through a second, immiscible liquid.

sublingual Under the tongue.

otic Relating to the ear.

intravenous Drug administration that utilizes injection into a vein.

- Elixirs, tinctures, and other ethanol-based preparations
- Suspensions and emulsions
- Rectal suppositories, made with a semisolid base that melts at body temperature

Although parenteral administration technically includes any route of administration that does not depend on the GI tract, the phrase is most commonly used to refer to administration by injection. Sublingual administration is considered parenteral because it is absorbed through the mucous membranes of the mouth directly into the systemic circulation. In sublingual administration, a rapidly dissolving tablet is placed under the tongue. As the tablet dissolves, the drug is quickly absorbed into the bloodstream. Not every drug can be given this way, but the sublingual route results in a rapid onset of action useful for a few drugs. Nitroglycerin, used for chest pain, is the most important example of a drug given sublingually. Drug formulations for topical, transdermal, sublingual, or injectable administration include, but are not limited to:

- Lotions, creams, and gels
- Nonsterile solutions and shampoos
- Ointments
- Patches for transdermal administration
- Tablets and sprays for sublingual use
- Tablets or suppositories for vaginal administration
- Sterile suspensions, solutions, and ointments for ophthalmic use
- Suspensions and solutions for otic (in the ear) use
- Sterile solutions and suspensions for injection

New technological advances are creating exciting new delivery systems for drugs that have typically been given by injection or by mouth. There are a number of devices available that can be implanted under the skin to deliver a drug at a constant or variable rate. These include insulin and chemotherapy pumps as well as implantable drug wafers. Very recently, the FDA approved a form of insulin that can be delivered by inhalation. Delivery systems that will deliver pain medication by transporting it across the skin using low-voltage electrical current are currently being investigated.

For each patient, the chosen route of administration is selected based on the available formulations of the drug and on the objective of the drug treatment. In a situation where a patient is critically ill and a rapid drug response is needed, a physician may order a drug to be given by the intravenous (IV) route, resulting in a nearly immediate onset of action.

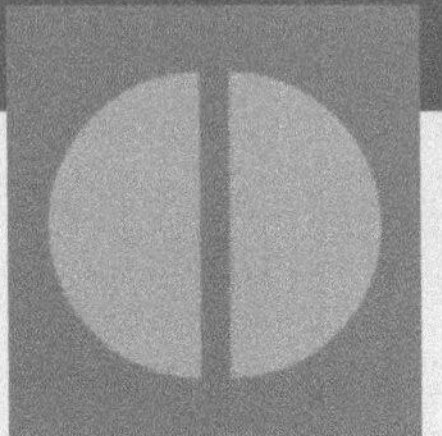

## Case 2.1

Parents of toddlers are often faced with the dilemma of how to get medication down the mouths of their children. Some toddlers take any opportunity to spit out whatever Mommy or Daddy really wants them to swallow, especially if it tastes bad. Capsules or tablets constitute a choking risk in toddlers. Most 2 to 3 year olds can usually be induced to take a chewable tablet. Injectable medications are painful, and more expensive, but are an option. If you were the parent of a toddler who was diagnosed with a throat infection that required treatment with penicillin, and your child could receive the antibiotic via a one-time IM injection, or by taking a suspension 4 times a day for 10 days, which would you choose and why?

Intramuscular (IM) or subcutaneous (SC) injections result in a more rapid response than orally administered medications, but the response is more delayed than IV injection because the drug must cross tissues to get into the blood stream. Medications cannot be given by mouth when a patient is unconscious, and a parenteral route is usually chosen. If a drug is poorly absorbed through the gastrointestinal tract, one of the few available options is to give it by injection. The disadvantages of giving a medication by injection include cost of the product, pain to the patient, and because the integrity of the skin is disrupted, a risk of infection. Unlike administration into the GI tract, which can be emptied if a large dosing error is discovered soon enough, dose errors made with injectable medications are irreversible, except in the rare cases where a specific antidote is available.

intramuscular A route of drug administration that utilizes injection into the muscle.

subcutaneous Beneath the skin.

Administration of a drug by injection (IV, IM, or SC) or the oral route usually results in dispersal of the drug throughout the body, and is said to be systemic treatment. If a disease affects the body as a whole, then the drug treatment must be given systemically. When administered systemically, drugs work at multiple sites of action. When drugs disperse throughout the body, they are more likely to cause undesirable effects than when they are used locally.

systemic Affecting the entire body.

Giving a drug by mouth is the most common route of administration, but also the most circuitous route to the ultimate site of action. Generally the onset of drug action after oral administration occurs about 30 to 60 minutes after a medication is taken. In order for an orally administered drug to take effect it must pass from the GI tract into the systemic circulation, a process referred to as absorption. Some drugs are absorbed from the stomach, but more often the small intestine is the major site of entry into the systemic circulation because of its large surface area for absorption. The stomach contents empty into the small intestines about every 15 to 20 minutes. The presence of food in the stomach delays the stomach emptying time and may delay the onset of action. If a drug is acid labile it is broken down by stomach acid. The presence of food in the stomach can significantly reduce the effectiveness of an acid labile drug due to delayed gastric emptying and increased exposure to stomach acid. Enteric coating or other delayed-release drug formulations protect drugs from the acidic environment of the stomach and may prevent gastric irritation, but will also delay the onset of action. Delayed-release formulations are also used to prolong the effects of a drug, allowing the patient to take oral medications less frequently.

absorption The movement and uptake of substances into cells or across tissues, as with the absorption of nutrients or drugs in the small intestine.

acid labile Chemically unstable in the presence of acid.

The topical route of administration restricts the drug to a certain area of the body because of minimal systemic absorption, and greater localized drug action. Because of reduced systemic absorption, local administration is associated with fewer side effects. Although applied topically, the transdermal route of administration delivers drugs systemically. Medications given by this route are often imbedded in a bandage-type delivery system called a transdermal patch. Patches are designed to deliver medications into the blood stream at a fairly constant level over a period of hours or days. They are well accepted by many patients because of convenience and ease of use.

enteric coating Coating used on drugs to prevent their dissolution until they leave the stomach and enter the small intestine.

The inhaled route of administration is sometimes used to deliver drugs to the lungs. This route is particularly effective and convenient for patients with respiratory complaints (for example, asthma or chronic obstructive pulmonary disease), because the drug is delivered directly to the site of action, and systemic side effects are minimized. Medications administered intranasally and by inhalation may, in some cases, be absorbed systemically. The anesthetic gases are examples of drugs that are inhaled for their systemic effects. **Table 2.1** describes these and other routes of administration.

topical Drug formulation designed for, or involving, application to and action on the surface of a body part, especially the skin, eyes, and ears.

## Drug Dosing and Expected Response

Paracelsus, one of the few scientists from the Middle Ages to make a significant contribution to health care, is credited with saying, "All substances are poisons—there is none which is not. The right dose differentiates a poison and a remedy." As with most aspects of

transdermal Absorption through the skin into the bloodstream, or a drug formulation that supplies active ingredient for absorption through the skin.

**Table 2.1** Available routes of drug administration, their advantages and disadvantages, and most common uses

| Route | Relative Speed of Onset | Advantages | Disadvantages | Application |
|---|---|---|---|---|
| Oral | Delayed, usually 30–60 minutes | Safe, easy, inexpensive | Difficult for very young, delay in onset, some drugs not absorbed | The route most often used |
| Sublingual, buccal | Rapid, 3–5 min | Rapid onset, avoids 1st pass through liver | Inconsistent absorption, bad taste | Nitroglycerin tabs and others |
| Rectal | Varies, 5–30 min | Useful for very young, or when oral route not possible | Variable absorption, unacceptable to many patients | Suppositories for nausea, laxatives, for pain/fever relief in infants |
| Intravenous | Very rapid, a minute or less | No absorption required, no swallowing required | Invasive, infection risk, can be irritating to tissues and painful. Requires trained personnel to administer. | Rapid treatment of serious illness |
| Intramuscular | Moderate, ≥10 minutes | Avoids GI tract, safer than IV | Pain on administration, invasive, slower than IV. Requires trained personnel to administer. | Post-op treatment of pain, useful when patient cannot swallow. |
| Subcutaneous | Moderate | Most patients can learn to self-administer | Invasive, infection, pain. Patient must use sterile technique. | Insulin, TNF inhibitors |
| Intrathecal, intra-articular | Moderate | Local effects in spinal cord and joints | Invasive, risk of infection, risk of damage to nearby tissues | Anesthesia, anti-inflammatory injections, and other uses |
| Inhalation | Rapid | Most drugs exert local effects | Administration requires coordination, pt teaching | Treatment of asthma |
| Transdermal | Varies, minutes–hours | Convenient, drug absorbed over hours–days | Systemic effects continue after patch removal, may peel off or leave adhesive on skin | Many uses, pain relief, birth control, tobacco cessation |
| Topical | Delayed | Drug effect localized, easy and noninvasive | Can be messy, local effect may be inadequate | Treatment of eyes, ears, skin |

GI, gastrointestinal; IV, intravenous; TNF, tumor necrosis factor.

life, "if a little is good, then more is better" is a rule that does not apply to drug therapy. Using the correct dose of a drug is a key part of proper medication use. For every drug, there is a relationship between a given dose and the expected response. This relationship is determined by biochemical reactions in the body, by the interaction of drugs with tissues in the body, and by individual variations that can occur. Some drugs are so safe that close attention to individual variation is unnecessary. For most drugs, however, pharmacists and physicians must understand dose-response relationships and the potential for individual variations that result in atypical responses.

## Effective Doses, Toxic Doses, and Therapeutic Index

If a research pharmacologist was to study incrementally increasing doses of a sedative in a large group of normal, healthy, average sized people, and measure the response to each increase in dose of the medication, a few people would become drowsy at low doses and some would require high doses, but most would respond somewhere in the middle. In this sample of people, the dose of drug needed to cause the desired response in half the group (50%) is known as the effective dose, or ED 50. In the same sample of normal healthy people, as the dose is increased, there will be a correlated increase in therapeutic effect up to a point where no further increase in therapeutic effect is seen. The range of doses that cause an increasing desired therapeutic effect is considered the effective dose range. Doses below this range are ineffective and above this range will not result in an increased response, but will cause an increased risk of toxicity. Within this effective dose range, there is the possibility of significant variation between patients because of their genetic make-up, physical condition, age, or other reasons. These variations can have a significant impact on any single individual's response to a drug.

effective dose range Range of drug doses that cause an increase in the desired pharmacologic effect with increasing dose.

The degree of the response to different doses of medication in a group of individuals can be measured and graphed against the dose of the drug used. The resulting curve is called a dose-response curve (see **Fig. 2.2**). Dose-response curves can be used to compare two drugs with similar actions. By comparing dose-response curves, the pharmacologist can determine the relative efficacy of the two drugs and the relative potency of the two drugs. It is important to differentiate between the concepts of potency and efficacy. Potency is a measure of how much drug is needed to cause a given response, whereas efficacy is a description of how thoroughly a drug causes a response. Drug X may be equally, more, or less potent than drug Y, but more effective (see **Fig. 2.3**). A case in point is acetaminophen (Tylenol®), a nonprescription analgesic and antipyretic, with a therapeutic dose similar to that of aspirin. These two drugs can be said to be equally potent because their effective doses are about equivalent. Aspirin, however, has anti-inflammatory properties that acetaminophen does not possess. Therefore aspirin is considered an effective anti-inflammatory agent (acetaminophen is not), and when inflammation contributes to pain, a more effective analgesic than acetaminophen.

dose-response curve A graph that shows the relationship between the dose of a drug and the degree of response it causes.

potency Refers to the relative amount of drug required to produce the desired response; related to strength of a drug, not efficacy.

efficacy The ability of a drug to treat or cure a disease.

Besides efficacy and potency, it is important to consider the relationship between toxicity and the dose of a drug. Toxicity occurs when doses of a drug are increased to the point that it becomes poisonous. If the sedative we discussed before was given in continuously increasing doses to the same group of average adults, they would eventually begin to show signs of toxicity caused by the drug. Just as the relationship between dose and therapeutic effect can be represented on a graph, the relationship between dose and toxic effects can also be measured and graphed. The dose at which half the people would be anticipated to succumb to toxic effects of the drug is called the lethal dose, or LD 50. When the dose-response curve for a drug is placed on the same graph with the curve generated by studying the relationship between toxic and therapeutic dose for that drug, the space between the two can be observed. The relationship between the effective dose and lethal dose of a drug is called the therapeutic index. The wider the space between a therapeutic and toxic dose, the wider the therapeutic index and the safer the drug is considered to be. **Figure 2.4** compares a drug with a narrow therapeutic index and a wide therapeutic index.

toxicity Relative degree of being poisonous.

therapeutic index The ratio of the dose expected to cause toxicity in half the population (LD 50) to the lowest effective dose in half the population (ED 50), important in comparing drug safety.

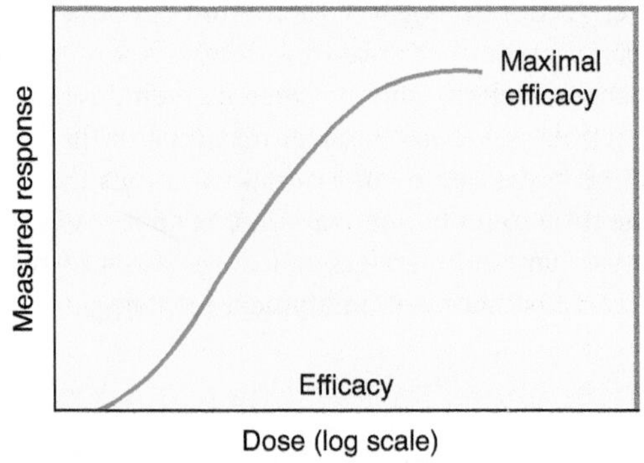

Measured response
Maximal efficacy
Efficacy
Dose (log scale)

**Figure 2.2** A dose-response curve demonstrates the relationship between an increasing dose of a drug and the measured drug response in a population of average people.

## Drug Response and Drug Receptors

enzyme A type of protein produced by a living organism that catalyzes biochemical reactions without itself being destroyed or altered.

The human body and other living organisms function because of the constant production, interaction, and metabolism of organic compounds. Within the body, chemical messengers carry information and cause a response; enzymes catalyze reactions, electrolytes flow in and out of cells, nutrients feed into systems that create new compounds, and hormones direct distant organs to respond. Drugs work because they mimic one or more of the naturally occurring chemicals in the body.

Effective drugs cause a response in the body when they interact with something called a drug receptor. A drug receptor is a target molecule, usually a protein, and may be found on cell surfaces, or inside cells (enzymes inside of cells can be target molecules, for example). Drug receptors exist on or within cells throughout the body and also on cells that are foreign to the body, such as microscopic organisms. Each drug receptor molecule has a specialized conformation, or shape, that allows interaction with a specific drug. This specificity allows each drug to exert its effect on certain target cells rather than affecting every cell in the body. When a drug binds to a drug receptor, this drug-receptor complex stimulates the cell to respond (see **Fig. 2.5**). The more tightly a drug attaches to the receptor, and the more efficiently the activated receptor responds, the more long lasting and greater the effect the drug will cause.

agonist A drug capable of combining with a receptor on a cell and initiating the same reaction produced by an endogenous substance.

A drug that causes a biological response when it attaches to the drug receptor is called an agonist. Some drugs bind to receptors but have no inherent ability to cause a biologi-

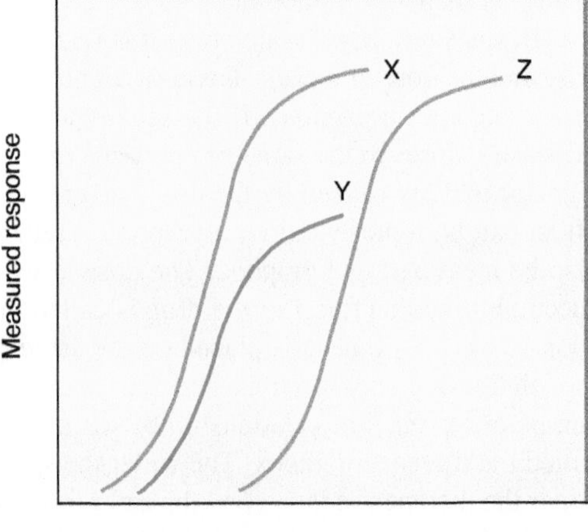


**Figure 2.3** Drug X causes a response at a lower dose than either drug Y or Z, and is therefore more potent. Drug X and Z are equally effective because they reach the same maximal response point. Although drug Y is more potent than drug Z (requires a lower dose to see an effect) it never can achieve the same response, and is therefore less effective than drug Z.

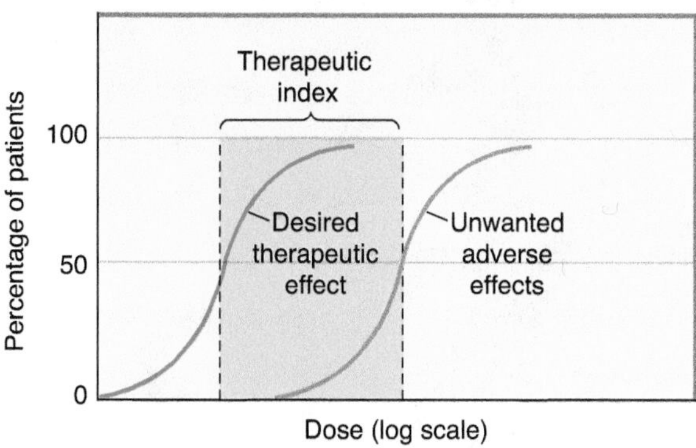


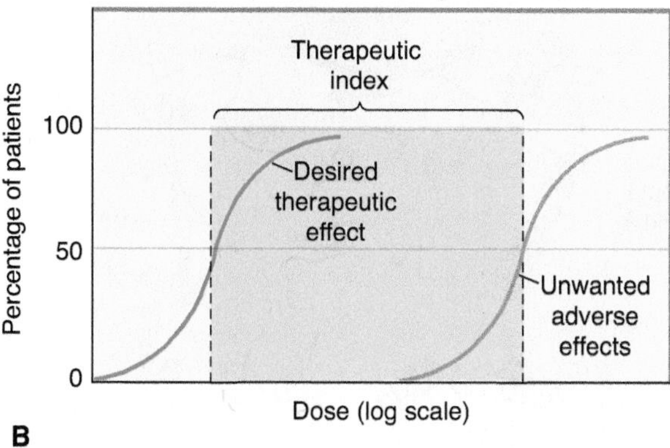


**Figure 2.4** Drugs with a narrow therapeutic index, such as warfarin, have a small difference between safe doses and toxic doses. Drugs with a wide therapeutic index, such as penicillin, have a much wider range of nontoxic doses. (Adapted with permission from Howland RD, Mycek MJ, Harvey RA, et al. *Lippincott's Illustrated Reviews: Pharmacology,* 3rd ed. Baltimore: Lippincott Williams & Wilkins, 2006.)

cal response; however, as long as these drugs remain bound to their receptors, they prevent other drugs or chemicals from attaching. This type of drug is called an antagonist. In some instances a drug may have antagonist properties while still stimulating the drug receptor to some degree and these drugs are considered to have mixed agonist and antagonist properties.

antagonist A drug that acts within the body to oppose the action of another drug, or a substance occurring naturally in the body, by blocking its receptor.

Pharmaceutical chemists use their knowledge of the molecular structure of known drugs and naturally occurring chemicals, combined with an understanding of drug receptor physiology to design new drugs (**Fig. 2.6**). Understanding structure-activity relationships (SAR) allows researchers to add an aromatic ring here or a side chain there and create potentially promising new compounds that may react more specifically with certain receptors,

structure-activity relationships Relationship between the chemical structure or make-up of a compound and its pharmacologic activity.

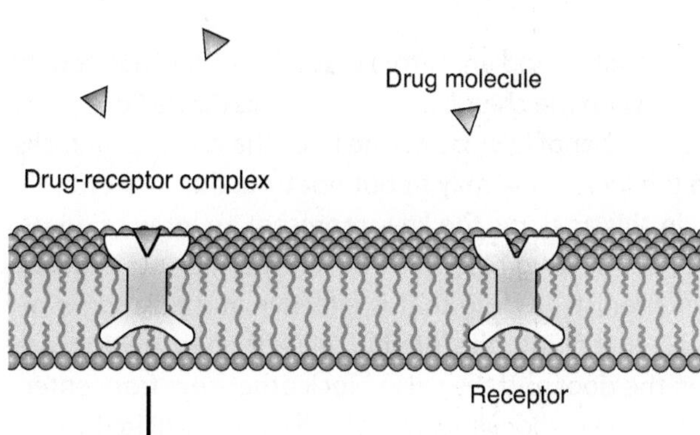


**Figure 2.5** A drug, represented by the orange triangle, binds to a specific receptor site to cause a cellular response.

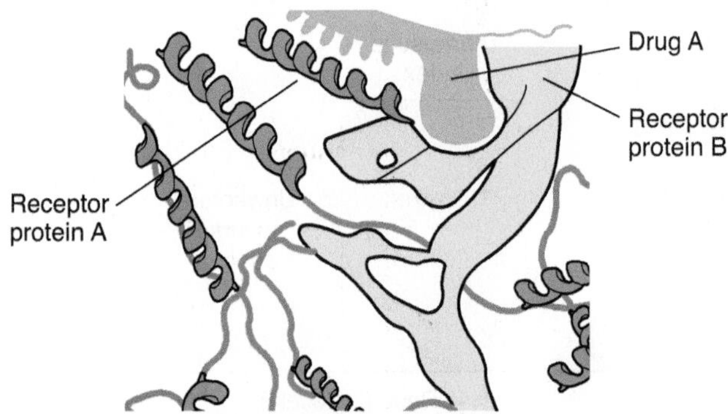
Drug A interacts with receptor proteins A and B to cause a response.
Drug A
Receptor protein B
Receptor protein A

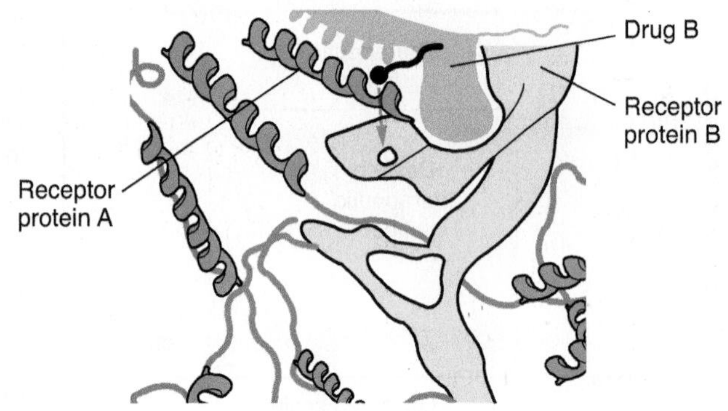
Drug B has a side chain that interacts with a part of the receptor to cause an additional side effect.
Drug B
Receptor protein B
Receptor protein A

**Figure 2.6** Pharmaceutical chemists use their knowledge of drug receptors and structure-activity relationships to modify medications, perhaps to bind more tightly to receptors, or to have fewer side effects.

therefore causing fewer unwanted effects. This same knowledge can be used to alter physical and chemical properties of a drug to make the effects last longer or make it more easily absorbed or otherwise change it so administration is easier for the consumer, without changing the essential therapeutic activity of the drug. Drugs that have similar chemical structures and similar therapeutic effects are described as being members of the same drug class. Just as pharmacologists use their knowledge of the chemistry of drug classes to create new compounds, technicians who understand general concepts about drug classes can easily understand new drugs in a class as they are developed.

## Analogy

Imagine for a moment the typical school custodian, carrying keys to fit the classrooms and offices for an entire high school. When the chemistry teacher locks himself out of his classroom, the custodian may try a number of keys before he finds the one that unlocks the door. Some keys will not fit in the lock, some may fit but not turn, but only one will fit in the lock and open the door. In this analogy, the keys represent an array of drugs. The lock on the door represents a specific drug receptor. The key that fits into the lock and opens the door represents an agonist—a drug that is effective at mediating a response at that specific receptor. Keys that fit into the lock but will not open the door are like antagonists; they will not open the door and they also block other keys from entering the lock, thereby blocking an effective response. Keys that will not even fit in the lock represent drugs with no affinity for the specific receptor.

# Review Questions

## Multiple Choice

Choose the best answer to the following questions:

1. If you wanted to find out how Tylenol is eliminated from the body (in the urine, feces, metabolized, etc.), you would be interested in which of the following information on Tylenol:
   a. Pharmacodynamics
   b. Effective dose
   c. Dose-response curve
   d. Pharmacokinetics
   e. Indications and contraindications

2. Which statement is correct?
   a. If a drug is contraindicated in pregnancy, it will be beneficial for pregnant women to take it.
   b. Drug formulation and available routes of administration are not considered when selecting a medication for a patient.
   c. Parenteral administration means drug administration by a route unassociated with the gastrointestinal tract.
   d. A syrup is a drug formulation that is administered parenterally.
   e. None of the above is correct.

3. In an emergency situation where a rapid drug response is needed, the route of administration that would give the quickest response is:
   a. Oral
   b. Intramuscular
   c. Intravenous
   d. Subcutaneous
   e. All of the above have equal response times

one answer

4. Given the following effective dose ranges and LD 50 data, which drug is probably the **least** safe?

| Drug A | 200–800 mg | LD 50 = 7 g |
|---|---|---|
| Drug B | 375–400 mg | LD 50 = 1 g |
| Drug C | 25–175 mg | LD 50 = 900 mg |
| Drug D | 800–1,200 mg | LD 50 = 6 g |

   a. Drug A
   b. Drug B
   c. Drug C
   d. Drug D

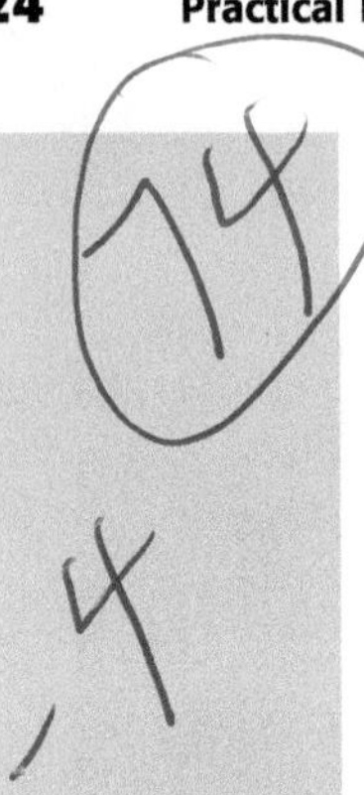

5. Which of the following is false concerning drug receptors?
   a. They can be found on bacteria within an infected tissue
   b. They are often proteins.
   c. They are found on cell surfaces but are not found on the inside of cells.
   d. The specialized conformation of each drug receptor allows a specific drug-receptor interaction.
   e. None of the above statements are false.

## True/False

6. Chemical and physical properties of a drug are important factors in determining what formulations are available.
   a. True
   b. False

7. A drug that is administered by injection remains localized at the site of administration.
   a. True
   b. False

8. Enteric coating on a tablet shortens the time to onset of drug action.
   a. True
   b. False

9. An agonist is a drug that causes a biological response when it attaches to a drug receptor.
   a. True
   b. False

10. If two drugs are of equal potency, then they must also have equal efficacy.
    a. True
    b. False

## Matching

For numbers 11 to 15, match the incomplete statement with the correct lettered choice from the list below. Choices will not be used more than once and may not be used at all.

11. A molecule found on cell surfaces and within cells that has a specific interaction with a drug is called a(n) _____.
12. In order to achieve _____ of a drug, the drug could be administered either orally, by injection, or via transdermal patch.
13. A(n) _____ compares different doses of a drug with the magnitude of the response for each given dose.
14. The relationship between the toxic dose and the effective dose of a drug is called the _____.
15. Topical administration is a route that results in _____ of the drug.

a. systemic distribution
b. dose-response curve
c. drug receptor
d. therapeutic index
e. LD 50
f. concentration-time curve
g. local distribution

## Short Answer

16. Mrs. Smith is a 28-year-old woman who is in her second trimester of pregnancy. She is healthy other than the fact that she has several known drug allergies. Mrs. Smith has been having some trouble breathing lately and her doctor has just diagnosed allergic asthma. Mrs. Smith is currently taking several herbal supplements. What are some of the factors in Mrs. Smith's case that would affect the choice of medication to control her asthma?

17. Shown below are the dose-response curves (black) and the curve demonstrating the occurrence of toxic effects (red) for two different drugs used to treat the same condition. If you were asked which drug to choose for treatment of the condition based on the data in the graphs, what would you say? Explain your reasoning.

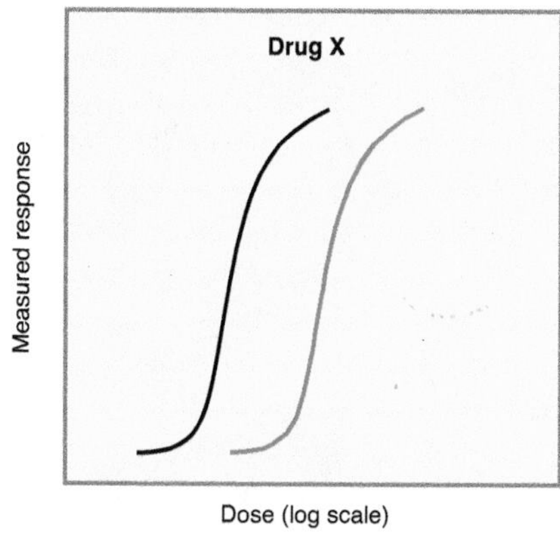


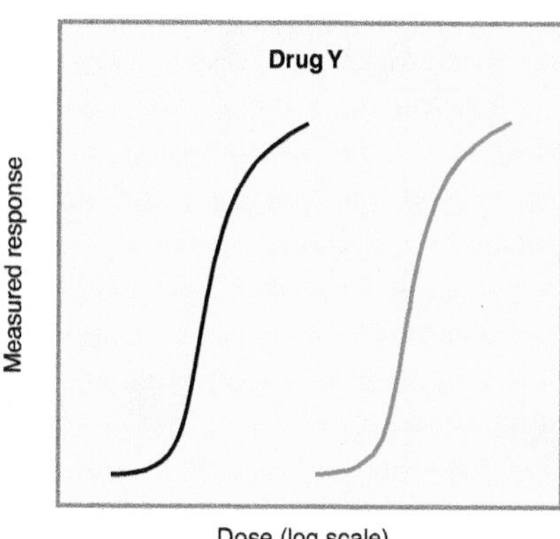


18. Discuss some of the benefits and drawbacks of the oral route of drug administration.

19. What information does the data below give you about the two drugs?

| | Drug Z (therapeutic dose = 600–1,200 mg) | Drug X (therapeutic dose = 400–800 mg) |
|---|---|---|
| Average amount of drug needed to reduce fever by 2 degrees in 50% of patients | 600 mg | 400 mg |
| Average degrees of fever reduction in patients given the drug throughout the therapeutic range | 4 | 2 |

20. Why is the specificity of drug-receptor interactions important? How can understanding these interactions lead to advancements in the field of medicine?

## FOR FURTHER INQUIRY

Use the Internet to find more information on one of the topics listed below. Find out if there is any new research or information on the topic. What practical application might this new information have on drug therapy and how might it impact patient care?

Drug receptors
Experimental methods of drug administration
New drug formulations to prolong absorption

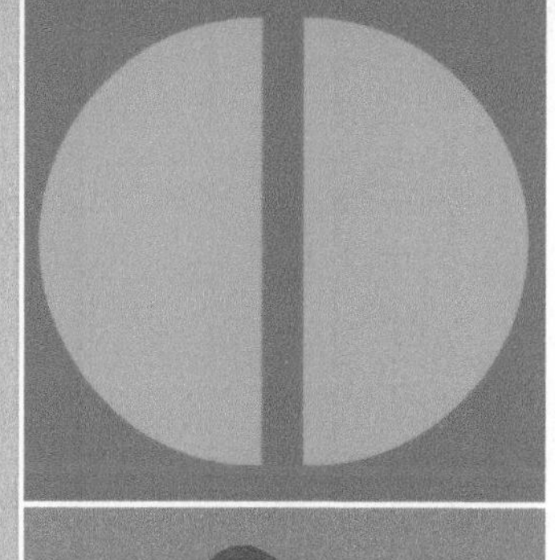

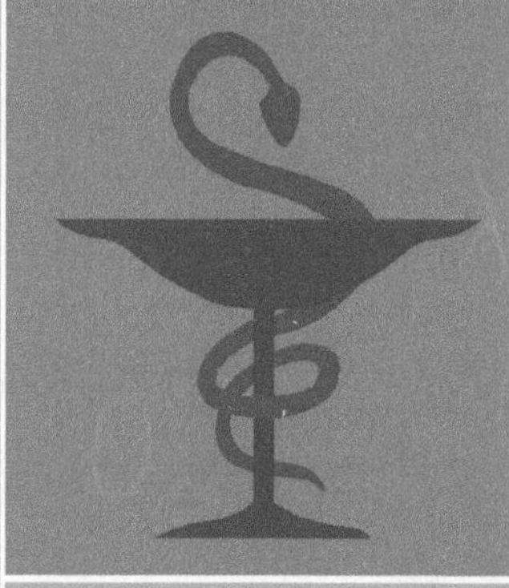

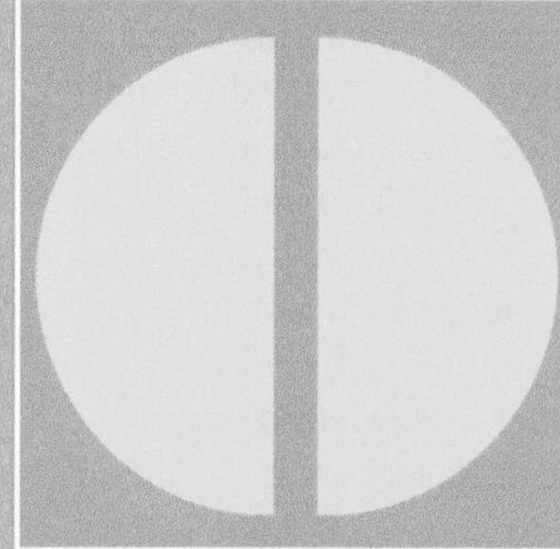

*KEY TERMS*

- achlorhydria
- adipose
- albumin
- aqueous
- bioavailability
- bioequivalent
- biotransformation
- blood-brain barrier
- capillary permeability
- cardiac decompensation
- carrier-mediated transport
- catalyze
- concentration gradient
- dissolution
- distribution
- epithelium
- equilibrium
- excretion

Chapter **3**

# Pharmacokinetics: The Absorption, Distribution, and Excretion of Drugs

## OBJECTIVES

After studying this chapter, the reader should be able to:

- Explain the meaning of the terms absorption, distribution, metabolism, and excretion.
- List two physiologic factors that can alter each of the processes of absorption, distribution, and excretion.
- Explain how bioavailability can impact drug response and product selection.
- Compare the roles of passive diffusion and carrier-mediated transport in drug absorption.
- Describe two types of drug interaction and explain how they might affect drug response and safety.

- extracellular
- first-pass effect
- hydrophilic
- interstitial
- intracellular
- lipids
- metabolism
- metabolite
- passive diffusion
- prodrug
- saturable process
- steady state
- volume of distribution

distribution The process by which a drug is carried to sites of action throughout the body by the bloodstream.

metabolism The total of all processes used by organisms to produce and maintain all cells and systems; also all processes used to handle consumed substances, whether nutrients, drugs, or toxins.

metabolite A product or byproduct of metabolism.

excretion The act or process of excreting; one form of elimination from the body.

Safe and effective drug treatment is not only a function of the physical and chemical properties of drugs, but also a function of how the human body responds to the administration of medication. The study of the bodily processes that affect the movement of a drug in the body is referred to as pharmacokinetics. To understand the pharmacology of drugs, the pharmacy technician must also understand the four fundamental pathways of drug movement and modification in the body (**Fig. 3.1**). First, drug absorption from the site of administration permits entry of the compound into the blood stream. Once absorbed, the drug may then leave the blood stream and disperse into the tissues and intracellular fluids where it can reversibly bind to receptors. This dispersal is called distribution. While some drug molecules are binding to receptors, others may be released from the receptors and be picked up again by the bloodstream. Drug particles in the blood stream are available to undergo biochemical changes, referred to as metabolism, in the liver or other tissues. Finally, the drug and its metabolites are excreted from the body in urine or feces. Metabolism and excretion are both pathways of drug elimination from the body.

Absorption, distribution, metabolism, and excretion are sometimes referred to collectively as ADME processes. These processes determine when the drug appears in the blood stream and for how long it remains there. In order for a drug to cause a therapeutic response, it must reach adequate concentrations in the blood so that it can reach and interact with drug receptors in adequate numbers to trigger a noticeable action. The course of drug action is, therefore, directly correlated with the concentration of the drug in the blood stream, and is dependent upon the ADME processes.

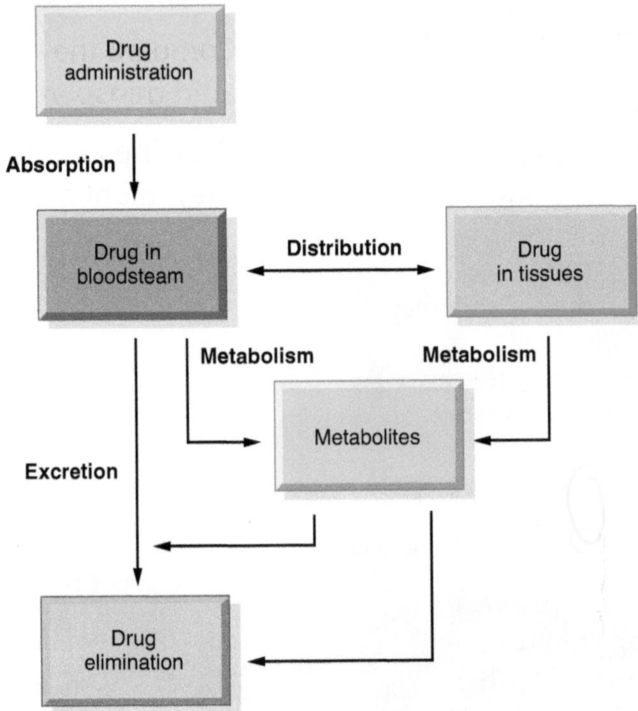


**Figure 3.1** A representation of the four fundamental pathways of drug movement and modification in the body, the ADME processes.

Knowledge of these processes and the ways that they can vary between individuals is an important part of understanding how and why a drug is selected for a patient. To investigate the pharmacokinetic characteristics of a study drug (drug X), researchers will give a group of healthy adults a standard dose of drug X intravenously (IV) or orally at the start of the study. Blood is drawn from the study subjects repeatedly, at predetermined times, and analyzed for the amount of drug per volume of blood at each point in time. The value obtained is the serum or plasma concentration of the drug at the time the blood was drawn. When serum drug concentrations are graphed versus time, the result is the serum concentration versus time curve illustrated in **Figure 3.2**.

Urine is also collected from the study subjects to monitor for the appearance of drug x or related metabolites. Immediately after intravenous administration and at a later time after oral or other routes of administration, the amount of drug in the blood will reach a peak (peak serum concentration) and then begin to fall off, eventually disappearing from the blood completely. The time it takes for the serum concentration to fall by one half is called the t½, or half-life, of elimination.

At some point after the drug is no longer detectable in the blood, the last of the drug and its metabolites, which have been filtered out by the kidneys, will also disappear from the urine. Plasma concentration data collected from this type of study is plotted against time and analyzed in order to understand the behavior of a specific drug in the body. This type of pharmacokinetic data, collected from average adults, is the basis for determining dose, dosing intervals, and limitations on the safe use of a drug. However, it is important for the technician student to remember that individuals do not always behave the way the average adult does. It is individual differences in ADME processes that create the need to modify doses or select different drugs in order to prevent poor treatment outcomes and adverse effects.

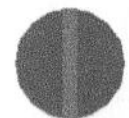

# Absorption

Absorption is the transfer of a drug from its site of administration to the bloodstream. The rate and extent of absorption depends on the route of administration, the formulation and chemical properties of the drug, and physiologic factors that can impact the site of absorp-

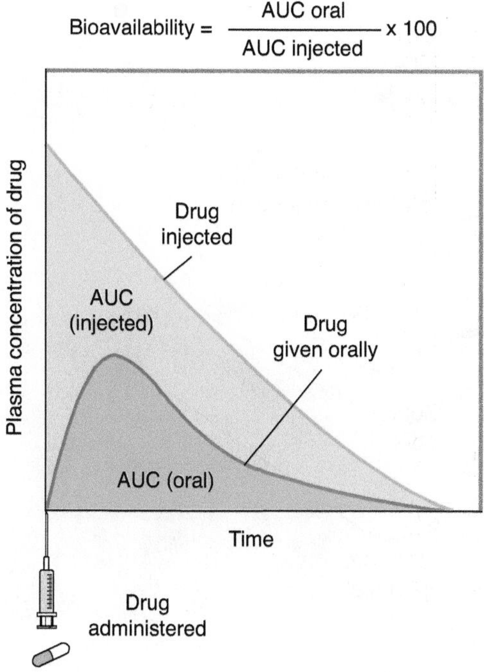


**Figure 3.2** Serum concentration versus time curves for oral and IV administration of a drug. The time it takes for the serum concentration to fall by one half is called the t½, or half-life of elimination. The bioavailability of the drug is determined by comparing the area under the two curves. AUC, area under curve. (Adapted with permission from Harvey RA, Champe PC, Howland RD, et al. *Lippincott's Illustrated Reviews: Pharmacology,* 3rd ed. Baltimore: Lippincott Williams & Wilkins, 2006.)

dissolution Process of dissolving or separating into component parts.

passive diffusion The process whereby particles become evenly spread solely as a result of spontaneous movement caused by their random thermal motion.

carrier-mediated transport Movement of a chemical substance, using a carrier protein and with the expenditure of energy, against a concentration gradient.

concentration gradient A variation in the concentration of a solute with regard to position; in pharmacology, especially in relationship to a semipermeable membrane.

epithelium Membranous cellular tissue that lines internal and external body surfaces, and is classified in types according to cell shapes and layers.

tion. When a drug is administered intravenously, absorption is not required because the drug is transferred from the administration device directly into the bloodstream. In the case of intravenous administration, the entire dose of the drug is available to move to the sites of drug action. Administration by other routes may result in less availability due to incomplete absorption. When this occurs, less of the drug is delivered by the bloodstream to the site of action. When a tablet or capsule is swallowed it must dissolve before it can be absorbed. The dissolving of a tablet or capsule is referred to as dissolution. Manufacturing processes and the water solubility of the drug affect dissolution rates. Highly water-soluble medications dissolve more readily in the gastrointestinal (GI) tract, while fat-soluble drugs dissolve more slowly. Drugs with smaller particle sizes go into solution more readily. The inert ingredients added to formulations can also affect their dissolution. Manufacturers must avoid producing tablets so compacted that they pass through the GI tract without ever dissolving. Tablets that dissolve too early are also problematic, because they taste bad and are difficult to swallow. Special formulations or coatings can be used to delay dissolution, thereby protecting the drug from stomach acid or allowing the gradual release of the drug to intentionally lengthen the absorption process. These are referred to as delayed or sustained release formulations. Liquid preparations do not require the step of dissolution. This explains the more rapid onset of action seen with liquid formulations as compared with the same drug given in tablet or capsule form.

Once dissolution has occurred, the drug molecules must pass through the selectively permeable membranes of the cells lining the gastrointestinal tract to reach the bloodstream. Depending on their chemical and physical properties, drugs will be absorbed either by passive diffusion or carrier-mediated transport across these membranes. Passive diffusion occurs when there is a high concentration of the drug on one side of the membrane and a low concentration on the other side. This difference from one side of the membrane to the other is called a concentration gradient. It is the natural tendency of substances to move from a region of higher concentration to a region of lower concentration; in other words, substances move down the concentration gradient. Drug molecules move across membranes or move through pores between the epithelial cells (**Fig. 3.3**). Diffusion is most efficient with

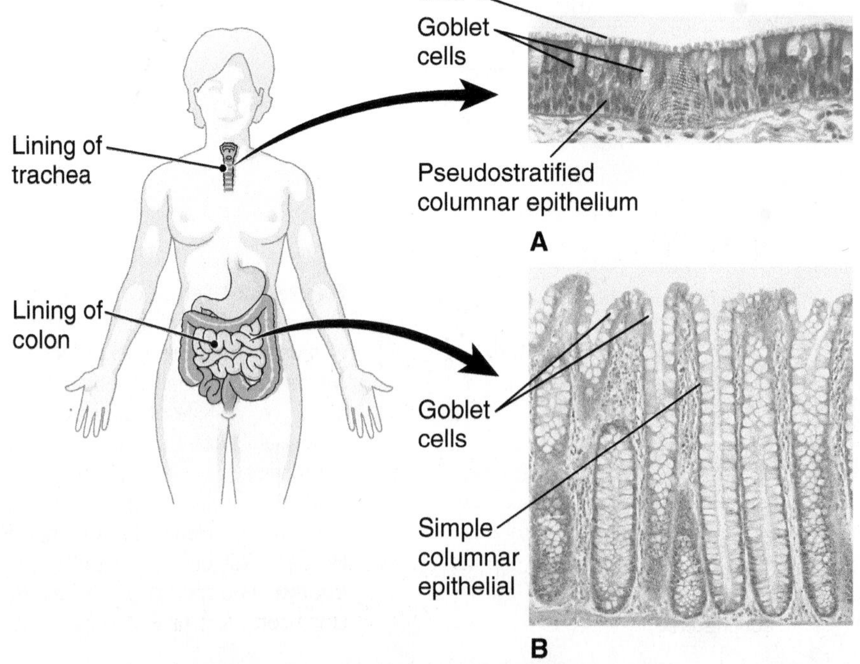


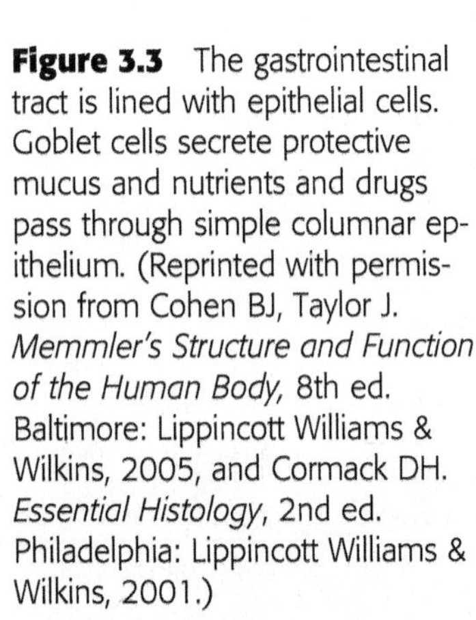
**Figure 3.3** The gastrointestinal tract is lined with epithelial cells. Goblet cells secrete protective mucus and nutrients and drugs pass through simple columnar epithelium. (Reprinted with permission from Cohen BJ, Taylor J. *Memmler's Structure and Function of the Human Body,* 8th ed. Baltimore: Lippincott Williams & Wilkins, 2005, and Cormack DH. *Essential Histology,* 2nd ed. Philadelphia: Lippincott Williams & Wilkins, 2001.)

drugs that are small molecules. This movement is solely driven by the kinetic energy within molecules, and continues until concentrations reach equilibrium. When equilibrium exists, the concentration of the substance is approximately equal on both sides of the membrane.

equilibrium A state of balance where no significant change occurs.

Passive diffusion does not involve a carrier molecule and the process is not a saturable process. Saturable processes are limited to a certain rate of activity by some aspect of the process. The vast majority of drugs gain access to the blood stream by diffusion. Drugs, which are usually somewhat lipid-soluble (fat-soluble), readily move across most biological membranes. Those drugs that are highly water-soluble penetrate the cell membrane through aqueous channels.

saturable process A process with a limited capacity; i.e., in drug metabolism there is a limited supply of drug metabolizing enzymes that must be free in order to proceed.

A few drugs that closely resemble naturally occurring compounds are absorbed via carrier-mediated transport. This process requires carrier proteins that attach to and actively carry the drug molecules across the membrane, utilizing a natural "pump" mechanism. This method of absorption is limited by the availability of the carrier protein and is therefore, saturable. Carrier-mediated transport requires energy and can move molecules against the concentration gradient. For an illustration of passive diffusion and carrier-mediated transport see **Figure 3.4**.

lipids Water insoluble, biologically active substances that are important components of living cells, sources of energy; includes fats, steroids, and related compounds.

## Bioavailability

The relationship between the drug dose and the amount ultimately delivered to the bloodstream is defined as bioavailability and is generally expressed as a percentage. If a 1 gram dose of a drug is administered by mouth, and half of that reaches the systemic circulation, the drug is 50% bioavailable. Bioavailability is calculated, not measured directly. Previously, the half-life of elimination and how it is determined was discussed. The same graph of serum concentrations against time also provides the data necessary to derive bioavailability. The area under the plasma concentration versus time curve represents the total amount of the drug reaching the circulatory system (see Fig. 3.2).

aqueous Made from or with water.

bioavailability Rate at which a drug is absorbed and becomes available to the target tissue.

This curve will have a different shape depending on the route of drug administration. The curve obtained from plotting values after intravenous administration of a drug serves as a reference for complete bioavailability. To determine bioavailability for nonintravenous formulations, the area under the curve obtained after drug administration is compared with the area achieved when the same dose is given intravenously. The ratio of the two is the bioavailability of the formulation tested.

The acid environment or presence of food in the stomach, the solubility and other chemical properties of the drug, and the effect of the initial exposure to metabolic processes in the liver may all reduce the amount of drug that reaches the systemic circulation after oral administration, thereby reducing the bioavailability of the drug. When a drug is absorbed through the GI tract, it must travel through the liver before entering the systemic cir-

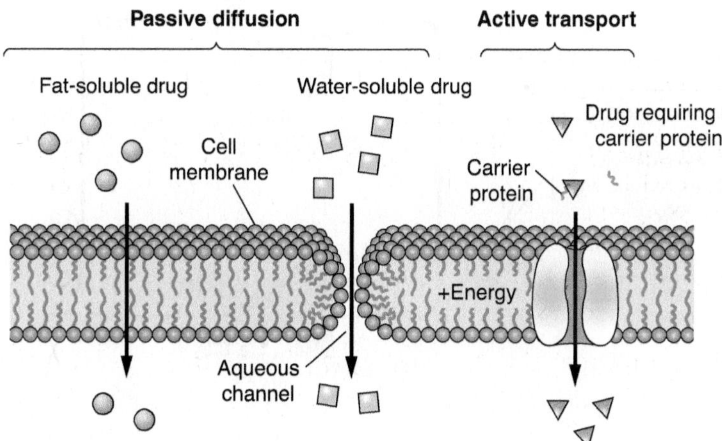


**Figure 3.4** Drugs are absorbed through the epithelium of the GI tract by both passive diffusion and carrier-mediated transport. Fat-soluble drugs pass through membranes easily, highly water soluble drugs pass through aqueous channels, and carrier-mediated transport requires a pump process and the expenditure of energy.

culation (see **Fig. 3.5**). If the drug is subject to metabolism by the liver, the amount of drug that reaches the systemic circulation is decreased. Some drugs, such as propranolol or enalapril, undergo significant metabolism during a single passage through the liver. This is called the first-pass effect. When drugs are highly susceptible to the first-pass effect, the oral dose needed to cause a response will be significantly higher than the intravenous dose used to cause the same response.

first-pass effect Biotransformation of a drug before it reaches the systemic circulation.

bioequivalent Two different drug formulations with identical active ingredients that possess similar bioavailability and produce the same effect at the site of action.

Bioavailability becomes important in drug product selection. While two generic products may contain the same active ingredients, they may not have the same dissolution or absorption characteristics and therefore cannot be considered bioequivalent. In the case of extended-release products, the change in dissolution characteristics is intentional. In some cases, however, products are simply poorly manufactured and should be avoided. Generic equivalent products approved by the Food and Drug Administration (FDA) must meet a standard of less than 20% variation from the comparison product, an amount that does not significantly affect therapeutic efficacy or safety in most cases. In practice, however, most generic products typically vary from the original by less than 5%. Bioequivalency data is published by the FDA's Center for Drug Evaluation and Research in the "Approved Drug Products with Therapeutic Equivalence Evaluations" publication, universally referred to as the "Orange Book" and available on the web.

## Factors Affecting Absorption

A number of patient-specific factors can affect absorption. Absorption from any site of administration requires blood flow. A patient who is in shock or cardiopulmonary arrest will need to have medications administered intravenously to achieve the desired response because of the reduced blood circulation in these situations. Most absorption after oral administration occurs in the small intestine because of its larger surface area and therefore greater blood flow. Significant impairment of absorption can result when sections of the small intestine are removed for medical reasons.

Contact time with the epithelial lining of the GI tract is also an important factor in drug absorption. In people with a very rapid transit time through the GI tract, due to severe diarrhea for example, medication cannot be effectively absorbed. Conversely, anything that delays stomach emptying (for instance, a large meal) will also delay and potentially reduce absorption.

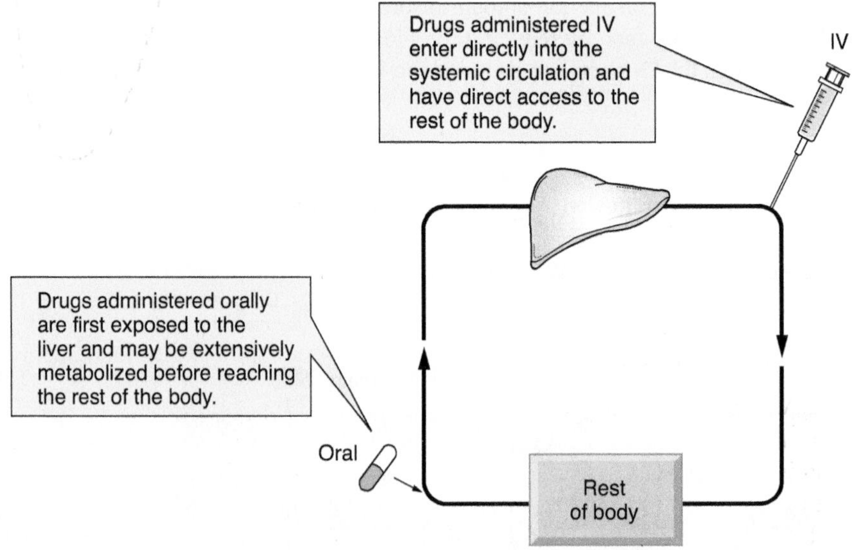
Drugs administered IV enter directly into the systemic circulation and have direct access to the rest of the body.
IV
Drugs administered orally are first exposed to the liver and may be extensively metabolized before reaching the rest of the body.
Oral
Rest of body

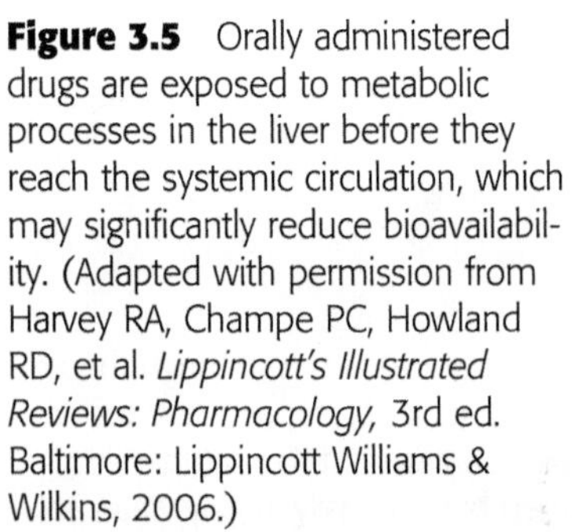

**Figure 3.5** Orally administered drugs are exposed to metabolic processes in the liver before they reach the systemic circulation, which may significantly reduce bioavailability. (Adapted with permission from Harvey RA, Champe PC, Howland RD, et al. *Lippincott's Illustrated Reviews: Pharmacology,* 3rd ed. Baltimore: Lippincott Williams & Wilkins, 2006.)

Some medications exhibit drug-food or drug-drug interactions with other compounds present in the GI tract. Specific foods or other drugs may bind a drug and prevent absorption. The interaction between tetracycline and dairy products or antacids is a good example of this effect.

achlorhydria The absence of hydrochloric acid from the gastric juices.

Although excess exposure to stomach acid may negatively impact some drugs, patients with very low levels of stomach acid (achlorhydria) may experience inadequate tablet dissolution and therefore poor drug absorption. Achlorhydria is most common in the elderly population.

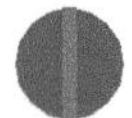

# Distribution

Once a drug is absorbed into the bloodstream it can be carried throughout the body. This process is called distribution, and is a reversible process; while some molecules may be interacting with receptors on cell membranes or inside of cells, other molecules may move back into the bloodstream. The delivery of a drug from the bloodstream to the site of drug action primarily depends on blood flow, capillary permeability, the degree of binding (attachment) of the drug to blood and tissue proteins, and the relative lipid-solubility of the drug molecule.

capillary permeability Property of capillary walls that allows for exchange of specific, fat-soluble molecules.

Blood flow to different organs of the body is not equal. The most vitally important organs of the body receive the greatest supply of blood. These organs include the brain, liver, and kidneys. Skeletal muscle and bone receive less blood, and adipose tissue (fat) receives the least. If blood flow were the only factor affecting distribution, it would be reasonable to expect that high concentrations of administered medications would always appear in the brain and liver. In reality, few drugs exhibit good penetration of the central nervous system. The anatomical structure of the capillary network in the brain creates a significant barrier to the passage of many drugs and is commonly referred to as the blood-brain barrier. This barrier is an adaptation that for the most part protects brain tissue from invasion by foreign substances. To readily penetrate into the brain, drugs must be fairly small and lipid-soluble or must be picked up by the carrier-mediated transport mechanism in the central nervous system. This explains why the small and highly fat-soluble anesthetic gases quickly and easily penetrate the brain to cause anesthesia, while other larger and water soluble molecules like penicillin antibiotics penetrate the central nervous system to a much lesser degree.

adipose Fat, or tissue containing fat cells.

blood-brain barrier An anatomical barrier that prevents many substance from entering the brain, created as a result of the relative impermeability of capillaries in the brain.

Compare the fairly impermeable capillaries of the brain to the highly permeable capillary walls in the liver and spleen (**Fig. 3.6**). These capillaries have gaps between their cells that allow large proteins to pass through to the capillary basement membrane. Capillary structure here is well adapted to the function of the liver, the key protein producer in the body and a center for chemical change of other compounds. In order to function, the liver must have access to amino acids, sugars, and other large molecules from the bloodstream. These molecules undergo chemical processing in the liver, and then must be moved out of the hepatic cells and back to the bloodstream.

## Factors Affecting Distribution

albumin Any of a number of water-soluble proteins that occur in blood plasma or serum, and other animal substances.

The blood is composed of a number of elements, including plasma, red and white blood cells, and plasma proteins. Most drugs reversibly bind to plasma proteins in varying degrees. Albumin is the plasma protein with the greatest capacity for binding drugs. Binding to plasma proteins affects drug distribution into tissues, because only drug that is not bound is available to penetrate tissues, bind to receptors, and exert activity. As free drug leaves the bloodstream, more bound drug is released from binding sites. In this way, drugs maintain a balance between free and bound drug that is unique to each compound, based

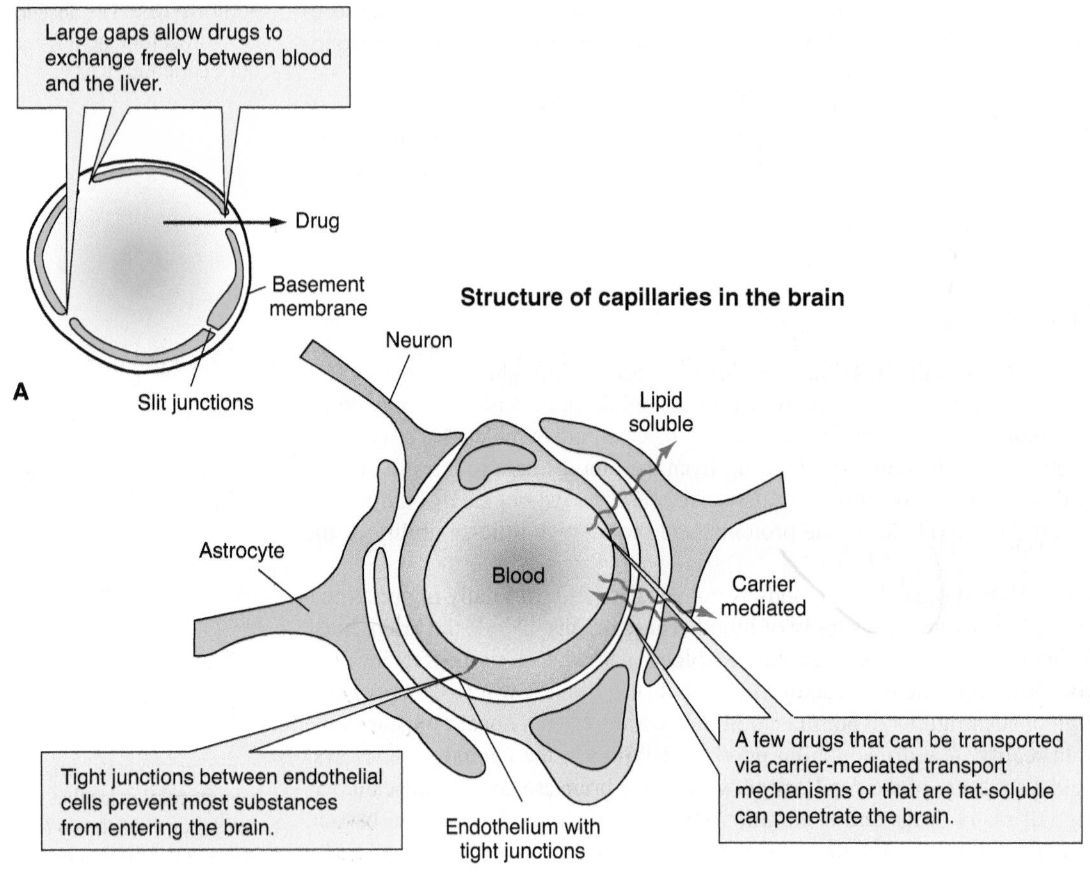


**Figure 3.6** Diagram demonstrating the difference in the anatomy of brain and liver capillaries. The tight junctions in brain capillaries prevent passage of most drugs into the brain. (Adapted with permission from Harvey RA, Champe PC, Howland RD, et al. *Lippincott's Illustrated Reviews: Pharmacology,* 3rd ed. Baltimore: Lippincott Williams & Wilkins, 2006.)

on its affinity for plasma proteins. Albumin, then, acts as a reservoir of an administered drug.

Some drugs have a high affinity for binding to serum proteins and may be 95% to 98% protein bound. With highly protein bound drugs, low albumin levels (as in protein-calorie malnutrition, or chronic illness) may lead to toxicity because there are fewer than the normal sites for the drug to bind. The amount of free drug is significantly increased in that case. The physician or pharmacist must consider the patient's serum albumin level when the dose of a highly protein bound medication is selected.

cardiac decompensation Failure of the heart to maintain adequate blood circulation; symptoms include shortness of breath and edema.

Competition for binding sites is one important way that drugs might interact. If a patient is using two highly protein bound drugs at the same time, there will be competition for binding sites on the albumin. The drug with the greatest affinity for the albumin will bind, and is thought to disrupt the normal ratio of free to bound drug for the second medication. As a result, the second medication will be more available to distribute to the site of action and potentially cause side effects.

volume of distribution The hypothetical volume required if the amount of drug in the body was distributed throughout the body at the same concentration measured in the blood.

Other patient variables that can affect distribution include body composition, cardiac decompensation (heart failure), and age of the patient. These factors all affect the apparent volume of distribution ($V_d$) of a drug and ultimately play a role in determining the appropriate dose of a drug. Volume of distribution is the hypothetical volume needed to account for all of the drug in the body based on the serum concentration in a blood sample. For example, assume that a 1-gram dose of drug X is given by IV injection to a patient. Thirty minutes later the serum concentration ($C_p$) is 25mcg/ml. If the drug were evenly distributed through the body, the apparent volume of distribution would have to be 40 liters (L) to account for the entire dose of the drug.

$C_p$ = Dose (amount in the body)/$V_d$

The adult human body is about 60% water. Therefore, the body of an average adult who weighs 70 kg (about 150 lbs) contains 42 L, or 10 gallons, of water. Total body water can be conceptually divided into three spaces or compartments. The fluid contained in the bloodstream makes up about 5 L, or about 9% of the volume of an average sized adult. The total water outside of the cells (extracellular fluid) includes the plasma volume plus the fluid in the interstitial space and is about 14 L. Intracellular fluid makes up the remaining 28 L. Drugs with high molecular weights or drugs that are extremely hydrophilic (with a strong affinity for water) tend to stay within the circulatory system and organs with a rich blood supply, and have a smaller apparent volume of distribution. Small, highly lipophilic drugs have a large apparent volume of distribution.

extracellular Outside of the cell or cells.

interstitial Situated within or between parts of a particular organ or tissue.

intracellular Existing or functioning inside a cell or cells.

hydrophilic Having an affinity for, readily absorbing, or mixing with water.

lipophilic Having an affinity for, or ability to absorb or dissolve in, fats.

### Case 3.1

John Q. Brewer was a frequent flyer in the emergency room. John had an alcohol addiction problem, and one night he came to the emergency room with seizures. John's wife said that he had been sober for 2 days. This afternoon she said he began to see things, and then the seizures began. The ER physician controlled the seizures with the benzodiazepine lorazepam, and wanted to follow that with a large oral dose of the anticonvulsant phenytoin and a prescription for ongoing phenytoin to be used for 6 months. The ER pharmacist suggested that because John was an alcoholic his albumin levels were probably low, and therefore he needed a reduced dose of albumin. The two conferred and decided to give John half the usual dose and check his albumin level.

Volume of distribution often becomes important when dosing calculations are made based on weight. A short, obese woman who weighs 250 lbs cannot handle the same dose of an aminoglycoside antibiotic that a tall, muscular man of the same weight would require. This is because a greater portion of the woman's body is made up of fat. Aminoglycoside drugs are water-soluble and stay mainly in extracellular fluid, therefore dosing must be based on adjusted body weight, which will more correctly reflect the true volume of extracellular fluid in the body.

Dosing of medications in infants and children requires special consideration. It is the often-repeated wisdom of pediatric health care specialists that "children are not simply small adults." This means that dosing cannot simply be adjusted based on the lower weight of children. The body composition of children is very different from adults. Their bodies contain a much higher percentage of water and a lower percentage of muscle and fat. Albumin levels may also be lower, especially in neonates. These variations result in different values for volume of distribution and significantly affect drug dosing.

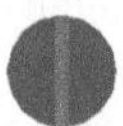

## Metabolism

Drugs are eliminated from the body either unchanged through the kidneys and bile, or they may undergo chemical changes that allow them to be more easily excreted. The process of undergoing chemical changes is called biotransformation, or metabolism. As previously noted, anything absorbed through the GI tract goes directly into the portal circula-

biotransformation Chemical alterations of a compound that occur within the body, as in drug metabolism.

tion that feeds into the liver. The liver is adapted to clear toxins from the body and is the major site for drug metabolism, but specific drugs may undergo biotransformation in other tissues.

The kidneys cannot efficiently excrete highly fat-soluble drugs that readily cross cell membranes because they are reabsorbed in the last stages of filtration. These compounds must first be metabolized in the liver to more water-soluble compounds and then removed. There are two types of metabolic processes drugs undergo in the liver. Most undergo one or both types of reactions.

catalyze To accelerate, or bring about an increase in, the rate of a chemical reaction.

In the first type of reaction drugs are made more polar through oxidation-reduction reactions or hydrolysis. These reactions use metabolic enzymes, most often those of the cytochrome P450 enzyme system, to catalyze the biotransformation. In enzyme-catalyzed reactions, the rate of the reaction is accelerated by the presence of enzymes. A limited amount of enzyme is present at any given time in the liver. Since the rate of enzyme-catalyzed drug metabolism is limited by the quantity of available enzyme, metabolism in these cases is considered a saturable process. This means that the rate of conversion will only continue at the normal pace until the available supply of enzyme is used. At that point, metabolism is slowed until enzyme becomes available again. For the usual doses of most drugs, these reactions never reach saturation. There are a few drugs where doses may reach the saturation point of the enzymes. Once enzymes become saturated, blood levels increase exponentially toward toxicity. Examples include metabolism of alcohol and phenytoin.

The second type of metabolism involves conjugation reactions. In this type of reaction the drug undergoing change is joined with another substance, such as glucuronic acid, sulfuric acid, acetic acid, or an amino acid. Glucuronidation is the most common conjugation reaction. The result of conjugation is a more water-soluble compound that is easier for the kidneys to excrete. These metabolites are most often therapeutically inactive.

prodrug An inactive drug precursor that is converted in the body to the active drug form.

Some agents are initially administered as an inactive compound (prodrug) in order to improve availability or reduce side effects. Metabolism converts the prodrug to the active form. Fosphenytoin, for example, is a prodrug of phenytoin, a drug used for seizure disorders. Fosphenytoin is more completely and quickly absorbed when given by IM injection than phenytoin and can be used in critical situations with greater ease because it dose not require insertion of an intravenous catheter.

## Factors Affecting Metabolism

Metabolism of drugs can vary widely between population groups. Deficiency of some drug metabolizing enzymes is genetic and will result in poor tolerance of certain drugs. For example, many Asians and Native Americans have difficulty metabolizing drugs that require acetylation, such as ethanol. These individuals will exhibit a low tolerance of such drugs, and can suffer adverse drug reactions at a much higher rate than the average population. Age is another important variable that has a bearing on metabolism. Organ function gradually declines with age and the elderly may poorly tolerate drugs that require metabolism. The very young require special consideration of drug dosing because of immaturity of their organ systems. This subject matter is worthy of further study for those technicians who will be serving these special populations.

Drug interactions may occur between two drugs that are metabolized by the same enzyme systems in the liver. Because there is a limit on available enzymes for metabolism, excess drug will remain active and free to exert an effect elsewhere in the body. Usually, of two drugs that are metabolized by the same enzyme system, one has a higher affinity for the enzyme, and levels of the second drug build up. In some cases, the drug being metabolized will induce the production of more of the enzymes. Enzyme induction sets the stage for another type of drug interaction, because the increased production of metabolizing enzymes may result in higher rates of removal and the need for an increased dose of the second drug. A good example of a drug that stimulates production of metabolizing enzymes is phenobarbital, a drug used to treat some forms of epilepsy.

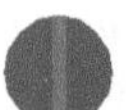

# Excretion

When a drug is taken into and distributed throughout the body, it must be subsequently removed, or concentrations of the drug would continue to rise with each successive dose. The complete removal of the drug from the body is referred to as elimination. Elimination of the drug encompasses both the metabolism of the drug, and excretion of the drug through the kidneys, and to a much lesser degree into the bile. Excretion into the urine is one of the most important mechanisms of drug removal.

The kidneys act as a filter for the blood and create urine as a vehicle for removal of waste. Blood enters the kidney through renal arteries and then is filtered by the glomerulus (see Chapter 21). The glomerular filtrate becomes concentrated and substances are removed as it passes through the renal tubule and eventually becomes urine. Drug molecules in the bloodstream that are not bound to albumin are also filtered out into the glomerular filtrate. When drugs have not been converted to water soluble compounds in the liver, they are likely to be reabsorbed back into the bloodstream at the end of the filtration process, and will cycle through the body again. If they are water soluble, they will end up in the urine and be excreted.

When a medication is given repeatedly, as most are in real patients, the total amount of drug in the body will increase up to a point and then stabilize. At this point, the amount being taken in by the patient is equal to the amount being removed by the liver and kidneys (**Fig. 3.7**). This state of equilibrium is called steady state, and drug levels will remain fairly constant unless there is a dose change, an interruption in treatment, or failure of the organs of elimination. The therapeutic effects of many drugs are closely correlated to a specific range of steady state serum drug levels, and physicians or clinical pharmacists will monitor these levels and adjust doses when necessary so that patients obtain the appropriate drug response.

steady state A state of equilibrium; especially related to drug serum levels.

## Factors Affecting Excretion

The complete elimination of a drug from the body is dependent on normal liver and kidney function. The kidney is the major organ of excretion; however, the liver also contributes to elimination through metabolism and excretion into the feces via the bile. When a patient has reduced kidney function or another problem that lengthens the half-life of a drug, dosage adjustment is required. If the dosage is not adjusted, the drug will accumulate in the body.

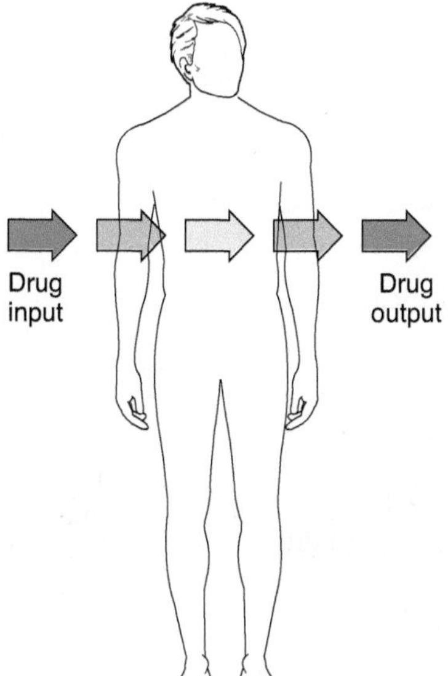


**Figure 3.7** At steady state, the input of the drug equals the elimination of the drug. (Adapted with permission from Harvey RA, Champe PC, Howland RD, et al. *Lippincott's Illustrated Reviews: Pharmacology,* 3rd ed. Baltimore: Lippincott Williams & Wilkins, 2006.)

Kidney or liver failure, or conditions where blood flow to these organs is reduced, complicate drug and dose selection. Drugs that are dependent upon excretion through the kidneys are not the best choice for patients with renal failure. Patients with liver disease will better tolerate drugs that can be cleared exclusively through the kidneys. Age must be considered in a discussion of drug excretion. The very young and very old will have lower rates of excretion; the old because of deterioration in organ function and the very young, because the kidneys have not reached full maturity. Doses often require reduction in these patients. Drug interactions, such as when multiple drugs compete for metabolic processes, can also reduce drug removal.

Clearly, the interactions between a drug and the human body are incredibly complex. This makes choosing the most appropriate medication and dose complicated, and that choice becomes more obscure when a patient is taking many other medications. This complexity makes it all the more essential that prescriptions be filled carefully and accurately at all times.

# Review Questions

## Multiple Choice

Choose the best answer to the following questions:

1. Which of the following is not one of the four fundamental pathways of drug movement and modification in the body?
   a. distribution
   b. metabolism
   c. absorption
   d. dissolution
   e. elimination

2. Which is correct regarding the process of passive diffusion?
   a. It requires a carrier protein molecule.
   b. It occurs when a concentration gradient exists from one side of a membrane to the other.
   c. It is a saturable process.
   d. The only drugs that can enter cells via passive diffusion are antibiotics.
   e. None of the above are correct.

3. Which of the following factors has the potential to affect absorption of an orally administered drug?
   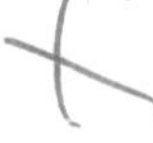
   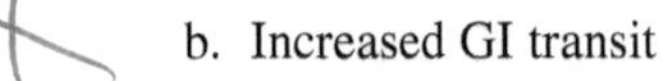
   a. Reduction in blood flow to the intestines
   b. Increased GI transit time
   c. Extremely low levels of stomach acid
   d. Eating a large meal just prior to taking an oral medication
   e. All of the above

4. Choose the incorrect statement.
   a. Most drugs reversibly bind to plasma proteins.
   b. Albumin is the most important drug binding plasma protein.
   c. Low albumin levels can lead to drug toxicity in the case of drugs that are highly protein bound.
   d. Only a drug that is protein bound can penetrate tissues.
   e. None of the above is incorrect.

5. Elimination of drugs from the body is dependent on which of the following?
   a. Biotransformation in the liver
   b. Filtration or secretion in the kidney
   c. Sufficient blood flow to the liver and kidneys
   d. Only a and b
   e. a, b, and c

## True/False

6. Enzymes facilitate chemical transformation reactions in drug metabolism.
   a. True
   b. False

7. After oral administration, drugs pass through the liver before they ever reach the circulation, with the potential for significantly reducing the amount of drug to reach the site of action.
   a. True
   b. False

8. Body weight is more important than age when determining the appropriate dose of a drug because a 6-month-old is just a smaller version of a 16-year-old child.
   a. True
   b. False

9. Before a tablet can be absorbed through the GI tract it must dissolve.
   a. True
   b. False

10. Half-life is defined as the time it takes for the serum concentration of a drug to drop to 0.
    a. True
    b. False

## Matching

Match each numbered phrase to the best corresponding answer listed below.

11. Oral absorption
12. Distribution
13. Protein binding
14. Enzyme catalyzed metabolism
15. Excretion

a. Albumin
b. Carrier-mediated transport
c. Blood flow
d. Small intestine
e. Kidneys
f. Cytochrome p450
g. Serum concentration

## Short Answer

16. Compare the two mechanisms of drug transfer across cell membranes, passive diffusion, and carrier-mediated transport.

17. How might the physiology of brain capillaries affect the choice of antibiotics for treatment of meningitis, an infection of the lining of the brain and spinal cord?

18. Briefly describe the process of metabolism and explain how individual patient differences can affect metabolism and, therefore, drug selection.

19. Drug P is an experimental drug that is known to be 98% eliminated as the active, unmetabolized drug in the urine. How would a significant loss of renal function likely affect the elimination, $t\frac{1}{2}$, and dose of this drug?

20. Describe two mechanisms for drug interactions.

## FOR FURTHER INQUIRY

Consider what you have learned about the ADME processes, and use additional references if necessary, to answer one of the following questions:

1. How do the absorption characteristics and rate of elimination ($t^1/_2$) of a drug affect patient acceptability and compliance with the physician's instructions for use of that drug?

2. Do you think it is important for pharmacists to have access to specific patient information when reviewing prescriptions for appropriateness of the drug and dose? What kind of information should the patient profile contain?

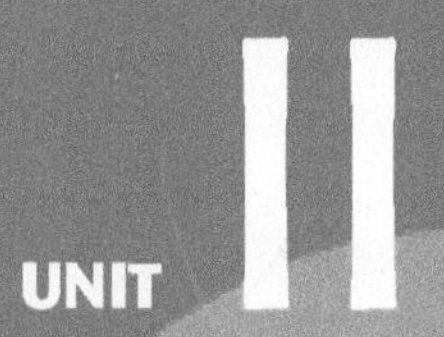

UNIT II

# Drugs Affecting the Nervous System

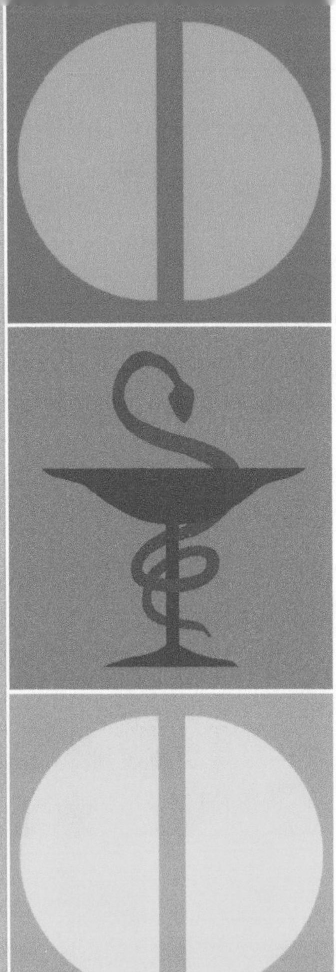

Chapter **4**

# The Anatomy and Physiology of the Nervous System

*KEY TERMS*

- action potential
- afferent
- autonomic
- axon
- central nervous system
- cerebellum
- cerebral cortex
- cerebrospinal fluid
- dendrite
- depolarization
- diencephalon
- effector
- efferent
- ganglia
- glial cells
- homeostasis
- innervate
- ion
- limbic system
- meninges

## OBJECTIVES

After studying this chapter, the reader should be able to:

- Explain, in brief, what occurs when a nerve impulse in a presynaptic nerve reaches the synapse.
- List the major neurotransmitters in the peripheral and central nervous systems.
- Describe the main anatomical features of the central nervous system.
- Describe the function of the peripheral nervous system.
- Compare and contrast the effect of nerve stimulation in the parasympathetic and sympathetic divisions of the autonomic nervous system.

- myelin
- neuromuscular junction
- neurons
- neurotransmission
- neurotransmitter
- parasympathetic
- peripheral nervous system
- postsynaptic
- presynaptic
- reflex arc
- resting membrane potential
- somatic
- sympathetic synapse
- synaptic cleft
- vestibular system

The human nervous system is incredibly complex, amazingly adaptable, and brilliantly efficient, but it is incompletely understood. The nervous system has been compared to a computer system, an analogy that is still insufficient to explain its complexity. Compare the computer systems required to monitor a space flight to the nervous system. As with the human body, data from the internal environment of the spacecraft, along with the trajectory and speed of the craft, and even the vital signs of the astronauts, are all collected and entered from onboard systems into the processing units of the computer on the ground. This data is analyzed for variation from desirable parameters. If variations are detected, then the computer will direct the equipment on board to make adjustments to the environmental, propulsion, and navigational systems as needed to maintain the normal ranges and keep the craft on the proper flight path. In the body, the nervous system is prepared to respond to input from the heart, kidneys, sensory, and other organs and make adjustments to maintain the status quo.

The nervous system of the body, like the computer system for a space flight, is responsible for homeostasis in the body. The brain is analogous to the processing units for a computer system. Data from every body system is constantly being sent via afferent nerves to the brain where it is analyzed. Instructions for adjustments to body systems are sent out via the efferent nerves. The central nervous system, composed of the brain and spinal cord, makes adjustments in breathing rate, heart rate, blood pressure, and other essential functions automatically, without any conscious deliberation. But unlike a computer system, the higher level thought processes of the brain are able to analyze a variety of types of input and use intellect, creativity, and stored memory to ponder external dilemmas and come up with solutions that are not automatic, and that require thought. Not only that, but our nervous system is faster, smaller, more durable, and able to learn and adapt to change.

Whereas a computer uses wires and chips to transfer and store messages, the nervous system uses cells. The human nervous system can pass information back and forth in fractions of a second because of the highly specialized nature of the cells of the nervous system. These cells have the ability, through the exchange of chemicals, to move tiny electrical impulses down the length of the cell, and across gaps to the adjoining cell.

homeostasis Relatively stable internal physiological conditions (as body temperature or the pH of blood) under fluctuating environmental conditions.

afferent Moving or conducting inwardly. Refers to vessels, nerves, etc.

efferent Moving or carrying outward or away from a central part. Refers to vessels, nerves, etc.

central nervous system Part of the nervous system consisting of the brain and spinal cord, which supervises and coordinates the activity of the nervous system.

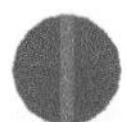

## Cells of the Nervous System

There are two main types of cells in the nervous system, neurons and glial cells. Neurons are highly specialized cells that conduct electrical impulses that are later translated into information or commands by effector cells, the tissue that responds to the nerve impulse. There are three types of neurons: sensory neurons, motor neurons, and interneurons. Sensory neurons bring information from organs or tissues toward the central nervous system (CNS), and motor neurons bring the stimulus for a response to effector cells (for example, muscle cells). Interneurons connect sensory and motor neurons and are found only within the CNS.

A neuron is composed of the cell body, where the nucleus and other cellular organelles are found, and two types of fibers for the conduction of impulses (**Fig. 4.1**). The cell body has multiple dendrites, branched fibers that bring information to the cell body. Each neu-

neurons Any of the cells of the nervous system that have the property of transmitting and receiving nervous impulses.

effector A molecule that activates, controls, or inactivates a process or action.

dendrite Threadlike extensions of the cytoplasm of a neuron that conduct impulses toward the body of a nerve cell.

ron usually has a single axon, a long fiber with minimal branching, which conducts impulses away from the cell body towards the synapse, the connection between two nerve cells. In the efferent (moving away from the brain) neurons of the peripheral nervous system (all nerve tissues located outside the CNS), cell bodies are found either in the CNS or in the ganglia. Ganglia are clusters of cell bodies originating outside of the CNS. Preganglionic fibers arise in the brainstem or spinal cord and then connect with the second group of cells that originate in the ganglia, called postganglionic fibers.

Glial cells provide support and serve in maintenance capacities for neurons. This support can be physical, where glial cells provide structure to cover and protect the neurons, or functional, where glial cells provide nutrients and are responsible for removing dead or damaged neurons. The axons of many neurons in the CNS are covered with a protective lipid sheath called myelin. A type of glial cell, called Schwann cells, produce myelin. In the central nervous system, nerves covered with myelin are white in color and make up the white matter. The gray matter of the CNS is unmyelinated tissue.

axon A long projection of the nerve cell that conducts efferent impulses from the cell body toward target cells.

synapse The connection between two neurons at which a nervous impulse passes from one to the other.

peripheral nervous system The part of the nervous system that is outside the central nervous system.

ganglia A group of nerve cell bodies located outside of the central nervous system.

glial cells Specialized cells that surround neurons and provide insulation, mechanical, and physical support.

myelin A soft, somewhat fatty material that forms a thick protective sheath around nerve axons.

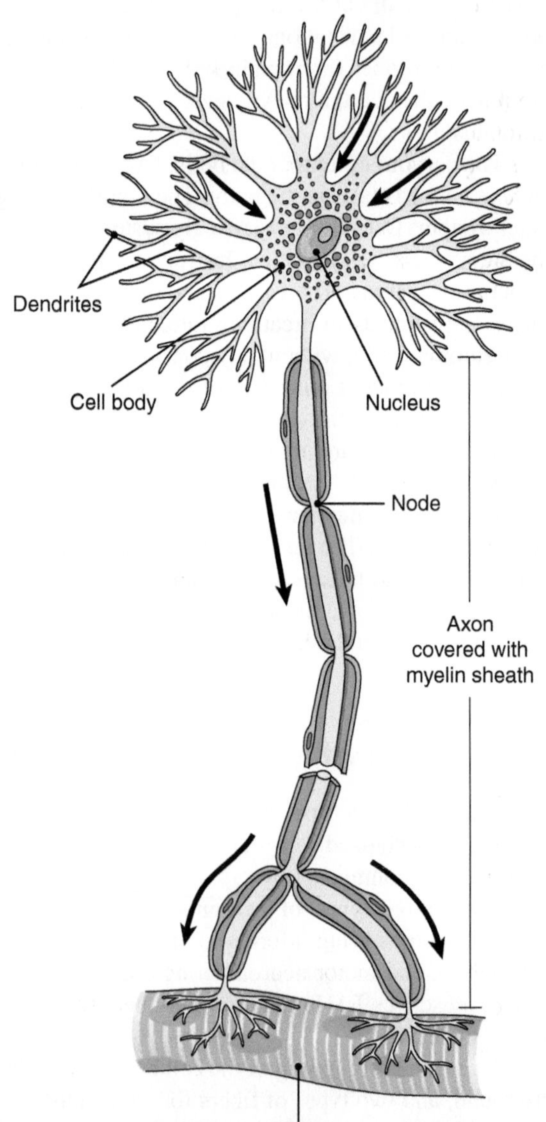


**Figure 4.1** An illustration of an efferent neuron showing the synapse with the effector cell, in this case, a muscle cell. (Adapted with permission from Cohen BJ, Taylor J. *Memmler's Structure and Function of the Human Body,* 8th ed. Baltimore: Lippincott Williams & Wilkins, 2005.)

## The Synapse

A single neuron usually does not span the entire distance between the cells of target tissues and the central nervous system. Neurons of varying length are strung together to form a connection between the CNS and the target tissue. Groups of these fibers are bundled together to form a nerve. For an impulse to travel rapidly down the nerve it must be passed from neuron to neuron in a continuous and efficient manner. Impulse transmission requires both chemical and electrical activity.

The membranes of cells that transmit nerve impulses carry a slight electrical charge while at rest. This occurs because there are more positively charged sodium particles, called ions, concentrated on the outside of the cell membrane, than there are positively charged potassium ions concentrated on the inside, causing the interior of the cell to have a negative charge with respect to the exterior. Just as a magnet or a battery is called "polarized" because it has positively and negatively charged poles, we say that excitable cells (nerve cells and muscle cells) are polarized. This electrical voltage is known as the resting membrane potential, and it creates the possibility for flow of electrical current in the cell. When the cell receives a stimulus, channels within the cell membrane open, and sodium ions flow rapidly into the cell, creating a tiny current. This is called depolarization, and is the process that allows minute electrical impulses, the action potential, to travel the length of the nerve fiber. Once the impulse passes, the ions are actively pumped back to their former positions and the nerve is ready to carry the next electrical message (**Fig. 4.2**).

At the end of the nerve fiber there is a junction that the electrical charge must cross. The junction between two neurons is called a synapse, and it is a significant and elegant anatomical structure. The conduction of the electrical impulse down the nerve and across the synapse is called neurotransmission. Neurotransmission occurs from the presynaptic nerve, across a tiny gap called the synaptic cleft, to the postsynaptic nerve.

In order for the nerve impulse to cross the synaptic cleft, chemical mediators called neurotransmitters are released by the presynaptic neuron, as shown in **Figure 4.3**. These chemicals are contained in tiny packets or vesicles, which move toward and release their contents into the synaptic cleft when an impulse arrives. Neurotransmitters diffuse across the gap and bind to specific receptors on the postsynaptic cell. The neurotransmitter-receptor complex initiates a response in the postsynaptic cell. The neurotransmitter is then either picked up by the presynaptic neuron to be recycled, or is destroyed by enzymes in the synapse.

Synapses occur in both the peripheral and central nervous systems. A similar sort of connection exists between nerves and effector cells. The connection between a nerve and muscle cell is called the neuromuscular junction and impulse transmission across this junction works similarly to synaptic transmission.

ion An atom or group of atoms that carries a positive or negative electric charge as a result of having lost or gained one or more electrons

resting membrane potential The tiny electrical charge that exists in excitable membranes at rest.

depolarization The loss of the difference in charge between the inside and outside of a cell, due to a change in permeability and migration of sodium ions to the interior.

action potential The sequential polarization and depolarization that travels across membranes of excitable tissue (such as nerve or muscle cells), in response to stimulation.

neurotransmission Passage of signals from one nerve cell to another via chemical substances and electrical signals.

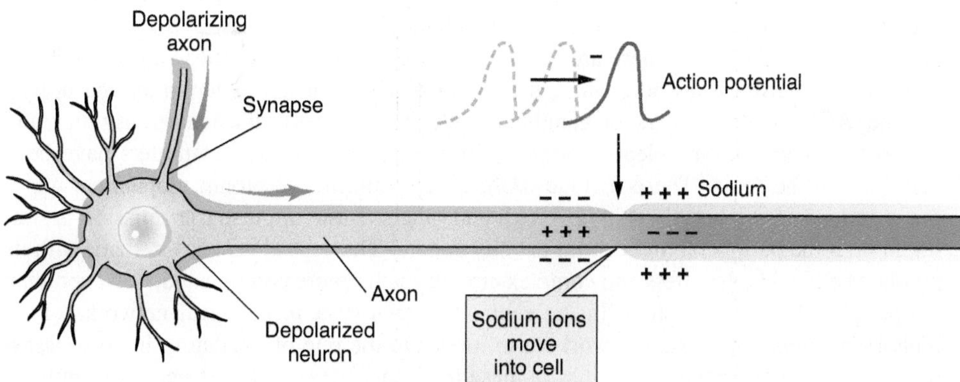


**Figure 4.2** A depiction of the movement of a nerve impulse, or action potential. At the moment the action potential passes, sodium rapidly moves into cells, then potassium moves out.

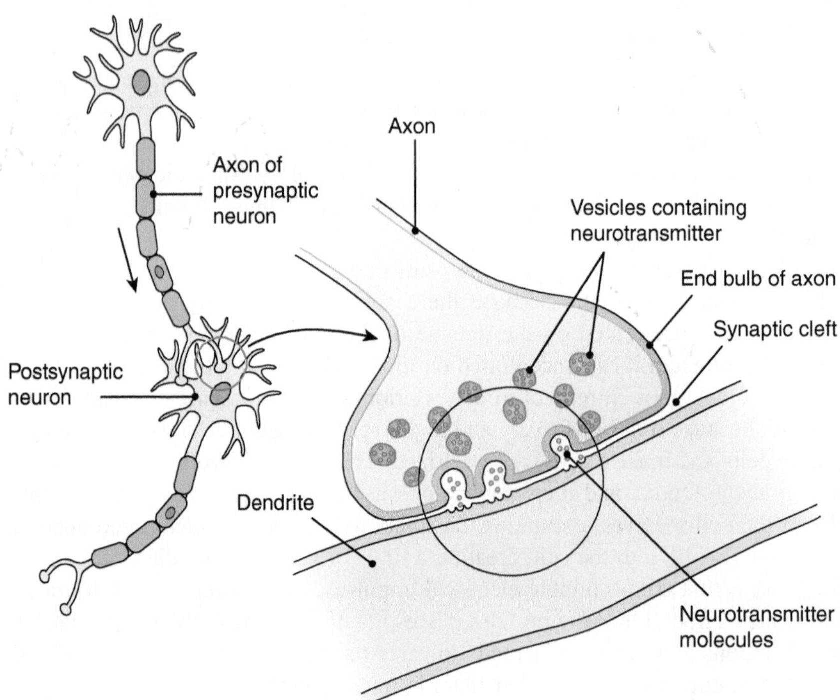


**Figure 4.3** The synapse. (Adapted with permission from Cohen BJ, Taylor J. *Memmler's Structure and Function of the Human Body*, 8th ed. Baltimore: Lippincott Williams & Wilkins, 2005.)

presynaptic Pertaining to or occurring before the synapse.

synaptic cleft The narrow space between neurons at a nerve synapse.

postsynaptic Pertaining to or occurring after the synapse.

neurotransmitter An endogenous substance that carries a nerve impulse across a synapse.

neuromuscular junction The junction of an efferent nerve fiber and a muscle fiber.

New information about the synapse suggests that these connections are far more complex than initially understood. Not only may any nerve ending have thousands of synapses, but also any one synapse may contain vesicles of different neurotransmitters. Researchers think that some of the neurotransmitters may modulate the release of the others. This means that propagation of nerve impulses in the healthy individual requires an exquisitely balanced interplay between excitatory and inhibitory impulses. It is easy to imagine that when the nervous system is out of balance, for whatever reason, the effects can impact not only our emotional, but also our physical well-being.

## Neurotransmitters

Currently, there are more than 50 known neurotransmitters that are classified into four chemical groups: acetylcholine, the biogenic amines (the catecholamines, including epinephrine and norepinephrine, histamine, and serotonin for example), the excitatory amino acids (L-glutamate, the major excitatory neurotransmitter in the brain, and others), and the neuropeptides (such as the endorphins). Undoubtedly many others await discovery. In the peripheral nervous system there are three major neurotransmitters. These are epinephrine (sometimes referred to as adrenalin), the chemically similar norepinephrine, and acetylcholine (ACh). At the presynaptic ganglia, acetylcholine serves as the neurotransmitter, and the postsynaptic neurons release norepinephrine. Numerous neurotransmitters have been identified in the brain. These include ACh, norepinephrine, serotonin, dopamine, glutamate, gamma amino butyric acid (GABA), and others. Basic impulse transmission is similar in both the peripheral and central nevous system. The central nervous system, with its myriad chemical transmitters and complex circuitry is far more complicated, however, than the peripheral nervous system. In the central nervous system, powerful networks of inhibitory neurons are constantly working to modulate the rate of excitatory impulse transmission. GABA is a neurotransmitter in these inhibitory neurons. Some neurotransmitters, however, may be involved in either inhibitory or excitatory capacity. The response they cause depends on which receptors they activate.

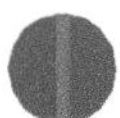

# Divisions Within the Nervous System

There are both structural (anatomical) and functional (physiological) divisions within the nervous system. The nervous system is made up of the brain, the spinal cord, and afferent and efferent nerves connecting the brain and spinal cord to the body systems (**Fig. 4.4**). As previously stated, the central nervous system includes the brain and the spinal cord. The peripheral nervous system (PNS) is made up of all the nerves outside the central nervous system. The peripheral nervous system is subdivided into two divisions. The efferent division consists of the neurons that carry signals away from the brain and spinal cord to the organ systems and other tissues. The third cranial nerve, the oculomotor nerve, controls most of the muscles of the eye, and the movement of the upper lid, and is an efferent nerve. The afferent division consists of the neurons that bring information from these tissues to the CNS. A good example of an afferent nerve is the second cranial nerve, the optic nerve, which carries visual information from the retina to the brain. **Figure 4.5** is a schematic diagram of the organization of the nervous system. The efferent portion of the peripheral nervous system is further divided into two major functional subdivisions, the somatic and the autonomic systems. The somatic nervous system is involved in the voluntary control of func-

somatic Of, relating to, supplying, or involving skeletal muscles.

autonomic Acting or occurring involuntarily; self-controlling.

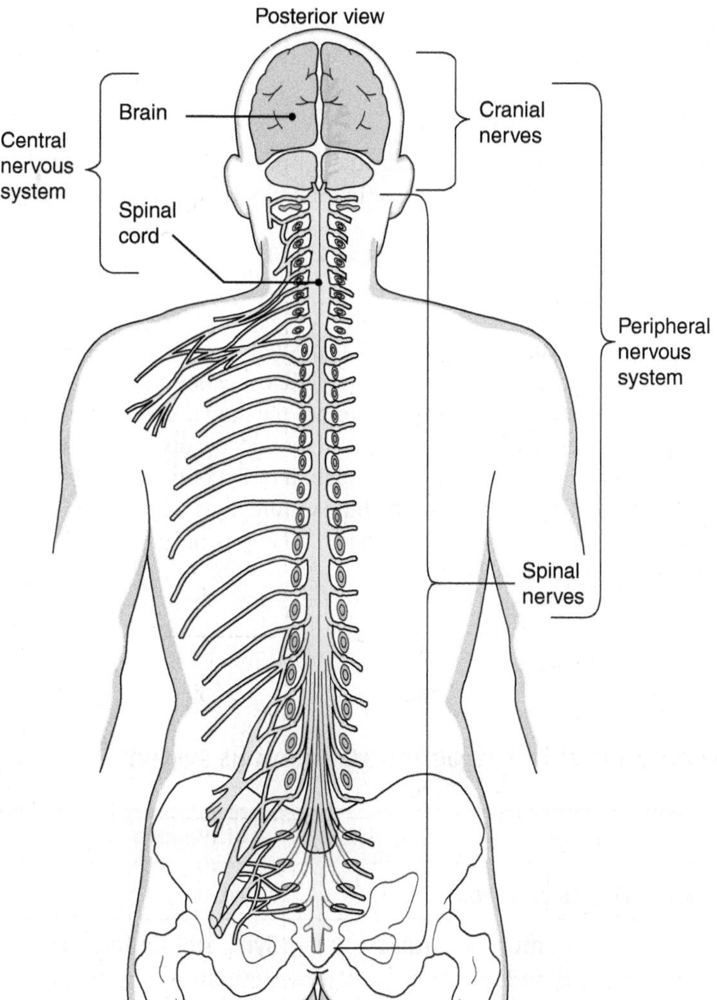


**Figure 4.4** The major anatomical divisions of the nervous system, including the locations of the cranial and spinal nerves. (Reprinted with permission from Cohen BJ. *Memmler's The Human Body in Health and Disease,* 10th ed. Baltimore: Lippincott Williams & Wilkins, 2005.)

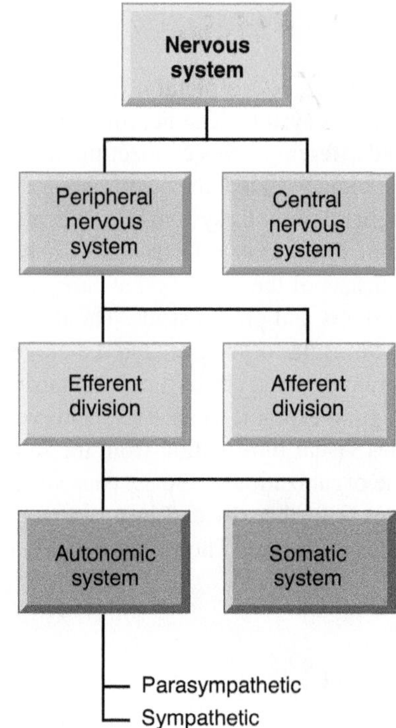


**Figure 4.5** Schematic representation of the organization of the nervous system. (Adapted with permission from Harvey RA, Champe PC, Howland RD, et al. *Lippincott's Illustrated Reviews: Pharmacology,* 3rd ed. Baltimore: Lippincott Williams & Wilkins, 2006.)

meninges The membranes that surround the brain and spinal cord: the dura mater (outer layer), arachnoid membrane (middle layer), and the pia mater (inner layer).

cerebrospinal fluid The fluid that fills the ventricles of the brain and the central canal of the spinal cord; serves to maintain uniform pressure within the CNS and cushion the brain and spinal cord.

tions such as contraction of the skeletal muscles essential for movement. On the other hand, the autonomic nervous system regulates automatic or involuntary functions like blood pressure or heart rate (**Table 4.1**).

## The Central Nervous System

The brain occupies the cranium and is covered and protected by membranes and fluid within the cavity of the cranium. These same tough membranes, called the meninges, and fluid, called cerebrospinal fluid, also surround and protect the spinal cord. Although the brain and spinal cord function as a coordinated unit, they can be divided into distinct anatomical regions. On examination of a longitudinal section of the brain, taken from front to back, it becomes apparent that the more evolved human functions of the brain are carried out in the upper regions, and the lowest, most basic functions occur in the lower regions closest to the spinal cord (**Table 4.2**).

**Table 4.1** Functional division of the efferent nerves of the peripheral nervous system

| Division | Control | Effectors | Subdivisions |
|---|---|---|---|
| Somatic nervous system | Voluntary | Skeletal muscle | None |
| Autonomic nervous system | Involuntary | Smooth muscle, cardiac muscle, and glands | Sympathetic and parasympathetic systems |

Reprinted with permission from Cohen BJ. *Memmler's The Human Body in Health and Disease,* 10th ed. Baltimore: Lippincott Williams & Wilkins, 2005.

**Table 4.2** Anatomical features and functions of the brain

| Division | Description | Functions |
|---|---|---|
| Cerebrum | Largest and uppermost portion of the brain<br>Divided into two hemispheres, each subdivided into lobes | Cortex (outer layer) is site for conscious thought, memory, reasoning, and abstract mental functions, all localized within specific lobes |
| Diencephalon | Between the cerebrum and the brain stem<br>Contains the thalamus and hypothalamus | Thalamus sorts and redirects sensory input; hypothalamus maintains homeostasis, controls autonomic nervous system and pituitary gland |
| Brain Stem | Anterior region below the cerebrum | Connects cerebrum and diencephalon with spinal cord |
| Midbrain | Below the center of the cerebrum | Has reflex centers concerned with vision and hearing; connects cerebrum with lower portions of the brain |
| Pons | Anterior to the cerebellum | Connects cerebellum with other portions of the brain; helps to regulate respiration |
| Medulla oblongata | Between the pons and the spinal cord | Links the brain with the spinal cord; has centers for control of vital functions, such as respiration and the heartbeat |
| Cerebellum | Below the posterior portion of the cerebellum<br>Divided into two hemispheres | Coordinates voluntary muscles; maintains balance and muscle tone |

Reprinted with permission from Cohen BJ. *Memmler's The Human Body in Health and Disease*, 10th ed. Baltimore: Lippincott Williams & Wilkins, 2005.

cerebral cortex The outer portion of the brain that is the part of the brain in which thought processes take place.

cerebellum Part of the posterior division of the brain. Concerned primarily with motor functions, coordination, and balance.

vestibular system The vestibule of the inner ear with the end organs and nerve fibers that function in mediating the sense of balance.

diencephalon Posterior portion of the forebrain that houses the thalamus and hypothalamus.

limbic system The parts of the brain that are concerned especially with emotion and motivation.

innervate To supply with nerves; to stimulate an organ to activity.

reflex arc The pathway followed by a nerve impulse that produces a reflex.

The outer layer of the brain, the cerebral cortex, is responsible for the development and comprehension of speech and written language, memory, learning, and creativity, and the ability to analyze all sensory input. The cerebral cortex is amazingly adaptable. When the brain is developing in early childhood, positive experiences such as exposure to reading and music actually cause more rapid development of areas of the brain responsible for comprehending and creating language and music. Likewise, infants and toddlers who are exposed to stress and maltreatment have brains that become "practiced" in reacting to this environment, and less capable of learning in areas that will be more likely to help them in adulthood.

Although it is well accepted that tissue in the central nervous system does not regenerate, some recovery from brain injury often occurs. Individuals who have suffered brain injury in confined areas are sometimes able to recover function. This is thought to be due to the ability of the brain to redirect impulses through adjacent tissue, creating new pathways for impulse transmission.

At the back of the head, below the cerebrum, is the cerebellum. The cerebellum is responsible for muscle tone and coordination, as well as balance. The cerebellum works in tandem with the vestibular system (the organ of the inner ear and associated nerves responsible for balance) and sensors in the muscles and tendons to coordinate these functions.

The diencephalon lies beneath the cerebrum and is composed of the thalamus and hypothalamus. The thalamus is responsible for directing sensory input to the areas of the cerebral cortex responsible for analyzing that input. The hypothalamus is the center for homeostasis and regulates many body functions. Regulation of temperature, appetite, circadian rhythm, and fluid and electrolyte balance occur here, as well as some part of the perception of fear and pleasure. The hypothalamus feeds information to the peripheral nervous system and the pituitary gland to effect change and maintain balance in these areas. At the border between the cerebrum and the diencephalon is the limbic system, which plays a role in memory formation and is the site where the experience of pleasure and emotions arise.

The brain stem connects the upper parts of the brain with the spinal cord. Besides being essential for the conduction of incoming and outgoing impulses to and from the higher centers of the brain, the brain stem is responsible for reflexive control of heart rate, respiration, and blood pressure. The brain stem is also the site of origin for 10 of the 12 pairs of cranial nerves.

The spinal cord begins directly below the brain stem. The cord passes through the 26 linked vertebrae of the spine, which protect it. There are 31 pairs of spinal nerves that branch off of the cord. The spinal cord is the pathway for sensory impulses coming into the brain. They reach the spinal cord via the sensory nerve endings that innervate everything from the neck down to the toes. Similarly, outgoing motor impulses travel down from the brain, through the cord, to the motor nerves that activate a response. This complete pathway from sensation to response is called a reflex arc. The simplest reflex arcs are called spinal reflexes and do not involve the brain at all. They consist of a stimulus received by a nerve ending, which is passed up the sensory neuron to the spine, where a response arises within the spinal cord. The stretch reflex is an example of this type of reflex. The stretch reflex is one of the fastest of the reflexes and requires only about 50 milliseconds reaction time (**Fig. 4.6**).

## The Peripheral Nervous System

The peripheral nervous system includes all nerve tissue outside of the central nervous system. It is further subdivided into the efferent and afferent divisions. The efferent can be further subdivided into the somatic and autonomic divisions as previously indicated. These distinctions are based partly on anatomy but mainly on function of the nerve fibers.

Within the somatic nervous system, each myelinated motor neuron originates in the CNS and travels directly to skeletal muscle. This differs from the autonomic nervous system, in which more than one neuron (preganglionic and postganglionic) is necessary to connect the central nervous system and target tissue. The result is more rapid impulse trans-

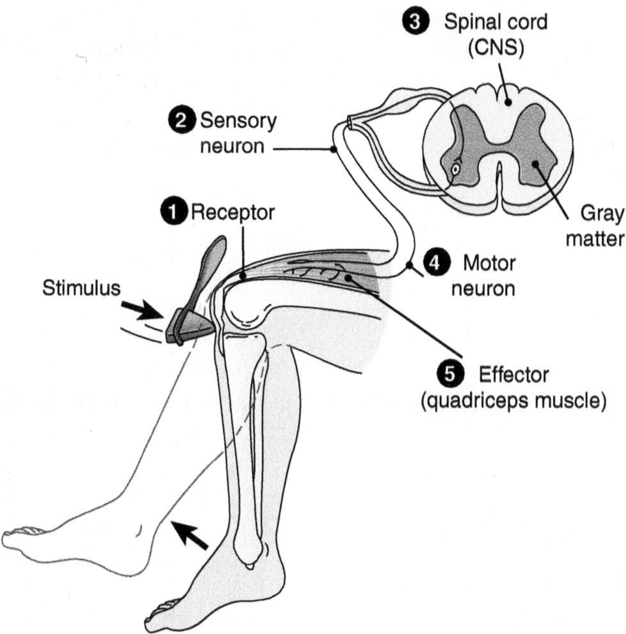


**Figure 4.6** A typical stretch reflex, in this case the patellar (knee) reflex, is a simple spinal reflex, and one of the fastest in the body. (Reprinted with permission from Cohen BJ. *Memmler's The Human Body in Health and Disease,* 10th ed. Baltimore: Lippincott Williams & Wilkins, 2005.)

mission in the somatic nervous system, because synapses slow the transmission of impulses. Unlike the autonomic system, the somatic nervous system is under voluntary control.

The autonomic nervous system is further subdivided into the sympathetic and the parasympathetic nervous systems. On the sympathetic side of the system, norepinephrine and epinephrine are the major neurotransmitters. In the parasympathetic system, acetylcholine is the only neurotransmitter. Although the nerves originate from up and down the central nervous system, the fibers emerge from the CNS in two different spinal cord regions. The neurons of the sympathetic system emerge from thoracic and lumbar regions of the spinal cord, and the parasympathetic fibers emerge from the cranium and from the sacral areas of the spinal cord (**Fig. 4.7**). Most organs receive nerve input from both the sympathetic and parasympathetic systems, and the actions of the two often oppose each other.

sympathetic Referring to the sympathetic division of the autonomic nervous system

parasympathetic Referring to the parasympathetic division of the autonomic nervous system

## The Sympathetic Division

Although it is continually active to some degree, the main role of the sympathetic division is to adjust baseline body functions in response to stressful situations, such as blood loss, fear, stress, low blood sugar, or exercise. The effect of sympathetic output is to increase heart rate and blood pressure, to cause the release of glucose from energy stores of the body, and to increase blood flow to the brain and skeletal muscles, among other changes. The changes experienced by the body during emergencies have been referred to as the "fight or flight" response. These reactions are triggered both by direct sympathetic input to the organs, and by stimulation of the adrenal gland to release epinephrine and lesser amounts of norepinephrine. The sympathetic nervous system tends to function as a unit, and it often discharges as a complete system, for example, during severe exercise or in reaction to fear.

## The Parasympathetic Division

The parasympathetic division maintains essential bodily functions, such as digestive processes and emptying of the bowels and bladder, and is required for life. It usually acts to oppose or balance the actions of the sympathetic division and is generally dominant over

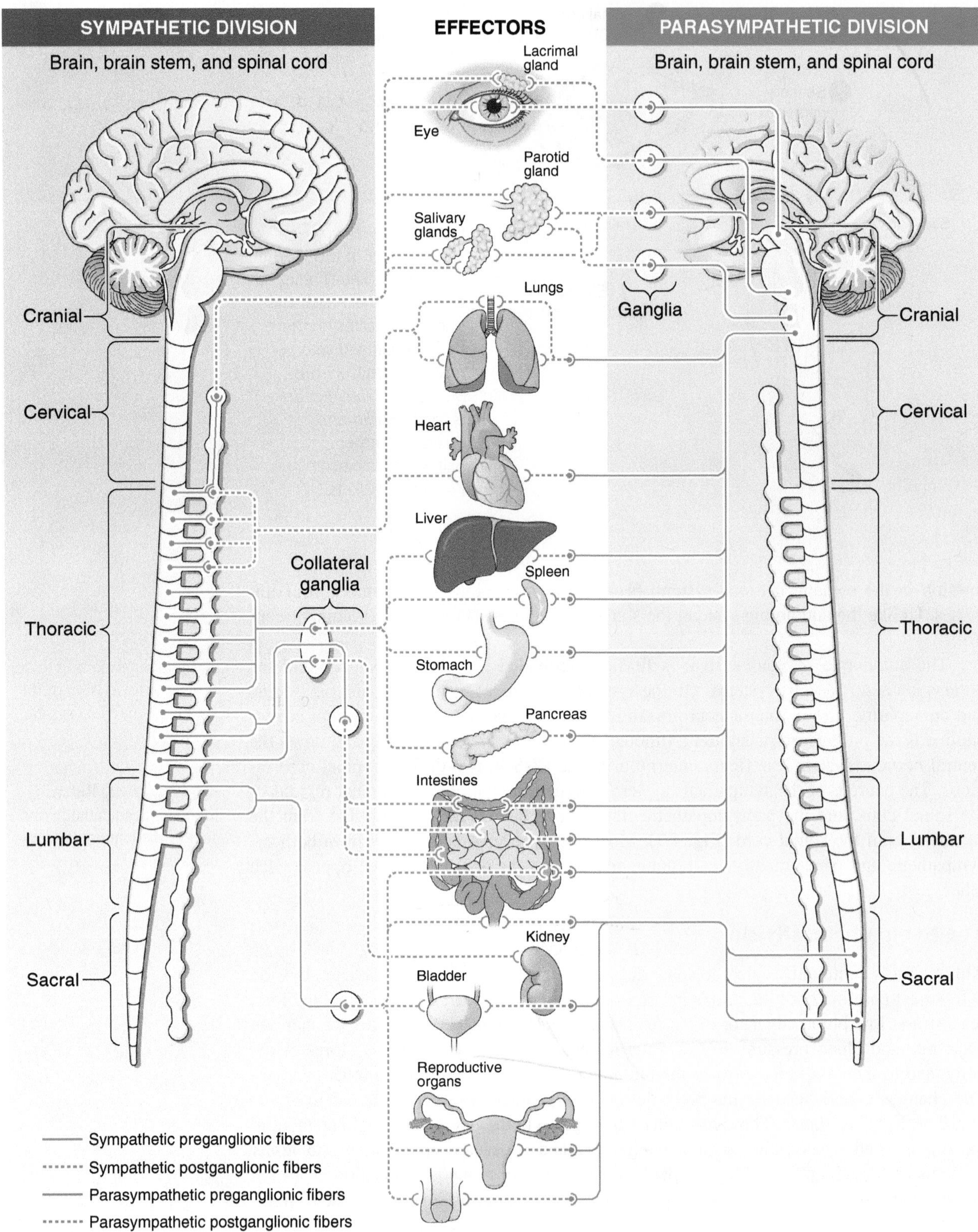


**Figure 4.7** The origins of the sympathetic and parasympathetic nerves and the corresponding effector tissues. (Reprinted with permission from Cohen BJ. *Memmler's The Human Body in Health and Disease,* 10th ed. Baltimore: Lippincott Williams & Wilkins, 2005.)

## Case 4.1

Imagine that you are walking to your parking spot, down a dark alley, very late on a moonless night. You hear some clanging and a loud crash coming from behind the fence. The thought of coming face to face with a burglar flashes through your head. While you're looking around to find an escape route and thinking about how to get out of there, what is happening to your body? Because your adrenal glands are secreting epinephrine and other stress hormones, your heart rate is up. Your blood pressure is probably elevated too, providing your brain and other essential organs with the necessary oxygen and glucose for quick responses. Your muscles are tense, and ready for running. Your eyes (if you could look in a mirror) are dilated to take advantage of all available light. Your airways are open so that when you run, you'll be able to maximize the oxygen you can take in. Just as you are ready to flee, you see a big mangy tomcat hop up to the top of the fence and give you a loud meow in greeting. False alarm, but your sympathetic nervous system had you primed for a "fight or flight."

the sympathetic system in normal resting conditions. The parasympathetic system is not a single functional unit, and never discharges as a complete system. If it did, it would produce massive, undesirable, and unpleasant results, including excessive salivation, constricted airways, diarrhea, and uncontrollable urination, among other effects. Instead, discrete parasympathetic fibers are activated separately, and the system functions to affect specific organs, such as the stomach or eye.

### The Autonomic Nervous System and Body Function

Conditions in the body are monitored with a variety of sensors and receptors located throughout. Specialized sensing cells are embedded within the circulatory system, the brain, and other tissues to collect data about the state of the body. This sensory input then travels to the spinal cord, brain stem, and hypothalamus where the data is integrated. When the central nervous system receives information about blood pressure, heart rate, concentration of oxygen, and other data from receptors throughout the body, the data is analyzed and a response is generated through the autonomic nervous system.

Both divisions of the autonomic nervous system innervate most organs in the body. For example, parasympathetic innervation slows the heart rate, and sympathetic innervation increases the heart rate. Despite this dual innervation, one system usually predominates in controlling the activity of a given organ. In the heart, the vagus (parasympathetic) nerve

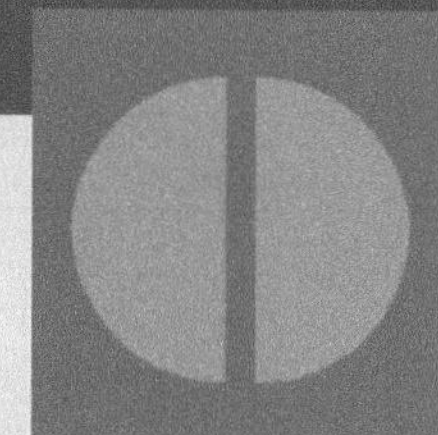

## Case 4.2

You are at home on a warm and sunny summer weekend. You've just finished mowing the lawn and sweeping the patio and now its time for lunch. You manage to get around a good-sized sandwich and a glass of iced tea, and the couch is looking mighty good. You open wide and yawn, but before you sprawl out on the couch for an afternoon siesta you need to visit the bathroom. What is going on in your body? You are in a resting state, with no unnecessary secretion of stress hormones. Your heart rate and blood pressure are normal. You've eaten, so your gastrointestinal tract is moving to process your meal. Your bladder sphincter is relaxed, so you can empty it. Your airways are in their normal, mucous-producing state. Your eyes are in the normal state of accommodating to near vision. You're ready to lie down on the couch and "rest and digest."

is the predominant factor for controlling heart rate. Although most tissues receive dual innervation, some organs, such as the adrenal medulla, kidneys, and sweat glands, receive innervation only from the sympathetic system. The control of blood pressure is also mainly a sympathetic activity, with essentially no participation by the parasympathetic system. (See **Figure 4.8** for a description of the effect of sympathetic and parasympathetic innervation on the body.)

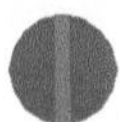

## The Nervous System and Medications

Although achieving even a basic understanding of the nervous system can seem like a daunting task, it is important for the pharmacy technician student to appreciate the relationship between the nervous system and organ function, and the relationship between neurotransmission and drug action. Neurotransmission across synapses serves as a model for understanding the general processes of chemical signaling between all cells. Chemical signaling is necessary for the body to make adjustments to changes in the external and internal environment. Although chemical signaling can occur from a distance, the same principle, of a chemical binding to a receptor to cause a response, exists. Each natural chemical, and there are likely hundreds of them, binds to a specific family of receptors. We know



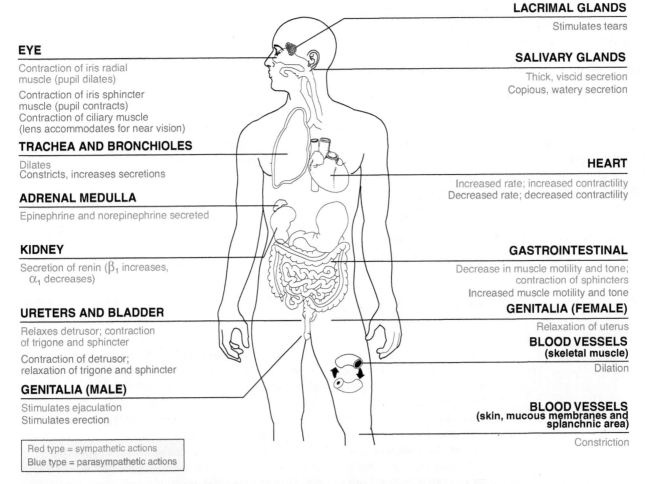

**Figure 4.8** The action of sympathetic and parasympathetic nerves on effector organs. (Adapted with permission from Harvey RA, Champe PC, Howland RD, et al. *Lippincott's Illustrated Reviews: Pharmacology,* 3rd ed. Baltimore: Lippincott Williams & Wilkins, 2006.)

that receptors for the biogenic amines, hormones, and peptides are distributed throughout the body. By understanding neurotransmission and chemical signaling, we can begin to understand the way drugs work.

Our understanding of drug action developed alongside our unravelling of the workings of the synapse and receptors in the nervous system. Most drugs exert their effect by either mimicking neurotransmitters or other agents of chemical signaling, affecting their synthesis or release, contributing to their breakdown, or by blocking their activity. As researchers learn more about receptors in the body, new drugs are specifically designed to alter the response at these receptors. Although these processes are complex and may be difficult for the novice to grasp, a basic understanding of the synapse and appreciation of neurotransmission is essential to understanding pharmacology.

# Review Questions

## Multiple Choice

Choose the best answer to the following questions:

1. Which of the following is not a division or subdivision of the nervous system?
   a. Central nervous system
   b. Somatic nervous system
   c. Systemic nervous system
   d. Peripheral nervous system

2. Regarding the human brain, which of the following anatomical-functional pairings is most correct?
   a. Cerebellum; muscle tone and coordination
   b. Cerebral cortex; spinal reflexes
   c. Thalamus; speech, vision, memory
   d. Spinal cord; regulation of body temperature and appetite

3. Which is a possible correct path for normal nerve impulse conduction?
   a. Cell body → dendrites → axon → ganglion
   b. Dendrites → cell body → axon → synapse
   c. Axon → cell body → synapse
   d. Cell body → synapse → axon → dendrites
   e. All of these are possible

4. When a nerve impulse crosses a synapse, the utilization of __________ is essential.
   a. Glial cells
   b. Neurotransmitters
   c. Schwann cells
   d. Electricity
   e. All of the above

5. Which statement about the autonomic nervous system and/or its divisions is correct?
   a. The autonomic nervous system is subdivided into the parasympathetic and the sympathetic nervous systems.
   b. Most organs in the body have some autonomic innervation.
   c. The parasympathetic nervous system helps the body adjust to stressful situations.
   d. Both a and b are correct.

## True/False

6. The brain is protected and supported by the cranium, the meninges, and the cerebrospinal fluid.
   a. True
   b. False

7. Neurons are specialized cells of the nervous system that relay information between the CNS and the tissues of the body.
   a. True
   b. False

8. The three major neurotransmitters in the peripheral nervous system are acetylcholine, epinephrine, and serotonin.
   a. True
   b. False

9. While sitting on the couch watching television, your parasympathetic nervous system is likely more active than your sympathetic nervous system.
   a. True
   b. False

10. Discoveries that reveal more information about neurotransmitters and their receptors are probably irrelevant to the creation of more effective and more specific therapeutic agents.
    a. True
    b. False

## Matching

For numbers 11 to 15, match the word or phrase with the correct lettered choice from the list below. Choices will not be used more than once and may not be used at all.

11. Sympathetic nervous system output
12. Hypothalamus
13. A junction between two neurons
14. Classes of neurotransmitters
15. Preganglionic neuron

a. Synapse
b. Type of neuron within the somatic nervous system
c. Regulation of temperature, appetite, circadian rhythm
d. Neuron complex
e. Increased blood pressure and heart rate, increased blood flow to the brain and skeletal muscles
f. Type of neuron within the autonomic nervous system
g. Biogenic amines and excitatory amino acids
h. Lipids, vitamins, and enzymes

## Short Answer

16. Diagram the conduction pathway of a spinal reflex arc, beginning with the initial stimulus.

17. Discuss any differences and similarities that exist between the autonomic nervous system and the somatic nervous system.

18. Keeping in mind what you have learned about the functions of the sympathetic nervous system, list some basic medical conditions in which treatment regimens might involve drugs that affect (stimulate or inhibit) the sympathetic nervous system.

19. Neurons are not the only cells in the nervous system. What other cells are part of the nervous system and why are they important?

20. Why is it important for pharmacy technician students to understand the basic functioning of the nervous system?

## FOR FURTHER INQUIRY

Choose one of the following topics to further investigate on your own.

1. Each of the 12 cranial nerves has a specific name and well-defined functions. Some of these nerves have both afferent and efferent functions, and some have one or the other. Investigate the names and roles of the twelve cranial nerves, and learn whether they bring data to the brain, operate an effector cell, or both. There are a number of mnemonic devices (some of them quite off-color) to help you learn the names, in case you wish to master their names.

2. Pick one of the neurotransmitters listed and see if you can find, searching the Internet, one or more drugs that work by mimicking or inhibiting that neurotransmitter. What conditions are the drugs you discovered used to treat?

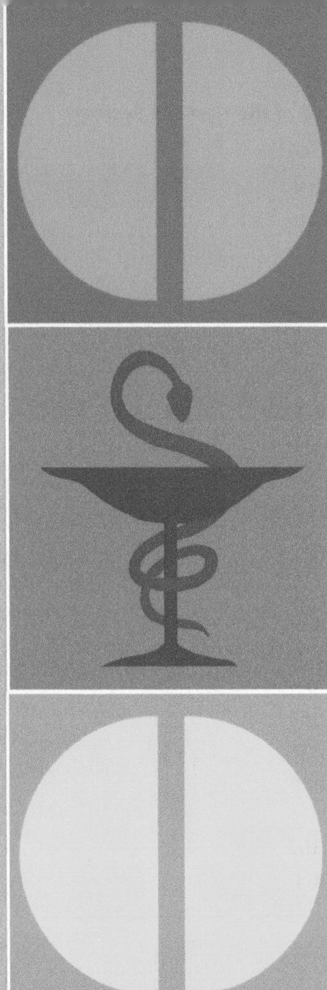

Chapter **5**

# The Autonomic Nervous System: Cholinergic Agonists and Antagonists

*KEY TERMS*

- acetyl-cholinesterase
- alkaloid
- anticholinergic
- aspirate
- bradycardia
- cholinergic
- hepatotoxicity
- intrinsic activity
- motility
- muscarinic receptor
- mydriasis
- myopic
- neurogenic
- nicotinic receptor
- patient package insert
- prototype
- stomatitis

## OBJECTIVES

After studying this chapter, the reader should be able to:

- Compare and contrast the direct-acting and indirect-acting cholinergic agents.
- List two conditions each for which cholinergic agonists and anticholinergic drugs might be used.
- Identify an important contraindication for use of both the cholinergic agonists and anticholinergic drugs.
- Describe the difference in action between the nondepolarizing neuromuscular blocking agents and succinylcholine and why this difference results in different side effects.
- Explain two ways that the technician can help to prevent medication errors with the neuromuscular blocking agents.

## DRUGS COVERED IN THIS CHAPTER*

| Cholinergic Agonists | | Cholinergic Antagonists | |
|---|---|---|---|
| **Direct Acting** | **Indirect Acting** | **Anticholinergic Agents** | **Neuromuscular Blockers** |
| Acetylcholine | Ambenomium | Atropine | Atracurium |
| Bethanechol | Demecarium | Scopolamine | Cisatracurium |
| Carbachol | Donepezil | | Mivacurium |
| Pilocarpine | Edrophonium | | Pancuronium |
| Nicotine | Galantamine | | Rocuronium |
| | Neostigmine | | Succinylcholine |
| | Physostigmine | | Vecuronium |
| | Pyridostigmine | | |
| | Rivastigmine | | |
| | Tacrine | | |
| | Echothiophate | | |

**The drugs covered in this chapter are active at cholinergic receptors. The most important of these are used for the treatment of glaucoma, Alzheimer's disease, and sometimes before, during, or after surgery.*

cholinergic Resembling acetylcholine in pharmacological action, stimulated by or releasing acetylcholine or a related compound.

Drugs affecting the autonomic nervous system are divided into two subgroups according to the type of receptor at which they exert their effect. Adrenergic agonists and antagonists (see Chapter 6) act on receptors where norepinephrine and other adrenergic agents act as neurotransmitters. The cholinergic drugs, described in this chapter, act on receptors where acetylcholine activates the receptor. Receptors where acetylcholine (ACh) is the predominant neurotransmitter are called cholinergic receptors, and include the sympathetic and parasympathetic ganglia, the clusters of cell bodies for the autonomic nervous system. The effector (postganglionic) neurons of the parasympathetic system and the somatic nerves that control skeletal muscle are also cholinergic. In addition, acetylcholine plays an important role as a neurotransmitter in the central nervous system.

There are five or six processes involving neurotransmitters that must occur to make the normal transmission of a nerve impulse in the peripheral nervous system possible. The neurotransmitter must be synthesized in the nerve, stored in vesicles, released into the synapse, and bound by the receptor. Unbound neurotransmitter must be removed from the synaptic cleft. It can be broken down by enzymes or taken back up into the nerve endings. Recycling of parts or all of the neurotransmitter can occur. For example, an enzyme breaks down free acetylcholine, and one component, the choline, is recycled. Each of these steps (illustrated in **Fig. 5.1**) is a potential target for drug action.

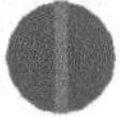

# Cholinergic Agonists

acetylcholinesterase An enzyme that breaks down unused acetylcholine in the synaptic cleft.

There are two kinds of cholinergic agonists, direct and indirect. Direct-acting agonists bind to the cholinergic receptor where, because they mimic ACh, they cause a response. Indirect agonists prevent the destruction of acetylcholine by acetylcholinesterase in the synapse.

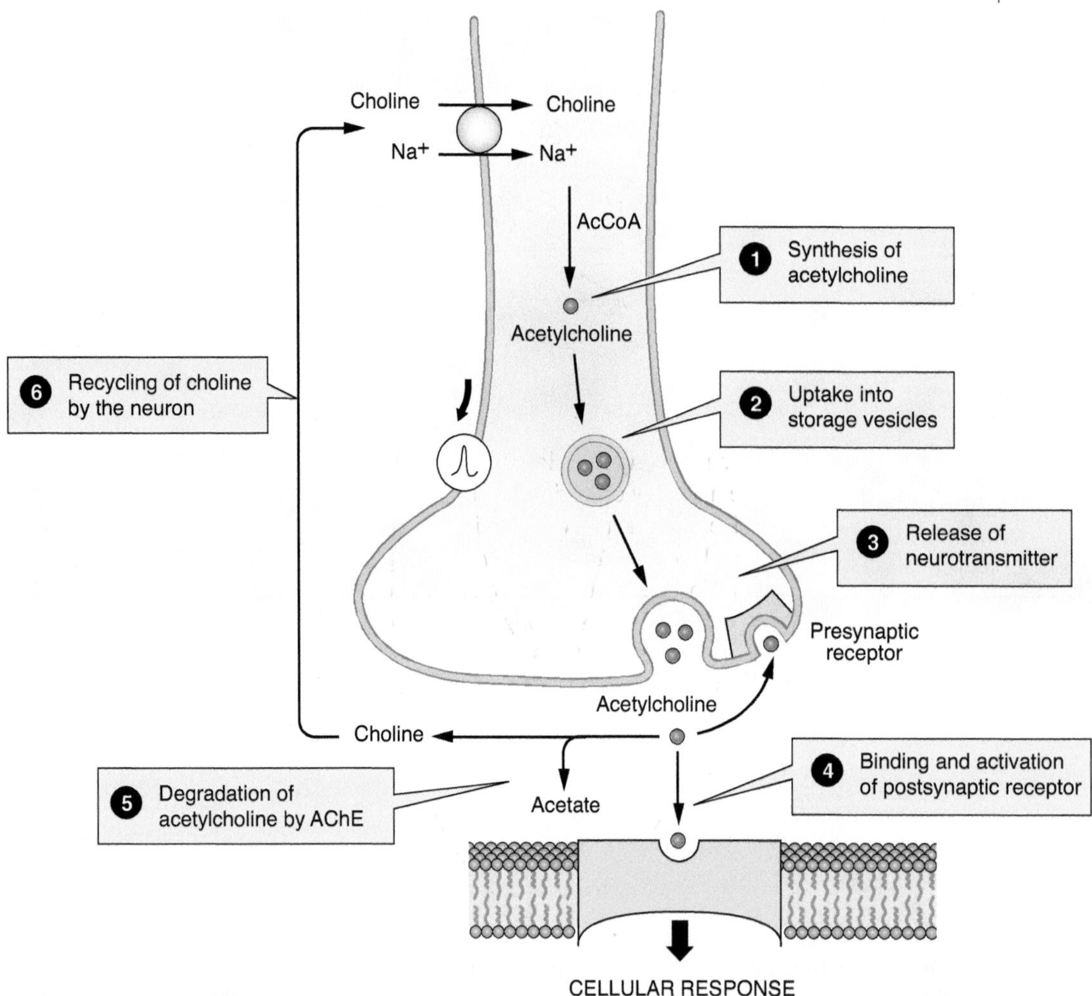


**Figure 5.1** A representation of the steps involved in synthesis, release, and degradation of acetylcholine in the parasympathetic synapse. (Adapted with permission from Harvey RA, Champe PC, Howland RD, et al. *Lippincott's Illustrated Reviews: Pharmacology,* 3rd ed. Baltimore: Lippincott Williams & Wilkins, 2006.)

This enzyme is responsible for breaking down ACh, and as a result arresting ACh action at the receptor. When the enzyme is inactivated it is prevented from breaking down ACh and consequently there is more acetylcholine available to stimulate receptors. Drugs that inhibit cholinesterase are called anticholinesterases.

Stimulation of cholinergic receptors in the parasympathetic nervous system causes physiologic changes throughout the body. Cholinergic innervation of the heart, via the vagus nerve, slows the heart rate. Mucus production is increased and bronchioles constrict in the pulmonary system. The tear and salivary glands increase production of secretions. In the gastrointestinal tract, the smooth muscle of the bowel is stimulated and gastrointestinal (GI) motility (movement) is increased. The sphincter muscle in the bladder relaxes, allowing urination.

motility Spontaneous movement, as in the movement of the gastrointestinal tract.

Stimulation of the neuromuscular junction in the somatic nervous system releases acetylcholine, and is required for the voluntary use of skeletal muscle. Cholinergic receptors here, in the adrenal glands and in the autonomic ganglia, are slightly different from those in the parasympathetic nervous system (**Fig. 5.2**). ACh stimulates both types of cholinergic receptors, identified as nicotinic and muscarinic receptors. Besides acetylcholine, nicotine also stimulates the receptors in the ganglia, adrenal glands, and skeletal muscle. Years ago, pharmacologists used nicotine to study the responses in the autonomic ganglia, so these cholinergic receptors were named nicotinic receptors. Likewise, muscarine, a substance taken from the highly toxic mushroom species *Amanita muscaria,* was used to study the parasympathetic nervous system. These cholinergic receptors are referred to as muscarinic receptors. Muscarinic receptors are located in the heart and smooth muscle, including the GI tract, bladder, and salivary glands. The slight differences between the two receptors allow pharmaceutical chemists to design drugs that will stimulate one receptor type and not the other.

nicotinic receptor One type of cholinergic receptor, found in the skeletal muscle, adrenal glands, and ganglia.

muscarinic receptor One of two types of cholinergic receptor, muscarinic receptors are found in the smooth muscle.

## Direct-Acting Agonists

The direct-acting cholinergic agonists are all chemically similar to acetylcholine. Pilocarpine (Pilocar®) and nicotine (Nicotrol®) are naturally occurring alkaloids (pharmacologically active nitrogenous compounds synthesized by plants) with cholinergic agonist properties. Bethanechol (Urecholine®) and carbachol (Miostat®) are synthetic drugs that are also cholinergic agonists. Acetylcholine is not absorbed orally, and would not be very useful even if it were. It not only activates cholinergic receptors throughout the body, a property that is not desirable when trying to treat specific symptoms, but it is also very short acting because it is rapidly inactivated by cholinesterases. Nevertheless, acetylcholine is considered the prototype of direct-acting cholinergic agents.

alkaloid Any one of the many pharmacologically active, complex, nitrogenous compounds found in plants.

prototype The first example of a drug class to which subsequent members of the class bear significant chemical and pharmacologic similarities.

### Actions and Indications

In general, the direct-acting cholinergic agents are used when constriction of the smooth muscle of the pupil, bladder, or bowel is desirable. One of the major uses of the direct-acting cholinergic (muscarinic) agents is local administration in the eye for the treatment

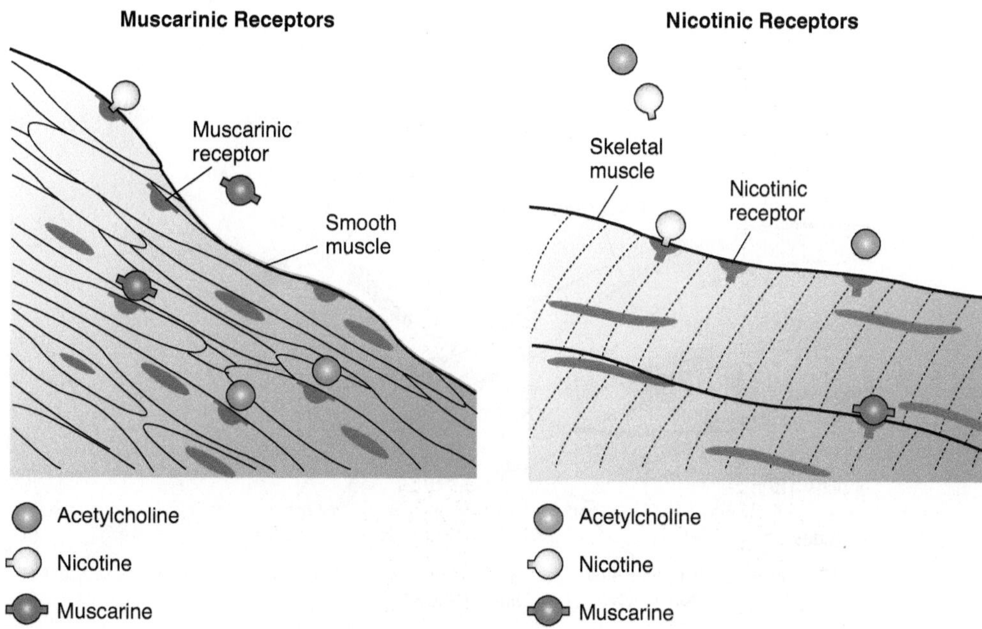


**Figure 5.2** The muscarinic and nicotinic receptors are configured such that acetylcholine is able to stimulate each. However, nicotine is unable to cause a response at the muscarinic receptor and muscarine likewise does not "fit" the nicotinic receptor.

of glaucoma. In glaucoma, an increase in intraocular pressure causes damage to the eye, and if left untreated, loss of vision occurs. The increase in intraocular pressure is usually due to inadequate drainage of the aqueous humor through the microscopic drainage system of the eye. The direct-acting cholinergic agonists, acetylcholine, pilocarpine, and carbachol, reduce intraocular pressure by causing constriction of the pupils. This allows aqueous humor to flow out of the chamber of the eye where its accumulation is responsible for the increased intraocular pressure (**Fig. 5.3**). Pilocarpine is a first line drug for emergency reduction of intraocular pressure in patients with glaucoma. Because the effects of acetylcholine are very short lived, acetylcholine ophthalmic is only used during surgery on the eye, when rapid pupillary constriction is needed.

The effects of pilocarpine and carbachol last considerably longer than the effects of acetylcholine. For this reason, these drugs are useful in the long-term treatment of glaucoma, either alone or in combination with other drugs. Up until recently, the direct-acting cholinergic agonists were considered drugs of first choice for the maintenance treatment of glaucoma. Now, use of other agents with fewer side effects has supplanted the use of these drugs to a significant extent.

The actions of bethanechol, another direct-acting agonist, are more specific for the cholinergic receptors of the GI and urinary tract than acetylcholine and other cholinergic agonists, making it suitable for systemic use. Bethanechol has little effect on the neuromuscular junction or the ganglia in usual doses. It is indicated for treatment of urinary retention caused by medications used in surgery, or by childbirth. It is also useful in treating neurogenic bladder, with urine retention. Neurogenic bladder occurs when there is a malfunction of the autonomic innervation of the bladder. Patients with spinal cord injury, for instance, may have difficulty completely emptying the bladder, a problem that would be amenable to treatment with bethanechol. Bethanechol stimulates the cholinergic receptors in the bladder, causing the sphincter to relax and increasing bladder tone, thereby allowing the initiation of urination and complete bladder emptying.

neurogenic Arising from, or caused by, the nervous system.

Nicotine, a cholinergic (nicotinic) agonist, stimulates sympathetic and parasympathetic ganglia to cause increased heart rate and blood pressure. Nicotine causes release of stress hormones from the adrenal glands. Central nervous system stimulation also occurs and is responsible for the addictive nature of nicotine. Clearly, the pharmacologic effects

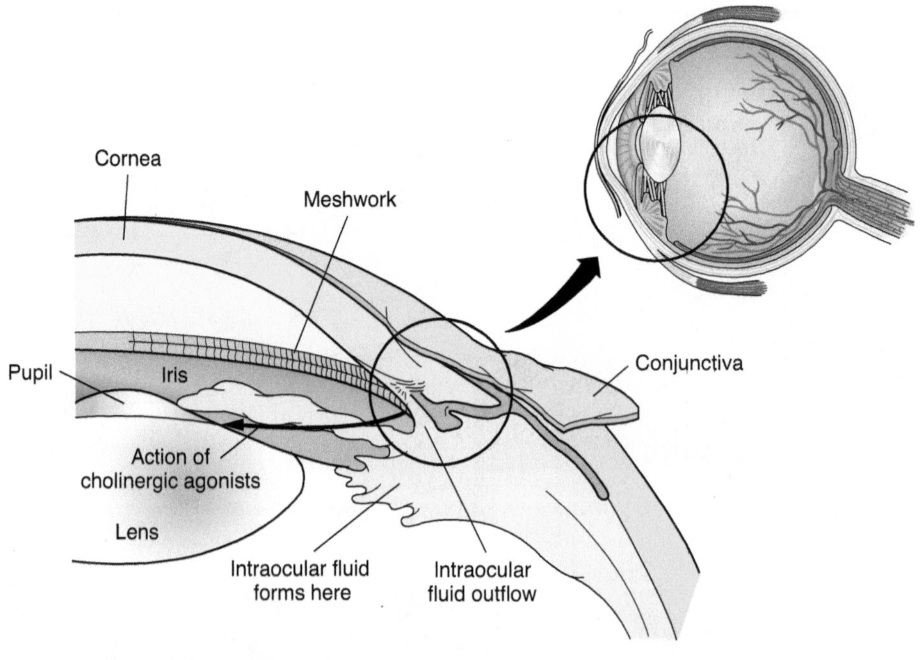

**Figure 5.3** In glaucoma, the cholinergic agonists work by constricting the pupil, thus allowing greater outflow of intraocular fluid.

of nicotine are undesirable, and the only therapeutic use for nicotine is as an aid in cessation of the use of tobacco. Nicotine is available in a number of preparations for this use. Nicotine products relieve nicotine withdrawal symptoms and cravings. The dose and frequency of use should gradually be reduced until it can be completely discontinued.

## Administration

The direct-acting cholinergic agents are available in a variety of formulations suited to their appropriate use, including formulations for injection, topical, and oral use. Acetylcholine and carbachol are both available for direct instillation into the eye, during surgery. Carbachol is sold as a sterile solution and acetylcholine is a sterile powder that requires reconstitution, using sterile technique, before use. **Table 5.1** lists the drugs covered in the chapter by generic and brand name, and includes the most common formulations.

Carbachol and pilocarpine are available as sterile ophthalmic solutions in a dropper container. Typically, carbachol drops are administered up to three times a day and pilocarpine is administered three to four times daily. In addition, pilocarpine is available as a sterile gel for the eye, administered once daily at bedtime, and as a sterile ocular insert. The Ocusert® system is placed and removed by the patient, much like a contact lens. It is placed in the corner of the eye where it releases a fairly constant dose of pilocarpine. This system is more convenient for patients because it only needs to be replaced on a weekly basis. However, it has the disadvantage of sometimes falling out of the eye. If the insert falls out and is undamaged, it should be rinsed with cool tap water and replaced.

Bethanechol is administered orally or by subcutaneous injection to stimulate urination. When given subcutaneously, the drug is rapidly and completely absorbed, and a much lower dose is needed than when given orally, because the first pass effect is avoided. The initial subcutaneous dose of 2.5 mg may be repeated if the patient does not respond. Oral doses start at 10 mg and are repeated every hour (to a maximum of 50 mg) until the appropriate dose is determined, based on response.

Nicotine is available in a variety of dosage forms, including nicotine gum, lozenges, transdermal patches, nasal spray, and an inhalation system. No matter which drug form is selected for use, the dose should be tapered in a systematic way until it can be discontinued. Most manufacturers recommend that tapering begin when the patient has been completely tobacco free for 8 to 12 weeks. At that time the nicotine product is gradually tapered over the recommended interval. Nicotine in any form should not be used if the client continues to smoke.

## Side Effects

It is worth noting here that all drugs share this common finding: side effects are very often unwanted pharmacologic actions of the drug being administered. Of course, all drugs may have additional, unexpected adverse affects as well. Knowledge of the physical response to cholinergic receptor stimulation provides clues to the side effects patients might anticipate while taking these medications. For example, increased GI motility could result in diarrhea, and contraction of bladder smooth muscle could result in urinary urgency (**Fig. 5.4**).

Although systemic absorption of ophthalmic products is unlikely, it can occur when high, frequent doses are being used or when the cornea is damaged. Systemic adverse effects that can be seen with acetylcholine, carbachol, and pilocarpine include low heart rate, low blood pressure, breathing difficulty, sweating or flushing, increased salivation, diarrhea and other GI distress, and urinary urgency and frequency. Typical local adverse effects are similar for all the direct-acting cholinergic ophthalmic products and include burning, irritation and redness of the eyes, corneal clouding, and temporary loss of visual acuity due to the inability of the pupil to accommodate to low light levels. Patients become temporarily myopic, or nearsighted, for a few hours after a new pilocarpine Ocusert® is placed in the eye, so bedtime administration is recommended. Side effects for bethanechol are similar to the systemic side effects sometimes seen with use of the cholinergic eye drops, except that the parasympathetic system effects may be more problematic since the drug is de-

myopic Suffering from nearsightedness.

**Table 5.1** Examples of the most commonly used cholinergic agonists*

| Generic Name | Brand Name | Indications | Available as | Notes |
|---|---|---|---|---|
| **Direct-Acting Cholinergic Agents** | | | | |
| Acetylcholine | Miochol-E | Ophthalmic Surgery | Injection | Prepared immediately before use |
| Bethanechol | Urecholine | Urinary retention | Tablets, injection | |
| Carbachol | Miostat, Isopto carbachol, & others | Glaucoma | Injection, ophthalmic drops | Maintain sterility of eye medications |
| Pilocarpine | Pilocar & others | Glaucoma | Ophthalmic drops, gel, inserts | Maintain sterility of eye medications |
| Nicotine | Nicotrol, NicoDerm, and others | Smoking cessation | Transdermal patch, gum, nasal spray, and inhaler | Dispose of properly |
| **Acetylcholinesterase Inhibitors** | | | | |
| Ambenonium | Mytelase | Myasthenia gravis | Tablets | |
| Demecarium | Humorsol | Glaucoma | Ophthalmic drops | Maintain sterility of eye medications |
| Donepezil | Aricept | Alzheimer's syndrome | Tablets | |
| Edrophonium | Tensilon & others | Diagnosis of myasthenia gravis | Injection | |
| Galantamine | Reminyl | Alzheimer's syndrome | Tablets, oral solution | |
| Neostigmine | Prostigmin | Antidote for NM blockers, myasthenia gravis | Injection, tablets | |
| Physostigmine | Antilirium | Antidote for NM blockers, atropine toxicity | Injection | |
| Pyridostigmine | Mestinon | Myasthenia gravis | Tablets, syrup, injection | |
| Rivastigmine | Exelon | Alzheimer's syndrome | Capsules, oral solution | |
| Tacrine | Cognex | Alzheimer's syndrome | Capsules | |
| Echothiophate | Phospholine Iodide | Glaucoma | Ophthalmic | Maintain sterility of eye medications |

* Listed by brand and generic names and including indications and available formulations.

signed for systemic absorption. Fortunately, bethanechol is most often used on a short-term basis.

Nicotine is quite toxic and has many undesirable effects. Children and pets are especially vulnerable, and all nicotine products should be kept out of the reach of children and pets. Signs and symptoms of nicotine poisoning include pallor, cold sweats, excess saliva-

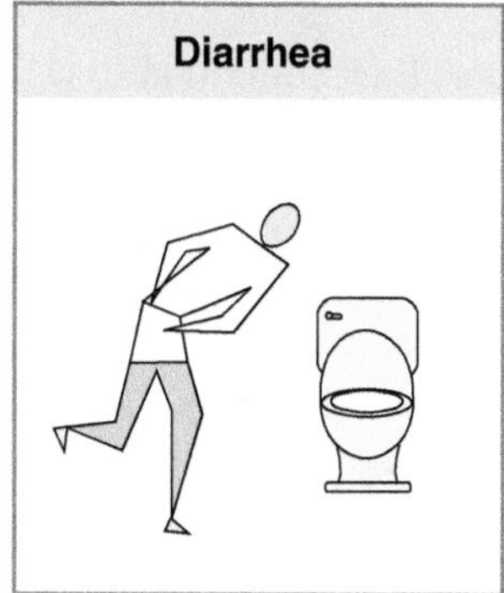


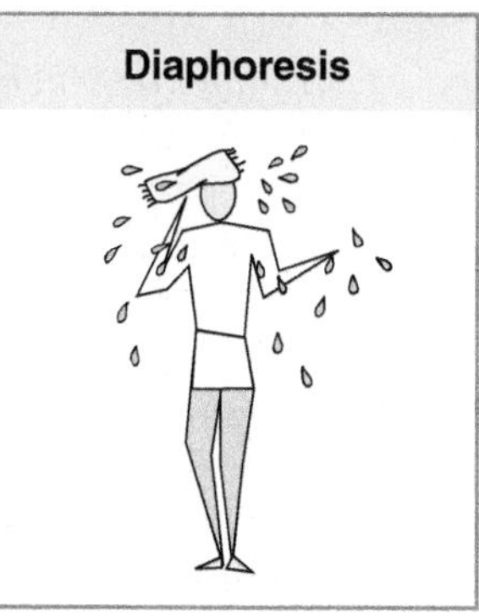


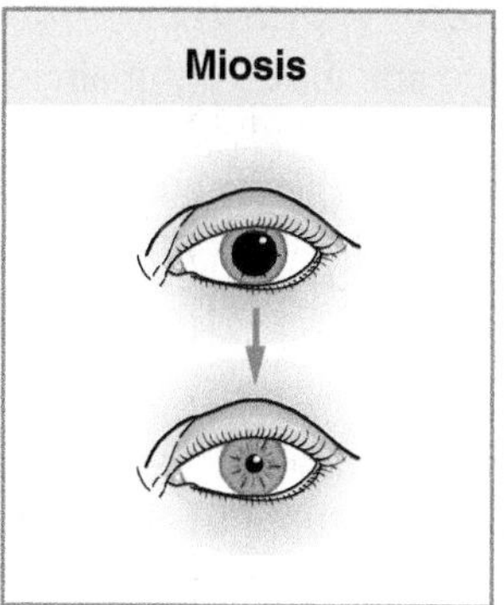


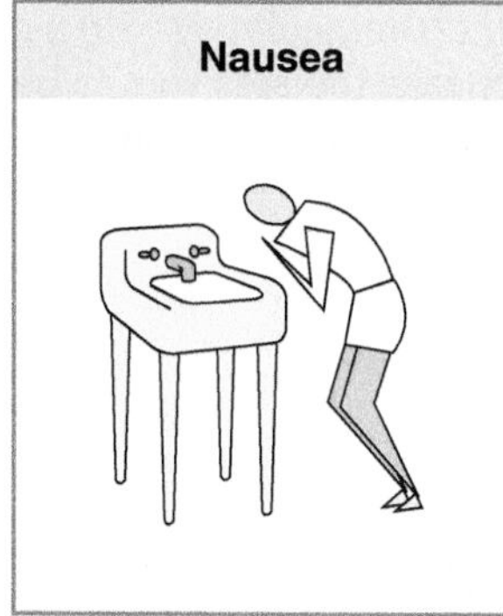


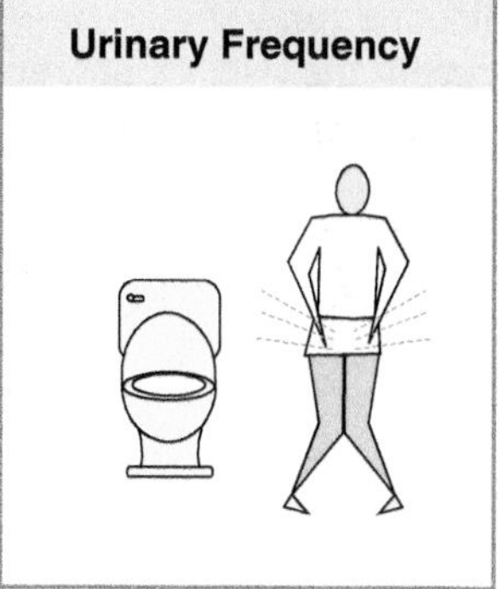


**Figure 5.4** Adverse effects most frequently associated with cholinergic drugs. (Adapted with permission from Harvey RA, Champe PC, Howland RD, et al. *Lippincott's Illustrated Reviews: Pharmacology,* 3rd ed. Baltimore: Lippincott Williams & Wilkins, 2006.)

tion, nausea and vomiting, abdominal pain and diarrhea, headache, confusion, and dizziness. Users of nicotine transdermal patches should be informed that absorption into the blood stream continues for some time after the patch has been removed

Common complaints associated with nicotine either inhaled or sprayed in the nose include chest tightness, upset stomach and stomatitis, a condition of inflammation of the epithelium of the mouth. Patients with pulmonary disease should use a different route of administration. Because nicotine raises blood pressure and affects the heart, physicians should evaluate the risk of nicotine cessation therapy as compared with other methods of quitting and also consider chance of success with various methods. Nicotine delays healing of peptic ulcers and causes GI irritation. Nicotine is also addictive; patients may experience withdrawal symptoms when abruptly discontinuing nicotine products.

stomatitis Inflammation of the mucous membranes of the oral cavity.

## Tips for the Technician

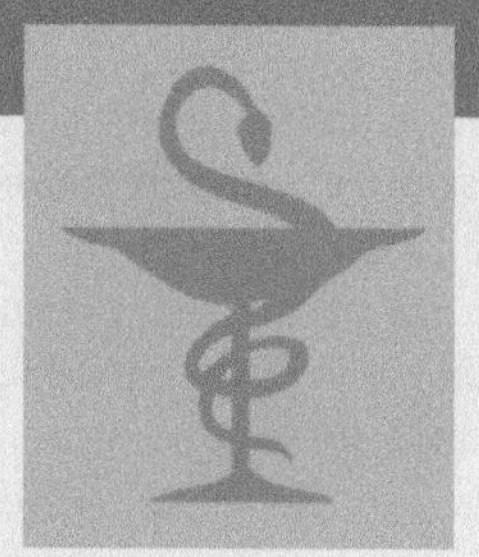

It is very important for hospital-based technicians to be aware that the intramuscular and intravenous (IV) routes are never used for administration of bethanechol. The technician must direct any orders received indicating administration by these routes to the pharmacist for clarification.

In outpatient pharmacy practice settings, technicians preparing prescriptions for ophthalmic use should apply an auxiliary label indicating the prescription is "for the eye." (See auxiliary prescription labels in Appendix C.) All ophthalmic preparations are sterile, and it is the responsibility of the pharmacist to make sure patients know

patient package insert A drug insert sometimes required by the FDA designed specifically to inform patients about risks associated with specific medications.

how to administer ophthalmic products in a manner that ensures their continued sterility. It is helpful, however, for technicians to determine whether or not the patient has been educated about ophthalmic preparations in the past, and pass this information on to the pharmacist. Technicians should make sure that each patient with a pilocarpine Ocusert® prescription receives the patient package insert that comes with the product.

Clients using nicotine preparations for smoking cessation need be made aware that nicotine is a potent drug and that dose recommendations should be carefully followed. Nicotine preparations should not be used while the patient continues to smoke. Nicotine can be absorbed through the skin and eyes and can be especially dangerous to children. Some drug will remain in the patch after removal; therefore, safe disposal is essential. Nicotine patches should be destroyed according to the manufacturer's recommendations. Any spills of the nicotine spray should be wiped up immediately with a paper towel. If the solution comes in contact with the skin, mouth, eyes or ears, the area should be flushed repeatedly with water. To prevent accidental ingestion by children or pets, carefully dispose of used nicotine gum in the garbage.

## Indirect-Acting Cholinergic Agonists

Acetylcholinesterase is the enzyme that terminates the action of acetylcholine by cleaving it into the components acetate and choline. It is located in the pre- and postsynaptic nerve terminals. Indirect-acting cholinergic agonists inhibit the action of acetylcholinesterase so that the lifespan of acetylcholine is extended and the cholinergic action is prolonged. Accumulation of acetylcholine in the synaptic cleft occurs as a result of the disruption of this process (**Fig. 5.5**). Assuming they penetrate the central nervous system, drugs that inhibit acetylcholinesterase can increase the cholinergic response at any cholinergic receptor in the body.

Anticholinesterase agents bind to cholinesterase reversibly or irreversibly. Irreversible binding results in a long-lasting increase in acetylcholine at all sites where it is released. Drugs that bind irreversibly are extremely toxic and many were developed by the military as weapons ("nerve gases"). Related compounds, such as parathion, are used as insecticides and are referred to as organophosphate compounds. Because of their toxicity, these compounds lack significant therapeutic usefulness. In fact, most hospital pharmacies must carry antidotes (see pralidoxime, Chapter 36) to organophosphate poisoning, which is most often seen in agricultural areas. Systemic exposure to irreversibly binding anticholinesterases cause cholinergic crisis, a situation where the continuous presence of ACh causes nerves and effector cells to be stimulated repeatedly to the point of paralysis. The end result is respiratory paralysis and death.

### Actions and Indications

Physostigmine (Antilirium®), another plant alkaloid, is the prototype of the reversible anticholinesterase drugs. Physostigmine is used for reversing excess effects of anticholinergic agents and other drugs with anticholinergic properties (covered later in this chapter). It easily penetrates the central nervous system, allowing for the reversal of unwanted central, as well as peripheral, effects. This can be useful after surgery, or in cases of toxicity due to overdose with atropine or other drugs, such as the tricyclic antidepressants. Although physostigmine was used in the past for glaucoma, newer agents with fewer side effects have supplanted its use.

Other reversible anticholinesterase agents are used for treatment of myasthenia gravis, a serious and progressive autoimmune neuromuscular disease that is characterized by a reduced number of working cholinergic receptors, and as a result, insufficient cholinergic activity at the neuromuscular junction. The early symptoms of the disease include weakness

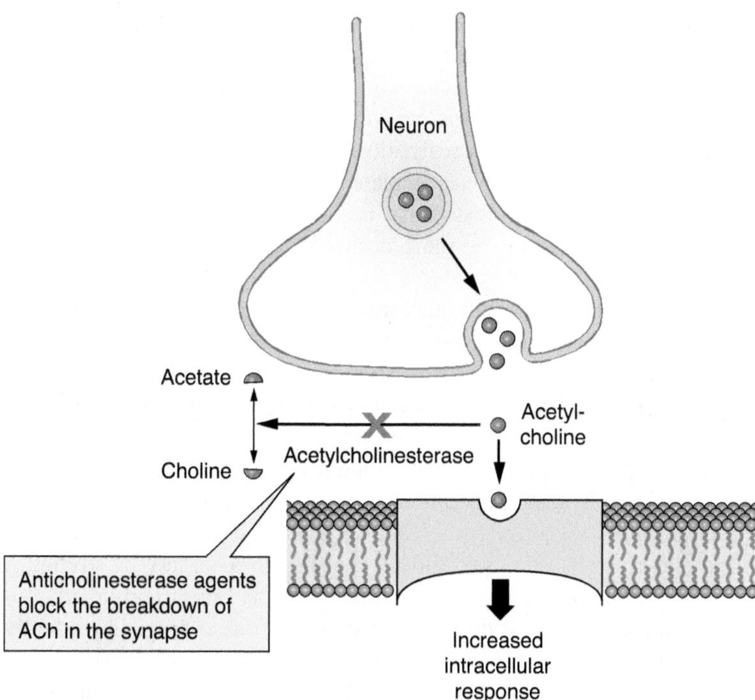


**Figure 5.5** Mechanism of action of the anticholinesterase drugs. (Adapted with permission from Harvey RA, Champe PC, Howland RD, et al. *Lippincott's Illustrated Reviews: Pharmacology,* 3rd ed. Baltimore: Lippincott Williams & Wilkins, 2006.)

of the eye muscles or difficulty swallowing. Myasthenia gravis progresses to generalized weakness of the skeletal muscles, and if left untreated, can end in death from respiratory failure. The anticholinesterase agents help to temporarily restore some cholinergic activity by increasing the amount of acetylcholine in the synapse. The most useful drugs for this condition have a longer duration of activity that will allow the patient to take the medication less frequently. Ambenonium (Mytelase®), neostigmine (Prostigmin®), and pyridostigmine (Mestinon®) are used to treat this disease, and edrophonium (Tensilon®) is used in its diagnosis. Because of their activity at the neuromuscular junction, these drugs are also useful to reverse the effects of neuromuscular blocking agents, used during surgery with general anesthesia (see cholinergic antagonists, below). Like bethanechol, the anticholinesterase drugs can be used to stimulate the bladder after surgery.

Echothiophate (Phospholine Iodide®) is the only irreversibly binding anticholinesterase agents used therapeutically. Although demecarium (Humorsol®) is a reversible cholinesterase inhibitor, its duration of action is as long as that of echothiophate. Both of these drugs are used topically in the treatment of glaucoma. Echothiophate is most useful in glaucoma that occurs after eye surgery. Echothiophate and demecarium are not considered first line treatment for glaucoma and are used only when other options have failed.

Research studies indicate that the progressive loss of cholinergic neurons is the likely cause of the memory loss that is a hallmark symptom of Alzheimer's disease. Inhibition of acetylcholinesterase within the central nervous system (CNS) is thought to improve cholinergic transmission at those neurons that are still functioning. A number of reversible anticholinesterase drugs that penetrate the CNS are approved for the treatment of mild to moderate Alzheimer's disease. They are donepezil (Aricept®), galantamine (Razadyne®), rivastigmine (Exelon®), and tacrine (Cognex®). All of these agents appear to have some selectivity for acetylcholinesterase in the CNS. These compounds provide a reduction in the rate of loss of cognitive functioning in Alzheimer's patients. Unfortunately, no drugs are available to prevent or cure this disease. There is very little understanding of what causes the loss of receptors in the first place.

## Administration

The cholinesterase inhibitors are available in a variety of formulations appropriate to their uses. Because it is indicated for reversing toxicity or for postoperative use, physostigmine is available only as a sterile solution for injection. It is administered by IV or intramuscular injection and repeated at 10 to 30 minute intervals if necessary until an adequate reversal of symptoms occurs. Anticholinesterase agents used for myasthenia gravis are available for oral use. The dose must be individualized because this disease waxes and wanes. In any patient, the dose necessary to control symptoms can vary on a daily basis. Ambenonium chloride tablets are usually given every 4 hours. Pyridostigmine is available in a syrup, as immediate release tablets, and as extended release tablets. The frequency of administration is dependent on the formulation used. Pyridostigmine is shorter acting than ambenonium; therefore, the extended release tablets may be more desirable for most patients. They are normally administered twice daily.

Edrophonium chloride is available for administration by injection only. It is very short acting and is used for diagnostic purposes in cases of suspected myasthenia gravis and to reverse the effects of neuromuscular blockade. However, pyridostigmine and neostigmine injection are more useful for reversal of the nondepolarizing neuromuscular blocking agents because of their longer durations of action. Neostigmine has a moderate duration of action, usually 30 minutes to 2 hours, and pyridostigmine lasts up to 4 hours. Atropine is generally given along with these drugs to prevent some of the more troubling side effects.

The cholinesterase inhibitors used to treat Alzheimer's disease are given orally. The oldest of these, tacrine and rivastigmine, are sold as capsules in a variety of strengths. Donepezil and galantamine are marketed as tablets. Galantamine and rivastigmine are also available as liquids. With the exception of donepezil, the dose of these drugs is gradually increased to the maximum recommended dose.

Echothiophate and demecarium are both used as ophthalmic drops. Echothiophate is provided as a sterile powder that must be reconstituted, using sterile technique, before dispensing. Demecarium may require dosing from daily to weekly, depending on the response. Echothiophate is generally administered on a daily basis, but can be administered every other day.

## Side Effects

Most side effects of these drugs are similar to those of the direct acting cholinergic agonists, and result from cholinergic stimulation. Common adverse effects include nausea, diarrhea, vomiting, urinary frequency, and slowed heart rate, all of which can be predicted by the pharmacologic actions of the drugs. The effects of physostigmine on the CNS may lead to convulsions when high doses are used.

Use of the locally administered ophthalmic agents will be accompanied by myopia (nearsightedness) due to the action of the drugs on the pupils. This effect is often prolonged because of the duration of effect of these drugs. Eye irritation and redness are not uncommon.

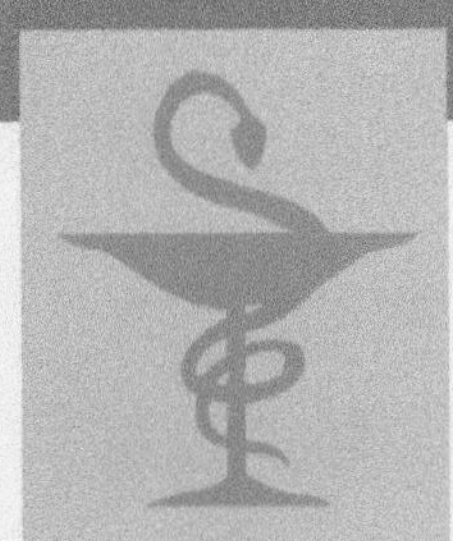

### Tips for the Technician

Patients with myasthenia gravis will usually adjust their own doses of the anticholinesterase drugs. For this reason, they need to be warned that symptoms of toxicity can mimic symptoms of their disease. Patients should be instructed to notify their physician if excess salivation, nausea, vomiting, or diarrhea occurs. The diagnostic drug edrophonium contains sulfites, which may cause allergic reactions in some people.

Caregivers of Alzheimer's patients may need instruction in the proper way to measure and administer liquid medications using an oral syringe. If medications are discontinued, a fairly rapid decline in cognitive function can occur. If treatment is interrupted, patients or caregivers should check with their pharmacist or physician before restarting therapy, since many drugs require a gradual dose increase over time.

All of the cholinesterase inhibitors used to treat Alzheimer's disease have a potential for interactions with drugs metabolized by cytochrome P450 enzymes, except rivastigmine. They can also interact with anticholinergic agents. Unlike the others, tacrine is associated with hepatotoxicity, or toxicity to the liver.

hepatotoxicity Liver toxicity or damage.

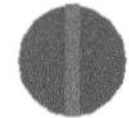

# Cholinergic Antagonists

The cholinergic antagonists that work at the muscarinic receptors, that is, the receptors in the parasympathetic nervous system, are called anticholinergic drugs. They work by competing with acetylcholine for attachment to the receptor. Anticholinergic drugs have no intrinsic ability to stimulate the cholinergic receptor, but prevent ACh from attaching. At the blocked receptor, effects of acetylcholine are inhibited, and the actions of sympathetic stimulation are left unopposed. Drugs that block the action of acetylcholine at the nicotinic receptors of the autonomic ganglia are called ganglionic blocking agents. Clinically, they are the least important of the cholinergic antagonists. A third family of compounds, the neuromuscular blocking agents, interfere with transmission of efferent impulses to skeletal muscle.

anticholinergic Opposing or blocking the physiological action of acetylcholine.

## Anticholinergic Agents

The anticholinergic agents block receptors in the parasympathetic system and reduce cholinergic input (**Fig. 5.6**). In addition, these drugs block the few sympathetic neurons that are cholinergic, such as those innervating salivary and sweat glands. Because they do not block nicotinic receptors, the anticholinergic drugs have little or no action at skeletal neuromuscular junctions or autonomic ganglia. A number of antihistamines and antidepressant drugs also have anticholinergic activity, and therefore side effects similar to those caused by these drugs.

There are numerous anticholinergic agents with a long list of indications for use (**Table 5.2**). They are inhaled for asthma, taken orally for urinary urgency, GI distress, Parkinson's disease, and are used locally in the eye to cause mydriasis, or dilation of the pupil. They are given preoperatively to dry secretions during surgery. Atropine, as the prototype of these drugs, and its close relatives, scopolamine (Transderm Scop®), and hyoscyamine are emphasized in this chapter. Other anticholinergic drugs, including homatropine and glycopyrrolate (Robinul®), are very similar in their pharmacologic action and side effects to atropine. Ipratropium and dicyclomine will be discussed in the chapters on the respiratory and renal systems, respectively.

mydriasis Excessive or prolonged dilation of the pupil.

Atropine, scopolamine, and hyoscyamine are alkaloids derived from the plant family Solanaceae, or the nightshade family. This plant has been used for centuries, both for its medicinal uses and for more nefarious purposes, since it is a highly toxic poison. The alkaloids from this plant family are referred to as the belladonna alkaloids. Mediterranean women instilled extracts from the plant into their eyes for the alluring effect of enlarged pupils; thus the name *belladonna*, or beautiful lady.

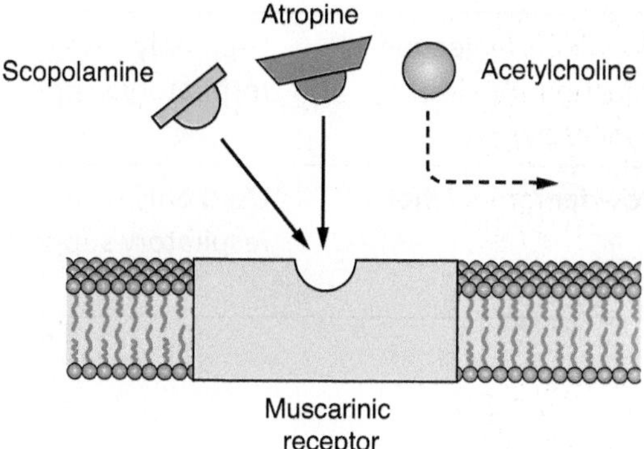


**Figure 5.6** Drugs such as atropine and scopolamine compete with acetylcholine to block the muscarinic receptor and prevent its activation. (Adapted with permission from Harvey RA, Champe PC, Howland RD, et al. *Lippincott's Illustrated Reviews: Pharmacology,* 3rd ed. Baltimore: Lippincott Williams & Wilkins, 2006.)

**Table 5.2** Examples of the most commonly used anticholinergic agents*

| Generic Name | Brand Name | Indications | Supplied as | Notes |
|---|---|---|---|---|
| **Anticholinergics** | | | | |
| Atropine | | Preoperative medication, cardiac emergencies, to slow GI motility, glaucoma | Tablets, injection (various concentrations), prefilled syringes, combinations for oral use, ophthalmic solution | Must always be available for emergency use in hospitals |
| Glycopyrrolate | Robinul | Preoperatively to reduce secretions | Tablets and injection | |
| Hyoscyamine | Anaspaz, Levsin | Irritible bowel, infant colic, to dry secretions | Tablets, solution, and injection | |
| Scopolamine | Transderm Scop | Preoperative medication, motion sickness | Tablets, injection (various concentrations), transdermal patch | |
| **Neuromuscular Blocking Agents** | | | | |
| Atracurium | Tracrium | Adjunct to anesthesia, to facilitate ventilator use | Injection | Used only with respiratory support |
| Cisatracurium | Nimbex | Adjunct to anesthesia, to facilitate ventilator use | Injection | Used only with respiratory support |
| Mivacurium | Mivacron | Adjunct to anesthesia, to facilitate ventilator use | Injection | Used only with respiratory support |
| Pancuronium | | Adjunct to anesthesia, to facilitate ventilator use | Injection, varying concentrations | Used only with respiratory support |
| Rocuronium | Zemuron | Adjunct to anesthesia, to facilitate ventilator use | Injection | Used only with respiratory support |
| Succinylcholine | Anectine, Quelicin | Adjunct to anesthesia, to facilitate ventilator use | Powder for injection, injection, varying concentrations | Used only with respiratory support |
| Vecuronium | Norcuron | Adjunct to anesthesia, to facilitate ventilator use | Powder for injection | Used only with respiratory support |

* Listed by brand and generic names and including indications and available formulations.

## Actions and Indications

The effects of atropine vary, depending on dose (**Fig. 5.7**). Atropine blocks cholinergic activity throughout the body and administration results in drying of secretions, reduced sweating, slowed heart rate, reduced movement of the GI tract, and mydriasis. Administration in the eye results in persistent mydriasis, or dilation of the pupil, and inability to focus for near vision (**Fig. 5.8**). This effect is useful to ophthalmologists because it helps them to visualize the retina and the inside of the eye.

The belladonna alkaloids can be used as an antispasmodic to reduce activity of the GI tract. Atropine, scopolamine and hyoscyamine are three potent drugs that produce this effect. They are often combined with the mild sedative phenobarbital for this purpose. Although gastric motility is reduced, hydrochloric acid production is not significantly affected, so these drugs do not promoting healing of peptic ulcers.

Atropine-like drugs are used to reduce overactive states of the urinary bladder that result in frequent urination or inability to retain the urine. Atropine blocks the salivary glands, producing a drying effect on the oral mucus membranes. The salivary glands are exquisitely sensitive to atropine. This effect of anticholinergic drugs is useful for patients who are undergoing general anesthesia. When patients are anesthetized secretions cannot be swallowed, and pose a risk to the patient if they are aspirated. Glycopyrrolate is a synthetic anticholinergic frequently used for its drying effects.

aspirate To draw in by breathing; inhale.

Atropine produces effects on the cardiovascular system that are useful in cardiac emergencies. It causes a modest increase in heart rate due to blockade of the vagus nerve, and is useful for the emergency treatment of bradycardia (slow heart beat). Atropine is also indicated as an antidote for the injudicious use of cholinergic agents, such as the anticholinesterase drugs discussed above, and as an antidote for poisoning by some insecticides. It is indicated as an antidote in mushroom poisoning for certain species of mushrooms. The advice of a poison control center or toxicologist should always be sought before using atropine as an antidote.

bradycardia A slowness of the heart beat, as evidenced by slowing of the pulse rate to less than 60 beats per minute.

Scopolamine produces peripheral effects similar to those of atropine. However, scopolamine has greater action on the CNS and a longer duration of action. Scopolamine is especially useful for preventing motion sickness. It can cause short-term amnesia and sedation as a result of its penetration into the central nervous system.

## Administration

Atropine is readily absorbed when given by mouth, and is partially metabolized by the liver but removed primarily by the kidneys. It has a half-life of about 4 hours. Atropine, scopolamine, hyoscyamine, or other anticholinergic agents are found in a variety of orally admin-

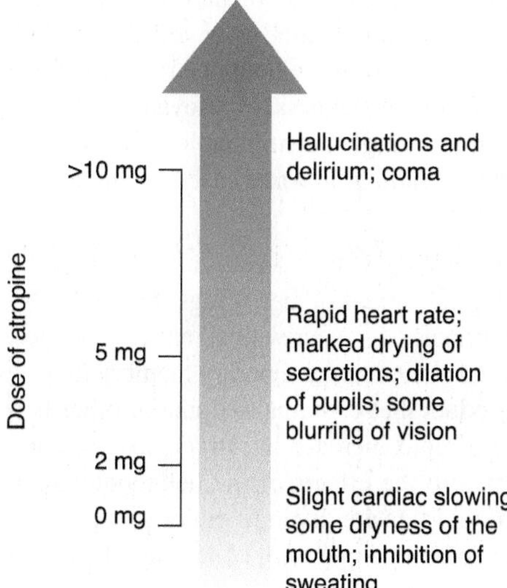


**Figure 5.7** The effects of atropine are dependent upon the dose administered. (Adapted with permission from Harvey RA, Champe PC, Howland RD, et al. *Lippincott's Illustrated Reviews: Pharmacology,* 3rd ed. Baltimore: Lippincott Williams & Wilkins, 2006.)

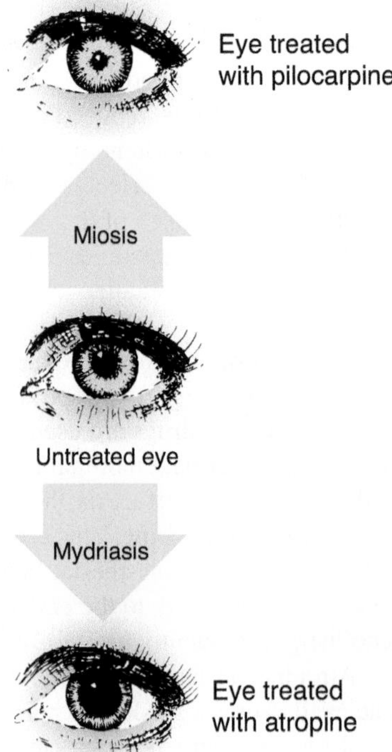


**Figure 5.8** Comparative effects of cholinergic and anticholinergic agents on the iris and pupil. (Adapted with permission from Harvey RA, Champe PC, Howland RD, et al. *Lippincott's Illustrated Reviews: Pharmacology,* 3rd ed. Baltimore: Lippincott Williams & Wilkins, 2006.)

istered combination products for colds and allergies, where they are added for their drying effect on secretions, and in products for GI upset, where they are added to slow gastrointestinal motility.

Atropine for injection is available in prefilled syringes and single or multiple dose vials. Prefilled syringes are useful in cardiac emergencies because they are ready to use. The usual adult dose for emergency treatment of bradycardia is 0.5 to 1 mg given intravenously, but prefilled syringes come in different concentrations and doses. Atropine and glycopyrrolate are generally given by intramuscular injection as preanesthetic medication. They are often given along with a sedative to relax the patient before surgery.

Atropine (0.5%, 1%, and 2%) and scopolamine (0.25%) are both available as sterile solutions for ophthalmic use. Atropine is also available as an ophthalmic ointment. Other products are preferable for diagnostic purposes because complete recovery from the mydriasis induced by topical atropine takes several days.

Scopolamine is available as a transdermal patch for prevention of motion sickness in adults. Transderm-Scop® delivers a consistent dose of scopolamine over a 3-day period. Patients apply the patch in the hairless area behind the ear 4 or more hours before they travel when they anticipate they will have a problem with motion sickness. Hyoscyamine is marketed in combination oral products for GI upset, and as a single agent in tablets and solution for the treatment of GI disorders that involve spasm, including, in some cases, infant colic.

## Side Effects

Side effects are predictable, based on the pharmacological actions of these drugs (**Fig. 5.9**). Dry mouth, constipation, blurred vision, and inability to urinate can occur with all anticholinergics. Scopolamine can cause drowsiness and confusion, and sometimes, temporary memory loss.

Patients with glaucoma should not use any product that contains atropine or other belladonna alkaloids, because these drugs can cause a rapid increase in intraocular pressure. Children and elderly people are especially sensitive to the effects of the belladonna alkaloids and special caution should be used when these drugs are given to either group of patients. Anticholinergic medication should not be used by people with obstructive bowel or bladder conditions, or in patients with Myasthenia gravis.

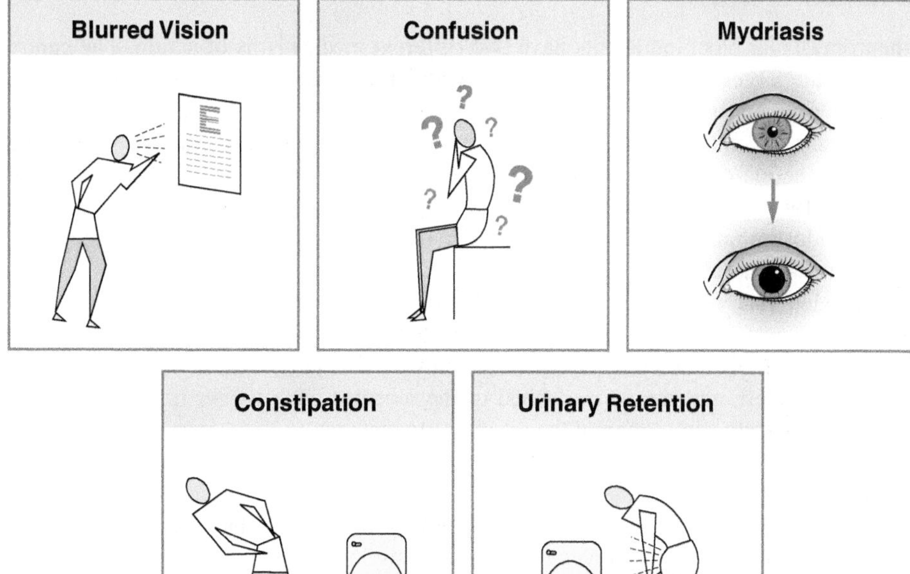


**Figure 5.9** Adverse effects most frequently associated with anticholinergic drugs. (Adapted with permission from Harvey RA, Champe PC, Howland RD, et al. *Lippincott's Illustrated Reviews: Pharmacology,* 3rd ed. Baltimore: Lippincott Williams & Wilkins, 2006.)

## Tips for the Technician

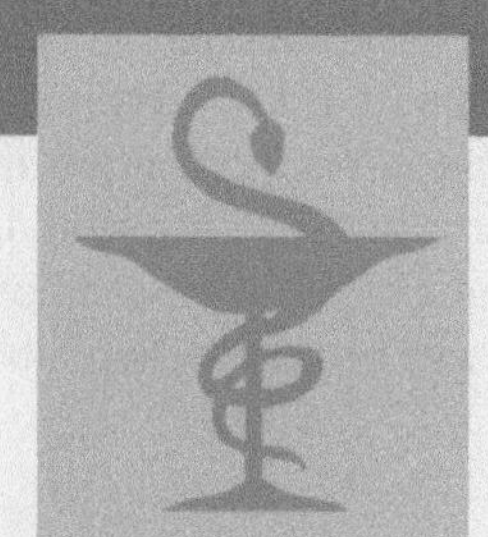

Patient profiles usually contain information about clients' diagnoses. It is important to alert the pharmacist of a diagnosis of glaucoma or benign prostatic hypertrophy (a common condition in men that causes bladder obstruction) on the profile of a patient that brings in a prescription for a product containing belladonna alkaloids, or other anticholinergic agents. These drugs are contraindicated in glaucoma and benign prostatic hypertrophy.

Hospital pharmacy technicians are often responsible for setting up the trays of emergency medications that are kept in "crash carts," the carts equipped with emergency supplies that are wheeled to cardiac and respiratory emergencies. Atropine is always included, but a number of strengths and sizes are available from manufacturers. To avoid errors, use a double-checking process before the pharmacist checks the trays.

# Neuromuscular Blocking Agents

Early in the nineteenth century, Sir Walter Raleigh and other European explorers witnessed the use of poisoned arrows and darts for hunting by the native people of South America. The tips of the arrows were dipped in a dark, sticky paste made from the bark of native plants of the loganaceae family. Minutes after the arrows pierced the animals they were dead. Much later, pharmacologists identified the plant alkaloids in arrow poisons as curare and tubocurarine, examples of neuromuscular blocking agents. The arrow poison works by paralyzing skeletal muscles (including the muscles involved in respiration) until the animals die of lack of oxygen.

## Action and Indications

intrinsic activity Inherent ability of a drug to bind to and activate a receptor, especially as compared to the endogenous compound that activates it; i.e., agonists have greater intrinsic activity than partial agonists.

The neuromuscular blocking agents have two different mechanisms of action. The curare type drugs (the largest group), compete with acetylcholine at the receptor on the skeletal muscle and bind, but have no intrinsic activity. They prevent depolarization of the muscle cell membrane and inhibit muscular contraction, and are referred to as nondepolarizing agents. Their action can be overcome by increasing the concentration of acetylcholine in the synapse, for example by administration of cholinesterase inhibitors, such as neostigmine or pyridostigmine. Anesthesiologists often employ this strategy to shorten the duration of the neuromuscular blockade.

Succinylcholine works differently than the nondepolarizing agents. It binds to the receptor on the muscle and acts like acetylcholine. Rather than rapidly releasing from the receptor and being broken down by enzymes, succinylcholine persists in high concentrations in the synaptic cleft, and remains attached to the receptor for a longer time than acetylcholine. This constant stimulation of the receptor prevents return to the normal, depolarized state and results in muscle paralysis. Succinylcholine is called a depolarizing neuromuscular blocking agent.

Different groups of muscles respond differently to neuromuscular blockade. The muscles responsible for fine motor movement, like the muscles of the eyes, eyelids and fingers, are the most sensitive. The muscles between the ribs and the diaphragm, both essential for breathing, are the last to be paralyzed. It is important to remember that these drugs do not affect the senses, or the ability to think. People can still hear, feel, and if someone lifts their eyelids, see, while their muscles are paralyzed. They simply cannot respond.

These drugs are indicated for use as an adjunct to anesthesia during surgery. Because they cause paralysis of skeletal muscles, much less anesthetic is required. They are also used prior to and sometimes after placing an endotracheal tube in patients who require a ventilator, so the patient does not fight against the ventilator.

## Administration

All of the neuromuscular blocking agents are administered by IV injection only. They are not adequately absorbed after oral administration. Dose is adjusted based on individual response. The duration of neuromuscular blockade after the drug is stopped varies, and ranges from about 5 minutes for succinylcholine to an hour or more for pancuronium. Only a physician who is experienced in intubation should administer these medications. Respiratory and life support equipment and personnel must always be readily available.

## Side Effects

The most common adverse effects unrelated to the action of the drugs include flushing, skin rashes, low blood pressure, and wheezing. These effects have been noted with all the nondepolarizing agents. The frequency and severity of the reactions vary between the related drugs. These reactions are due to the release of histamine from cells in the body.

malignant hyperthermia Rapidly rising fever and hypermetabolic state that occurs as a reaction to some neuromuscular blocking agents and anesthetic agents that is often fatal.

Use of succinylcholine is sometimes associated with muscle weakness and pain because it causes skeletal muscle contraction before blockade occurs. It may also trigger malignant hyperthermia, a life-threatening syndrome associated with increased need for oxygen, muscle rigidity, and high fevers. This is an extremely rare condition that sometimes occurs during surgery. Succinylcholine can also cause irregular heart rhythms.

These agents can all cause residual muscle weakness. Patients given these drugs before they are asleep can be traumatized; although fully aware of their surroundings, they are completely unable to make any response. However, the greatest risk to the patient occurs when these drugs are mistakenly given without adequate respiratory support, often resulting in death.

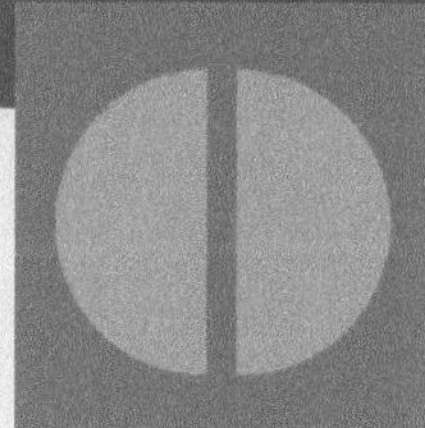

## Case 5.1

Mrs. Gale Windham, a 42-year-old woman, was in a terrible automobile accident. Fortunately, she was wearing her seatbelt, so she had no serious injuries to her neck and spinal cord, although she had some head trauma and was unconscious when she was brought by ambulance to the hospital. There, doctors placed an endotracheal tube so she could have ventilator support during surgical repair of several fractures in her ankle and shin on her right leg. After surgery she was admitted to the ICU. The doctor wrote numerous medication orders, including oral Vicodin® if able to swallow, or IV morphine sulfate for pain, and an order for pancuronium 2 mg IV for agitation (because she was on the ventilator). Happily, although still in some pain, by the second postoperative day Mrs. Windham was awake, almost completely alert, and off of the ventilator. She was to be transferred to a room outside the ICU. The medication orders from the ICU read:

1. Discontinue mechanical ventilation
2. Transfer to post-ICU
3. Continue same medications

Mrs. Windham's nurse, Fawn Young, brought the orders to the pharmacy and asked for the medications. Nurse Young was a brand new graduate, and she was concerned because her patient was quite agitated and in pain. She requested that the technician, Alden Wise, at least give her the pancuronium and the morphine. Alden knew about the patient's discomfort, but was also aware there was no pharmacist available to check his work at the moment. He thought for a moment and then gave her an answer. What do you think the answer was, and why? What are the potential problems with the orders in this situation, and what could be done to prevent them in the future?

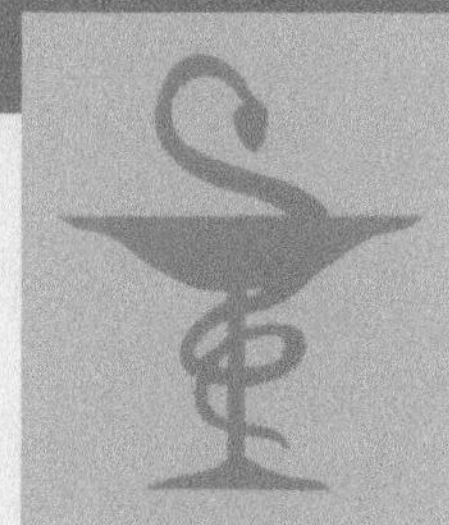

## Tips for the Technician

Because they are high-risk medications, it makes sense for hospital pharmacies to have special procedures to guard against inappropriate dispensing of the neuromuscular blocking agents. These medications are usually used only in operating rooms, emergency rooms, and intensive care units. Know and follow the dispensing procedures at your workplace and question the pharmacist about any orders or requests for these drugs that fall outside of the usual parameters. Never dispense the neuromuscular blocking agents without a check by the pharmacist.

A number of these products have special storage requirements. Atracurium, cisatracurium, rocuronium, pancuronium, and succinylcholine all require refrigeration. Generally, hospital pharmacies will keep these medications separated in some way from other medications. Know and follow the storage policy at the workplace.

# Review Questions

## Multiple Choice

Choose the best answer to the following questions:

1. Which of the following best summarizes the processes involving acetylcholine at the cholinergic synapse?
   a. Acetylcholine is synthesized, released, binds the receptor, and free ACh is taken back up for recycling.
   b. Acetylcholine is synthesized, stored, released in response to an impulse, binds the receptor, and free ACh is broken down by the enzyme acetylcholinesterase.
   c. Acetylcholine is synthesized, stored, released in response to an impulse, binds the receptor, and free ACh is taken back up for recycling.
   d. Acetylcholine is synthesized, stored, released in response to an impulse, binds the receptor, and free ACh is broken down by the enzyme acetylcholinesterase. Choline can then be recycled by the neuron.
   e. Acetylcholine is synthesized, released, binds the receptor, and free ACh is broken down by the enzyme catechol-o-methyltransferase.

2. In which of the following conditions might a direct-acting cholinergic agent be used?
   a. Tobacco cessation therapy
   b. Postoperative urinary retention
   c. Glaucoma
   d. b and c only
   e. All of the above

3. Of the side effects below, which one is not likely to be seen with the administration of a cholinesterase inhibitor?
   a. Constipation
   b. Increased salivation
   c. Constriction of pupils
   d. Reduced heart rate
   e. Exacerbation of asthma symptoms

4. Which of the following drugs is indicated for the treatment of myasthenia gravis?
   a. Pilocarpine
   b. Atropine
   c. Ambenonium chloride
   d. Pancuronium bromide
   e. Nicotine

5. Which of the following are considered common adverse effects of anticholinergic use?
   a. Excess salivation, bronchoconstriction, and pin-point pupils
   b. Dry mouth, constipation, and enlarged pupils
   c. Rapid heart rate, difficulty breathing, and reduced blood pressure
   d. Confusion, GI irritation, and headache
   e. None of the above

## True/False

6. Succinylcholine is a nondepolarizing neuromuscular blocking agent.
   a. True
   b. False

7. Neuromuscular blocking agents are safe to use throughout a hospital, without regard to personnel or available ventilation equipment.
   a. True
   b. False

8. Anticholinergic drugs can be found in many combination products for treatment of GI upset or cough and colds.
   a. True
   b. False

9. Historically, women used the belladonna (beautiful lady) alkaloids to enlarge their pupils, an effect that ophthalmologists exploit to allow better visualization of the retina during eye exams.
   a. True
   b. False

10. When patients treated with neuromuscular blocking agents become paralyzed, they can no longer hear what goes on around them.
    a. True
    b. False

## Matching

For numbers 11 to 15, match the word or phrase with the correct lettered choice from the list below. Some choices may not be used at all.

11. Atropine
12. Rivastigmine
13. Neostigmine
14. Scopolamine
15. Mivacurium

a. Indicated for the treatment of Alzheimer's disease
b. Indicated for the prevention of motion sickness
c. Useful to reverse effects of the neuromuscular blocking agents
d. Indicated for some insecticide poisoning
e. Useful as a decongestant
f. Indicated during surgery for muscle relaxation

## Short Answer

16. Compare the mechanisms of action of the direct-acting cholinergic drugs with the cholinesterase inhibitors. Why are side effects for the two groups similar?

17. Explain why it is important to properly dispose of the nicotine patch and gum products, especially when a household includes children or pets.

18. Esther has recently been diagnosed with glaucoma and her ophthalmologist has written a prescription for pilocarpine Ocusert® inserts. What are the important points the pharmacist will discuss with her? As the technician, what will you be responsible for?

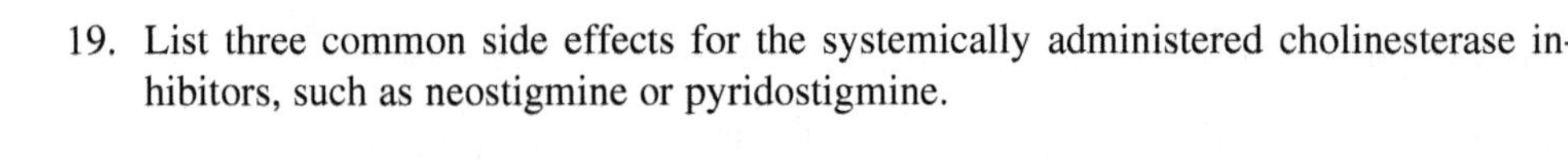

19. List three common side effects for the systemically administered cholinesterase inhibitors, such as neostigmine or pyridostigmine.

20. Why is it essential that technicians understand and follow policies and procedures related to the use and dispensing of neuromuscular blocking agents?

## FOR FURTHER INQUIRY

Learn more about either glaucoma or myasthenia gravis by visiting the web sites of either the Glaucoma Foundation, or another nonprofit group that supports glaucoma research, or the Myasthenia Gravis Foundation of America. Find out what research is being conducted on these diseases, and what improvements in treatment are on the horizon.

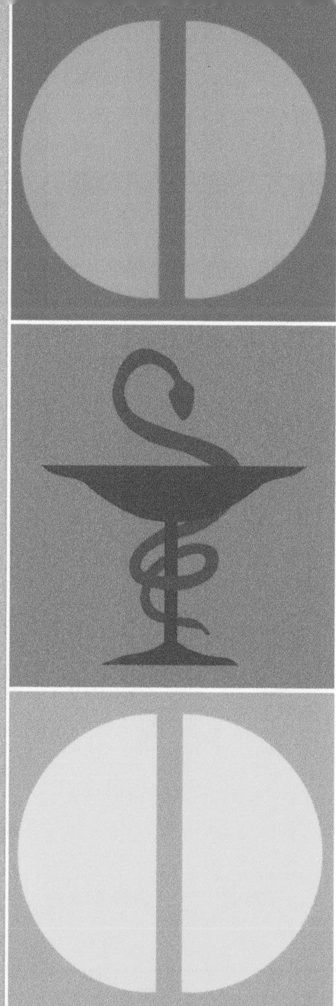

*KEY TERMS*

- adrenergic
- anaphylaxis
- arrhythmia
- benign prostatic hypertrophy
- bronchoconstriction
- catecholamine
- endogenous
- hypertension
- hypovolemia
- monoamine
- necrosis
- postural hypotension
- pressor
- priapism
- reuptake
- shock
- sympatholytic
- sympathomimetic
- vasoconstriction
- vasodilation
- vasopressor

Chapter **6**

# The Autonomic Nervous System: Adrenergic Agonists and Antagonists

## OBJECTIVES

After studying this chapter, the reader should be able to:

- Explain neurotransmission at the adrenergic receptor, including the steps involved in the action and inactivation of norepinephrine.
- List the effect of epinephrine and norepinephrine on the blood vessels, heart, and bronchioles, and explain why the actions of these drugs differ.
- Name three important adrenergic agonists, conditions for which they can be used, and typical adverse effects.
- Name three important adrenergic antagonists, conditions for which they can be used, and typical adverse effects.
- Compare and contrast a nonselective β blocker with a selective β blocker, listing advantages (if any), indications, and risks associated with each.

## DRUGS COVERED IN THIS CHAPTER

### Adrenergic Agonists

| Alpha agonists | Beta Agonists | Mixed Agonists |
|---|---|---|
| Clonidine | Albuterol | Epinephrine |
| Midodrine | Dobutamine | Ephedrine |
| Norepinephrine | Dopamine | |
| Phenylephrine | Formoterol | |
| | Isoproterenol | |
| | Metaproterenol | |
| | Ritodrine | |
| | Salmeterol | |
| | Terbutaline | |

### Adrenergic Antagonists

| Alpha Blockers | Beta Blockers | Mixed Antagonists |
|---|---|---|
| Doxazosin | Acebutolol | Carvedilol |
| Phenoxybenz-amine | Atenolol | Labetalol |
| Phentolamine | Esmolol | |
| Prazosin | Metoprolol | |
| Tamsulosin | Nadolol | |
| Terazosin | Propranolol | |
| | Timolol | |

adrenergic Neurons that are activated by, or secrete, norepinephrine or another chemically similar catecholamine.

sympathomimetic Drug that mimics, or an effect similar to, the actions of the sympathetic nervous action.

sympatholytic Agents that oppose the actions of the sympathetic nervous system or of sympathomimetic drugs.

The adrenergic drugs affect receptors in the sympathetic nervous system activated by norepinephrine (NE), epinephrine (Epi), or dopamine. Some adrenergic drugs act directly on the receptor by activating it, and are said to be sympathomimetic. Others block the action of the neurotransmitters, and are referred to as sympatholytic, or as adrenergic antagonists. These drugs have an affinity for the adrenergic receptor, but no intrinsic ability to activate it. Still other drugs affect adrenergic function by altering the release of neurotransmitter from adrenergic neurons. Most of the drugs described in this chapter exert their effect by mimicking norepinephrine (noradrenaline) or epinephrine (adrenaline), or by inhibiting the action of the neurotransmitter at the adrenergic receptor. See the list of adrenergic drugs at the beginning of this chapter; the complete explanation of some of the drugs is found in later chapters where discussion of their major indications is more appropriate.

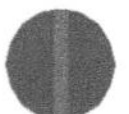

# The Adrenergic Synapse

Norepinephrine is the major neurotransmitter at adrenergic neurons. These neurons are found in the central nervous system (CNS) and also in the sympathetic division of the autonomic nervous system. Recall that the sympathetic nervous system is activated in times of stress, and regulates essential organ systems. It causes the fight or flight response.

Neurotransmission at sympathetic synapses shares similarities to transmission in cholinergic nerves. Norepinephrine and other transmitters in the sympathetic system are synthesized from the amino acid tyrosine and stored in the neuron. The endogenous (originating in the body) sympathetic neurotransmitters norepinephrine, epinephrine, and dopamine are related in their chemical structure and are sometimes referred to as catecholamines, or monoamines.

endogenous Developing or growing within or arising from internal causes.

When a nerve impulse arrives, the neurotransmitter is released into the synapse where it binds to the receptor. There are three mechanisms of removal from the synapse. The first is removal by diffusion out of the synapse back into the general circulation. The neurotransmitter can also be metabolized in the synapse, where it is broken down by the enzyme catechol-o-methyltransferase (COMT). The neurotransmitter can be pumped back into the neuron where it will either be broken down or reused. This removal mechanism is referred to as reuptake**.** The enzyme responsible for metabolism in the neuron is monoamine oxidase. There are a number of drugs that work by affecting one or more of these steps (see **Fig. 6.1**).

catecholamine A biogenic amine, derived from the amino acid tyrosine, that functions as a neurotransmitter or hormone.

monoamine An organic compound containing only one amino group; examples include the neurotransmitters epinephrine, norepinephrine, dopamine, and others.

The response to stimulation of the adrenergic receptor depends upon the type and location of the activated receptor. In the sympathetic nervous system, there are two families of receptors, called alpha ($\alpha$) and beta ($\beta$) receptors. Although both families of receptors may occur in any organ with adrenergic input, organs and tissues tend to have a predominance of one type of receptor. For example, tissues such as the blood vessels in skeletal muscle have both $\alpha$ and $\beta$ receptors, but the $\beta$ receptors predominate. Other tissues may have one type of receptor exclusively, with no significant numbers of other adrenergic receptors. For example, the heart muscle almost exclusively contains $\beta$ receptors.

reuptake Reabsorption of a neurotransmitter following the movement of a nerve impulse across a synapse.

The adrenergic neurotransmitters noradrenaline and epinephrine cause different responses because each is able to interact with the adrenergic receptor families to different degrees. Norepinephrine, the major neurotransmitter of the sympathetic nervous system, exerts its most significant stimulatory effect at alpha receptors, but causes some stimulation of beta receptors, while epinephrine is more active at beta receptors. The study of the action of epinephrine and norepinephrine by pharmacologists is the basis for our understanding of adrenergic receptors.

The adrenergic receptor families are further divided into subtypes, such as $\beta_1$ or $\beta_2$. The subtypes help to further explain the predominant action of Epi, NE, and other drugs on certain tissues. The heart contains mainly $\beta_1$ receptors, and in the bronchioles and blood vessels $\beta_2$ receptors predominate. Norepinephrine has little or no effect on the $\beta_2$ receptors, but significantly activates the $\alpha$ receptors of the smooth muscle in blood vessels and the $\beta_1$ receptors in the heart. When stimulated, the $\alpha$ receptors in blood vessels cause the smooth muscle to constrict, increasing blood pressure. In contrast, the activated $\beta_2$ receptors in the blood vessels cause relaxation of smooth muscle and blood pressure drops. Since norepinephrine has no effect on $\beta_2$ receptors, the anticipated response is an increase in blood pressure ($\alpha$ stimulation) and increased stimulation of the heart muscle ($\beta_1$ stimulation), exactly what occurs. Epinephrine interacts with both types of $\beta$ receptors, and as might be anticipated, increases heart rate, and causes dilation of the smooth muscle of blood vessels and bronchioles. Refer to **Table 6.1** for a description of the effects of receptor activation.

By learning something about the action of the adrenergic neurotransmitters, it may have become apparent that some of their actions could be therapeutically useful. In fact, each of the known adrenergic neurotransmitters has been synthesized for use in medicine. Pharmacologists and pharmaceutical chemists used their understanding of the type and distribution of the receptors, and the effects of the adrenergic neurotransmitters to create drugs useful for the treatment of asthma, cardiac emergencies, and many other conditions.

**Figure 6.1** The synthesis and release of norepinephrine in the adrenergic neuron. (Adapted with permission from Harvey RA, Champe PC, Howland RD, et al. *Lippincott's Illustrated Reviews: Pharmacology,* 3rd ed. Baltimore: Lippincott Williams & Wilkins, 2006.)

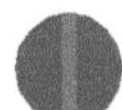

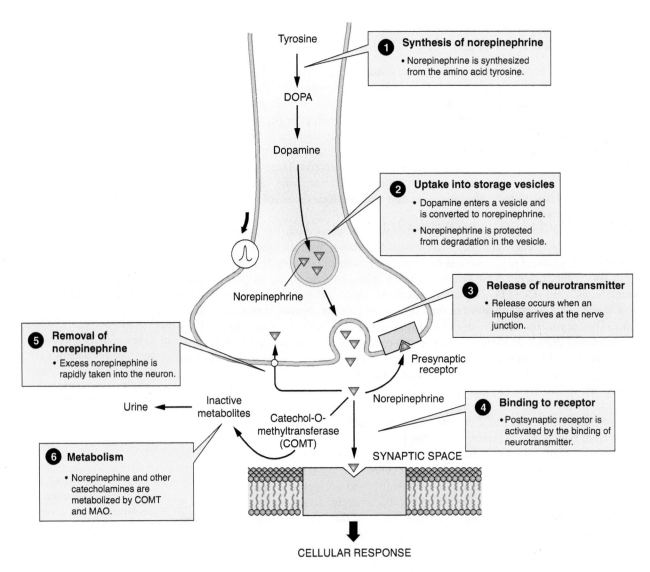

# Adrenergic Agonists

Most of the adrenergic agonists are chemically similar to epinephrine, norepinephrine, dopamine (Intropin®), or isoproterenol (Isuprel®). Norepinephrine (Levophed®) is considered the prototype α adrenergic agonist. Epinephrine (Adrenalin®) is a mixed adrenergic agonist. At low doses the beta effects predominate, but at higher doses, alpha effects are greater. Isoproterenol is a nearly pure beta agonist, and is considered the prototype β agonist.

The catecholamine type drugs are generally fast acting, because they directly stimulate adrenergic receptors. They do not penetrate the central nervous system well because they are not particularly fat-soluble. By substituting different chemical groups onto the basic structure, pharmaceutical chemists produce a variety of compounds with varying pharmacokinetic profiles, selectivity of activation of α and β receptors, and ability to penetrate the CNS. Some drugs activate the adrenergic receptor by causing the release of norepinephrine

**Table 6.1** Physiologic results of alpha and beta receptor stimulation

| Adrenoceptors |
|---|
| $\alpha$ |
| Vasoconstriction |
| Increased blood pressure |
| Mydriasis |
| Increased closure of internal sphincter of the bladder |
| $\beta_1$ |
| Rapid heart rate |
| Increased myocardial contractility |
| $\beta_2$ |
| Vasodilation |
| Bronchodilation |
| Increased production of glucose by liver and muscle |
| Relaxed uterine smooth muscle |

and are therefore considered indirect acting agonists. Others both directly stimulate the adrenergic receptor and cause the release of neurotransmitters (**Fig. 6.2**).

## Actions and Indications

The adrenergic agonists are used in a number of emergency situations, including the treatment of shock and cardiac arrest. From the perspective of lives affected however, use of beta agonists in the treatment of asthma would have to be considered the most important clinical application of these drugs.

shock Profound disruption of hemodynamic and metabolic processes, characterized by pallor, rapid but weak pulse, rapid but shallow respirations, and low blood pressure.

### Alpha Agonists

Drugs with predominantly alpha agonist activity, such as norepinephrine and phenylephrine (Neo-Synephrine®) are used to raise blood pressure in cases of hypovolemic shock, or other conditions where blood pressure urgently needs to be increased. Drugs that raise blood pressure are referred to as vasopressors. Outpatients whose lives are negatively impacted by chronically low blood pressure can take midodrine (ProAmatine®), an orally active vasopressor. Other uses of alpha agonists include topical or oral administration to induce vasoconstriction, constriction of blood vessels. When small blood vessels in the mucous membranes are dilated, fluid leaks out and the surrounding tissues swell. Decongestants work by constricting the vessels, thereby reducing congestion. These drugs are used for nasal or ophthalmic decongestion, and in the treatment of glaucoma. Pseudoephedrine (Sudafed®) and phenylephrine are alpha agonists useful as nasal decongestants.

hypovolemia Abnormally low volume of the circulating blood.

vasopressor A drug that causes contraction of the smooth muscle of the vasculature.

vasoconstriction Constriction of vascular smooth muscle, causing the inside of the vessel to narrow.

Some alpha agonists work in the central nervous system where stimulation of $\alpha$ receptors feeds back to reduce sympathetic stimulation in the periphery. This is the proposed

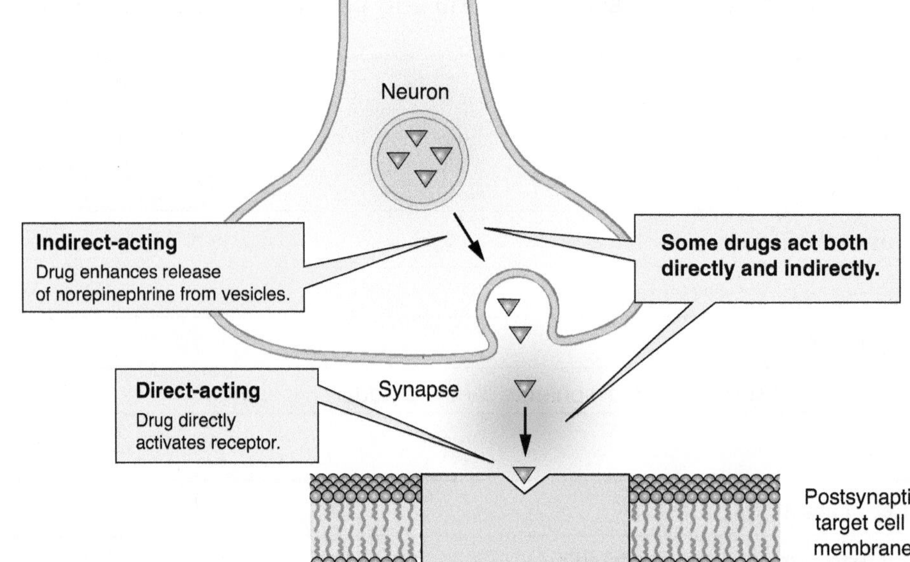


**Figure 6.2** A representation of the mechanisms of action of the adrenergic agonists. (Adapted with permission from Harvey RA, Champe PC, Howland RD, et al. *Lippincott's Illustrated Reviews: Pharmacology,* 3rd ed. Baltimore: Lippincott Williams & Wilkins, 2006.)

mechanism for the blood pressure lowering effects of clonidine (Catapres®), and probably methyldopa (Aldomet®; see Chapter 17).

## Beta Agonists

Beta agonists are used to stimulate the heart in cardiac arrest. Isoproterenol and dopamine are strong cardiac stimulants. They increase heart rate and strength of contraction without causing constriction of blood vessels. Dopamine has the additional benefit of stimulating peripheral dopamine receptors. This results in increased blood flow to the kidneys. In cases of shock, getting additional blood flow to the kidneys can be a significant advantage, since without blood flow they cannot function. Dobutamine (Dobutrex®) is a synthetic $\beta_1$ agonist that causes increased contractility of the heart without a large increase in heart rate.

In the past, isoproterenol was inhaled for treatment of asthma because it is a potent bronchodilator. Now there are many beta agonist drugs that are much more specific for $\beta_2$ receptors in the bronchioles and do not cause the tremendous cardiac stimulation seen with isoproterenol. The use of the beta agonists albuterol, formoterol, metaproterenol, pirbuterol, and salmeterol in the treatment of asthma is discussed in Chapter 20. Terbutaline (Brethine®) was developed as a selective $\beta_2$ agonist for use in asthma, but now other, more selective, drugs are more widely used.

Besides being located in bronchioles and blood vessels, $\beta_2$ receptors are also found in the smooth muscle of the uterus. As it does elsewhere, stimulation of these receptors results in relaxation of the smooth muscle. Ritodrine (Yutopar®) and sometimes terbutaline are used to stop preterm labor.

## Mixed Agonists

anaphylaxis An acute, life-threatening allergic reaction caused by release of histamine that can result in bronchoconstriction and hypotension.

In life-threatening allergic reactions, called anaphylaxis, epinephrine is a life saving drug. It raises blood pressure and causes bronchodilation. Epinephrine opposes the effects of histamine release. It is the release of endogenous histamine that causes the drop in blood pressure and bronchoconstriction (tightening of airways) seen in severe allergic reactions. Epinephrine is a potent cardiac stimulant kept on crash carts for use in cardiac emergencies.

bronchoconstriction Narrowing of bronchioles.

Local anesthetics are often combined with epinephrine. The epinephrine causes local vasoconstriction during repair of wounds or in minor surgery. This provides the double benefit of reducing bleeding and prolonging the effect of the local anesthetics, because they move out to the general circulation more slowly.

Still other adrenergic agonists, specifically the amphetamine derivatives, are used legally and illegally as central nervous system stimulants. Legally, they are used to treat narcolepsy, attention deficit disorder and, for short-term use, as appetite suppressants. Ephedrine, from the herb ma huang (ephedra), was available without prescription in many dieting aids until recently. The FDA banned these products in 2004 because of cardiovascular risks. Ephedrine was also used as a performance-enhancing drug, for which it has been banned for decades. The CNS stimulant drugs are covered in more detail in Chapter 10.

## Administration

Alpha agonists and mixed agonists are administered intravenously (IV) for their pressor effect in shock. Norepinephrine and metaraminol (Aramine®) are available for IV use only. Intravenous, intramuscular (IM), or subcutaneous injection of phenylephrine is indicated for treatment of shock or to maintain blood pressure during some procedures. Ephedrine is available as a sterile solution for IV administration as a vasopressor, and also for nasal administration as a decongestant. Phenylephrine is frequently used as a nasal spray for its decongestant effects, and comes in a variety of strengths. Although ephedrine and pseudoephedrine were often included as decongestants in oral cough, cold, or allergy preparations, many companies are replacing these with phenylephrine because of growing restrictions on their sale, and in the case of ephedrine, negative publicity. There are a variety of products that employ alpha agonists for topical nasal or ophthalmic decongestion. Examples include Afrin® Nasal Spray and Opcon A® ophthalmic drops.

pressor Tending to raise blood pressure or producing vasoconstriction.

Epinephrine is available for intravenous or subcutaneous injection, and for inhalation. Epinephrine injectable comes in a variety of concentrations in ampules, vials, and in prefilled syringes. Epinephrine appropriate for personal use is sold by prescription in prefilled syringes for people who are highly allergic to bee stings or have other serious allergies. It is given by IM injection into the thigh.

Dopamine and dobutamine are manufactured for intravenous use only. Dopamine is manufactured in concentrated form in both vials and ampules, in prefilled syringes, and diluted in ready to hang IV bags. Isoproterenol is usually given intravenously as well. Both epinephrine and isoproterenol can be administered directly into the heart when no IV access is available. Refer to **Table 6.2** for a listing of adrenergic agonists, their uses, and available formulations.

Ritodrine and sometimes terbutaline are given parenterally or orally to stop preterm labor. Terbutaline can be administered subcutaneously for acute bronchoconstriction. Other $\beta_2$ agonists used in asthma are available in a variety of forms. Although many are marketed for oral use, administration by inhalation is preferred. Inhalation is much more advantageous because the active ingredient is delivered directly to the bronchioles and unwanted systemic effects are reduced.

## Side Effects

The main side effects of the alpha adrenergic agonists are directly related to their pharmacologic effect. Intravenous catheters, which are inserted for the delivery of IV fluids, can sometimes become displaced from the patient's vein. When this happens, fluid is delivered into the surrounding tissues, and is referred to as infiltration. Infiltration with alpha agonists is dangerous because it causes severe local vasoconstriction and tissue death (necrosis), which can lead to gangrene.

necrosis Death of living tissue in a structure or organ.

When adrenergic agonists are used repeatedly as ophthalmic or nasal decongestants, patients may notice rebound congestion after the effect of the drug wears off. Rebound congestion often leads to long-term use of the medication and, as a result, chronically congested and dry eyes or nasal mucous membranes.

Elevation of blood pressure can result from vasoconstriction. When adrenergic agonists are used systemically, they can cause an undesirable increase in blood pressure in

**Table 6.2** Most important adrenergic agonists, their brand names, indications, and available formulations

| Generic Name | Brand Name | Indications | Available as | Notes |
|---|---|---|---|---|
| **Alpha agonists** | | | | |
| Metaraminol | Aramine | Hypovolemic shock[1] | Injection | Leakage into tissues can cause cell death |
| Midodrine | ProAmatine | Orthostatic hypotension | Tablets | |
| Norepinephrine | Levophed | Hypovolemic shock | Injection | Leakage into tissues can cause cell death |
| Phenylephrine | Neo-Synephrine | Vasopressor, decongestant | Injection, nasal solution, oral combinations, ophthalmic solution | |
| **Beta agonists** | | | | |
| Dobutamine | Dobutrex | Cardiac arrest, failure | Injection | |
| Dopamine | Intropin | Cardiac emergencies | Injection, premix[2] | |
| Isoproterenol | Isuprel | Cardiac, respiratory emergencies[1] | Injection | |
| Ritodrine | Yutopar | Halt preterm labor | Injectable, premix | |
| Terbutaline | Brethine | Halt preterm labor, asthma | Injection, tablets | |
| **Mixed agonists** | | | | |
| Epinephrine | Adrenalin, Epifrin | Cardiac and respiratory emergencies, anaphylaxis, glaucoma | Injection, topical, aerosol, Inhalation solution, ophthalmic solution | |
| Ephedrine | | Vasopressor, decongestant | Injection, some oral combinations | Many companies are removing ephedrine from combinations |

[1] rarely used, safer alternatives available; [2] available premixed in IV bags ready to use.

arrhythmia Any variation from the normal rhythm of the heart beat.

vasodilation Relaxation of vascular smooth muscle, causing the inside of the vessel to widen.

some people. Excessively high blood pressure can result in stroke or strain on the heart. Patients with high blood pressure should avoid these medications if at all possible. Adrenergic agonists may also cause tremors, headache, wakefulness, and irritability.

Beta-agonist administration carries the risk of excess cardiac stimulation and cardiac arrhythmia, or abnormal heart rhythm. Even selective $\beta_2$ agonists used repeatedly or in high doses can have deleterious cardiac effects. Beta agonists can produce adverse CNS effects that include anxiety, fear, tension, headache, and tremor. Activation of the beta receptors in blood vessels results in vasodilation and can cause blood pressure to fall. This is not a problem in most people, but can be problematic when used in cardiac emergencies. This is one reason why isoproterenol is less frequently used to stimulate the heart than epinephrine. See **Figure 6.3** for a pictorial summary of side effects seen with adrenergic drug use.

## Tips for the Technician

Hospital-based technicians are often responsible for replacing crash cart medications after the cart is used in an emergency. Be sure that stock is rotated so that fresh stock is always available. Check expiration dates regularly. Prefilled emergency medication syringes usually have relatively short shelf lives. Maintain adequate stock levels in case of multiple or prolonged emergencies.

EpiPen® and EpiPen Jr.® are prefilled syringes of epinephrine for use by patients who are highly allergic. EpiPen Jr.® is a lower concentration formulation for young children. Double-check the dose before dispensing. Remind clients that the product dating should be checked frequently and replaced before the drug expires. EpiPen kits should be stored in a cool, dark place. They should not be left in the glove compartment of the car.

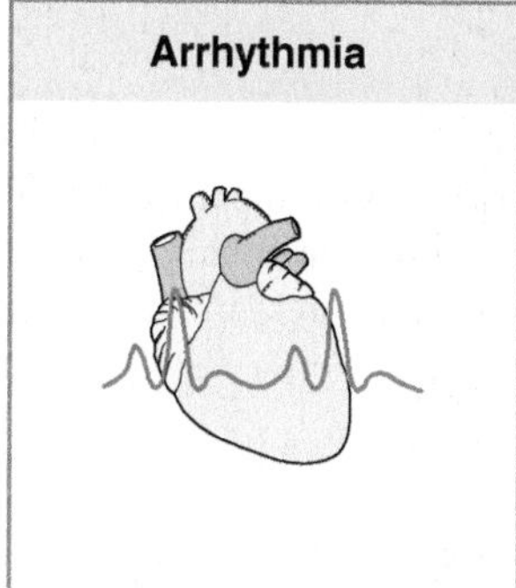

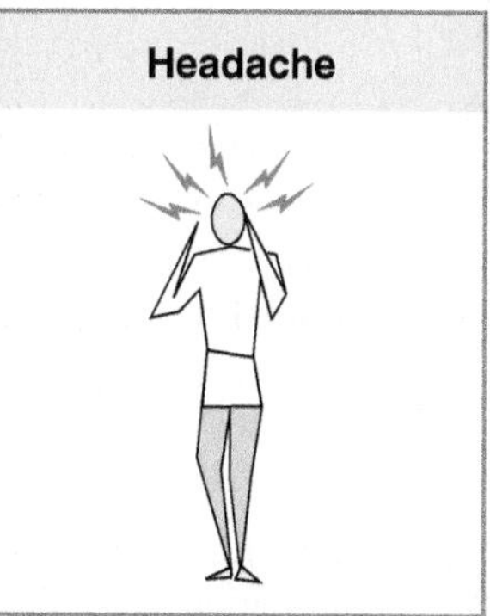

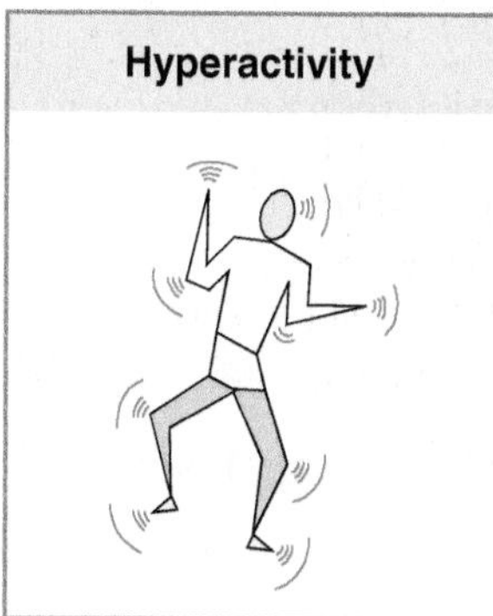

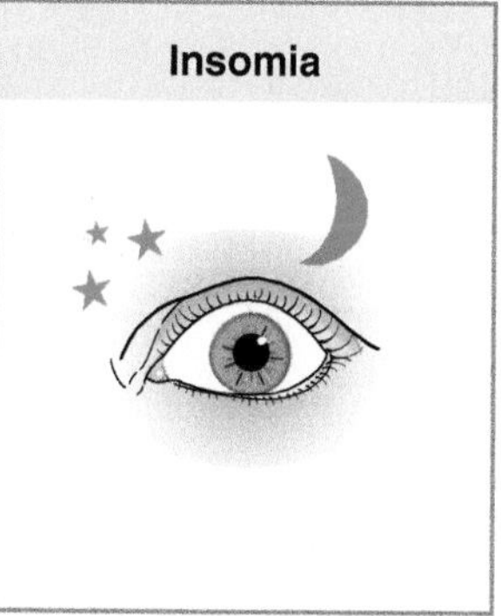

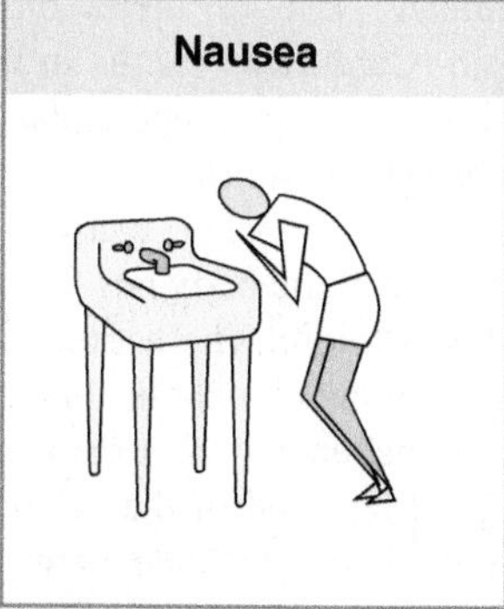

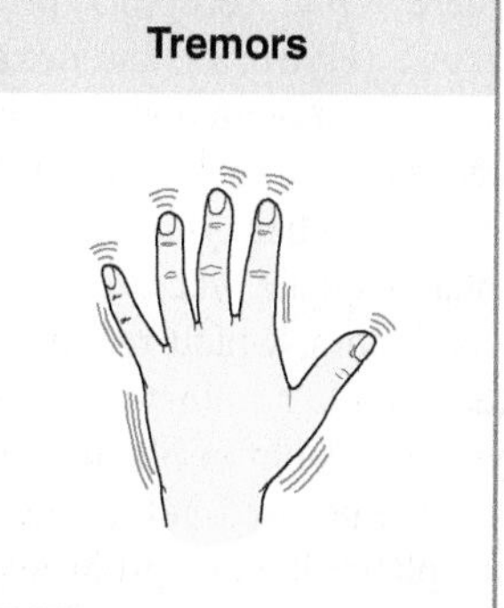

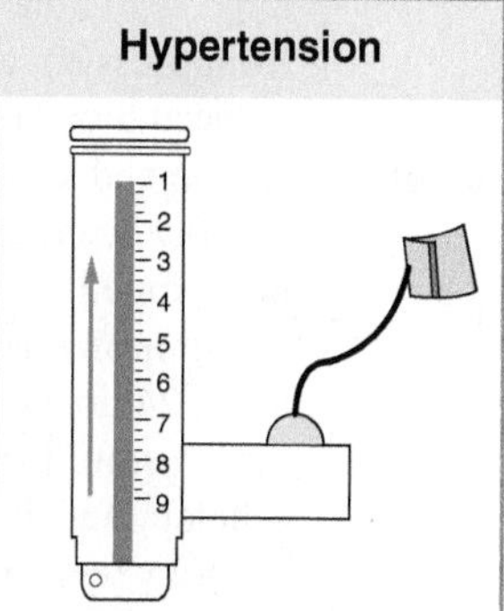


**Figure 6.3** A representation of some of the adverse effects seen with adrenergic agonists. (Adapted with permission from Harvey RA, Champe PC, Howland RD, et al. *Lippincott's Illustrated Reviews: Pharmacology,* 3rd ed. Baltimore: Lippincott Williams & Wilkins, 2006.)

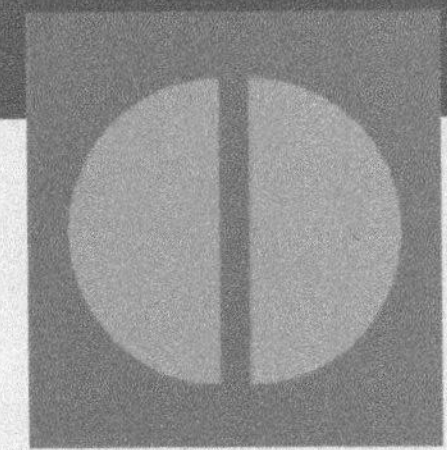

## Case 6.1

Tom Jefferson was the pharmacy technician who got stuck with working on the Fourth of July. Just as he was getting ready to sit down and eat his lunch he received a frantic telephone call from a mother named Betsy Ross who said her son was highly allergic to peanut butter. She told Tom they were enjoying a neighborhood picnic when her 6-year-old son ate a peanut butter cookie before she could stop him. Her EpiPen Jr.® was recently outdated. It looked clear, but had a slight yellow tinge. She told Tom she was at least 10 minutes from the nearest pharmacy and 15 minutes or more from the nearest hospital. Tom put her on hold for a moment to find the pharmacist, but she had somehow temporarily disappeared. When Tom got back on the line, Mrs. Ross said her son was starting to wheeze. What should Tom have advised the mother to do? What other potential options does he have in this situation?

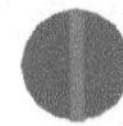

# Adrenergic Antagonists

The adrenergic antagonists (also called alpha blockers or beta blockers) bind to adrenergic receptors but do not trigger the usual response. These drugs act by attaching to the receptor and preventing its activation by neurotransmitters. Like the agonists, the adrenergic antagonists are classified according to their relative affinities for α or β receptors in the peripheral nervous system.

## Actions and Indications

Alpha and beta blockers are used in a variety of situations where excess sympathetic input results in disease. The usual use of these drugs is in treatment of cardiac arrhythmias or elevated blood pressure. The discussion of heart disease, elevated blood pressure, and their treatment continues in Unit III.

### Alpha Antagonists

Alpha blockers compete with norepinephrine for attachment to alpha receptor sites. The result of this binding is less sympathetic stimulation to the tissues. Blood vessels are the most important area where alpha receptors predominate. Use of alpha blockers prazosin (Minipress®), terazosin (Hytrin®), and doxazosin (Cardura®) results in vasodilation and reduced blood pressure. Although not considered first line treatment, alpha blockers are effective and indicated for hypertension (elevated blood pressure).

hypertension Persistently elevated blood pressure.

Phenoxybenzamine (Dibenzyline®), a potent alpha blocker, causes irreversible and noncompetitive alpha blockade, and the only mechanism the body has for overcoming it is to synthesize new receptors, which requires a day or more. The actions of this drug last about 24 hours after a single administration. It has limited clinical usefulness, but is sometimes useful for symptom relief in pheochromocytoma, an adrenal tumor that secretes catecholamines. It can also be used before the surgical removal of the tumor. In contrast to phenoxybenzamine, phentolamine produces competitive blockade of α receptors. This drug's action lasts for approximately 4 hours after a single administration and it is used to aid in the diagnosis of pheochromocytoma. Phenoxybenzamine or phentolamine are sometimes effective in treating Raynaud's phenomenon, a condition where spastic constriction of small blood vessels of the fingers and toes causes cell death, and sometimes necrosis of the involved areas.

The alpha antagonists tamsulosin (Flomax®) and terazosin (Hytrin®) are used as an alternative to surgery in patients with symptomatic benign prostatic hypertrophy (BPH). In BPH urine outflow is partially blocked when the enlarged prostate gland puts pressure on the neck of the bladder and the urethra. Blockade of the α receptors decreases tone in the smooth muscle of the bladder neck and prostate and improves urine outflow. Tamsulosin is not indicated for treatment of hypertension.

benign prostatic hypertrophy Benign enlargement of the prostate gland common in older men.

## Beta Antagonists

The beta blockers are classified as either selective or nonselective antagonists (**Table 6.3**). Nonselective antagonists block both $\beta_1$and $\beta_2$ receptors, whereas selective beta antagonists block $\beta_1$ receptors exclusively or nearly exclusively. Propranolol (Inderal®), nadolol (Corgard®), and timolol (Blocadren®) are nonspecific beta blockers. The cardioselective $\beta_1$ antagonists include atenolol (Tenormin®), metoprolol (Lopressor®), and esmolol (Brevibloc®). Acebutolol (Sectral®) is not a pure antagonist; instead, it has the ability to weakly stimulate both $\beta_1$ and $\beta_2$ receptors. It is effective because it prevents the more active catecholamines from binding (see **Fig. 6.4**). The administration of beta blockers causes reduced sympathetic tone in the cardiac muscle. Beta blockade reduces heart rate and force of contraction, and depresses electical conduction in the heart. Cardiac output, work, and oxygen consumption are decreased, and blood pressure is reduced. These effects are helpful in hypertension, arrhythmias, and chest pain, and in early cases of heart failure. Some of the beta blockers are indicated after heart attack to reduce injury to the heart muscle. Beta blockers are also used topically in the treatment of glaucoma. Nonspecific beta blockers may be extremely useful to protect patients with severe hyperthyroidism (thyrotoxicosis) from the effects of exaggerated sympathetic stimulation. **Figure 6.5** summarizes the clinical applications of beta blockers.

**Table 6.3** Receptor specificity of the beta antagonists

| Drug | Receptor Specificity | Uses |
|---|---|---|
| Propanolol | $\beta_1$, $\beta_2$ | Hypertension<br>Glaucoma<br>Migraine<br>Hyperthyroidism<br>Angina pectoris<br>Myocardial infarction |
| Nadolol | $\beta_1$, $\beta_2$ | Glaucoma<br>Hypertension |
| Atenolo<br>Esmolol<br>Metoprolol | $\beta_1$ | Hypertension |
| Pindolol | $\beta_1$, $\beta_2$ | Hypertension |
| Carvedilol<br>Labetalol | α, $\beta_1$, $\beta_2$ | Hypertension<br>Congestive heart failure |

Adapted with permission from Harvey RA, Champe PC, Howland RD, et al. *Lippincott's Illustrated Reviews: Pharmacology*, 3rd ed. Baltimore: Lippincott Williams & Wilkins, 2006.

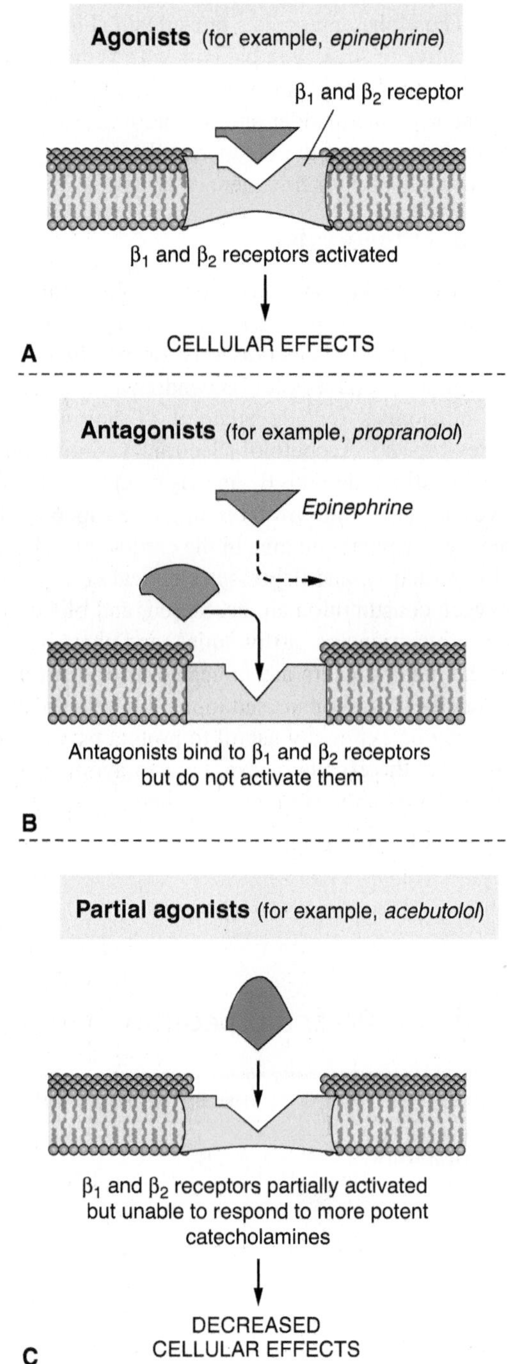


**Figure 6.4** Representations of the mechanisms of action of adrenergic antagonists, agonists, and partial agonists. (Adapted with permission from Harvey RA, Champe PC, Howland RD, et al. *Lippincott's Illustrated Reviews: Pharmacology*, 3rd ed. Baltimore: Lippincott Williams & Wilkins, 2006.)

### Mixed Antagonists

Mixed antagonists are able to affect both alpha and beta receptors to some degree. The mixed antagonists carvedilol (Coreg®) and labetalol (Normodyne®) are used much like the beta blockers in the treatment of hypertension. In addition, carvedilol is indicated for heart failure and in patients who have had recent heart attacks.

## Administration

The alpha blockers prazosin, terazosin, doxazosin, and tamsulosin are all available for oral use only, as either tablets or capsules. The dose of these drugs should be gradually in-

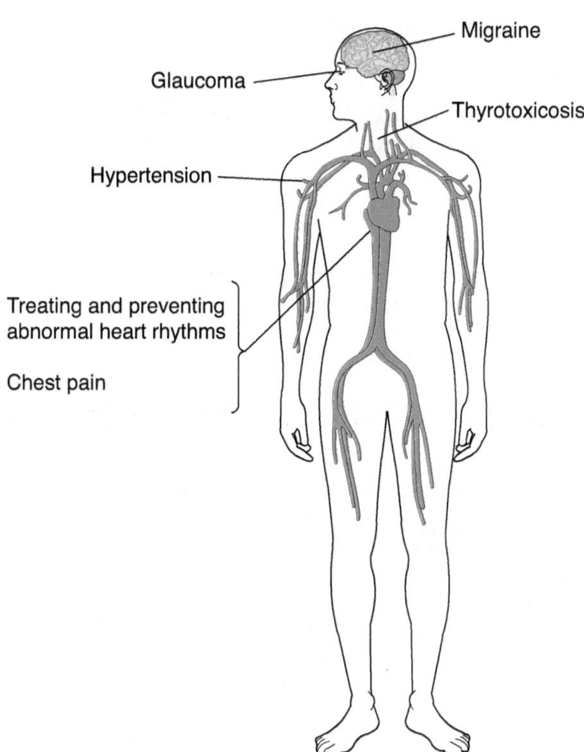


**Figure 6.5** Indications for use of some beta blockers. (Adapted with permission from Harvey RA, Champe PC, Howland RD, et al. *Lippincott's Illustrated Reviews: Pharmacology,* 3rd ed. Baltimore: Lippincott Williams & Wilkins, 2006.)

creased when initiated to avoid side effects. Phentolamine is available as a powder to be reconstituted for intravenous or intramuscular injection in the diagnosis of pheochromocytoma. Phenoxybenzamine is given orally.

Beta blockers are available in a variety of formulations appropriate to their indications. Acebutolol, atenolol, nadolol, and sotalol, as well as the mixed blocker carvedilol, are available for oral use only in either tablets or capsules. Beta blockers atenolol, propranolol, metoprolol, and the mixed blocker labetalol are available for oral administration and intravenous injection. Timolol is available for oral and topical ophthalmic use. Esmolol is only available for IV use for serious arrhythmias. **Table 6.4** is a listing of important adrenergic blockers by brand and generic name, indication, and formulations.

## Side Effects

It will come as no surprise that side effects of these drugs are often related to pharmacologic activity. It is worth noting that where two control systems balance each other in the body, blocking one causes the effect of the other to become more prominent. Thus, blocking sympathetic input to the heart causes an exaggeration of parasympathetic input, resulting, for example, in a slowed heart rate.

Use of alpha blocking drugs prazosin, terazosin, and doxazosin may result in blood pressures low enough to cause dizziness or even loss of consciousness. This problem occurs on arising and is referred to as postural hypotension. It is particularly significant during the first few doses of the medication. It is generally recommended that doses be gradually increased to avoid this problem.

postural hypotension Low blood pressure that occurs upon arising from a bed or chair.

Additional effects of alpha blockers include blurred vision, GI upset, and nasal congestion (**Fig. 6.6**). These drugs may also rarely cause priapism in males. Drowsiness, especially early in therapy, is not uncommon. Most of these medications can cause some weight gain, probably related to fluid retention. Many of these drugs are metabolized in the liver to some degree. Therefore, they are used cautiously or not at all in patients with serious liver dysfunction.

priapism A persistent, often painful erection that is a result of injury, disease, or an unwanted effect of medication.

**Table 6.4** The most important adrenergic antagonists, their brand names, indications, and available formulations

| Generic Name | Brand Name | Available as | Indications | Notes |
|---|---|---|---|---|
| **Alpha Blockers** | | | | |
| Phenoxybenzamine | Dibenzyline® | Capsules | Pheochromocytoma | |
| Phentolamine | | Powder for injection | Pheochromocytoma | |
| Prazosin | Minipress | Capsules | Hypertension | Risk of dizziness on arising |
| Tamsulosin | Flomax | Capsules | Benign Prostatic Hypertrophy (BPH) | Risk of dizziness on arising |
| Terazosin | Hytrin | Tablets and capsules | Hypertension, BPH | Risk of dizziness on arising |
| **Beta Blockers** | | | | |
| Acebutolol | Sectral | Capsules | Hypertension, arrhythmias | Do not abruptly DC |
| Atenolol | Tenormin | Tablets | Hypertension, angina | Do not abruptly DC |
| Metoprolol | Lopressor, Toprol XL | Tablets, extended-release tablets | Hypertension, angina | Do not abruptly DC |
| Propranolol | Inderal | Tablets, extended-release capsules, injection, oral solution | Hypertension, arrhythmias, MI, thyrotoxicosis | Do not abruptly DC |
| Timolol | Timoptic, Blocadren | Ophth soln, tablets | Glaucoma, hypertension | Do not abruptly DC |
| **Mixed Antagonists** | | | | |
| Carvedilol | Coreg | Tablets | Hypertension, CHF | |
| Labetalol | Trandate, Normodyne | Tablets, injection | Hypertension | |

Recall that stimulation of $\beta_2$ receptors in the bronchioles causes dilation, or opening of the airways. Blocking these receptors may result in bronchoconstriction and exacerbation of lung conditions like asthma or emphysema. This is a disadvantage of the use of nonspecific beta antagonists, and to a lesser degree, even cardiac specific drugs (**Fig. 6.7**). Although beta blockers are important therapy in the early stages of heart failure, they can exacerbate more advanced stages of heart failure because they reduce cardiac output.

Beta blockers can also interfere with metabolism of glucose. This may result in reduced blood sugar (hypoglycemia) that occurs without the symptom of rapid heart rate, which usually alerts the diabetic patient to the need for food. Carbohydrate metabolism is less affected with acebutolol and pindolol than it is with propranolol. Other side effects include drowsiness, especially early in therapy, GI upset, and rarely, sexual side effects.

One of the ways the body maintains equilibrium of heart rate and blood pressure is through reflex changes. For example, if the blood pressure temporarily drops, systems in the body correct the reduction in pressure by raising the heart rate, and constricting blood

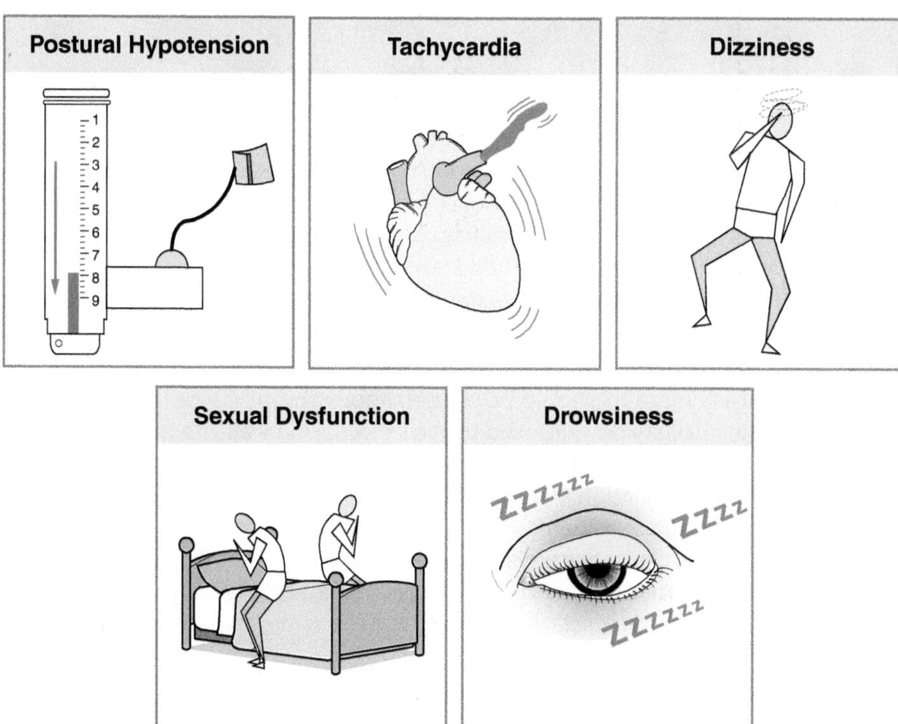


**Figure 6.6** Important side effects known to occur with alpha blocking agents. (Adapted with permission from Harvey RA, Champe PC, Howland RD, et al. *Lippincott's Illustrated Reviews: Pharmacology,* 3rd ed. Baltimore: Lippincott Williams & Wilkins, 2006.)

vessels. Adrenergic blockade at least partially prevents the reflexive correction of low blood pressure or reduced heart rate. This becomes even more problematic when a second drug is given that accentuates these effects. An example of this type of drug interaction occurs when the calcium channel blockers, which slow heart rate, are used in patients receiving beta blockers. The combination can exacerbate heart failure or other heart conditions. A similar situation can occur when the cardiac muscle is depressed by general anesthesia. Anesthesiologists may want patients to discontinue beta blockers before surgery. Abrupt withdrawal of beta antagonists can be dangerous, however, because of the possibility of sympathetic hypersensitivity, so gradual discontinuation is advisable.

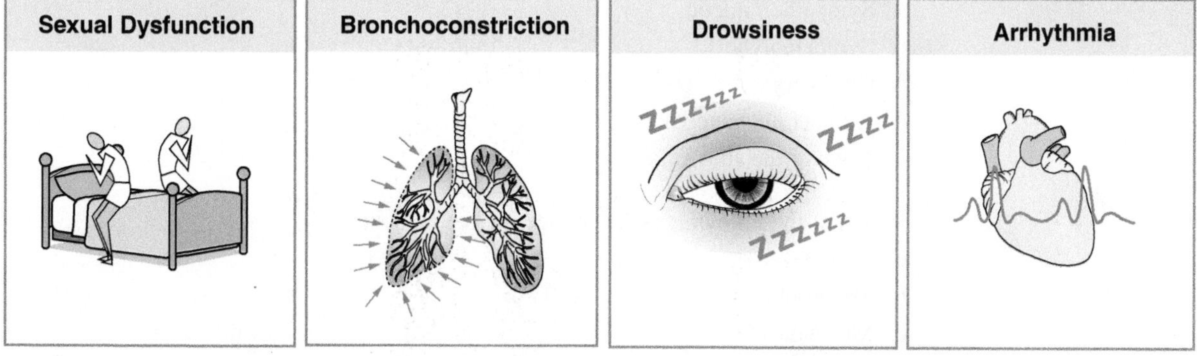


**Figure 6.7** Some of the side effects known to occur with use of nonspecific beta blockers. (Adapted with permission from Harvey RA, Champe PC, Howland RD, et al. *Lippincott's Illustrated Reviews: Pharmacology,* 3rd ed. Baltimore: Lippincott Williams & Wilkins, 2006.)

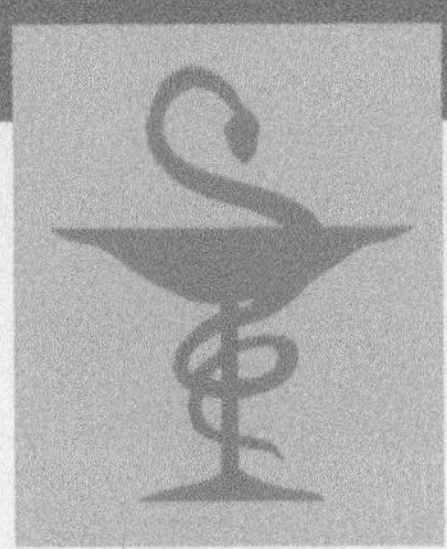

## Tips for the Technician

The pharmacist should counsel patients about the use of all new prescriptions; this is doubly important for the patient in whom alpha blockers are being initiated. They should be warned about the possibility of low blood pressure on arising, dizziness, and drowsiness, especially early in therapy. The same advice is applicable after a dose increase or when therapy is resumed after an interruption. Patients may be more prone to postural hypotension after standing for long periods, when alcohol is consumed, or in hot weather. Auxiliary labels advising caution when driving or consuming alcohol should be applied to the prescription container.

Patients taking beta blockers should be warned about abrupt discontinuation and the appropriate auxiliary label applied to the prescription vial. The beta antagonists are involved in a number of drug interactions, including potential interactions with over-the-counter medication and the pharmacist should be consulted before starting any new medications. Patients with diabetes should be warned that these drugs could mask signs of hypoglycemia and alter blood sugar levels. Food may reduce the absorption of sotalol and it should be taken on an empty stomach. Drowsiness may occur and technicians should attach the appropriate warning label.

# Review Questions

## Multiple Choice

Choose the best answer to the following questions:

1. The main function of the sympathetic nervous system is to
   a. Maintain essential organ function in normal or resting state.
   b. Regulate essential organ function during periods of severe physical or other stress.
   c. Regulate vital signs during sleep.
   d. Regulate digestive and metabolic processes.
   e. Maintain sensory organs and regulate their input to the brain.

2. A drug that acts directly to stimulate the adrenergic receptor is described as a
   a. Sympathomimetic
   b. Sympatholytic
   c. Cholinergic
   d. Adrenergic antagonist
   e. None of the above

3. Which of the following is a nonselective beta blocker?
   a. Atenolol
   b. Metoprolol
   c. Mebendazole
   d. Propranolol
   e. All of the above

4. What are some side effects of alpha agonists?
   a. Decrease in blood pressure
   b. Hypertension
   c. Headache
   d. Hearing loss
   e. b and c

5. Which of the following is not an indication for beta agonists?
   a. Asthma
   b. Halt preterm labor
   c. Viral pneumonia
   d. Cardiac arrest

## True/False

6. Epinephrine is a mixed adrenergic agonist used to reverse the effects of histamine in life-threatening allergic reactions.
   a. True
   b. False

7. Beta blockers can be discontinued without regard to tapering the dose.
   a. True
   b. False

8. When therapy with alpha blockers is initiated, pharmacists should caution patients about the possibility of dizziness due to low blood pressure on arising.
   a. True
   b. False

9. Prazosin is available as a tablet, liquid, and rectal suppository.
   a. True
   b. False

10. Nasal decongestants work by dilating the blood vessels so more air can pass through them.
    a. True
    b. False

## Matching

For numbers 11 to 15, match the drug name to the correct lettered indication, from the list below, for which it can be used. Choices will not be used more than once and may not be used at all.

11. Norepinephrine
12. Terazosin
13. Timolol
14. Metoprolol
15. Albuterol

a. Benign Prostatic Hypertrophy
b. Diabetes
c. Hypovolemic shock
d. Glaucoma
e. Hypertension
f. Asthma
g. Influenza

### Short Answer

16. Describe the steps involved in the action and inactivation of norepinephrine at the adrenergic receptor.

17. Explain the difference between $\beta_1$ and $\beta_2$ receptors.

18. Epinephrine and norepinephrine are chemically similar neurotransmitters. Compare and contrast the pharmacologic effects of epinephrine and norepinephrine and explain the differences between the two.

19. List four side effects seen with beta blockers.

20. Name an indication in which propranolol, a nonspecific beta blocker, is preferred and an indication where atenolol would be preferred and explain why.

## FOR FURTHER INQUIRY

Ephedrine, phenylephrine, and pseudoephedrine have been in the national news lately because of problems associated with their sale or use. Investigate one of these three products to find out what the fuss is all about. How have the laws controlling the sale of ephedrine and pseudoephedrine changed in the last year and why?

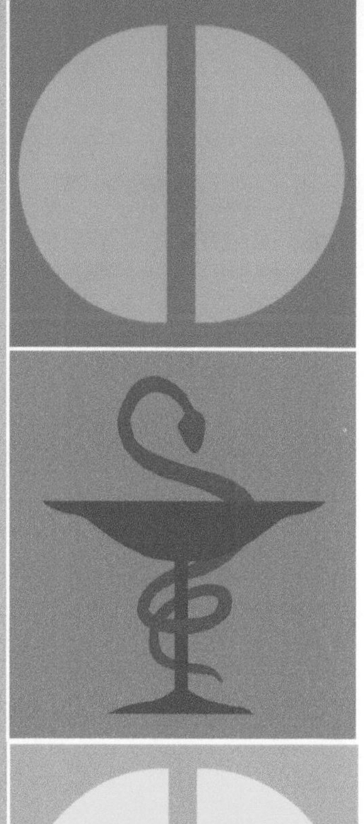

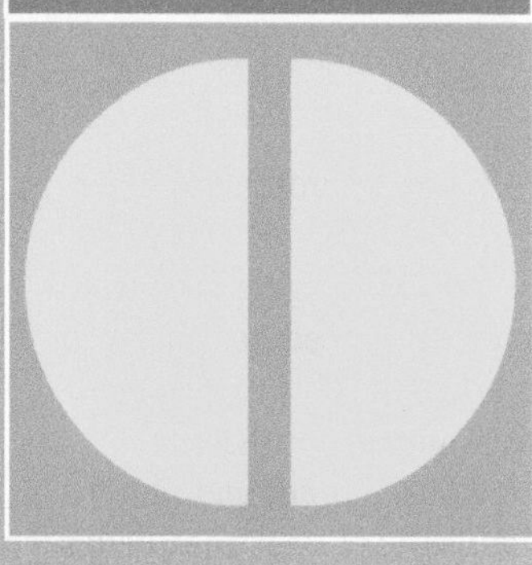

Chapter **7**

# Anesthetic Agents

## KEY TERMS

- amnesia
- black box warning
- hypersensitivity
- hypoxia
- malignant hyperthermia
- tachycardia
- vital signs
- volatile

## OBJECTIVES

After studying this chapter, the reader should be able to:

- Define general anesthesia and local anesthesia.
- Compare and contrast general anesthesia and conscious sedation and describe a situation when each might be used.
- List two inhaled and two injectable anesthetics and an indication for each.
- Name two undesirable effects sometimes seen with the use of local anesthetics.
- Discuss the difference between the ester and amide subclasses of local anesthetics and name two of each subclass.

## DRUGS COVERED IN THIS CHAPTER

| Inhaled Anesthetics | Injectable Anesthetics | Local Anesthetics |
|---|---|---|
| Desflurane | Barbiturates | Benzocaine |
| Enflurane | Thiopental | Bupivacaine |
| Halothane | Methohexital | Cocaine |
| Isoflurane | Etomidate | Lidocaine |
| Nitrous Oxide | Ketamine | Mepivacaine |
| Sevoflurane | Midazolam | Procaine |
| | Propofol | Tetracaine |

Anesthesia is essential for patients undergoing major surgery. When appropriately anesthetized, patients are unconsciousness, and while unconscious, they should not experience pain or anxiety, nor should they move reflexively. Unfortunately, no single agent is capable of rapidly inducing this state, safely maintaining it throughout extended procedures, and also producing analgesia. For best results, combinations of anesthetics are used. This type of anesthesia is referred to as general anesthesia, because the entire body is under anesthesia.

When minor procedures are being done, unconsciousness is not required, and may be unnecessarily risky. In these situations, local anesthetics can be useful. Local anesthetics reversibly abolish sensation in a limited area of the body without producing unconsciousness. By administering local anesthetics in combination with analgesics, antianxiety medications, or injectable anesthetics, analgesia and amnesia can be induced, much like the early stage of general anesthesia. This state is referred to as conscious sedation, because the patient can still be aroused. The idea of conscious sedation is to prevent pain, movement, and anxiety during short surgical procedures, or procedures that might cause anxiety or discomfort in the patient, such as colonoscopy.

amnesia Loss of memory; in some cases related to the use of anesthesia or other medications.

Combinations of several different categories of drugs are used to produce adequate anesthesia while limiting side effects. Preanesthetic medications, such as sedatives, narcotics, antiemetics, and anticholinergics, serve to calm the patient, prevent pain, reduce the risk of postoperative nausea and vomiting, and protect against other undesirable effects of the anesthetic. Use of preanesthetic agents often reduces the amount of anesthetic required (**Fig. 7.1**). Neuromuscular blockade facilitates intubation and suppresses muscle tone. Potent general anesthetics are delivered via inhalation or intravenous (IV) injection. With the exception of nitrous oxide, modern inhaled anesthetics are all volatile, halogenated hydrocarbons that were developed as a result of research and earlier experience with ether and chloroform. A number of chemically unrelated drugs, given intravenously, can also be used to induce general anesthesia.

volatile Readily changes state from liquid to vapor at relatively low temperatures.

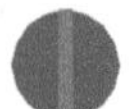

# General Anesthesia

General anesthesia can be divided into three stages: induction, maintenance, and recovery. Induction is the period of time from the start of administration of the anesthetic to the point where adequate surgical anesthesia is established. Following induction, the anesthesiologist may switch to a different anesthetic to maintain anesthesia. Recovery is the time from discontinuation of the anesthetic until consciousness and normal physiologic reflexes return.

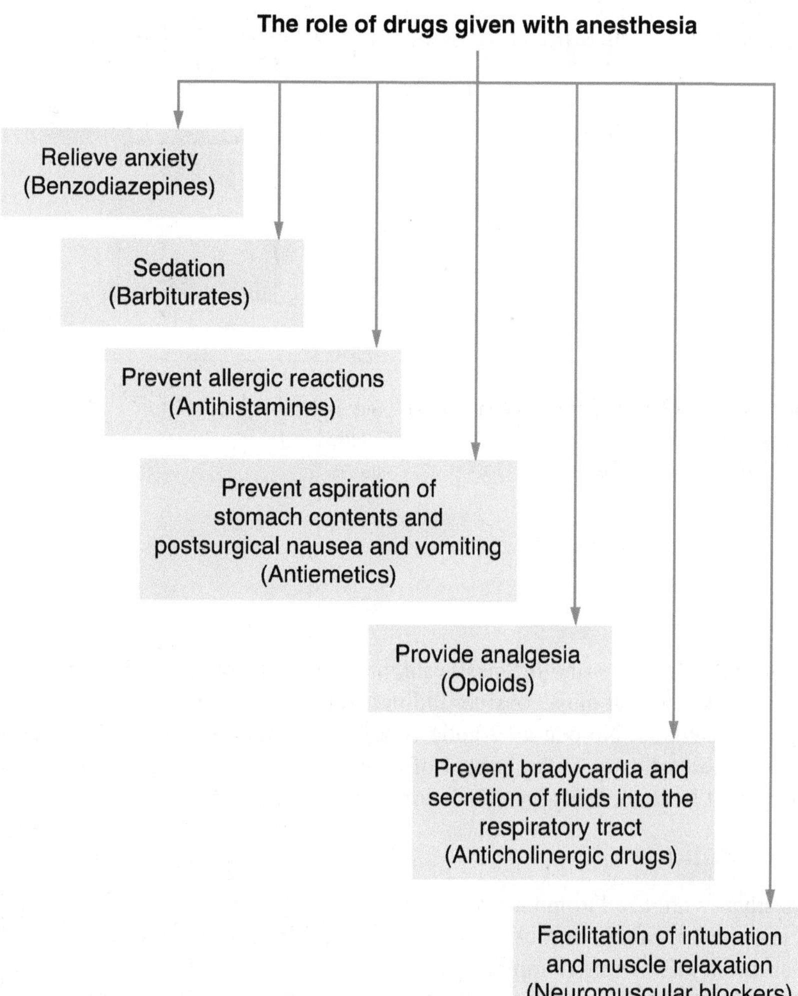


**Figure 7.1** Drugs commonly given before and during anesthesia to prevent adverse effects and minimize the amount of anesthetic used. (Adapted with permission from Harvey RA, Champe PC, Howland RD, et al. *Lippincott's Illustrated Reviews: Pharmacology,* 3rd ed. Baltimore: Lippincott Williams & Wilkins, 2006.)

Speed of induction of anesthesia depends on how quickly effective concentrations of the anesthetic drug reach the brain; recovery is the reverse of induction, and depends on how fast the anesthetic drug diffuses out of the brain.

General anesthesia is normally induced with an intravenous anesthetic like thiopental, which produces unconsciousness within 25 seconds after injection. At that time, additional intravenous or inhalation drugs are given to produce the desired depth of anesthesia. The anesthesiologist monitors the patient's vital signs and response to stimuli throughout the surgical procedure to carefully balance the amount of drug inhaled or infused with the depth of anesthesia.

There are four levels or stages that describe the depth of anesthesia. Stage I involves loss of pain sensation and loss of consciousness. Stage II is an excitatory stage that anesthesiologists try to minimize by using rapid induction with intravenous drugs. Patients can become quite agitated during this phase if induction isn't rapid. Stage III is considered surgical anesthesia, and stage IV anesthesia indicates brain stem paralysis and leads to death if not recognized (**Fig. 7.2**).

Anesthesia is usually maintained with the volatile anesthetics. These agents are short acting and offer minute-to-minute control over the depth of anesthesia. Narcotic analgesics, such as fentanyl (Sublimaze®), are often used with these agents because the anesthetic gases are not true analgesics. After surgery the anesthesiologist withdraws the anesthetic mixture and monitors the patient's return to consciousness.

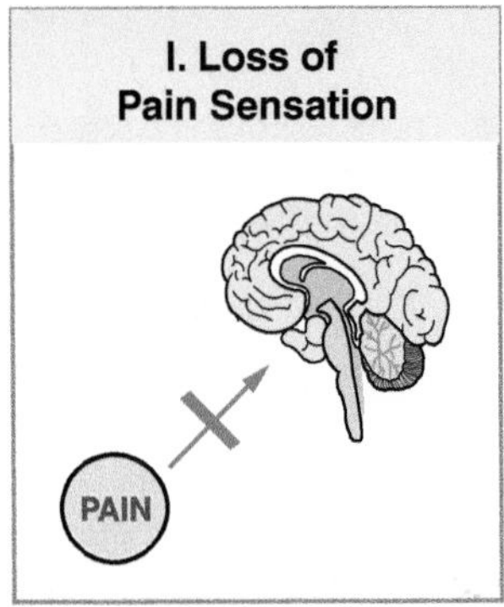


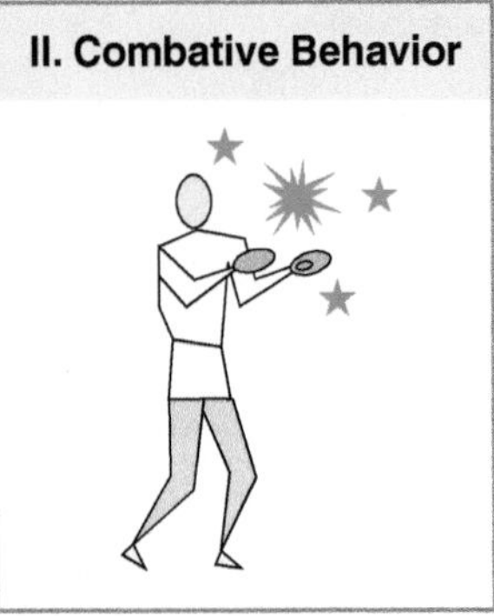


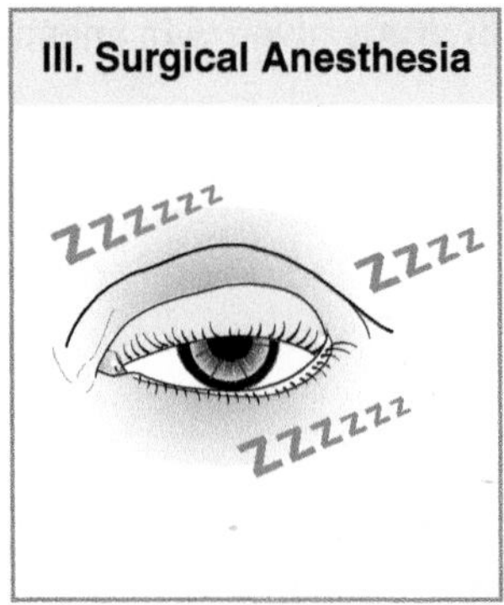


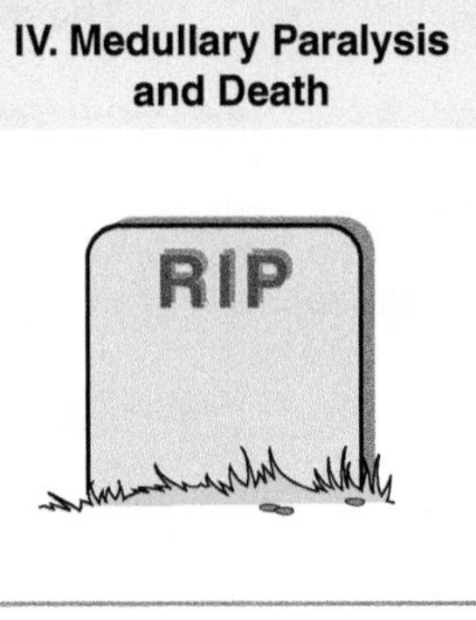


**Figure 7.2** The four stages that represent the depth of anesthesia, from initial loss of pain sensation to coma and eventual death. (Adapted with permission from Harvey RA, Champe PC, Howland RD, et al. *Lippincott's Illustrated Reviews: Pharmacology,* 3rd ed. Baltimore: Lippincott Williams & Wilkins, 2006.)

## Inhaled Anesthetics

Anesthetic gases are the cornerstone of anesthesia, and are used for the maintenance of anesthesia. The anesthesiologist must consider individual patient variables and conditions when choosing an anesthetic. No one anesthetic is superior to another under all circumstances. Inhalation anesthetics have the benefit of being rapidly reversible because most are quickly eliminated from the body by exhalation.

### Action and Indications

The inhaled anesthetics are used to maintain general, or surgical, anesthesia. Although all of the inhaled anesthetics, except nitrous oxide, are able to induce and maintain this level of anesthesia, an agent that can more rapidly induce anesthesia is usually preferred for induction. The mechanisms of action of these drugs are not clearly understood, but are probably related to an effect, either direct or indirect, on inhibitory ion channels and other inhibitory systems of the central nervous system (CNS). All the inhaled anesthetics, whether closely related chemically or not, induce similar physical states.

Anesthetic gases vary in their analgesic effect. While all anesthetics cause depression of the CNS, and as a result, relaxation of skeletal muscles, some anesthetics have greater muscle relaxation effects and potentiate the neuromuscular blocking agents. Some of the anesthetic gases are metabolized in the liver or eliminated to some degree by the kidneys. Most are eliminated by exhalation. See **Table 7.1** for a comparison of anesthetic effects. All of these factors are considered by anesthesiologists when selecting an anesthetic.

Nitrous oxide is an excellent analgesic, is odorless, and has no irritant effects on the respiratory tract. However, it does not cause muscle relaxation and cannot produce surgical anesthesia. It has little or no effect on the heart or liver. Its safety makes it an ideal choice for use by dentists for office procedures, in combination with local anesthetics. Anesthesiologists also use it in combination with other inhaled anesthetics because of its safety and other attributes.

hypoxia Inadequate oxygen supply to tissues due to low oxygen levels in the blood.

vital signs The signs of life, specifically the pulse rate, respiratory rate, body temperature, and blood pressure.

### Administration

General anesthetics are administered only by an anesthesiologist or other trained professionals working under the supervision of an anesthesiologist. The inhaled anesthetics are delivered via facemask in a mixture that contains adequate oxygen to prevent hypoxia. The patient's vital signs (heart rate, blood pressure, respiration, temperature) and oxygen levels are monitored throughout anesthesia and adjustments to the anesthetic mixture are made when needed.

**Table 7.1** Characteristics of frequently used inhaled anesthetics

| Generic Name | Brand Name | Indications | Cardiac effects | Respiratory effects | Notes |
|---|---|---|---|---|---|
| Desflurane | Suprane® | Induction and maintenance | Avoid in patients with heart disease | Irritating, avoid in children | Requires special vaporizer, MH risk |
| Enflurane | Ethrane® | Induction and maintenance | Some risk of arrhythmias | Reduced respiratory response to $CO_2$ | Low risk of liver toxicity, avoid in kidney or seizure disorders, MH risk |
| Halothane | | Induction and maintenance | Increased risk of arrhythmia, reduced BP | Nonirritating, Reduced response to $CO_2$ | Risk of liver toxicity, MH risk |
| Isoflurane | Forane® | Induction and maintenance | Low risk of arrhythmias, some hypotension | Reduced response to $CO_2$ | Low risk of liver toxicity, MH risk |
| Nitrous Oxide | | Outpatient procedures, as supplement to other drugs | None | Nonirritating | Hypoxia risk |
| Sevoflurane | Ultane® | Induction and maintenance | Reduced BP, avoid in certain patients | Nonirritating | Requires special vaporizer, avoid in kidney disease, MH risk |

BP, blood pressure; MH, malignant hyperthermia.
With the exception of nitrous oxide, these products are volatile liquids that are vaporized for inhalation.

Inhalation of the vaporized anesthetic provides rapid movement into the blood and from there into the CNS. These drugs are all small molecules that are highly fat-soluble, a factor that increases penetration into the brain. The degree of CNS depression is directly related to the concentration of anesthetic in the brain.

The inhaled anesthetics, except nitrous oxide, are actually manufactured as liquids. These liquids are volatile, meaning they evaporate quickly at room temperature unless kept in a tightly closed container. Two of the newer anesthetics, sevoflurane (Ultane®) and desflurane (Suprane®), are less volatile and require the use of special vaporizing equipment for administration. Nitrous oxide is a gas at room temperature and is supplied in pressurized cylinders. The pharmacy department is not generally responsible for purchasing or storing nitrous oxide.

## Side Effects

Halothane is metabolized to some degree in the liver, resulting in the formation of toxic byproducts, and its use is largely being replaced in the United States because it can produce severe liver toxicity. In some patients (probably about 1 in 20,000 or more), liver failure is fulminant and fatal. This is more likely in women who have been anesthetized with halothane in the recent past. Other halogenated anesthetics that are partially metabolized or are cleared through the kidneys also cause some organ toxicity, but at a much lower rate.

Enflurane causes kidney toxicity and, because it is metabolized in a similar way, so may sevoflurane.

Individual anesthetics have other characteristic adverse effects to be aware of. Because of noxious odors, some of the inhaled anesthetics are particularly irritating to the respiratory tissues and GI tract. Desflurane (Suprane®) is an example of a highly irritating anesthetic. Use of this type of anesthetic is associated with excess mucous production and postoperative nausea and vomiting. The most serious side effect seen with nitrous oxide is hypoxia. If adequate oxygen is not administered with the nitrous oxide, nitrogen can replace oxygen in the tissues, which, if not corrected, can lead to death.

Some of the inhaled anesthetics have the potential to cause cardiac arrhythmias by virtue of increasing the heart muscle's sensitivity to sympathetic input. The anesthetics can also depress cardiac tissue and reduce cardiac output. This can result in a reduction of blood pressure. See Table 7.1 for a comparison of side effects from the inhaled anesthetics.

tachycardia Rapid heart rate; usually applied to rates >100 beats/minute.

All volatile inhaled anesthetics and the depolarizing neuromuscular blocking agents have been associated with malignant hyperthermia. This is a very rare, but often fatal, syndrome of tachycardia (rapid heart rate), muscle rigidity, increased oxygen demand and carbon dioxide production, high fever, and other metabolic changes. There is a genetically linked predisposition for this syndrome. Hospitals where surgery is performed must keep a supply of dantrium, an intravenously administered skeletal muscle relaxant that is the only specific drug treatment approved for the syndrome.

### Tips for the Technician

Hospital pharmacies are sometimes responsible for the purchase of volatile anesthetics. Technicians need to be aware that ether and cyclopropane, although rarely used, are flammable and require special storage conditions. Flammable anesthetics should have a separate, fire-resistant storage space that is vented to the outside.

Pharmacies are likely to be responsible for keeping special medication carts stocked for treating emergencies in the operating room. These can include a malignant hyperthermia cart, which is stocked with medications to support the patient and treat this condition. Although this syndrome occurs very rarely, adequate supplies of in date dantrolene must be maintained.

## Injectable Anesthetics

The injectable anesthetics are CNS depressants with a rapid onset of action. They are usually administered intravenously. These drugs are highly fat-soluble and distribute quickly into the CNS. They also move out of the CNS rapidly and tend to collect in adipose (fat) tissue. Recovery from intravenous anesthetics is due to redistribution out of the CNS. Eventually, the drugs are metabolized and eliminated via the urine and feces. There are representatives from a number of classes in this group of drugs, including barbiturates, a benzodiazepine, and several miscellaneous compounds. The comparative advantages and disadvantages of the agents used for general anesthesia are shown in **Table 7.2**.

### Actions and Indications

Injectable anesthetics are indicated for the rapid induction of anesthesia, which is then maintained with an appropriate inhalation agent. They work through a direct depressant action on the CNS. The barbiturates, thiopental (Pentothal®) and methohexital (Brevital®), also depress respiratory function. Most injectable anesthetics have no analgesic properties.

**Table 7.2** Advantages and disadvantages of the drugs most commonly administered for general anesthesia

| Drug | Disadvantages | Advantages |
|---|---|---|
| **Inhaled Anesthetics** | | |
| Desflurane | • Requires special vaporizer<br>• irritating | (none) |
| Halothane | • Lowers BP and increases risk of arrhythmia<br>• Rare but serious liver toxicity | • Useful in children<br>• Relaxes bronchi |
| Isoflurane | (none) | • No sensitization of heart muscle<br>• Rapid recovery |
| Nitrous oxide | • Must be combined with other anesthetics | • Good analgesia<br>• Rapid onset and recovery<br>• Safe |
| Sevoflurane | • Requires special vaporizer | • Rapid onset and recovery<br>• Nonirritating<br>• Useful in children |
| **Intravenous Anesthetics** | | |
| Thiopental | • Not analgesic<br>• Causes respiratory depression | • Rapid onset<br>• Effective anesthetic |
| Ketamine | • Emergence reactions in adults | • Good analgesia |
| Propofol | • Painful injection<br>• Lowers BP | • Rapid onset |

BP, blood pressure.

The exception is ketamine (Ketalar®), which causes significant analgesia and amnesia. Etomidate (Amidate®) is useful in patients with cardiac disease because it has little depressant effect on the heart or respiratory center.

Some of these agents can be used in combination with nitrous oxide and narcotic analgesics for short procedures, without the use of other inhaled anesthetics. Midazolam (Versed®) causes amnesia, which is considered an advantage, especially in children. Midazolam has the additional advantage of being reversible with use of flumazenil, a benzodiazepine antidote. Midazolam is often used for conscious sedation.

Propofol (Diprivan®) is widely used and has replaced thiopental as the first choice for anesthesia induction. It can also be used in intensive care units for sedation. Propofol is a popular choice for anesthesia in adults and children because it produces a euphoric feeling in the patient and does not cause postanesthetic nausea and vomiting

As with all anesthetics, the injectable anesthetics should be administered only by personnel trained in their use. The intravenous route can be used to administer all of these drugs. Some can be given by direct IV injection and some must be diluted and infused slowly.

Thiopental and methohexital are available as powders that must be reconstituted and diluted for IV infusion. Ketamine and etomidate are given by slow IV injection. Ketamine can also be administered intramuscularly. Propofol is a sterile emulsion, given by IV infusion or by slow IV injection. Midazolam is given by slow IV injection, or intramuscular injection. Now an oral preparation is available for use as a preprocedure sedative in children. **Table 7.3** summarizes product information for the injectable anesthetics.

**Table 7.3** Comparison of commonly used injectable anesthetic agents

| Generic Name | Brand Name | Indications | Available as | Notes |
|---|---|---|---|---|
| Methohexital | Brevital | Induction, supplement to other agents, outpatient anesthesia | Powder for Injection | CIV<br>Respiratory depression, additive to other depressants |
| Thiopental | Pentothal | Induction, supplement to other agents, status epilepticus | Powder for Injection | CIII<br>Respiratory depression, additive to other depressants |
| Ketamine | Ketalar | Induction, as supplement to $NO_2$, as sole agent in short procedures | Injection | CIII<br>Available in multiple concentrations, emergence reactions common in adults |
| Midazolam | Versed | Conscious sedation, outpatient procedures, induction and pre-op, as supplement to other agents | Injection, syrup | CIV<br>Available in two concentrations, additive CNS depression[1] |
| Propofol | Diprivan | Induction, supplement to other agents, ICU patient sedation | Injectable emulsion | Additive CNS depression, pain at injection site, causes hypotension |

[1]effects reversed with flumazenil

## Side Effects

All short-acting barbiturates are known for their depressant effect on respiration, and the injectable anesthetics thiopental and methohexital are no exception. Midazolam can cause respiratory depression too, but not as frequently or as significantly as the barbiturates. Whenever injectable anesthetics are used, resuscitation equipment should be available. Adipose tissue acts as a repository for these drugs and gradual diffusion from the fat into the blood stream causes a post-anesthesia "hangover."

Both etomidate and propofol can cause skeletal muscle stimulation and movement. Propofol can cause cardiac arrhythmias and can lower blood pressure. Propofol can cause discoloration of the urine, usually to a pinkish color. Ketamine is known to cause significant psychological reactions as patients come out of anesthesia, called emergence reactions. They are less frequent in younger patients. These reactions can range from a dream-like state to vivid hallucinations, and even delirium, agitation, confusion, and irrational behavior. For this reason, use of this drug in adults is infrequent. Sevoflurane, which is non-irritating to the airways, and propofol are gradually replacing the use of ketamine in children.

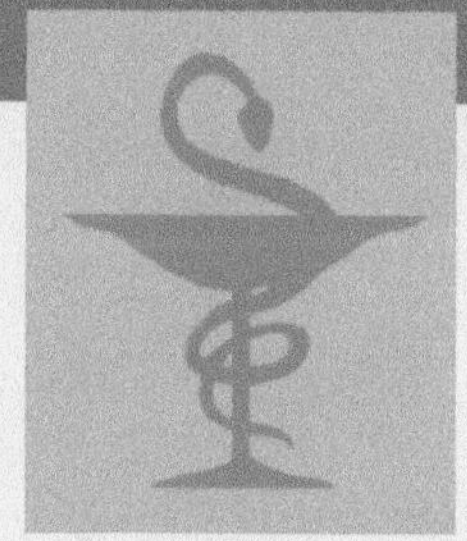

## Tips for the Technician

These drugs are not routinely stocked by retail pharmacies. In hospital pharmacies, the technician may be ordering these medications and supplying them to operating rooms. It is important to know the pharmacy policy on providing and keeping track of injectable anesthetics. Note that thiopental, methohexital, ketamine, and midazolam are all controlled substances. Because of its hallucinogenic effects, the illicit use of ketamine is becoming more common and is usually associated with raves—all night dance parties where illicit drugs are frequently found. Because they are drugs with abuse potential, controlled substances have special record keeping and storage requirements. Technicians should make certain that meticulous records and inventories of controlled substances are kept at all times.

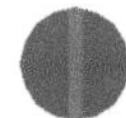

# Local Anesthesia

The first local anesthetic discovered and purified for medical use is an alkaloid found in the leaves of the plant genus Erythroxylum. South American natives were observed chewing these leaves in 1571 by the Spanish explorer and conquistador Pizarro, as had been their practice for thousands of years. It wasn't until the late 1800s that European scientists isolated the active ingredient from coca leaves and named it cocaine. It became the first local anesthetic available.

By the first part of the 20th century, safer alternatives to cocaine were beginning to be produced. Procaine (Novocaine®) was the first of these. Today there are numerous local anesthetics of two subclasses, the amides and esters. These two groups differ in the intermediate chain linkage component of their structure.

The most frequently used local anesthetics are members of the amide family, and include bupivacaine (Marcaine®), lidocaine (Xylocaine®), and mepivacaine (Carbocaine®), among others. These are generally considered safer than the esters because they are less likely to cause allergic reactions. The esters include benzocaine (Lanacane® and many others), cocaine, procaine ,and tetracaine (Pontocaine®). Because of its high abuse and addiction potential (cocaine is a schedule II controlled substance), other drugs have mostly replaced the use of cocaine.

## Actions and Indications

Local anesthetics work by preventing the sensory nerves from transmitting pain sensations to the brain. They temporarily block the sensation of pain in a limited area of the body without producing unconsciousness. The small, unmyelinated nerve fibers that conduct impulses for pain, temperature, and autonomic activity are most sensitive to actions of local anesthetics. Only in much higher concentrations are other nerves affected. These effects are reversible. Once the drug distributes away from the area, normal impulse transmission resumes.

The onset and duration of action, as well as activity when applied topically, determine the route of administration and use of most local anesthetics (**Fig. 7.3**). Lidocaine is an effective amide anesthetic, available in a number of topical preparations, that works fairly quickly. Generally, however, the ester anesthetics are more effective, and have a more rapid onset when applied topically than the amides. When it is used as a local anesthetic, cocaine

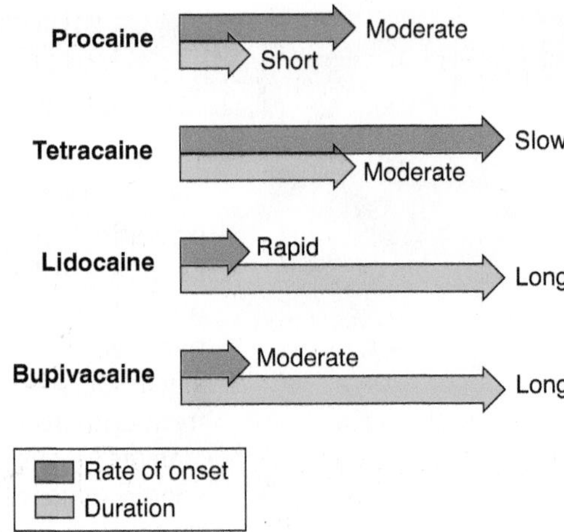


**Figure 7.3** Relative onset and duration of action of some local anesthetic drugs. (Adapted with permission from Harvey RA, Champe PC, Howland RD, et al. *Lippincott's Illustrated Reviews: Pharmacology*, 3rd ed. Baltimore: Lippincott Williams & Wilkins, 2006.)

is used topically, often in the oropharynx. It may also be combined with tetracine and epinephrine, in an extemporaneous compound called T.A.C., for topical use in children who have wounds that require suturing. This combination deadens the area without the additional trauma of being injected with anesthetic. Benzocaine is found in over-the-counter products intended to treat everything from insect bites to sunburns to minor wounds.

Local anesthetics can be injected to produce peripheral nerve block in a limited area for minor surgical procedures, such as dental work or before suturing a superficial wound. These products are often combined with epinephrine for peripheral nerve block, because the epinephrine slows the diffusion of the anesthetic away from the site of injection by causing vasoconstriction.

Some local anesthetics are indicated for blocking the spinal nerves so that a large area of the body is anesthetized, but the patient is still awake. This is sometimes referred to as central nerve block and includes epidural, caudal, and spinal anesthesia. It is possible and sometimes desirable to do major surgeries under local anesthesia. Patients who, because of concomitant illnesses, are not candidates for general anesthesia may be able to undergo the necessary surgery with spinal or epidural anesthesia combined with sedation. Caesarean section deliveries are almost always done with local anesthesia to avoid CNS depression in the newborn infant. Patients with severe pain may benefit from injections of lower doses of local anesthetics into the regions of the spinal cord. Only preservative free anesthetics without epinephrine should be used for spinal, caudal, or epidural injection.

Injectable local anesthetics include bupivacaine, lidocaine, mepivacaine, procaine, and tetracaine. Lidocaine is by far the most frequently used injectable agent. It is also used as an antiarrhythmic agent, but this application will be covered in Chapter 15. Lidocaine and mepivacaine are indicated for spinal and epidural anesthesia as well as for local nerve block in dental and other minor procedures.

Both procaine and tetracaine are members of the ester group of local anesthetics. Procaine was the second local anesthetic available, but is almost never used anymore because safer alternatives exist. Tetracaine is available for topical ophthalmic use and also as an injection for spinal anesthesia. See **Table 7.4** for a comparison of the local anesthetics.

## Side Effects

hypersensitivity A state of exaggerated immune system reactivity to foreign substances.

Adverse effects of the local anesthetics are related to the release of histamine and sensitivity reactions, and the effects on the cardiovascular system when systemic absorption occurs. Histamine release commonly occurs when local anesthetics are injected and can result in redness and itching at the injection site. Clients who frequently use topical anesthetics are more likely to develop hypersensitivity (allergy) to the product. The ester

**Table 7.4** Comparison of commonly used local anesthetics

| Generic Name | Brand Name | Use Indication | Available as | Onset (min)* | Duration (hr)* |
|---|---|---|---|---|---|
| **Esters** | | | | | |
| Cocaine | | Topical anesthesia—in T.A.C. for wounds, also to nasal, oral mucosa | 4%–10% Topical solution | 1–5 | 0.5–1 |
| Benzocaine | D Dermoplast, Solarcaine, Orajel | Sunburns, insect bites, mouth pain | Creams, sprays, ointments | <5 | 0.25–0.75 |
| Tetracaine | Pontocaine, others | Topical—in T.A.C., ophthalmic, central block | Solutions for injection, ophthalmic | 3-8 | 2–3 |
| **Amides** | | | | | |
| Bupivacaine | Marcaine | Peripheral nerve block, epidural and caudal (0.25%) | 0.25%–0.75% soln for injection, plain or with epi | 5 | 2–4 |
| Lidocaine | Xylocaine | Peripheral and central nerve block, topical, pain management | 0.5%–4% soln for injection, plain or with epi | <2 | 0.5–2, plain<br>2–6, with Epi |
| Mepivacaine | Carbocaine, Polocaine | Peripheral, central nerve block, pain management | 1%–3%<br>3% with levonordefrin | 3–5 | 0.75–1.5 |

* Varies with route of administration.

anesthetics are especially allergenic. To avoid systemic absorption, these drugs should not be applied to large areas of blistered or broken skin. Adverse systemic effects, including hypotension, can occur if the drug gains access to the systemic circulation. Parents need to be especially careful when using local anesthetics in children. Topical application in children results in a higher degree of systemic absorption than in adults.

Topical anesthetic products intended for use on the oral mucosa, such as viscous lidocaine and Orajel® are not meant to be swallowed. These drugs suppress the normal gag reflex, enhance the risk of aspiration (inhalation) and are absorbed into the systemic circulation if swallowed.

Although bupivacaine (and the levo isomer levobupivacaine) have been safely used for spinal and epidural block in obstetrics, its use has also been associated with serious adverse effects. Inadvertent intravenous administration has resulted in cardiac emergencies in the mother, and fetal death has occurred when used for paracervical block. Bupivacaine carries a black box warning recommending against use of the 0.75% strength in obstetrics.

At high doses the local anesthetics depress all nerve tissue, and toxicity is a direct result of these effects. They can penetrate the CNS where the initial effect is excitatory, and agitation and tremors are seen. Seizures, and eventually coma and death, follow. Negative cardiac effects include hypotension and cardiac arrhythmias.

black box warning The strongest type of side effect warning, required by the Food and Drug Administration to appear on some drugs that cause significant risk of serious or life-threatening side effects.

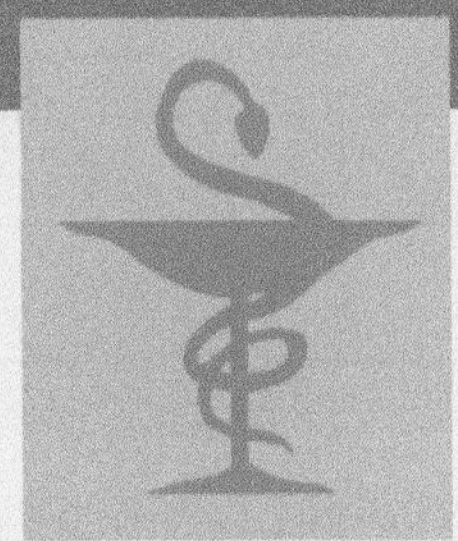

## Tips for the Technician

Pharmacy technicians should make certain that all allergies are recorded in patient profiles, including reactions to over-the-counter preparations. Check the labels of over-the-counter anti-itch medications, sunburn relief products, and other topical pain or itch relieving products so that you are aware of the presence of local anesthetics, especially benzocaine. Inform clients purchasing these products that they contain local anesthetic drugs. Suggest consultation with a pharmacist before using these products on very young children.

Injectable local anesthetics come in a variety of concentrations, with and without preservatives and with and without epinephrine. It is important that pharmacy technicians employed in inpatient care settings understand when each of these preparations should be used. Product labels for different concentrations of the same drug look similar, so always have products double or triple checked before dispensing. Remember that any vial without a preservative is considered a single-use vial.

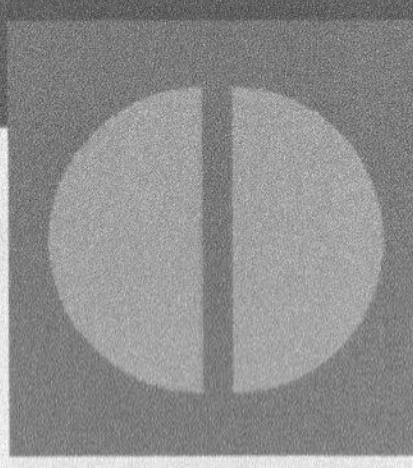

## Case 7.1

It is early in the morning and surgical technician Ernest Cutter calls the OR satellite pharmacy and says that he needs lidocaine PF, right away for an epidural. You have refilled the OR stock list, but the pharmacist hasn't checked them yet, and he just stepped out of the pharmacy. Ernest says he has a partial vial left over from the last case yesterday, but that is all that he can find in the OR, and you can hear the anesthesiologist yelling in the background because he does not want to be late for his wife's birthday party. What do you do?

# Review Questions

## Multiple Choice

Choose the best answer to the following:

1. Which of the following is not one of the stages of general anesthesia?
   a. Induction
   b. Metabolism
   c. Maintenance
   d. Recovery
   e. All are stages of anesthetics

2. Why are preanesthetic medications used before general anesthesia?
   a. To reduce the amount of anesthetic needed
   b. For improved pain control
   c. To reduce anesthetic side effects after recovery from anesthesia
   d. All of the above

3. Of the following statements about the inhaled anesthetics, which is correct?
   a. Recovery occurs when the anesthetic distributes out of the CNS.
   b. Some anesthetics are metabolized to compounds toxic to the liver or kidneys.
   c. Anesthetic gases are mainly eliminated by the kidneys.
   d. All of the above are correct.
   e. a and b are correct.

4. The injectable anesthetics are often used for
   a. Induction of anesthesia
   b. During anesthesia recovery
   c. Local anesthesia
   d. None of the above

5. Which of the following drug combinations might be used in conscious sedation?
   a. Local anesthetics and thiopental
   b. Midazolam, local anesthetics, and narcotics
   c. Halothane and atropine
   d. Sevoflurane and Nitrous Oxide

## True/False

6. Ketamine produces emergence reaction in adults that may include nightmares, delirium, and hallucinations. Because these can be unpleasant, the risk of ketamine abuse is very low.
   a. True
   b. False

7. Local anesthesia temporarily abolishes sensation in a limited area of the body without producing unconsciousness.
   a. True
   b. False

8. Of the local anesthetics, the ester family (which includes benzocaine and procaine) is the least likely to cause allergic reactions with frequent use.
   a. True
   b. False

9. Cocaine, discovered when Europeans invaded South America, was the first drug to be isolated and used for local anesthesia.
   a. True
   b. False

10. Epinephrine is sometimes added to local anesthetics to prolong their action. The epinephrine causes vasoconstriction and thus prevents the distribution of the local anesthetic away from the site of injection.
    a. True
    b. False

## Matching

For numbers 11 to 15, match the word or phrase with the correct lettered choice from the list below. Some choices may not be used.

11. May cause rare, but potentially fatal, liver toxicity
12. Can be gargled, but not swallowed
13. A drug that reverses its effects is available
14. Useful for peripheral nerve block
15. Should never be used for obstetrical anesthesia

a. Lidocaine viscous
b. Propofol
c. Halothane
d. Nitrous oxide
e. Lidocaine 1% plus epinephrine
f. Midazolam
g. Bupivacaine 0.75%

## Short Answer

16. Describe some of the attributes and any disadvantages of nitrous oxide and explain why it is a useful anesthetic in outpatient settings.
17. What combination of drugs could be used to provide conscious sedation for removal of wisdom teeth?
18. List and explain the adverse reactions to local anesthetic agents.
19. What special procedures do technicians need to be aware of when dispensing ketamine, midazolam, cocaine, and thiopental?
20. List three situations in which the local anesthetics might be useful.

# FOR FURTHER INQUIRY

Investigate the historical use of anesthetics in an area of interest to you, such as surgical, dental, or obstetrical anesthesia. Consider narrowing your search by choosing to learn about either the inhaled anesthetics or injectable anesthetics. See if you can find a trend in anesthesia practice towards more frequent or less frequent use of anesthesia in some settings (dentistry or obstetrics, for example), or a trend toward use of more or less general anesthesia (during surgery, for example).

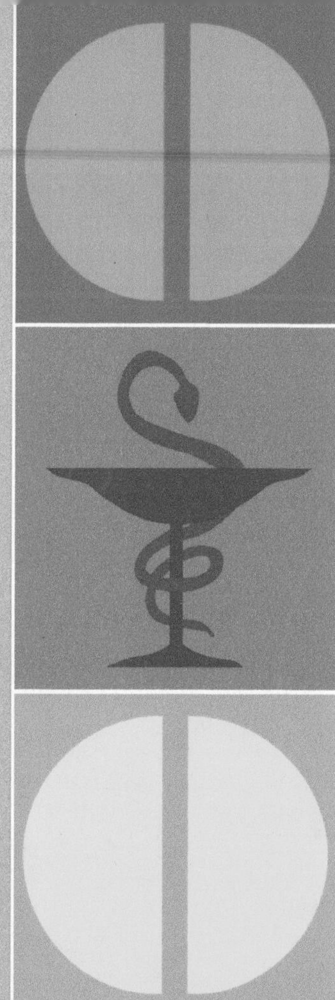

Chapter **8**

# Central Nervous System Depressants: The Anxiolytic and Hypnotic Drugs

## OBJECTIVES

After studying this chapter, the reader should be able to:

- Define the terms *anxiety, anxiolytic, insomnia, tolerance, dependence*, and *hypnotic* and explain why treatment for anxiety and insomnia is reserved for chronic cases.
- Compare and contrast the benzodiazepines and the barbiturates and explain why the benzodiazepines are considered safer drugs.
- Explain why patients taking any anxiolytic or sedative-hypnotic drug should be warned to avoid the consumption of alcohol.
- List the common side effects of buspirone and describe a situation when it would be advantageous to use buspirone in preference to the benzodiazepine antianxiety drugs.
- Describe three characteristics of the ideal hypnotic drug.

## KEY TERMS

- antianxiety
- ataxia
- anxiety
- anxiolytic
- dependence
- exfoliative dermatitis
- hypnotic
- insomnia
- lethargy
- palpitations
- status epilepticus
- Stevens-Johnson syndrome
- tolerance

## DRUGS COVERED IN THIS CHAPTER

### Anxiolytic Drugs—Benzodiazepines

Alprazolam
Chlordiazepoxide
Clonazepam
Diazepam
Lorazepam
Oxazepam

### Other Anxiolytic Drugs

Buspirone
Hydroxyzine

### Sedative Drugs—Benzodiazepines

Estazolam
Flurazepam
Temazepam
Triazolam

### Other Sedatives

Chloral Hydrate
Eszopiclone
Zaleplon
Zolpidem

### Sedative Drugs—Barbiturates

Mephobarbital
Methohexital
Phenobarbital
Pentobarbital
Secobarbital
Thiopental

anxiety An abnormal sense of apprehension and fear, often including physical signs such as sweating or racing pulse, that is a disproportionate response to an event.

antianxiety Intended to prevent or relieve anxiety.

palpitations Unpleasant sensation of irregular or abnormal heart beat, which may or may not be symptomatic of heart disease.

anxiolytic A medication used to treat or relieve anxiety.

Anxiety is an unpleasant state of tension, worry, or uneasiness. It is disproportional to actual life events and arises from an unknown source. Anxiety is one of the most commonly diagnosed and treated mental disorders, which explains the plethora of antianxiety medications available. The symptoms of severe anxiety are similar to those of fear (such as tachycardia, sweating, trembling, and palpitations), and involve sympathetic activation. As already noted, in some situations it is normal for the sympathetic system and the adrenal glands to be activated in the fight or flight reaction, or stress response. In anxiety conditions, the stress response is abnormal and may be triggered by something as insignificant as having to walk out into the backyard in broad daylight, or being introduced to an unfamiliar person.

Episodes of mild anxiety in response to new or strange experiences (for example, starting a new job) are common and do not warrant treatment, because they pass quickly and generally do not affect lifestyle. However, the symptoms of severe, chronic anxiety should be treated because they can be severely debilitating and can have a deleterious effect on relationships and jobs. Treatment options include psychological treatment, antianxiety drugs (sometimes called anxiolytic drugs), or both. Unfortunately, drug therapy is not curative in these conditions, and drugs should be used only for symptomatic relief. In some cases, anxiety accompanies depression. There are a number of chronic anxiety disorders, including panic disorder, social anxiety disorder, and posttraumatic stress disorder. Use of antidepressant medications may be indicated in some of these situations.

Because nearly all of the antianxiety drugs also cause some sedation, the same drugs often function clinically as both anxiolytic and hypnotic (sleep-inducing) agents. Hypnotic drugs are used to treat insomnia. As with mild, occasional anxiety, occasional sleepless nights do not require treatment, but untreated chronic insomnia can lead to other health problems.

hypnotic Drug used to induce sleep.

Insomnia is the inability to fall asleep or the inability to stay asleep. This includes early awakening without falling back to sleep. Chronic insomnia is defined by symptoms lasting 4 or more weeks. When insomnia is chronic, the patient's sleep habits and other medications should be assessed before hypnotic drugs are prescribed. Some medications cause wakefulness as can certain daytime habits and activities. **Table 8.1** is a list of drugs and practices that may cause wakefulness. Drug therapy for insomnia is generally recommended for only a limited duration, while the causes of the insomnia are determined. The following nonpharmacologic approaches may improve sleep hygiene:

insomnia Recurring inability to fall asleep or stay asleep.

- Regular exercise
- Eat a lighter evening meal, well before bedtime
- Create a comfortable, quiet environment for sleeping
- Stick to a regular sleep schedule
- Establish the bed as the place for sleep
- If unable to sleep get up and do something relaxing until sleepy.
- Allow a time for relaxing activities before bed, such as a warm shower or bath, listen to quiet music, read, or have a massage.
- No caffeinated beverages within 4 hours of bedtime
- Use relaxation techniques
- Avoid watching the clock

Normal sleep follows predictable patterns called the sleep cycle. Sleep is generally divided into two types: nonrapid eye movement sleep (NREM) and rapid eye movement sleep (REM). Based on brain wave studies, NREM is divided further into 4 stages (stage I, II, III, and IV). In the healthy young adult, NREM sleep accounts for 75% to 90% of sleep time (3% to 5% stage I, 50% to 60% stage II, and 10% to 20% stages III and IV) and REM sleep accounts for 10% to 25% of sleep time. In stage I sleep, the individual is actually aware of his surroundings. Although no longer aware of the surroundings, individuals in stage II sleep are still easily aroused. Stages III and IV NREM sleep are the stages of deep sleep and are thought to be important for physical rest and restoration. REM sleep follows NREM sleep and is considered most important for reinvigorating the mind. An individual will experience several complete sleep cycles every night. The ideal hypnotic does not interfere with sleep patterns, will induce sleep quickly, allow the patient to awaken feeling refreshed, and not cause dependence (reliance upon the medication) or tolerance (increasing doses are required for to achieve the same effect).

dependence Refers to habituation to the use of a drug that will result in withdrawal symptoms if the drug is discontinued.

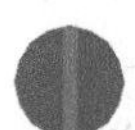

# Benzodiazepines

The benzodiazepines are among the most frequently used medications in the world. Originally marketed in the United States in the early 1960s, the first benzodiazepine to win FDA approval was chlordiazepoxide (Librium®). This was followed three years later by the approval of diazepam (Valium®). Because of their relative safety, use of the benzodiazepines has almost entirely replaced use of the barbiturates in the treatment of anxiety and insomnia. There were 5 benzodiazepines on the list of the top 100 most prescribed drugs in the United States in 2004.

tolerance A need for increasing doses of a drug to achieve the same response.

## Actions and Indications

Benzodiazepines penetrate the central nervous system (CNS) where they exert their effect. Gamma aminobutyric acid (often referred to as GABA) is an inhibitory neurotransmitter.

**Table 8.1** Drugs, conditions, and practices known to cause insomnia

| **Medical Conditions** |
|---|
| • Pain or painful conditions, such as arthritis |
| • COPD |
| • Heart conditions, such as angina, CHF |
| • GI conditions: ulcer disease, irritable bowel syndrome, and others |
| • Urinary frequency caused by BPH or incontinence |
| • Depression and anxiety |
| • Alzheimer's syndrome or other dementia |
| • Hyperthyroidism |
| • Menopause |
| **Medications** |
| • Asthma Medications—theophylline, beta agonists |
| • Diuretics |
| • Antiarrhythmic agents |
| • Antidepressants |
| • Amphetamines |
| • Decongestants |
| • Thyroid supplements |
| • Caffeine |
| • Alcohol |
| • Nicotine |
| **Practices** |
| • Cigarette Smoking |
| • Consumption of caffeinated beverages close to bedtime |
| • Napping during the day |
| • Eating excessively at night |

BPH, benign prostatic hyperplasia; CHF, congestive heart failure; COPD, chronic obstructive pulmonary disease; GI, gastrointestinal.

## Analogy

Most lamps have a simple on and off switch, but some have a dimmer switch, called a rheostat. Rheostats control the brightness of lamps by reducing the amount of power reaching the bulb. The inhibitory systems in the CNS could be compared to a rheostat in a lighting system. In the CNS, inhibition and excitation are balanced, and just the right amount of stimulation (electrical power and illumination) is the result. Sometimes, the CNS has an overabundance of electrical stimulation going on, either because of excess CNS stimulation or because of problems in the "wiring." As a result, disease states such as insomnia, anxiety, and seizure disorders (where electrical activity is uncontrolled, like lightning) can occur. When the inhibitory GABA receptors are stimulated, excessive electrical activity is turned down, and a more balanced state ensues.

This means that stimulation of GABA receptors dampens excitatory responses in the CNS. GABA receptors are complex clusters composed of separate units. One of these units is the site of benzodiazepine attachment and is sometimes referred to as a benzodiazepine receptor. By binding, the benzodiazepines enhance the affinity of GABA for the receptors, and therefore increase the level of CNS inhibition.

These drugs are most often used for the treatment of anxiety and insomnia, but are indicated for other illnesses as well. Diazepam is useful in the treatment of skeletal muscle spasms, including muscle strain, and in treating spasticity from degenerative disorders, such as multiple sclerosis and cerebral palsy. Lorazepam (Ativan®) and diazepam are administered intravenously (IV) to stop seizures and are considered drugs of choice for this purpose. Clonazepam (Klonopin®) is prescribed to prevent seizures in certain seizure disorders. Some benzodiazepines are used for presurgical sedation, involuntary movement disorders, and detoxification from alcohol and other substances. At low doses, the benzodiazepines are thought to reduce anxiety by inhibiting input to the limbic system of the brain, the center of emotions. Patients become calmer and less emotional. They are better able to realistically assess situations that otherwise might trigger stress. These effects are distinct from the general CNS depressant effects that are responsible for sedation and some of the side effects seen with these drugs. The benzodiazepines are reserved for continued severe anxiety, and then preferably for short periods of time because of addiction potential. The benzodiazepines most frequently used as anxiolytics are alprazolam and lorazepam. See **Table 8.2** for a comparison of the names, uses, and available formulations of the benzodiazepines.

Benzodiazepines also act in the spinal cord, where they cause muscle relaxation, and in the brain stem, where they exert anticonvulsant effects. At different doses, all benzodiazepines can cause some degree of amnesia. This is considered useful when the drug is given before surgery or other procedures, but can be disturbing if the drug is used for routine sedation, and dangerous when in the hands of unscrupulous individuals. The date rape drug, Rohypnol, used to sedate and cause amnesia in unsuspecting victims, is a benzodiazepine.

The most important differences between the individual benzodiazepines are not so much related to their action as to differing pharmacokinetic profiles. They can be roughly divided into short-, intermediate-, and long-acting groups (**Fig. 8.1**). Many benzodiazepines have very long half-lives and are metabolized in the liver to active metabolites. Patients with serious liver disease can safely use a short acting drug without active metabolites only, such as oxazepam (Serax®). Oxazepam is useful because it is metabolized to an inactive by-product and is partially cleared by the kidneys.

Although all benzodiazepines can help induce sleep, ideally a hypnotic will rapidly induce sleep without causing excessive drowsiness in the morning, or "hangover." Therefore,

**Table 8.2** Comparison of benzodiazepine drugs*

| Generic Name | Brand Name | Indications | Available as | Notes |
|---|---|---|---|---|
| **Sedatives** | | | | |
| Alprazolam | Xanax® | Anxiety, panic disorders | Tablets, ER tabs, solution, oral disintegrating tabs | Active metabolites, CIV |
| Chlordia-zepoxide | Librium® | Anxiety, alcohol with-drawals, pre-op | Capsules, injection | Active metabolites, CIV |
| Diazepam | Valium® | Anxiety, muscle relaxation, seizures, pre-op | Tablets, oral liquid, oral concentrate, injection, rectal gel | Active metabolites, CIV |
| Lorazepam | Ativan® | Anxiety, acute treatment of seizures, pre-op | Tablets, injection, oral concentrate | CIV |
| Oxazepam | Serax® | Anxiety, alcohol with-drawals | Capsules, tablets | CIV |
| **Hypnotics** | | | | |
| Estazolam | ProSom® | Insomnia, short term | Tablets | CIV |
| Flurazepam | Dalmane® | Insomnia, short term | Capsules | Active metabolites, CIV |
| Temazepam | Restoril® | Insomnia, short term | Capsules | CIV |
| Triazolam | Halcion® | Insomnia, short term | Tablets | CIV |

* Including brand names, indications, and available formulations.

benzodiazepines with more rapid onset, shorter half-life, and metabolism to inactive compounds make the most desirable hypnotic drugs. For the most part, benzodiazepines do not alter REM sleep and have minor effects on NREM sleep. Flurazepam (Dalmane®), estazolam (ProSom®), temazepam (Restoril®), and triazolam (Halcion®) are all indicated for short-term treatment of insomnia.

## Administration

Benzodiazepines are highly fat soluble and are readily absorbed after oral administration. Because of their fat solubility, the three injectable preparations require the use of propylene glycol as the diluent, a very viscous substance that can be difficult to administer and can cause a drop in blood pressure if administered too rapidly. Absorption of diazepam and chlordiazepoxide from intramuscular (IM) injection is both slow and incomplete, and generally not recommended. Lorazepam absorption after IM administration is more rapid. When IV administration is desired, the undiluted drug should be given by slow IV injection to avoid compatibility problems.

All of the benzodiazepines used for anxiety are available as tablets, capsules, or both, and some are also available in solution. Alprazolam, diazepam, and lorazepam are available as oral solutions. The hypnotic benzodiazepines are available as tablets or capsules only.

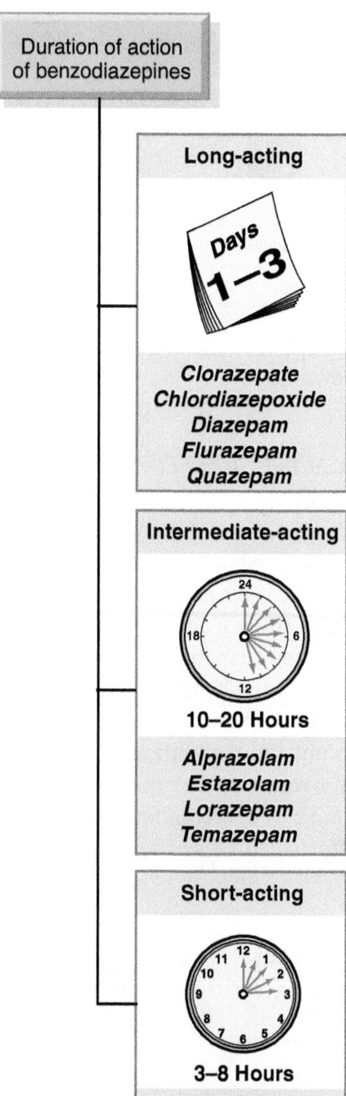


**Figure 8.1** Classification of the benzodiazepines based on the duration of their effect. (Adapted with permission from Harvey RA, Champe PC, Howland RD, et al. *Lippincott's Illustrated Reviews: Pharmacology,* 3rd ed. Baltimore: Lippincott Williams & Wilkins, 2006.)

## Side Effects

All of the benzodiazepines can induce tolerance and dependence. Dependence occurs with long-term use of the benzodiazepines, but the withdrawal syndrome is not as difficult or as severe as with narcotics or barbiturates. All of the benzodiazepines are CIV controlled substances (on a scale of CI to CV), meaning that although their use is associated with some risk of abuse and dependence, that risk is fairly low.

Other side effects are predictable extensions of therapeutic effects. Drowsiness is common and patients should be warned to be especially cautious when operating cars or other machinery. Ataxia (lack of coordination, especially noticeable when walking or standing) and confusion can occur with higher doses or in elderly patients who are more sensitive to these drugs (**Fig. 8.2**). The benzodiazepines with long half-lives should be avoided in the elderly because of the greater accumulation of the drug. This is due to the gradually deteriorating organ function found in the elderly, and is especially problematic when the metabolism of the drug produces active metabolites. Because of this, prescribers usually use lower doses in the elderly than those given to younger adults. Accumulation of the drug and

ataxia Inability to coordinate voluntary muscle movements that can be an adverse drug effect or a symptom of some neurologic disorders.

Drowsiness

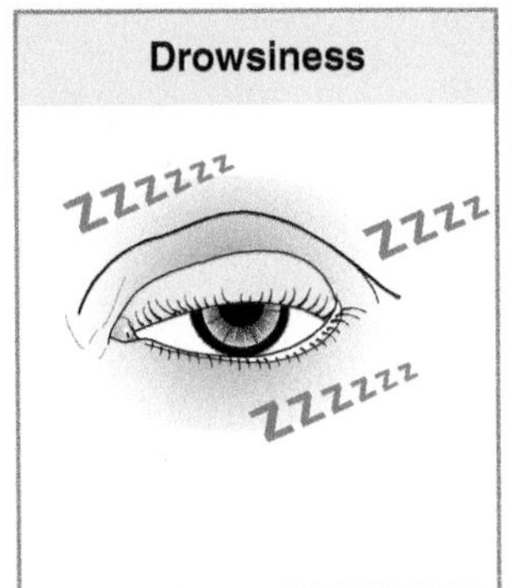


Ataxia

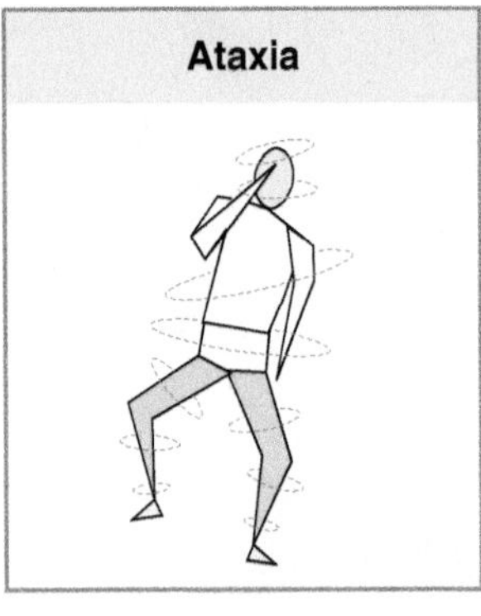

Drug-Alcohol Interaction

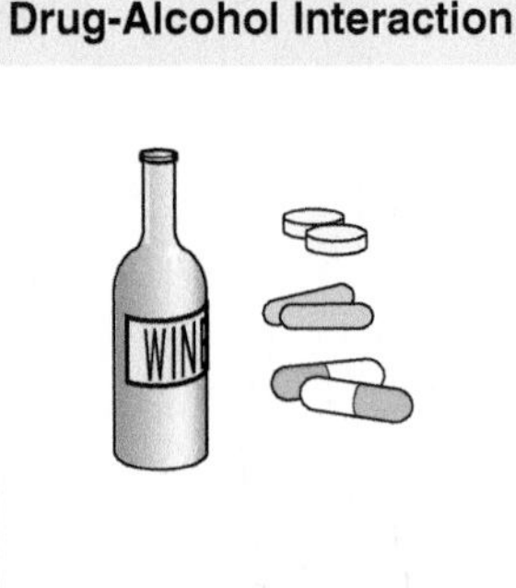


Potential for Addiction

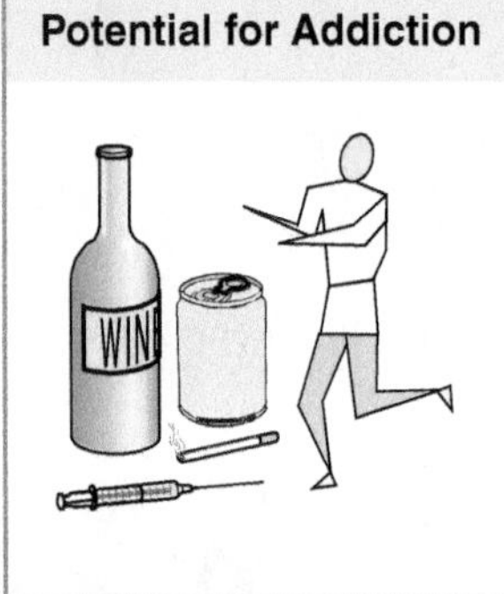


**Figure 8.2** Representation of the most well-known of the benzodiazepine side effects. (Adapted with permission from Harvey RA, Champe PC, Howland RD, et al. *Lippincott's Illustrated Reviews: Pharmacology,* 3rd ed. Baltimore: Lippincott Williams & Wilkins, 2006.)

possible ataxia combine to dramatically increase the risk of falls in the elderly, who may already have difficulty with balance and walking.

Amnesia can occur with higher doses of the benzodiazepines, especially triazolam (Halcion®). When Halcion® was introduced, recommended doses were higher than now. This drug was touted as being so safe that travelers could use it to ease their jet lag. There were reports of people taking this sedative before long airplane flights so they could rest, and awakening without any recollection of boarding the aircraft. Patients may experience drug hangover and lack of coordination on awakening when taking the longer acting benzodiazepines.

The most serious side effects occur when these drugs are taken with other CNS depressants, such as alcohol. In general, the benzodiazepines do not cause significant respiratory depression when taken alone, even with large, intentional overdoses. For this reason, they are considered the safest of the CNS depressants (**Fig. 8.3**). When combined with other CNS depressants, however, the respiratory depressant effects can be serious and in overdose situations, lethal.

## Tips for the Technician

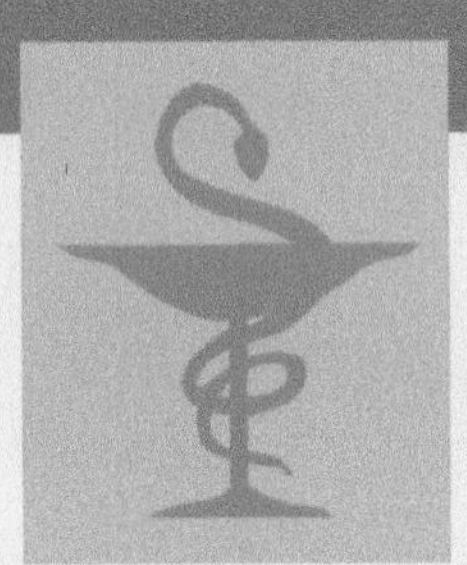

Technicians filling outpatient prescriptions must be very careful to attach the appropriate accessory warning labels to these prescription medications before they are dispensed. All benzodiazepines need a label cautioning against the consumption of alcoholic beverages while taking these medications. Medications prescribed for anxiety should also carry a drowsiness warning. Some pharmacists prefer to not include a warning regarding the potential for drowsiness on prescription hypnotic drugs because drowsiness is the desired result of taking the medication. Others feel patients need to be warned about the risk of operating machinery while taking these medications because of the possibility that the patient might decide to get into the car even after he has taken his medication for sleep. Pharmacy employees may be liable if a patient is not properly warned about the risk of taking prescription medication and a problem results. The benzodiazepines can be taken without regard to meals. Patients who take benzodiazepines, or any medications, for seizure disorders should be encouraged to wear or carry medication alert information.

Benzodiazepines should not be diluted for intravenous use. Although this makes IV administration a little more difficult, IV admixtures with benzodiazepines are not stable. When given IV, nurses need to be aware that rapid administration may result in hypotension.

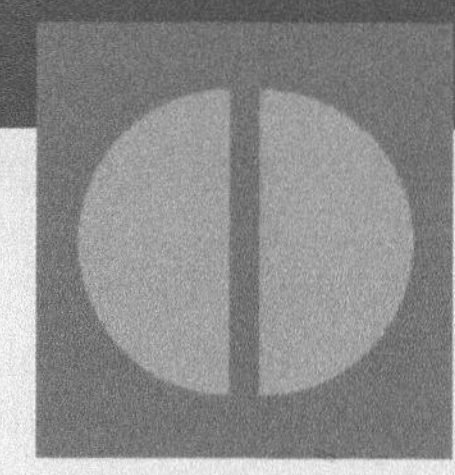

## Case 8.1

Long ago and far away, an eager intern pharmacist, excited about practicing clinical pharmacy, took it upon herself to counsel every patient about all new prescriptions she dispensed in the pharmacy where she worked, although the law did not require this at the time. Her employer barely tolerated this practice and the pharmacy clerk routinely smirked during her discussions with patients, until the Valium® incident.

On this occasion, a patient (call him Mr. Sweet) came in with a new prescription for diazepam, which the intern carefully filled and had checked. She reviewed the risks of taking the medication with the patient, including the possibility of drowsiness and the additive effect of taking other CNS depressants, and especially warned him about alcohol. Mr. Sweet appeared unimpressed and only half listened, and claimed he wasn't much of a drinker.

The following Monday Mr. Sweet came back into the pharmacy, looking rather sheepish. He asked to speak to the pharmacist in charge, and thanked him effusively for the intern's warning, which unfortunately, he disregarded. That weekend he had taken his diazepam as directed, but went to visit friends for a barbecue, and consumed a couple of beers. On his way home he made a right turn into his driveway, or so he thought. Actually, he missed the driveway, ran over the curb, and on through his neighbor's living room window. Fortunately, no one was hurt. Nobody in the pharmacy ever snickered about the intern's enthusiasm again either.

What could have been the result in this situation if the patient had not been counseled? Whose responsibility is it to make sure patients are informed about the risks of taking prescription medications?

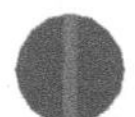

# Barbiturates

The barbiturates were formerly the mainstay of treatment of anxiety and insomnia. Today, they have been largely replaced by the benzodiazepines. This is because the barbiturates induce tolerance, and cause physical dependence associated with severe withdrawal symptoms when the drug is discontinued. Furthermore, they cause coma in toxic doses. For many years they were the agents of choice for people trying to commit suicide. Now, prescribing and dispensing of the most dangerous barbiturates is tightly controlled. Three barbiturates are still widely used in medicine for conditions other than anxiety or as sedatives. Thiopental and methohexital (Brevital®) are used for anesthesia, and phenobarbital is often prescribed for the treatment of seizure disorders.

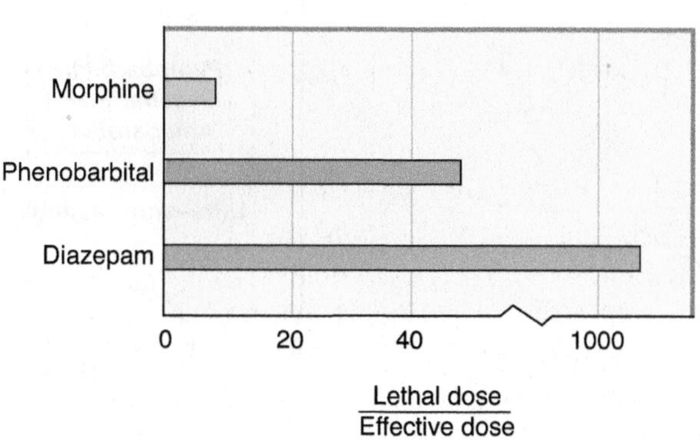


**Figure 8.3** The relative safety of the benzodiazepines as compared to morphine and phenobarbital. The graph shows the relationship between lethal dose and effective dose. The lethal dose of diazepam is more than 1,000 times the effective dose. (Adapted with permission from Harvey RA, Champe PC, Howland RD, et al. *Lippincott's Illustrated Reviews: Pharmacology,* 3rd ed. Baltimore: Lippincott Williams & Wilkins, 2006.)

## Actions and Indications

Barbiturates may be prescribed for daytime sedation (phenobarbital and mephobarbital), for their hypnotic effects (secobarbital or Seconal®, pentobarbital or Nembutal®, and phenobarbital), as anticonvulsants, or as anesthetic or pre-anesthetic agents. They are general CNS depressants that can, in cases of overdose, produce anesthesia and death. In low doses they increase the actions of GABA, and have antianxiety and hypnotic properties. Unlike the benzodiazepines, they cause increasing generalized CNS depression with increasing doses. All barbiturates have anticonvulsant properties in doses sufficient to cause anesthesia. In extreme cases of persistent seizures, called status epilepticus, barbiturate induced coma may be used for therapeutic purposes. Two drugs, phenobarbital (Luminal®) and mephobarbital (Mebaral®), have anticonvulsant properties at doses that do not induce sleep. Phenobarbital is indicated for treatment of a variety of kinds of seizures and is also sometimes given by injection for acute seizures or status epilepticus.

status epilepticus A prolonged series of seizures without complete recovery of consciousness between them.

Comparisons of the barbiturates are usually based on the duration of their effects (**Fig. 8.4** for a comparison of barbiturate drugs). The duration of effect is related to fat solubility of the drugs. The shortest acting agents are highly lipid soluble and are rapidly distributed into and out of the CNS. Phenobarbital is the longest acting and the least fat-soluble, while thiopental, used for anesthesia, is ultra-short acting. As much as half of a phenobarbital dose may be removed unchanged by the kidneys. The other barbiturates are primarily cleared by metabolism in the liver.

The barbiturates induce the drug metabolizing enzymes in the liver. Consequently, they will gradually begin to reduce their own and some other drugs effectiveness after a few days

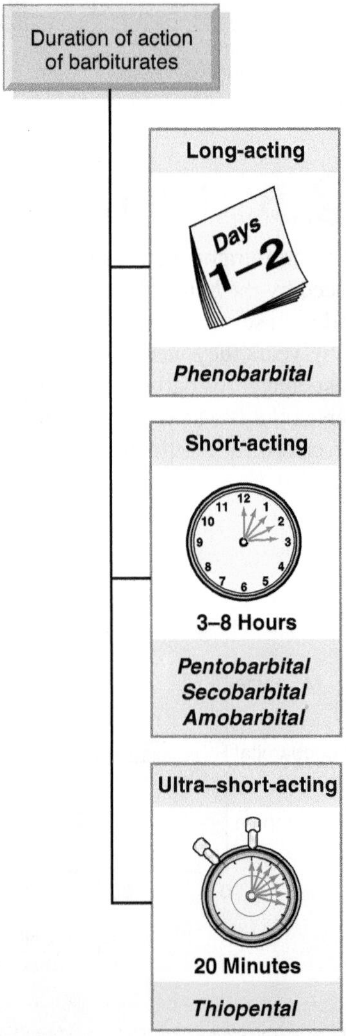

Duration of action of barbiturates

Long-acting
Days 1–2
*Phenobarbital*

Short-acting
3–8 Hours
*Pentobarbital*
*Secobarbital*
*Amobarbital*

Ultra-short-acting
20 Minutes
*Thiopental*

**Figure 8.4** Classification of the barbiturates based on the duration of their effects. (Adapted with permission from Harvey RA, Champe PC, Howland RD, et al. *Lippincott's Illustrated Reviews: Pharmacology,* 3rd ed. Baltimore: Lippincott Williams & Wilkins, 2006.)

of therapy. This results in gradually increasing dosage requirements in order to achieve the same effect. This effect is called tolerance. In the case of phenobarbital, serum drug levels are monitored so that dose adjustments can be made that continue to provide adequate anticonvulsant effect.

## Administration

The barbiturates are well absorbed orally. Thiopental and methohexital are available only for injection, which reflects their uses in anesthesia. Of all the barbiturates, phenobarbital and thiopental are probably the most widely used. Phenobarbital is available as tablets, capsules, and elixir for oral use and as 30, 60, 65, and 130 mg/mL sterile solution for injection. Because phenobarbital is such an old and thoroughly studied medication, it is indicated for use in children. Doses vary widely for different indications and patient ages. Phenobarbital is a long-acting barbiturate, with a half-life of 2 days or more. This drug can sometimes be given only once daily, although twice daily administration is more common for the prevention of seizures.

Secobarbital and pentobarbital are rarely used because of the dangers associated with their use (see side effects). When administered for insomnia, they are given at bedtime and generally are not repeated. Nightly administration of these medications should not exceed 2 weeks. Seconal is available as capsules and pentobarbital is available as an injection. Refer to **Table 8.3** for a summary of the barbiturates and other nonbenzodiazepine sedatives and hypnotics and their available formulations.

**Table 8.3** Nonbenzodiazepine sedative-hypnotic agents*

| Generic Name | Brand Name | Indications | Available as | Notes |
|---|---|---|---|---|
| **Barbiturates** | | | | |
| Mephobarbital | Mebaral® | Sedative, anticonvulsant | Tablets | CIV |
| Phenobarbital | Luminal® | Sedative, hypnotic, anticonvulsant | Tablets, liquid, injection | CIV |
| Pentobarbital | Nembutal® | Hypnotic, status epilepticus | Injection | CII |
| Secobarbital | Seconal® | Hypnotic | Capsules | CII<br>Short-term use |
| **Other Anxiolytic and Hypnotic Drugs** | | | | |
| Buspirone | BuSpar® | Anxiety disorders | Tablets | |
| Hydroxyzine | Atarax®<br>Vistaril® | Anxiety, anti-itch, pre-op med | Capsules, tablets, injection, syrup, suspension | Look alike-sound alike drug |
| Chloral Hydrate | Aquachloral® | Preprocedure sedative | Capsule, syrup, suppository | CIV |
| Eszopiclone | Lunesta® | Insomnia | Tablets | CIV |
| Zaleplon | Sonata® | Insomnia | Capsules | CIV<br>Short-term use |
| Zolpidem | Ambien® | Insomnia | Tablets | CIV<br>Short-term use |

* By brand and generic name, with indications and available formulations.

## Side Effects

lethargy Abnormal drowsiness or sluggishness.

exfoliative dermatitis Generalized shedding of the skin in layers; often a drug reaction.

Stevens-Johnson syndrome A severe and often life-threatening allergic drug reaction that causes inflammation and sometimes sloughing of the skin and mucous membranes.

Drowsiness, lethargy, ataxia, and drug hangover are the most frequent side effects associated with barbiturate usage. Impaired judgment and lack of coordination occurs in patients who have not developed tolerance to the effects or who are taking excessive doses. Barbiturates may rarely cause serious forms of anemia. Very rarely, use of phenobarbital is known to cause serious and sometimes fatal allergic skin reactions called exfoliative dermatitis. In exfoliative dermatitis the outer layers of the skin peel off and is associated with loss of fluids and electrolytes. Stevens-Johnson syndrome is one form of exfoliative dermatitis. See **Figure 8.5** for a summary representation of barbiturate side effects. All barbiturates are respiratory depressants. At hypnotic doses this effect is similar to the normal respiratory slowing that occurs with sleep. Excessive doses lead to coma and respiratory failure. The short-acting agents have the most significant respiratory depressant effects. These become even more significant, and dangerous, when combined with other CNS depressants such as alcohol. Treatment of barbiturate poisoning is difficult because there is no antidote for these drugs. In barbiturate toxicity, depression of the CNS results in reduced blood flow to vital organs and eventual organ failure. Immediate treatment requires emptying of the gastrointestinal (GI) tract to remove any unabsorbed drug, followed by support of respiration and blood pressure.

The Drug Enforcement Administration (DEA) lists these drugs as controlled substances because of the risk of abuse and addiction, particularly with the shorter acting barbiturates. Classifications range from CIV (phenobarbital, mephobarbital and methohexital) to CII (secobarbital, pentobarbital, and amobarbital). Abrupt discontinuation after chronic use can precipitate withdrawals.

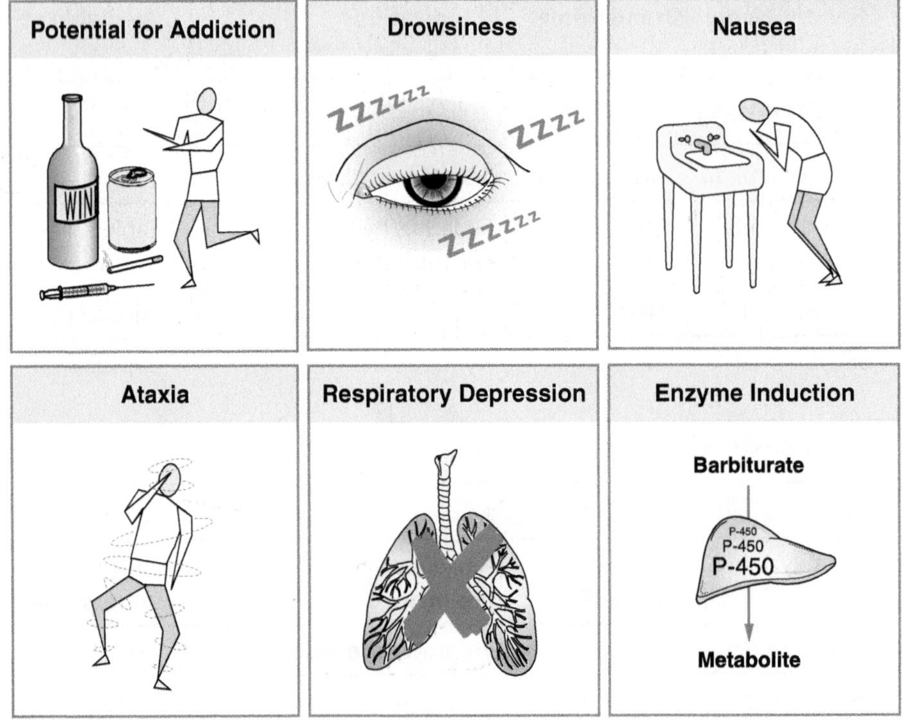


**Figure 8.5** A review of the most well known side effects caused by the barbiturates. (Adapted with permission from Harvey RA, Champe PC, Howland RD, et al. *Lippincott's Illustrated Reviews: Pharmacology,* 3rd ed. Baltimore: Lippincott Williams & Wilkins, 2006.)

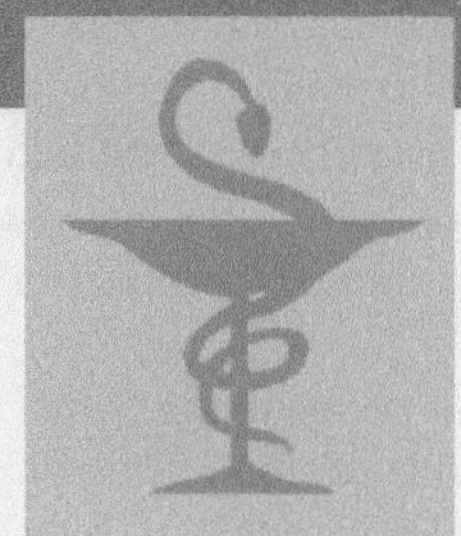

### Tips for the Technician

Special caution needs to be used when filling prescriptions for any controlled substances, but especially for those classified as CII controlled substances. This classification indicates that the drug is associated with a high risk of addiction and potential for abuse. Technicians should always carefully screen CII prescriptions for evidence of tampering or alteration. Become familiar with record-keeping requirements where you practice and make sure records are complete and accurate.

As previously noted, all sedatives require the application of accessory labels warning of the risk of operating dangerous machinery while taking the medication. The barbiturates also require labels warning against the consumption of alcoholic beverages. For safety reasons, physicians are encouraged to prescribe these drugs in limited quantities.

When drugs are prescribed for children, doses are often calculated based on body weight. Physicians may want pharmacists to make the calculation themselves, using the child's current weight. For example, the physician may write "phenobarbital 5 mg/kg/day in two divided doses." However the order is written, the pharmacist should verify that doses are within the established dose range, especially when ordered for children. It is important that the technician ascertains that the patient's profile contains the accurate weight.

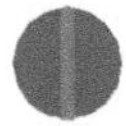

# Other Drugs

There are a number of anxiolytic and sedative hypnotic drugs that are neither benzodiazepines nor barbiturates. Included in this miscellaneous category are the antianxiety drugs buspirone (BuSpar®) and hydroxyzine (Vistaril, Atarax®). Miscellaneous hypnotic agents include the very old drug chloral hydrate, and the newer agents eszopiclone (Lunesta®), zaleplon (Sonata®), and zolpidem (Ambien®). The cost of the newer hypnotic agents is as much as four or more times higher than a generic benzodiazepine hypnotic.

## Actions and Indications

Buspirone is not related to any other antianxiety drugs. Its mechanism of action is unknown. It does have some affinity for the benzodiazepine receptor, but does not affect GABA binding. Buspirone lacks the muscle relaxant and anticonvulsant effects of the benzodiazepines. The antianxiety effects of buspirone are generally not associated with excessive sedation. It is indicated in the treatment of anxiety disorders.

An antihistamine with antianxiety properties, hydroxyzine is indicated in the symptomatic treatment of anxiety associated with psychoneurosis, and anxiety associated with other diseases. For example, hydroxyzine might be used with other drugs in the treatment of alcoholism, in allergic conditions with anxiety components such as chronic urticaria, or in anxious patients with cardiac disease.

Chloral hydrate is an old sedative hypnotic not prescribed extensively. In hypnotic doses, it produces very deep and quiet sleep, which makes it useful as a sedative before x-ray or other diagnostic procedures in pediatric patients. Very little is known about the mechanism of action. There is no antidote for chloral hydrate effects, and for this reason midazolam has supplanted the use of chloral hydrate in nearly all cases.

Zaleplon, zolpidem, and eszopiclone (the S isomer of zopiclone) are not members of the same chemical family. They are not chemically related to the benzodiazepines, but are thought to work by binding to a part of the GABA–benzodiazepine receptor complex. These drugs lack the muscle relaxant and anticonvulsant properties of the benzodiazepines and are classified as CIV controlled substances. They have CNS depressant effects that are additive with other, similar drugs. These sedatives are metabolized in the liver.

Zaleplon and zolpidem are indicated for short-term treatment of insomnia, while eszopiclone is indicated for insomnia with no restriction in regards to duration. This difference is related to the clinical trials submitted to the FDA. The company that markets eszopiclone studied the drug in longer clinical trials, thereby gaining the advantage of a unique indication. However, experts have agreed that treatment for insomnia should be short lived, because all of the drugs available for use can be habituating.

## Administration

All of the miscellaneous compounds for treatment of anxiety or insomnia are absorbed orally. Buspirone is available as tablets ranging in strengths from 5 to 30 mg. Hydroxyzine is available as two different salts, hydroxyzine hydrochloride and pamoate. Dose and indications are similar. The pamoate salt is available in capsule and suspension form and the hydrochloride in tablet, syrup, and injectable form. The injectable form is indicated for control of nausea and will be discussed in Chapter 21.

Chloral hydrate is available as a syrup, capsule, and rectal suppository. Generally, the oral route is preferred for more predictable absorption. The suppositories contain tartrazine, a compound that can cause sensitivity reactions.

Zolpidem and eszopiclone are available as tablets and zaleplon is provided as capsules. It is important to note that the recommended dose of all sedating drugs for elderly patients is generally about half the recommended dose for younger adults. The onset of action is delayed when these drugs are taken with food, so it is recommended that they be taken on an empty stomach.

## Side Effects

A comparison of common side effects of buspirone and the benzodiazepines demonstrates both advantages and disadvantages to buspirone therapy. Buspirone causes less drowsiness and has less effect on ability to concentrate. This can be a significant advantage in treatment of elderly people. Buspirone may cause headaches and dizziness, and a significant number of patients experience nausea. Buspirone is subject to a variety of drug interactions, because it is metabolized by the cytochrome P450 enzyme system. Interacting compounds include erythromycin and related drugs, oral antifungal agents, phenytoin (and several other anticonvulsants), and many other drugs.

Side effects from chloral hydrate include excessive sedation, GI irritation, which can be severe, and allergic skin reactions. Tolerance rapidly develops when chloral hydrate is taken regularly, but it produces much less respiratory depression than the barbiturates. Because tolerance can occur with all the sedative-hypnotic drugs, long-term use is not recommended. Withdrawal symptoms may occur on abrupt discontinuation of chloral hydrate after long-term use. The hypnotics are also associated with rebound sleep disturbances when taken nightly for more than the recommended duration. With the newer agents, sleep disturbances generally do not persist for more than a day or two.

As with the benzodiazepines, the newer hypnotic agents are associated with loss of coordination and morning drowsiness. In addition, headache and dizziness are common side effects with the newer nonbenzodiazepine drugs. Eszopiclone is also associated with an unpleasant taste in the mouth.

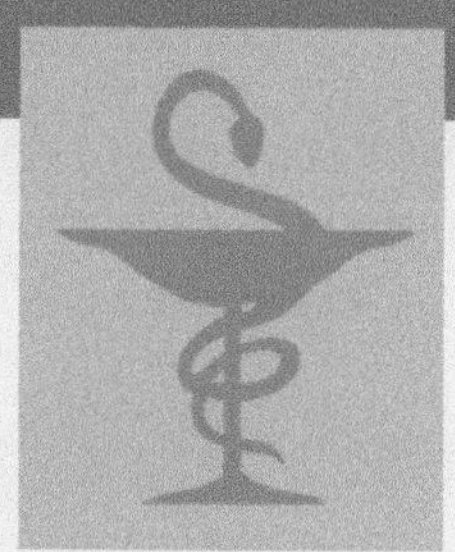

## Tips for the Technician

As with any CNS depressants, patients must be warned about the additive effects seen when these drugs are combined with alcohol or CNS depressants. Accessory labels warning patients to avoid alcohol and to avoid driving or operating other dangerous machinery need to be applied to outpatient prescriptions. Because the nonbenzodiazepine sedatives are all controlled substances, technicians need to be careful that record-keeping is accurate and complete, as well as remaining alert to alterations to written prescriptions.

While absorption of buspirone may be delayed by taking it with meals, patients may do so to avoid GI upset. It is important, however, that patients take the medication consistently, either with or without meals, so that effects remain fairly constant from day to day. Be aware of the risk of drug interactions with buspirone.

# Review Questions

## Multiple Choice

Choose the best answer to the following questions:

1. Anxiolytics are drugs that might be prescribed for all of the following reasons except:
   a. Irrational fear of other people
   b. Posttraumatic stress disorder
   c. Lethargy and loss of appetite
   d. Panic attacks
   e. All of the above are indications for anxiolytics

2. Which are indications for the use of barbiturates?
   a. Treatment of seizures, use as a weight loss agent, treatment of depression
   b. Anesthesia, treatment of allergic skin reactions, treatment of respiratory distress
   c. Treatment of diazepam addiction, treatment of depression, treatment of liver disease
   d. Anesthesia, preanesthetic medication, treatment of seizures
   e. None of the above

3. Typical side effects of the benzodiazepines include:
   a. Excitation, inability to sleep, seizures
   b. Drowsiness, loss of coordination, amnesia at high doses
   c. Significant respiratory depression at usual doses, headache, GI irritation
   d. Life-threatening skin reactions, anemia
   e. Itching, tolerance, diarrhea

4. Which of the following is not a characteristic of the ideal hypnotic drug?
   a. The ideal hypnotic induces sleep quickly.
   b. An ideal hypnotic should maintain sleep throughout the night.
   c. Tolerance and dependence are not caused by the ideal hypnotic agent.
   d. The patient awakes with no morning grogginess after taking the ideal hypnotic.
   e. All of the above are characteristics of the ideal hypnotic drug.

5. Which of the following changes could significantly improve a patient's ability to fall asleep at night?
   a. Avoid drinking caffeinated beverages and use of nicotine and other stimulants within 4 to 6 hours of bedtime.
   b. Make strenuous exercise a habit immediately before bedtime.
   c. Eat a big meal right before bed, so you won't be hungry in the middle of the night.
   d. Leave a clock right by the bed, so you can see how many hours you've been awake.

## True/False

6. Anxiety is an unpleasant state of unease, often associated with physical findings such as tachycardia, that is disproportional to triggering life events.
   a. True
   b. False

7. Anxiety of any duration is best treated with drugs. Other therapies are not recognized as effective.
   a. True
   b. False

8. Technicians should always apply an ancillary label warning against the consumption of alcoholic beverages to any prescription vial of benzodiazepines.
   a. True
   b. False

9. The newer nonbenzodiazepine hypnotic agents, such as Ambien® and Sonata®, are a better choice for patients with chronic insomnia because they are safe to use for longer periods of time and are less expensive.
   a. True
   b. False

10. Buspirone is less likely to cause nausea than the benzodiazepines.
    a. True
    b. False

## Matching

For numbers 11 to 15, match the side effect with the drug most likely to cause it from the lettered choices in the list to the right.

11. GI irritation
12. Dangerous allergic skin reactions
13. Morning grogginess or drug "hangover"
14. Respiratory depression
15. Nausea and headache

a. Flurazepam
b. Phenobarbital
c. Buspirone
d. Chloral Hydrate
e. Secobarbital

### Short Answer

16. Describe the relationship between the benzodiazepine drugs and the inhibitory neurotransmitter GABA.

17. Why are shorter-acting sedative-hypnotics generally more desirable for use in the elderly?

18. Explain the sleep cycle and the difference between REM and NREM sleep.

19. Why is it important for the pharmacist to counsel patients receiving new prescriptions for any anxiolytic or hypnotic drug?

20. Why are most of the drugs in this chapter designated as controlled substances?

## FOR FURTHER INQUIRY

There are five major types of anxiety disorder, including generalized anxiety disorder (GAD), obsessive compulsive disorder (OCD), panic disorder, post-traumatic stress disorder (PTSD), and social anxiety disorder (SAD). Visit the National Institute of Mental Health web site (www.nimh.nih.gov) to learn more about one of these types of anxiety. Investigate other classes of drugs or other types of therapy that might be used for treatment.

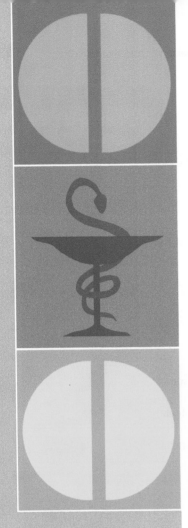

Chapter **9**

# Central Nervous System Depressants: The Opioid Analgesics and Antagonists

*KEY TERMS*

- addiction
- antitussive
- dysphoria
- dyspnea
- endorphins
- enkephalins
- euphoria
- expectorant
- hyperalgesia
- narcotic
- neuropathic
- opiate
- opioids
- peptide
- somatic
- visceral

## OBJECTIVES

After studying this chapter, the reader should be able to:

- Define the terms opiate and opioid.
- Describe the mechanism of action of the opioid analgesics in the treatment of pain.
- List the most common side effects of the opioid analgesics.
- Compare and contrast the effects of morphine or another opioid with those of a commonly used opioid agonist-antagonist used for analgesia.
- Explain the special requirements for dispensing controlled substances (such as opioids) of which technicians need to be aware.

## DRUGS COVERED IN THIS CHAPTER

| Opioid Agonists | | Opioid Antagonists | |
|---|---|---|---|
| ***Strong Agonists*** | ***Moderate to Weak Agonists*** | ***Pure Antagonists*** | ***Mixed and Partial Agonist/Antagonists and Other Analgesics*** |
| Alfentanyl | Codeine | Naloxone | Buprenorphine |
| Fentanyl | Oxycodone | Naltrexone | Butorphanol |
| Meperidine | Hydrocodone | | Nalbuphine |
| Methadone | Propoxyphene | | Pentazocine |
| Morphine | | | Tramadol |
| Sufentanil | | | |

From the beginning of time humankind has suffered with, and tried to relieve, pain. Very early in human history, the analgesia and euphoria (an exaggerated sense of well-being) caused by the resin of the opium poppy were discovered. For centuries people have used opium for pain relief and misused it for its euphoric effects. Opium derivatives are the most effective pain relievers known. Because of the demand for these drugs, both licit and illicit, the opium trade was and is highly profitable. In the 18th and 19th centuries opium was one of the world's most profitable commodities. The opium trade was the cause of wars, political upheaval, and social conflict. In spite of the well-known risks of opium use, most nations, including the United States, did nothing to control the purchase of opium and its derivatives until the twentieth century. Now, every nation in the world has laws controlling the sales of opium and its powerful analgesic derivatives. This chapter discusses the drugs derived from or chemically related to the compounds found in the resin of the opium poppy and their use. These drugs commonly known as the narcotic (drugs with characteristics similar to morphine) analgesics and antagonists.

euphoria A feeling of well-being or elation; in pharmacology, the "high" associated with drugs of abuse.

The narcotic analgesics include the opiates and opioids. The opiates are naturally occurring alkaloids, such as morphine and codeine, that are derived from the opium poppy, *Papaver somniferum* (**Fig. 9.1**). The opiods are synthetic or semisynthetic compounds that produce morphine-like effects. The word opioid is now more often used as a general term for both synthetic and naturally occurring drugs, but the term opiate refers specifically to naturally occurring drugs. The usage of the term opioids in this text refers to the entire class of narcotic agonists.

narcotic A drug that in moderate doses reduces the sensation of pain and other senses and causes sedation, usually applied to opioids.

opiate Drug derived from the opium poppy.

The production of euphoria is an important component of the pharmacologic action of some opioids. On the other hand, it is the euphoric effect that causes some of these drugs to have a high potential for abuse. Narcotic antagonists reverse the effects of the opioids. The antagonists play an important role in treatment of overdose, a common result of the illicit use of narcotics. Mixed agonist-antagonists have analgesic properties in addition to blocking the effect of euphoria.

opioids Originally used to describe synthetic drugs resembling opiates; now more commonly used to include both natural opiates and synthetic relatives.

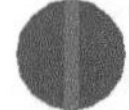

# Pain and Its Treatment

The relief of pain remains one of the greatest challenges to health care providers today. Pain is the body's way of signaling the brain that something is amiss. It is defined as an unpleasant sensory and emotional experience associated with actual or potential tissue damage. Pain can be either acute or chronic, and is a consequence of complex processes in the

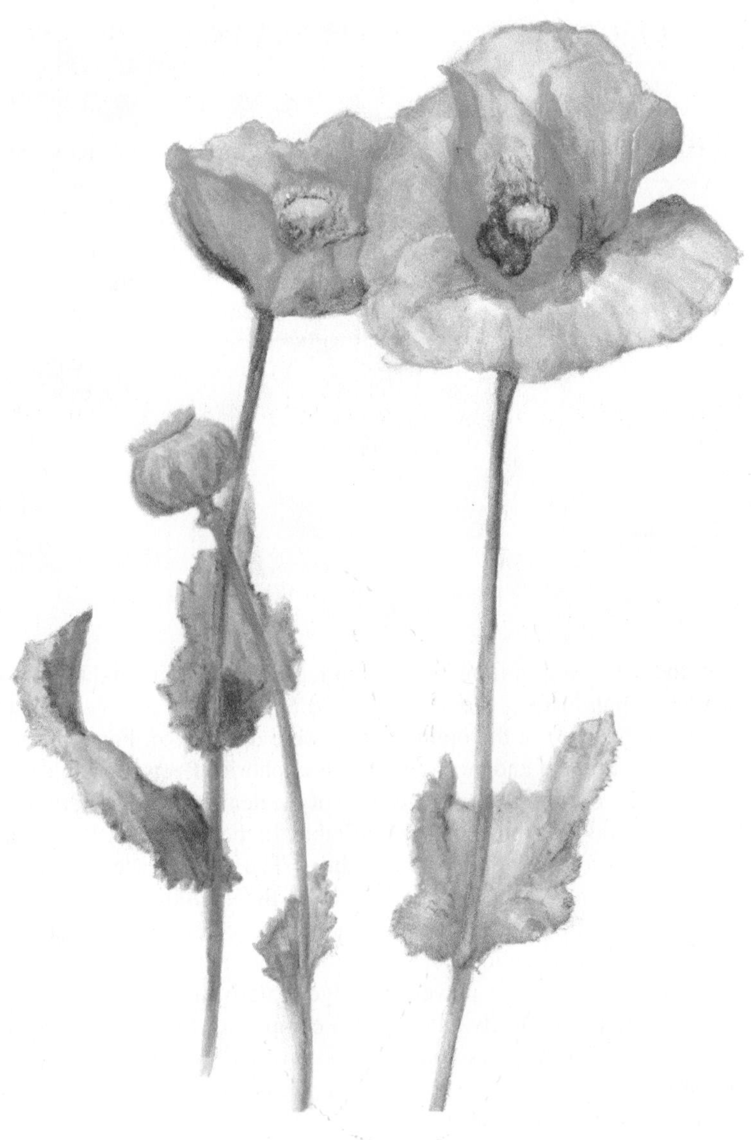

**Figure 9.1** The resin of the opium poppy, *Papaver somniferum*, provides humankind with our most potent pain relievers, the opioid analgesics. (Image by Rachel Sakai.)

peripheral and central nervous systems (CNS). The immediate pain that occurs with an injury or after surgery is acute pain. When tissue injury occurs, sensory signals are sent to the brain. Locally, tissue injury releases chemicals that begin the inflammatory process, and attract a variety of cells to the site of the injury. Depending on the extent of the injury, muscles in the region may contract, providing extra support and protection to the injured tissues. As tissues heal and inflammation resolves, the sensation of pain dissipates. In some cases, however, pain can become chronic, either because of some permanent damage, or even when damage has resolved.

When health professionals assess pain, they classify it according to its source, severity, and chronicity. Visceral pain is associated with injury to the internal organs, somatic pain with injury to the body, and neuropathic pain is a result of damage to, or abnormal function of, the nerves. The perception of pain is a highly individualized experience. Factors such as fear, anxiety, and past experience with pain contribute to its perception. Physicians must rely on the patient's sensation and description of pain in order to properly treat it. Studies of the pathogenesis and biology of pain indicate that some patients who have experienced significant acute pain become sensitized to it. Researchers believe that

visceral Of, relating to, or located in, the organs of the abdominal cavity.

somatic 1. Of, relating to, supplying, or involving skeletal muscles. 2. Of, relating to, or affecting the body.

neuropathic Of or relating to pathology of the nervous system.

actual changes develop in the CNS that result in an exaggerated neurological response called hyperalgesia, or a lowered pain threshold. Even though their old injury may be healed, the pain these patients experience is real, and very difficult to treat. Pain specialists may use a variety of treatment options to control pain and minimize the use of narcotics. These can include nondrug treatments like biofeedback, distraction techniques, and acupuncture, and nonnarcotic drugs.

hyperalgesia Increased sensitivity to pain.

The appropriate treatment of pain depends on its type (**Fig. 9.2**). People usually can adequately treat minor pain on their own. In many cases such as headache, minor sports injuries, or mild pain from osteoarthritis, acetaminophen (Tylenol®) or nonsteroidal anti-inflammatory agents (NSAIDs, see Chapter 23) such as ibuprofen (Motrin®), are sufficient to treat the pain. Neuropathic pain often responds well to gabapentin (Neurontin®) or amitriptyline (Elavil®), two drugs used for other neurologic disorders that add to the effects of analgesics. For moderate to severe acute or chronic pain, such as acute postoperative pain or chronic back pain, narcotic analgesics are usually the drugs of choice. No class of drugs available is more effective for treating pain than the opioid agonist analgesics.

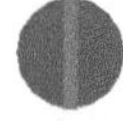

# Opioid Agonists

Although the opioids have a broad range of actions, their most important use is to relieve intense pain and the anxiety that accompanies it, whether that pain is from surgery, a result of injury, or related to a disease such as cancer. The opioids vary in efficacy, but they share the common characteristic of relieving pain by altering the perception of pain. They do not affect other sensory functions and do nothing to treat the underlying cause of the pain.

peptide A compound made up of two or more amino acids; many biologically active compounds are peptides.

## Actions and Indications

The opioid agonists act at receptors in the nervous system that are activated by endogenous peptides, the enkephalins, and endorphins, which are native compounds that alter the perception of pain. These receptors are commonly referred to as opioid receptors, and are widely distributed throughout the CNS (**Fig. 9.3**). They are also found in sensory nerves of the peripheral nervous system. There are three different families of opioid receptors and each drug has a different affinity for the receptor families. The mu ($\mu$) receptors are the most widely studied and are most closely associated with typical opiate effects, including pain relief, euphoria, and respiratory depression.

enkephalins Endogenous pentapeptides that bind to and activate opiate receptors in the CNS.

When opioid drugs activate the opioid receptors in different regions of the nervous system, different responses occur. For example, opioid receptors in the brain stem regulate respiration rate, blood pressure, cough, pupil diameter, and nausea and vomiting. The opioid agonists will (depending on the drug, dose, and patient variables) inhibit the cough reflex, reduce the respiratory rate and blood pressure, cause constriction of pupils, and trigger the receptors in the brain that cause nausea and vomiting. The opioid receptors in the limbic system are involved in the experience of pleasure and are important for the role they play in addiction.

endorphins A group of endogenous opioid-type peptides found in the CNS that bind to opiate receptors and produce effects similar to the opioids.

| Body Pain | Organ Pain | Neuropathic Pain |
|---|---|---|
| • Tactile stimulation<br>• Cold packs<br>• Acetaminophen or NSAIDs<br>• Opioids<br>• Local anesthetics | • Opioids<br>• NSAIDs<br>• Intraspinal local anesthetics | • Anticonvulsants, such as gabapentin<br>• Tricyclics<br>• Nerve block<br>• Opioids |

**Figure 9.2** Recommendations for the treatment of acute pain.

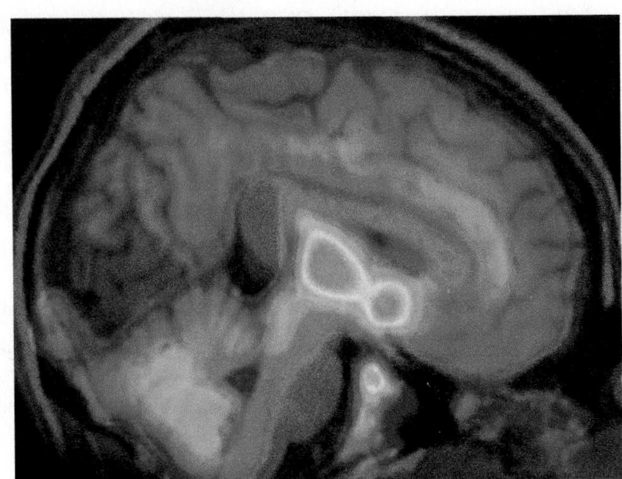

**Figure 9.3** An image depicting opioid receptor distribution in the brain. (Copyright University of Michigan. Used with permission.)

Morphine is the prototype of the strong opioid analgesics against which all other analgesic drugs are measured. It relieves pain without the loss of consciousness. Opioids relieve pain both by raising the pain threshold at the spinal cord level and, more importantly, by altering the perception of pain. Patients treated with morphine are still aware of the presence of pain, but they are no longer disabled by it. Heroin is a close chemical and pharmacologic relative of morphine. In the United States, because of its extreme potential for abuse, heroin is not considered to have any justifiable medical use. Oral methadone (Dolophine®), another strong opioid agonist, is used as a replacement for heroin in substance abuse programs.

Other strong agonists include hydromorphone (Dilaudid®), fentanyl (Sublimaze®, Duragesic®) and closely related compounds, and meperidine (Demerol®). When used as analgesics, these highly effective opioid agonists are reserved for the treatment of severe pain, such as postoperative pain or the pain associated with heart attacks, kidney stones, traumatic injuries, or certain types of cancer. Because the opioid agonists do more than modify the perception of pain, they are useful in other conditions and situations besides the treatment of pain. For example, sufentanil (Sufenta®), alfentanil (Alfenta®), and other compounds related to fentanyl, are used almost exclusively as the analgesic component of anesthesia.

dyspnea Shortness of breath; difficulty breathing.

Morphine dramatically relieves dyspnea (difficulty breathing) caused by excess fluid in the lungs from heart failure or other causes. Morphine dilates blood vessels, which causes the pressure of the venous blood returning to the heart to fall. When this pressure falls, the failing heart is better able to squeeze the blood out of its chambers and back into circulation. As a result, less fluid backs up into the lungs, and breathing becomes easier.

antitussive A drug that relieves or suppresses cough.

expectorant Drug that encourages (usually by thinning secretions) the removal of mucus from the respiratory tract.

Morphine, codeine, and their derivatives have antitussive (cough suppressant) properties. For the treatment of cough, codeine and hydrocodone are generally combined with expectorants (agents that promote removal of mucous), or other ingredients. Not all opioids are equally effective as antitussives.

Dextromethorphan, a drug found in many nonprescription cough suppressants, is a synthetic opioid. When dextromethorphan is given in normal cough-suppressant doses, it has no euphoric or respiratory depressant effects, and can be purchased without a prescription. In high doses, however, it produces vomiting and can cause respiratory problems, hallucinations, psychosis, seizures, and death. Some individuals abuse it for its hallucinogenic properties at extremely high doses, and it has been involved in numerous deaths.

The opioid agonists relieve diarrhea and dysentery by decreasing the motility (movement) and increasing the tone of the intestinal smooth muscle. All opioids decrease GI motility, but only a few are indicated for treatment of diarrhea. Diphenoxylate is an opioid drug that is combined with atropine in Lomotil®, a commonly used antidiarrheal agent.

Codeine, its derivative hydrocodone, and propoxyphene (Darvon®) are opioid agonists with potential to relieve mild to moderate pain. These drugs are most often given in combination with acetaminophen, which further improves pain relief. They are less effective than morphine at relieving pain, but cause less euphoria, making them ideal for use by patients with mild to moderate pain. Oxycodone, another drug related to codeine, is useful for moderate to severe pain. Oxycodone has a higher potential for abuse than the other codeine relatives. Oxycodone abusers crush the sustained-release tablets (OxyContin®) in order to cause the immediate release of the drug, which then reaches excessive blood levels and causes a high. **Table 9.1** compares the pharmacology of the opioids discussed here.

The opioid drugs vary in their onset of action and duration of effect. They distribute widely into tissues, including the CNS. As a family, most opioids undergo significant metabolism in the liver, but some breakdown also occurs in the CNS. They and their metabolites are excreted mainly in the urine.

## Administration

The choice of analgesic and route of administration is determined by the acuity, cause, and severity of the pain, as well as the ability of the patient to swallow medications. The opioids are most effective for acute, severe pain when they are given by injection. All of the strong agonists are available for parenteral administration. When administered for pain they are most often given by intramuscular (IM) or intravenous (IV) injection. The preservative-free formulations of morphine and sufentanil may be administered into the epidural space.

**Table 9.1** Comparison of the pharmacology of opioid agonists

| Generic Name | Analgesic Effect | Antitussive Effect | Respiratory Depression | Abuse Potential | Nausea/ Vomiting Risk |
|---|---|---|---|---|---|
| Alfentanil | strong | undetermined | undetermined | undetermined | undetermined |
| Codeine | weak | strong | low | low | low |
| Fentanyl | strong | undetermined | low-moderate | undetermined | undetermined |
| Hydrocodone | weak | strong | low | low | low |
| Hydromorphone | strong | strong | moderate | moderately high | low |
| Meperidine | strong | weak | moderate | moderately high | moderate |
| Methadone | strong | moderate | moderate | low | low |
| Morphine | strong | strong | moderate | moderately high | moderate |
| Oxycodone | moderate | strong | moderate | moderately high | moderate |
| Propoxyphene | weak | undetermined | low | low | low |
| Sufentanil | very strong | undetermined | undetermined | undetermined | undetermined |

Adapted from Drug Facts and Comparison. St. Louis, MO: Wolters Kluwer Health, 2005. Available online at http://www.factsandcomparisons.com/, accessed October 31, 2007.

Many hospitals provide postsurgical and other alert patients with the ability to control the administration of their own analgesia, with a patient-controlled analgesia (PCA) pump. These are computerized syringe pumps that allow nursing staff to program in parameters that include the size of each dose, the time between doses, and a limit to the total amount the patient can inject in a given time period. Patients activate the pump when they are feeling pain. This improves pain control and usually results in less total use of narcotics in a given patient.

Absorption after oral administration is erratic and slow for many of the opioids. For example, GI absorption of fentanyl is slow and incomplete and no oral fentanyl tablets or capsules are available. However, fentanyl is fairly quickly absorbed from the buccal mucosa (mucous membranes of the mouth). Oralet® is a fentanyl sucker that takes advantage of the fast buccal absorption combined with the slower GI absorption for treatment of pain in children. Fentanyl is also available as a transdermal patch that provides a sustained level of drug and is changed every 72 hours. In spite of variable absorption, many of the strong agonists are available as tablets, capsules or liquid preparations and are useful for treatment of severe chronic pain. Often the oral dose requirements are much higher than the IM or IV dose because of poor absorption and first-pass metabolism. Refer to **Table 9.2** for a summary of available products.

Codeine and related drugs are well absorbed orally, adding to their suitability for use in outpatients. Codeine is available as a single agent in tablet form, oral solution, and injection. As mentioned previously, codeine and its derivatives are frequently combined with other drugs in analgesic and antitussive preparations.

## Side Effects

The narcotic analgesics cause respiratory depression by reducing the sensitivity of the respiratory center to carbon dioxide ($CO_2$). Normally, the presence of increased levels of $CO_2$ is a powerful stimulus to breathing. Mild respiratory depression occurs with ordinary doses of morphine and is accentuated as the dose increases until, ultimately, breathing stops. Respiratory depression is the most common cause of death in acute opioid overdose. Because of respiratory depression and carbon dioxide retention, blood vessels in the brain dilate and increase the cerebrospinal fluid (CSF) pressure. For this reason, morphine and other opioids are avoided or used with extreme caution in individuals with acute, severe brain injury.

The opioids can cause drowsiness, mental clouding, and dizziness related to CNS depression. All opioids are constipating to some degree. Constipation is a direct result of the pharmacological effects of the opioids on the gastrointestinal tract. The opioids also cause release of histamine. Histamine release results in itching, sweating, and flushing. When people with lung disease are given opioids, they are monitored carefully because of the potential for histamine release and respiratory depression.

Certain patients are particularly vulnerable to the nausea and vomiting that can occur with opioid use. Patients may report that they are allergic to the opioids because they experienced nausea or itching in response to taking one of them, but these are pharmacologic effects, not true drug allergies. **Figure 9.4** illustrates the most common side effects associated with opioid administration.

addiction Compulsive use of a habit-forming substance known by the user to be physically, psychologically, or socially harmful.

All of the opioids can cause physical dependence when taken regularly. Physical dependence is different than addiction. Addiction is characterized by compulsive drug use and cravings, and implies psychological dependence. On the other hand, physical dependence connotes tolerance, requiring increasing doses to elicit the same response. Patients who are dependant will develop a withdrawal syndrome if the medication is abruptly discontinued. Fear of causing addiction often prevents physicians from prescribing adequate treatment for patients who need opioids for pain control. While they may become tolerant of the effects of opioids, patients who are in pain and have no social history indicative of addictive behavior will not become addicts simply because their pain is treated with these drugs.

**Table 9.2** Opioid agonist and antagonist drugs, formulations, and indications

| Generic Name | Brand Name | Available as | Indications | Notes |
|---|---|---|---|---|
| **Opioid Agonists** | | | | |
| Codeine | | Tablets, oral solution, injection, combination products | Cough, pain | CII – alone<br>CIII – CV in combination |
| Hydrocodone | Vicodin®, Hycodan® | In combination products only, tablets and liquids | Cough, Pain | CIII |
| Hydromorphone | Dilaudid® | Tablets, injection, liquid, suppository | Pain | CII |
| Morphine | MS Contin®, Roxanol®, Duramorph® | Injection, sustained-release tablets, oral solution, suppositories, preservative-free injection | Pain, pre-op, respiratory distress associated with heart failure | CII |
| Oxycodone | OxyContin®, Percocet® | Tablets, capsules, sustained-release tablets | Pain | CII |
| Alfentanil | Alfenta® | Injection | Anesthesia, pain | CII |
| Fentanyl | Sublimaze®, Actiq®, Duragesic® | Injection, sucker, transdermal patch | Adjunct to anesthesia, pain | CII |
| Meperidine | Demerol® | Injection, tablets, syrup | Preoperative med, pain | CII |
| Sufentanil | Sufenta® | Injection | Anesthesia, analgesia | CII |
| Methadone | Dolophine® | Injection, tablets, dispersible tablets, oral solution, oral concentrate | Pain, treatment of heroin addiction | CII |
| Propoxyphene | Darvon®, Darvocet® | Capsules, combination tablets, and capsules | Pain | CIV |
| **Agonist/Antagonists, Mixed Agonists, and Partial Agonists** | | | | |
| Buprenorphine | Subutex®, Buprenex® Suboxone® | Sublingual tablet, SL tablet combination and injection | Pain, opioid dependence | CIV- injection<br>CIII - others |
| Butorphanol | Stadol® | Injection, nasal spray | Pain, preoperative analgesia | CIV |
| Nalbuphine | Nubain® | Injection | Pain, preoperative analgesia | |
| Pentazocine | Talwin® | Tablets, injection | Pain | CIV |
| Tramadol | Ultram® | Tablets | Pain | |
| **Opioid Antagonists** | | | | |
| Naloxone | Narcan® | Injection, two concentrations | Reversal of opioid effects, overdose | |
| Naltrexone | ReVia® | Tablets | Alcoholism, treatment of narcotic addiction | |

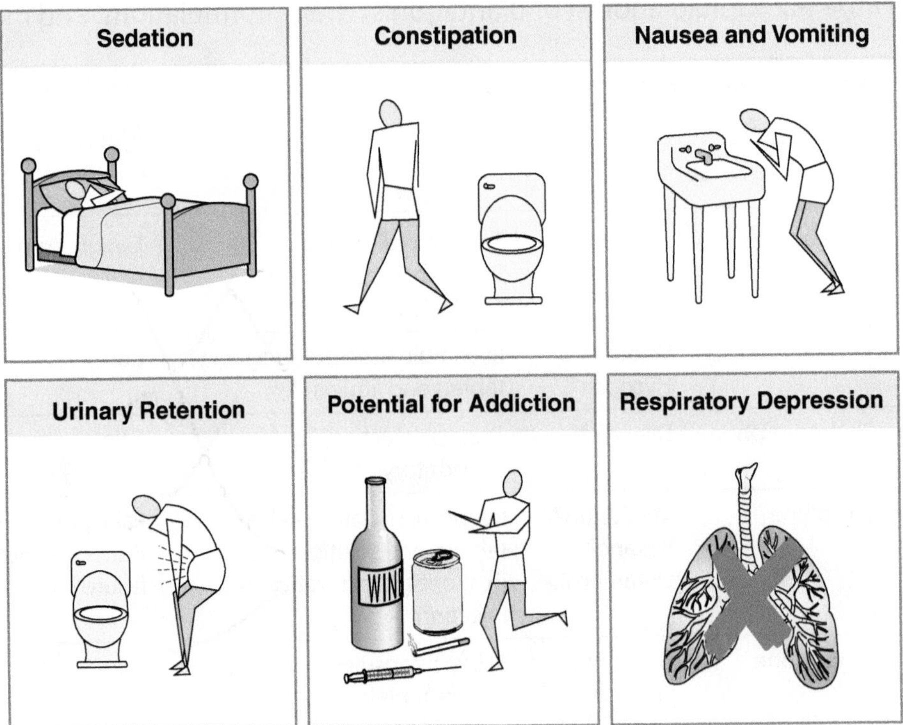


**Figure 9.4** Common adverse effects of the opioid analgesics. (Adapted with permission from Harvey RA, Champe PC, Howland RD, et al. *Lippincott's Illustrated Reviews: Pharmacology,* 3rd ed. Baltimore: Lippincott Williams & Wilkins, 2006.)

The opioids are involved in a number of well-documented drug interactions. They should not be given to a patient who has received a monoamine oxidase inhibiter (MAOI) antidepressant in the prior 2 weeks. The coadministration of meperidine and the MAOIs have resulted in death. Propoxyphene should be avoided in patients receiving the anticonvulsant medication carbamazepine. Propoxyphene can cause a significant elevation in the blood levels of carbamazepine leading to adverse effects or toxicity. Because the opioids are CNS depressants, patients must be warned against drinking alcohol and combining the opioids with other sedating medications.

Norpropoxyphene, a propoxyphene metabolite, is associated with cardiac side effects. Because of its long half-life, this metabolite can accumulate in the body when multiple doses of propoxyphene are administered. This is especially problematic in elderly patients or patients with kidney impairment. Because of the weak analgesic effect of propoxyphene and the risks associated with its use, some hospitals no longer include propoxyphene-containing drugs on their formularies.

Meperidine was, until recently, one of the most frequently used of the strong agonists. Now, however, most experts encourage a reduction in its use. This is because of increasing awareness of the risks associated with one of its metabolites, normeperidine. Normeperidine is eliminated by the kidneys, and in the elderly or patients with poor kidney function, it accumulates in the body. Normeperidine can cause CNS toxicity, including seizures. Meperidine is generally considered less effective as an analgesic than morphine and is associated with greater risks.

## Tips for the Technician

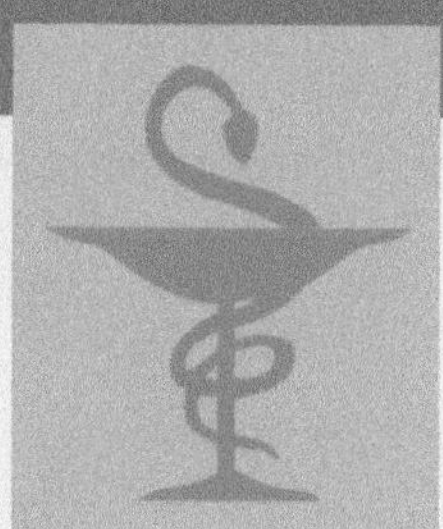

All of the opioids are controlled substances. Federal law requires that all prescriptions for controlled substance must be issued for a legitimate medical purpose. Pharmacies are held accountable for determining that prescriptions are legitimate before they fill them. To help assure legitimacy, it is important that staff members know the ordering physician. The legitimacy of prescriptions written by an unknown physician or brought to the pharmacy by an unknown individual should be verified before dispensing.

Keeping accurate controlled substance records is a job that often falls to the technician. All records pertaining to dispensing CII controlled substances including the prescriptions themselves, must be kept separately from other records. A complete inventory of controlled substances is required on a biennial basis. Any loss of a controlled substance must be reported to the Drug Enforcement Administration (DEA). It is important for technicians in both hospital and retail pharmacies to be familiar with both the federal and state laws regulating controlled substances.

There are a number of opioid names that can be confused because they look and sound similar, for example hydromorphone and morphine, or hydromorphone and hydrocodone. Always verify drug names with the pharmacist if any confusion exists. Packaging of different drug products may look very similar and cause confusion. There is often little to differentiate between the package of a drug formulated in an immediate-release preparation, and the packaging of the drug with an extended-release formulation. Technicians who are confused about which medication to use should remember the saying, "When in doubt, check it out."

The strong opioids, codeine as a single agent, and oxycodone alone or in combination, are class II controlled substances and subject to the most rigid prescribing and dispensing restrictions. Prescriptions for schedule II controlled substances must be hand written by the physician. These prescriptions must be correct as written, and cannot be changed, except in limited circumstances, by the pharmacist. Prescriptions for CII controlled substances cannot be refilled.

When opiod drugs are dispensed in the retail setting, patients must be warned about drug interactions, especially with other CNS depressants. Auxiliary labels warning against alcohol consumption, and of the risks of operating dangerous machinery while taking the opioid agonists should be attached to prescription vials. Patients can take the oral opioids with food to reduce nausea. This can delay onset of action, however. Clients should also be advised to increase the intake of fiber and liquids in their diets to help reduce the severity of constipation associated with use of these agents.

The well-prepared pharmacy technician is aware that his or her duty, ethically and legally, is to support the pharmacist in providing the safest and most effective drug therapy to patients. The ultimate responsibility of every person who works in pharmacy is the best care for patients. This charge can only be met when employees are alert, clearheaded, and unimpaired. Because health care workers have ready access to controlled substances, drug abuse in health professionals can, unfortunately, occur. Therefore, any technician who reasonably believes that someone with whom he or she works is impaired because of the use of drugs, either legal or illicit, must report these suspicions to the appropriate authority.

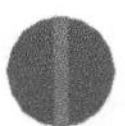

# Opioid Antagonists and Other Drugs

The term opioid antagonist is imprecise. Within this group of drugs are the nearly pure opioid antagonists, mixed agonist-antagonist drugs, and partial agonists. Suffice it to say that these drugs vary in their ability to block or stimulate the different opioid receptors, resulting in variation in their activity.

## Actions and Indications

### Opioid Antagonists

The pure or nearly pure opioid antagonists bind tightly to opioid receptors, but do not activate the receptor. There are no noticeable effects when a dose of a pure opioid antagonist is given to a person who has not taken an opioid. However, in patients receiving opioids, pure antagonists rapidly reverse opioid effects. In dependent individuals they abruptly precipitate the symptoms of opiate withdrawal. The most important use of these drugs is as an antidote in opioid overdose.

Naloxone (Narcan®) is used to reverse the coma and respiratory depression of opioid overdose. It rapidly displaces all receptor-bound opioid molecules and is able to reverse respiratory depression and loss of consciousness in moments after administration. This is useful both in the emergency room, where a narcotic overdose in a drug abuser would be treated, and in the hospital, where overzealous treatment with opioids can occur.

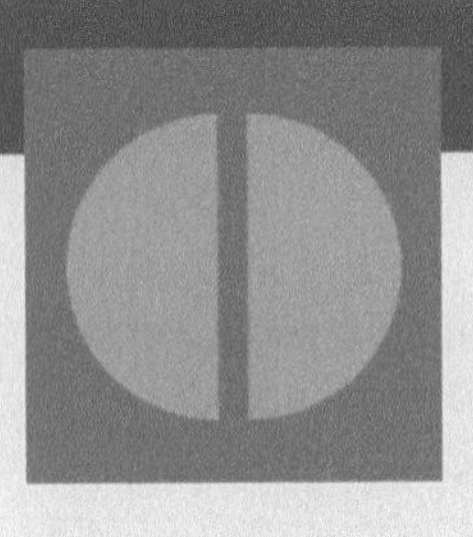

**Case 9.1**

Nurse Poppy La Roux from the Emergency Department calls to say she is out of naloxone in her automated dispensing machine. She wonders if you can come and fill it for her. You tell her, yes, the pharmacist is checking the refill drugs now, and you'll be over in a few minutes. Ten minutes later, the Pharmacy Director comes storming out of his office. He grabs 6 ampules of naloxone and tells the pharmacist to take it immediately to the Emergency Room. He tells you to come to his office. You think to yourself, what did I do? What did you do, and how might you have prevented getting called into the office?

Naltrexone (ReVia®) has actions similar to those of naloxone. It has a longer duration of action than naloxone, and a single oral dose of naltrexone blocks the effect of injected heroin for up to 2 days. Naltrexone is used in conjunction with other drugs in opioid abstinence programs. It is also used for the treatment of alcohol dependence, where its mechanism of action is incompletely understood.

### Opioid Agonist-Antagonists

The opioid agonist-antagonists activate opioid receptors variably and can be antagonists at one group and agonists at another. The result of this mixed activity is that, although they are analgesics, they can also trigger the withdrawal syndrome in patients dependent on opioids. These agents cause less euphoria than pure opioid agonists, and as a result are less likely to be abused. Butorphanol (Stadol®), nalbuphine (Nubain®), and pentazocine (Talwin®) are agonist-antagonists indicated for pain management, including pre- and post-operative use. These drugs are useful for women in labor because they cause less respiratory depression in the newborn.

Buprenorphine (Buprenex®) is considered a partial agonist. It produces opioid agonist effects such as analgesia and sedation, but these reach a plateau. In opioid-dependent individuals, buprenorphine prevents the onset of withdrawal at usual therapeutic doses. In high doses, however, it can precipitate withdrawal. Because of these unique characteristics, buprenorphine plays an important role in the treatment of opium dependence. The injectable formulation is also indicated for pain relief.

### Other Drugs

Tramadol (Ultram®) is a synthetic drug that is chemically distinct from the opioids. Its mechanism of action is incompletely understood, but it does act in the CNS and is thought to trigger opioid receptors. It is used to manage moderate to moderately severe pain. Although it can cause some euphoria, risk of abuse is considered low and it is not, as yet, designated as a controlled substance.

## Administration

Naloxone is not absorbed orally. It is administered by injection only and can be given IV, subcutaneously, or by IM injection. It has a shorter duration of action than most of the drugs it is used to reverse. Patients must, therefore, be monitored closely and doses of naloxone repeated until the symptoms of overdose no longer recur. Initial doses may be given every 2 to 3 minutes until a response is seen and repeat doses may be needed in 20 minutes to an hour, depending on the route of administration. Naltrexone is available only as a tablet, administered daily.

Most of the agonist-antagonist drugs are not given orally. Butorphanol, nalbuphine and pentazocine can all be given intravenously or intramuscularly. Butorphanol is available as a nasal spray that can be used to relieve the pain associated with migraine headaches, or for other chronic pain control. Pentazocine is available as both an injection and as tablets in combination with other ingredients. Because of the risk of abuse of the tablets, the pharmaceutical company that produces Talwin® tablets began adding a small amount of naloxone. Since naloxone is not absorbed orally, it has no effect when the tablets are taken as prescribed. If tablets are crushed and injected, however, the naloxone triggers withdrawals in addicted individuals.

Buprenorphine is available as a sublingual tablet for the treatment of opioid dependence, either as a single agent or combined with naloxone. Chewing or swallowing the tablets will reduce their absorption. Under the Drug Addiction Treatment Act, qualified physicians in private practice can administer buprenorphine to opioid addicts in an office-based addiction treatment program. This is an advantage over the use of methadone, because it can only be administered in tightly regulated methadone maintenance programs that may not be available in all areas.

Tramadol is well absorbed after oral administration, and undergoes extensive metabolism in the liver. It is available as a tablet only. The duration of effect after an oral dose is about 6 hours. It is sold as a single agent, or in combination with acetaminophen.

## Side Effects

Pentazocine, butorphanol, and nalbuphine produce less euphoria than the opioid agonists, however dependence can still occur. At higher doses, these drugs can cause respiratory depression, but not to the degree of the pure opioid agonists. The most common side effects include drowsiness and dizziness, or a lightheaded sensation. Along with these typical side effects, they can also cause unpleasant CNS sensations of anguish and restlessness called dysphoria. Abnormal dreams or nightmares are not uncommon. They can cause dry mouth and urinary retention in some patients. High doses can have negative cardiovascular effects such as elevated blood pressure and rapid heartbeat, and can induce withdrawal in addicts.

dysphoria A state of feeling disquiet, agitated, or unwell; opposite of euphoria.

Buprenorphine can cause CNS side effects that are similar to those seen with other opioids, but to a lesser degree. Respiratory depression can occur with higher doses, but it is less likely to be life threatening unless combined with other respiratory depressant drugs. Buprenorphine use in addicts is associated with a variety of liver problems. There is not enough data available to know if this is a toxic effect of the drug or is a result of the known risks to the liver associated with intravenous drug abuse. It may be a combination of both. High dose buprenorphine can precipitate withdrawal symptoms in opioid-dependent individuals. Because it is a partial agonist with a very long half-life, the withdrawal syndrome associated with discontinuation of buprenorphine is mild.

Tramadol causes many of the same side effects seen with the opioids. Typical side effects include drowsiness, dizziness, constipation, and nausea. This drug can also cause CNS stimulation and seizures. For this reason, tramadol is generally avoided in patients with a history of seizure activity.

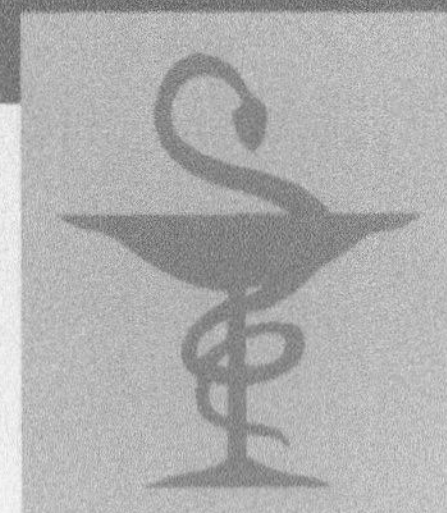

## Tips for the Technician

Butorphanol and pentazocine are CIV controlled substances, but nalbuphine is not a controlled substance. Buprenorphine is a CIII controlled substance. Technicians should always be alert to the possibility of prescription tampering when any controlled substance is prescribed. Screen all controlled substance prescriptions for indications that the quantity of the drug has been changed, or that the prescription has been forged.

Opioid agonist-antagonist prescription vials should be labeled with auxiliary labels warning against the consumption of alcohol or other CNS depressants. Patients need to be cautioned against driving while taking these medications. Taking these medications with food may reduce nausea, but can slow the onset of action.

# Review Questions

## Multiple Choice

Choose the best answer for the following questions:

1. Which is incorrect regarding narcotic analgesics?
   a. These are the drugs of choice for moderate to severe acute or chronic pain.
   b. Some drugs in this class produce euphoria.
   c. These are used in treatment of pain associated with some types of cancer.
   d. Hydromorphone, fentanyl, and phenylbutazone are all narcotic analgesics.
   e. None of the above is incorrect.

2. Which best describes the mechanism of analgesia produced by the opioid agonists?
   a. Action at receptors in the CNS and sensory peripheral nerves blocks the transmission of painful stimuli to the cerebral cortex.
   b. Action at receptors in the CNS and sensory peripheral nerves alters the perception of pain and raises the pain threshold at the level of the spinal cord.
   c. Action destroys neurotransmitters produced by sensory peripheral nerves so pain signals cannot be transmitted to the brain.
   d. Both b and c are part of the correct mechanism.
   e. None of these are the correct mechanism.

3. Which of the following choices lists effects that can result from morphine administration?
   a. Respiratory depression, decreased blood pressure, decreased intestinal motility
   b. Increased cardiac workload, respiratory depression, constriction of blood vessels
   c. Diarrhea, cough suppression, constriction of blood vessels
   d. Nausea, CNS stimulation, diarrhea
   e. All of the above are effects that can be caused by morphine

4. Which of these is a reason for cautious use or altogether avoidance of meperidine?
   a. Patient currently taking a monoamine oxidase inhibitor antidepressant.
   b. Treating pain with meperidine usually leads to physical dependence in the patient.
   c. Metabolism of meperidine generates a toxic metabolite that can accumulate in eldrly patients or patients with renal dysfunction.
   d. Metabolism of meperidine generates a toxic metabolite that causes heart failure.
   e. Both a and c are correct.

5. Which of these is not something that should be done when dispensing a schedule II controlled substance?
   a. Schedule II drug records should be kept separately from other drug records.
   b. Check to make sure the prescription is handwritten by the physician.
   c. When dispensing to outpatients, warn them of the risks of possible drug interactions.
   d. Allow refills on the prescription, but only up to 2 refills per prescription.
   e. Call physician's office to verify the prescription if it is brought in to the pharmacy by an unknown individual or was written by an unknown physician.

## True/False

6. The euphoric effect produced by some of the opioids results in a high potential for abuse.
   a. True
   b. False

7. Narcotic analgesics are indicated for the treatment of pain resulting from headaches, muscle soreness after exercise, or mild arthritic pain.
   a. True
   b. False

8. Morphine, a strong opioid agonist, is frequently used because it produces analgesia as well as loss of consciousness.
   a. True
   b. False

9. Opioids are controlled substances with the exception of codeine and its derivatives, which are not controlled substances.
   a. True
   b. False

10. In addition to the more common side effects of dizziness, drowsiness, and light-headedness, dysphoria is an unpleasant state of anguish and agitation that is a potential side effect of the opioid agonist-antagonist drugs.
    a. True
    b. False

## Matching

For questions 11 to 15, match each drug name with the lettered choice that contains correct information about that drug. Answer choices may be used once or not at all. No answer choice will be used more than once.

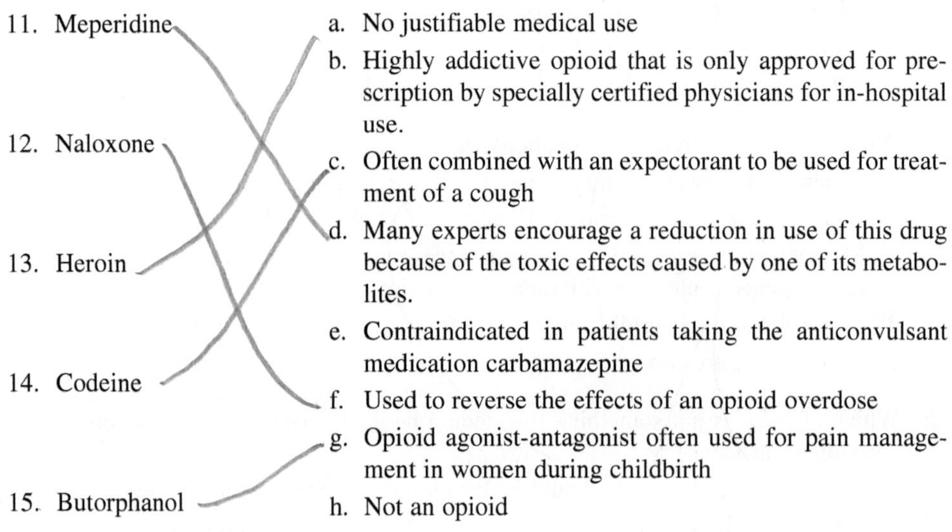

11. Meperidine
12. Naloxone
13. Heroin
14. Codeine
15. Butorphanol

a. No justifiable medical use
b. Highly addictive opioid that is only approved for prescription by specially certified physicians for in-hospital use.
c. Often combined with an expectorant to be used for treatment of a cough
d. Many experts encourage a reduction in use of this drug because of the toxic effects caused by one of its metabolites.
e. Contraindicated in patients taking the anticonvulsant medication carbamazepine
f. Used to reverse the effects of an opioid overdose
g. Opioid agonist-antagonist often used for pain management in women during childbirth
h. Not an opioid

## Short Answer

16. What is an opioid agonist-antagonist and what are some indications for use of these drugs? Why might agonist-antagonists be used instead of pure opioid agonists?

17. What would you do if a new customer came to the pharmacy with a prescription for oxycodone from an out-of-town physician? What if the prescription was typewritten and allowed for three refills?

18. List one specific opioid that has a high potential for abuse as well as one that has a lower potential for abuse and briefly explain why there is a difference in abuse potential between the two.

19. Why do different opioids have varying actions and effects? Briefly discuss some of the opioid receptors that are present in the body and the effects produced by stimulation at different receptors.

20. List the common side effects seen with the use of tramadol, and describe a situation in which it would not be the best choice for treatment of pain.

## FOR FURTHER INQUIRY

Use the Internet or the library to investigate one of the topics listed below. For Internet research, be selective about the web sites you use. Look for research-based information and websites of reputable organizations.

1. Because of the ready availability of controlled substances in health care, substance abuse by health care professionals can be a problem. What are the consequences of narcotic abuse for pharmacy technicians and pharmacists where you live? Investigate resources for the treatment of narcotic addiction. What are the most successful current practices?

2. Avoidance of adverse drug events is a national priority. Since narcotic analgesics are frequently used in hospital settings and can cause significant respiratory depression, these are considered high-risk/high-use drugs, and hospital-based health care personnel must take special precautions to avoid adverse events. What are some of the practices used in hospitals to prevent improper use of opioid analgesics and prevent adverse drug events?

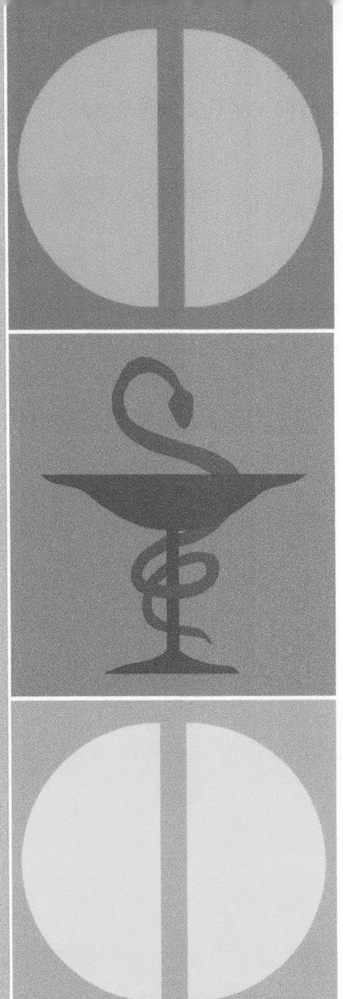

Chapter **10**

# Central Nervous System Stimulants and Hallucinogens

## OBJECTIVES

After studying this chapter, the reader should be able to:

- Describe the impact of drug abuse on society.
- List three indications for use of psychomotor stimulants.
- Describe the symptoms of ADHD and the recommendations for treatment.
- Compare the unwanted side effects of caffeine with those of the amphetamine-type stimulants.
- Name three drugs of abuse and describe typical symptoms associated with their use.

### *KEY TERMS*

- analeptic
- angina pectoris
- angioedema
- cerebrovascular accident
- hyperkinesia
- narcolepsy
- over-the-counter
- psychomotor
- psychotomimetic

## DRUGS COVERED IN THIS CHAPTER

| Psychomotor stimulants | Hallucinogens |
|---|---|
| Amphetamines | Lysergic acid diethylamide |
| Atomoxetine | Marijuana (Tetrahydrocannabinol) |
| Caffeine | Phencyclidine |
| Cocaine | |
| Pemoline | |
| Phentermine | |
| Modafinil | |
| Methylphenidate | |
| Sibutramine | |
| Theobromine | |
| Theophylline | |

The illicit use of drugs creates a tremendous financial drain on society, from the cost of law enforcement to the treatment of addiction. According to the White House drug policy clearinghouse, the cost of drug abuse in the United States in the year 2000 was over $160 billion. Included in this number are the costs of drug-related crime and the numerous health problems that occur in abusers. It does not include the increased health care costs for infants that are exposed to drugs in utero. Illicit drug use impacts the profession of pharmacy, too. Increased regulations, nonreimbursed costs to health care facilities for the care of indigent patients, and the risk of drug-related crimes to pharmacies are just some of the results of illegal drug use. It is useful for individuals who work in pharmacy to be familiar with drug abuse, so that if it is encountered, it is recognized. In this chapter, students will be introduced to both the legal and illegal uses of the central nervous system (CNS) stimulants, and the actions of the hallucinogens.

CNS stimulants increase mental alertness and can improve physical performance. The central nervous system stimulants include one of the most frequently used drugs in the world and some of the most frequently abused drugs in the world. Although these medications are not widely prescribed, their illicit use has a financial and social impact on society. The psychomotor stimulants include the methylxanthines, amphetamine, and other centrally acting adrenergic stimulant drugs, such as cocaine. The hallucinogens, or psychotomimetic, drugs are also discussed in this chapter. Although not chemically related to each other or to the CNS stimulants, all of these drugs produce profound changes in thought patterns and mood. Included in this group are lysergic acid diethylamide (LSD), phencyclidine (PCP), and tetrahydrocannabinol (THC). Because of the illicit nature of many of the drugs covered in this chapter, the format of this chapter will vary slightly from that of other chapters.

psychomotor Pertaining to motor effects of cerebral or psychic activity.

psychotomimetic Inducing psychoses or psychotic behavior.

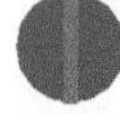

# Psychomotor Stimulants

Legend holds that the Chinese have been drinking tea for 5,000 years. Shen Nung, an early emperor, was an amateur scientist who believed that all drinking water should be boiled for health reasons. One day while resting from his travels, the servants began to boil water for the emperor. Dried leaves from a nearby bush fell into the boiling water. According to the story, the Emperor was interested in this new liquid, drank some, and found it to be delightful. From China, the use of tea spread to Japan and throughout Asia. With the evolution of shipping, tea quickly became a prominent item of trade and was the most popular beverage in Great Britain by the turn of the 18th century.

Coffee plants are thought to have originated in northern Africa. There are records of its use as a beverage that date back as far as 800 BC. By the 16th century there was a growing market for coffee throughout Europe and in the 18th century its use spread throughout the world. People around the world continue to drink caffeinated beverages for their mild stimulant effect. Because of the consumption of tea and coffee, caffeine is the most widely used stimulant and possibly the most widely used drug in the world.

Caffeine, theobromine, and theophylline are naturally occurring plant alkaloids called methylxanthines. Both coffee berries (**Fig. 10.1**) and tea leaves contain caffeine and other methylxanthines. A cup of coffee contains from 80 to 135 mg of caffeine on average, while tea contains about 50 mg of caffeine, as well as a small amount of theophylline and theobromine. Chocolate contains a very small amount of caffeine and theobromine. Refer to **Table 10.1** for caffeine content of these and other familiar products. The methylxanthine drugs have many similar actions and were used historically to treat asthma, for their effect of relaxing the smooth muscle of the bronchioles, as diuretics, and of course, as central nervous system stimulants.

Amphetamine and related compounds make up the other group of psychomotor stimulants. These drugs have significant potential for abuse and their use is tightly regulated. Although there are some legitimate uses for these agents, their use as performance-enhancing drugs and street drugs is probably more widely known.

## Actions and Indications

analeptic A drug that acts as a restorative or stimulant in the central nervous system; for example, caffeine.

Of the methylxanthines, only caffeine and theophylline are used as medications. Theophylline, a drug used to treat asthma, is no longer considered a drug of first choice because of the availability of medications that are safer and more effective in most situations (Chapter 20). Caffeine is considered an analeptic, or a medication used to restore alertness, and it is an additive in a variety of soft drinks and "energy" drinks. The caffeine contained in one to two cups of coffee causes a temporary decrease in fatigue and increased mental alertness as a result of stimulating the cortex and other areas of the brain.

Caffeine and other methylxanthines relax the smooth muscles of the bronchioles. Before the modern treatment of asthma, people with this disease would drink coffee to help resolve asthma attacks. In the past, caffeine was used in cases of central nervous system depression from drug overdose. With the availability of reversing agents for narcotics and benzodiazepines and the reduction in use of the short acting barbiturates, this treatment is rarely used. Caffeine is used as a respiratory stimulant in preterm infants. Its use replaced the use of theophylline in these patients because of a better safety record.

Caffeine has a mild diuretic action. It is combined with acetaminophen and with other ingredients in numerous nonprescription products for relief of pain. Caffeine has no analgesic activity, but is used for its analeptic effect to counteract any sedative properties of the drugs with which it is combined, and for the mild diuretic effects.

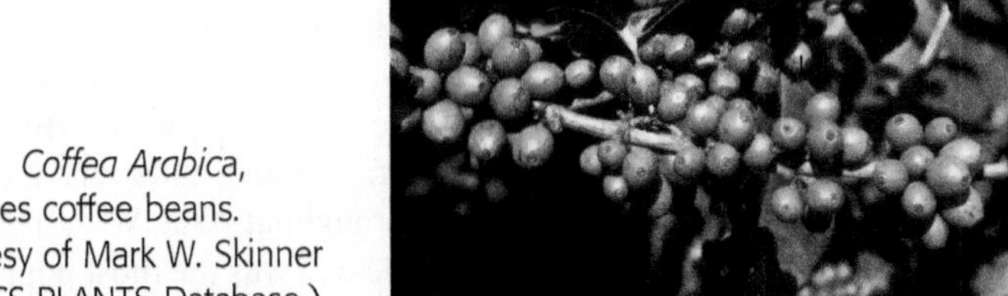

**Figure 10.1** *Coffea Arabica*, which produces coffee beans. (Photo courtesy of Mark W. Skinner @ USDA-NRCS PLANTS Database.)

**Table 10.1** The caffeine content of familiar products

| Product | Serving Size | Typical Caffeine Content |
|---|---|---|
| **Coffee** | | |
| Brewed | 6 oz | 100 mg |
| Espresso | 1 oz | 40 mg |
| **Starbucks Frappuccino** | 9.5 oz | 80–96 mg |
| **Coffee Ice Cream** | 8 oz | 50 mg |
| **Tea** | | |
| Brewed | 6 oz | 40 mg |
| Bottled | 6 oz | 20 mg |
| **Caffeinated Soft drinks** | 12 oz | 22–70 mg |
| **Energy Drinks** | | |
| No Fear | 8 oz | 83 mg |
| Red Bull | 250 ml (about 8 oz) | 80 mg |
| **Chocolate** | | |
| Milk Chocolate | 1.5 oz | 10 mg |
| Dark Chocolate | 1.5 oz | 30 mg |
| **Hot Cocoa** | 6 oz | 7 mg |
| **OTC Medications** | | |
| Analgesics | 1 tablet | 32–64 mg |
| Stimulants | 1 tablet | 100–200 mg |

Amphetamine and the other related CNS stimulants are sympathomimetic amines that act by releasing intracellular stores of catecholamines, including norepinephrine and dopamine, in the brain. This leads to increased alertness, decreased fatigue, depressed appetite, and insomnia. People who abuse the amphetamines and other CNS stimulants may become very thin, and develop a haggard appearance from the lack of sleep.

Although the CNS stimulation is similar, cocaine apparently exerts its effect in the CNS by both preventing the reuptake of the catecholamines and potentiating their action. The effect of accentuated dopamine activity caused by cocaine is especially important in the limbic system, where it is responsible for the euphoria experienced with cocaine use and the resultant craving when the pharmacologic effect wears off. Cocaine is sometimes used legally as a topical anesthetic. When combined with other agents (usually tetracaine and adrenalin), it can prevent further trauma and pain in children who are injured if it is used to numb their wounds before suturing. In adults, cocaine is used as a local anesthetic in the nose or oral cavity after trauma or surgery.

The legitimate uses and indication for amphetamines and related drugs are limited. They are indicated for attention deficit hyperactivity disorder (ADHD), the treatment of narcolepsy A sleep disorder that includes involuntary sleep episodes in the daytime and disturbed sleep patterns at night.

hyperkinesia Abnormally increased and sometimes uncontrollable motor activity.

narcolepsy, a neurological disorder that disrupts the normal patterns of wakefulness and sleep, and for short-term use to assist in weight loss.

ADHD is a syndrome that appears in childhood and can continue into adulthood. Children with this disorder frequently have difficulty in school because of their inability to focus on a subject for more than a few moments. Their impulsivity results in behavior problems at school and causes stress at home. Increased motor activity, called hyperkinesia, typically accompanies this inability to concentrate. A multimodal approach to treatment is recommended by most experts and usually includes behavioral therapy for the child, family counseling and support, educational interventions, and drug treatment.

The action of the centrally acting sympathomimetic amines is paradoxical in these children, and may result from an accentuated stimulation effect on inhibitory neurons. The amphetamine derivatives are able to alleviate many of the behavioral problems, and reduce the hyperkinesia associated with this syndrome. The patient's attention span is prolonged, allowing him or her to function better both at school and at home. Drugs indicated for treatment of ADHD include methylphenidate (Ritalin®), dextroamphetamine (Dexedrine®), pemoline (Cylert®) and a newer agent, atomoxetine (Strattera®). Atomoxetine is chemically dissimilar to the amphetamines and is indicated for ADHD in both children and adults. It increases the levels of norepinephrine by inhibiting its reuptake, and has little or no effect on dopamine. As a result, atomoxetine does not cause significant CNS stimulation.

Narcolepsy is a rare neurological syndrome characterized by uncontrollable daytime sleeping. Patients fall asleep without warning and are unable to move or speak although they maintain awareness of their surroundings. Nighttime sleep patterns are disrupted, and patients may awaken frequently. Standard treatments include the amphetamines and related drugs. Modafinil (Provigil®) is a newer drug now available to treat narcolepsy. Modafinil produces stimulant and euphoric effects typical of other CNS stimulants. The mechanism of action is as yet undefined, but it is possible that it blocks dopamine reuptake in the CNS.

Although most health care professionals do not encourage their use, a number of amphetamine derivatives and related drugs are available for short-term use as appetite suppressants. Examples include sibutramine and phentermine. Tolerance to the appetite suppressant effect develops within a matter of a few weeks. These drugs should only be used in conjunction with dietary changes and exercise, and only for a short period of time in otherwise healthy adults.

## Administration

over-the-counter Sold without a prescription.

All of the methylxanthines are rapidly and well absorbed orally. Caffeine distributes throughout the body and passes readily into the central nervous system and all tissues. It is metabolized in the liver. Caffeine is available in over-the-counter (nonprescription) products such as NoDoz® and Vivarin®. It is manufactured as tablets, capsules, and lozenges. For use as a respiratory stimulant, caffeine citrate is available as an oral solution and an injection for intravenous (IV) administration.

The amphetamines and pharmacologically related compounds are also well absorbed orally. They are formulated as tablets and capsules. Methylphenidate and pemoline are both available as chewable tablets. Adderall® is a combination of several amphetamine salts designed to provide an even level of drug effect. Some products are available in sustained-release preparations for use in ADHD, narcolepsy, and as appetite suppressants (see **Table 10.2**). Atomoxetine is rapidly absorbed after oral administration. It is metabolized in the liver, and the kidneys are mainly responsible for excretion of the metabolites. Atomoxetine is sold as capsules in a wide variety of strengths. Modafinil is available as a tablet and is administered once daily.

Cocaine is well absorbed through mucous membranes. The leaves of the coca plant are chewed by mountain dwelling South American Indians as a stimulant to counteract the effects of altitude. Abusers self-administer cocaine by intranasal snorting, smoking, or intravenous (IV) injection. The peak effect occurs at 15 to 20 minutes after intranasal intake of

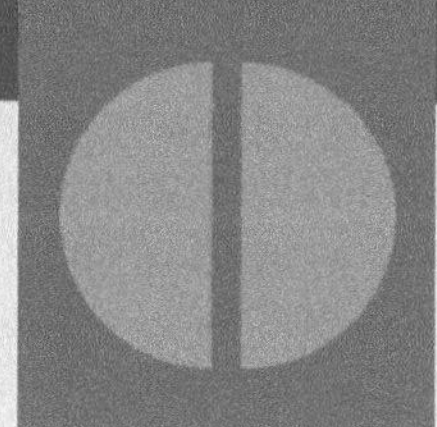

## Case 10.1

Dee Pitts, pharmacy technician, is working behind the prescription counter when she receives a telephone call from Betty Bohm, a mother who just picked up her son's prescription for ADHD. She states that the drug name on the label doesn't sound like what the doctor said he was prescribing. She spells the name for Dee, and Dee places the call on hold for just a moment while she takes a look at the prescription. Dee's heart sinks as she sees that she filled the sloppily written prescription, which now looks as though it is for Adderall 10 mg, with Inderal 10 mg, and the pharmacist missed the error. What is Dee to do? What could she have done to prevent this mistake?

**Table 10.2** Comparison of available psychomotor stimulants and indications for use

| Generic Name | Brand Name | Available as | Indications | Notes |
|---|---|---|---|---|
| Caffeine | Cafcit®, Vivarin®, others | Injection, oral solution, tablets, capsules, lozenge | Apnea of prematurity, fatigue | Rx, OTC, & in beverages |
| Atomoxetine | Strattera® | Capsules | Attention deficit hyperactivity disorder | |
| Dextro-amphetamine | Dexedrine® | Tablets, sustained-release capsules | Narcolepsy, attention deficit disorder | CII |
| Meth-amphetamine | Desoxyn® | Tablets | Attention deficit disorder, obesity | CII |
| Amphetamine Mixtures | Adderall® | Tablets, sustained-release capsules | Narcolepsy, attention deficit disorder | CII |
| Methylphenidate | Ritalin®, Concerta®, others | Tablets, chewable tablets, sustained-release tablets and capsules | Attention deficit disorder, narcolepsy | CII |
| Modafinil | Provigil® | Tablets | Narcolepsy | CIV |
| Pemoline | Cylert® | Tablets, chewable tablets | Attention deficit hyperactivity disorder | CIV |
| Phentermine | Ionamin®, Pro-Fast® | Tablets and capsules, regular and sustained release | Obesity | CIV |
| Sibutramine | Meridia® | Capsules | Obesity | CIV |

cocaine, and the "high" disappears in about an hour. Rapid but short-lived effects are achieved following IV injection of cocaine or by smoking the freebase form of the drug known as "crack."

Chronic abuse of methamphetamine (speed, crystal meth, or crank) is becoming epidemic in the United States because it is inexpensive and can be easily made in home "labs" from pseudoephedrine, a commonly available decongestant. State and federal laws now restrict the sale of pseudoephedrine in an effort to control the flow of methamphetamine. Methamphetamine produces euphoria that ensues quickly and is fairly long lasting, making it highly addictive.

## Side Effects

angina pectoris Irregular attacks of crushing chest pain, symptomatic of a lack of oxygen to the myocardium and usually precipitated by effort or emotion.

In high doses, caffeine can significantly increase heart rate and strength of contraction of the heart. This can be detrimental in a patient with angina, severe chest pain associated with inadequate delivery of oxygen to the heart. All methylxanthines stimulate secretion of hydrochloric acid from the gastric mucosa, which can cause gastrointestinal (GI) irritation and acid reflux commonly referred to as "heartburn." Individuals with peptic ulcers should avoid beverages containing methylxanthines. Modest doses of caffeine can cause insomnia and exacerbate anxiety. A high dosage is required for toxicity, which is manifested by vomiting and seizures. The lethal dose is 10 g or about 100 cups of coffee, which makes death by caffeine highly unlikely.

Caffeine is now added to about 70% of all soft drinks, and the consumption of caffeine by children as well as adults is increasing. When as little as 200 mg, the amount in 2 cups of coffee or 2 to 3 caffeinated soft drinks, is regularly consumed, a withdrawal syndrome can ensue after abrupt discontinuation. Feelings of fatigue, irritability, inability to concentrate, and headache occur in users who have routinely consumed caffeinated beverages daily and then suddenly stop.

Cocaine is one of the most highly psychologically addictive drugs, and it is currently abused daily by more than 3 million people in the United States. Crack cocaine is possibly the most addictive of all drugs of abuse. The intense euphoria characteristic of cocaine use is caused by prolonged effect of dopamine in the pleasure system (limbic system) of the brain. Cocaine abusers know that the more rapidly cocaine gets into the body, through intravenous administration or by smoking freebase cocaine, the more intense this euphoria is. Chronic intake of cocaine, however, rapidly depletes dopamine. The depletion of dopamine results in a vicious cycle of intense craving and use, followed by a rapid and dramatic low that leads to further cocaine intake, which is necessary to return the user to a feeling of normalcy. When cocaine use stops, dopamine levels may take years to normalize, and some experts say levels may never return to normal. This makes recovery from cocaine addiction particularly difficult.

Systemic cocaine use can precipitate an anxiety reaction that includes tachycardia, sweating, and paranoia. Use can induce seizures, cardiac arrhythmias, hypertension, and can lead to heart attacks or other life-threatening cardiac emergencies. The high after use of cocaine or amphetamines is followed by physical and emotional depression.

The physical and emotional symptoms of amphetamine abuse are very similar to those of cocaine. The amphetamines, including methamphetamine, can produce a psychotic state that resembles an acute schizophrenic attack. These drugs pass through the placenta and cause abnormalities in infants born to mothers who abuse them. Changes to the infant brain can affect the child throughout life.

cerebrovascular accident General term used to describe an acute loss of oxygen to some part of the brain due to an embolus or rupture of a blood vessel.

Methamphetamine is especially dangerous because it is so readily available and inexpensive. The extreme elevations of blood pressure in meth users can cause bleeding into the brain known as a cerebrovascular accident (CVA), or stroke. Strokes are not rare in the elderly or people with poorly controlled hypertension. But in areas where meth use is common, strokes are seen in 20- and 30-year-olds as a result of their methamphetamine abuse. Amphetamine overdose is characterized by agitation, fever, assaultive behavior, hypertension, and hallucinations. In fatal overdoses, seizures are usually followed by coma and death.

Methylenedioxymethamphetamine (MDMA), or ecstasy, is a more recent addition to the long list of drugs of abuse. MDMA is an amphetamine derivative that shares similar actions with the amphetamines. Like the amphetamines and cocaine, it rapidly releases quantities of neurotransmitter in the CNS. It is unique in that along with release of norepinephrine, it causes extensive release of serotonin. Serotonin is a neurotransmitter that mediates mood. It also plays a significant role in memory and learning, temperature regulation, and behavior. People who take MDMA report nausea and vomiting, fever, dehydration, teeth grinding, and euphoria described as an ecstatic feeling of belonging. There is evidence that ecstasy use does long-term damage to neurons and affects the brain's capacity to synthesize serotonin. Users may develop depression and impaired memory. Deaths from ecstasy use are usually related to hyperpyrexia, dehydration, and seizures, and are becoming more frequent with increasing use of the drug.

The legal use of the amphetamine type drugs for treatment of narcolepsy, appetite suppression, or ADHD can cause insomnia, rapid heart rate, nausea, anxiety, and elevated blood pressure (**Fig. 10.2**). Special caution is used when physicians prescribe these drugs for patients who are morbidly obese, because hypertension and heart failure can be underlying problems. The amphetamine-like drugs have been associated with pulmonary hypertension, a frequently fatal disease more likely to occur when the cardiovascular system is already compromised.

Use of these drugs in children with ADHD is associated with slowed growth rates, probably related to the effect of appetite suppression. It is thought that children may regain some or most of the growth if the medication is discontinued in adolescence. Long-term use of atomoxetine has not been well studied, but use over 12 months was also associated with growth slowing in children. Atomoxetine caused urinary retention in some adults treated for ADHD. Its use is contraindicated in glaucoma, and in any patient taking monoamine oxidase inhibitor drugs.

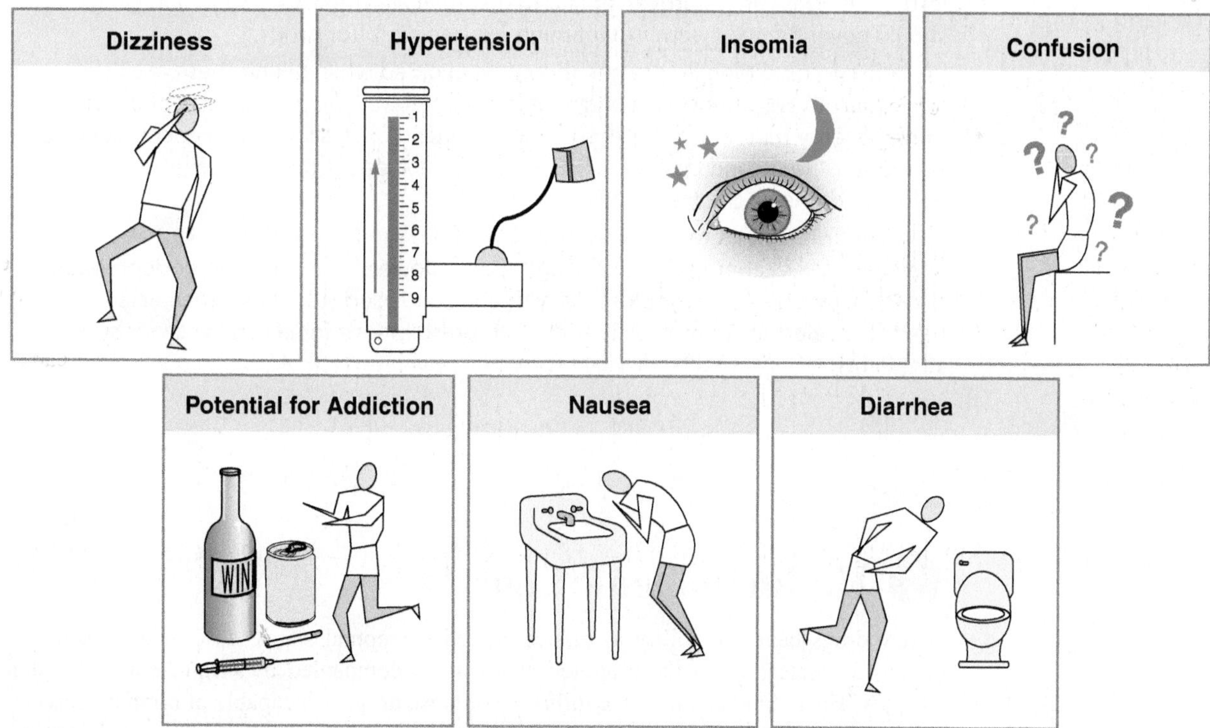


**Figure 10.2** Adverse effects seen with the use of the amphetamines. (Adapted with permission from Harvey RA, Champe PC, Howland RD, et al. *Lippincott's Illustrated Reviews: Pharmacology,* 3rd ed. Baltimore: Lippincott Williams & Wilkins, 2006.)

angioedema An often serious allergic skin reaction characterized by wheals and edema of the skin and the mucous membranes.

Modafinil use has caused sensitivity reactions, including angioedema, inflammation and swelling of subcutaneous tissue, and urticaria, or hives. More common are symptoms of anxiety, insomnia, headache, and stomach upset. Because it can cause chest pain and increased heart rate, it is used cautiously or not at all in patients with heart conditions.

### Tips for the Technician

Both the oral solution and injectable caffeine citrate (Cafcit®), used for apnea in neonates, are packaged in identical vials with labels that differ only slightly. In spite of numerous requests from pharmacists and technicians for a change in the packaging, the manufacturer does not plan any changes in the near future. Although they both are packaged as sterile solutions, once the vial of the oral solution is opened, sterility is no longer assured. This means that technicians need to be very careful not to use a vial of the oral solution for an intravenous preparation by mistake.

All the amphetamines and related drugs are controlled substances. The technician must take special precautions when ordering, receiving, storing, and dispensing these drugs. Class II controlled substances can only be ordered by the pharmacist, and require use of a special form. As with the opioids, meticulous inventory records must be maintained.

Patients taking stimulant drugs for narcolepsy should be warned that the medications might not eliminate the tendency to fall asleep unexpectedly. Therefore, avoidance of driving or other tasks requiring alertness must continue until the medication demonstrates a proven ability to maintain alertness. CNS stimulant drugs should never be taken with monoamine oxidase inhibitor drugs.

Caffeine-containing beverages should be avoided while taking these medications. Alert those parents who may not be aware that caffeine is prevalent in soft drinks, energy bars, and other foods or beverages. Parents should be encouraged to administer the second dose of ADHD medication, if one is ordered, several hours before bedtime so children can fall asleep.

It is important that technicians be aware of the symptoms of stimulant abuse; excitement, excess energy or unusual agitation followed by exhaustion or depression, and in many people, weight loss. As with any controlled substance, technicians need to be alert to signs of tampering with prescriptions for central nervous system stimulants.

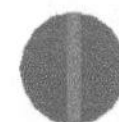

## Hallucinogenic Agents

A few drugs have the ability to induce altered perceptual states, described by some as dream-like states. Often these altered states are accompanied by bright, colorful visual changes. The individual under the influence of these drugs is incapable of normal decision-making, because the drug interferes with rational thought. These compounds are known as hallucinogens or psychotomimetic drugs. With the exception of THC, these drugs have no accepted medical use or value. They are briefly discussed because of the health, social, and financial costs of their use.

## Use and Adverse Effects of Lysergic Acid Diethylamide and Phencyclidine

Lysergic acid diethylamide (LSD, acid) was first synthesized as part of a large research program searching for medically useful ergot derivatives. Ergot alkaloids come from the rye-infesting fungus, *Claviceps purpurea.* Widespread infection of grains occurred in the Middle Ages and resulted in ergot poisoning, or Saint Anthony's fire. Ergot is a powerful vasoconstrictor and consumption of contaminated bread caused bizarre CNS disturbances, gangrene of the limbs, and death. Experimentation with ergot derivatives resulted in early use (1600–1800) as an oxytocic, to stimulate uterine contractions, and later use as a treatment for migraine headaches.

After the synthesis of LSD researchers used the drug for a few years in psychotherapy studies, thinking that it would help them to better understand and treat psychoses and schizophrenia. In the 1960s recreational use of LSD spread, and at the same time admissions to emergency rooms for adverse reactions brought on by LSD use increased. LSD was outlawed in the United States in 1967.

LSD stimulates a number of receptors in the CNS, but serotonin and dopamine receptors are believed to be most closely involved with its actions. Activation of the sympathetic nervous system occurs, which causes dilation of the pupils, increased blood pressure, and increased body temperature. Adverse effects include nausea, muscular weakness, and an exaggeration of muscle reflexes. In some individuals, the drug may produce long-lasting psychotic changes. Delusions have led users to attempt feats that result in physical harm. Some users have extraordinarily negative and frightening experiences, described in slang usage as "bad trips." Users can also experience "flashbacks," an unexpected return of the effects of the drug at a much later date. Antipsychotic agents, such as haloperidol, may be useful to treat patients with untoward effects from LSD.

LSD is absorbed orally. It is an extremely potent hallucinogen; the minimum hallucinogenic dose is about 25 mcg. It is often sold on decorative blotter paper saturated with multiple doses of the drug (**Fig. 10.3**). As with any illicit drug, there are no controls or safeguards in the production of this drug. Users risk potential adulteration and variation in dosage strength.

Phencyclidine, or PCP (angel dust), inhibits the reuptake of dopamine, serotonin, and norepinephrine in the central nervous system. It is most frequently smoked, but is also absorbed orally and through the mucous membranes. Tolerance develops after repeated use. PCP is an analog of ketamine, and causes hallucinations, amnesia, feelings of isolation, insensitivity to pain without loss of consciousness, and analgesia. It produces numbness of extremities, staggered gait, slurred speech, and muscular rigidity. Sometimes, hostile and bizarre behavior occurs, and agitated patients under the influence of this drug may exhibit exaggerated strength. Chronic use can result in prolonged and severe behavioral disturbances, chronically impaired speech, social withdrawal, and thoughts of suicide.

## Tetrahydrocannabinol (THC)

The main psychoactive alkaloid contained in marijuana is tetrahydrocannabinol, or THC. When marijuana is smoked, peak plasma levels of THC occur within about 10 minutes and effects last for about 2 to 3 hours. Marijuana typically produces euphoria, followed by drowsiness and relaxation. There are no accepted therapeutic indications for the use of marijuana, and it is classified as a CI controlled substance. THC alone, known as dronabinol, is used therapeutically.

### Actions and Indications

Use of marijuana is associated with a wide range of effects, including euphoria, appetite stimulation, visual hallucinations, impaired memory, and delusions. The action of THC is mediated through a unique receptor system, found in the CNS and in the periphery, called

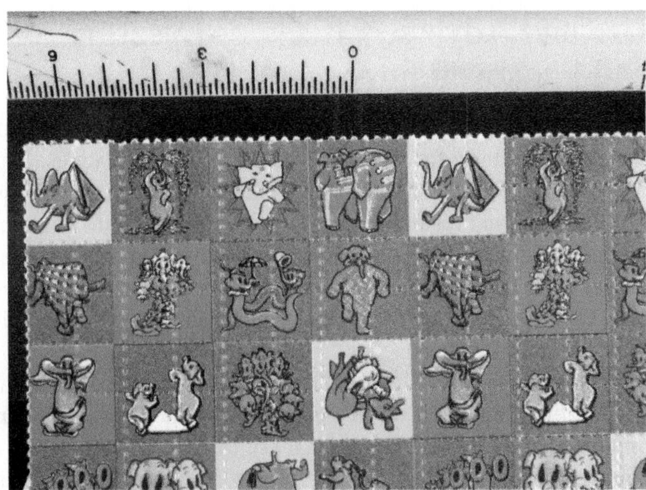

**Figure 10.3** Decorative blotter paper, used to deliver multiple doses of LSD. (Courtesy of the U.S. Drug Enforcement Administration.)

the cannabinoid receptors. In the CNS, these receptors are found in the cerebellum and the part of the limbic system involved in memory. When the receptors were identified, scientists looked for and found a naturally occurring cannabinoid produced by the body. Anandamide, the endogenous substance that attaches to the cannabinoid receptor, is a much shorter lived and fragile molecule than THC. This explains why THC causes cognitive (related to intellectual activity) impairment while the natural compound does not. A high concentration of cannabinoid receptors is found in the uterus, where researchers believe anandamide may have an effect in establishing pregnancy. There is a concern that marijuana (THC) use could interfere with signaling between the uterus and the embryo, with potential to negatively affect the pregnancy or fetus.

The FDA approved dronabinol (Marinol®), synthetically produced THC, for marketing in 1985. It is indicated in the treatment of nausea and vomiting associated with cancer chemotherapy, and as an appetite stimulant in patients with AIDS. Efforts have been made to legalize marijuana for these same uses. Legalization of marijuana is a long-standing political agenda for some special-interest groups, who base their legalization efforts on the therapeutic effects of THC as an antiemetic, appetite stimulant, and for the treatment of glaucoma. Although marijuana has some positive therapeutic effects in these situation, no study has shown that its effects are superior to or even equal to dronabinol, which is readily available, and manufactured under rigorous quality controls.

## Administration

Dronabinol is available for oral use only and is well absorbed after oral administration. It is available as a gelatin capsule that requires refrigeration. Drug interactions with alcohol and other CNS depressants are likely, and these combinations are generally avoided.

## Side Effects

In addition to negatively affecting short-term memory and cognitive ability, marijuana (THC) decreases muscle strength, distorts perception, and impairs judgment and skilled motor activity, such as that required to drive a car. These effects seem to last much longer than the 2- to 3-hour "high." Long-term effects occur as a result of the smoke inhaled, and can include narrowing of the airways, bronchitis, and increased risk of lung infections. The National Institute of Health states that smoking five marijuana cigarettes per week is comparable to smoking a pack of cigarettes daily because of the increased amount of tar. Although still controversial, there is concern that chronic marijuana use may lead to lasting cognitive changes and "amotivational syndrome," especially when use begins in adolescence.

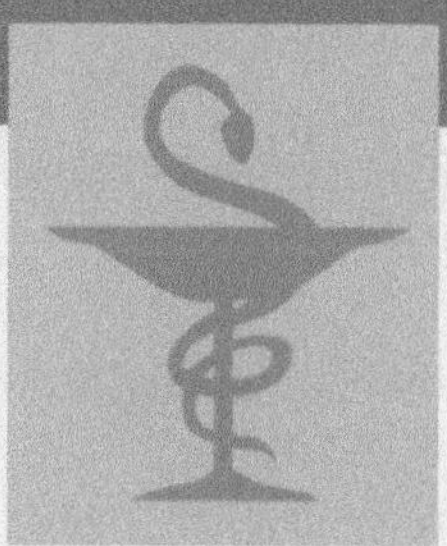

## Tips for the Technician

Dronabinol (THC) is a CIII controlled substance. The soft gelatin capsules need to be kept dry to prevent them from sticking together, but they also need to be stored at temperatures less than 60°F. Therefore, storage in a tightly sealed container, in the refrigerator, is generally recommended. Prescriptions for dronabinol should be labelled with auxiliary cautions to avoid driving while taking this medication, and avoid alcohol consumption.

# Review Questions

## Multiple Choice

Choose the best answer for the following questions:

1. Which statement is *incorrect* regarding the use of caffeine?
   a. Caffeine is a naturally occurring plant alkaloid found in coffee beans, tea leaves, and cacao beans.
   b. Caffeine is the most frequently used stimulant in the world.
   c. The methylxanthines cause CNS stimulation, relaxation of the bronchioles, and an increase in gastric acid production.
   d. Tea and hot cocoa contain greater amounts of caffeine per volume than does espresso.
   e. Caffeine can cause a mild withdrawal syndrome if it is discontinued after routine use of moderate doses (200 mg or more per day).
2. Which of the following is *not* an FDA approved indication for use of an amphetamine derivative?
   a. Narcolepsy
   b. Use as an analeptic
   c. Attention deficit hyperactivity disorder
   d. Short-term use for weight loss in obesity
   e. All of the above are indications
3. Circle the answer that best describes the mechanism of action of the amphetamine derivatives.
   a. They act by releasing intracellular stores of catecholamines in the brain.
   b. They act as agonists at sympathetic receptors in the brain.
   c. They act by releasing intracellular stores of norepinephrine in the peripheral nervous system.
   d. They increase cerebral blood flow, providing more oxygen to the brain.
   e. B and C are correct
4. Which of the following choices lists effects that are most commonly associated with abuse of amphetamines?
   a. Postural hypotension, hallucinations, appetite stimulation, loss of coordination
   b. Constipation, high fever, loss of appetite, feelings of calm and euphoria

c. Agitation, hypertension, anorexia, insomnia, depression
d. Chest pain, joint pain, high fever, visual hallucinations
e. Weight loss, improved concentration, feelings of calm and euphoria

5. Circle the statement below that is correct regarding both phencyclidine and lysergic acid diethylamide.
   a. Both drugs require intravenous administration because they are poorly absorbed orally.
   b. Phencyclidine is a more potent hallucinogen than LSD.
   c. Use of these drugs has never resulted in death.
   d. PCP is known for causing muscle weakness and LSD is known for causing "flashbacks."
   e. Neither drug has any accepted medical use in humans.

## True/False

6. The amphetamine derivative appetite stimulants can be used for obesity without regard to the patient's cardiac status because they will only be used for two to three weeks.
   a. True
   b. False

7. Marijuana should be legalized for medical use because double-blind clinical studies have shown it to be equal to or superior to other treatments for glaucoma and anorexia associated with AIDS.
   a. True
   b. False

8. Lysergic acid diethylamide (LSD) is a highly potent hallucinogen that was first synthesized as part of a large research program searching for medically useful ergot derivatives.
   a. True
   b. False

9. Use of psychomotor stimulant drugs in children with ADHD is associated with slower growth rates, probably related to the effect of appetite suppression.
   a. True
   b. False

10. Modafinil use has been associated with sensitivity reactions, including angioedema and hives.
    a. True
    b. False

## Matching

For questions 11 to 15, match each drug name with the lettered choice that contains correct information about that drug. Answer choices may be used once or not at all. No answer choices will be used more than once.

11. Cocaine
12. Marijuana
13. Phencyclidine
14. Methamphetamine
15. LSD

a. Abuse of this relatively inexpensive drug is associated with hypertensive emergencies and stroke.
b. Acts by releasing intracellular stores of catecholamines in the central nervous system.
c. Associated with increased appetite, lack of coordination, euphoria, and hallucinations.
d. Known to cause delusions and long-term psychotic changes in some users.
e. Frequently associated with the rave scene, this drug is a common cause of hyperpyrexia, dehydration, and nausea and vomiting.
f. One of the most highly psychologically addictive drugs.

## Short Answer

16. Why do technicians need to be extra cautious when preparing intravenous admixtures containing Cafcit®?
17. Briefly describe narcolepsy and typical treatment for this disease.
18. Briefly describe ADHD and the recommended treatment of this disorder.
19. Explain why cocaine is extremely psychologically addictive and why the addiction is so difficult to recover from.
20. What is PCP and what are some typical results of is use?

# FOR FURTHER INQUIRY

The battle against drug abuse in this country consumes billions of dollars in resources and lost productivity every year. Using reputable Internet web pages and other references, research the topic of legalizing a drug or all drugs. Develop your position either supporting or opposing legalization of the drug(s) based on your research. Once you have decided where you stand, consider the topic from the perspective you are not naturally inclined to support, so that you have a thorough understanding of the issue.

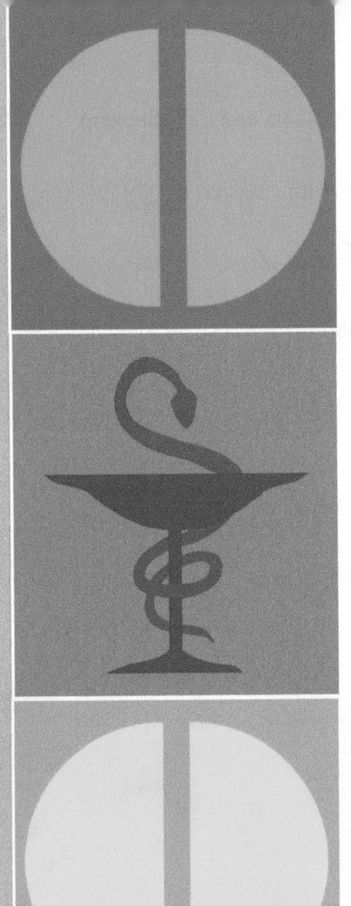

Chapter **11**

# Antidepressants

## KEY TERMS

- bipolar disorder
- cation
- depression
- enuresis
- hypertensive crisis
- mania
- oxidation
- polyuria
- schizophrenia

## OBJECTIVES

After studying this chapter, the reader should be able to:

- Describe major depression, and compare its treatment with the treatment of reactive depression.
- Compare and contrast the common side effects caused by the tricyclic antidepressants with those caused by the selective serotonin reuptake inhibitors.
- List three indications for use of a serotonin reuptake inhibitor.
- Explain the dietary restrictions required of patients taking monoamine oxidase inhibitors and why they are necessary.
- Explain why it is important for patients taking lithium to have frequent laboratory monitoring done.

## DRUGS COVERED IN THIS CHAPTER

### Tricyclic and Related Antidepressant Drugs

Amitriptyline
Amoxapine
Desipramine
Doxepin
Imipramine
Mirtazapine
Nortriptyline
Protriptyline

### Monoamine Oxidase Inhibitors

Phenelzine
Tranylcypromine
Isocarboxazid

### Selective Serotonin Reuptake Inhibitors

Citalopram
Fluoxetine
Fluvoxamine
Paroxetine
Sertraline

### Miscellaneous Antidepressants

Bupropion
Duloxetine
Nefazodone
Trazodone
Venlafaxine

Depression is the most common of all psychiatric disorders. Even in ancient times depression existed and was described in ancient writings, such as the Ebers Papyrus found in Egypt, one of the world's oldest medical documents. King Saul of the Old Testament very likely suffered from depression. The Greeks referred to depression as melancholia, and Cato of Rome described the depressed man as a man with an afflicted soul. "The man with an afflicted soul is like a man trapped in a tunnel. He knows that the sky is blue and the earth is full of life, but he feels like he cannot see. He knows the glories of the night sky and the brightness of the stars, but they give him no joy." Treatment of psychiatric ailments, including depression, is vastly improved over past eras, which often depended on banishing evil spirits, or confining victims to prevent self-harm. However, there is enough room for improvement that new medications continue to be developed.

depression A mood disorder; typical symptoms range from sadness, inactivity, and changes in sleep and eating patterns to anger, guilt, and suicidal thoughts.

bipolar disorder A mood disorder characterized by alternating episodes of excitement and depression.

schizophrenia Major psychotic disorder characterized by disturbances in thought and mood.

mania Excitement and mood elevation of excessive proportions, marked by mental hyperactivity and irrational behavior.

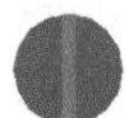

## Depression

Depression can take many forms. The sadness experienced as a result of outside events, such as death of a loved one or loss of a job, is referred to as reactive depression. This condition is generally self-limited, and with time and family support will resolve. Major depression and bipolar disorder are chronic illnesses that affect mood, energy, sleep, appetite, sex drive, and the ability to function. Depression is different from schizophrenia, which produces disturbances in thought. The symptoms of depression are intense feelings of sadness, hopelessness, despair, and the inability to experience pleasure in usual activities. Sleeplessness and loss of appetite may also occur. Mania, which occurs along with depression in bipolar disorder, is characterized by the opposite behavior, that is, enthusiasm, rapid thought and speech patterns, extreme self-confidence, and impaired judgment. Bipolar disorder is sometimes referred to as manic-depressive disorder.

Major depression and bipolar disorder are not associated with any external cause and routinely require drug therapy and psychotherapy for adequate treatment. All clinically useful antidepressant drugs work by mimicking the actions, or increasing the activity of one or more of the major neurotransmitters (norepinephrine, dopamine, and serotonin) in the brain. An understanding of antidepressant drug action, along with other evidence, led to the biogenic amine theory. This theory proposes that depression is caused by reduced activity of one or more of the major neurotransmitters, in areas of the brain responsible for mood. Although this theory of depression may be overly simplistic, it does correctly conclude that these illnesses are related to an imbalance of chemical transmitters in the brain.

The antidepressant drugs fall into three main classes: the tricyclic antidepressants (TCAs) and related drugs, the selective serotonin reuptake inhibitors (SSRIs), and the monoamine oxidase inhibitors (MAOIs). The drugs in each class are chemically similar to each other and have similar actions and side effects. In addition to these drugs, there are several effective antidepressants chemically unrelated to the three main groups. These miscellaneous antidepressants will be discussed separately. Lithium, used to treat bipolar disorder, is classified as a mood stabilizer, but will be discussed in this chapter.

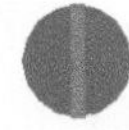

# Tricyclic Antidepressants and Related Drugs

The tricyclic antidepressant drugs derive their name from their three-ringed chemical structure. The related drugs also have ringed structures, some with two rings and others with four rings. These similarities account for the similar actions and side effects within the group. Because the tricyclic antidepressants have been around since 1957, when they were the first class of drugs marketed for the treatment of depression, their use is very well understood and they are relatively inexpensive to use.

## Actions and Indications

In normal nerve activity an impulse is carried from one cell to another by release of chemicals (neurotransmitters) from the nerve ending. These transmitters cross the synapse, the gap between nerve cells, and bind and activate the receptors on the next cell, causing the electrical "message" to be carried forward. The neurotransmitter molecules are then taken back up into the first cell, where they are broken down or recycled for later release. In depression, the activity of the chemical messengers is reduced. The tricyclic antidepressant drugs work by blocking the reuptake of norepinephrine and serotonin (see **Fig. 11.1**). As a result, the quantity of neurotransmitter in the synapse is restored to a more normal level. This action takes place immediately, but the full antidepressant effect from these drugs takes several weeks. The long delay before full antidepressant effect develops is typical of all antidepressants (see **Fig. 11.2**). One explanation suggests that the receptors themselves are altered over time, making them more sensitive to the neurotransmitters. Besides increasing the activity of neurotransmitters, the TCAs block some receptors, including cholinergic receptors. This accounts for many of the side effects associated with this group of drugs. Receptor blockade may play a role in the therapeutic benefits of these drugs, but this is still unclear.

All of the TCAs and related drugs are similarly effective in the treatment of depression. They elevate mood, improve alertness, increase physical activity, and reduce thoughts of suicide. In therapeutic doses, they do not cause central nervous system stimulation or mood elevation in healthy people. All of the tricyclics and related drugs are indicated for the treatment of major depression. The decision of which medication to prescribe is made by considering side effects, how well the drug is tolerated, the convenience of use, and the cost. Refer to **Table 11.1** for a comparison of antidepressants, the available formulations, and indications for their use.

enuresis Involuntary urination that occurs after the age where bladder control should have developed.

In addition to treatment of depression, imipramine (Tofranil®) has been successfully used to treat enuresis, or bed-wetting, in children 6 years of age and older. The tricyclics

A synapse in the brain before treatment for depression
Receptors on the presynaptic neuron inhibit the production and release of neurotransmitter.
Neurotransmitter
Reuptake removes available neurotransmitter from the synapse. As a result, stimulation at postsynaptic neuron is reduced.
Synaptic cleft
A
A synapse in the brain after treatment for depression
Neurotransmitter
SSRI and tricyclic antidepressants normalize production and inhibit reuptake of neurotransmitter. Increased neurotransmitter in the synapse leads to enhanced stimulation of the postsynaptic neuron.
B

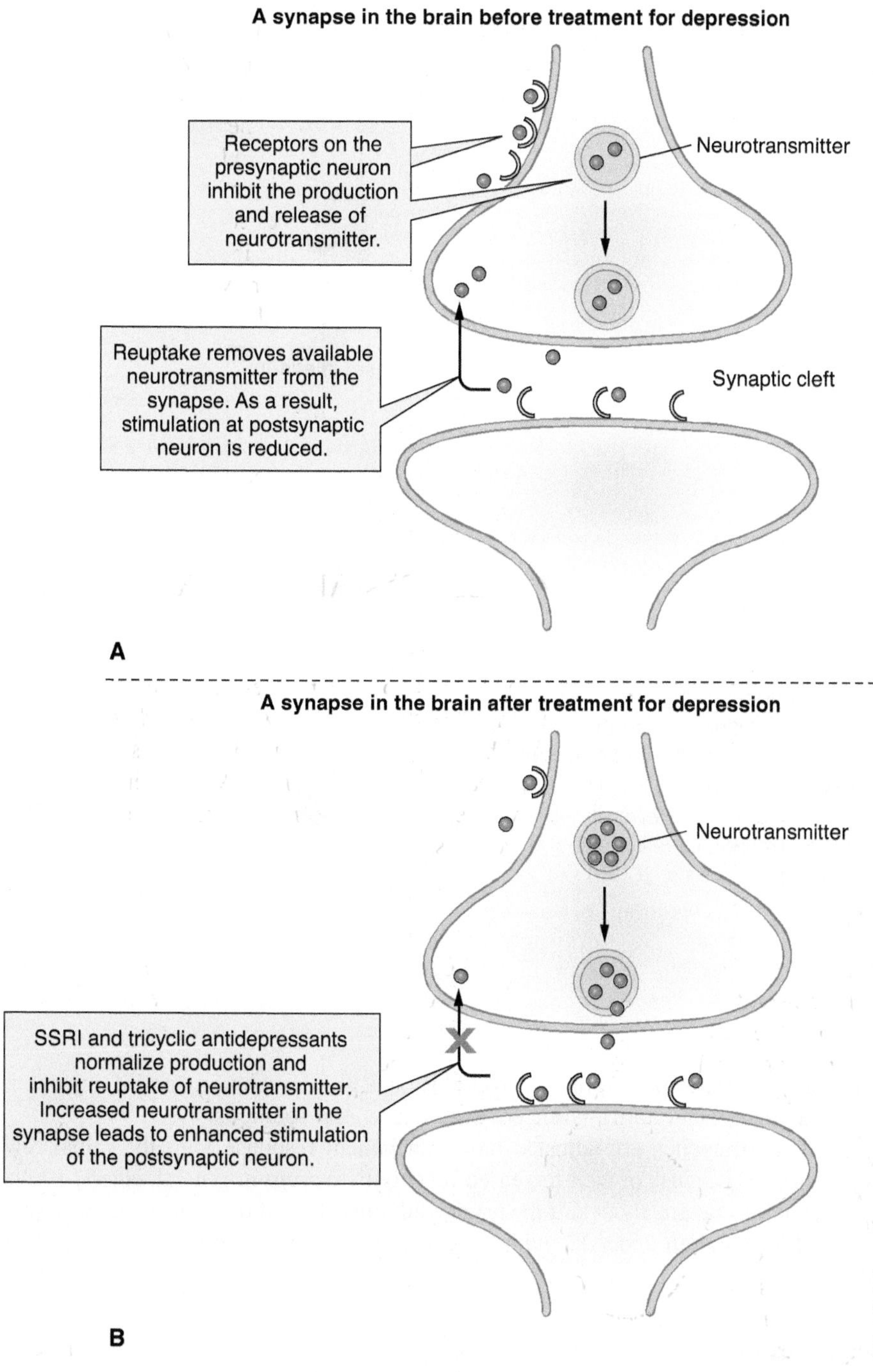

**Figure 11.1** The mechanism of action of the most important antidepressant agents.

are sometimes used to augment the pain relief of analgesics in the treatment of neuropathic pain. Amitriptyline (Elavil®) and nortriptyline (Pamelor®) are the drugs most likely to be used in this way. Experts believe the TCAs work by increasing activity of norepinephrine in the neuron pathways that inhibit pain.

## Administration

The tricyclic antidepressants are well absorbed when taken orally. They are available as immediate-release tablets and capsules and are typically given once a day at bedtime. Because these drugs have long durations of effect and half-lives, delayed-release formula-

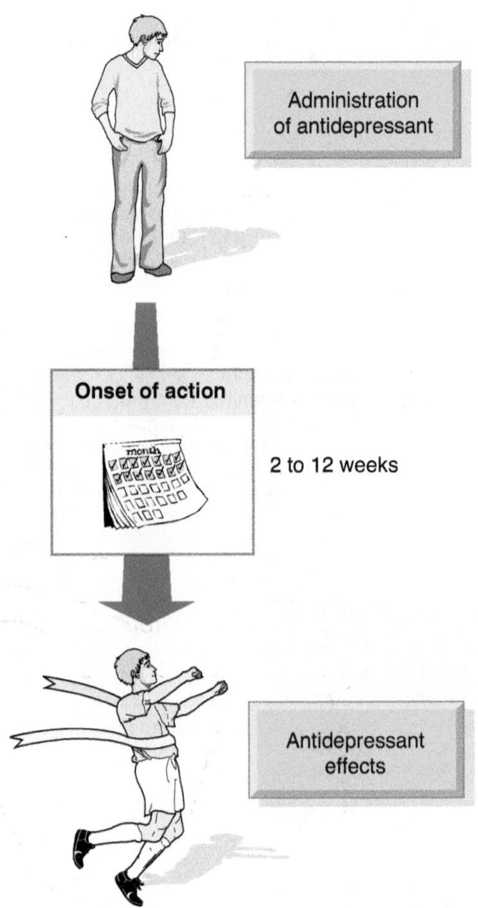


**Figure 11.2** Maximum therapeutic effect of antidepressants requires more than 2 weeks of therapy. (Adapted with permission from Harvey RA, Champe PC, Howland RD, et al. *Lippincott's Illustrated Reviews: Pharmacology,* 3rd edition. Baltimore: Lippincott Williams & Wilkins, 2006.)

tions are unnecessary. Amitriptyline is available in a sterile solution for IM injection. Doxepin (Sinequan®) and nortriptyline are available as oral solutions.

Doses of the tricyclics are adjusted based on patient response after the initial few weeks of treatment. Because of their increased sensitivity to drugs in general, elderly adults are started on doses that are about half the usual adult dose. Use of tricyclic antidepressants is not advised for children under 12, with the exception of the use of imipramine to treat enuresis.

## Side Effects

The cholinergic receptor blocking activity of this drug class is responsible for the most commonly observed side effects. These include dry mouth, constipation, urinary retention, and blurred vision. Urinary retention may be especially problematic in middle-aged or older men who are more likely to have enlarged prostate glands, a frequent cause of urinary retention. These drugs should be used cautiously or not at all in patients with epilepsy or glaucoma, because the tricyclics may aggravate these diseases. Sedation may be a problem, especially early in therapy (see **Fig. 11.3**).

Serious cardiac side effects, a result of increased stimulation of adrenergic receptors, may also occur. These drugs may cause cardiac arrhythmias and low blood pressure, especially when the dose is excessive. Tricyclic antidepressants have a narrow therapeutic index. Overdoses can result in life-threatening cardiac arrhythmias, CNS overstimulation,

**Table 11.1** Antidepressant Medications, Formulations, and Indications

| Generic Name | Brand Name | Available as | Indications | Notes |
|---|---|---|---|---|
| **Tricyclic & others** | | | | |
| Amitriptyline | Elavil® | Tablets, injection | Depression | Drowsiness risk |
| Amoxapine | | Tablets | Depression | Drowsiness risk |
| Desipramine | Norpramin® | Tablets | Depression | |
| Doxepin | Sinequan® | Capsules, oral concentrate | Depression | Drowsiness risk |
| Imipramine HCl & pamoate | Tofranil® | Tablets, capsules | Depression, childhood enuresis | Drowsiness risk |
| Nortriptyline | Pamelor®, Aventyl® | Capsules, solution | Depression | |
| Protriptyline | Vivactil® | Tablets | Depression | Drowsiness risk |
| Mirtazapine | Remeron® | Tablets, orally disintegrating tabs | Major depression | Drowsiness risk |
| **SSRI drugs** | | | | |
| Citalopram | Celexa® | Tablets, solution | Major depression | |
| Fluoxetine | Prozac® | Tablets, capsules, ER tabs*, solution | Major depression, anxiety disorders, premenstrual syndrome, bulimia | ER tabs cannot be crushed |
| Fluvoxamine | Luvox® | Tablets | Obsessive-compulsive disorder | |
| Paroxetine | Paxil® | Tablets, suspension, ER tabs* | Major depression, anxiety disorders, premenstrual syndrome | ER tabs cannot be crushed |
| Sertraline | Zoloft® | Tablets | Major depression, anxiety disorders, premenstrual syndrome | |
| **MAOI drugs** | | | | |
| Isocarboxazid | Marplan® | Tablets | Depression not responsive to other agents | Many drug interactions & diet restrictions |
| Phenelzine | Nardil® | Tablets | Depression not responsive to other agents | Many drug interactions & diet restrictions |
| Tranylcypromine | Parnate® | Tablets | Depression not responsive to other agents | Many drug interactions & diet restrictions |
| **Miscellaneous** | | | | |
| Bupropion | Wellbutrin® | Tablets, ER tablets*, 12 and 24 hr | Major depression, adjunct in smoking cessation | ER tabs cannot be crushed |
| Duloxetine | Cymbalta® | ER capsules* | Major depression, pain from diabetic neuropathy | |
| Nefazodone | Serzone® | Tablets | Major depression | |
| Trazodone | Desyrel® | Tablets | Major depression | May cause drowsiness |
| Venlafaxine | Effexor® | Tablets, ER capsules* | Major depression, anxiety disorders | |

*ER, extended-release formulations are formulated to release over a specific number of hours, usually 12 or 24.

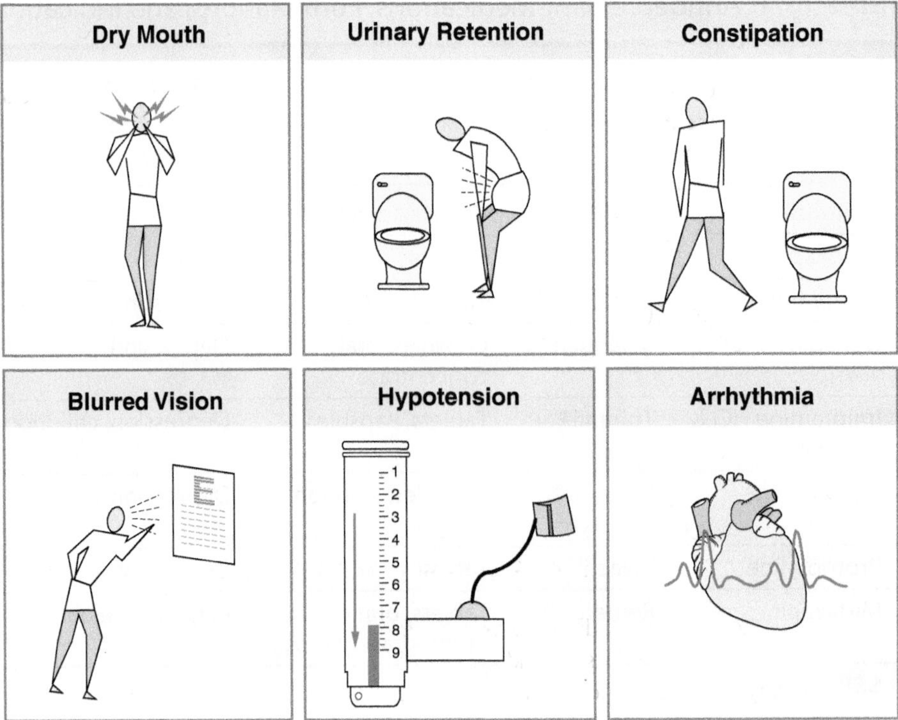


**Figure 11.3** Common side effects observed during treatment with the tricyclic-type drugs.

seizures, and coma. Poisonings with TCAs are extremely dangerous, difficult to manage, and may result in death. For this reason, depressed patients who are or could become suicidal are prescribed small quantities of antidepressant medications, especially early in treatment.

## Tips for the Technician

A number of other medications may interact with the tricyclic antidepressant drugs in well-described and clinically important ways. Tell the pharmacist if there are other sedating drugs on the patient's prescription profile because the effects will be additive to the CNS depressant effects of the TCAs. There is also an additive effect with CNS stimulants, such as the amphetamines. Tricyclics should never be given with the monoamine oxidase inhibitors. This combination of drugs can cause profound stimulation, elevated blood pressure and temperature, seizures, and in some cases, death.

These drugs can impair the consumer's ability to drive or operate other equipment. Auxiliary labels warning of drowsiness and cautioning against use of alcohol or other sedatives should be affixed to TCA prescription vials. Additional auxiliary labels warning clients about the risk of photosensitivity, and cautioning against discontinuing the medication without the advice of the physician should also be attached before dispensing.

# 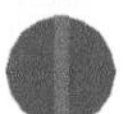 Selective Serotonin Reuptake Inhibitors

The selective serotonin reuptake inhibitors (SSRIs) are the newest class of antidepressants. The prototype, fluoxetine (Prozac®), became commercially available in 1987. In the ensuing years, the SSRIs have become by far the most frequently prescribed antidepressant drug class. Their popularity is a result of more specific action, and fewer, less serious side effects. SSRIs are much safer in cases of overdose. There are five chemically distinct SSRI drugs available in the United States and all are similarly effective at equivalent doses (refer back to the beginning of this chapter for the summary of drugs covered in this chapter). A sixth drug, escitalopram (Lexapro®), is an isomer of citalopram (Celexa®), with identical effects and side effects.

## Actions and Indications

The selective serotonin reuptake inhibitors work by inhibiting the reuptake of serotonin into the nerve ending, leaving more available in the synapse for neurotransmission. As with the tricyclics, researchers believe that this higher lever of available neurotransmitter may alter the receptors on the postsynaptic nerve to make them respond more normally to the neurotransmitter.

Although there are minor differences between the SSRIs, they are about equally effective in the treatment of depression and are as effective as the tricyclic and related antidepressants. Many of these medications have been used in children. In addition to indications for use in major depression, the SSRIs have been successfully used in a variety of anxiety disorders, including panic disorder, social anxiety disorder, obsessive-compulsive disorder and posttraumatic stress disorder, in eating disorders, and premenstrual syndrome.

## Administration

The SSRIs are administered by the oral route, and are available as tablets or capsules. Citalopram, fluoxetine, and sertraline (Zoloft®) are also available in liquid form. As with the tricyclic group, these drugs require several weeks of treatment to achieve full affect. Typically, these drugs are administered once daily in the morning.

Because SSRIs are metabolized in the liver, no dosage adjustment is required for patients with kidney disease. The SSRIs inhibit enzymes in the liver responsible for the elimination of tricyclic antidepressant drugs, antipsychotic drugs, antiarrhythmics, and beta blockers, among others. This can result in a slower rate of removal of these drugs, and result in additional side effects. Drugs in this class are highly bound to proteins found in the blood. If the patient is taking other highly protein-bound drugs (for example, warfarin or phenytoin), the SSRIs could, in theory, displace them, causing an increased risk of side effects. As a result of these effects and others, this class of drugs is implicated in a number of potentially significant drug interactions.

## Side Effects

This drug class is relatively free of most of the unwanted side effects of the TCAs, including effects on the heart, low blood pressure, dry mouth, constipation, and urinary retention. The most common side effects caused by the SSRI drugs include stomach upset, agitation and insomnia (sometimes referred to as activation), loss of appetite, weight loss, and reduced libido or other sexual side effects (**Fig. 11.4**). Weight loss is usually not excessive and after long-term use, some patients report weight gain.

There is some controversy over the use of these medications in children because of several reported deaths from suicide in children. With all antidepressants, suicidal patients must be monitored very carefully early in treatment, and when medication is changed or discontinued. The FDA warned that there is a potential for increased thoughts of suicide

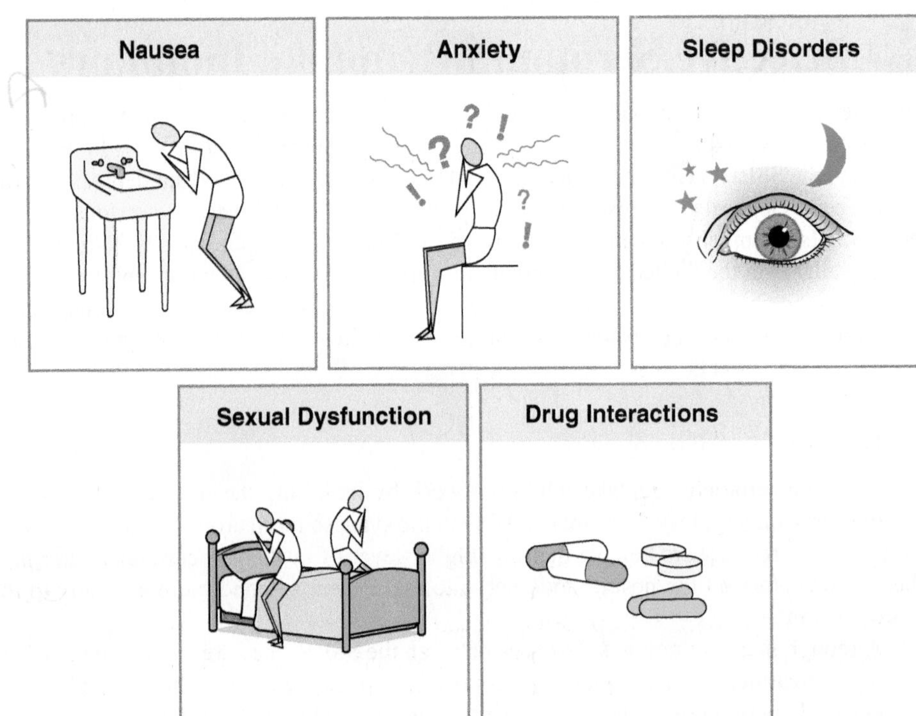


**Figure 11.4** Common side effects observed during treatment with the SSRI antidepressants. (Adapted with permission from Harvey RA, Champe PC, Howland RD, et al. *Lippincott's Illustrated Reviews: Pharmacology,* 3rd edition. Baltimore: Lippincott Williams & Wilkins, 2006.)

and risk of suicide early in the treatment of children with major depression no matter what medications they are taking. The underlying cause of this phenomenon is not completely understood.

Serotonin syndrome may occur as a result of excessively high doses, including intentional overdose, or with some drug interactions. Serotonin syndrome may be life threatening in extreme cases. Symptoms of this syndrome include diarrhea, changes in mental status, fever, exaggerated reflexes, agitation, tremor, sweating, and shivering.

## Tips for the Technician

Patients should be advised to check with the pharmacist or their physician before taking any new medications, because of the potential for interactions with these drugs. The SSRIs are usually given in the morning to avoid insomnia. Although most SSRIs do not cause drowsiness, as a general rule it is recommended that patients avoid alcohol while taking them.

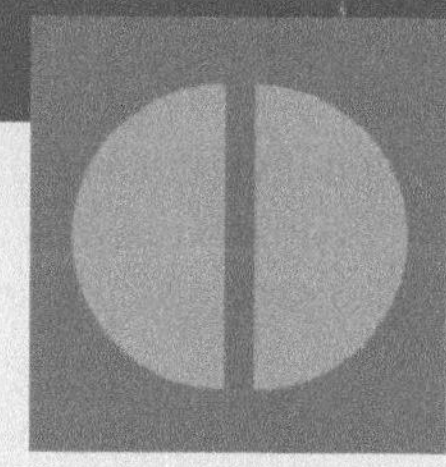

**Case 11.1**

Mrs. Judy Blue picked up her first Marplan® prescription about 2 weeks ago, after trying several other antidepressants with disappointing results. The pharmacist counseled her at that time with regard to dietary restrictions, side effects, and drug interactions. Now she is back at Bell's Drug Store, where you work, complaining of a cold and holding two cough and cold preparations, Tylenol® Multisymptom Cold Formula and Robitussin® DM syrup. She wants you to advise her on which will be safe to take with her MAOI antidepressant. What do you tell her?

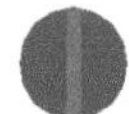

# Monoamine Oxidase Inhibitors

The monoamine oxidase (MAO) inhibitor iproniazid was the second antidepressant in the United States, and was approved shortly after imipramine. Three MAOIs are currently available for treatment of depression: phenelzine, isocarboxazid, and tranylcypromine. Because of the risk of side effects and serious drug interactions, and the requirements for complicated dietary restrictions, these drugs are rarely prescribed today.

## Actions and Indications

Monoamine oxidase is an enzyme found in nerves and many other tissues, such as the intestine and liver. It is one of the enzymes responsible for the breakdown of excess monoamines, including norepinephrine, serotonin, and dopamine, in the synapse. Most MAOIs form complexes with monoamine oxidase and irreversibly inactivate it. The inhibition of the enzyme permits neurotransmitter molecules to accumulate within a few days of starting the medication. The increased presence of the neurotransmitters results in activation of norepinephrine and serotonin receptors, and may be responsible for the antidepressant action of these drugs. Peak antidepressant effect takes several weeks, as with the other classes of antidepressants.

The lack of specificity of the MAOIs results in an increase in monoamines that is not restricted to the central nervous system. As a consequence, their usefulness is limited. MAOIs are indicated for major depression in patients who are unresponsive or allergic to other antidepressants, or those who may benefit from the CNS stimulation caused by the MAOIs.

## Administration

All three medications available in this class are sold only as tablets. Administration schedules vary, but all are given in divided doses, generally two or three times daily. Patients need to be well educated about the use of these medicines so that they will avoid potential drug interactions.

## Side effects

The MAOIs inactivate MAO throughout the body, where it is crucial to the oxidation of other compounds besides neurotransmitters. Oxidation is an important mechanism for preventing the accumulation of some medications and other substances that can be toxic. For example, tyramine, an amino acid found in some foods, requires oxidation in the intestine to prevent accumulation. Tyramine mimics adrenergic compounds like norepinephrine and can cause a hypertensive crisis (critically high elevation of blood pressure), tachycardia (rapid heart rate), and extreme central nervous system stimulation when it accumulates.

oxidation Removal of one or more electrons from a compound through interaction with oxygen.

hypertensive crisis Sudden onset of dangerously high blood pressure requiring immediate treatment to prevent organ damage.

Patients on MAO inhibitors must limit their consumption of foods high in tyramine (see **Fig. 11.5**). Foods high in tyramine include red wine, beer, liver, sausages and dried, pickled or cured fish, among others.

Other possible side effects include drowsiness, postural hypotension, hypertension, arrhythmias, dry mouth, constipation, and urinary retention. The MAOIs are sometimes associated with nausea, vomiting, and malaise when they are abruptly discontinued. Patients should always be gradually withdrawn from these medications.

These drugs should not be used with other antidepressants, and a wash-out period of several weeks is recommended when switching from another antidepressant to an MAOI. Patients should be warned against taking any over the counter medications without consulting the pharmacist or their physician, or any medications containing decongestants such as pseudoephedrine. Prescription adrenergic agonists, such as albuterol inhalers, or combinations of antihistamines and decongestants, must also be avoided.

**Some Foods High in Tyramine***

| Cheeses | Meats | Alcoholic Beverages | Fruits/Veggies |
|---|---|---|---|
| Blue cheese | Chicken livers | Red wine, especially Chianti | Sauerkraut |
| Boursault | Salami | Sherry | Dried fruits |
| Camembert | Bologna | Dark beers | Marmite |
| Emmenthaler | Pepperoni | | Avocados, ripe |
| Stilton | Game meat | | Figs, ripe |
| Swiss | Caviar | | |
| ... and others | Smoked or pickled fish | | |

*In addition, people taking MAOIs should avoid coffee, tea, chocolate, and other foods and medications containing ingredients that could raise blood pressure.

**Figure 11.5** Patients taking MAOIs must avoid foods high in tyramine or other ingredients that could precipitate a hypertensive crisis.

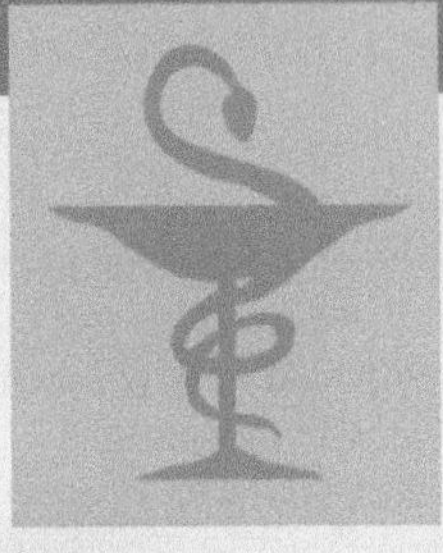

## Tips for the Technician

The pharmacist must adequately counsel patients who receive medications from this class of drugs. Besides the important dietary restrictions, patients must be warned about drug interactions. Complete lists of potentially interacting drugs are available in most drug references, such as *Drug Facts and Comparisons*. Alcohol should not be consumed while taking MAOIs. Patients, especially the elderly, should be warned about a potential drop in blood pressure on standing that can occur with these drugs.

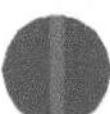

# Miscellaneous Antidepressants

Trazodone, nefazodone, bupropion, venlafaxine, and duloxetine are antidepressants that are chemically unrelated to the tricyclic antidepressant group, the selective serotonin reuptake inhibitors, or the monoamine oxidase inhibitors. Their mechanisms of action are less well described than other antidepressants.

## Actions and Indications

Trazodone and nefazodone have effects similar to 5-hydroxytryptophan, a serotonin precursor. Trazodone may selectively inhibit serotonin reuptake. Because of its sedative properties, trazodone can be quite useful in patients where insomnia and anxiety is a problem.

Bupropion is a weak reuptake inhibitor of norepinephrine, serotonin, and dopamine. Its mechanism of action is unknown. It is indicated in depression and as an aid in smoking cessation therapy. Venlafaxine and duloxetine are inhibitors of the reuptake of serotonin and norepinephrine.

## Administration

All of the miscellaneous antidepressants are available only for oral administration. With the exception of bupropion, they are generally administered at bedtime, because of their propensity to cause sedation. Venlafaxine is available as both immediate-release tablets and extended-release capsules.

## Side Effects

Both trazodone and nefazodone may cause drowsiness, dizziness, and hypotension. The usefulness of nefazodone is seriously limited by the rare, but life-threatening, liver failure that it can cause. A substantial number of patients taking bupropion will experience restlessness and insomnia from its use. Bupropion use is associated with a risk of seizures, so it should be avoided in people with seizure disorders. Venlafaxine and duloxetine cause dry mouth, urinary retention, and other symptoms of cholinergic blockade similar to the tricyclic antidepressants, as well as anxiety and sexual side effects comparable to the SSRI drugs. Duloxetine can cause an increase in heart rate and blood pressure.

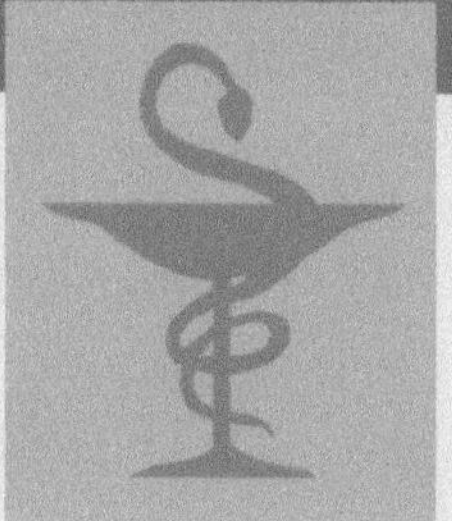

### Tips for the Technician

Patients should be cautioned to avoid other sedating medications or alcohol, which may impair judgment or ability to drive. Be sure to apply warning labels cautioning against abrupt discontinuation of these medications. Technicians should be aware that there are many potential drug interactions between these drugs, and a number of other drugs including the MAOIs. There is an increased risk of serotonin syndrome when any of these drugs are used along with SSRIs. Always report any drug interaction messages that appear while prescriptions are entered into the pharmacy computer system to the pharmacist.

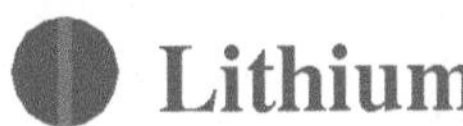

# Lithium

## Actions and Indications

cation Positively charged ion.

Lithium carbonate is used to treat manic episodes associated with bipolar disorder, and as maintenance therapy, to reduce the rate of recurrences. This drug is not a sedative or CNS depressant and should only be used in bipolar disorder. The exact way that lithium exerts its antimanic activity is unknown. Experts believe that it shifts the balance of the monoamines out of the synapse by accentuating their reuptake. Lithium competes with other positively charged ions (cations) in the body, such as sodium and potassium, in ion transport processes. Ion transport is important for impulse transmission in nerve cells and muscle contraction. This widespread competition with body cations explains the systemic nature of side effects caused by lithium.

## Administration

Lithium carbonate is available as immediate-release capsules or tablets and sustained-release tablets, and syrup. It is given in divided doses. The therapeutic and toxic effects of lithium are closely correlated to serum levels. It is essential that drug serum levels be monitored.

## Side Effects

polyuria Excessive secretion of urine.

Because lithium distributes throughout the body and competes with other cations in processes where ion flow is important, the range of potential side effects is impressive. Adverse reactions include diarrhea, nausea, thirst, increased urine production, called polyuria, kidney toxicity with long-term use, elevated white blood cell count, goiter and hypothyroidism, and drowsiness and other CNS side effects. The most common side effects are drowsiness, weakness, nausea, fatigue, hand tremor, and increased thirst and urination. Weight gain can occur with chronic lithium use and may be related to a reduced metabolic rate.

Lithium has a very narrow therapeutic index, and must be individually dosed based upon the concentration of the drug in the serum after a few days of initial therapy. Signs of toxicity may occur at serum levels very near those that are considered therapeutic and include tremors, confusion, muscle weakness, diarrhea, nausea and vomiting, and dehydration. As toxicity worsens, seizures, cardiac arrhythmias, vascular collapse, and coma may occur.

### Tips for the Technician

The pharmacist needs to counsel patients about the importance of having the prescribed laboratory work done. It is important that patients be aware of the signs of lithium overdose. They should be instructed to call their physician if signs of toxicity occur.

# Review Questions

## Multiple Choice

Choose the best answer for the following questions

1. Which of the following is not a symptom commonly associated with major depression?
   a. Intense feelings of sadness and hopelessness
   b. Insomnia
   c. Loss of interest in pleasurable activities
   d. Loss of appetite
   e. All of the above can be symptoms of major depression

2. None of the following tricyclic antidepressants is approved for use in children under twelve except
   a. Amitriptyline
   b. Imipramine
   c. Protriptyline
   d. Nortriptyline
   e. All of the above are approved for use in children

3. Circle the side effect that is not associated with use of tricyclic antidepressant drugs.
   a. Dry mouth
   b. Constipation
   c. Blurred vision
   d. Serotonin syndrome
   e. Urinary retention

4. Which of the following side effects are commonly seen with the SSRI drugs?
   a. Weight gain, drowsiness, and cardiac arrhythmia
   b. Weight loss, dry mouth, and drowsiness
   c. Insomnia, stomach upset, and loss of libido
   d. Rash, headache, drowsiness, and cough
   e. A and B are both correct

5. Which of the following foods should be avoided while taking the monoamine oxidase inhibitors?
   a. Swiss cheese
   b. Salami
   c. Caviar and smoked oysters
   d. Chianti wine
   e. All of the above

## True/False

6. All clinically useful antidepressant drugs work by mimicking the actions or increasing the activity of one or more of the major neurotransmitters.
   a. True
   b. False

7. Mania is characterized by excessive lethargy, rapid thought and speech patterns, extreme lack of self-confidence, and impaired judgment.
   a. True
   b. False

8. Drug treatment of depression generally reaches peak effectiveness in a matter of days.
   a. True
   b. False

9. Bupropion is indicated in depression and as an aid in rehabilitation programs for alcoholism.
   a. True
   b. False

10. Because it causes sedation, trazodone can be useful in depressed patients with a high degree of associated anxiety.
    a. True
    b. False

## Matching

For questions 11 to 15, match the following generic drug names to the correct brand name. Some names may not be used.

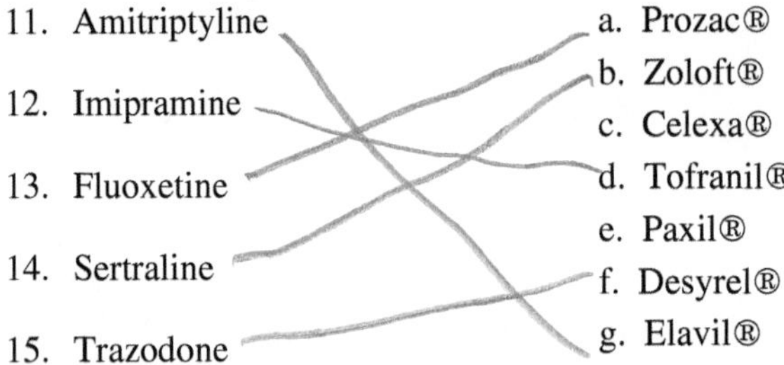

| | |
|---|---|
| 11. Amitriptyline | a. Prozac® |
| 12. Imipramine | b. Zoloft® |
| 13. Fluoxetine | c. Celexa® |
| 14. Sertraline | d. Tofranil® |
| 15. Trazodone | e. Paxil® |
| | f. Desyrel® |
| | g. Elavil® |

## Short Answer

16. Briefly describe the difference between reactive depression and major depression.

17. Why is it important for physicians to prescribe small quantities of tricyclic antidepressant drugs to patients with major depression?

18. Why is it necessary for patients taking lithium to have lithium serum levels checked?

19. Which medications would not be the best choice to treat depression in an elderly man who also has benign prostatic hypertrophy, and why?

20. What are three of the indications for use of the SSRI antidepressants?

# FOR FURTHER INQUIRY

Use the Internet or the library to investigate bipolar disorder, posttraumatic stress disorder, or another disorder for which one of the drugs discussed in this chapter is indicated. Learn about the disease, symptoms, and treatments.

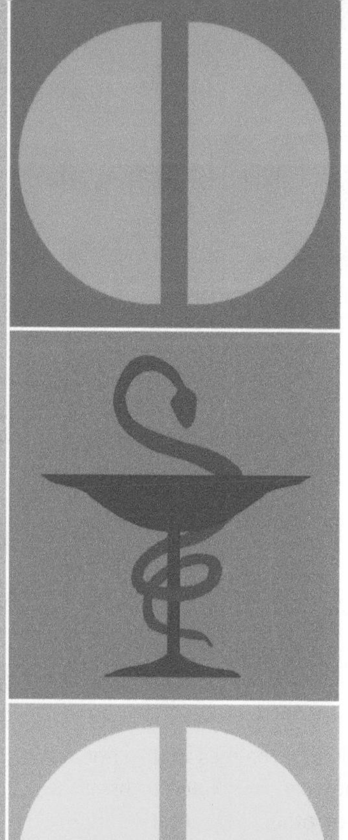

Chapter **12**

# The Antipsychotic Drugs

## KEY TERMS

- agranulocytosis
- akathisia
- antipsychotic
- delirium
- dystonia
- extrapyramidal symptoms
- gynecomastia
- hyperglycemia
- neuroleptic
- neuroleptic malignant syndrome
- off-label
- tardive dyskinesia
- torticollis
- Tourette syndrome

## OBJECTIVES

After studying this chapter, the reader should be able to:

- Describe schizophrenia, including the suspected biochemical cause, and explain why treatment with antipsychotic medication has become so important.
- Explain the mechanism of antipsychotic action common to all antipsychotic drugs, and explain why they differ in their other effects.
- List a unique indication for three different phenothiazine drugs.
- Compare and contrast the side effects associated with use of conventional antipsychotic drugs with those associated with the atypical antipsychotic drugs.
- List three warning labels that should be applied to prescription vials for both conventional and atypical antipsychotic drugs.

## DRUGS COVERED IN THIS CHAPTER

| Conventional Antipsychotic Medications | Atypical Antipsychotic Medications |
|---|---|
| Chlorpromazine | Aripiprazole |
| Fluphenazine | Clozapine |
| Haloperidol | Olanzapine |
| Pimozide | Quetiapine |
| Prochlorperazine | Risperidone |
| Promethazine | Ziprasidone |
| Thiothixene | |
| Thioridazine | |

Psychoses are a group of personality disorders characterized by disturbances in thought and mood, often accompanied by hallucinations and delusions. They can be related to brain injury from a variety of causes, including Alzheimer's disease or other degenerative neurological diseases, to drug therapy, or to specific disorders, such as schizophrenia. Psychotic episodes can sometimes occur in conjunction with severe depression, in bipolar disorder, and with posttraumatic stress disorder.

Schizophrenia is the most common form of psychosis and is a tremendously debilitating disease. Typically, the illness first appears in adolescence or young adulthood; it is a chronic disorder. Patients lose contact with reality and undergo personality changes that prevent them from having normal interpersonal relationships and leading productive work lives. Schizophrenia is an old and historically misunderstood disorder that people believed was caused by possession of the body by demons or evil spirits.

We now know that schizophrenia has a strong genetic component and is probably caused by fundamental biochemical abnormalities involving the production of dopamine and dopamine receptors, possibly triggered by some change or cellular injury early in life. This disease is described as having both positive and negative symptoms. Positive symptoms are behaviors that normal people do not demonstrate, and include thought disturbances, delusions (such as paranoia or delusions of grandeur), hallucinations, and other bizarre behavior. Negative symptoms are behaviors that normal people have, but people with schizophrenia lack. Schizophrenic people have a lack of ability to empathize, have difficulty expressing emotions, are often apathetic, and lose their sense of self.

antipsychotic A drug that is indicated for and effective in the treatment of psychosis.

neuroleptic Antipsychotic.

The drugs used to treat psychoses are referred to as antipsychotic or neuroleptic drugs. These drugs are further divided into the conventional antipsychotic medications and the atypical antipsychotic medications. The atypical antipsychotic medications became widely available in the 1990s. To date, most studies suggest that the atypical drugs offer an advantage over the conventional drugs because they are better tolerated and may provide better control of the negative symptoms of schizophrenia. However, there is no body of evidence to suggest that any one drug from either group demonstrates consistently superior efficacy over any other in the treatment of psychoses.

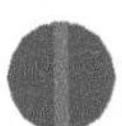

## Conventional Antipsychotic Drugs

Most of the conventional antipsychotic agents are chemically related and are called phenothiazines. They became widely available in the 1950s and they transformed the treatment of schizophrenia. Before drug therapy was available, schizophrenic patients were confined to mental institutions, such as the Bethlem Royal Hospital in London, the world's oldest psychiatric hospital. The word bedlam, defined as a disturbing uproar, is derived from a nickname of this historic facility. Psychiatric institutions, especially those built before the era of modern medical practice, were notorious for the terrible conditions in which patients were kept. Since the advent of drug treatment for psychosis, the number of patients confined to mental institutions has been reduced to about 10% of the institutionalized population of the 1950's.

The first drug used for psychosis was chlorpromazine (Thorazine®), and it is considered the prototype of the phenothiazines. These drugs share some characteristics in common with the antihistamines. Two of the phenothiazines, promethazine and prochlorperazine, are used more often as antiemetic agents than as antipsychotic agents. Haloperidol (Haldol®) is a very important conventional antipsychotic drug that is not chemically related to the phenothiazines, but acts similarly. Pimozide (Orap®) is a conventional agent with characteristics similar to the others, but with limited indications. Molindone (Moban®), another conventional antipsychotic agent, offers no advantages over other drugs and is rarely used.

## Actions and Indications

All of the antipsychotic drugs, including the atypical agents, exert their effect by blocking dopamine receptors (**Fig. 12.1**). Five types of dopamine receptors have been identified and are named D1, D2 and so on through D5. The antipsychotic drugs bind to these receptors in varying degrees. The clinical efficacy of the conventional antipsychotic agents correlates closely with their relative ability to block D2 receptors in the brain. Most of these agents also block acetylcholine, adrenergic, histamine, and serotonin receptors to varying degrees (**Fig. 12.2**). Because the drugs distribute widely, they cause widespread effects by binding dopamine and other receptors. This explains the wide range of both desirable and unwanted effects. Several phenothiazines have significant antiemetic and antihistaminic activity because of their interaction with ACh and histamine receptors.

The conventional antipsychotic drugs, with the exception of promethazine, are very effective at treating the positive symptoms of schizophrenia, such as hallucinations and delu-

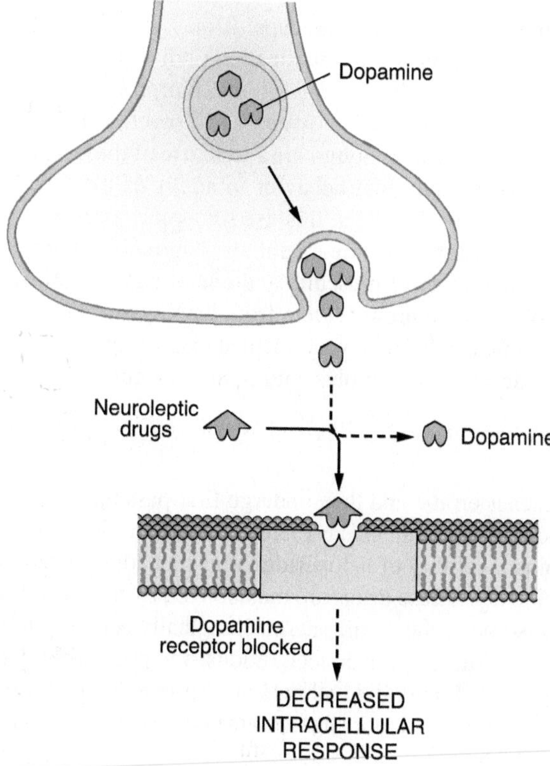


**Figure 12.1** All of the antipsychotic medications act by blocking dopamine receptors. (Adapted with permission from Harvey RA, Champe PC, Howland RD et al. *Lippincott's Illustrated Reviews: Pharmacology*, 3rd edition. Baltimore: Lippincott Williams & Wilkins, 2006.)

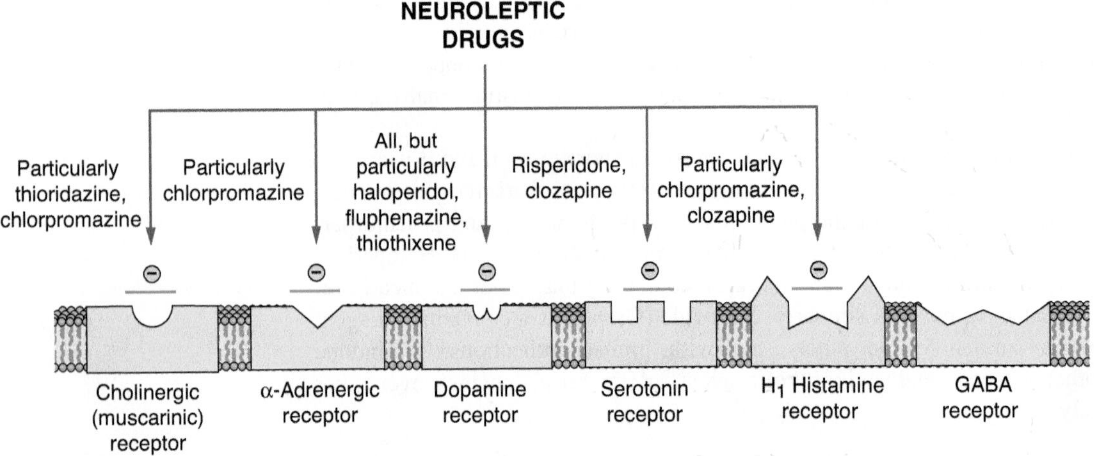


**Figure 12.2** Affinity for other receptors explains the variety of other effects these drugs exert. (Adapted with permission from Harvey RA, Champe PC, Howland RD, et al. *Lippincott's Illustrated Reviews: Pharmacology,* 3rd edition. Baltimore: Lippincott Williams & Wilkins, 2006.)

sions. They are sedating, and reduce excess movement when it occurs. The negative symptoms of schizophrenia are less responsive to treatment with the conventional drugs.

Promethazine (Phenergan®) is a drug with significant antihistaminic and anticholinergic effect and little or no antipsychotic activity. It is useful for the treatment of nausea and vomiting, especially when the underlying problem is associated with anxiety. It is often used postoperatively and in patients undergoing cancer chemotherapy. It is highly sedating. Because of its antihistaminic effects, promethazine may be used alone or combined with other drugs for treatment of allergies, itching, or cough. Prochlorperazine, although it has antipsychotic properties, is nearly always used to treat nausea and vomiting. Both of these drugs work on the nausea center in the brain and do not prevent motion sickness.

Chlorpromazine is effective treatment for intractable hiccups. It may also be used to treat delirium, an acute state of confusion associated with intoxication with hallucinogenic drugs, alcohol withdrawals, and many other disorders of the brain. Chlorpromazine and haloperidol are sometimes used in children to control combativeness and severe behavioral problems that are unresponsive to other treatments. Although long-term use of these agents is considered inappropriate for the control of abnormal behavior in adults or the elderly who suffer from brain disorders, brain injury, or dementia, this use sometimes occurs.

delirium An acute, reversible mental disorder often due to illness or medications with symptoms of confusion, incoherent speech, and hallucinations.

Haloperidol and pimozide are indicated for the treatment of Tourette syndrome. Patients with Tourette syndrome exhibit a number of muscular and one or more vocal tics that cause the patient emotional distress and often prevent them from having normal social and occupational lives. People with Tourette can become very adept at disguising the motor tics, but the vocal tics, which may include shouting out obscenities, are difficult to hide.

Tourette syndrome A neuropsychiatric disorder that is characterized by involuntary motor and vocal tics.

## Administration

The oral absorption of the phenothiazines is erratic and they undergo first-pass metabolism in the liver. For acute psychotic episodes, the intramuscular route of administration is generally preferred. The absorption and bioavailability of haloperidol after oral administration is significantly better than the phenothiazines. These drugs are metabolized by the enzymes of the liver to a number of compounds, some of them still pharmacologically active. There is no correlation between the dose of these drugs, serum concentrations, and pharmacologic effect. Both drug selection and dosing is based on individual patient response. Special caution must be exercised when these medications are administered to the elderly, who are particularly sensitive to both the therapeutic and adverse effects of these drugs. In elderly patients, the usual initial dose is half of the recommended adult dose.

The conventional antipsychotic medications are available in a variety of different dosage forms. Most are available as tablets or capsules, as liquid concentrates, and in an injectable form. Haloperidol and fluphenazine (Prolixin®) are available in long-acting, depot injections. See **Table 12.1** for a summary of products and indications.

**Table 12.1** Antipsychotic Drugs, Formulations, and Indications

| Generic | Brand Name | Available as | Indications | Notes |
|---|---|---|---|---|
| **Conventional Drugs** | | | | |
| Chlorpromazine | Thorazine® | Tablets, oral concentrate, suppositories, injection | Intractable hiccups, nausea & vomiting, psychoses, severe behavioral disorder in children | Significant EPS[1] risk |
| Fluphenazine | Prolixin® | Tablets & depot injection† | Psychotic disorders | Significant EPS risk |
| Haloperidol | Haldol® | Tablets, oral concentrate, injection, depot injection† | Psychosis, Tourette syndrome, severe behavioral disorder in children | Significant EPS risk |
| Pimozide | Orap® | Tablets | Tourette syndrome | |
| Prochlorperazine | Compazine® | Tablets, ER* capsules, syrup, suppositories | Nausea and vomiting, schizophrenia | Significant EPS risk with chronic use |
| Thiothixene | Navane® | Capsules | Schizophrenia | Significant EPS risk |
| Thioridazine | Mellaril® | Tablets, oral concentrate | Schizophrenia | Significant EPS risk |
| **Atypical Drugs** | | | | |
| Aripiprazole | Abilify® | Tablets, oral solution | Schizophrenia, bipolar disorder | |
| Clozapine | Clozaril® | Tablets, orally disintegrating tablets | Schizophrenia | Restricted dispensing, labs required |
| Olanzapine | Zyprexa® | Tablets, injection, orally disintegrating tablets | Schizophrenia, bipolar disorder | Causes significant wt. gain |
| Quetiapine | Seroquel® | Tablets | Schizophrenia, bipolar disorder | Causes wt. gain |
| Risperidone | Risperdal® | Tablets, injection, orally disintegrating tablets, solution | Schizophrenia, bipolar disorder | Causes wt. gain |
| Ziprasidone | Geodon® | Capsules, injection | Schizophrenia | |

[1]EPS, extrapyramidal symptoms; †a long-acting injection; *ER, extended release.

## Side Effects

While the pharmacologic action of the phenothiazines is directly related to blockade of dopamine receptors, their wide range of adverse effects is due to action at the dopamine receptors as well as their anticholinergic and antiadrenergic effects. Differences in the side effect profiles exist among the conventional antipsychotic agents, and also between the conventional drugs and the atypical agents. These differences are mainly due to differences in binding affinities at other receptors.

Possibly the most troubling side effects caused by these drugs are a number of abnormal motor symptoms, referred to as extrapyramidal symptoms. Akathisia (uncontrollable motor restlessness), torticollis (involuntary contraction of neck muscles and twisting of the neck), and dystonia (a lack of or abnormal muscle tone) can occur early in treatment. Parkinson-like symptoms and tardive dyskinesia (involuntary postures of the face, neck, trunk, and limbs) occur with chronic treatment. The bizarre movements of tardive dyskinesia can include facial grimacing, lip smacking, and disturbance of gait, and are seen late in treatment. They are not reversible.

extrapyramidal symptoms Motor or movement abnormalities usually related to medication use.

akathisia A condition of motor restlessness or an urge to move about that is a common extrapyramidal effect due to antipsychotic medication.

In untreated people, the effects of dopaminergic neurons are balanced by the actions of cholinergic neurons. Blocking dopamine receptors alters this balance, causing a relative excess of cholinergic influence, which results in extrapyramidal motor effects. If cholinergic activity is blocked in the patient receiving these drugs, a more nearly normal balance is maintained, and extrapyramidal effects are minimized. Many psychiatrists prescribe anticholinergic drugs, such as benztropine, to prevent these symptoms. This is not always completely effective and does produce additional side effects. The antipsychotic agents with strong anticholinergic activity, such as thioridazine, cause few extrapyramidal disturbances. This is probably related to dampening of cholinergic activity by the drug. This contrasts with haloperidol and fluphenazine, which have low anticholinergic activity and frequently produce extrapyramidal effects.

torticollis Abnormal contraction of the muscles of the neck that results in abnormal carriage of the head; sometimes a reaction to the phenothiazine antipsychotics.

Other side effects are similar to those caused by the tricyclic antidepressant drugs. They often produce dry mouth, urinary retention, and blurred vision. Constipation can be a significant problem with these agents, especially in patients taking high doses. The conventional antipsychotic drugs have the potential to cause seizures, a side effect more commonly seen in patients with a seizure disorder. Drowsiness can occur, especially during the first two weeks of treatment, but tolerance to the drowsiness usually develops (**Fig. 12.3**). Both the phenothiazine type drugs and haloperidol can alter hormone levels in men and women resulting in gynecomastia (development of breast tissue in men) and altered menses in women. Ocular changes, especially retinal pigmentation with thioridazine, can occur with long-term use.

dystonia Abnormal tone of muscles.

tardive dyskinesia Neurological disorder with involuntary movements of the mouth, tongue, and limbs; often as a side effect of chronic use of antipsychotic drugs.

Some of the phenothiazines are irritating to the skin and mucous membranes and can cause GI upset. Medical personnel, including pharmacy technicians, can develop contact dermatitis from repeated skin contact with phenothiazines. For some patients, photosensitivity or skin rashes can occur as a result of taking these medications.

gynecomastia Excessive development of the male mammary gland.

These medications are prescribed with caution in patients with underlying cardiovascular disease because they can cause adverse cardiovascular effects. They block $\alpha$-adrenergic receptors, resulting in lowered blood pressure and orthostatic hypotension. Some of the phenothiazines, such as thioridazine, have a greater potential for causing cardiac side effects, such as arrhythmias.

Neuroleptic malignant syndrome A reaction to the use of antipsychotic drugs that includes rigidity, stupor, fever, and unstable blood pressure, among other symptoms.

Neuroleptic malignant syndrome is a rare, but very serious condition that occurs most frequently after intramuscular administration of one of the conventional antipsychotic agents. Signs of this syndrome include fever, muscle rigidity, mental confusion, unstable heart rate and blood pressure, sweating, and possibly arrhythmias. The condition can progress to breakdown of muscle tissue, renal failure, and death.

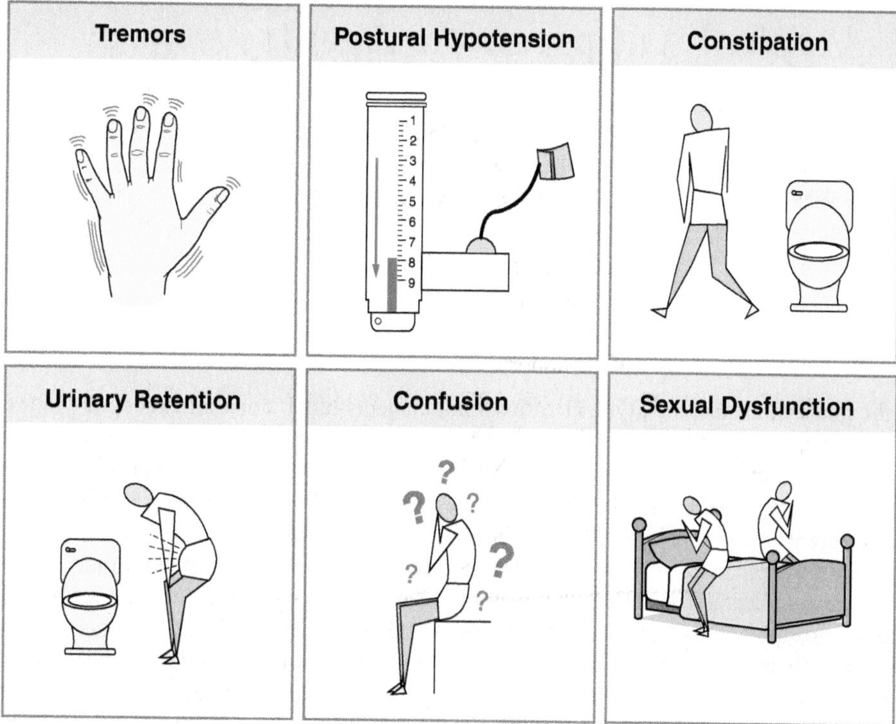


**Figure 12.3** Side effects commonly observed in people taking the conventional antipsychotic medications. (Adapted with permission from Harvey RA, Champe PC, Howland RD, et al. *Lippincott's Illustrated Reviews: Pharmacology*, 3rd edition. Baltimore: Lippincott Williams & Wilkins, 2006.)

## Tips for the Technician

These medications have numerous side effects, and should not be used chronically for agitation or anxiety. Because of the high risk of unpleasant side effects, noncompliance is an important reason for inadequate treatment when these drugs are truly needed in the treatment of psychoses. Technicians can make sure that patients or caregivers know they have a right to speak to a pharmacist if they have questions or concerns about their medications.

A number of auxiliary warning labels are applied to outpatient's prescription vials. These include warnings for the risk of drowsiness and avoidance of alcohol. Patients should also be warned against unprotected exposure to sunlight and against discontinuing their medication, except on the advice of their physician. Abrupt discontinuation can result in a rebound of symptoms. To avoid GI distress, patients should be advised to take these medications with food or milk. Patients should be advised to get up slowly when first awakening in the morning to avoid dizziness caused by postural hypotension.

Anyone handling the phenothiazines should be made aware of the potential for skin irritation or contact dermatitis. When unit-dosing these drugs, especially the concentrated liquid formulations, it is advisable for the technician to wear gloves and wash hands thoroughly before and after handling medications. Advise patients, nurses, or other caregivers that extended-release preparations cannot be crushed for administration.

# 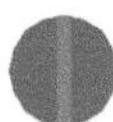 Atypical Antipsychotic Agents

Although clozapine was marketed in the Unites States in 1990, risperidone, which was released in 1994, was the first of several atypical antipsychotic agents made available without any prescribing restrictions. These drugs are promoted for their equal or superior effectiveness in treating psychosis, with a safer side effect profile than conventional antipsychotic agents. Recently, some experts have questioned whether or not these advantages are great enough to be worth the tenfold cost difference between the atypical drugs and the conventional antipsychotic agents.

## Actions and Indications

Like the phenothiazines, the atypical antipsychotic agents block dopamine receptors in the central nervous system. They are unique for their greater selectivity for dopamine receptors in the limbic system and for their affinity for serotonin receptors. Within the group of atypical agents, there is considerable variation with regard to affinity for other receptor types. These differences may explain differing actions and side effects within the group.

As with the phenothiazines, these drugs are indicated for schizophrenia. Some of the drugs are also indicated for bipolar disorder, both for maintenance treatment and for manic episodes. Clozapine (Clozaril®) may be the most effective of all the atypical agents, but its use is generally reserved for schizophrenia that is refractory to other treatments because of the high risk of serious side effects associated with this drug. Only pharmacies registered with the company that makes this medication can dispense it. Refer to Table 12.1 for a summary of products, indications, and dosage forms. Because they are perceived to be relatively safe, the atypical antipsychotic drugs have been widely used off-label (without an official FDA indication) for the symptoms of psychosis and behavioral problems associated with Alzheimer's and other forms of dementia in the elderly. They are also used with some success in Tourette syndrome.

off-label Use of a drug for an indication or use other than those approved by the FDA.

## Administration

All of the atypical antipsychotics are well absorbed orally. They are metabolized by the enzyme systems of the liver. In patients with significant liver disease, a reduced dose may be needed. Metabolism of aripiprazole (Abilify®), clozapine, and risperidone (Risperdal®) produces active metabolites. In the case of risperidone, the metabolites are excreted in the urine, so that in patients with kidney disease the dose of risperidone is less than in healthy patients.

Because organ function gradually deteriorates with age, special caution must be used when administering these drugs to the elderly, and doses are generally reduced. Women may require a lower dose of some of these drugs than men. Pharmacokinetics studies indicate that women have a slower clearance of olanzapine and aripiprazole. Smoking increases the rate of removal of olanzapine.

The atypical antipsychotic drugs are available in a variety of formulations for oral administration. Depending on their duration of action, these drugs are administered either on a daily or twice daily basis. Three agents, risperidone, ziprasidone (Geodon®), and olanzapine (Zyprexa®), are available as sterile powders to be reconstituted for IM injection.

## Side Effects

The atypical antipsychotic drugs are much less likely to cause extrapyramidal effects, and tardive dyskinesia is rare. Of the atypical agents, risperidone and ziprasidone are associated with the highest risk of extrapyramidal effects. Refer to **Figure 12.4** for a comparison of extrapyramidal symptoms related to use of some of the conventional and atypical antipsychotic drugs. Neuroleptic malignant syndrome is very rare with the atypical drugs. Cardiac arrhythmias and EKG changes are less common than with the conventional antipsychotic agents. However, although safer in many respects, the atypical antipsychotic medications are not without troubling side effects.

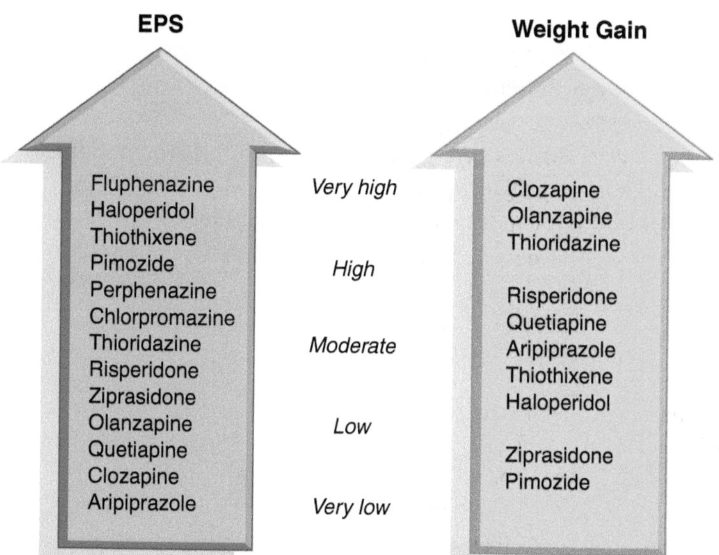


**Figure 12.4** A comparison of two types of troubling side effects observed during treatment with antipsychotic drugs

The atypical antipsychotic agents can cause significant weight gain (Fig. 12.4) and alter glucose and lipid metabolism. New onset of diabetes occurs in some patients, probably related to the excessive weight gain. Diabetic patients taking these drugs can develop severe hyperglycemia (abnormal elevations of blood sugar) that may result in the need for hospitalization. Evidence suggests these effects place some patients at greater risk for cardiovascular disease. Clozapine and olanzapine are associated with the most significant weight gain.

hyperglycemia Abnormally elevated serum glucose level.

Recently the FDA concluded that the elderly treated with these drugs are at greater risk of death from cardiac complications and pneumonia. They have alerted physicians and other health care providers to use caution when using these drugs in the elderly. Since these drugs have only been available for about 10 years, the full range of long-term adverse effects is probably incompletely understood.

Constipation, nausea, and vomiting are not uncommon side effects. While dry mouth is a side effect reported for most of the atypical drugs, excessive salivation occurs more frequently with clozapine. Skin reactions occur infrequently. Although sedation occurs with some of these drugs, insomnia has been reported with others.

Use of clozapine is tightly regulated because of the high incidence of side effects seen with its use. Clozapine causes agranulocytosis, a kind of anemia characterized by a lack of white blood cells necessary for fighting infection. The drug is only provided to patients when proof of required laboratory studies of the blood are submitted. Agranulocytosis is reversible if treatment is stopped. Clozapine use is accompanied by a risk of seizures, which are more frequently seen with higher doses of the drug. Serious adverse cardiovascular effects have been noted with clozapine, including severe orthostatic hypotension, rarely resulting in respiratory or cardiac arrest. Inflammation of the cardiac muscle is rare, but can be fatal.

agranulocytosis An acute condition, often caused by drug therapy, characterized by a marked decrease in the number of granulocytes and associated with signs of infection.

## Tips for the Technician

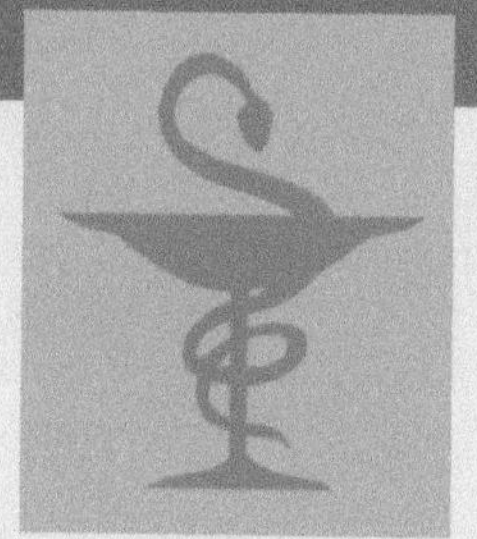

It is important for the technician to be aware that there may be a wide range of acceptable doses of the atypical antipsychotic drugs for different patient populations. Elderly patients are generally started on a dose about half that recommended for younger adults. There are a number of reported drug interactions and patients should be warned about taking any OTC products without first checking with the pharmacist.

Attach auxiliary precaution labels to all outpatient prescription vials warning the patient to avoid consumption of alcoholic beverages while taking these medications. Labels warning the patient of the potential for drowsiness and cautioning against abrupt discontinuation of the drug should also be affixed to the vial. Patients should take care to rise slowly upon awakening to avoid dizziness due to orthostatic hypotension.

Storage requirements for injectable products vary. Risperidone powder for injection is stored in the refrigerator and protected from light until it is dispensed. Olanzapine and ziprasidone powder for injection can be left on the shelf at room temperature until reconstituted. Products for oral use are stored at room temperature.

## Case 12.1

Your best friend's grandmother, Mrs. Delores Luna, was recently moved into a nursing home because her dementia has progressed to the point that she can no longer care for herself. Her doctor and the nursing home staff would like to treat Grandma Luna with olanzapine, but your friend has some concerns about that. She heard on the news that the FDA warned of increased risk of cardiac complications in elderly people who take olanzapine. She wants your advice. What will you tell her?

# Review Questions

## Multiple Choice

Choose the best answer for the following questions:

1. Which of the following factors is not known to contribute to or cause psychoses?
   a. Some drug therapies
   b. Alzheimer's disease
   c. Schizophrenia
   d. Posttraumatic stress disorder
   e. All of the above can be associated with psychosis

2. Which of the following drug and indication combinations is not correct?
   a. Haloperidol – Tourette syndrome
   b. Promethazine – nausea and vomiting
   c. Clozapine – intractable hiccups
   d. Risperdal – schizophrenia
   e. Prochlorperazine – nausea and vomiting

3. Why is frequent laboratory monitoring a requirement for use of clozapine for schizophrenia?
   a. Clozapine can cause a serious form of anemia called agranulocytosis.
   b. Clozapine can cause drowsiness.
   c. Clozapine can cause seizures.
   d. Clozaril can cause myocarditis.
   e. Clozaril can cause allergic reactions.

4. Which of the following atypical antipsychotics is most frequently associated with extrapyramidal symptoms?
   a. Risperidone
   b. Quetiapine
   c. Ziprasidone
   d. Olanzapine
   e. A and C

5. Which of the following statements about the storage of risperidone powder for injection is correct?
   a. It can be kept at room temperature until reconstitution if it is protected from light.
   b. It should be refrigerated and protected from light until it is dispensed.
   c. It should be frozen.
   d. There are no special storage requirements.
   e. It should be stored in a warm, moist place.

## True/False

6. An auxiliary label warning the patient to avoid consumption of alcoholic beverages should be affixed to outpatient prescriptions for antipsychotic medications.
   a. True
   b. False

7. Patients taking antipsychotic medications should be warned not to discontinue them except on the advise of their physician.
   a. True
   b. False

8. There is no special cause for concern with regard to using any of the antipsychotic drugs for dementia in the elderly.
   a. True
   b. False

9. Use of the conventional antipsychotic agents carry a greater risk of causing weight gain and diabetes than do the atypical drugs.
   a. True
   b. False

10. Patients using the phenothiazines and haloperidol are at greater risk of developing tardive dyskinesia than those taking atypical drugs.
    a. True
    b. False

## Matching

For questions 11 to 15, match each term with the lettered choice that contains the correct definition or description. Answer choices may be used once or not at all. No answer choices will be used more than once.

11. Positive schizophrenic symptoms
12. Neuroleptic malignant syndrome
13. Tardive dyskinesia
14. Akathisia
15. Dystonia

a. Uncontrollable restlessness, urge to move
b. Involuntary contraction of neck muscles and twisting of the neck
c. A syndrome involving motor and vocal tics
d. Involuntary posturing of the face, lip smacking, and other movements of the neck, trunk, and limbs
e. Hallucinations, paranoia, and delusions
f. A condition that includes fever, muscle rigidity, mental confusion, unstable heart rate, and blood pressure
g. Abnormal muscle tone

## Short Answer

16. How and why would the initial dose of olanzapine differ in an elderly person versus a young adult?
17. What mechanism of action do all antipsychotic medications share? Why are other drug effects different?
18. Why is it advisable for health care workers handling the phenothiazine drugs to wear gloves, and wash their hands carefully afterwards?
19. Why would use of the atypical antipsychotic drugs be of concern in a diabetic patient?
20. List three phenothiazine drugs and three indications for their use that are not related to psychiatric disturbances.

# FOR FURTHER INQUIRY

Investigate one of the topics below, using Internet or print resources.

1. Research other nondrug forms of treatment of schizophrenia and think about what role they play in the overall treatment of the disease. What services are available for schizophrenic patients and their families in your community?
2. Find out more about Tourette syndrome and the drugs available to treat it. What are nondrug treatment alternatives? Are there Tourette syndrome support groups and, if so, what service do they provide?

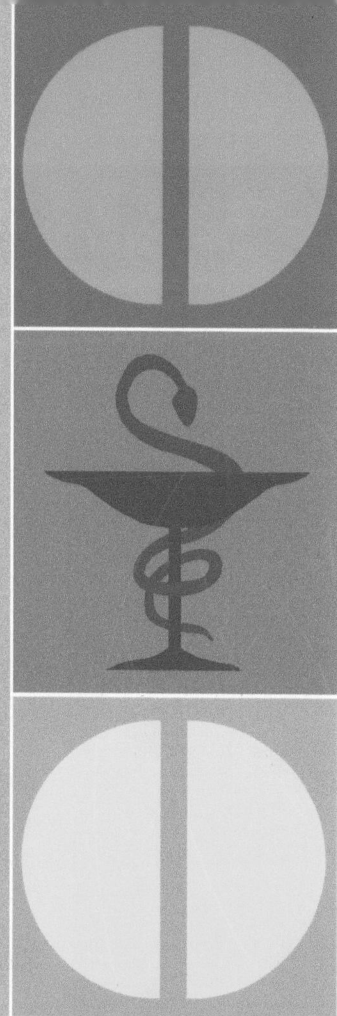

# Chapter 13

# Drugs Used to Treat Parkinson's Disease, Epilepsy, and Migraines

## OBJECTIVES

After studying this chapter, the reader should be able to:

- Explain why symptoms of tremor, shuffling gait, and other abnormal movements occur in Parkinson's disease.
- List three different drugs used to treat Parkinson's disease and explain how their mechanisms of action relate to dopamine balance in the central nervous system.
- Describe the underlying cause of epilepsy and explain why seizures can vary in their presentation.
- List three drugs used for epilepsy and specify for which type of epilepsy they would be indicated.
- Describe migraine headaches and list two drugs used to treat migraine headache pain, and an important side effect of each.

## KEY TERMS

- absence
- aplastic anemia
- aura
- compliance
- dyskinesia
- electroencephalogram
- febrile seizure
- gingival hyperplasia
- myoclonic
- nystagmus
- petit mal
- psychomotor seizure
- seizure
- substantia nigra
- tonic-clonic
- trigeminal neuralgia

## MEDICATIONS COVERED IN THIS CHAPTER

### Anti-Parkinson's Drugs

Levodopa
Bromocriptine
Pergolide
Pramipexole
Ropinirole
Amantadine
Carbidopa
Entacapone
Selegiline
Tolcapone
Benztropine
Trihexyphenidyl

### Drugs Used to Treat Epilepsy

| Primary Drugs | Adjunct Drugs |
|---|---|
| Carbamazepine | Felbamate |
| Clonazepam | Gabapentin |
| Diazepam | Lamotrigine |
| Lorazepam | Levetiracetam |
| Ethosuximide | Oxcarbazepine |
| Phenytoin | Topiramate |
| Fosphenytoin | |
| Phenobarbital | |
| Primidone | |
| Valproic Acid | |

### Drugs for Migraines

| Triptans | Ergot Alkaloids |
|---|---|
| Almotriptan | Dihydroergotamine |
| Rizatriptan | ErgotamineGuaifenesin |
| Sumatriptan | Pseudoephedrine |
| Zolmitriptan | Oxymetazoline |

There are many important neurological diseases that affect large numbers of the American public each year. Three of the most common neurological disorders and their treatment are discussed here: Parkinson's disease, epilepsy, and migraine headaches. These illnesses arise from different pathological changes in the central nervous system and are not related except for their frequent occurrence. Epilepsy is the second most common neurologic disease in North America, and typically affects children. Nearly one out of one hundred older Americans are afflicted with Parkinson's syndrome. More than twenty-eight million Americans suffer from migraine headaches. For each of these diseases, drug treatment is available. Clearly, an understanding of the medications used to treat these diseases is important for any pharmacy technician.

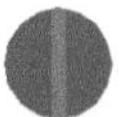

## Parkinson's Disease

Parkinson's disease is one of several incurable neurodegenerative diseases. Other examples include Huntington's disease, amyotrophic lateral sclerosis (ALS, Lou Gehrig's disease), and Alzheimer's disease. These devastating illnesses are characterized by the progressive loss of selected neurons in specific brain areas, resulting in disruption of motor, sensory, or cognitive functioning. Alzheimer's disease (Chapter 5) is characterized by the loss of cholinergic neurons in one region of the brain, whereas Parkinson's disease is associated with a loss of dopaminergic neurons in another. Parkinson's disease is second only to Alzheimer's syndrome as the most common neurodegenerative disease, affecting approximately 1.5 million Americans. Unfortunately, there are no drugs available that can significantly alter the inevitable outcome of ALS or Huntington's disease, but treatment of

Parkinson's disease can significantly lengthen and improve the quality of life for these patients.

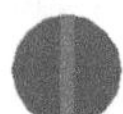

## Drugs Used to Treat Parkinson's Disease

A part of the cerebrum called the basal ganglia contains cells, referred to as the substantia nigra, that are responsible for producing dopamine. In this area of the brain, dopaminergic neurons are responsible for modulating nerve impulses to another area of the brain to assure smooth and purposeful muscle activity. In Parkinson's disease, these cells degenerate and can no longer produce dopamine (see **Fig. 13.1**). Symptoms of the disease do not occur until 60% to 80% of the cells are damaged or destroyed. Without the modulating effect of dopamine in this region of the brain, there is a relative excess of the excitatory effects of acetylcholine. The result of the imbalance is rigidity (sometimes referred to as cogwheel rigidity), a distinctive shuffling gait, tremors, and other findings typical of the disease.

substantia nigra Layer of pigmented gray matter in the midbrain that contains dopamine-producing nerve cells.

Why the degeneration of dopamine producing cells occurs is not known, but drug treatment is aimed at restoring the normal neurotransmitter balance caused by reduction of dopamine producing cells. Treatments include drugs that replace dopamine, drugs that are dopamine agonists, and drugs that inhibit the breakdown of dopamine in the neuron. Anticholinergic drugs are also sometimes used to even out the dopamine-acetylcholine balance.

Typically levodopa (Larodopa®), a precursor to dopamine, is combined with carbidopa to increase dopamine levels in the CNS. This combination (Sinemet®) is the cornerstone of treatment in Parkinson's disease. Dopamine agonists can also be used as first steps in treatment. Anticholinergics and drugs that slow the metabolism of dopamine may be used to supplement primary drug therapy. Relief provided by these drugs is only symptomatic, and it lasts only while the drug is present in the body. There is no known cure for Parkinson's disease and as yet no drug to delay the progression of neuronal destruction.

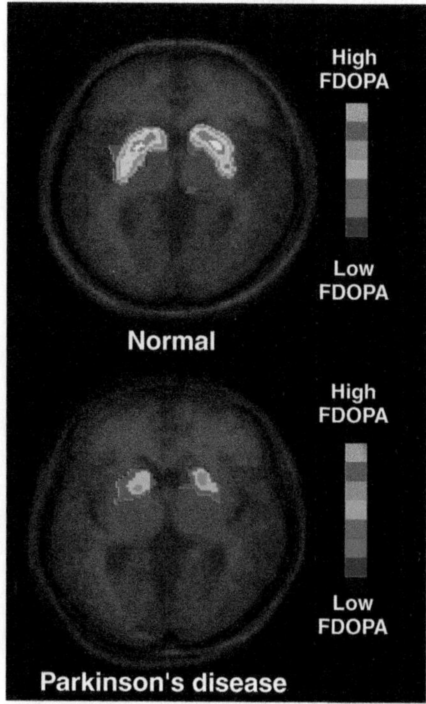


**Figure 13.1** Positron-emission tomography (PET) scan of the brain shows the difference in dopamine production in the brains of those with and without Parkinson's disease. (Reprinted with permission from Harvey RA, Champe PC, Howland RD, et al. *Lippincott's Illustrated Reviews: Pharmacology*, 3rd edition. Baltimore: Lippincott Williams & Wilkins, 2006.)

## Action and Indications

Levodopa is a precursor of dopamine. Unlike dopamine, levodopa passes readily into the central nervous system. Once inside the CNS, it restores dopamine levels in the area of the brain that atrophies in Parkinson's syndrome. The residual dopaminergic neurons in the substantia nigra are responsible for converting levodopa to dopamine. Levodopa decreases the rigidity, tremors, and other symptoms of this illness and is indicated for the treatment of Parkinson's disease.

Levodopa is transformed to dopamine by neurons that contain the necessary enzyme, dopa decarboxylase. This occurs in the central nervous system, but the conversion can also take place in the GI tract and other tissues, thereby reducing the amount of levodopa that penetrates the brain where it is needed. Giving levodopa with carbidopa, a drug that inhibits the enzymatic conversion of levodopa to dopamine, can significantly increase the amount of levodopa that reaches the CNS. Carbidopa does not cross the blood-brain barrier. When given with levodopa, it reduces the conversion to the active form in the gastrointestinal tract and peripheral tissues only, and therefore enhances the action of levodopa in the CNS.

Besides levodopa, there are four other agents that can activate dopamine receptors in the CNS. These four dopamine agonists include two older ergot derivatives, bromocriptine (Parlodel®), and pergolide (Permax®) and two newer, nonergot agonists. The actions of the dopamine agonists are similar to those of levodopa, and are especially useful later in therapy as the ability to convert levodopa to the active dopamine becomes affected. The two newer dopamine agonists, pramipexole (Mirapex®) and ropinirole (Requip®), alleviate motor deficits in patients who have never been treated with levodopa as well as patients with advanced Parkinson's disease who are taking levodopa. They may delay the need for levodopa therapy early in the disease, and may decrease the dose of levodopa in advanced disease. Some experts recommend them as the first step in the treatment of younger patients newly diagnosed with Parkinson's disease, because this group of patients is likely to be better able to tolerate the CNS side effects of the dopamine agonists than elderly patients.

Other drugs found to be useful in the treatment of Parkinson's disease work by preventing the breakdown of endogenous or replaced dopamine. At normal doses, selegiline (Eldepryl®) selectively inhibits monoamine oxidase B, an enzyme that metabolizes dopamine, but does not inhibit monoamine oxidase A, the enzyme responsible for breaking down norepinephrine and serotonin. By decreasing the metabolism of dopamine, selegiline has been found to increase dopamine levels in the brain. When it is administered together with levodopa and carbidopa, selegiline reduces the required dose of levodopa. Selegiline can be useful when given alone in the early stages of the disease.

As described in Chapter 6, catecholamines, including dopamine, can also be metabolized by the enzyme catechol-o-methyltransferase (COMT). Two newer drugs, entacapone (Comtan®) and tolcapone (Tasmar®), selectively and reversibly inhibit COMT and lead to increased concentrations of dopamine in the brain. Both of these agents have been demonstrated to reduce the "on-off" phenomena (described under administration) seen in patients on maintenance levodopa–carbidopa combination therapy.

The anticholinergic drugs, trihexyphenidyl and benztropine mesylate (Cogentin®), do not act directly on the dopaminergic system. Instead they decrease the activity of acetylcholine, which acts as an excitatory neurotransmitter involved with movement in the same area of the brain affected by Parkinson's disease. They are limited in their usefulness and anticholinergic side effects of constipation and urinary retention can be problematic, especially in the elderly. They are used mainly for treating tremors associated with mild Parkinson's disease, and are less effective than levodopa or the dopamine agonists. Amantadine (Symmetrel®) is an antiviral drug that was fortuitously discovered to be helpful in the treatment of Parkinson's disease. It is thought to stimulate the release of dopamine, although its effects are short-lived.

## Administration

All of the medications discussed in this chapter are available for oral administration only. Levodopa and carbidopa are available in combination, in different ratios of carbidopa to levodopa. The combination is also marketed as an extended-release product. Refer to **Table 13.1** for a comparison of products, formulations, and indications.

In newly diagnosed patients, the therapeutic response to levodopa is consistent, because there are adequate dopaminergic neurons available to convert levodopa to dopamine. Unfortunately, with time, the number of neurons decreases, and fewer cells are capable of converting levodopa to dopamine. Consequently, inconsistent muscle control develops. This means that early in the disease, administration of the medications is fairly straightforward and generally successful, but as the disease progresses, the effect of the drugs may begin to wear off before the next dose is due. The state of oscillating response to levodopa is called the "on-off " phenomenon. To compensate for it, complex administration schedules may be devised to maximize the effect of drug therapy, and stretch the periods of adequate control.

High-protein meals interfere with the transport of levodopa into the CNS. Levodopa and levodopa combinations should be taken on an empty stomach, typically 30 minutes be-

**Table 13.1** A Comparison of Drug Formulations and Indications for Drugs to Treat Parkinson's Disease

| Generic | Brand Name | Available As | Indications | Notes |
|---|---|---|---|---|
| Levodopa | Larodopa®<br>Sinemet®† | Tablets, plain tabs, ER* combined | Parkinson's disease (PD) | Most often combined with carbidopa in 1:10 or 1:4 ration carbi:l-dopa |
| Bromocriptine | Parlodel® | Tablets, capsules | PD, female infertility, prevents lactation | Dopamine agonist |
| Pergolide | Permax® | Tablets | Adjunct to carbi-levodopa in PD | Dopamine agonist |
| Pramipexole | Mirapex® | Tablets | PD | Dopamine agonist |
| Ropinirole | Requip® | Tablets | PD | Dopamine agonist |
| Amantadine | Symmetrel® | Capsules, syrup | PD, antiviral | Not primary therapy |
| Carbidopa | Lodosyn® | Tablets | PD, only given with L-dopa | For individual titration of carbi–levodopa ratios |
| Entacapone | Comtan® | Tablets | Adjunct to carbi-levodopa in PD | Reduces the wearing-off phenomenon |
| Selegiline | Eldepryl®, Carbex® | Tablets, capsules | Adjunct to carbi-levodopa in PD | MAOI, dietary, and drug interaction precautions |
| Tolcapone | Tasmar® | Tablets | Adjunct, when others don't work | Risk of potentially fatal liver failure |
| Benztropine | Cogentin® | Tablets, injection | Adjunct in PD, to control EPS‡ | Anticholinergic |
| Trihexyphenidyl | | Tablets | Adjunct in PD, to control EPS | Anticholinergic |

† Brand name of the carbidopa/levodopa combination; *ER, extended-release; ‡EPS, extrapyramidal symptoms.

fore a meal. Patients can eat fifteen to twenty minutes after the dose if GI upset is a problem. Other drugs can be given without regard to food.

Initial doses of these drugs are generally lower for the elderly than for younger adults. Dose adjustments are made based on symptom control, and are not related to serum levels of the drugs. When a patient has poor renal function, adjustment in the dosage of amantadine and pramipexole is necessary. Discontinuation of the drugs used to treat Parkinson's disease must be gradual, over a period of days. Abrupt discontinuation can result in a rebound of the disease or a syndrome that resembles neuroleptic malignant syndrome. Therefore, abrupt discontinuation of any treatment of Parkinson's disease is avoided.

## Side Effects

Drugs that increase dopamine levels in the brain and in the peripheral nervous system have some central and peripheral side effects in common (**Fig. 13.2**). Central side effects include a lack of muscle tone resulting in slow or weak movement and dyskinesia, a lack of control over voluntary movements. Other central side effects include behavioral changes, seizures, mood changes, and hallucinations. Common side effects related to peripheral dopamine excess include nausea, vomiting, loss of appetite, and dry mouth. Side effects are less common when levodopa is combined with carbidopa than when it is given alone.

Selegiline, levodopa, bromocriptine, and pergolide have been associated with cardiac arrhythmias. Postural hypotension is a side effect of all drug therapy for Parkinson's disease. Levodopa, alone or in combination, and entacapone can cause darkening of the urine. Pergolide, bromocriptine, and selegiline can cause drowsiness. Tolcapone packaging carries an FDA required warning regarding the risk of acute, fulminant liver failure. This tox-

dyskinesia Impairment of normal voluntary muscle movement that results in halting or jerky movement.

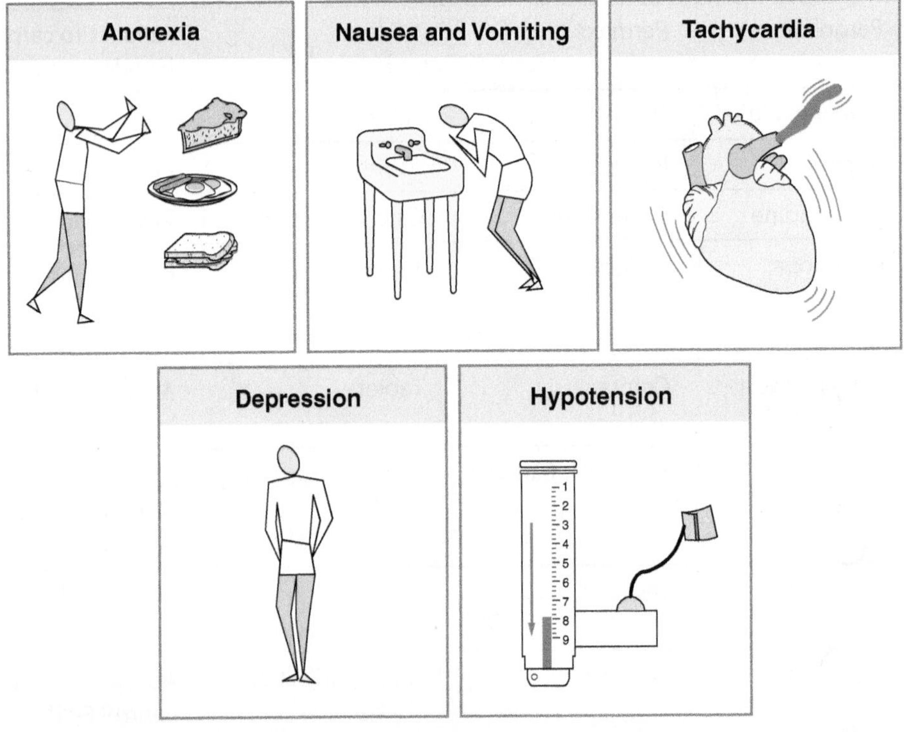


**Figure 13.2** Common adverse effects of drugs that increase dopamine activity. (Adapted with permission from Harvey RA, Champe PC, Howland RD, et al. *Lippincott's Illustrated Reviews: Pharmacology*, 3rd edition. Baltimore: Lippincott Williams & Wilkins, 2006.)

icity is potentially fatal. Tolcapone is, therefore, reserved for patients who have not responded adequately to other medications, and it is discontinued if a significant response to the drug is not seen within three weeks of the start of treatment. Frequent laboratory monitoring of liver function tests must be conducted.

There are a number of important drug interactions noted with these medications. The phenothiazine and other antipsychotic medications reduce the effectiveness of Parkinson's treatments by their blockade of dopamine receptors. The drugs for Parkinson's disease must be given cautiously with blood pressure lowering medications, because they can have an additive hypotensive effect. Although it is a specific MAO B inhibitor, selegiline should never be given with meperidine, and other drug–drug and drug–food combinations of concern should also be avoided (see MAOIs, Chapter 11).

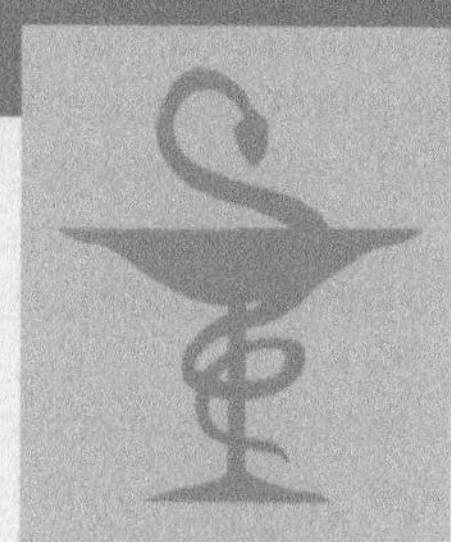

## Tips for the Technician

Drug therapy for Parkinson's disease can be complex and confusing, even for people who work in pharmacy. Younger patients with the disease may not have difficulty managing their drug therapy, but the elderly might find compliance, or adherence to the prescribed medication regimen, very difficult. They might benefit from tablet dispenser systems that help organize medications according to the time of day at which they should be taken. Patients should be encouraged to get all of their medications from one pharmacy, so that the pharmacist can assist with medication schedule organization, and drug interactions can be avoided.

compliance The process of following a prescribed regimen of treatment.

Outpatient prescription vials should bear auxiliary labels cautioning against the consumption of alcohol while taking the medications for Parkinson's disease, and against abrupt discontinuation of these medications. Apply the appropriate auxiliary label to all levodopa containing products and entacapone in order to alert patients that some of their drugs can discolor the urine. Affix cautionary labels warning patients about the potential for impairment of their ability to drive or operate machinery to all vials containing medications for Parkinson's disease. Warn patients who receive pergolide, bromocriptine, and selegiline about the potential for these medications to cause drowsiness by attaching the appropriate auxiliary label to the prescription vials.

During consultation with the pharmacist, patients should be warned to avoid driving until they are comfortable that these medications will not impair their driving ability. The pharmacist should also advise patients to sit up gradually in the morning to avoid dizziness from postural hypotension.

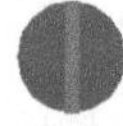

# Epilepsy

Epilepsy is widespread among the general population, with more than 2.5 million individuals affected in the United States. It is the second most common neurologic disorder after stroke. Epilepsy is not a single disease, but rather a family of different seizure disorders classified by their origin within the brain. The sudden, excessive, and simultaneous discharge of cerebral neurons is common to all forms of epilepsy. This discharge results in abnormal movements or perceptions that are of short duration but tend to recur, referred to as seizures.

seizure Abnormal electrical discharge in the brain.

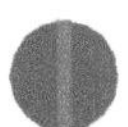

# Drugs Used to Treat Epilepsy

Although drug therapy is the most successful mode of treatment for epilepsy, it is not completely effective in all patients. Antiepileptic medications are chosen based on the origin and type of seizures, so the correct diagnosis is fundamental to successful drug therapy. A list of the antiepileptic medications discussed here is at the beginning of the chapter.

Drug treatment completely controls epilepsy in only about half the cases, but it provides significant improvement in another 25%. One of the impediments to better results is a lack of patient compliance to treatment regimens. There are many reasons for poor compliance, and this is an area where pharmacists and technicians can make a positive impact on the treatment of this troubling disease.

The site of the electric discharge determines the symptoms that are produced. For example, electrical discharge in the motor cortex will result in generalized tonic-clonic or grand mal seizures. Some seizures result in visual, auditory, or olfactory hallucinations if the parietal or occipital cortex plays a role. The electrical discharge that initiates a seizure results from the firing of a small population of neurons in a specific area of the brain that is referred to as the primary focus. Anatomically, this focal area may appear to be perfectly normal. If there are brain abnormalities, they can often be identified using neuroimaging techniques (see **Fig. 13.3**). An electroencephalogram (EEG), or a recording of the brain's electrical activity, can be useful in diagnosing and classifying the type of seizures, especially when a seizure is observed during the EEG (**Fig. 13.4**).

electroencephalogram A diagnostic test that measures and records electrical activity of the brain.

tonic-clonic A generalized seizure (also known as grand mal seizure) with muscle rigidity, followed by shaking, ending with confusion and drowsiness.

Seizures have been classified into two broad groups: partial (or focal) and generalized. Some of the most common forms (and the type discussed in this chapter) are generalized seizures. In a generalized seizure the abnormal electrical discharge spreads rapidly and affects the entire brain. Tonic-clonic seizures result in loss of consciousness, followed by tonic (continuous muscle contraction) and then clonic (rapid muscle contraction and relaxation) phases. Absence (petit mal) seizures are characterized by brief, abrupt, and self-limiting loss of consciousness where the patient stares and exhibits rapid eye blinking, which lasts for three to five seconds. In this form of epilepsy, onset occurs in childhood, often beginning at three to five years of age and usually lasting until puberty. Myoclonic seizures consist of short episodes of muscle twitching. This type of seizure is rare and usually occurs as a result of some organic brain injury. Very young children can experience a generalized tonic clonic seizure in association with a rapidly rising fever. These are called febrile seizures and although frightening to parents rarely cause any kind of long-term problem to the child.

absence A generalized seizure that is marked by the transient loss of consciousness, usually with a blank stare, that begins and ends abruptly; also known as petit mal.

myoclonic Related to, or describing, uncontrollable muscle twitching; i.e., a myoclonic seizure.

febrile seizure A seizure, usually seen in infants, caused by a rapid rise in body temperature.

## Action and Indications

Drugs that are effective in seizure reduction can either block the initiation of the electrical discharge within the focal area, or more commonly, prevent the proliferation of the abnormal electrical discharge to adjacent brain areas. They accomplish this most often by interference with sodium and calcium ion movement that is required for nerve impulse generation, by enhancing the inhibitory action of GABA, or by interfering with excitatory neurotransmission. Phenytoin (Dilantin®) is one of the most important antiepileptic agents and is a member of the hydantoin group. Phenytoin affects the influx of sodium in the neuron, and slows the recovery time after an impulse passes, thereby reducing the propagation of abnormal impulses throughout the brain. It is effective for both partial and generalized seizures.

Other hydantoin drugs include ethotoin (Peganone®) and fosphenytoin (Cerebyx®). Fosphenytoin is a prodrug of phenytoin that, unlike phenytoin, is appropriate for intramuscular use. After administration, fosphenytoin is immediately converted to phenytoin. It is indicated for the short-term control or prevention of seizures when other methods are unavailable or inappropriate.

Phenytoin is metabolized in the liver by the cytochrome P450 drug metabolizing enzyme system, as are phenobarbital and carbamazepine. These drugs can induce their own and other drugs' metabolism. The therapeutic effects of many of the antiepileptic drugs, in-

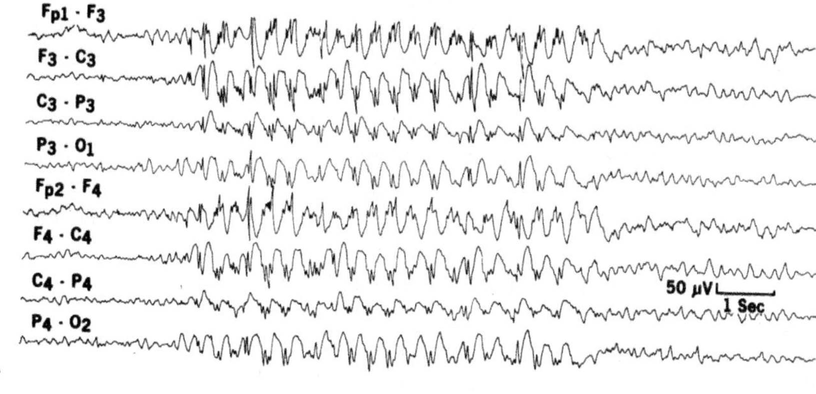


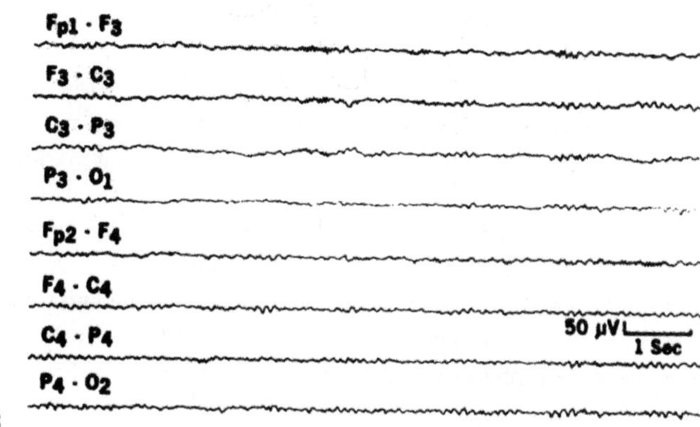


**Figure 13.3** An abnormal electroencephalogram (A), demonstrating spike and wave activity typical of absence seizures and a normal EEG (B). Each line is a recording of electrical activity picked up by an electrode placed according to a standard procedure and indicated by the numbers and letters on the left. (© 2007 Epilepsy Foundation of America, Inc. Reprinted with permission.)

cluding phenytoin, carbamazepine (Tegretol®), phenobarbital, and valproic acid (Depakene® and other), are directly related to serum concentrations of the drugs. Serum concentration levels are monitored to determine dose adjustments. The metabolism of phenytoin is saturable. For practical purposes, this means that above a certain, unpredictable dose, small dose increases will result in large increases in serum concentration. The half-life of elimination also increases, making dosing difficult in some patients and increasing the need for monitoring of drug levels.

The mechanism of action of carbamazepine is similar to that of the hydantoins. It inhibits the spread of abnormal electrical discharge by interference with the movement of sodium ions. Carbamazepine is useful in partial or generalized seizures, including psy-

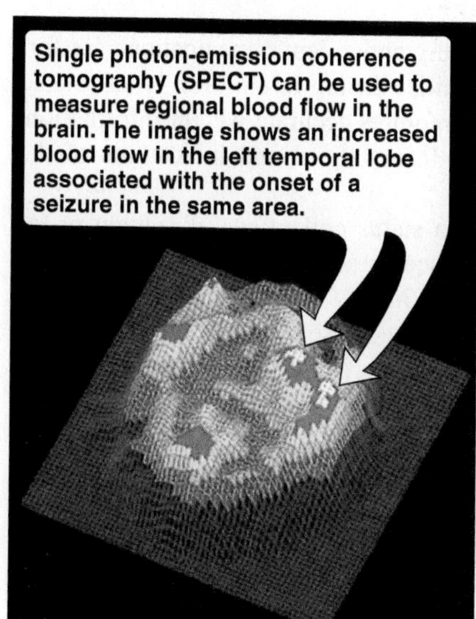


**Figure 13.4** Anatomical abnormalities can sometimes be identified in the brain of the patient with epilepsy by using neuroimaging techniques. (Reprinted with permission from Harvey RA, Champe PC, Howland RD, et al. *Lippincott's Illustrated Reviews: Pharmacology*, 3rd edition. Baltimore: Lippincott Williams & Wilkins, 2006.)

chomotor seizures, complex seizures with psychic, sensory, and motor components. It is also indicated for the treatment of trigeminal neuralgia, a very painful condition associated with localized demyelination of the trigeminal nerve, one of the twelve cranial nerves.

psychomotor seizure
Seizure type marked by complex sensory, motor, and psychic components.

trigeminal neuralgia
Excruciating, intermittent pain in the areas of the face enervated by the trigeminal nerve.

Phenobarbital limits the spread of abnormal electrical discharge in the brain and elevates the seizure threshold. The barbiturates act by enhancing the effects of the inhibitory neurotransmitter GABA, at the GABA receptor. Phenobarbital is useful in treating generalized seizures, including status epilepticus, a series of rapidly recurring seizures that is often resistant to drug therapy, and some focal seizures. Primidone (Mysoline®) is a prodrug that is converted to phenobarbital, and it resembles phenobarbital in its antiepileptic activity. Primidone is an alternative choice in partial seizures and tonic-clonic seizures.

The succinimides are a group of drugs useful only for treating petit mal, or absence seizures. Ethosuximide (Zarontin®) reduces propagation of abnormal electrical activity in the brain by inhibiting calcium channels in a manner similar to the action of phenytoin on sodium channels. It is only indicated for absence seizures, where it is the drug of choice.

The importance of the role of the benzodiazepines in the treatment of seizure disorders cannot be overemphasized. Diazepam and lorazepam are the first line of treatment in acute seizure episodes and status epilepticus. Clonazepam is indicated for absence and myoclonic seizures.

Valproic acid is a widely used antiepileptic drug that is active in many types of epilepsy. It works both by impeding sodium ion influx and by enhancing the effects of the inhibitory neurotransmitter, GABA. This drug is effective in myoclonic, absence and tonic-clonic seizures, but is usually used as adjunct therapy. Valproic acid is almost entirely metabolized in the liver, but unlike phenytoin, phenobarbital, and carbamazepine, it does not seem to induce drug-metabolizing enzymes.

Several newer antiepileptic drugs were developed and marketed in the last decade. They are used as secondary drugs in refractory epilepsies and are FDA approved as adjunctive therapy. Some of them are also effective as single agents for the treatment of epilepsy. Important newer agents include gabapentin (Neurontin®), oxcarbazepine (Trileptal®), lamotrigine (Lamictal®), topiramate (Topamax®), and levetiracetam (Keppra®). Felbamate (Felbatol®), another newer agent, has limited usefulness because of serious side effects. Lamotrigine inhibits the excitatory amino acid glutamine and inhibits sodium influx. Topiramate and levetiracetam may also inhibit sodium channels. Gabapentin, which is structurally related to GABA, is also useful for the treatment of neuropathic pain.

## Administration

Because epilepsy is often a disease of childhood, many antiepileptic medications are formulated for administration by a variety of routes. Initial dosing in children is calculated based on weight, therefore safe and effective dosing requires accurate weight information. Refer to **Table 13.2** for a comparison of available formulations and indications of the antiepileptic drugs discussed.

For rapid control of acute seizure episodes or in status epilepticus, diazepam or lorazepam is given by intravenous injection. Intramuscular administration is not recommended because absorption from the muscle is slow. When IV access is not available, diazepam can be given rectally and lorazepam tablets have been used sublingually. Phenytoin is available for IV injection, but must be given slowly. Neither diazepam nor phenytoin should be diluted for IV administration because of stability problems when diluted. Fosphenytoin can be given IV or IM.

Carbamazepine suspension provides higher serum levels than the same dose taken as a tablet. When converting from suspension to tablets, some dosing adjustment may be needed. Phenytoin suspension requires vigorous shaking to evenly distribute the drug before administration. Valproic acid and phenytoin can be taken with food to reduce GI irritation. Some drugs are available as chewable or quick dissolving oral tablets, and as sprinkle capsules. The content of sprinkle caps can be emptied into a small amount of soft food such as pudding or applesauce and swallowed. Mixtures should not be stored for later use.

Because gabapentin is not metabolized by the liver and is excreted by the kidneys, the dose is adjusted in patients with renal failure. It is not implicated in any drug interactions. Dosage reduction of topiramate and levetiracetam are also recommended in renal failure.

**Table 13.2** Comparison of Available Products, Indications, and Related Information for the Antiepileptic Medications

| Generic | Brand Name | Available as | Indications | Notes |
|---|---|---|---|---|
| **First-Choice Drugs** | | | | |
| Carbamazepine | Tegretol® | Tablets, chewable tabs, suspension, ER* tabs, & caps | Partial, generalized, & mixed seizures | Lab monitoring required, induces enzymes |
| Clonazepam | Klonopin® | Tablets, orally disintegrating tabs | Petit mal, myoclonic seizures | Controlled—CIV |
| Diazepam | Valium® | Injection, tablets, rectal gel, oral solution, oral concentrate | Status epilepticus (SE), acute seizures, all types | Controlled—CIV |
| Lorazepam | Ativan® | Injection, tablets | SE | Controlled—CIV |
| Ethosuximide | Zarontin® | Capsules, syrup | Absence seizures | |
| Phenytoin | Dilantin® | Injectable, suspension chewable tablets, capsules, ER caps | Grand mal, psycho-motor, SE | Shake suspension very well, induces enzymes |
| Fosphenytoin | Cerebyx® | Injection | SE, phenytoin loading dose | Converted to phenytoin |
| Phenobarbital | Luminal® | Injection, tablets, capsules, elixir | SE, generalized, & febrile seizures in infants and children | Controlled - CIV, induces enzymes |
| Primidone | Mysoline® | Tablets | Grand mal, psycho-motor or focal | |
| Valproic acid, divalproex | Depakene®, Depakote® | Tablets, suspension, ER tabs, sprinkle caps | Partial, mixed, and absence seizures | Also used in behavior disorders and migraines |
| **Adjunct Agents** | | | | |
| Felbamate | Felbatol® | Tablets, suspension | For resistant cases only | Liver failure, anemia |
| Gabapentin | Neurontin® | Capsules, tablets, solution | Adjunct therapy, partial seizures | Adjust dose in renal failure |
| Lamotrigine | Lamictal® | Tablets, chewable tabs | Partial seizures | Serious skin rashes |
| Levetiracetam | Keppra® | Tablets, oral solution | Adjunct therapy, partial seizures | Adjust dose in renal failure |
| Oxcarbazepine | Trileptal® | Tablets, suspension | Adjunct therapy, partial seizures | Induces enzymes, carbamazepine relative |
| Topiramate | Topamax® | Tablets, sprinkle capsules | Adjunct therapy, partial & generalized | Adjust dose in renal failure |

*ER, extended release.

Dosing adjustments may be required when additional antiepileptic medications are added, because of induction of drug metabolizing enzymes. The anticonvulsant medications cannot be abruptly discontinued without the risk of precipitating seizures.

nystagmus Involuntary, rapid side to side or up and down eye movement that may be an adverse drug effect.

gingival hyperplasia Proliferation of gum tissue, sometimes related to drug therapy.

aplastic anemia A form of anemia, often caused by toxic agents or drugs, that occurs when the bone marrow ceases to produce sufficient red and white blood cells.

## Side Effects

Most of the antiepileptic medications are considered central nervous system depressants and sedation, confusion, and ataxia (uncoordination) are known to occur, especially when therapy is initiated, or with higher doses. High phenytoin levels are associated with nystagmus, a rapid and involuntary movement of the eyeball. Nausea and vomiting are common reactions to phenytoin, carbamazepine, ethosuximide, and valproic acid. Gingival hyperplasia may cause the gums to grow over the teeth after long-term use of phenytoin. Because of interference with vitamin $B_{12}$ utilization, phenytoin can also cause anemia over time.

More serious adverse effects, although rare, can also occur. Carbamazepine can cause a reduction in white blood cells, as well as liver toxicity, and laboratory monitoring is necessary for the safe use of this drug. Oxcarbazepine side effects are similar to those of carbamazepine. Rare but serious toxicity to the liver can occur with administration of valproic acid. Felbamate has caused fatal liver failure and aplastic anemia, a kind of anemia that has a high risk of fatality. Phenobarbital and lamotrigine have caused very serious blistering rashes, including Stevens-Johnson syndrome. These rashes can cause extensive skin sloughing and fluid loss and in some cases are fatal. Topiramate is associated with an increased risk of kidney stones and patients should be encouraged to drink plenty of water as a preventative measure.

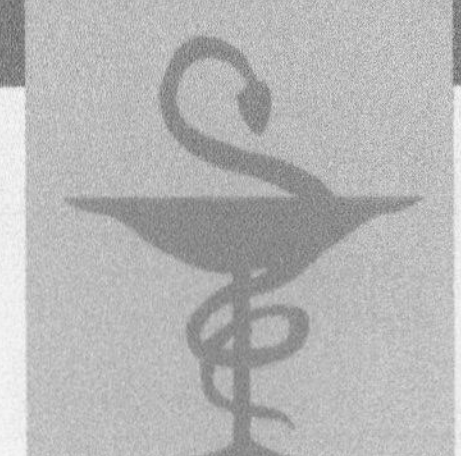

### Tips for the Technician

All suspensions must be shaken before administration and the technician should be sure that containers of suspensions are labelled "shake well." Phenytoin suspension is particularly susceptible to settling and parents need to be aware that therapeutic effects can be compromised if the drug is not evenly dispersed. Gabapentin solution must be refrigerated and "keep in the refrigerator" auxiliary labelling must be included on the final product. These medications can be taken with food to avoid GI upset. Topiramate prescriptions should be labelled with auxiliary directions encouraging the patient to take the medication with plenty of water. Alcohol consumption should be avoided in patients taking antiepileptic medications because it can contribute to sedation and, in some patients, can precipitate seizures.

The pharmacist's advice to clients should include the serious nature of the adverse effects associated with some of these drugs. Patients need to be instructed to report rashes immediately and to report sore throats that do not resolve in a few days time to their physicians. Patients with seizure disorders should be encouraged to wear medication alert bracelets, so that in the case of an acute seizure, emergency room personnel will have ready access to the patient's medication information.

Hospital pharmacy technicians may be asked to dilute phenytoin for use as an IV piggyback. Although some hospitals do mix phenytoin for immediate use in a small volume IV, compatibility data indicate that the stability of these admixtures in most solutions and concentrations is unreliable. Make sure you know and follow the policy where you work. Some facilities avoid the phenytoin dilution problem by only allowing fosphenytoin to be used for intravenous infusion. However, this drug is more expensive, and the brand name, Cerebyx®, can be confused with Celebrex® and Celexa®. Double-check the drug name before you prepare an admixture with this expensive product.

## Case 13.1

Mr. Dusty Rhodes asks to speak to the pharmacist about his son Rocky's seizure medication. The pharmacist notes that Rocky takes Dilantin® suspension, and he asks Mr. Rhodes how he can help. Rhodes states that his boy seems to get more drowsy and uncoordinated as they use the medication. When they get the new prescription, the drowsiness lets up a bit. He wants to know if there is something wrong with the medicine. What do you think might be happening? How can it be corrected?

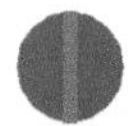

# Migraine Headaches

Although any headache is disagreeable, migraine headaches can be incapacitating. About 10% of the population suffers from migraines, and they are three times more likely to occur in women than men. Patients typically describe migraine headaches as causing moderate to severe pain, usually with a pulsing or throbbing quality, and often on only one side of the head. In a significant number of migraine sufferers, headaches are accompanied by nausea (sometimes with vomiting) and sensitivity to light and sound. In some patients, migraines are preceded by a prodrome, or sometimes by an aura. A prodrome is a set of symptoms that occur as much as a day before the headache begins that tip victims off to the coming headache. These symptoms may include tiredness, irritability, thirst, and a craving for sweets, among others. Auras are a set of sensory signs that usually begin minutes before a headache. These can include flashes of light, dazzling lines through the field of vision or other visual changes, or tingling in one arm or leg.

aura A subjective sensation that precedes an attack of a neurological disorder, such as epilepsy or migraine headache.

All headache pain can be triggered by stress or hormonal changes, and migraine headaches are no exception. In addition, some patients report that certain foods trigger their headaches. Although the pathology of migraine headaches is not completely understood, researchers believe that abnormalities in trigeminal nerve (one of the twelve cranial nerves) function are involved. Experts do know that serotonin levels fall during a headache. These falling serotonin levels are thought to trigger an inflammatory process that results in vasodilation and pain.

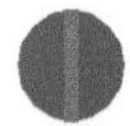

# Treatment of Migraine Headaches

The goal of treating migraine headaches is to reduce their frequency and severity, and to restore the patient's ability to function by controlling pain and shortening the duration of the headaches. Available treatments include drugs that may prevent headaches from occurring and drugs to treat the pain associated with migraines. Preventative medications include beta-blockers, usually used for the treatment of cardiovascular disease and high blood pressure, tricyclic and SSRI antidepressants, anti-inflammatory drugs such as ibuprofen, and the antiseizure medicines valproic acid and gabapentin. Refer to the appropriate chapters for more information on these drugs.

The ergot alkaloids and triptans are drugs used to treat migraine headache pain. Sumatriptan (Imitrex®) was the first drug specifically developed to treat migraines. The ergot alkaloids are very old drugs derived from the rye fungus, Claviceps purpurea. Their actions are less specific than the triptans, and therefore can cause a greater variety of adverse effects.

## Triptans

Although sumatriptan is the prototype of this drug class, several related drugs are available. Three of these are almotriptan (Axert®), rizatriptan (Maxalt®), and zolmitriptan (Zomig®). These migraine-specific treatments are used in people with moderately to severely disabling migraines.

### Actions and Indications

The triptans are indicated for the acute treatment of migraines headaches. They are reserved for patients with disabling headaches that are not responsive to other pain-relieving drugs. Although not approved by the FDA for use in children, there have been clinical trials of these drugs in pediatric and adolescent populations where they were shown to be effective. These drugs are selective agonists at serotonin receptors. By activating serotonin receptors in the cranial arteries, the triptans cause vasoconstriction and reduce inflammation.

### Administration

Some of the triptans can be administered by injection or by nasal spray. This is an advantage, since many headache sufferers have nausea along with their headaches. Injectable formulations are much faster acting, with relief occurring in less than 30 minutes. Sumatriptan and zolmitriptan are available for subcutaneous injection, as tablets, and as a nasal spray. Refer to **Table 13.3** for a summary of the drugs used to treat acute migraine headaches.

**Table 13.3** A Comparison of Available Product Formulations and Indications for Drugs Used to Treat Acute Migraine Headaches

| Generic | Brand Name | Available as | Indications | Notes |
|---|---|---|---|---|
| **Triptans** | | | | |
| Almotriptan | Axert® | Tablet | Acute migraine headaches | |
| Rizatriptan | Maxalt® | Tablet, buccal tablet | Acute migraine headaches | |
| Sumatriptan | Imitrex® | Injection, tablets, nasal spray | Acute migraine headaches | Single-use nasal spray |
| Zolmitriptan | Zomig® | Injection, tablets, buccal tablets, nasal spray | Acute migraine headaches | Single-use nasal spray |
| **Ergot alkaloids** | | | | |
| Dihydroergotamine | D.H.E. 45®, Migranal® | Injection, intranasal | Acute migraine headaches | Keep cool, protect from light |
| Ergotamine | Cafergot®, Ergomar® | Combined with caffeine in supps or tabs, alone in SL tabs | Acute migraine headaches | |

SL, sublingual.

### Side Effects

Although these drugs are fairly well tolerated by most headache patients, there are some side effects and some contraindications to their use. The triptans should not be used in people with coronary artery diseases, such as chest pain, poorly controlled high blood pressure, or recent heart attack. Their use is avoided in people who have risk factors for stroke. People who have taken an ergot alkaloid, an SSRI, or another serotonin agonist for migraine within the past day cannot use these drugs.

When they occur, side effects are likely to include flushing or a feeling of warmth, dizziness, or tingling in the arms or legs. Less frequently, changes in blood pressure can occur. People with a history of heart disease can develop chest pain or palpitations. Use of the nasal spray is associated with a bad taste in the mouth and sometimes throat or mouth irritation or pain.

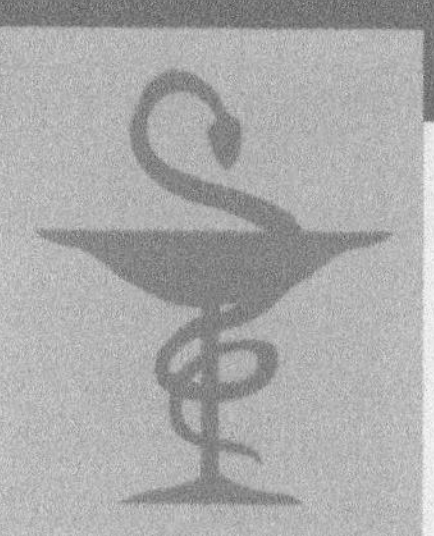

**Tips for the Technician**

Some of the triptans are given by injection. It is important to verify with patients that they know how to prepare the skin and use the injection device. If they are not familiar with the product, be certain they speak to a pharmacist. The pharmaceutical companies that make Imitrex® and Zomig® have patient information leaflets on the use of their devices available for downloading from their websites.

## Ergot Alkaloids

The vasoconstrictive action of the ergot alkaloids has been known for centuries. During the Middle Ages, bread made from flour contaminated with Claviceps purpurea was known to cause ergotism, ergot toxicity associated with vasoconstriction so severe the limbs became gangrenous. During the twentieth century the ergot alkaloids were shown to be helpful for the treatment of migraines. They were considered the standard of care for treatment of acute migraines for many years. The ergot derivatives were traditionally combined with other ingredients, including aspirin, sometimes a sedative, and caffeine. A number of ergot alkaloid products are still available. Although they are effective, their use has declined because of their lack of specificity.

### Actions and Indication

Ergot alkaloids are nonspecific alpha-adrenergic, dopaminergic, and serotonin agonists. They cause vasoconstriction in the cranial arteries and in the peripheral blood vessels, and they are highly active uterine muscle stimulants. Ergotamine (Ergomar®, Cafergot®) and dihydroergotamine (Migranal®, D.H.E. 45®) are indicated for the treatment of acute migraine headaches. Although not the drug of first choice, ergotamine is also indicated for prevention of migraine headaches. Caffeine is added to some ergot derivatives because it, too, is a cranial vasoconstrictor.

### Administration

Dihydroergotamine can be administered by the intravenous, intramuscular, or subcutaneous route for treatment of a migraine attack. Migranal® is dihydroergotamine in a preparation for nasal administration. Ergomar® tablets are sublingual tablets used at the first signs of an impending attack to prevent the oncoming headache. Use of these tablets is limited to three in 1 day and five total in a week in order to prevent rebound headaches. Cafergot® rectal suppositories contain ergotamine and caffeine, and are used to treat migraine headaches.

### Side Effects

Because they are potent uterine stimulants, ergot alkaloids cannot be given to pregnant women with migraines. Ergot derivatives are contraindicated for use in people with peripheral vascular disease and coronary artery disease, or individuals with poorly controlled high blood pressure. The ergot alkaloids frequently cause nausea or vomiting. Tingling of the fingers, weakness in the legs, and itching occur less frequently. Rarely, these drugs can be associated with heart attack and abnormal rhythms. The nasal spray causes a bad taste in the mouth, nausea, and runny nose in 10% or more of cases. Patients who take the ergot derivatives can develop a type of dependence where headaches return more frequently and the dose required for relief increases.

The ergot derivatives are implicated in a number of important drug interactions. They should not be taken with the serotonin agonists, certain antifungals, some antiviral medications, or the macrolide antibiotics because of the increased risk of excessive vasoconstriction.

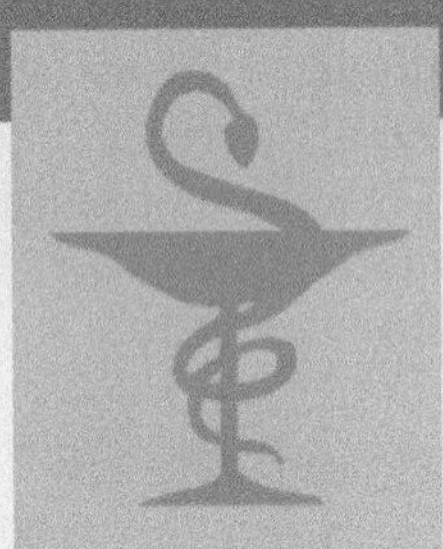

### Tips for the Technician

Dihydroergotamine products must be kept cool (less than 77°F) and protected from light. While the injection can be refrigerated, the nasal spray cannot. When dispensing the nasal spray, be certain to include the patient information booklet. Cafergot suppositories should be stored in the refrigerator. Be sure to label all ergot products with auxiliary instructions warning patients to avoid taking these drugs during pregnancy.

# Review Questions

## Multiple Choice

For the following questions, choose the best answer.

1. Treatment for Parkinson's disease is directed at which of the following?
   a. Restoring levels of norepinephrine by blocking breakdown in the synapse
   b. Restoring the balance between serotonin and dopamine
   c. Restoring the balance between acetylcholine and dopamine by increasing levels of acetylcholine
   d. Increasing levels of serotonin
   e. Restoring relative levels of dopamine by replacing it, preventing its destruction, or by reducing cholinergic input

2. Which of the following characterizes Parkinson's disease?
   a. Tardive dyskinesia, akathisia, dystonia
   b. Delusions, hallucinations, cognitive impairment
   c. Inability to stay awake, eye blinking, muscle wasting
   d. Tremors, shuffling gait, and muscle rigidity
   e. None of the above

3. Which of the following are typical side effects of drugs that increase dopamine levels?
   a. Nausea, vomiting, loss of appetite, hypotension
   b. Constipation, weight gain, euphoria
   c. Vivid dreams, dry eyes, hypertension
   d. Ringing in the ears, elevated blood glucose
   e. All of the above

4. Which of the following mechanisms is not one by which antiepileptic medications exert their effect?
   a. Interference with sodium and calcium ion movement in neurons
   b. Potentiation of the inhibitory effects of GABA
   c. Block reuptake of dopamine
   d. Inhibition of excitatory input
   e. Agonist activity at the benzodiazepine receptor

5. Migraine sufferers should avoid which of the following medications while receiving ergot derivatives for their migraine headaches?
   a. Valproic acid derivatives
   b. Caffeine
   c. Erythromycin
   d. Lamotrigine
   e. None of the above

## True/False

6. There is no treatment at present that halts the destruction of dopamine producing cells in the basal ganglia, which is the underlying cause of Parkinson's disease.
   a. True
   b. False

7. Abrupt discontinuation of dopamine-agonists should be avoided because of the potential for causing a syndrome similar to neuroleptic malignant syndrome.
   a. True
   b. False

8. The sudden, excessive, and simultaneous discharge of cerebral neurons is common to generalized forms of epilepsy only.
   a. True
   b. False

9. The pharmacist does not need to counsel new patients with epilepsy because the medications are all quite safe and effective.
   a. True
   b. False

10. Chronic use of the ergot derivatives is dangerous because it causes the frequency of headaches and the dosage required for successful treatment to increase.
   a. True
   b. False

### Matching

For questions 11 to 15, match each drug name with the lettered choice that lists correct information associated with that drug. Answer choices may be used once or not at all.

11. Ethosuximide
12. Valproic Acid
13. Primidone
14. Phenytoin
15. Gabapentin

a. Induces its own and other drugs metabolism
b. Indicated only for the treatment of petit mal
c. Excreted unchanged by the kidneys
d. Metabolized to phenytoin
e. Can cause rare, but serious liver toxicity
f. Converted to phenobarbital
g. Indicated for migraine headaches

### Short Answer

16. What is status epilepticus and what are the drugs likely to be used to treat it?
17. Describe the goal of treatment of Parkinson's disease and the different classes of drugs available for treatment.
18. List four side effects that can be attributed to excess dopamine concentrations outside of the central nervous system.
19. Why should antiepileptic drugs not be abruptly discontinued?
20. After initial dosing, on what basis are dose adjustments made in patients taking phenytoin? What are the characteristics of phenytoin that can make it difficult adjust?

## FOR FURTHER INQUIRY

Read the book *The Spirit Catches You and You Fall Down* by Anne Fadiman. If you can convince some classmates to read it with you, spend an hour discussing it. Does the book change your impression of health care as it is delivered in the United States? How do you think it will affect the way you interact with people who are sick?

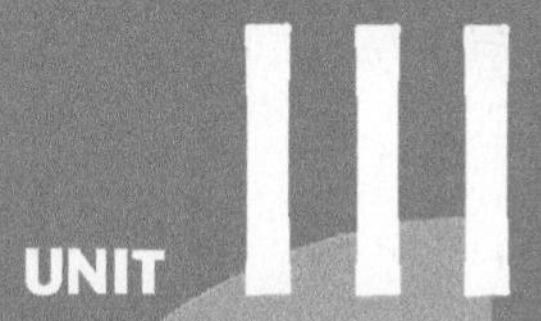

UNIT III

# Drugs Affecting the Cardiovascular System

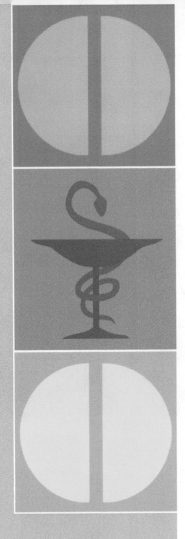

Chapter **14**

# The Anatomy and Physiology of the Cardiovascular System

## OBJECTIVES

After studying this chapter, the reader should be able to:

- Explain the physiologic function of the cardiovascular system and list its anatomical components.
- Describe the conduction of a normal electrical impulse through the heart and a factor that could change the rate of contraction of the heart.
- Trace the pathway of a drop of blood from the left ventricle around the body and back to the left atrium, including a description of how the how blood perfuses organs.
- List the components of the blood and describe the function of each.
- List three diseases of the cardiovascular system and one preventative measure for each that would reduce the incidence or severity of the disease.

*KEY TERMS*

- aggregate
- anemia
- aorta
- atherosclerosis
- atrioventricular node
- baroreceptors
- cardiac output
- complement
- conduction system
- diastole
- edema
- endothelium
- erythrocytes
- glucose
- granulocyte
- heart failure
- hemolysis
- leukemia
- leukocytes
- myocardial infarction

- myocarditis
- myocardium
- normal sinus rhythm
- perfuse
- pericardium
- plasma proteins
- platelets
- sinoatrial node
- systole
- thalassemia
- thrombocytopenia
- vasculature

The heart has been the subject of study since the beginning of recorded history. Most of the ancient studies of the heart were highly inaccurate because they were undertaken with prejudices stemming from misinformation. A perfect example of this was the extensive work of Galen, the Greek physician and philosopher. He lived during the second century AD and his studies on anatomy were groundbreaking at the time, but rife with errors. Galen proposed that arteries were responsible for pumping blood. His work was so influential that his erroneous conclusions regarding the cardiovascular system were virtually cast in stone for the next 1,500 years. It wasn't until 1533, when the great anatomist Vesalius was a medical student, that the true nature and function of the heart finally began to be examined. Later, the British physician William Harvey used observation and experimentation to accurately explain the contraction of the heart and the circulation of the blood through the body.

Today, not only are the anatomical features of the cardiovascular system well described, we also have an excellent understanding of its physiology. The cardiovascular system is made up of the heart, blood vessels, and the blood, and it is intimately connected with the lungs, both structurally and in function. Within this system the heart acts as a pump, and is responsible for moving oxygenated blood and nutrients to the organs and tissues, and returning deoxygenated blood to the lungs for removal of carbon dioxide and for reoxygenation.

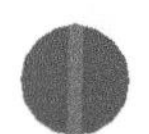

## The Heart

The human heart beats unceasingly, at a rate of about 70 strokes every minute. This occurs without conscious thought for our entire lives. As William Harvey wrote, "The heart is the foundation of life, the sovereign of everything within, that upon which all growth depends, from which all power proceeds." A normal adult heart is about the size of an adult's fist and is located between the lungs and to the left of the midline of the body. The heart is divided into two halves, and each half contains two chambers. The uppermost chambers are called the right and left atria, and the lower chambers are the right and left ventricles. One-way valves are located at the junction between the two chambers and at the outlet of the ventricles. The valves prevent the backflow of blood, which allows for efficient, unidirectional circulation. **Figure 14.1** illustrates the heart and its chambers, the orientation of the major vessels, and the flow of blood.

The walls of the heart are made up of muscle, called the myocardium, which is anatomically similar to skeletal muscle. The outer wall of the heart is lined with a thin but tough tissue called the pericardium. A small quantity of fluid between the sac formed by the pericardium and the myocardium reduces friction between the two surfaces during muscle contraction. Like all muscles, the heart requires a continuous supply of oxygen and the removal of the waste products produced by consumption of energy. The myocardium is perfused with oxygenated blood by the coronary arteries and drained of deoxygena blood and the waste products of metabolism by the coronary veins.

myocardium The muscular walls of the heart.

pericardium The membranous sac that encloses the

Although the heart is divided into right and left halves, the two halves contract sim taneously. The contraction cycle of the myocardium begins in the atria. When the atria c tract they push blood through one-way valves, forcing it into the ventricles. Immediat thereafter, the ventricles contract. The contraction of the right ventricle sends deoxygena blood into the pulmonary circulation, where the lungs remove carbon dioxide and resup the blood with oxygen. The contraction of the left ventricle forces oxygenated blood i the aorta to enter the systemic circulation. This not quite simultaneous contraction of t upper and lower chambers of the heart results in the "lub-dub" sound of a heartbeat. T contraction of the chambers, referred to as systole, is followed by the relaxation of the at and then the ventricles during diastole.

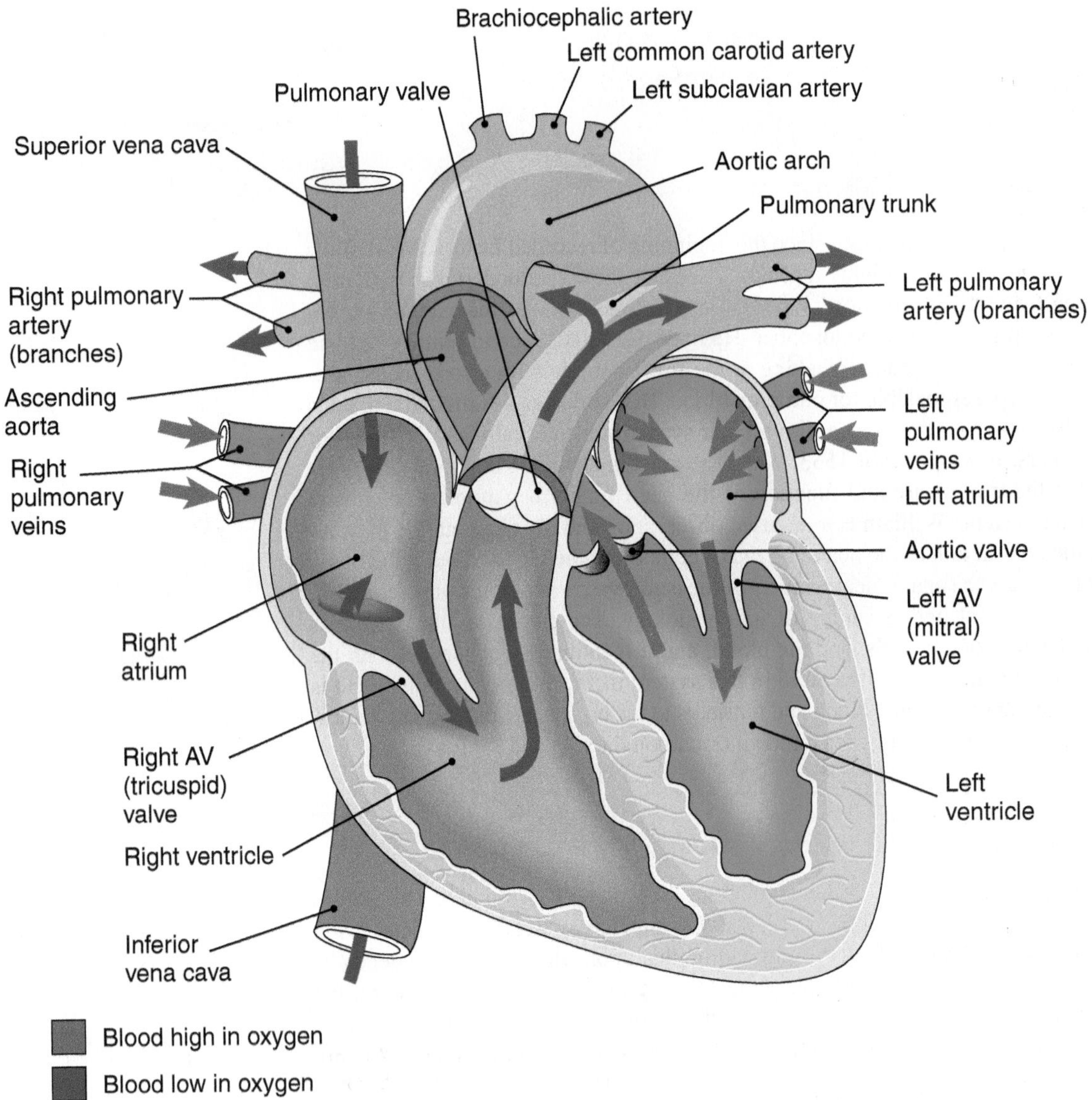


**Figure 14.1** The heart and major vessels. Arrows show the flow of blood. (Adapted with permission from Cohen BJ. *Memmler's The Human Body in Health and Disease,* 10th edition. Baltimore: Lippincott Williams & Wilkins, 2005.)

conduction system The system in the heart responsible for moving electrical impulses from the atria to the ventricles; responsible for cardiac muscle contraction.

sinoatrial node Tissue that is the site of origin of the mpulses that stimulate the rtbeat.

ricular node conduction eart that ceived de

The heart functions automatically, and is under the control of the autonomic nervous system. The myocardium is stimulated to contract by electrical impulses that travel through specialized tissue of the cardiac conduction system. Contraction begins at the sinoatrial node (SA node), a small area of tissue located in the upper wall of the right atrium. The SA node automatically generates an electrical impulse, or action potential, at a rate of about 70 per minute, and is the heart's pacemaker. This electrical impulse causes the atria to contract. The action potential travels down specialized fibers to a second node, the atrioventricular node (AV node). Here, the electrical impulse causes the AV node to fire. This secondary impulse continues downward through conducting fibers called the Bundle of His to cause the contraction of the ventricles. A tracing of the electrical activity of the heart can by recorded by means of an electrocardiograph (EKG or ECG), an instrument that picks up and records the electrical activity of the heart. A normal EKG tracing is illustrated in **Figure 14.2**.

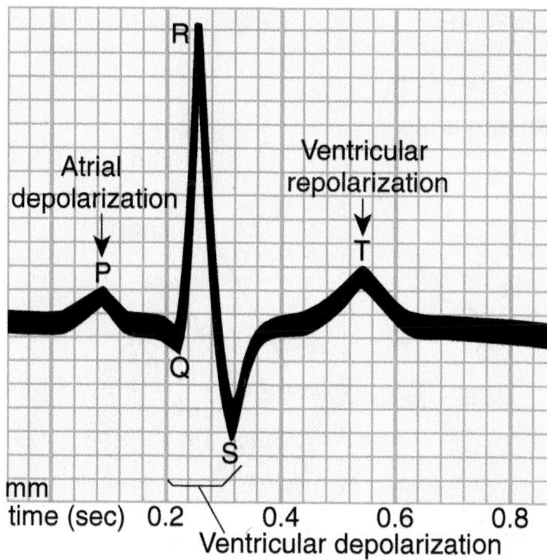


**Figure 14.2** A normal EKG tracing of a single cardiac cycle. (Adapted with permission from Cohen BJ. *Memmler's The Human Body in Health and Disease,* 10th edition. Baltimore: Lippincott Williams & Wilkins, 2005.)

The normal and regular beat of the heart, which is initiated at the SA node and travels down through the AV node to the ventricles, is called normal sinus rhythm. The rate of the heartbeat is modified by input from the autonomic nervous system. Sympathetic stimulation, such as during the fight or flight response or when blood pressure falls, can dramatically increase the heart rate and the force of contraction. The result is increased output of blood, or cardiac output, in response to an increased need perceived by the nervous system. Cardiac output is described as the total volume of blood the heart pumps in one minute. Along with blood pressure and heart rate, cardiac output is maintained in a normal range through feedback from the autonomic nervous system. During periods of rest, the parasympathetic nervous system input maintains the firing of the SA node, and therefore the heart rate, at the resting pace.

normal sinus rhythm The normal and regular heart rhythm, generated by the sinoatrial node.

cardiac output Measurement of the volume of blood ejected by the heart to the systemic circulation, expressed as liters per minute.

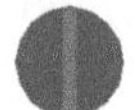

## The Blood Vessels

The blood vessels of the cardiovascular system form two circuits, the pulmonary and systemic circulation, which carry deoxygenated blood to the lungs and oxygenated blood to the body, respectively. **Figure 14.3** is a schematic drawing of the cardiovascular system. There are three general categories of vessels in the body: arteries, capillaries, and veins. The size and characteristics of blood vessels in the body vary with their function.

The walls of both arteries and veins are made up of an outer layer of connective tissue, smooth muscle for elasticity, and a thin layer of endothelium lining the inside. The walls of arteries are thicker and tougher than veins because they carry blood pumped under about fifty times the pressure found inside of veins. The smooth muscle of the blood vessels is under autonomic nervous system control, and alpha adrenergic receptors predominate (refer to Chapter 6 for a review of alpha receptors). Elasticity of blood vessels is an important factor in the ability of the body to regulate blood pressure and maintain adequate blood flow.

endothelium Type of epithelial cells that line blood vessels and the cavities of the heart.

Pressure sensors called baroreceptors are located in the walls of the aorta, the large artery that carries blood away from the left ventricle, and in other crucial locations. These receptors trigger a rapid response in the case of a significant change in blood pressure. Feedback from these sensors goes to the central nervous system, where increased sympathetic activity causes vessel walls to constrict (vasoconstriction) and decreased sympathetic activity causes vessels to dilate (vasodilation). This ability to quickly respond to significant changes in blood pressure can be lifesaving in certain situations (significant blood loss, for example), where vasoconstriction or vasodilation can assure at least temporary blood flow to vital organs. These same receptors play a role in maintaining blood pressure in the normal range when the body is in a normal state.

baroreceptors Specialized tissue in the walls of the large arteries and the atria that senses changes in blood pressure.

aorta The largest artery in the body, the aorta originates in the heart and branches to carry the blood through the body.

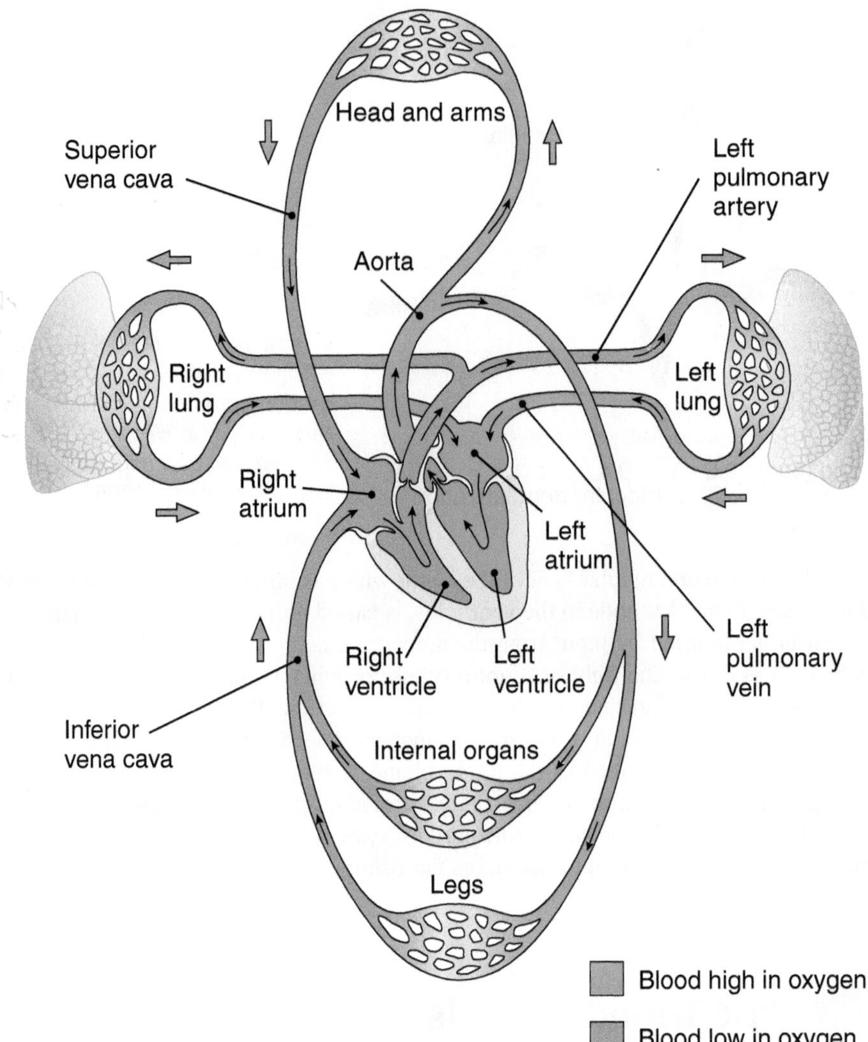


**Figure 14.3** This schematic representation of the circulatory system demonstrates that the right side of the heart pumps blood into the lungs to be oxygenated and the left side pumps oxygenated blood to the systemic circulation. (Reprinted with permission from Cohen BJ. *Memmler's The Human Body in Health and Disease*, 10th edition. Baltimore: Lippincott Williams & Wilkins, 2005.)

The pressure that blood exerts against the walls of blood vessels varies depending on blood volume, cardiac output, and the degree of resistance of the blood vessels. Blood vessels that are constricted because of increased sympathetic activity, or are less elastic due to other factors, present more resistance to blood flow. Blood pressures are reported as two numbers, systolic and diastolic pressures. Systolic pressure is measured during contraction of the heart and diastolic during the relaxation phase. Normal resting blood pressure in adults should be less than 135 systolic and less than 80 diastolic. Blood pressure is expressed in millimeters of mercury (mmHg).

perfuse To force a fluid through tissue, especially by way of the blood vessels.

The aorta carries oxygenated blood away from the left side of the heart. Blood moves from the aorta, the largest artery in the body at about one inch in diameter, to smaller arteries and then to arterioles. Arterioles deliver blood to the capillary beds. Essential organs, such as the brain, liver and kidneys, as well as other tissues, are perfused with nutrient rich blood via the capillaries.

glucose The sugar that is the end product of carbohydrate metabolism and the main source of energy for living things.

Capillaries form a sort of netting between the arteries and veins. Capillaries are extremely thin walled; the walls are made of a single endothelial cell layer and basement membrane. Their diameter is so small that blood cells must move through them single file. It is in the capillary beds that the work of cellular respiration occurs. Here, oxygen needed for metabolic processes in the tissues is exchanged for carbon dioxide, the byproduct of metabolic processes. Fluids, white blood cells, glucose (a sugar that is a readily utilizable source of energy for the body), endogenous chemical messengers involved in immune and other responses, and drugs can move in and out between the gaps in the capillary walls too. The exchange of fluids and small compounds occurs mainly by diffusion.

### Analogy

The circulatory system can be compared to the nation's highway system. The roadways allow vehicles that carry important products to reach small towns and big cities all over the country. We can compare the vehicles, carrying produce and other essentials, to the blood and blood cells, which carry oxygen and nutrients to our organs and tissues. In this analogy, the system of roads is comparable to the circulatory system of the human body. In the cities and towns (our tissues), where the number of roads increases and the size of the roads decrease, the exchange of goods takes place, as it does in the capillary beds. Just as there are thousands of miles of roads in this country, there are also thousands of miles of blood vessels in every human body. If all the blood vessels of an adult human were strung end to end, it is estimated they would extend 60,000 miles, enough to circumnavigate the globe twice!

After blood circulates through the capillary beds, it returns via the veins. Capillaries return blood containing waste products to the venules, which are smaller diameter veins, then into veins, which in turn carry the blood on its way back to the heart. Because veins must push blood against the force of gravity, they usually contain valves that prevent backflow of blood. **Figure 14.4** illustrates the anatomy of arteries, veins and capillaries.

Two large-diameter veins, the superior and inferior vena cava, empty deoxygenated blood directly into the right atrium. This deoxygenated blood moves into the right ventricle, where it enters the pulmonary circulation via the right and left pulmonary arteries. In the lungs, carbon dioxide is removed and oxygen is absorbed into the pulmonary vasculature, or network of blood vessels. Oxygenated blood is returned via the pulmonary veins to begin the process of circulation all over again.

vasculature The arrangement of blood vessels in an organ or area.

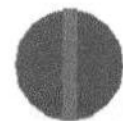

## The Blood

The blood serves the crucial role of transporting all of the many elements needed for life to every part of the body. It carries nutrients away from the GI tract to the organs responsible for converting these nutrients into proteins and tissues, and carries oxygen to every tissue of the body. The blood is crucial for defending the body against invaders and catastrophes of all sorts. It brings the antibodies and cells necessary for immune defences to where they are needed, and carries drugs, toxins, and waste products of metabolism to the lungs, liver, and kidneys for removal. Blood contains constituents called clotting factors that keep us from bleeding to death when we cut ourselves. Many of the regulatory systems of the human body are dependant on blood flow, including regulation of body temperature. Hormones, water, salts, proteins, and other compounds carried by the blood affect fluid balance, the acidity of the blood, and the function of organs.

### Components of the Blood

The blood is composed of both solids and fluid. The solid, or formed, elements of the blood include the various blood cells. The fluid portion of the blood is called plasma, and is made up of about 90% water. Of the total blood volume, a little more than half is plasma. Besides

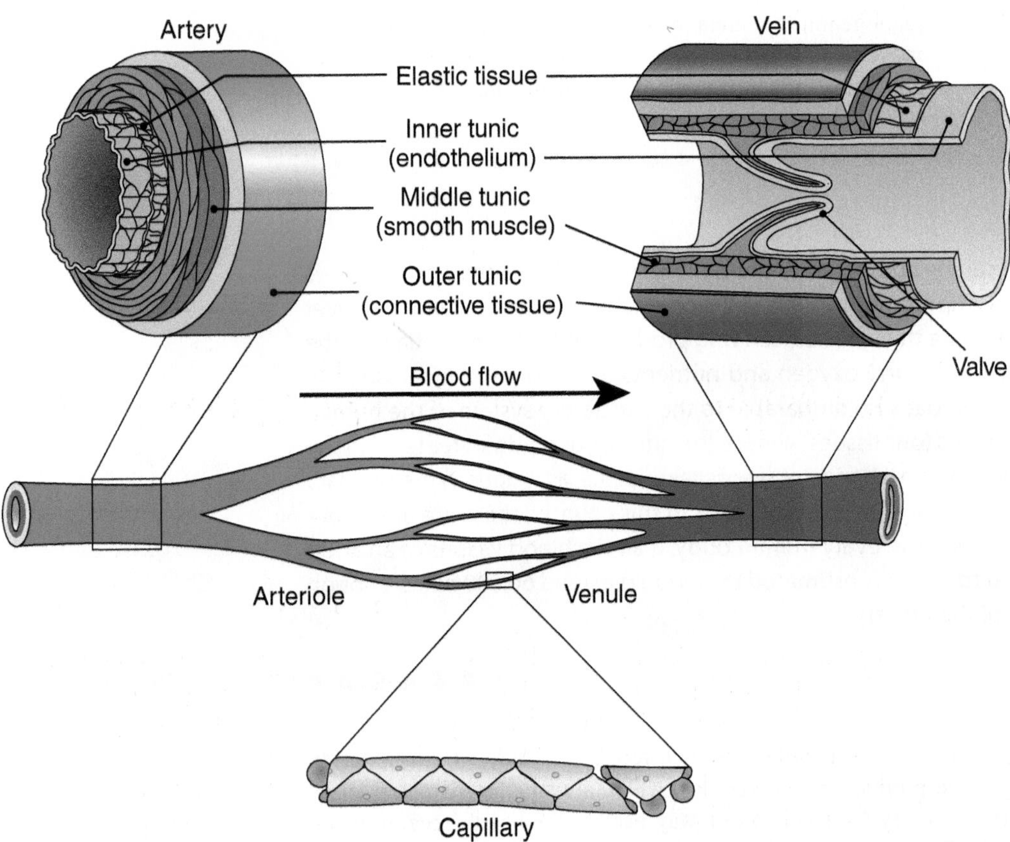


**Figure 14.4** Illustration compares the anatomy of the thick-walled artery, the vein, with valves, and the single-cell layered wall of the capillary. (Reprinted with permission from Cohen BJ. *Memmler's The Human Body in Health and Disease,* 10th edition. Baltimore: Lippincott Williams & Wilkins, 2005.)

plasma proteins Dissolved proteins of blood plasma including mainly albumin and antibodies.

complement A group of about 20 serum proteins which, working in tandem with other parts of the immune system, activate pathways that cause the destruction of specific antigens.

leukocytes General term for any type of white blood cells.

granulocyte White blood cells that contain granules in the cytoplasm.

water, plasma contains other substances, including glucose, electrolytes, lipids such as cholesterol and triglycerides, and a variety of proteins referred to as plasma proteins (see **Fig. 14.5**).

The most abundant plasma protein is albumin. Albumin is important for keeping fluid within the blood vessels, and carrying drugs and other compounds to their destinations. Levels of albumin in the blood serve as a marker for nutritional status. Clotting factors are proteins that are essential to the normal blood clotting mechanism and include thrombin and fibrin. Albumin and clotting factors are synthesized in the liver. Antibodies and complement, a group of proteins that cause the destruction of some "foreign" cells, make up another important portion of the plasma protein. Antibodies are produced by specialized white blood cells, and function to identify foreign cells, bacteria, or other proteins. When antibodies attach to invading substances, they trigger the complement system, a group of about 30 enzymes, most of which are synthesized in the liver, that help to carry out the destruction of the identified substances.

There are three types of blood cells, all produced in the bone marrow. Leukocytes, or white blood cells (**Fig. 14.6**), are specialized cells essential to combating disease and closely involved with inflammation and allergic reactions. There are a variety of types of white blood cells. The granulocytes are white blood cells that contain packets of enzymes that are stained by dyes used for identification in laboratories. Granulocytes include the neutrophils, which are the most abundant type of white blood cell, the eosinophils, whose

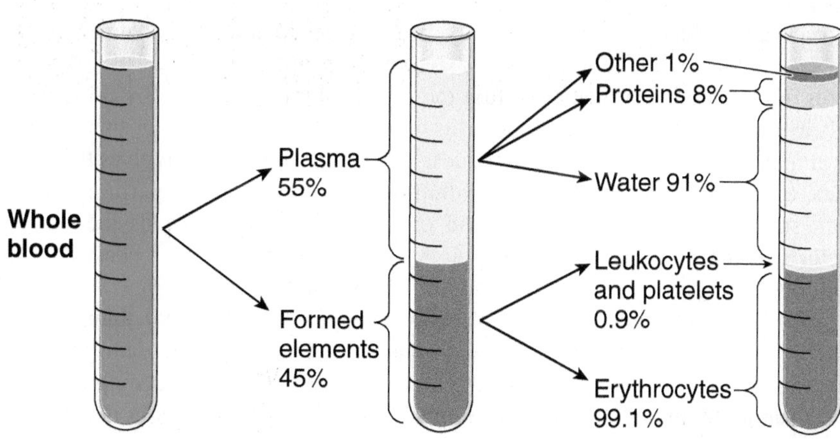


**Figure 14.5** The composition of whole blood with the normal proportions of the formed elements and components of plasma. (Reprinted with permission from Cohen BJ. *Memmler's The Human Body in Health and Disease,* 10th edition. Baltimore: Lippincott Williams & Wilkins, 2005.)

numbers increase in allergic reactions and parasitic diseases, and the basophils. After the physical barrier provided by the skin, the neutrophils are the body's first line of defense against infection. Lymphocytes are the next most common white blood cell form and are important in recognition of foreign proteins and production of antibody. Production of white blood cells is increased when there is infection, and also in some types of leukemia.

Erythrocytes, or red blood cells, are rich in hemoglobin, the iron-containing protein that carries oxygen to the tissues. Mature red blood cells have no nucleus and therefore cannot divide. They are by far the most numerous of all the cellular components of the blood and they only last about 120 days in the systemic circulation before they are removed. In order to keep up with the necessary production of erythrocytes, the bone marrow requires an adequate supply of protein, iron, folic acid and other nutrients. Production of red blood cells in the bone marrow is stimulated by erythropoietin, a hormone produced by the kidneys.

erythrocytes Red blood cells.

Platelets, or thrombocytes, are the smallest of the formed elements. Platelets are not cells in the classic sense of containing a nucleus and other cellular components. They are irregularly shaped bodies produced in the bone marrow that play a crucial role in blood clotting. When the blood comes into contact with any tissue other than the smooth endothelial lining of the normal blood vessel, chemical signals from the damaged tissues cause platelets to collect. The activated platelets become sticky and form a seal over the damaged tissues. This, in turn, activates other processes that begin the formation of a clot.

platelets A tiny, disk-shaped, non-nucleated body found in the bloodstream that plays a key role in blood clotting.

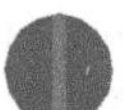

# Diseases of the Cardiovascular System

Diseases of the cardiovascular system are the most common causes of death in industrialized nations. Cardiovascular diseases affect every process within the cardiovascular system, and often affect multiple processes. Primary diseases of the heart can cause direct damage to the myocardium, such as with myocarditis (inflammation of the myocardium),

myocarditis Inflammation of the muscular walls of the heart.

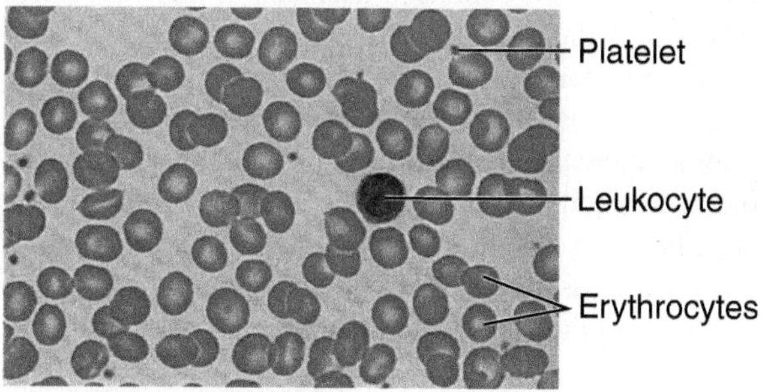


**Figure 14.6** Erythrocytes, leukocytes, and platelets as viewed through a microscope. (Reprinted with permission from Cohen BJ. *Memmler's The Human Body in Health and Disease,* 10th edition. Baltimore: Lippincott Williams & Wilkins, 2005.)

damage to the valves, such as rheumatic heart disease or endocarditis, or damage to the conduction system that results in arrhythmias, abnormal heart rhythms.

atherosclerosis The progressive narrowing of the arteries caused by fatty deposits and fibrosis of the vessels.

Diseases of the blood vessels that perfuse the myocardium can eventually cause damage to the heart. In atherosclerosis, fatty deposits narrow the arteries, and can significantly reduce the amount of oxygen delivered to tissues. When atherosclerosis involves the coronary arteries, oxygen delivered to the myocardium is reduced in the area perfused by the artery in question. When the oxygen demand of the myocardium exceeds the supply, angina pectoris, or chest pain, occurs. A typical angina patient describes chest pain as crushing or constricting, as though an elephant is standing on his chest.

aggregate To collect or gather into a mass, as when platelets aggregate to form a thrombus.

myocardial infarction An area of tissue death in the myocardium resulting from obstruction of the local circulation due to a blood clot; heart attack.

As atherosclerotic changes progress, deposits damage the endothelial lining of the blood vessels, causing platelets to aggregate, or gather at the site of the damage. Once platelets aggregate, clots are likely to form. A clot in a coronary artery can completely cut off the blood supply to an area of the myocardium. When the oxygen supply is cut off, a portion of the myocardium dies. This is referred to as myocardial infarction (MI), or heart attack. Symptoms of an MI include severe, crushing pain that may seem to radiate down the left arm or into the neck or jaw, shortness of breath, sweating, and nausea and vomiting. Some people experiencing an MI may develop shock, lose consciousness, or die before they can receive treatment. Survival depends on the speed of treatment and the extent of damage to the cardiac muscle. People who survive MI often end up with cardiac arrhythmias or heart failure.

heart failure Condition where inefficient contraction of the heart muscle results in reduced blood circulation; compensatory mechanisms lead to fluid retention and further deterioration.

Heart failure (HF) occurs when the heart cannot keep up with the demand for perfusion and can be a result of MI, arrhythmia, or high blood pressure. If the heart is damaged or has to constantly pump against excessive pressure, the muscle will begin to stretch and weaken, and eventually fail. When the heart weakens, it no longer efficiently provides adequate oxygen to the tissues. Body mechanisms increase fluid retention in an attempt to increase perfusion of tissues, and the strain on the heart increases further. The heart eventually stretches beyond its capacity to efficiently pump, and fluid backs up, causing congestion of tissues with fluid, referred to as edema. This stage of heart failure is referred to as congestive heart failure (CHF). Edema that collects in the lungs is called pulmonary edema and is a very serious condition.

edema Abnormal accumulation of fluid in the spaces between cells, especially subcutaneous tissue.

hypertension Persistently elevated blood pressure.

Hypertension, chronically elevated blood pressure, is estimated to affect 50 million Americans. Most people with hypertension never experience any symptoms, and may never be diagnosed or treated for the condition. Untreated hypertension can have disastrous results, including stroke and heart failure. Hypertension is more common in African-American people, and people who smoke. Other risk factors include age, family history, and other conditions, such as diabetes.

Strokes, or cerebrovascular accidents (CVA), are caused when the oxygen supply to an area of the brain is cut off. This can happen when a blood vessel in the brain ruptures, causing blood to flood an area of the brain tissue, which results in damage from increased pressure and lack of oxygen, or when a blood clot cuts off circulation and oxygen supply. Stroke is the third-leading cause of death in the United States, and is usually directly related to atherosclerotic vessel disease, hypertension, or drug abuse. People who survive strokes often have significant residual disability, including paralysis, inability to speak, or loss of cognitive abilities.

Prediction and prevention of cardiovascular disease depends on the identification of risk factors, and modification of those factors that can be changed. Age, gender, and heredity play an important role in prediction, but obviously cannot be altered. Three very important, health-related behaviors that can be modified are tobacco use, lack of physical activity, and poor nutrition. These three factors contribute significantly to cardiovascular disease and play a direct role in the development of hypertension and atherosclerosis. Nicotine directly stimulates the autonomic ganglia to increase heart rate and blood pressure. In addition, the other chemicals in tobacco smoke increase the plaque deposits of atherosclerosis. Hypertension, or high blood pressure, when left untreated or incompletely treated, is a major risk factor in the development of heart disease. Lack of exercise and a diet high in saturated fats can contribute to obesity and increased lipid levels in the blood, which in turn contributes to atherosclerosis. Excess body weight can lead to diabetes, another significant risk factor for heart disease.

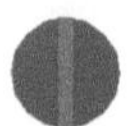

# Disorders of the Blood

Disorders of the blood can be divided into three broad categories: anemias, cancers of the blood, such as the leukemias, and clotting disorders. The leukemias are acute or chronic diseases characterized by an abnormal increase in the number of white blood cells, and classified by the type of white blood cells affected (Chapter 33). Anemia occurs when there are insufficient nutrients to form healthy blood cells, when there are inherited anomalies of the blood, when there is blood loss, as a result of unwanted drug effects, and when there is hemolysis, or rupture of red blood cells. The most common form of anemia is iron deficiency anemia, frequently seen in women of childbearing age. Anemia can also result from deficiency of folic acid or as a result of poor absorption of vitamin $B_{12}$. In patients with kidney disease, where erythropoietin production is reduced, anemia is quite common. Inherited forms of anemia include sickle cell anemia, and the thalassemias, a group of rare inherited anemias that occur more often in African, Asian, or Mediterranean people.

Clotting disorders are characterized by a disruption of the clotting process that can result in abnormal bleeding or enhanced clotting, depending on the disorder. In most inherited clotting disorders, some factor required for normal coagulation is missing, which results in abnormal bleeding. Good examples include hemophilia, where factor VIII is usually deficient, and Von Willebrand's disease, where there is a shortage of a plasma component necessary for platelet adhesion.

Thrombocytopenia is a blood disorder characterized by a shortage of platelets. This disorder results in a high risk of abnormal bleeding, because the platelets play such a crucial role in the clotting process. Thrombocytopenia can occur because platelets are being removed from the circulation in excessive numbers or because of reduced bone marrow production. Drug toxicity is a common cause of thrombocytopenia.

leukemia A malignancy of the blood forming tissues that occurs in people and other mammals and is characterized by excessive production of white blood cells.

anemia A condition that results from a lack of red blood cells, hemoglobin, or total blood volume.

hemolysis Rupture of red blood cells with resultant release of hemoglobin.

thalassemia Inherited anemias that occur due to an anomaly in hemoglobin; they tend to occur especially in people of Mediterranean, African, or Asian descent.

thrombocytopenia An abnormally low platelet count with an increased risk of bleeding.

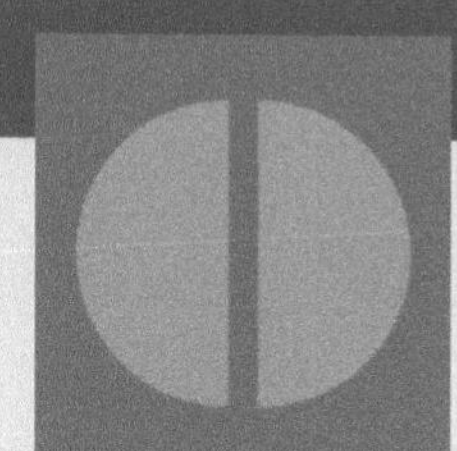

## Case 14.1

Your father is 58 years old, 5'9", and weighs 195 pounds. He smokes cigarettes, but recently cut back from smoking a pack per day to about two packs per week. His father died of heart failure when he was 67 years old. His total cholesterol level is 205. Your dad was diagnosed with high blood pressure about 5 years ago. He works as a flight controller in the tower at Los Angeles International Airport and is 4 years away from retirement. On his days off he enjoys relaxing in front of the television or playing a round of golf. Last weekend, for the first time, he experienced chest pain while out mowing the lawn. He is very worried and wants your opinion on what he should do to live a heart-healthy lifestyle.

# Review Questions

## Multiple Choice

Choose the best answer for the following questions:

1. Choose the correct statement regarding the path of blood flow in the normal heart.
   a. Blood flows from the inferior vena cava directly into the right ventricle.
   b. The left ventricle pumps blood into the pulmonary circulation.
   c. Blood flows from the left atrium to the right atrium, then into the right ventricle, then to the left ventricle and out into the systemic circulation.
   d. Oxygenated blood from the lungs re-enters the heart at the left atrium.
   e. None of these statements are correct.

2. Which statement about the anatomy of the heart is not correct?
   a. The heart has four chambers, including two atria and two ventricles.
   b. The pericardium is a thick sac that allows the myocardium to be bathed in blood, delivering oxygen and nutrients to the muscle cells.
   c. The myocardial cells are similar to skeletal muscle cells.
   d. There are one-way valves located between the atria and ventricles.
   e. b and c are both incorrect.

3. What essential function does the blood perform?
   a. Transports antibodies and cells needed for immune function
   b. Carries oxygen to all tissues in the body
   c. Plays a role in regulation of body temperature
   d. Contains clotting factors
   e. All of the above

4. Which of the following is not a normal blood component?
   a. Keratin
   b. Water
   c. Albumin
   d. Cholesterol
   e. Electrolytes

5. What changes would you suggest to a friend with a family history of cardiovascular disease?
   a. Exercise regularly
   b. Quit smoking, but only if you are not eating a healthy diet
   c. Have your doctor monitor your blood pressure so that hypertension does not go undetected.
   d. b and c
   e. a and c

## True/False

6. Electrical impulses originate at a rate of about 70 per minute from the atrioventricular node, which is the heart's pacemaker.
   a. True
   b. False

7. Following a massive hemorrhage, you would expect baroreceptors in the walls of the aorta to send signals to the central nervous system, resulting in increased sympathetic nervous system discharge causing vasoconstriction.
   a. True
   b. False

8. After oxygenated blood leaves the heart, it flows from the aorta to smaller arteries, then to veins, which deliver the oxygenated blood to the capillary beds within various tissues.
   a. True
   b. False

9. Leukocytes and erythrocytes are produced in the bone marrow but platelets are not.
   a. True
   b. False

10. Folic acid deficiency, iron deficiency, adverse drug effects, and blood loss are all possible causes of anemia.
    a. True
    b. False

## Matching

For numbers 11 to 15, match the word or phrase with the correct lettered choice. Choices will not be used more than once and may not be used at all.

11. Leukocytes
12. Cardiovascular System
13. Increased sympathetic nervous system stimulation
14. Capillaries
15. Myocardial infarction

a. Extremely thin-walled vessels that are the site of oxygen and carbon dioxide exchange between blood and tissues.
b. Cellular precursors of red blood cells
c. Consists of the heart, vessels, and the blood
d. Cells involved with inflammation, allergic reactions, and immune system function
f. Maintains firing of the sinoatrial node at resting heart rate
g. Lower incidence in individuals that eat a diet high in saturated fat and protein, and low in vegetables and carbohydrates
h. Causes vasoconstriction and increased cardiac output
i. Caused by a blood clot that cuts off blood supply to an area of the myocardium

## Short Answer

16. Outline the flow of blood from the left ventricle to the right atrium.
17. Describe the differences in the anatomical structures of arteries, veins, and capillaries.
18. What changes might you expect to see in the blood of a patient with liver disease and why? What about a patient with a bacterial infection?
19. Your friend's father has recently suffered a stroke. Your friend is now curious about what happened to his father and wants to know what happens when a person has a stroke. He also would like to know what he could do to reduce his own risk of having a stroke. What do you tell your friend?

20. Your 25-year-old sister has been feeling lethargic and drained lately so she goes to see her doctor about the problem. When she gets home she calls you and tells you that the doctor's office left a message saying she is anemic. Your sister is in a panic, assumes the worst, and is certain she has a serious disease. What can you say to allay her fears?

## FOR FURTHER INQUIRY

Not every person's cardiovascular anatomy is the same, and exercise physiologists know that we can train our hearts and lungs for better athletic performance. Use the Internet or the public library in your community to learn how Lance Armstrong's unique physiology, training routines, and competitive nature made him perfectly suited to win the coveted Tour de France bicycle race a record seven times. You can begin your search with an article by Edward F. Coyle in the *Journal of Applied Physiology, J Appl Physiol* 98: 2191–2196, 2005 or search (Lance Armstrong, physiology) on Google. If there is an opportunity to do so, share what you've learned with your class.

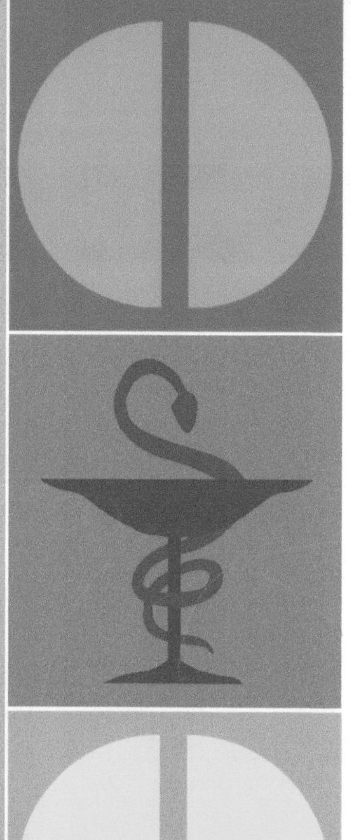

Chapter **15**

# Antiarrhythmic Drugs

## KEY TERMS

- atrial arrhythmia
- atrial flutter
- autoimmune
- automaticity
- cardioversion
- fibrillation
- heart block
- hemolytic anemia
- hypokalemia
- loading dose
- neuropathy
- neutropenia
- paroxysmal
- pathology
- premature ventricular contractions
- proarrhythmic
- refractory period
- supraventricular
- ventricular arrhythmia

## OBJECTIVES

After studying this chapter, the reader should be able to:

- List two atrial and two ventricular arrhythmias and describe the risks associated with each.
- Describe the Vaughan Williams classification of antiarrhythmic agents and list a drug from all six classes (1A–C, II, III, and IV).
- Explain when lidocaine is used, how it is administered and why, and describe the most serious potential side effect seen with its use.
- Compare and contrast the class II and class IV antiarrhythmic agents. State which class is used to suppress arrhythmias in patients who have recently experienced a heart attack and explain why.
- Describe one important role of the hospital pharmacy technician with regard to emergency medications.

## DRUGS COVERED IN THIS CHAPTER

### Class I Antiarrhythmic Agents (Sodium Channel Blockers)

Disopyramide
Flecainide
Lidocaine
Mexiletine
Propafenone
Procainamide
Quinidine

### Class II Antiarrhythmic Agents (Beta Antagonists)

Acebutolol
Atenolol
Esmolol
Metoprolol
Propranolol

### Class III Antiarrhythmic Agents (Potassium Channel Blockers)

Amiodarone
Bretylium
Sotalol

### Class IV Antiarrhythmic Agents (Calcium Channel Blockers)

Diltiazem
Verapamil

### Other Antiarrhythmic Agents

Digoxin
Adenosine

In contrast to skeletal muscle, which contracts when it receives a signal under voluntary nervous system control, the heart responds to specialized cells in the cardiac conduction system that automatically generate electrical impulses. These "pacemaker" cells generate a spontaneous electrical impulse. Both the SA node and the AV node contain pacemaker cells, but in normal conditions impulses from the SA node control the heart's rhythm. Normally an action potential begins in the SA node and travels down through the cardiac conduction system to cause the contraction of the heart. Abnormal impulse generation or conduction at any number of sites in the heart can cause an abnormality in cardiac rhythm, referred to as an arrhythmia.

pathology The study of diseases and the structural and functional changes produced by them.

automaticity The ability of a cell, organ, or system to initiate its own activity.

## The Cardiac Arrhythmias

When the cardiac conduction system is healthy, it generates about 70 electrical impulses per minute, which results in the regular contraction of the myocardium called normal sinus rhythm. Abnormal or irregular rhythms usually occur because of cardiac pathology (an abnormality, disease, or malfunction) or as a consequence of medication use or drug abuse. When they are damaged, cells outside of the conduction system can spontaneously generate electrical impulses. The spontaneous production of impulses is referred to as automatic-

## Analogy

When we were young, we played a game called "red light, green light." To play this game, a leader is chosen, who will act as the "light" and the rest of the players line up and follow directions. When the leader turns to face the group, she says "red light" and no one can move. When she turns her back on the group, she says "green light" and players can move forward at will. Now, imagine a cardiac version of this game. All the players (and there are thousands of them) are in a circle, and when the leader says "green light," everyone takes two steps, in unison, towards the center of the circle (contraction of the myocardium). When the leader says "red light" everyone takes two steps out, and rests for a moment before the green light (relaxation of the myocardium). But what if, after about the ten millionth round, a couple of wise-guys in the circle got bored and gave the "green light" signal between the leader's signals? Undoubtedly, some of the players who become confused will step forward at the wrong time and generate disorganization among the players. Perhaps the group nearest the leader would follow her commands, while the people near the troublemakers would follow their signal. Worst of all, mass confusion might ensue, with no one moving on command at all. In this analogy, the players represent myocardial cells and the leader represents the SA node. The players who try to take the leader's role represent cells with abnormal automaticity that can trigger arrhythmias, a form of myocardial confusion and disorganization.

ity. Impaired conduction of impulses due to cell damage can also cause abnormal rhythms. One or both kinds of pathology commonly occur after a heart attack, for example. Less often, arrhythmias arise without any known underlying cardiac condition. Classification of an arrhythmia is based on the area of its origin and the kind of rhythm pattern observed. Arrhythmias that arise in the atria or the AV node are called supraventricular (above the ventricles) or atrial arrhythmias, and those that arise in the ventricles are called ventricular arrhythmias.

supraventricular Originating or occurring above the ventricles.

Arrhythmias usually result in inefficient movement of blood, either because the cardiac muscle is not contracting uniformly, or because there is inadequate time between contractions for filling of the chambers. In some cases, blood may become static, and the risk of blood clots increases. If a blood clot forms and passes out of the atria, the result can be pulmonary embolus or stroke, either of which can have disastrous consequences. Ventricular arrhythmias are considered much more dangerous than atrial arrhythmias. When the ventricles cannot pump efficiently, all of the essential organs are at risk of damage from lack of oxygen.

atrial arrhythmia Abnormal heart rhythm caused by conduction disturbances in the atria.

ventricular arrhythmia An abnormal rhythm of the heart beat that arises in the ventricles.

The American Heart Association sets standards for the emergency treatment of arrhythmias and other cardiovascular emergencies. The ACLS guidelines provide recommendations for treatment that is often lifesaving. Cardioversion (the application of electric shock to the chest in order to restore normal sinus rhythm), not drug therapy, is often the first choice treatment of arrhythmias. Acute care hospital professional staff members are trained in advanced cardiac life support (ACLS), and hospitals are equipped with the drugs and equipment necessary for any cardiac emergency.

cardioversion Application of an electric shock, usually to the chest, in order to restore normal heartbeat.

## Supraventricular Tachycardia, Atrial Fibrillation, and Atrial Flutter

The supraventricular arrhythmias are considered fairly benign relative to ventricular arrhythmias, but patients must be protected from the risk of blood clots, and the rate of contraction of the ventricles must be controlled. Tachycardia, a heart rate of greater than 100

paroxysmal Episodic recurrences or attacks of a disease.

fibrillation Twitching or contraction of individual muscle fibers; in cardiology an arrhythmia characterized by contraction of individual fibers in a disorganized fashion.

atrial flutter A rapid, organized atrial arrhythmia, with atrial rate of >200, but a slower ventricular rate.

beats per minute (BPM), can produce inefficient pumping of the blood. Fortunately, most supraventricular tachycardias (SVT) are paroxysmal, meaning they come in spontaneous bursts that usually resolve without treatment (**Table 15.1**). Paroxysmal supraventricular tachycardia can be disconcerting and provoke anxiety, even though it is usually harmless. People with this disorder may feel like they are mildly short of breath and may experience palpitations. Caffeine consumption, tobacco use, and stress are common precipitants of this arrhythmia. Persistent or chronic SVT requires treatment.

Fibrillation is a type of arrhythmia characterized by disorganized contraction of myocardial fibers. In atrial fibrillation, instead of contracting simultaneously to force blood into the ventricles, atrial myocardial fibers contract individually. Fibrillating myocardium looks like a wriggling mass of muscle, and the result is an entirely inefficient contraction. The greatest risk to the patient in this situation is from blood clots that may form because blood is not circulating through the atria as efficiently as it should. Initial treatment of this disorder is directed at preventing blood clots, then converting the rhythm to normal sinus rhythm. Atrial fibrillation usually occurs in older people with underlying cardiovascular disease.

Atrial flutter most often occurs in the same types of patients that develop atrial fibrillation, but it can also occur in adults or children who have congenital heart defects or have undergone heart surgery for repair of defects. It is a much more regular, organized rhythm than atrial fibrillation. In flutter, instead of traveling from the SA node down through the conduction system to the ventricles, electrical impulses reach an area where conduction is disrupted or slowed and they circle back around through the atria to the SA node (**Fig. 15.1**). This sets up a circular conduction through the atria called reentry, and results in a rapid atrial rate of about 300 BPM. Fortunately, conduction through the AV node is slower than through the SA node, so ventricular rate of contraction is usually half the rate of atrial contraction.

**Table 15.1** Common Arrhythmias and Antiarrhythmic Drugs and Classes Recommended for Their Treatment

| | Antiarrhythmic Drugs | | | | |
|---|---|---|---|---|---|
| **Type of Arrhythmia** | **Class I** | **Class II** | **Class III** | **Class IV** | **Other** |
| **Atrial Arrhythmias** | | | | | |
| Atrial Flutter | | Propanolol | | Verapamil | Digoxin* |
| Atrial Fibrillation | Dofetilide* | Propanolol | Amiodarone | | Anticoagulant therapy |
| **Supraventricular Tachycardias** | | | | | |
| Paroxysmal supraventricular tachycardias | | | | Verapamil* | Adenosine |
| **Ventricular Arrhythmias** | | | | | |
| Acute ventricular tachycardia | Lidocaine | | Amiodarone | | |
| Ventricular fibrillation (not responding to electrical defibrillation) | Lidocaine* | | Amiodarone | | Epinephrine |

* denotes alternative drugs. Those without asterisks are commonly used drugs.

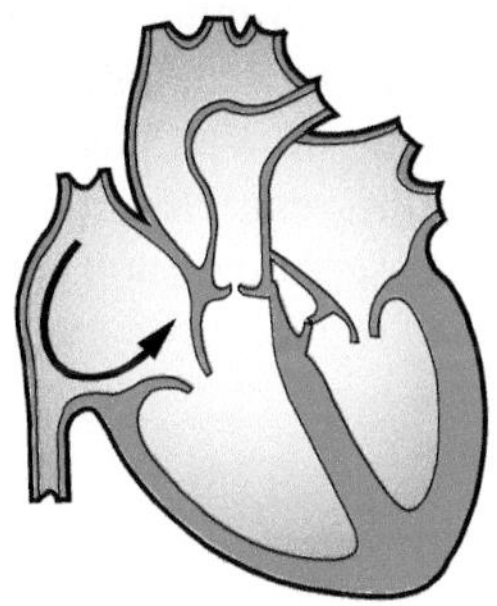

**Figure 15.1** An image of the heart with a re-entry pathway indicated in the atria.

## Ventricular Arrhythmias

Premature ventricular contractions (PVCs) are the most common form of ventricular arrhythmia. They occur when an impulse arises spontaneously within the ventricles and causes the ventricles to contract out of sequence with the normal rhythm. The seriousness of this arrhythmia depends upon the frequency of the PVCs and the underlying health of the individual experiencing them. They are not uncommon in perfectly healthy young adults, and are reported as feeling as though the heart has "skipped" a beat. They can occur as a result of MI, electrolyte imbalance, or drug use, including either illicit drugs such as cocaine, or prescription medications. In people who have recently experienced an MI, or when PVCs occur in clusters, or with frequency, there is a serious risk that they will cause ventricular tachycardia and sometimes ventricular fibrillation. Treatment is generally aimed at correcting underlying causes of the arrhythmia and suppressing spontaneous beats.

premature ventricular contractions Early contractions of the ventricles that occur because of abnormal electrical activity.

Sustained ventricular tachycardia (lasting more than 30 seconds) and ventricular fibrillation are life-threatening arrhythmias, and usually occur in patients with significant cardiac disease. Although ventricular tachycardia is an organized rhythm, it is inefficient because the ventricles cannot fill with blood between contractions. If it is not corrected, patients lose consciousness from lack of oxygen. Sometimes ventricular tachycardia spontaneously degenerates into ventricular fibrillation. Like atrial fibrillation, ventricular fibrillation is a disorganized rhythm (**Fig. 15.2**), and blood is not pushed out to the aorta or the pulmonary circulation at all. If ventricular fibrillation is not rapidly converted, death ensues quickly.

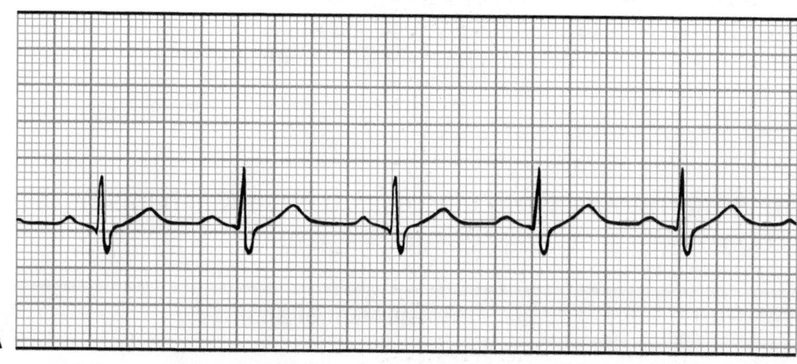


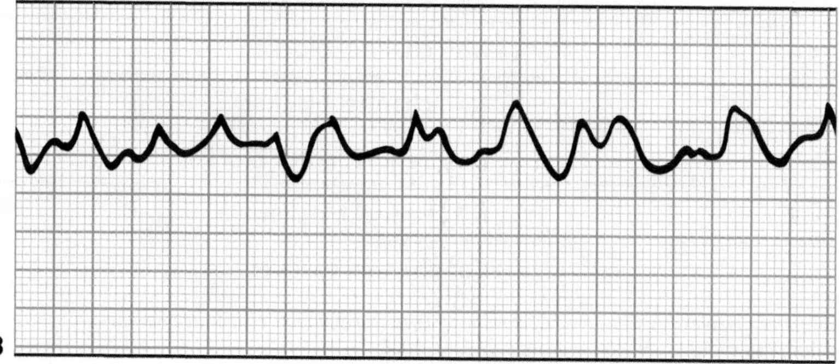


**Figure 15.2** (A) A normal EKG tracing compared with (B) an EKG tracing showing the disorganization of ventricular fibrillation. 

heart block Disturbance of cardiac impulse conduction that delays or completely prevents movement of the electrical impulse from the atria to the ventricles.

Bradycardia is a slow heart rate, usually defined as less than 60 beats per minute in an adult. Bradycardia does not usually cause symptoms, nor is it likely to be treated, until the heart rate is less than 50 BPM. Symptomatic bradycardia is likely a result of heart block, a reduction in the rate of conduction of impulses between the atria and the ventricles. It can usually be successfully treated with atropine. Atropine reduces the impact of the parasympathetic nervous system, and shifts the balance toward the stimulation produced by sympathetic input.

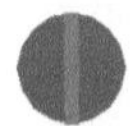

# Antiarrhythmic Medications

proarrhythmic A compound that causes or creates an environment that encourages arrhythmias.

The antiarrhythmic drugs work either by inhibiting the generation of electrical impulses, by slowing conduction, or both. Although many such drugs are available, their usefulness for chronic treatment of arrhythmias is limited. Several of the older agents are known to have dangerous proarrhythmic actions, meaning they actually may cause other arrhythmias. Implantable pacemakers and defibrillators are gaining favor for long-term control of arrhythmias, especially since numerous clinical studies have demonstrated that chronic use of antiarrhythmics does not seem to prolong life in patients with arrhythmia, and in some cases may increase the risk of death. Antiarrhythmic drug therapy does have proven usefulness in many situations, however. Examples in which antiarrhythmic therapy is proven to reduce unfavorable outcomes include the correction of ventricular tachycardia by lidocaine, the suppression of arrhythmias after an MI with beta blockers, and conversion of supraventricular tachycardia by adenosine or verapamil.

The antiarrhythmic drugs can be classified according to their predominant effects on the conduction mechanisms in the heart (**Table 15.2**) This classification system is referred to as the Vaughan Williams classification, named after the Oxford University physician who suggested it. Although it is convenient, it is not entirely clear-cut, because many of the drugs have actions that fit in more than one class or may have active metabolites with a different class of action. Two frequently used drugs, digoxin and adenosine, do not fit in any of the classes and will be discussed separately.

## Class I Antiarrhythmic Drugs

Drugs in this class include quinidine, procainamide, disopyramide (Norpace®), lidocaine (Xylocaine®), mexiletine (Mexitil®), flecainide (Tambocor®), and propafenone (Rythmol®). Although several of these drugs are local anesthetics or their derivatives (lidocaine, procainamide, and flecainide), they are not all chemically related. The use of

**Table 15.2** The Antiarrythmic Drug Classes and Their Mechanisms of Action

| Classification of drug | Mechanism of action |
|---|---|
| IA | $Na^+$ channel blocker |
| IB | $Na^+$ channel blocker |
| IC | $Na^+$ channel blocker |
| II | β-Adrenoreceptor blocker |
| III | $K^+$ channel blocker |
| IV | $Ca^2$ channel blocker |

Adapted with permission from Harvey RA, Champe PC, Howland RD, et al. *Lippincott's Illustrated Reviews: Pharmacology*, 3rd edition. Baltimore: Lippincott William & Wilkins, 2006.

sodium channel blockers is declining due to their possible proarrhythmic effects and other risks.

## Actions and Indications

Class I antiarrhythmic drugs act by blocking the flow of sodium ions into the cells of the conduction system in the same way that the local anesthetics do in nerves. The decreased rate of entry of sodium ions slows depolarization in the cell, slows conduction of the impulse, and consequently reduces the excitability of the myocardium. Based on their effect on the action potential, class I drugs are further subdivided into subsections. Those classified as 1A drugs (quinidine, procainamide and disopyramide) are mainly used for control of atrial arrhythmias, including atrial flutter and fibrillation, and paroxysmal supraventricular tachycardia (PSVT). They slow the rate of depolarization and the movement of impulses through the conduction system and reduce the excitability of the myocardium. Other, safer drugs are rapidly replacing the use of these drugs for maintenance therapy in atrial arrhythmias. Class IA drugs have some effect in ventricular arrhythmias, but are not routinely used because there are more effective agents.

Class 1B drugs include lidocaine and mexiletine. These drugs are used for ventricular arrhythmias only, and they work mainly by reducing the risk of an extra action potential spontaneously arising from myocardial cells. They exert little effect in the heart operating at a normal heart rate. Lidocaine is an important part of every emergency cart in hospitals, commonly referred to as "crash carts," and is a drug of choice to control life threatening ventricular tachycardia and fibrillation.

Class 1C drugs include flecainide and propafenone. These drugs have approved indications for atrial fibrillation, PSVT, and ventricular arrhythmias. However, because there are safer and more effective treatments, they are not drugs of choice for any arrhythmia. Their main clinical use is in treatment of life-threatening ventricular arrhythmias that have not responded to other drugs and treatments. They depress conduction through all cardiac tissue, and exert the greatest effect of the class I drugs on the influx of sodium through sodium channels.

## Administration

Quinidine is available as quinidine gluconate tablets for oral use, or as injection. The injectable form is almost never used, and is no longer part of the ACLS recommendations for any arrhythmias. Quinidine is well absorbed orally, and undergoes extensive metabolism in the liver. Disopyramide is available as capsules and extended release capsules for oral use, and it is well absorbed. Because the main route of elimination is via the kidneys, the dose of disopyramide must be adjusted in patients with renal failure and in older adults. Procainamide is available for injection and for oral administration. Procainamide is one option, under the ACLS protocols, for the drug treatment of life threatening ventricular arrhythmias. If procainamide is used, it is given by slow IV injection, followed by IV infusion for maintenance of arrhythmia control.

Lidocaine is given intravenously because extensive first-pass metabolism by the liver precludes oral administration. It is eliminated almost entirely via metabolism in the liver, and dosage adjustment may be necessary in patients with significant liver dysfunction. Lidocaine is frequently used in cardiac resuscitation efforts, where it is administered by direct IV injection, followed by continuous infusion. Lidocaine is packaged in prefilled syringes in standard adult and pediatric concentrations, and ready to hang IV bags in commonly used concentrations to facilitate rapid administration during emergency situations. It is a first line drug on ACLS protocols for the treatment of ventricular arrhythmias.

Mexiletine is structurally similar to lidocaine, but is administered orally and is nearly completely bioavailable. Because it is mainly metabolized, the dose may need to be reduced in patients with hepatic dysfunction. Flecainide and propafenone are both administered orally. Propafenone use is complicated by the fact that about ten percent of people are slow metabolizers of the drug. The physician must closely follow the effects of the drug to avoid toxicity. It is usually recommended that concomitant use with other antiarrhythmic agents should be avoided. Drug effects are closely related to serum drug concentrations for all of the drugs discussed in this section, and serum drug levels are used to adjust doses in outpatients. Refer to **Table 15.3** for a listing of drug names, products, and indications for all of the antiarrhythmic agents.

**Table 15.3** A Comparison of Commonly Prescribed Antiarrhythmic Agents, Formulations, and Indications

| Generic Name | Brand Name | Available As | Indications | Notes |
|---|---|---|---|---|
| **Class I Drugs** | | | | |
| Disopyramide | Norpace® | Capsules and ER capsules | Life-threatening ventricular arrhythmias | |
| Flecainide | Tambocor® | Tablets | Prevention of supra-ventricular and ventricular arrhythmias | Only indicated if benefits outweigh risks |
| Lidocaine | Xylocaine® | Injection: vials amps, PFS, IV bags | Acute management of ventricular arrhythmias | ACLS first-line treatment |
| Procainamide | | Capsules, ER tabs, injection | Life-threatening ventricular arrhythmias | Benefits must outweigh risks |
| Propafenone | Rythmol® | Tablets, ER capsules | Prevention of supra-ventricular and ventricular arrhythmias | Benefits must outweigh risks |
| Quinidine | | Tablets, ER tabs, injection | Prevention of supra-ventricular arrhythmias and V Tach | Rarely appropriate for ventricular arrhythmias |
| **Class II Drugs** | | | | |
| Acebutolol | Sectral® | Capsules | Management of PVCs | |
| Atenolol | Tenormin® | Tablets, injection | Hypertension, for rapid ventricular rate from atrial tachyarrhythmia | Especially useful after MI |
| Esmolol | Brevibloc® | Injection | Rapid control of SVT | Used for intra- and post-operative SVT |
| Metoprolol | Lopressor®, Toprol® | Tablets, ER tabs, injection | Atrial arrhythmias after MI, hypertension, angina | |
| Propranolol | Inderal® | Tablets, oral soln, injection ER capsules | Tachyarrhythmias, both SVT and VT, used after MI, hypertension, angina, others | For arrhythmias caused by digoxin toxicity, anesthesia |

*(continues)*

| Generic Name | Brand Name | Available As | Indications | Notes |
|---|---|---|---|---|
| **Class III Drugs** | | | | |
| Amiodarone | Cordarone®, Pacerone® | Tablets, injection | Ventricular arrhythmias | Off-label use for atrial fib and SVT |
| Bretylium | | Injection: vials amps, PFS, IV bags | Acute management of ventricular arrhythmias unresponsive to lidocaine | |
| Sotalol | Betapace®, Betapace AF | Tablets | Ventricular arrhythmias, maintenance of NSR after atrial fib/flutter | Different patient information for two preparations |
| **Class IV Drugs** | | | | |
| Diltiazem | Cardizem®, Dilacor® | Tablets, ER tabs and capsules, injection | Control of atrial fib/flutter, conversion of PSVT, hypertension, angina. | Injectable for arrhythmias |
| Verapamil | Calan, Isoptin | Tablets, ER tabs and capsules, injection | Acute control of atrial fib/flutter, conversion of PSVT, chronic control of afib/flutter, angina, hypertension | |
| **Miscellaneous Drugs** | | | | |
| Adenosine | Adenocard® | Injection | Conversion of PSVT | |
| Digoxin | Lanoxin® | Tablets, elixir, capsules, injection | Atrial fib/flutter, PAT, congestive heart failure | |

ER, extended release; MI, myocardial infarction; PAT, paroxysmal atrial tachycardia; PFS, pre-filled syringes; PSVT, paroxysmal supraventricular tachycardia; SVT, supraventricular tachycardia; VT, ventricular tachycardia.

## Side Effects

The most dangerous side effects associated with administration of all the class I drugs are the propensity to induce other, often very serious, arrhythmias. Other side effects vary, depending on the drug. Quinidine, which is related to quinine, can cause symptoms similar to those seen with quinine use, including diarrhea, nausea, and ringing in the ears. Another serious complication of quinidine use is thrombocytopenia. It can cause hemolytic anemia, an anemia caused by rupture of red blood cells, in people with an inherited enzyme deficiency called glucose-6-phosphate dehydrogenase deficiency (G6PD deficiency). Quinidine can increase the steady-state concentration of digoxin by displacement of digoxin from tissue-binding sites, and by decreasing digoxin renal clearance.

Procainamide is also known for causing anemias, including thrombocytopenia, hemolytic anemia, neutropenia (a shortage of neutrophils, one form of granulocyte), and agranulocytosis (a marked deficiency of granulocytes). Hypotension, fever, and seizures have occurred. Procainamide treatment is a well-documented and frequent cause of drug-induced systemic lupus erythematosus. Lupus is an autoimmune disorder, characterized by a typical skin rash, joint pain, and sometimes damage to vital organs. People with lupus produce antibodies that attack their own tissues. Along with the risk of inducing further arrhythmias, disopyramide can cause heart failure with chronic use. It commonly causes dry

hemolytic anemia Anemia caused by rupture of red blood cells.

neutropenia An abnormally low white blood cell count chiefly due to a shortage of neutrophils.

autoimmune Relating to conditions caused by antibodies or cells that react to tissues of the individual that produces them.

mouth, constipation, urinary retention in older males, and other symptoms related to its anticholinergic activity.

When compared with other antiarrhythmic agents, lidocaine has a fairly wide therapeutic index. It does not significantly reduce the cardiac output. CNS effects include sedation, slurred speech, sensation of numbness, confusion, and in excess doses, seizures. Cardiac arrhythmias can occur, however lidocaine is the least cardiotoxic of the class I drugs. Mexiletine is proarrhythmic and causes central nervous side effects similar to those seen with lidocaine. In addition it causes GI upset in about 40% of patients and is involved in a number of drug interactions. Antacids may reduce the absorption of mexiletine.

Flecainide and propafenone are among a number of antiarrhythmic drugs whose long-term use has not demonstrated benefit in clinical studies. In one study, use of class 1C antiarrhythmic drugs was actually associated with a higher risk of death. Flecainide and propafenone can cause dizziness, blurred vision, taste changes, and nausea, as well as significant cardiac toxicity.

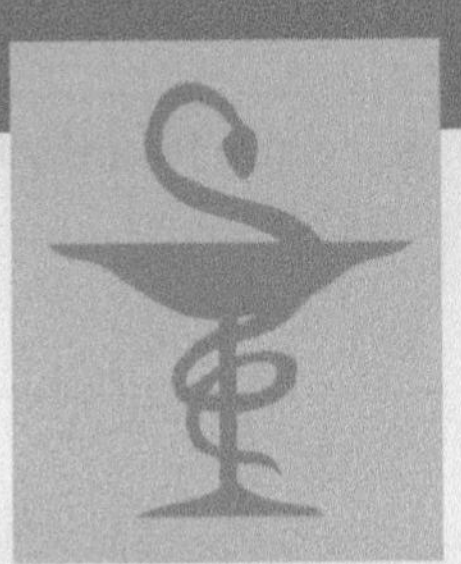

## Tips for the Technician

The hospital pharmacy technician needs to be familiar with drugs stocked on emergency carts and aware of stock levels of all medications used in emergency situations. Crash carts typically hold nondrug supplies that are stocked by other departments and a tray or drawer of drugs. Besides drugs for arrhythmias, they will contain atropine, epinephrine, dextrose, sodium bicarbonate, and other medications. Each hospital will determine what is to be included based on ACLS recommendations and physician preference. Adequate supplies must always be available for resupplying floor stock in appropriate areas and restocking crash carts. Some products, such as pre-filled syringes, have short shelf lives, and dating needs to be checked routinely. The job of restocking crash cart medications usually falls to the technician, and it is a vital role.

In retail pharmacy settings, it is important that all patients with prescriptions for antiarrhythmic drugs receive adequate consultation from the pharmacist on how to recognize side effects and when to report them to the physician. Patients should be instructed to follow directions exactly as written. In the case of the agents that cause drug-induced anemias, patients should report signs of excess bruising, or sore throat that does not resolve. A number of the class I antiarrhythmic agents are formulated as prolonged-release products. Although some prolonged-release products can be split in half, the vast majority must be swallowed whole. It is good practice to attach a "do not crush" label to these prescriptions.

## Class II Antiarrhythmic Drugs

Class II agents are β-adrenergic antagonists, previously discussed in some detail in Chapter 6. Many β-adrenergic antagonists, including acebutolol (Sectral®), atenolol (Tenormin®), esmolol (Brevibloc®), metoprolol (Lopressor®), and propranolol (Inderal®), are approved for use in treatment of arrhythmias. With the exception of acebutolol and esmolol, however, they are more likely to be encountered but most are used more often in the treatment of hypertension.

### Actions and Indications

The beta-blockers are general myocardial depressants. They slow conduction and reduce automaticity in the myocardium, and decrease the heart rate and the contractility of the heart muscle. Class II agents are useful in treating tachycardia caused by increased sympathetic activity. They are also used for atrial flutter and fibrillation. The beta-blockers have demonstrated the ability to reduce the risk of death after a myocardial infarction by 25% or more, especially when the drugs are initiated early and continued for several months. They prolong life after heart attack not only because they reduce the risk of arrhythmia, but also because they block the sympathetic stimulation that occurs as a result of a drop in blood pressure. Consequently, the beta-blockers inhibit potent endogenous chemicals that cause vasoconstriction, raise blood pressure, and encourage fluid retention. Many beta-blockers, including propranolol, are used for prevention of arrhythmias. However, agents that are more specific for beta receptors in the heart, such as metoprolol or timolol, are preferred in most patients. Esmolol is a very short-acting β-blocker used in acute arrhythmias that occur during surgery or emergency situations.

### Administration

Propranolol, metoprolol, and esmolol are available as injections for intravenous administration. Esmolol is only administered intravenously and is dosed based on body weight. Because it is very short acting, it must be administered as a larger initial dose to rapidly establish therapeutic drug levels, referred to as a loading dose, followed by a continuous infusion of a dilute solution. Propranolol, metoprolol, acebutolol, timolol, and atenolol are all available for oral administration.

loading dose Large initial dose or doses of a drug given at the start of therapy in order to rapidly achieve a therapeutic level.

### Adverse Effects

Adverse effects of the beta-blockers depend on their specificity. Drugs that are nonselective beta antagonists are associated with bronchoconstriction in patients with asthma, and are more likely to be associated with hypoglycemia in diabetics. Other adverse affects include fatigue, dizziness, and sexual dysfunction.

Adverse cardiovascular effects include the possibility of symptomatic hypotension. Bradycardia can occur as a result of the depressant effects of the beta-blockers on the conduction system. Because these drugs can reduce cardiac output, their use can aggravate advanced cardiac failure. Abrupt withdrawal of beta antagonists can result in angina, myocardial infarction, ventricular arrhythmia, and even death.

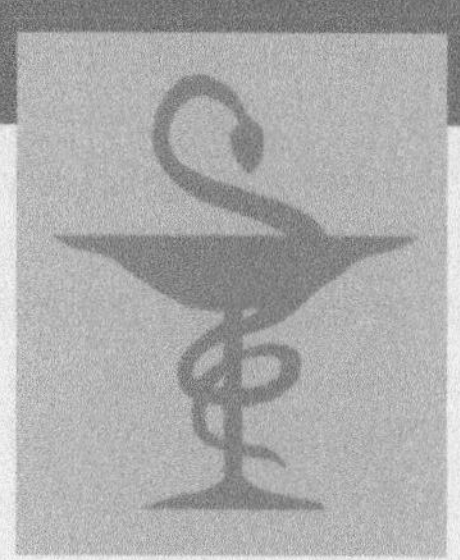

#### Tips for the Technician

Patients should be warned not to abruptly discontinue these medications, and prescription vials labelled accordingly. Prescription labelling ought to warn patients to be cautious while driving or performing other tasks that require alertness. The possibility of drowsiness is especially significant early in therapy. The pharmacist should ensure that patients know the signs of worsening heart failure, including shortness of breath, and edema or swelling in the legs and ankles.

It is important to be aware that because oral propranolol undergoes extensive first pass metabolism in the liver, the oral dose is ten or more times higher than the intravenous dose. The usual intravenous dose is 1 to 3 mg. Any order for intravenous propranolol in a dose higher than 3 mg should be brought to the attention of the pharmacist.

## Class III Antiarrhythmic Agents

Class III agents block the outflow of potassium from the myocardial cells. Drugs in the class include amiodarone (Cordarone®), bretylium, and sotalol (Betapace®). Amiodarone is the most widely used of these drugs. All class III drugs have the potential to induce arrhythmias.

## Actions and Indications

refractory period The interval after the passage of an action potential in an excitable cell and before the cell recovers the capacity to respond to another.

By slowing the outflow of potassium from myocardial cells, these drugs prolong the recovery time after an impulse has passed, called the refractory period. During the refractory period, the cell cannot conduct another impulse. By prolonging the refractory period, the class III drugs reduce the opportunity for excitable myocardial tissues to generate premature impulses.

Although amiodarone exerts action in all four Vaughan Williams classes, its predominant effect is prolongation of the refractory period. Amiodarone reduces angina as well as exerting antiarrhythmic activity. It is not as likely to promote ventricular tachycardias as the class I drugs and is recommended in ACLS protocols as a first-line drug, especially for some ventricular arrhythmias. Amiodarone is effective in the treatment of severe refractory supraventricular and ventricular tachyarrhythmias. Its chronic use is limited by its toxicity.

Bretylium is a second-line agent, following the use of lidocaine, in the ACLS protocol for the treatment of life-threatening ventricular arrhythmias. It is an adrenergic antagonist that works by inhibiting the release of norepinephrine. Bretylium effects have been referred to as a "chemical sympathectomy," meaning that peripheral sympathetic input is essentially shut down.

Although sotalol is a nonselective beta antagonist, its predominant effect is prolongation of the refractory period, and it is therefore considered a class III antiarrhythmic agent. It is used to help maintain normal sinus rhythm in patients with atrial fibrillation or flutter, and for treatment or prevention of ventricular arrhythmias, especially after myocardial infarction, where the use of β-blockers is known to reduce mortality.

## Administration

Amiodarone is administered intravenously or orally. Loading doses are given initially until the rhythm is stabilized and then a lower maintenance dose is used. Absorption of amiodarone is erratic, and the presence of food increases the rate and extent of drug absorption. It is completely metabolized in the liver, and has an extremely long elimination half-life of about 50 days. Because of these factors, doses are carefully adjusted based on individual response. Amiodarone is involved in a number of significant drug interactions. Concomitant use with other antiarrhythmic agents is not recommended. Amiodarone significantly increases the anticoagulant effects of warfarin. Cimetidine, a nonprescription product for GI irritation, can increase amiodarone levels, and should be avoided.

Because it is poorly absorbed after oral administration, bretylium is available only for injection. It can be administered intravenously or by intramuscular injection. It should not be used in combination with other antiarrhythmic agents, digoxin, or the MAO inhibitors.

Sotalol is only available for oral use in the United States. Food decreases the oral absorption of sotalol and it should be given on an empty stomach. This drug is removed entirely by the kidneys, so the dose of sotalol must be adjusted in renal failure. As with other drugs, coadministration with other antiarrhythmic agents is not advised.

## Adverse Effects

Amiodarone causes a variety of very serious adverse effects. After long-term use, more than half of patients receiving the drug have side effects that are severe enough to prompt its discontinuation. In some clinical studies, pulmonary toxicity occurred in 10% to 17% of patients. Pulmonary toxicity is fatal in about one of ten patients who develop it. Serious liver toxicity can also occur. Less serious adverse events include gastrointestinal tract intolerance, tremor, ataxia, dizziness, photosensitivity, and muscle weakness. Amiodarone can cause neuropathy (abnormal changes) in the optic nerve that can result in loss of vision. Because amiodarone contains iodine and is chemically similar to thyroxine, it can cause thyroid changes. Blue skin discoloration is caused by iodine accumulation in the skin. Serious toxicities occur less frequently in patients treated with low doses over shorter time periods.

neuropathy An abnormal state or condition of the nervous system.

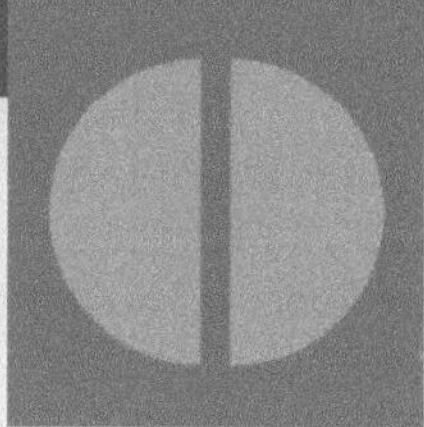

## Case 15.1

Mr. Harte is a kindly older gentleman who just got out of the hospital where he had coronary artery bypass grafting because of increasingly bad angina. Mr. Harte tells Cora, the pharmacy technician, that he had a close call with an arrhythmia during surgery, and will be taking amiodarone 200 mg twice daily, along with his other medications, enalapril, and nitroglycerin sublingual tablets if he needs them. Cora hands him the filled prescriptions, wishes him luck and says goodbye. Nine months later, Mr. Harte is in the pharmacy again while Cora is there. He has a new prescription for levothyroxine, and he is also refilling the amiodarone and enalapril. While the other tech works on the orders, Cora asks Mr. Harte how he is feeling. He says his chest pain is all gone, but now he is tired all the time, and apparently his thyroid gland is not working properly. He thinks his medication is causing the problem, and asks Cora what he should do. How should she respond? Are any of Mr. Harte's present medications likely to cause his new problem? What additional information should Cora give the pharmacist?

Adverse effects seen early in treatment with bretylium are related to an initial release of norepinephrine. This can lead to increased susceptibility to arrhythmia. Later side effects are due to the sympathetic blockade and include hypotension, which can be severe, and bradycardia.

Sotalol is associated with significant proarrhythmic risk. When therapy is initiated, patients are hospitalized for three days and their heart rhythms are monitored continuously because of the risk of other arrhythmias. Sotalol use is related to an increased chance of heart failure, as well. Other adverse effects are similar to the β-antagonists, and include drowsiness, dizziness, and decreased libido.

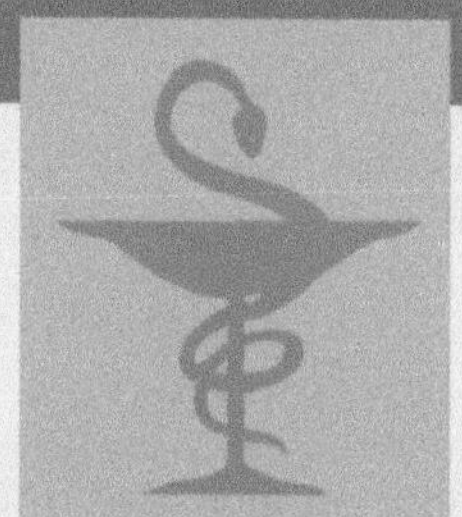

## Tips for the Technician

As previously mentioned, the pharmacy technician will need to monitor stock levels of all medications used in emergency situations, and be aware of alternative supply sources in the event of shortages. Adequate supplies of emergency drugs must always be available for restocking crash carts.

Be careful not to confuse amiodarone with amrinone, another drug that is used in cardiac emergencies. It is important that all outpatients on amiodarone receive adequate consultation from the pharmacist on how to recognize side effects and to report them to the physician. Pharmacy technicians need to be especially aware of potential drug interactions with amiodarone.

People who are taking sotalol must be warned about the danger of abrupt discontinuation of the drug. In addition, they should be cautious while driving or performing other tasks that require alertness. Technicians can assure that this information is conveyed to clients by affixing the appropriate auxiliary labels.

Sotalol is indicated for two different kinds of arrhythmia, ventricular arrhythmias and maintenance of normal sinus rhythm after atrial fibrillation. Although the products are identical, the manufacturer has two different patents for this drug. One, Betapace AF®, is only indicated for atrial fibrillation. The other, Betapace® is indicated only for ventricular arrhythmias. According to the company, the two cannot be interchanged because of significant differences in the patient education materials, dosing, and safety information.

## Class IV Antiarrhythmic Agents

Excitable tissues are able to generate electrical charges because of the movement of charged particles that creates a minute electrical flow. Class IV drugs inhibit the flow of calcium ions, important in the electrical activity of the heart. These drugs are known as calcium channel blockers. Verapamil (Calan®) and diltiazem (Cardizem®) are the calcium channel blockers indicated for arrhythmias. Chapter 17 includes additional information on the use of other calcium channel blockers in the treatment of hypertension.

### Actions and Indications

By decreasing the influx of calcium that occurs in myocardial cells, calcium channel blockers slow the rate of conduction in cardiac tissue. This same effect occurs in any tissue that is dependent on calcium channels. Although calcium channels occur in many different tissues, the major effect of calcium channel blockers is on the smooth muscle found in blood vessels, where it causes vasodilation, and on the heart. Verapamil has a greater effect on the heart than on vascular smooth muscle, whereas nifedipine, a calcium channel blocker used to treat hypertension, exerts a stronger effect on the vascular smooth muscle than on the heart. Diltiazem is intermediate in its actions. Verapamil and diltiazem are more effective against atrial arrhythmias than ventricular arrhythmias. They are useful in treating supraventricular tachycardia and in slowing the ventricular rate in atrial flutter and fibrillation. Because of their action on blood vessels, these drugs can be used to treat hypertension and angina as well.

### Administration

Verapamil and diltiazem are rapidly absorbed after oral administration. Both are available as immediate-release and extended-release formulations. The extended-release formulations allow for less frequent administration. Immediate release formulations need to be given as often as every six hours. Both drugs undergo significant first pass metabolism.

Verapamil and diltiazem injectable formulations can be given intravenously for treatment of arrhythmias. Because of the first-pass effect, the oral dose is many times higher than the intravenous dose. A typical oral dose of verapamil, for example, is 80 mg, while the intravenous dose is usually 5 or 10 mg. Verapamil is metabolized in the liver and it should be administered cautiously to patients with hepatic dysfunction. Both drugs should be used cautiously with digoxin, because they increase digoxin levels. If a patient is receiving digoxin, the digoxin dose must be reduced. Use of multiple antiarrhythmic agents should be avoided.

### Adverse Effects

Verapamil and diltiazem slow heart rate and can cause bradycardia. An increased risk of heart failure may result or cause deterioration of existing heart failure may result from use of these medications. Calcium channel blockers are usually avoided in patients with preexisting heart failure. Both drugs can also produce a decrease in blood pressure because of peripheral vasodilation, which can be worse on arising. Common adverse effects include headache, dizziness, and constipation.

#### Tips for the Technician

Patients should be cautioned about the risk of dizziness, especially on arising. Some people taking diltiazem may experience flushing or rash because of the effects of vasodilation.

The pharmacist should ensure that patients know the signs of worsening heart failure, including excessive weight gain, shortness of breath, and edema. Patients should report frequent or persistent dizziness and signs of heart failure to their physicians.

Auxiliary labels encouraging patients to take their prescription exactly as directed, and advising that these drugs not be discontinued except on the advice of the physician should be applied. The absorption of some of the calcium channel blockers is increased if they are taken with food, especially high-fat meals or grapefruit juice. Patients should be encouraged to take these drugs at the same time in relationship to eating every day.

## Other Drugs Used for Arrhythmia

Two other drugs, digoxin (Lanoxin®) and adenosine (Adenocard®), are used for arrhythmia, but do not fit any of the Vaughan Williams classifications. Adenosine is a naturally occurring compound chemically related to the nucleotide adenine. Digoxin is a cardiac glycoside used most often for congestive heart failure, and its use will be discussed more fully in Chapter 16.

### Actions and Indications

In the heart, adenosine acts on the AV node where it slows conduction and prolongs the refractory period. It also reduces automaticity and inhibits reentry pathways. Intravenous adenosine is the drug of choice for abolishing acute supraventricular tachycardia because it is the most effective and least toxic drug available.

Digoxin prolongs the effective refractory period and slows the rate of conduction within the conduction system of the heart. It improves contractility of the heart muscle and is used in infants and children with heart failure due to congenital heart defects. It is used to control the heart rate in atrial fibrillation and flutter. Although it can be used in paroxysmal supraventricular tachycardia, it is not the drug of choice.

### Administration

Adenosine is rapidly metabolized and has an extremely short duration of action of approximately ten to fifteen seconds. In order to achieve a therapeutic effect it must be administered by rapid IV injection. It needs to be administered directly into the vein if possible. If direct IV injection is not possible it is given into the IV port that is closest to the patient's arm. If the initial dose of 6 mg is not successful at restoring normal sinus rhythm within a minute or two, twelve milligrams can be given.

Digoxin can be administered either orally or by intravenous injection. When treating an acute atrial arrhythmia, patients who have not taken digoxin in the past may be given a loading dose over a period of hours to days. A loading dose is used to quickly get the patient's serum drug levels into the therapeutic range, and is determined based on patient specific pharmacokinetic parameters. It can be two or three times the usual dose of the drug. In the case of digoxin, the loading dose is divided and given in several doses so that the potential for toxicity is minimized.

### Side Effects

Because of its rapid metabolism, adenosine has a negligible risk of toxicity. It can cause brief symptoms, including flushing, chest pressure, shortness of breath and hypotension. These symptoms last only for minutes. It may cause ventricular bradycardia in patients with conduction abnormalities, so its use is avoided in these patients.

Digoxin has a narrow therapeutic index and drug levels are monitored during initiation of therapy. At toxic concentrations, digoxin causes premature ventricular contractions that may result in ventricular tachycardia and fibrillation. Digoxin is known to sometimes cause arrhythmias indistinguishable from the arrhythmia being treated. The presence of hypokalemia (low potassium levels) accentuates digoxin toxicity. The kidneys remove a significant proportion of a digoxin dose, and patients with renal failure require a reduced dose of the drug.

hypokalemia Unusually low serum potassium levels.

## Tips for the Technician

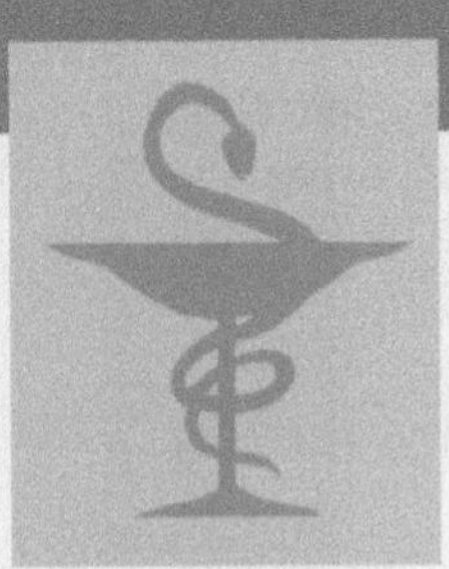

Adenosine injection may crystalize if vials become very cool. Check the vials for crystals before dispensing. If crystallization occurs, vials can be gently warmed to room temperature by holding them. Once they are clear, they may be dispensed. The methylxanthines, including caffeine and theophylline, antagonize the affects of adenosine.

# Review Questions

## Multiple Choice

Choose the best answer for the following questions:

1. Which of the following is the most likely cause for a ventricular arrhythmia?
   a. High blood pressure, controlled with medication
   b. Use of acetaminophen with codeine for postoperative pain
   c. A myocardial infarction
   d. Drinking two cups of coffee every day
   e. Playing basketball

2. The occurrence of which arrhythmia is not normally associated with any serious health consequences?
   a. Paroxysmal supraventricular tachycardia
   b. Atrial fibrillation
   c. Ventricular tachycardia
   d. Ventricular fibrillation
   e. Frequent runs of premature ventricular contractions

3. Which of the following is not considered a Class I antiarrhythmic drug?
   a. Lidocaine
   b. Mepivacaine
   c. Procainamide
   d. Flecainide
   e. Quinidine

4. Of the following statements about lidocaine, circle the one that is not correct.
   a. Lidocaine undergoes significant first-pass metabolism, and is therefore only given by intravenous injection for treatment of arrhythmia.
   b. By slowing the uptake of sodium into the cells, lidocaine prevents the initiation of extra action potentials.
   c. Lidocaine is the treatment of choice for life-threatening ventricular arrhythmias.
   d. Lidocaine treatment is not proarrhythmic.
   e. Typical side effects from lidocaine include sedation, feeling of numbness and slurred speech.

5. Which of the following treatments is clinically demonstrated to improve outcomes for patients with arrhythmias?
   a. Correction of ventricular tachycardia with lidocaine
   b. Suppression of arrhythmias after an MI with beta-blockers
   c. Conversion of supraventricular tachycardia by adenosine or verapamil
   d. None of the above
   e. All of the above

## True/False

6. A serious side effect common to all the class I antiarrhythmic agents is their potential to cause other, potentially more serious arrhythmias.
   a. True
   b. False
7. Class II agents are calcium channel blockers, including acebutolol, atenolol, esmolol, metoprolol, and propranolol.
   a. True
   b. False
8. Patients should be warned not to abruptly discontinue class II antiarrhythmic agents because of the potential for rebound sympathetic activity that could increase the risk of arrhythmia, angina, or other cardiovascular event.
   a. True
   b. False
9. Amiodarone is a very safe drug, especially in low doses, for long-term maintenance of normal sinus rhythm in patients with atrial fibrillation.
   a. True
   b. False
10. Adenosine acts to slow conduction through the AV node, prolong the refractory period, reduce automaticity, and inhibit reentry pathways. Intravenous adenosine is the drug of choice for converting supraventricular tachycardia to normal sinus rhythm.
    a. True
    b. False

## Matching

For questions 11 to 15, match each drug with the lettered choice that best describes its indication. Answer choices may be used once or not at all.

11. Digoxin
12. Verapamil
13. Bretylium
14. Lidocaine
15. Esmolol

a. Rapid control of SVT, especially during and after surgery
b. Prevention of supraventricular and ventricular arrhythmias
c. Treatment of third-degree heart block
d. Acute or chronic control of atrial fibrillation or flutter, angina, and hypertension
e. Acute management of ventricular arrhythmias unresponsive to lidocaine
f. Management of atrial fibrillation or flutter, paroxysmal atrial tachycardia, and congestive heart failure
g. Acute management of ventricular arrhythmias

### Short Answer

16. What is the Vaughan Williams classification, and why is it a less than perfect system? Give an example.

17. The calcium channel blockers can potentially contribute to heart failure in susceptible patients. Explain how this occurs, and give an example of a sign of worsening heart failure of which patients should be made aware.

18. Describe the use of lidocaine in cardiac emergencies. What products are available to make emergency use of lidocaine more efficient?

19. Select one drug from each of the four main antiarrhythmic classes and list an associated unique side effect other than a proarrhythmic effect.

20. What steps can the pharmacy technician take to assure the availability, at all times, of the antiarrhythmic agents necessary for emergency use.

## FOR FURTHER INQUIRY

Go to the American Heart Association web site and investigate the Advanced Cardiac Life Support treatment recommendations for one of the arrhythmias discussed here. What is always the first treatment instituted? If you found someone unconscious would you know what to do? Contact your local hospital, Red Cross, or Heart Association and find out if there are basic life support classes available to the public at no cost. If you do not already have a basic life support card, consider taking a class.

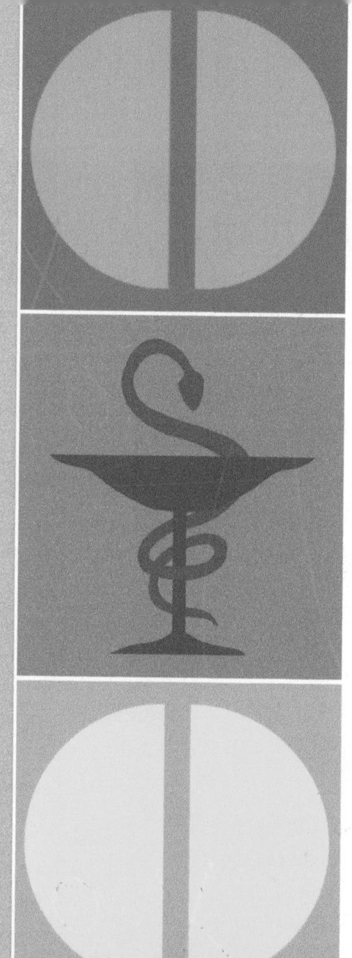

Chapter **16**

# Drugs Used to Treat Heart Failure and Angina Pectoris

## OBJECTIVES

After studying this chapter, the reader should be able to:

- Describe the causes and typical symptoms of heart failure and angina pectoris.
- List the goals of drug therapy and three of the most clinically useful drug classes in the treatment of heart failure.
- Explain how the ACE inhibitors improve hemodynamics in heart failure.
- List two potential side effects of digoxin therapy and describe how digitalis toxicity can be treated.
- List three nitrates used to treat angina, explain how they work, and list two common side effects.

### *KEY TERMS*

- aldosterone
- anorexia
- congestive heart failure
- dialysis
- diuretic
- hemodynamics
- inotropic
- intravenous bolus
- peripheral resistance
- placebo
- precipitate

## DRUGS COVERED IN THIS CHAPTER

### Drugs Used to Treat HF

| Diuretics | Beta Blockers | Renin Angiotensin System Antagonists: ACE Inhibitors | Renin Angiotensin System Antagonists: ARB Agents |
|---|---|---|---|
| Bumetanide | Carvedilol | Captopril | Losartan |
| Furosemide | Metoprolol | Enalapril | Valsartan |
| Hydrochlorothiazide | | Lisinopril | |
| Aldactone | | Quinapril | |
| | | Ramipril | |

| Inotropic Agents |
|---|
| Digoxin |
| Dobutamine |
| Inamrinone |
| Milrinone |

### Drugs Used to Treat Angina

| Nitrates | Beta-Blockers | Calcium Channel Blockers |
|---|---|---|
| Isosorbide dinitrate | Acebutolol | Amlodipine |
| Isosorbide mononitrate | Atenolol | Diltiazem |
| Nitroglycerin | Metoprolol | Nicardipine |
| | Propranolol | Nifedipine |
| | | Verapamil |

Heart failure (HF) is a progressive disorder involving the heart and systems in the body responsible for fluid balance. In failure, the heart is unable to pump sufficient blood to meet the needs of the body. The cardinal symptoms of heart failure are dyspnea (shortness of breath), fatigue, and fluid retention. Patients with heart failure are unable to tolerate exercise, and may have difficulty climbing a flight of stairs. Angina pectoris, or chest pain, can accompany heart failure, and when the patient is not in failure, angina is a harbinger of heart disease that can progress to failure. Angina occurs when the coronary arteries are unable to supply the heart with enough blood to meet its oxygen demands. This occurs because of atherosclerotic changes (narrowing or hardening) in the coronary arteries.

Drug therapy of heart failure and angina share some similarities. In both cases, treatments are intended to reduce the workload of the heart, and therefore reduce oxygen consumption by the myocardium. Many of the drugs used to treat heart failure are also effective in angina. In heart failure, treatment is aimed at improving the efficiency of the heart muscle, and in angina, dilating vessels can increase the supply of blood to the heart. Ultimately, the goals of treatment in both cases are to alleviate symptoms and improve the quality of life of the patient. By making lifestyle changes, the progression of both diseases is slowed, and the patient's lifespan can be prolonged. In heart failure, drugs that improve cardiac contractility, reduce fluid volume, and cause dilation of the blood vessels accomplish some of these objectives. In addition to the material found in the discussion of dugs used for heart failure, the diuretics, inhibitors of the renin-angiotensin hormone system, and the beta-blockers are covered in Chapters 21 and 17, respectively.

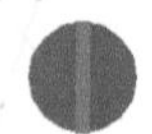

# Heart Failure and Angina

Heart failure occurs because the heart is unable to adequately fill with or eject blood. It is accompanied by abnormal increases in blood volume and interstitial (between the cells) fluid, or edema. The term congestive heart failure (CHF) refers to the later stages of heart failure, where fluid accumulation in the lungs causes difficulty breathing, and in the legs results in edema of the feet and ankles. Underlying causes of heart failure (HF) include atherosclerotic heart disease, myocardial infarction, hypertension, diseases of the heart valves, and pathology of the myocardium. The number of newly diagnosed patients with HF is increasing because more individuals now survive acute myocardial infarction and go on to develop HF.

congestive heart failure Inability of the heart to effectively pump returned venous blood, leading to accumulation of fluid in the lungs and lower extremities.

The reduced cardiac output that occurs as a result of early HF triggers three compensatory responses. First, the sympathetic nervous system is activated, which stimulates beta receptors in the heart and alpha receptors in the blood vessels. The heart rate is increased, the heart muscle contracts with greater force, and vasoconstriction increases the return of blood to the heart. The early drop in cardiac output also decreases blood flow to the kidney, and results in activation of the renin-angiotensin-aldosterone system, a second compensatory mechanism. Hormones important in fluid volume maintenance are released. This results in retention of sodium and water and increases vasoconstriction in the peripheral circulation. Blood volume increases, and more blood is returned to the heart. Lastly, the heart compensates by stretching, in order to accommodate the extra volume and increase the strength of contraction. In the short-term, these mechanisms improve cardiac output.

In the long-term, chronic activation of the sympathetic nervous system and fluid retention causes reshaping of cardiac tissue, and stretching of muscle fibers. Excessive elongation of the fibers eventually results in weaker contractions, and the change in the shape of the heart diminishes the ability to eject blood. All three compensatory responses ultimately increase the work the heart must do to supply blood to the body, they increase oxygen demand, and result in further deterioration of cardiac function over time (**Fig. 16.1**). The shape of the heart becomes more spherical, interfering with its ability to efficiently function as a pump. This prompts additional fluid retention, creating a vicious cycle that if left untreated, leads to death.

Angina pectoris is a characteristic sudden, severe, pressing chest pain radiating to the neck, jaw, back, and arms. It is caused by inadequate coronary blood supply, which is unable to meet the oxygen demands of the heart. When a healthy adult exerts, the heart rate increases, but the excess demand for oxygen by the myocardium is met through dilation of the coronary arteries and increased blood supply to the myocardium. In angina, atherosclerotic lesions in the coronary artery walls prevent vessels from dilating, and cause the imbalance between oxygen delivery and cardiac work. The transient chest pain of angina is not associated with myocardial cell death. Rather, it is a symptom of declining cardiovascular health, which can end in myocardial infarction or heart failure.

## Drug Therapy in Heart Failure

As a better understanding of the causes of HF and outcomes of drug treatments have developed, treatment guidelines have dramatically changed. The foundation of treatment of patients at risk of developing HF is prevention. Lifestyle changes (smoking cessation, diet), treatment of underlying conditions such as hypertension and diabetes, elimination of triggering factors such as drugs that may promote HF, and improvement of fitness are key to successful care in the early stages of the disease. Drug treatment of symptomatic HF includes judicious use of diuretics, inhibitors of the renin-angiotensin system, beta-blockers where indicated, and use of inotropic drugs (increase the force of heart contractions) in select patients. Direct vasodilators, such as hydralazine and isosorbide (orally) or nitroprusside (intravenous), are added in some cases to reduce the workload on the heart.

inotropic Altering or affecting the force of muscular contractions.

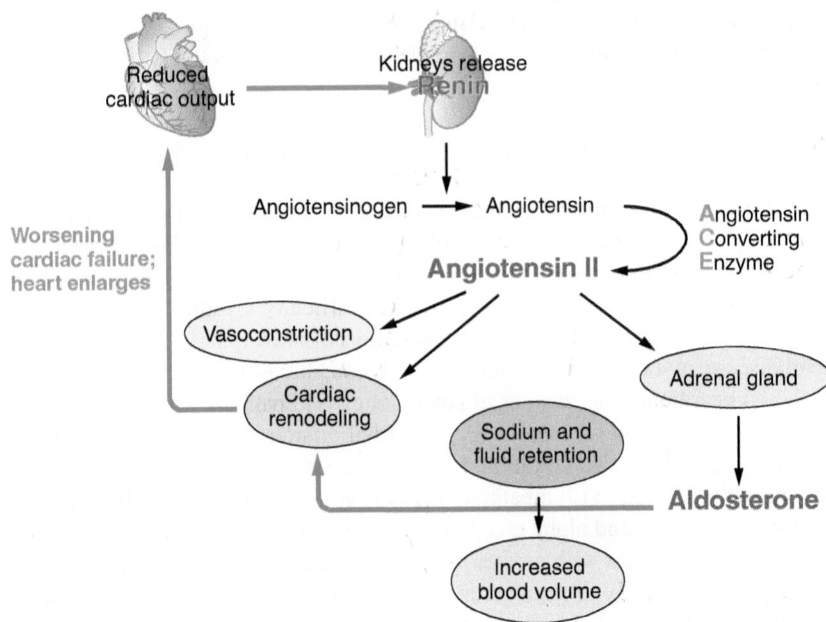


**Figure 16.1** The cycle of physiologic factors involved in the development of heart failure.

## Drug Treatment of Angina

Three classes of drugs, the nitrates, beta-blockers, and calcium channel blockers, used either alone or in combination, are effective in treating angina. Other nondrug interventions, such as cessation of smoking or weight loss in the overweight patient, are effective and important treatment strategies. Refer to Chapters 15 and 17 for additional discussion of the calcium channel blockers.

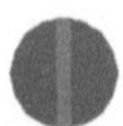

# Drugs That Reduce Cardiac Work: Diuretics, Beta Antagonists, Renin-Angiotensin System Inhibitors and Vasodilators

## Diuretics and Beta Antagonists

diuretic A drug that promotes the excretion of urine.

Diuretics are drugs that promote the formation and excretion of urine through their effects on the kidneys. In patients with CHF, diuretics relieve pulmonary congestion and peripheral edema, and also reduce blood pressure. Chapter 21 provides more detailed information on the diuretics. Beta antagonists counteract the chronic activation of the sympathetic nervous system, thereby helping to interrupt the cycle of deteriorating heart function.

### Actions and Indications

Diuretics decrease plasma volume and subsequently decrease the volume of blood returning to the heart. They exert their action by reducing the reabsorption of sodium and chloride during the formation of urine, thereby increasing the volume of fluid that must be excreted with the salts. As a result, diuretics relieve symptoms of shortness of breath, especially at night when patients are reclining. The reduction in blood volume decreases the cardiac workload and the oxygen demands of the myocardium. Diuretics reduce blood pressure, which, in turn, reduces cardiac work. The diuretics most often used for heart failure are furosemide (Lasix®), bumetanide (Bumex®), spironolactone (Aldactone®), and hydrochlorothiazide (HydroDIURIL®).

Spironolactone is especially useful because it is an aldosterone inhibitor. Aldosterone is a hormone produced by the adrenal glands that promotes the retention of sodium and water by the kidney (see Fig. 16.1). Spironolactone reduces the retention of sodium and increases the retention of potassium. It is most often used in conjunction with an inhibitor of the renin-angiotensin system.

aldosterone A steroid hormone produced by the adrenal glands that acts in the kidneys to contribute to the control of salt and water balance.

The beta-blockers metoprolol (Lopressor®), carvedilol (Coreg®) and bisoprolol (Zebeta®) have all been shown to be effective in heart failure, although carvedilol is the only one of the three that has an FDA approved indication for use in this particular disease (see **Fig. 16.2**). Researchers believe that the beta-blockers work because they block the negative effects of sympathetic stimulation, such as the increase in heart rate and cardiac workload. They also block the secretion of renin by the kidney, which in turn reduces the production of angiotensin and aldosterone. These benefits accrue in spite of the fact that beta blockers reduce total cardiac output.

## Administration

Bisoprolol and carvedilol are available as tablets for oral administration only. Metoprolol is available for intravenous injection and as oral tablets, both extended- and immediate-release formulations. These drugs should not be abruptly discontinued because of the risk of rebound sympathetic stimulation. Doses may need to be reduced in the elderly, and if side effects occur. The diuretics are adequately absorbed orally, and are available in a variety of formulations for oral use. In addition, furosemide and bumetanide can be given by intramuscular or intravenous injection.

## Side Effects

As an extension of their pharmacologic activity, the beta-blockers can reduce heart rate and cardiac output excessively and cause the patient in heart failure to deteriorate further. For this reason, these drugs are usually avoided in patients who have a very low heart rate, or other symptoms of worsening disease. They are most beneficial early in the course of the disease. Patients may note dizziness because of lowered blood pressure. Some patients may have worsening symptoms of asthma, and these should be reported to the physician.

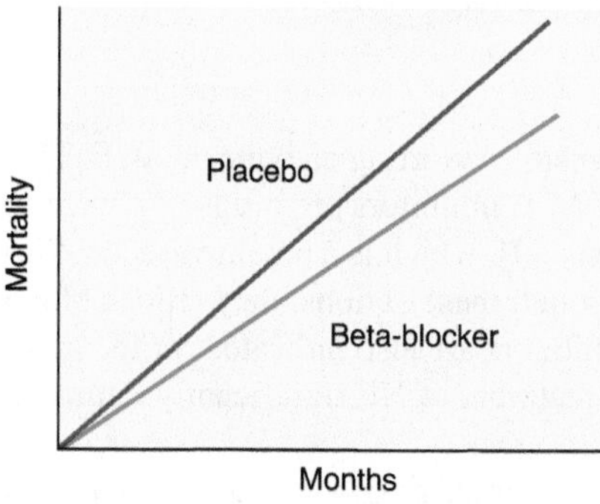


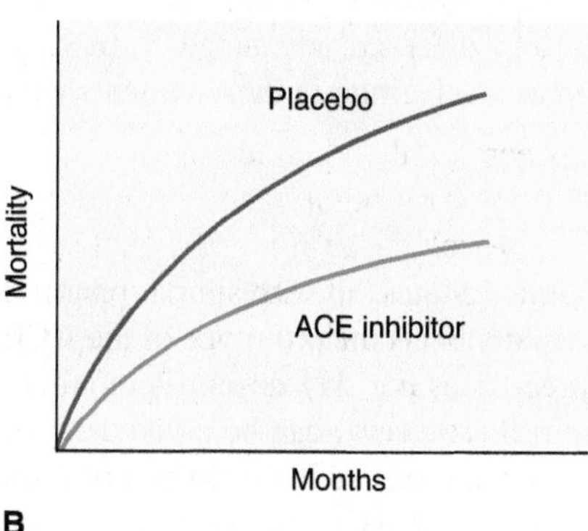


**Figure 16.2** Risk of death in heart failure patients who did not receive a beta-blocker or ACE inhibitor compared to those who did. Beta-blockers and ACE inhibitors reduce mortality in patients with heart failure.

Diuretics alter the concentration of electrolytes in the blood to varying degrees. Reduced blood levels of potassium are the most problematic of the electrolyte abnormalities that are likely to occur with diuretic therapy. Low potassium levels can result in weakness, muscle cramping, delirium, and arrhythmias. Hypokalemia is especially dangerous in patients who take digoxin, because it increases the risk of digoxin toxicity. Hypokalemia is not a problem in patients who take potassium-sparing diuretics. However, they can cause excess potassium levels in some people.

### Tips for the Technician

Patients should be cautioned about abrupt discontinuation of any of the drugs used to treat heart failure and prescription vials should be labelled accordingly. The beta-blockers can cause drowsiness, especially early in therapy, so auxiliary caution labels should be attached. All patients on diuretics should be warned about the possibility of dizziness on arising. Getting up slowly can prevent this problem. Patients should notify their physicians if they experience significant dizziness or worsening edema while on these medications.

## Renin-Angiotensin System Inhibitors

The renin-angiotensin-aldosterone system is one of many mechanisms in the body that promote the normal state of physiologic balance. This hormone system is important in regulating blood pressure and fluid volume. When specialized cells in the kidney sense reduced blood perfusion and increased sympathetic activity, the cells respond by increasing the release of renin, an enzyme responsible for converting the precursor angiotensinogen to angiotensin. This promotes the production of angiotensin II, a potent vasoconstrictor, and the release of aldosterone, which increases fluid retention (see Fig. 16.1). This mechanism improves hemodynamics (movement of the blood) in the short term, and can be lifesaving in situations where there is blood loss, but prolonged activation of the system will damage the heart over time.

hemodynamics Forces and mechanisms involved with blood circulation.

### Actions and Indications

Angiotensin is converted to angiotensin II by angiotensin converting enzyme or ACE. This enzyme is an important target for drug therapy. The ACE inhibitors are drugs of choice in heart failure because they block formation of angiotensin II, which is a potent vasoconstrictor and stimulates the production of aldosterone. Through these actions, they reduce blood pressure and the workload on the heart. The ACE inhibitors are also indicated for the treatment of hypertension. The use of these drugs in the treatment of HF significantly improves outcomes and prolongs patient's lives (Fig. 16.2).

Angiotensin receptor blockers (ARBs) are potent antagonists of the angiotensin receptor, with actions very similar to the ACE inhibitors. The ARBs, losartan (Cozaar®) and valsartan (Diovan®), are not considered first choice drugs however, because they are considerably more expensive than the ACE inhibitors, and offer no advantage in treating symptoms of HF or prolonging life. They can be used as a substitute in those patients who cannot tolerate ACE inhibitors.

### Administration

There are numerous ACE inhibitors available in the United States, all with similar pharmacologic profiles, and all absorbed orally. Captopril (Capoten®) is the prototype of the ACE inhibitors, but it is less likely to be used because three times per day dosing is required. Enalapril (Vasotec®), lisinopril (Prinivil®), and ramipril (Altace®) can be given daily or twice daily. Food significantly reduces the absorption of captopril so it should be given on an empty stomach. Although absorption of most of the other ACE inhibitors is slowed when taken with food, the extent of their absorption is unchanged, and they can be taken without regard to meals. Enalaprilat is the only ACE inhibitor available as an injection. Enalaprilat is the active metabolite of enalapril. Refer to **Table 16.1** for names, indications and available formulations of products used to treat HF.

Most of the ACE inhibitors undergo some combination of renal excretion, metabolism and elimination via the feces. Dosage adjustment in the presence of renal failure is required for captopril, lisinopril, and enalapril because the majority of elimination occurs via the kidneys. Fosinopril (Monopril®) and ramipril are significantly removed through metabolism, and patients with liver disease may require lower doses of these drugs. These drugs should never be administered to pregnant women. They are known to be highly toxic to the fetus in the second and third trimester of pregnancy.

The angiotensin receptor blockers are available for oral administration only. Absorption is variable and, in the case of valsartan, is significantly reduced in the presence of food. Elimination occurs mainly through metabolism in the liver. The dose of losartan is reduced in patients with renal failure so severe that it requires dialysis, a procedure that mechanically removes waste from the blood stream and adjusts fluid and electrolyte balance in place of the kidneys. As with the ACE inhibitors, these drugs should not be administered to pregnant women.

dialysis Medical procedure that uses a machine to filter waste products from the blood and adjust fluid and electrolyte imbalances in people with renal failure.

## Side Effects

All of the ACE inhibitors have side effects similar to the ARBs, with one exception. The ACE inhibitors are known for causing a dry and persistent cough that is not caused by the ARBs. In some of the less frequently used agents (not discussed here) the incidence of cough is as high as 25%. The more frequently used drugs, such as enalapril, benazepril (Lotensin®), lisinopril, and ramipril are associated with a lower, but still significant, frequency of cough of less than 10%. Although the cough is annoying, it is not dangerous and it resolves with discontinuation of the drug. These drugs can cause GI upset and an unpleasant taste in the mouth.

Other more serious side effects are possible. Since both the ACE inhibitors and the ARBs are antihypertensive agents, hypotension can be problematic. Doses are very gradually increased to avoid this problem. Hypotension can predispose patients to renal failure. The ACE inhibitors and ARBs are known to worsen renal function in some patients, especially when used in conjunction with diuretics. Both ACE inhibitors and ARBs can cause increases in serum potassium levels and must be used cautiously in patients taking spironolactone, other potassium-sparing diuretics, or potassium supplements. Both drug classes can cause a rare but potentially life-threatening swelling of the face, lips, tongue, and throat called angioedema. They can also cause thrombocytopenia, and depression of the production of neutrophils resulting in reduced neutrophil counts, or neutropenia.

### Tips for the Technician

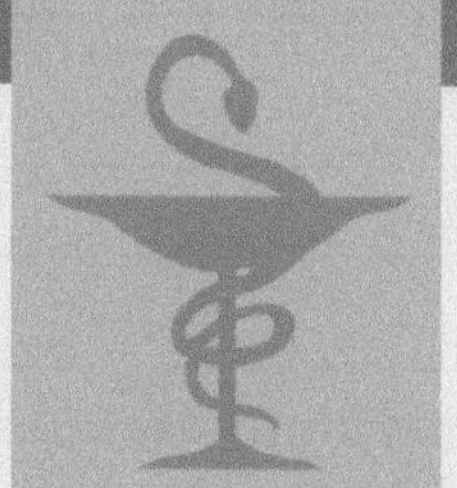

Patients should be advised regarding side effects, and encouraged to comply with the doctor's orders for laboratory monitoring. Women of childbearing age need to be informed about the risks of taking these drugs during pregnancy. Patients experiencing any kind of rash or facial edema should be advised to stop taking the medication and contact their physician immediately. Otherwise, medication should not be discontinued except on the advice of the physician. Patients taking captopril and valsartan should be cautioned to take these medications on an empty stomach. Apply the appropriate auxiliary labels to prescription vials containing these drugs. Absorption may be reduced when the ACE inhibitors or ARBs are taken with antacids or iron, and prescriptions should be labelled with instructions to avoid these products.

**Table 16.1** Comparison of Drugs Used for Heart Failure With Formulations and Indications.

| Generic | Brand Name | Available as | Indications | Notes |
|---|---|---|---|---|
| **Diuretics** | | | | |
| Bumetanide | Bumex® | Tablets, solution, injection | Edema of HF & renal failure | Causes profound diuresis |
| Furosemide | Lasix® | Tablets, solution, injection | Edema of HF & Renal failure, HTN | Causes profound diuresis |
| Hydrochloro-thiazide | HydroDIURIL® | Tablets, capsules, oral solution | Hypertension, edema due to HF | May be used in infants and children |
| Spironolactone | Aldactone® | Tablets | Hypertension, HF edema, primary hyperaldo-steronism | Antagonist of renin-angiotensin-aldosterone system |
| **Beta-Blockers** | | | | |
| Bisoprolol | Zebeta® | Tablets | Hypertension | Used for HF in clinical studies |
| Carvedilol | Coreg® | Tablets | HF, HTN treatment after MI | Alpha and beta antagonist |
| Atenolol | Tenormin® | Tablets, injection | HTN, Angina, Post MI | |
| Metoprolol | Lopressor®<br>Toprol XL®† | Tablets, ER tabs, injection | HTN, angina, post MI, HF – ER only | Used off-label for many conditions |
| **Renin-Angiotensin System Inhibitors** | | | | |
| ACE Inhibitors | | | | |
| Benazepril | Lotensin® | Tablets | HTN | QD – BID |
| Captopril | Capoten® | Tablets | HF, HTN, diabetic nephro-pathy, Post MI | q8h dosing<br>Avoid in pregnancy* |
| Enalapril | Vasotec® | Tablets, injection | HF, HTN | QD – BID |
| Lisinopril | Prinivil®, Zestril® | Tablets | HF, HTN, Post MI | QD |
| Quinapril | Accupril® | Tablets | HF, HTN | QD – BID |
| Ramipril | Altace® | Capsules | HF, HTN, Reduce risk of MI | QD |
| ARB Agents | | | | |
| Losartan | Cozaar® | Tablets | HTN, HTN with HF, diabetic nephropathy | |
| Valsartan | Diovan® | Tablets | HTN | |
| **Inotropic Agents** | | | | |
| Digoxin | Lanoxin® | Tablets, elixir, capsules, injection | Heart failure, arrhythmias | Narrow therapeutic index |
| Dobutamine | Dobutrex® | Injection | Cardiac decompensation | |
| Inamrinone | | Injection | Short-term IV therapy of CHF | |
| Milrinone | Primacor® | Injection, premixed bag | Short-term IV therapy of CHF | |

†Extended Release. ER, extended release; HF, heart failure; HTN, hypertension; MI, myocardial infarction. *All ACE inhibitors and ARBs are avoided in pregnancy.

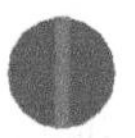

# Drugs That Improve the Efficiency of the Heart: Inotropic Agents

Agents that enhance the ability of the cardiac muscle to efficiently and completely contract will increase cardiac output. Although these drugs act by different mechanisms, in each case the result is enhanced contractility of cardiac muscle. Digoxin (Lanoxin®) is used in both hospital and outpatient settings, while dobutamine (Dobutrex®), inamrinone, and milrinone (Primacor®) are reserved for end-stage heart failure and are administered in hospital settings only.

## Cardiac Glycosides

The cardiac glycosides are often called digitalis glycosides, because the drugs come from the foxglove plant, *Digitalis purpurea.* They are a group of chemically similar compounds that can increase the contractility of the heart muscle. Because of this property they are widely used in the treatment of heart failure. Digoxin is now the only cardiac glycoside available in the United States.

### Actions and Indications

Like some of the antiarrhythmic drugs, the cardiac glycosides influence the flow of sodium and calcium ions in the cardiac muscle. By reducing the outflow of calcium, digoxin increases the force of cardiac contractility, causing the cardiac output to more closely resemble that of the normal heart (see **Fig. 16.3**). Stronger myocardial contraction leads to in-

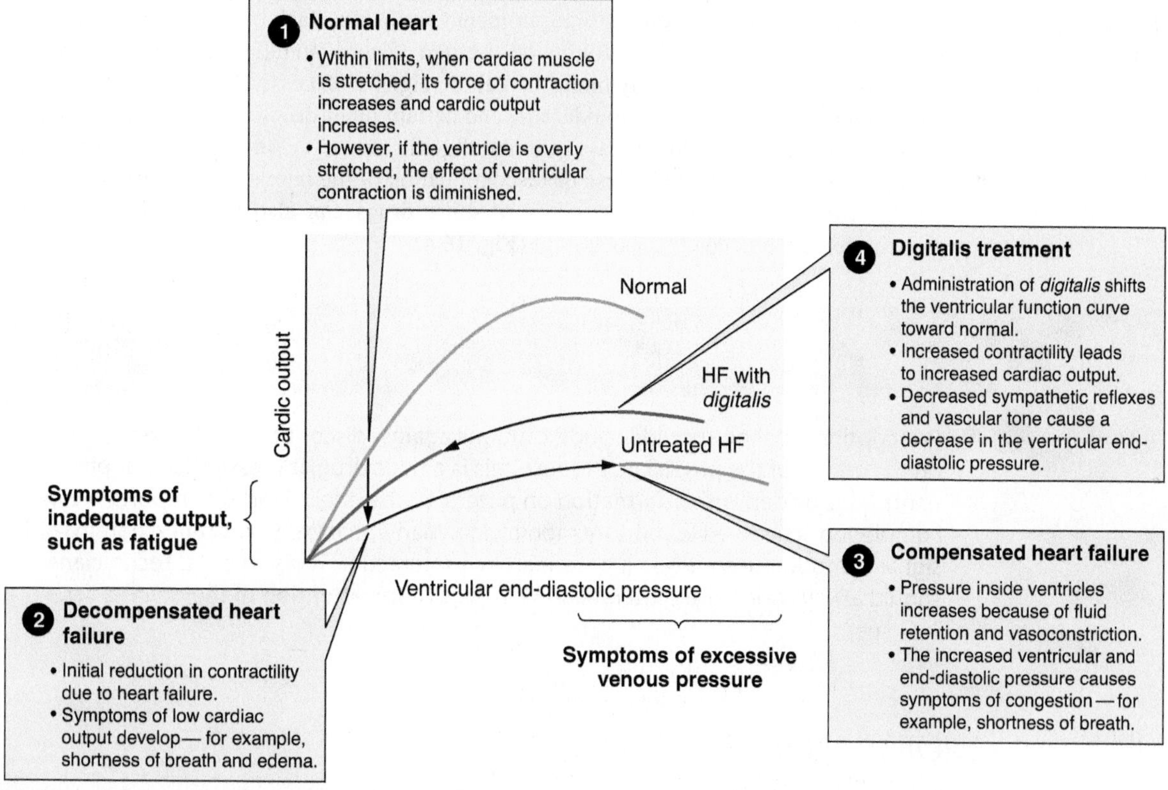


**Figure 16.3** Comparison of ventricular function in the normal heart, in decompensated heart failure and with digoxin treatment. (Adapted with permission from Harvey RA, Champe PC, Howland RD, et al. *Lippincott's Illustrated Reviews: Pharmacology,* 3rd edition. Baltimore: Lippincott Williams & Wilkins, 2006.)

creased efficiency of the heart. The resulting improvement in blood flow leads to reduced sympathetic activity, which in turn reduces peripheral resistance (the resistance to the flow of blood caused by the blood vessels). Together, these effects allow a reduction in heart rate, and reduce the workload on the heart. Digoxin therapy is indicated in some patients with severe, symptomatic HF after initiation of diuretic, ACE inhibitor, and beta-blocker therapy.

peripheral resistance Resistance to the flow of blood in peripheral arterial vessels.

### Administration

The therapeutic effects and adverse effects of digoxin are well correlated to serum levels. Because digoxin has such a narrow therapeutic window, serum levels are monitored to prevent toxicity. Digoxin is available as tablets, capsules, an elixir, and injection. The bioavailabilities of these different digoxin formulations vary. For example, the elixir is essentially completely absorbed, whereas the bioavailability of the tablets is only about 75%. Changing brands or formulations when filling prescriptions may result in changes in the patient's digoxin levels, so this practice is avoided. Digoxin is mainly eliminated unchanged in the urine, and patients with kidney failure may require a reduction in their daily dose.

### Side Effects

There is only a small difference between a therapeutically effective dose of digoxin and doses that are toxic or even fatal. Symptoms of digitalis toxicity are some of the more commonly encountered adverse results of treatment with this drug. Decreased serum levels of potassium predispose a patient to digoxin toxicity. When digoxin serum levels are elevated, but the patient has minor or no symptoms, the drug can simply be discontinued and restarted later at a lower dose. However, severe digoxin toxicity associated with cardiac arrhythmias requires treatment of the arrhythmia and the use of antibodies to digoxin (Digibind®), which bind and inactivate the drug.

anorexia Loss of appetite for food; sometimes a symptom of drug therapy.

Typical adverse reactions to digoxin include anorexia (lack of appetite), nausea, and vomiting. Slow pulse, fatigue, confusion, blurred vision, alteration of color perception, halos around objects, and arrhythmias can all be signs of excessively high serum digoxin levels. Quinidine, verapamil, amiodarone, and certain other drugs interact with digoxin to cause as much as a twofold increase in serum digoxin levels. These combinations generally require a reduction in digoxin dose or discontinuation of the interacting medication. Many diuretics, corticosteroids, and a variety of other drugs can also predispose patients to digoxin toxicity by depleting potassium (**Fig. 16.4**).

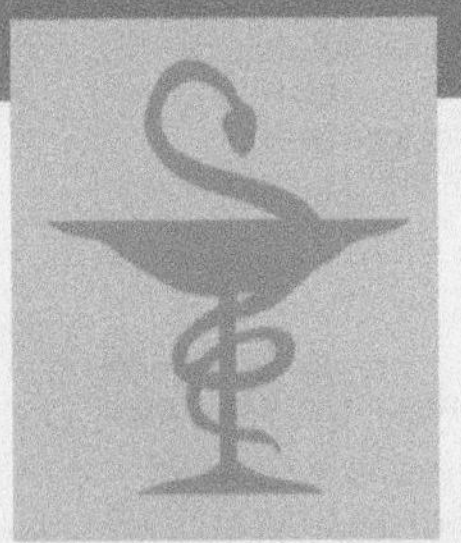

### Tips for the Technician

Prescription labeling should include cautions against discontinuing digoxin, except on the advice of the physician. Because this is a toxic drug, it is essential that patients be provided with information on potential side effects and the importance of completing scheduled laboratory monitoring. Many pharmacy computer systems signal computer users when a potential drug interaction is discovered. Technicians should always bring drug interaction warnings to the attention of the pharmacist.

## Other Inotropic Agents

Dobutamine, inamrinone, and milrinone are other inotropic drugs that are used in the hospital setting only, usually for patients with uncontrolled HF. Dobutamine is the most commonly used inotropic agent after digoxin. It is a beta adrenergic agonist chemically similar to dopamine. Inamrinone and milrinone are both phosphodiesterase inhibitors used in similar circumstances as dobutamine.

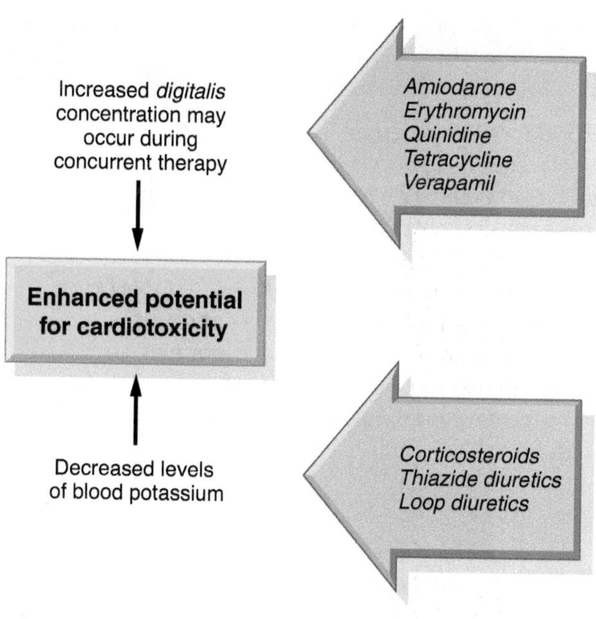


**Figure 16.4** Potential drug interactions between digitalis glycosides and other drugs. (Adapted with permission from Harvey RA, Champe PC, Howland RD, et al. Lippincott's Illustrated Reviews: *Pharmacology,* 3rd edition. Baltimore: Lippincott Williams & Wilkins, 2006.)

## Actions and Indications

Dobutamine, inamrinone, and milrinone are used for HF emergencies. Treatment with these drugs is limited to short-term use only. The phosphodiesterase inhibitors increase levels of intracellular calcium and, therefore, cardiac contractility. They also act on peripheral blood vessels to cause vasodilation. Dobutamine directly stimulates beta receptors in the heart to increase contractility and cardiac output, and reduces the workload on the heart by causing vasodilation.

## Administration

Dobutamine, inamrinone, and milrinone have short durations of action and are administered by intravenous infusion. An initial IV bolus (the injection of a large dose of a drug given at once) is recommended before beginning the IV infusion with inamrinone and milrinone. Doses of all three drugs are based on the patient's body weight, and dose is adjusted based on the response to the drug. It is because of the route of administration, the critically ill condition of the patients who receive these drugs, and the requirement for constant monitoring and dose adjustment that patients who receive these medications are always hospitalized. A number of injectable preparations are available for these drugs and are shown in Figure 16.3.

intravenous bolus A dose of a substance given by intravenous injection; includes large initial doses used to rapidly achieve the needed therapeutic blood levels.

## Side Effects

Side effect profiles are different for the phosphodiesterase inhibitors and dobutamine. Dobutamine causes side effects similar to other beta adrenergic agonists, including increased heart rate, hypertension related to increased cardiac output, palpitations, and possible arrhythmias. Dobutamine is prepared with a preservative called sodium metabisulfate that can cause asthma attacks in sensitive individuals. Adverse reactions due to dobutamine (not the preservative) generally resolve with dosage reduction or discontinuation of the drug.

Inamrinone and milrinone share some similarities in the side effects they cause. Both drugs can cause thrombocytopenia, although it is more common with inamrinone. Both drugs can cause hypotension related to their vasodilating effect. Both drugs can cause arrhythmias, although administration of milrinone is associated with a higher risk of ventricular and other arrhythmias. Some studies lasting more than a month and comparing milrinone to a placebo (an inert preparation used in controlled experiments) demonstrated no significant benefit from the drug and a higher risk of side effects and even death.

placebo A pharmacologically inert substance used in controlled trials to test the efficacy of a drug.

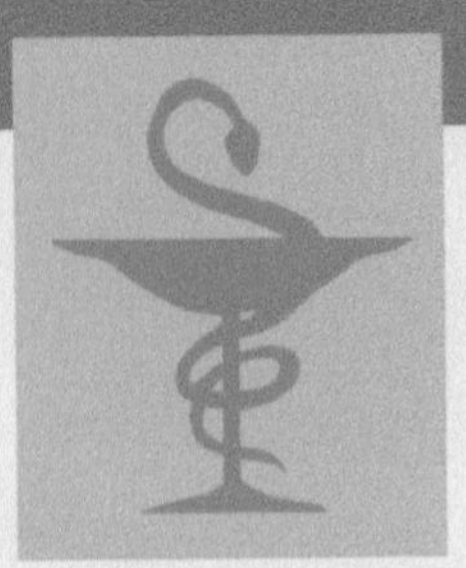

## Tips for the Technician

When one of these drugs is used for decompensated heart failure it is delivered by continuous IV infusion. Although premixed IV solutions are available for both dobutamine and milrinone, the hospital-based technician may be involved with compounding IV solutions of any of these drugs. Some drugs are incompatible with certain intravenous solutions. It is important to have a reliable reference source for compatibility information, such as Lawrence Trissel's *Handbook on Injectable Drugs*. Dobutamine is incompatible with alkaline solutions and a long list of drugs. Furosemide cannot be injected into an IV solution containing milrinone or inamrinone. This combination causes formation of a precipitate (a solid compound that results from a chemical reaction). Inamrinone should not be diluted with dextrose containing solutions.

precipitate An insoluble solid that settles out of a solution; also the formation of such a solid

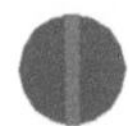

# Antianginal Drugs

## The Nitrates

The nitrates are a group of organic compounds long known to be effective in the treatment of angina pectoris. They are manufactured through a process that mixes nitric acid and glycerin. The nitric acid ionizes, and then binds to the glycerin that is added to the mixture. After nitroglycerin and its explosive potential was discovered in 1847 by Ascanio Sobrero, Alfred Nobel, of Nobel prize fame, developed a process for manufacturing this substance. When explosions killed many people during the manufacture and use of nitroglycerin, Nobel created a safer explosive by combining nitroglycerin with diatomaceous earth, a substance we now know as dynamite.

Serendipitously, during the discovery and later manufacturing processes, nitroglycerin was noted by its discoverer and factory workers to cause headaches if even a tiny amount came in contact with the skin. At about this same time, amyl nitrite was discovered to be useful for angina, but patients soon became resistant to its effects. The propensity of the two compounds to cause headaches, and other similarities were noted and soon thereafter, nitroglycerin, in minute quantities, began to be used for angina.

### Actions and Indications

Nitrates reduce workload on the heart and increase blood flow to the myocardium. They accomplish this by dilation of the large veins that feed back to the heart and by dilation of coronary arteries. When there is dilation of coronary arteries there is improved blood flow to the myocardium and therefore, increased oxygen delivery. By causing dilation of veins, they reduce the workload on the heart and consequently reduce the demand for oxygen by the cardiac muscle. The organic nitrates, such as nitroglycerin, are converted in the body to nitric oxide, which is naturally present in the body and is important in controlling vascular muscle relaxation.

All of the nitrates are effective, but they differ in their onset of action and rate of elimination. For prompt relief of an angina attack precipitated by exercise or emotional stress, nitroglycerin sublingual tablets (Nitrostat®), or nitroglycerin spray (Nitrolingual®) under the tongue is the drug of choice. Those drugs that have a longer delay in onset of action are used to help prevent angina attacks.

## Administration

The choice of the route of administration of the nitrates is determined by the need. The time to onset of nitrate action varies from one minute or less for immediate onset, sublingual nitroglycerin formulations to more than one hour for isosorbide products, which are given orally for prevention of attacks (**Fig. 16.5**). Nitroglycerin undergoes extensive first-pass metabolism in the liver after oral administration. It is rapidly absorbed through mucous membranes and even the skin, however. Drugs absorbed through the mucous membranes pass directly into the bloodstream, avoiding immediate metabolism in the liver. Nitroglycerin is usually administered either sublingually, topically as a cream, or via a transdermal patch, although long-acting oral preparations are available. It is administered by IV infusion in the treatment of congestive heart failure and acute hypertension.

Isosorbide products owe their improved bioavailability and long duration of action to stability against hepatic breakdown. There are two salts of isosorbide, dinitrate (Isordil®), and mononitrate (Imdur®). Oral isosorbide dinitrate undergoes metabolism to two mononitrates, both of which possess antianginal activity. The nitrates are available in a variety of formulations, both immediate and prolonged release. Refer to **Table 16.2** for a review of these products.

## Adverse Effects

The most common adverse effect of nitroglycerin, as well as of the other nitrates, is headache. A majority of patients will experience headaches, sometimes throbbing, especially early in therapy. The headaches are usually short-lived, and patients will develop tol-

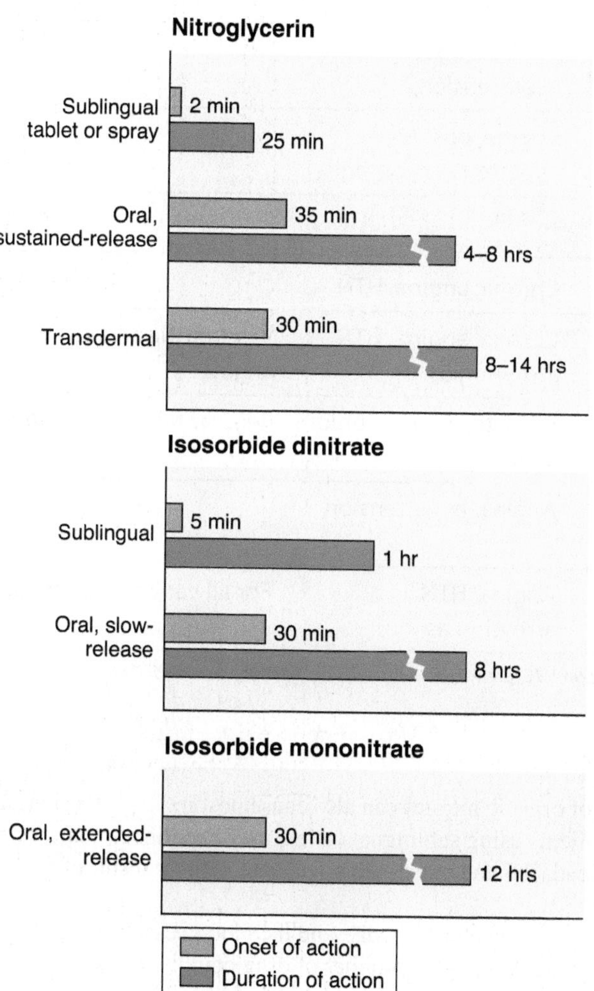


**Figure 16.5** Time to peak effect and duration of action of some nitrate preparations. (Adapted with permission from Harvey RA, Champe PC, Howland RD, et al. *Lippincott's Illustrated Reviews: Pharmacology,* 3rd edition. Baltimore: Lippincott Williams & Wilkins, 2006.)

**Table 16.2** Summary of Drugs Used for Angina, with Available Formulations and Indications.

| Generic | Brand Name | Available as | Indications | Notes |
|---|---|---|---|---|
| **Nitrates** | | | | |
| Isosorbide dinitrate | Isordil® | Tablets, ER tabs, ER capsules, chewable | Angina prophylaxis | Not for acute angina |
| Isosorbide mononitrate | Imdur®, Monoket® | Tablets, ER tablets | Angina prophylaxis | Not for acute angina |
| Nitroglycerin | Nitrostat®, Nitrodur®, others | Sublingual tabs, ER tabs and caps, ointment, IV transdermal patches, buccal tabs | Acute angina, Angina prophylaxis hypertension | Spray, sublingual for acute attacks, IV for HF |
| **Beta-Blockers** | | | | |
| Acebutolol | Sectral® | Capsules | PVCs, angina | Not 1st choice for angina |
| Atenolol | Tenormin® | Tablets, injection | HTN, angina, atrial arrhythmias | Useful after MI |
| Metoprolol | Lopressor®, Toprol® | Tablets, ER tabs, injection | Angina, post MI, hypertension, | |
| Propranolol | Inderal® | Tablets, oral soln, injection ER capsules | Angina, post MI, hypertension, others | |
| **Calcium Channel Blockers** | | | | |
| Amlodipine | Norvasc® | Tablets | Chronic angina, HTN | |
| Diltiazem | Dilacor®, Cardizem® | Tablets, ER tabs and capsules | Chronic angina, HTN, arrhythmias | Vasospastic and chronic angina |
| Nicardipine | Cardene® | Capsules, ER capsules, injection | Hypertension, chronic angina | Regular release for angina |
| Nifedipine | Procardia®, Adalat® | Capsules, ER tablets | Angina, hypertension | |
| Verapamil | Calan®, Isoptin® | Tablets, ER tabs & capsules, injection | Angina, HTN, arrhythmias | For all variants of angina |

ER, extended release; HF, heart failure; HTN, Hypertension; MI, Myocardial Infarction; PVC, premature ventricular contraction.

erance to this effect. High doses of organic nitrates can also cause postural hypotension, facial flushing, and tachycardia. Patients using sublingual tablets may experience some burning under the tongue with use. Headache and other side effects are a direct result of the vasodilation caused by the nitrates.

Tolerance to the actions of nitrates develops rapidly, and the blood vessels become less responsive to the vasodilating effects. Although a number of drug combinations have been used to try to prevent tolerance, the only sure way tolerance can be avoided is by providing a daily "nitrate-free interval" to restore sensitivity to the drug. This interval is typically eight to twelve hours, usually at night, because demand on the heart is decreased at that time. Nitroglycerin patches can be worn for twelve hours then removed for twelve hours. Nitroglycerin ointment can be removed at bedtime and then reapplied in the morning. Physicians have to consider other therapeutic options for patients who continue to have angina despite nitrate therapy.

There are a number of drug interactions of concern with the nitrates. Patients taking other medications that can cause orthostatic hypotension, such as alpha adrenergic blocking agents, the tricyclic antidepressants, alcoholic beverages, or the opioids, should be cautioned about the potential for dizziness or even fainting. Sildenafil potentiates the action of the nitrates. To prevent the dangerous hypotension that may occur with the combination, an interval of at least six hours between the ingestion of the two drugs is recommended.

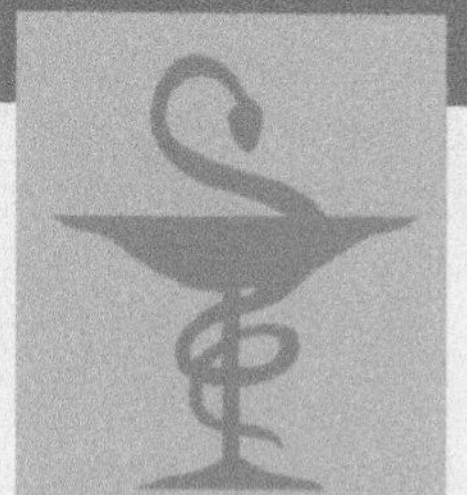

## Tips for the Technician

Pharmacy technicians need to be aware of the possibility of product confusion between Nicobid® and Nitro-Bid®, two brand name products that can look and sound alike. While Nitro-Bid® is a nitroglycerin product, Nicobid® is niacin. Confusion can occur between nitroglycerin and nitroprusside.

Nitroglycerin infusions must be prepared in glass IV bottles, because the drug binds to plastic. The manufacturer provides special IV tubing, which must be used. If it is prepared in plastic and the special tubing is not used, most of the nitroglycerin will never reach the patient. Nitroglycerin stability is of concern in the outpatient setting. Nitroglycerin must be stored in its original, amber glass container in order to preserve stability. It should never be stored in refrigerators, bathrooms, or other moist or warm places. Patients should keep a bottle of nitroglycerin with them at all times so that it is readily available when they experience chest pain.

Nitroglycerin patches or cream and isosorbide products should not be abruptly discontinued. When discontinuing these products, a dose-tapering plan is appropriate. People with sensitivity to adhesives may have reactions to nitroglycerin transdermal patches. If a patient has an allergy to tape, it should be brought to the attention of the pharmacist when nitroglycerin patches are ordered. Containers of nitrate products should be labelled, where appropriate, with warnings regarding product storage, abrupt discontinuation, avoiding other medications except on the advice of the physician, and avoiding alcohol.

# Beta-Blockers and Calcium Channel Blockers in Angina

Other treatments and drugs that reduce the oxygen demands of the heart can also be effective in the treatment of angina. The beta-blockers and calcium channel blockers are two additional drug classes that can be used to treat angina. Calcium channel blockers are avoided when the patient has heart failure.

## Actions and Indications

The beta adrenergic blocking agents decrease the oxygen demands of the heart by lowering the heart rate and the force of contraction of the heart and also by the resultant decrease in blood pressure. The demand for oxygen by the myocardium is reduced by beta-blockers both during exertion and at rest. Although propranolol is the prototype for this class of compounds, it does not selectively block the beta receptors in the heart. As a consequence, other beta-blockers such as metoprolol, or atenolol (Tenormin®), are preferred for the treatment of angina.

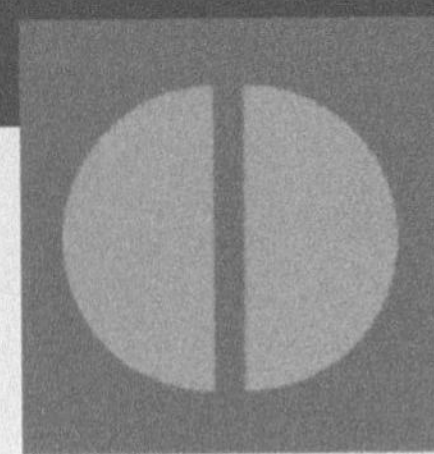

## Case 16.1

Mrs. Cordelia Valentine is an 83-year-old client at the clinic pharmacy where you work. She calls in for a refill of her nitroglycerin tablets, and requests that you give her two bottles. Mrs. Valentine says that she keeps one bottle at her bedside, one at her daughter's house, and one in the glove compartment of her car, so it will always be available when she needs it. She says the one at her daughter's house expired two months ago and the one she keeps at home is almost empty. What is wrong with Mrs. Valentine's approach to keeping nitroglycerin readily available, and how will you advise her regarding storage of nitroglycerin?

All calcium channel blockers cause a decrease in smooth and cardiac muscle tone. Vasodilation and reduced heart rate, strength of contraction, and blood pressure are reduced. This causes a reduction in cardiac workload. Nifedipine (Procardia®), nicardipine (Cardene®), amlodipine (Norvasc®), diltiazem (Cardizem®), and verapamil (Calan®) are all approved for use in angina. Nifedipine is the calcium channel blocker used most commonly because it has the greatest effect on vascular smooth muscle.

### Administration

The beta antagonists and calcium channel blockers are administered orally in the treatment of angina. They can be used in combination with the nitrates. Nifedipine and the other calcium channel blockers are often administered as extended-release formulations. As previously noted, it is important not to discontinue beta-blocker therapy abruptly. Although no rebound phenomenon has been documented to occur if calcium channel blockers are abruptly discontinued, most practitioners recommend that the dose should be gradually tapered off.

### Side Effects

Side effects of beta-blockers were covered in previous chapters, and most often include drowsiness early in therapy, dizziness, and hypotension. Calcium channel blockers, and especially nifedipine, can cause flushing, headache, hypotension, and peripheral edema as a result of vasodilation. All calcium channel blockers can cause constipation because of their relaxation of smooth muscle. Nifedipine may cause tachycardia as a reflex reaction to a significant decrease in blood pressure. All calcium channel blockers have the potential to exacerbate heart failure.

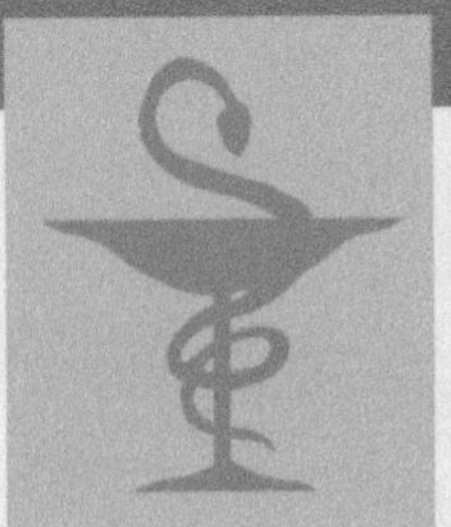

## Tips for the Technician

The pharmacist should ensure that patients know the signs of progressing heart failure, including shortness of breath and edema. Patients should be warned not to abruptly discontinue any of the medications used to treat angina, and prescription vials should be labelled accordingly. Beta-blockers should also be labelled with cautions regarding driving or performing other tasks that require alertness, because of the possibility of drowsiness, especially early in therapy. None of the extended-release formulations should be broken or crushed because this will cause the immediate-release of the contents. Pharmacy technicians should alert pharmacists to any automatic drug interaction warnings they note in the pharmacy computer system. Of special importance is the interaction between calcium channel blockers and digoxin previously covered in this chapter.

# Review Questions

## Multiple Choice

Choose the best answer for the following questions:

1. Which of the following is not one of the current recommendations for treating or preventing heart failure?
   a. Lifestyle changes, such as quitting smoking
   b. Treatment for other diseases that might predispose a patient to heart failure
   c. Diuretic therapy
   d. Negative inotropic drugs that decrease the force of contraction of the heart
   e. All of the above are excellent recommendations for treating or preventing heart failure

2. The ACE inhibitors and the angiotensin receptor blockers (ARBs) share many of the same effects. Which choice below correctly describes a difference between the two drug classes?
   a. The ARBs have been proven to be much more effective than the ACE inhibitors for the treatment of heart failure.
   b. The ACE inhibitors often cause a persistent dry cough, whereas the ARBs do not cause this side effect.
   c. The ACE inhibitors are much more expensive than the ARBs.
   d. The ACE inhibitors pose the risk of damage to the fetus in pregnant women and should not be administered to pregnant women. The ARBs, however, are safe for use in pregnant women.
   e. c and d are both correct.

3. Which of the following does not apply to the drug digoxin?
   a. Works by increasing the contractility of the heart
   b. Often the first drug prescribed when early signs of heart failure are detected
   c. Serum levels are monitored to prevent toxicity from developing
   d. Patients with kidney failure may require a reduced dose
   e. Severe toxicity can result in arrhythmias

4. What is angina pectoris?
   a. A defect of the pectoral muscles that puts excessive pressure on the chest cavity, resulting in severe chest pain.
   b. A chronic pain syndrome that is effectively treated with weight loss and digoxin therapy.
   c. A severe and sudden radiating chest pain that is a sign of declining cardiovascular health.
   d. A dull aching chest pain that is a characteristic symptom of myocardial cancer.
   e. A plant species from which several drugs that are useful in treating heart failure are derived.

5. Choose the incorrect statement regarding the nitrates
   a. Isosorbide dinitrate or mononitrate can be used for fast relief in an acute angina attack.
   b. Nitroglycerin is rapidly absorbed through mucous membranes and skin.

c. Nitroglycerin must be stored in its original amber glass bottle and IV infusions must be prepared in glass bottles rather than plastic bottles.
d. The most common side effect seen with nitrates is headache.
e. All of the above statements are correct.

## True/False

6. It is okay for patients to break their nifedipine extended-release tablet into pieces before swallowing if they think the tablet may be uncomfortably large to swallow.
   a. True
   b. False

7. In patients with chronic heart failure, long-term activation of the sympathetic nervous system and the renin-angiotensin-aldosterone system leads to stretching and reshaping of the heart.
   a. True
   b. False

8. Furosemide and bumetanide reduce blood pressure and relieve edema by promoting fluid excretion in the urine, which results in decreased plasma volume.
   a. True
   b. False

9. There is a high risk for serious drug interactions between the ACE inhibitors and quinidine, verapamil, or any of the diuretics.
   a. True
   b. False

10. When dobutamine, inamrinone, and milrinone must be compounded for intravenous use, preparations can be made using any available intravenous solution as long as the solution is not expired.
    a. True
    b. False

## Matching

For questions 11 to 15, match each number with the correct lettered choice.

11. Congestive heart failure
12. The only beta-blocker that is FDA approved for use in treating heart failure
13. Angioedema
14. Low serum potassium levels predispose patients to toxicity from this drug
15. Administered sublingually, topically, or transdermally

a. Spironolactone
b. A condition in which heart failure is accompanied by persistent upper respiratory infections
c. Carvedilol
d. Heart failure with accumulation of fluid, typically in lungs and extremities
e. A rare but potentially fatal side effect of the ACE inhibitors and ARBs that involves swelling of the face, lips, tongue, and throat
f. Metoprolol
g. Digoxin
h. A rare but potentially fatal side effect of the beta-blockers that involves swelling of the face, lips, tongue, and throat
i. Nitroglycerin

### Short Answer

16. What are the goals of drug treatment in congestive heart failure?

17. What role do the ACE inhibitors play in the treatment of heart failure?

18. What is the best strategy to prevent tolerance to the vasodilating effects of the nitrates?

19. Why is digoxin toxicity fairly common? What are some potential symptoms of an elevated digoxin level?

20. Your grandmother takes digoxin and furosemide, a diuretic, for her heart failure. She is scheduled to have blood drawn at the clinical laboratory today to check her electrolyte levels and her digoxin level, but she says she is too tired to go to the lab. What can you tell your grandmother to encourage her to go to her lab appointment?

## FOR FURTHER INQUIRY

Learn how the treatment of heart failure, once known as dropsy, has changed over the last 100 years. What were some of the drugs or other treatments used in the 1800s and early 1900s? What were the risks associated with their use?

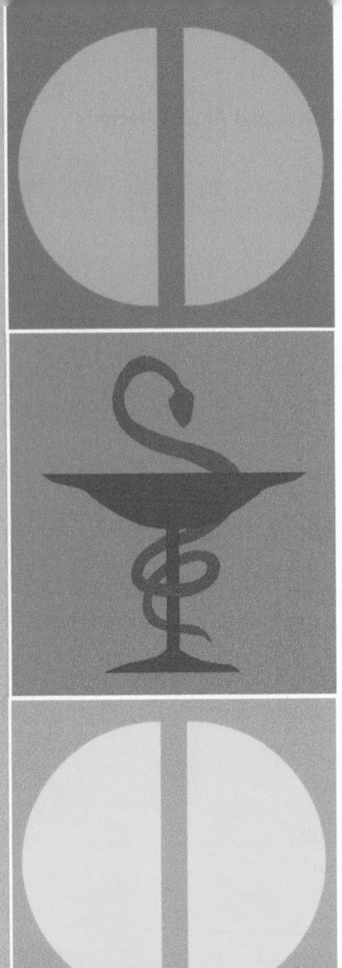

Chapter **17**

# Treatment of Hypertension

## KEY TERMS

- essential hypertension
- hyperkalemia
- hypertrichosis
- hyperuricemia
- ischemia
- syncope

## OBJECTIVES

After studying this chapter, the reader should be able to:

- Describe the goal of the treatment of hypertension and the risks associated with inadequately treated hypertension.
- List three lifestyle modifications that are most likely to result in significant reduction in blood pressure.
- Discuss the current recommendations for the treatment of hypertension, list the drug classes recommended for treatment in the order that they are added, and explain why noncompliance is so often responsible for treatment failure.
- List an example of a drug from each antihypertensive class and two side effects of each.
- Describe hypertensive crisis, list two drugs that are indicated for use in this situation, and explain a potential pitfall that technicians should take care to avoid for each.

## DRUGS COVERED IN THIS CHAPTER

### Antihypertensive Medications

| Diuretics | Beta-Blockers | ACE Inhibitors | AR II Blockers |
|---|---|---|---|
| Chlorothiazide | Atenolol | Benazepril | Candesartan |
| Hydrochlorothiazide | Labetalol | Captopril | Irbesartan |
| Metolazone | Metoprolol | Enalapril | Losartan |
| Furosemide | Nadolol | Fosinopril | Valsartan |
| Spironolactone | Propranolol | Lisinopril | |
| | | Quinapril | |
| | | Ramipril | |

| Calcium Channel Blockers | Alpha-Blockers | Miscellaneous Antihypertensives |
|---|---|---|
| Amlodipine | Doxazosin | Clonidine |
| Diltiazem | Prazosin | Hydralazine |
| Felodipine | Terazosin | Methyldopa |
| Nicardipine | | Minoxidil |
| Nisoldipine | | Nitroprusside |
| Verapamil | | |

The body regulates blood pressure within a narrow range of normal limits in order to guarantee adequate perfusion of the vital organs. This is achieved both through feedback from the baroreceptors, which are especially important in controlling blood pressure on a moment to moment basis, and via the renin-angiotensin-aldosterone system in the kidneys, which plays a significant role in maintaining pressure levels. Elevated blood pressure is an extremely common disorder, by some estimates affecting as many as 30 of every 100 Americans. Of these, one out of every three are unaware they have the disease, because typically hypertension causes no symptoms. Although it can be a result of underlying disease (such as kidney disease or pheochromocytoma) nine out of ten people with high blood pressure have essential hypertension, or hypertension without a known cause. No one knows why the normal regulating systems "reset" to maintain blood pressures at higher levels in those individuals with hypertension, but we do know that the damage done to the cardiovascular system by these chronically elevated pressures is devastating.

essential hypertension
High blood pressure that occurs without an identifiable cause.

Chronic hypertension that is left untreated can lead to congestive heart failure, myocardial infarction, kidney damage, and strokes. When high blood pressure is properly treated, the risk of stroke is reduced by about 40%, heart attacks by 25%, and heart failure by 50%. A family history of hypertension increases the likelihood that an individual will develop hypertensive disease. Essential hypertension is four times more common among African Americans than among Caucasians, and it occurs more often among middle-aged males than among middle-aged females. A stressful lifestyle, obesity, and smoking predispose an individual to hypertension.

Elevated blood pressure is classified according to severity, and classifications include prehypertension, Stage I, and Stage II hypertension. People with blood pressures greater than the desired 120/70 are considered to be in the prehypertension stage. Stage I hypertension includes people with a systolic pressure, the pressure during heart contraction, of >140 or a diastolic pressure, the pressure during heart relaxation, of >90. Patients with blood pressures >160 mm Hg systolic (top number) or >100 mm Hg diastolic (bottom number) are said to have stage II hypertension.

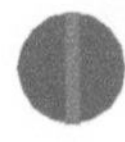

## Goals and Approaches to Successful Treatment

The goal of the treatment of hypertension is to prevent damage to the cardiovascular system by maintaining blood pressure below 140/90, and preferably 135/80 or less. In their seventh guideline for treatment of hypertension (JNC 7), the Joint National Committee on Prevention, Detection, Evaluation, and Treatment of High Blood Pressure recommends lifestyle changes as a first step in treatment of hypertension or "prehypertension," when blood pressure is above the desired range, but below the levels generally requiring drug treatment (Stage I). Major lifestyle modifications that consistently reduce blood pressure include weight loss in those who are obese, quitting smoking, and significant diet and exercise changes. When lifestyle modifications do not reduce blood pressure to the desired pressures of less than 140 systolic and less than 90 diastolic, medications are needed. The drug treatment of hypertension centers on five different drug classes and several miscellaneous medications. The thiazide diuretics have been the cornerstone of the treatment of hypertension for decades, and have repeatedly been proven to be safe, effective, and relatively inexpensive. Additional drugs are added to the diuretic regimen on an individual basis, but often include an ACE inhibitor, a beta antagonist, or a calcium channel-blocking agent as a second drug (**Fig. 17.1**). Sometimes a third drug will be needed to get the patient's blood pressure under adequate control. This third drug may include a drug from one of the classes listed previously (although not a drug from the same classes already in use), or it may be one of a number of other drugs, including direct acting vasodilators, alpha antagonists, and centrally acting alpha agonists.

### Treatment Failure in Hypertension

Poor compliance is a significant problem in the treatment of hypertension, and is the number one reason for treatment failure. Drug treatment in hypertension is directed at preventing future negative outcomes, rather than in relieving the patient's present discomfort. The hypertensive patient rarely experiences symptoms from this disease, but often experiences some, mostly minor, adverse effect from the drug regimen. The adverse effects associated with the hypertensive therapy may bother the patient enough to outweigh, in the patient's mind, the future benefits. For example, beta-blockers can decrease libido or cause other sexual side effects, particularly in middle-aged and elderly men. This drug-induced sexual dysfunction may prompt the patient to discontinue therapy.

An incomplete understanding of either hypertension or its treatment increases the likelihood of nonadherence to therapy. Some patients are naturally averse to taking medications because they interpret the need for medication as a symbol of weakness. Lack of patient involvement in the plan of care can also discourage compliance. For these reasons, effective communication with patients is essential, and encourages success in the treatment of hypertension.

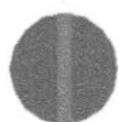

## Thiazide Diuretics

The current JNC 7 treatment recommendations are to begin treatment of hypertension with a thiazide diuretic unless there are compelling reasons to employ another drug class. Low-dose thiazide diuretic therapy is safe and effective in preventing all of the unwanted cardiovascular outcomes seen with untreated high blood pressure. Although all oral diuretics (including potassium sparing spironolactone and the loop diuretic, furosemide) can be used to lower blood pressure, the thiazides are the least expensive and consistently provide a significant reduction in blood pressure. Other diuretics will be discussed in Chapter 21.

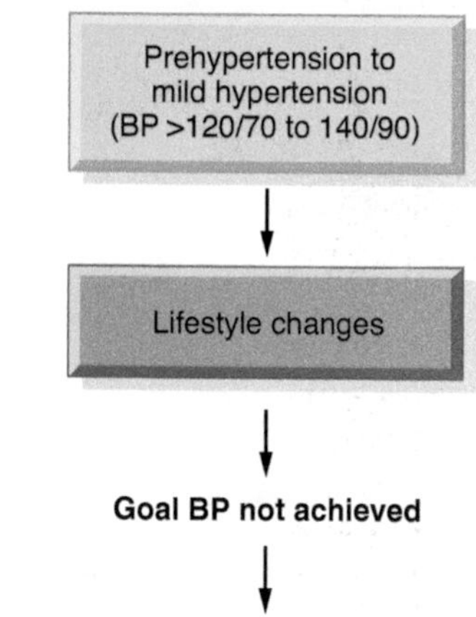


**An antihypertensive medication is started.**

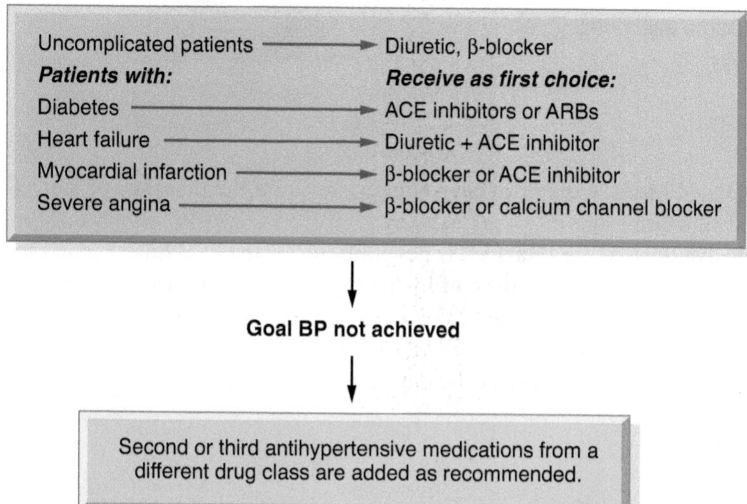


**Figure 17.1** Antihypertensive drug recommendations for otherwise healthy adults and those people with concomitant conditions.

## Actions and Indications

Thiazide diuretics, such as hydrochlorothiazide (HydroDIURIL®), lower blood pressure initially by increasing sodium and water excretion in the kidney. This causes a decrease in blood volume early in treatment and a reduction in peripheral resistance (**Fig. 17.2**). Spironolactone (Aldactone®), a potassium-sparing diuretic, can be combined with a thiazide diuretic. Spironolactone adds additional benefit in people with heart failure because it blocks aldosterone, a hormone that contributes to myocardial remodeling, which results in a less efficient heart shape. Thiazide diuretics lower blood pressure in both standing and reclining positions. They are used in combination with other antihypertensive drugs that may cause fluid or sodium retention (such as hydralazine or some of the calcium channel blockers) because they can offset these undesirable effects. In order for the thiazides to work, the kidney must be functioning normally or nearly normally. The thiazide-like diuretics, such as metolazone (Zaroxolyn®), are effective in the presence of significant kidney dysfunction.

## Administration

All of the thiazide diuretics are absorbed well when taken orally, can be taken without regard to food, and are available in a number of single agent and combination products. Only chlorothiazide (Diuril®) is available as an injectable product, and it is rarely used in adult patients. Hydrochlorothiazide is the most frequently used thiazide diuretic. Refer to **Table 17.1** for a comparison of available drugs and formulations. The loop diuretics, including furosemide (Lasix®) and bumetanide (Bumex®), are more frequently used when an in-

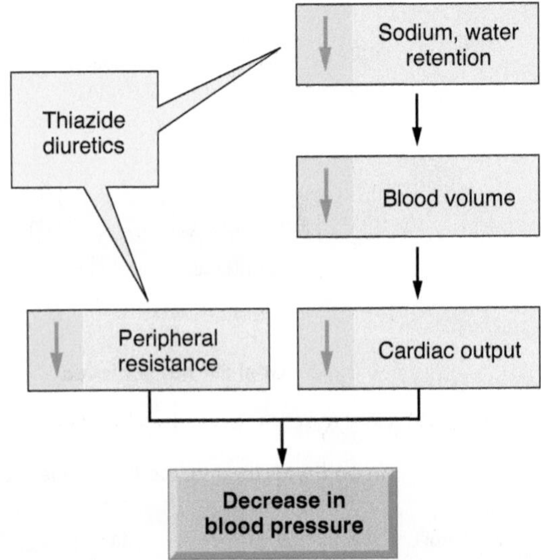


**Figure 17.2** The mechanism of antihypertensive actions of the thiazide diuretics. (Adapted with permission from Harvey RA, Champe PC, Howland RD, et al. *Lippincott's Illustrated Reviews: Pharmacology,* 3rd edition. Baltimore: Lippincott Williams & Wilkins, 2006.)

jectable diuretic is needed because they can cause diuresis even in the presence of significantly impaired renal function.

The antihypertensive dose of the thiazides is generally lower than the dose needed for the treatment of edema. For example, the dose of hydrochlorothiazide employed for edema is typically 25 to 100 mg daily. Adequate antihypertensive effect is usually seen with 12.5 to 50 mg daily. As is typical of most drugs, the elderly require lower doses of thiazide diuretics. These drugs should be taken early in the day to avoid frequent nighttime awakening to urinate.

## Table 17.1 Antihypertensive Medications and Representative Combination Products, Formulations, and Indications

| Generic | Brand Name | Available as | Indications | Notes |
|---|---|---|---|---|
| **Thiazide Diuretics** | | | | |
| Chlorothiazide | Diuril® | Tablets, oral susp, powder for injection | HTN, edema | May be used in infants and children |
| Hydrochlorothiazide | HydroDIURIL® | Tablets, capsules, oral solution | HTN, edema | May be used in infants and children |
| Metolazone | Zaroxolyn® | Tablets | Hypertension, HF, edema | |
| **Other Diuretics** | | | | |
| Furosemide | Lasix® | Tablets, oral solution, injection | Hypertension, HF, edema | |
| Spironolactone | Aldactone® | Tablets | HTN, HF, edema, primary hyperaldosteronism | Antialdosterone effect an advantage in heart failure |

*(continues)*

| Generic | Brand Name | Available as | Indications | Notes |
|---|---|---|---|---|
| **Beta-Blockers** | | | | |
| Atenolol | Tenormin® | Tablets, injection | HTN, Angina, Post MI | |
| Labetalol | Normodyne®<br>Trandate® | Tablets, injection | HTN, hypertensive crisis | Mixed alpha-beta blocker |
| Metoprolol | Lopressor®<br>Toprol XL® | Tablets, ER tabs, injection | HTN, angina, post MI, HF – ER only | Used off-label for many conditions |
| Nadolol | Corgard® | Tablets | HTN, Angina | Not specific for $beta_1$ receptors |
| Propranolol | Inderal® | Tablets, oral soln, injection ER capsules | HTN, post MI, angina, others | Not specific for $beta_1$ receptors |
| **ACE Inhibitors** | | | | |
| Benazepril | Lotensin® | Tablets | HTN | Avoid in pregnancy |
| Captopril | Capoten® | Tablets | HF, HTN, Post MI, diabetic nephropathy | Q8h administration<br>Avoid in pregnancy |
| Enalapril | Vasotec® | Tablets, injection | HF, HTN | Avoid in pregnancy |
| Lisinopril | Prinivil®, Zestril® | Tablets | HF, HTN, Post MI | Avoid in pregnancy |
| Quinapril | Accupril® | Tablets | HF, HTN | Avoid in pregnancy |
| Ramipril | Altace® | Capsules | HF, HTN, Reduce risk of MI | Avoid in pregnancy |
| **ARB agents** | | | | |
| Candesartan | Atacand® | Tablets | HTN | Avoid in pregnancy |
| Irbesartan | Avapro® | Tablets | HTN | Avoid in pregnancy |
| Losartan | Cozaar® | Tablets | HTN, HTN with HF, diabetic nephropathy | Avoid in pregnancy |
| Valsartan | Diovan® | Tablets | HTN | Avoid in pregnancy |
| **Calcium Channel Blockers** | | | | |
| Amlodipine | Norvasc® | Tablets | HTN, Chronic angina | |
| Diltiazem | Dilacor®,<br>Cardizem® | Tablets, ER tabs and capsules | Chronic angina, HTN, arrhythmias | |
| Felodipine | Plendil® | ER tablets | HTN | |
| Nicardipine | Cardene® | Capsules, ER capsules, injection | HTN, chronic angina | All forms indicated for HTN |
| Nifedipine | Procardia®,<br>Adalat® | Capsules, ER tabs | HTN, angina | |
| Verapamil | Calan, Isoptin | Tablets, ER tabs & capsules, injection | Angina, HTN, arrhythmias | |

*(continues)*

**Table 17.1** Antihypertensive Medications and Representative Combination Products, Formulations, and Indications *(continued)*

| Generic | Brand Name | Available as | Indications | Notes |
|---|---|---|---|---|
| **Alpha-Blockers** | | | | |
| Doxazosin | Cardura® | Tablets | HTN | |
| Prazosin | Minipress® | Capsules | HTN | |
| Terazosin | Hytrin® | Capsules | HTN, BPH | |
| **Miscellaneous Agents** | | | | |
| Clonidine | Catapres®, Catapres TTS® | Tablets, transdermal patch | HTN | Many off-label uses, including alcohol, drug withdrawal |
| Hydralazine | Apresoline® | Tablets, injection | HTN | Second-line drug |
| Methyldopa | Aldomet® | Tablets, injection | HTN, acute hypertensive crisis | |
| Minoxidil | Loniten® | Tablets | Severe HTN | Reserved for HTN unresponsive to other drugs |
| Nitroprusside | Nipride® | Injection | Hypertensive crisis | Protect from light |
| **Antihypertensive Combinations** | | | | |
| Bisoprolol/HCTZ | Ziac® | Tablets | HTN | Strength of bisoprolol varies |
| Benazepril/HCTZ | Lotensin HCT® | Tablets | HTN | Strength of both ingredients varies |
| Clonidine/ Chlorthalidone* | Combipres® | Tablets | HTN | Strength of clonidine varies |
| Losartan/HCTZ | Hyzaar® | Tablets | HTN | Constant ratio of losartan to HCTZ |

BPH, benign prostatic hypertrophy; ER, extended release; HCTZ, hydrochlorothiazide; HF, heart failure; HTN, hypertension; MI, myocardial infarction.
*Chlorthalidone is a thiazide diuretic.

## Side Effects

The most common adverse effects reported with use of thiazide diuretics are electrolyte abnormalities. Diuretics deplete electrolytes because they act by preventing the reabsorption of sodium and other electrolytes from the dilute urine, thereby impairing the kidneys' ability to concentrate the urine. Potassium depletion is one of the more common and problematic electrolyte abnormalities, and may require potassium replacement. Low levels of potassium are referred to as hypokalemia, and can result in symptoms of weakness, lethargy, and muscle cramps. Potassium and other electrolyte levels are usually monitored closely in all patients, but this is especially important in those who receive digoxin or are susceptible to arrhythmias, because hypokalemia predisposes patients to digoxin toxicity and arrhythmias. Thiazide diuretics can deplete sodium, chloride, and magnesium as well.

hyperuricemia
Abnormally elevated serum uric acid level.

Other adverse effects include elevated levels of uric acid, called hyperuricemia. Elevations of uric acid levels can predispose patients with gout to have acute gouty attacks, which include painful, red, and swollen joints. Thiazides compete with uric acid for excretion in the kidney, causing uric acid levels to be elevated. Although thiazide diuretics have been reported to increase serum glucose and lipid levels, metabolic abnormalities are uncommon with low doses of thiazides. In most patients, the benefit of blood pressure control outweighs the risks of the minor metabolic changes that occur. For people with diabetes or hyperlipidemia, however, these side effects can be significant enough to make a different class of drugs a better choice. Thiazides can also cause gastrointestinal upset, and in some patients, sun sensitivity.

### Tips for the Technician

The thiazide diuretics should be appropriately labelled with auxiliary labels encouraging patients to take their medication exactly as directed, to reinforce the importance of compliance. Other auxiliary labelling should include the recommendation that the drug be taken in the morning, as well as a warning about possible photosensitivity. People taking thiazide diuretics should be encouraged to wear sunscreen.

Clients should be educated about symptoms that might indicate electrolyte imbalance, such as weakness, fatigue, muscle cramps, dizziness or palpitations. Many pharmacies provide information about foods that are high in potassium and low in sodium, such as bananas, orange juice, apricots, avocados, fish, and potatoes. Patients on diuretics are encouraged to eat these foods because they will replenish potassium without intake of excess sodium.

Many retail pharmacies provide blood pressure screening and monitoring for their patients, as well as providing home blood pressure monitoring devices for sale. Home monitoring is usually recommended so that patients can take control of the management of their disease, and to improve compliance with their medication regime. It is advantageous for technicians to know about blood pressure monitoring and the available home blood pressure monitoring kits.

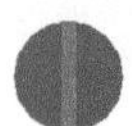

## Beta Receptor Antagonists

Beta-blockers are currently recommended as first-line drug therapy for hypertension in patients that also suffer from heart failure or severe angina. They are used along with diuretics in otherwise healthy patients that cannot attain goal blood pressure with a diuretic alone. Please refer back to Chapter 6 for additional information on the β-adrenergic antagonists.

### Actions and Indications

The administration of beta-blockers causes reduced sympathetic stimulation in the heart and elsewhere. Beta-blockade reduces heart rate and force of contraction and depresses conduction in the heart. Cardiac output, work, and oxygen consumption are decreased, and blood pressure is reduced. Beta-blockers inhibit the release of renin and the formation of angiotensin II, two mechanisms that contribute to the antihypertensive action. The cardioselective $\beta_1$ antagonists, including atenolol (Tenormin®) and metoprolol (Lopressor®), are the most frequently prescribed beta-blockers for hypertension. Labetalol (Normodyne®) is also quite useful because it has mixed alpha and beta antagonist activity, which results in an effect on the myocardium as well as on the vasculature.

The beta-blockers are more effective for treating hypertension in Caucasians than in African American patients, and in young compared to elderly patients. The beta-blockers are useful in treating patients that may have other conditions along with hypertension, such as supraventricular tachyarrhythmia, previous myocardial infarction, angina pectoris, chronic heart failure, or migraine headache. Treatment of hypertension is the most common use for the beta-blockers.

## Administration

Beta blockers are available in a variety of formulations, listed in Figure 17.2. Several beta-blockers are manufactured as combination products with diuretics, and a representative assortment of these combinations are also listed in Figure 17.2. Atenolol and nadolol (Corgard®) are available for oral use only, as tablets. Propranolol (Inderal®), metoprolol, and the mixed blocker labetalol are available for oral and intravenous injection. Atenolol and nadolol are administered on a once daily basis, while labetalol and metoprolol are administered twice daily. Metoprolol is available as an extended-release product for daily administration.

These drugs are used cautiously, if at all, in patients with very advanced heart failure, asthma, COPD, or diabetes. Once patients are maintained on beta-blockers, they should not be abruptly discontinued, because of the risk of rebound hypertension. The beta-blockers may take several weeks to develop their full effects.

## Side Effects

CNS side effects such as fatigue, lethargy, and dizziness are a common result of beta-blocker therapy (see **Fig. 17.3**). Unwanted cardiac effects include mild bradycardia, which is fairly common. Less frequent but more serious effects include progressive AV block along with severe bradycardia, or progression of congestive heart failure. The beta antagonists can also cause an excessive reduction in blood pressure, resulting in hypotension.

The beta antagonists can decrease libido and cause impotence, two side effects that can have a serious negative impact on patient compliance with the medication regime, and therefore interfere with control of hypertension. Along with changes in glucose metabolism, which can be problematic in diabetics, beta-blockers can also disturb lipid metabolism. The risk of bronchoconstriction, especially when nonspecific beta-blockers are used in patients with asthma, is worth repeating.

### Tips for the Technician

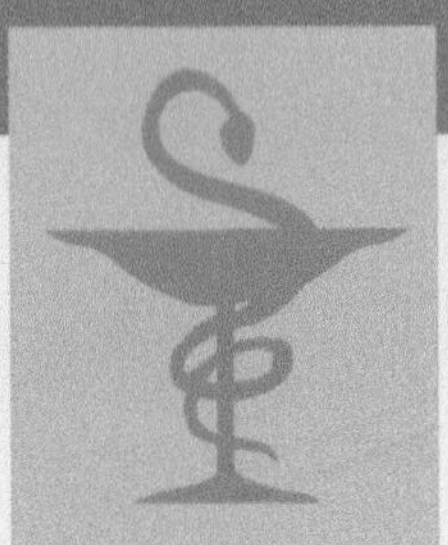

Patients taking beta-blockers should be warned about abrupt discontinuation and the appropriate accessory label should be applied to the prescription vial. Applying auxiliary labels that encourage patients to take their medication exactly as directed can reinforce the importance of compliance with the drug regimen. The beta antagonists are involved in a number of drug interactions, including potential interactions with over-the-counter medications. The pharmacist or physician should be consulted before starting any new medications.

Patients with diabetes should be warned that these drugs could mask signs of hypoglycemia and alter blood sugar levels. It is important for patients with congestive heart failure to monitor their weight on a regular basis since weight gain can be an indication of fluid retention in advancing heart failure. A gain of four or more pounds in a week is reason for the client to call the physician. Drowsiness can occur when taking beta-blockers and technicians should attach the appropriate warning label.

Beta-blockers can cause drug-induced sexual dysfunction. Some clients may feel more comfortable discussing side effect concerns such as this with the technician. It is very important that information of this nature be passed on to the pharmacist accurately so that he or she can assist the client or contact the doctor.

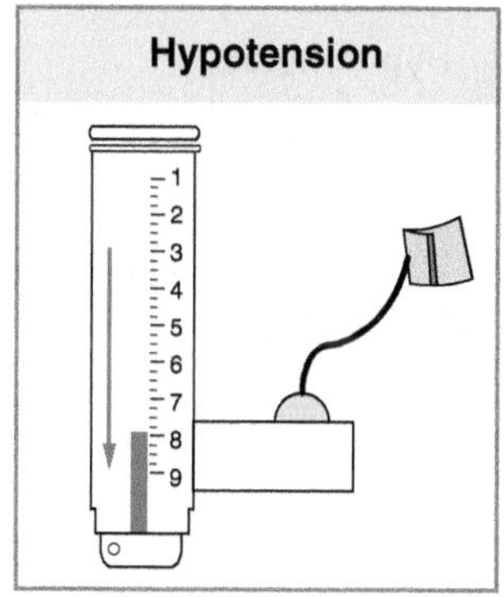


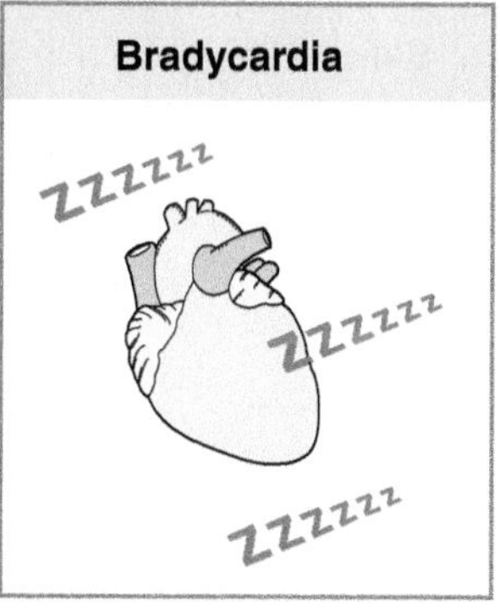


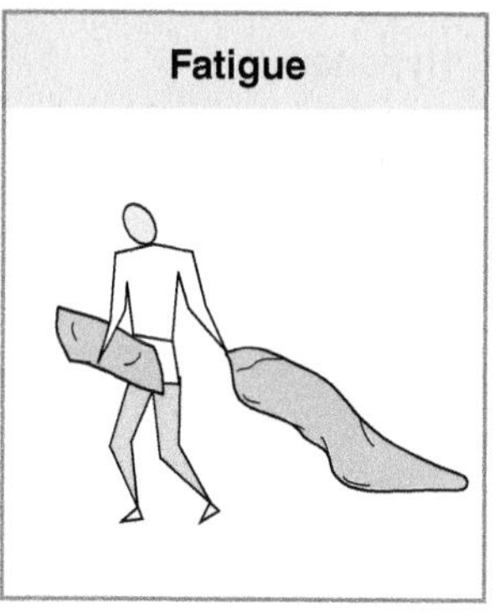


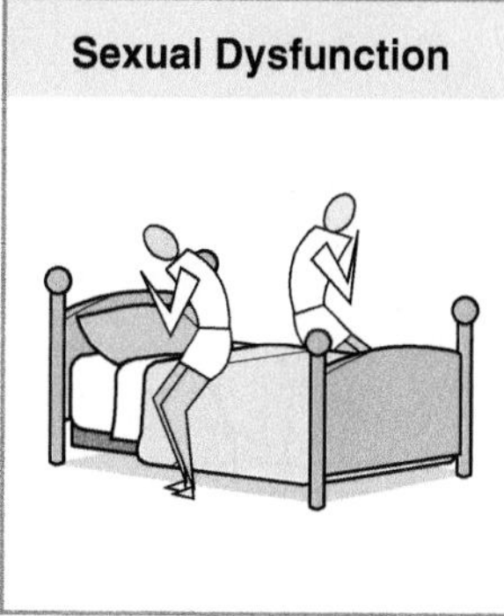


**Figure 17.3** Well recognized adverse effects of beta-blockers. (Adapted with permission from Harvey RA, Champe PC, Howland RD, et al. *Lippincott's Illustrated Reviews: Pharmacology,* 3rd edition. Baltimore: Lippincott Williams & Wilkins, 2006.)

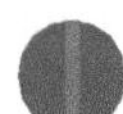

# The ACE Inhibitors

The ACE inhibitors are useful in the treatment of hypertension because they block formation of angiotensin II, a potent vasoconstrictor. Angiotensin II receptor blockers (ARBs) are compounds that are potent antagonists of the angiotensin receptor, with effects similar to those of the ACE inhibitors. These drugs offer no advantage in blood pressure control. They are considerably more expensive than the ACE inhibitors, but are used as a substitute in those patients who cannot tolerate the minor side effect differences.

## Actions and Indications

The ACE inhibitors lower blood pressure by reducing peripheral vascular resistance without reflexively increasing heart rate or contractility. These drugs block the enzyme that cleaves angiotensin I to form the potent vasoconstrictor angiotensin II. By reducing circulating angiotensin II levels, ACE inhibitors also decrease the secretion of aldosterone, resulting in decreased sodium and water retention.

ACE inhibitors are most effective in hypertensive patients who are Caucasian. However, when used in combination with a diuretic, the effectiveness of ACE inhibitors improves in African-American patients. Along with the ARBs, ACE inhibitors slow the progression of diabetic nephropathy and decrease the loss of protein through the kidneys. For this reason, ACE inhibitors are considered the first choice antihypertensive medication in diabetic patients. They are also effective in the management of patients with chronic heart failure and hypertension.

## Administration

The ACE inhibitors most frequently used for hypertension, such as enalapril, lisinopril, and ramipril, all have similar pharmacologic profiles, and are absorbed orally. Although captopril (Capoten®) is the prototype of the ACE inhibitors, it is less often used because it requires more frequent administration than most of the newer agents, which are given on a daily or twice daily basis. Food significantly reduces the absorption of captopril.

The ACE inhibitors are available as single agents and in a variety of combinations with thiazide diuretics (Table 17.1). Although enalapril (Vasotec®) is available in an injectable form, all of the other ACE inhibitors and the ARBs are available for oral use only.

## Side Effects

Common side effects include dry cough, rash, altered taste, and hyperkalemia, or elevations in potassium levels (**Fig. 17.4**). A dry cough occurs in about ten percent of patients, is re-

hyperkalemia Abnormally elevated serum potassium level.

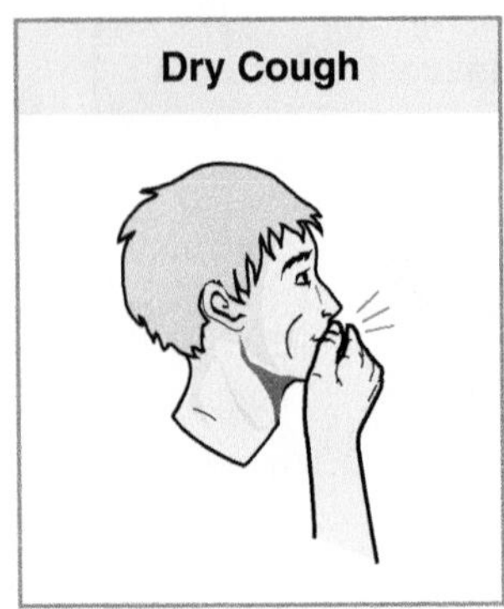


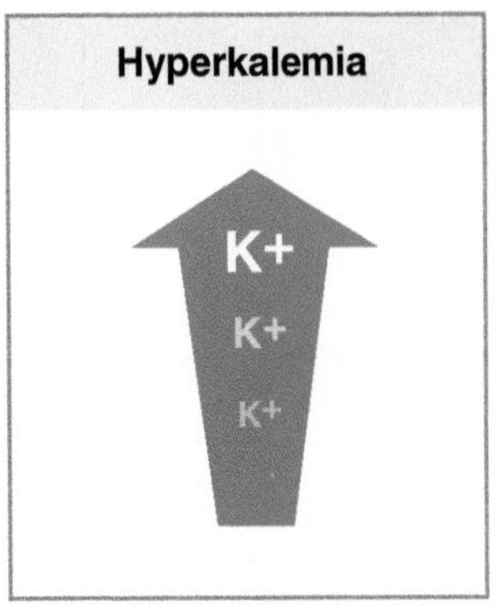


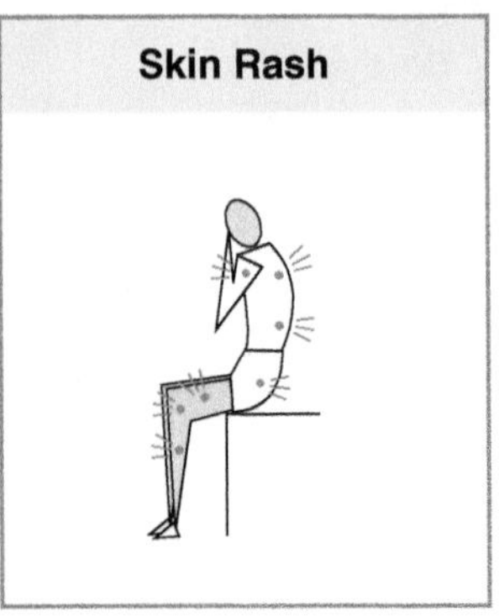


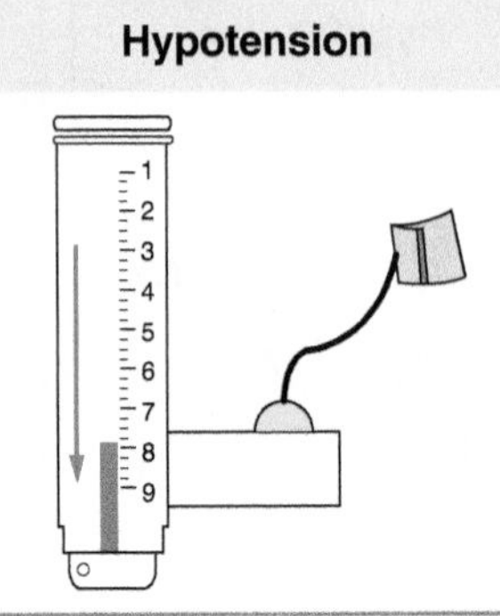


**Figure 17.4** Well-recognized adverse effects of the ACE inhibitors. (Adapted with permission from Harvey RA, Champe PC, Howland RD, et al. *Lippincott's Illustrated Reviews: Pharmacology*, 3rd edition. Baltimore: Lippincott Williams & Wilkins, 2006.)

versible with discontinuation of the drug, and although annoying, is harmless. Potassium levels are monitored in patients who take these medicationss. Typically, people taking diuretics need potassium supplements. If they are taking an ACE inhibitor and a diuretic, potassium supplementation may not be needed. When ACE inhibitors are given with spironolactone, dangerously high levels of potassium can result. Consequently, the combination is usually avoided. Angioedema is a rare but potentially life-threatening reaction seen with both the ACE inhibitors and the ARBs. Renal failure can be exacerbated or precipitated by the ACE inhibitors or the ARB's, especially in people taking diuretics, and in those who become dehydrated for other reasons. Women who are pregnant should not take any of the drugs from these two classes, because they can cause fetal harm or death in the second and third trimesters.

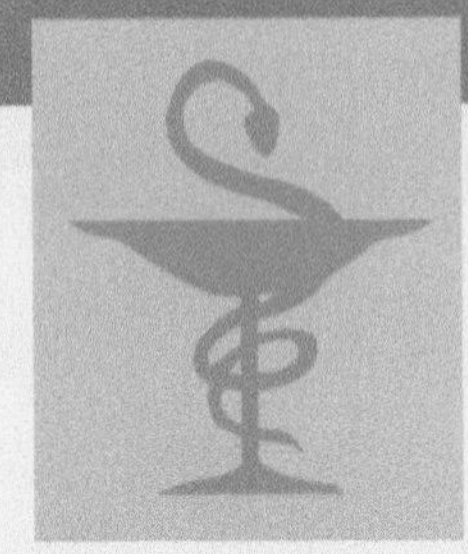

### Tips for the Technician

Pharmacists will counsel patients regarding side effects and the importance of complying with the physician's orders for laboratory monitoring. Women of childbearing age need to be told about the danger to the fetus that these drugs impose if taken during pregnancy. Any kind of rash or facial edema experienced during therapy is cause for discontinuing the medication and contacting the physician. Otherwise, medication should not be discontinued except on the advice of the physician. Prescription labels should include instructions to take captopril or moexipril (Univasc®, an infrequently used ACE inhibitor) on an empty stomach. Absorption may also be reduced when these drugs are taken with antacids or iron supplements, so prescriptions should be appropriately labelled with instructions to avoid these products.

## 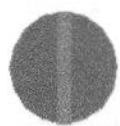 Calcium Channel Blockers

Although they are also useful as antiarrhythmic agents, the most important clinical application of the calcium channel blocking agents is in the treatment of hypertension. These drugs can be subdivided into three chemically related subgroups, but for general purposes it is easier to think of them as two subgroups. Verapamil (Calan®) and diltiazem (Cardizem®), considered as one group, cause vasodilation in addition to depressing cardiac tissues. The other group, the dihydropyridine drugs, mainly cause vasodilation. In this chapter, discussion will focus on the dihydropyridine drugs, including amlodipine (Norvasc®), felodipine (Plendil®), nicardipine (Cardene®), and the prototype of this group, nifedipine (Procardia®).

## Actions and Indications

Calcium channel blockers are recommended when the diuretics, beta-blockers, and ACE inhibitors are contraindicated or ineffective. Although they are not the first antihypertensive that should be selected in most patients, they are quite useful in treating hypertension in patients with angina. They are useful second drugs in patients with diabetes, and in early stages of renal failure. Calcium channel blockers are helpful in the treatment of hypertensive patients who have asthma, and they are more effective in African Americans than the ACE inhibitors.

Calcium channel antagonists block the movement of calcium into the myocardial cells and smooth muscle cells of the coronary and peripheral vasculature. This causes vascular smooth muscle to relax, dilating mainly arterioles, reducing peripheral vascular resistance and thereby reducing blood pressure. These drugs have a mild diuretic effect, which is helpful in managing hypertension.

## Administration

All of the calcium channel blockers used for hypertension are administered orally. Many of these agents have short half-lives (3 to 8 hours) following an oral dose and administration is required two to three times a day to maintain good blood pressure control. Sustained-release preparations permit once-daily dosing, and are available for felodipine, nicardipine and nifedipine (Table 17.1). Amlodipine can be given once daily in the immediate-release form.

Several of the calcium channel blockers are available in combination with either diuretics or ACE inhibitors. Some of the newer agents, such as amlodipine and nicardipine, have the advantage that they have a low risk of interacting with other cardiovascular drugs, such as digoxin or warfarin, which may be used concomitantly with calcium channel blockers.

## Side Effects

Because the calcium channel blockers can depress cardiac tissue to some degree, they can increase the risk of, or worsen existing heart failure. Calcium channel blockers are usually avoided in patients with preexisting heart failure. The dihydropyridine drugs are more likely to cause flushing, headaches, and light-headedness than diltiazem and verapamil. Constipation can be an issue with some of these agents. Hypotension can occur, especially early in therapy. This is most problematic with the immediate-release form of nifedipine because it causes the most significant vasodilation. When hypotension occurs, reflex tachycardia (caused when the baroreceptors sense a drop in blood pressure) can occur. For this reason, many experts recommend that only the extended release form of nifedipine be used. Refer to **Figure 17.5** for a pictorial summary of well-recognized side effects to the calcium channel blockers.

### Tips for the Technician

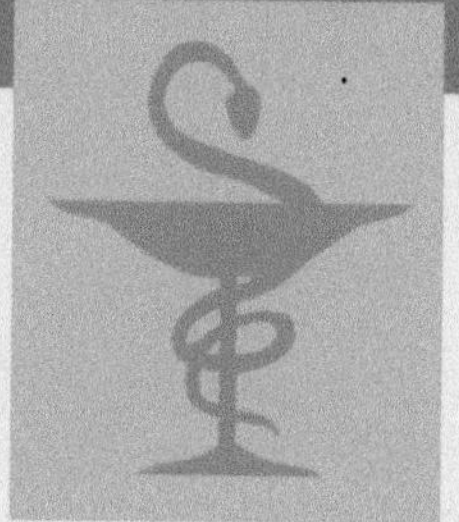

Patient counseling by the pharmacist is important with these drugs, because patients need to be familiar with signs that indicate progression of heart failure, including shortness of breath and edema. They should also be warned about the risk of dizziness, particularly on arising, and especially early in therapy. Persistent light-headedness or dizziness should be reported to the physician.

Auxiliary labels encouraging patients to take their prescription exactly as directed and advising that these drugs not be discontinued except on the advice of the physician should be applied. The absorption of the dihydropyridine drugs will be significantly increased when taken with fatty meals. Grapefruit juice may significantly increase the absorption of amlodipine, felodipine, nifedipine, and nicardipine. Patients should be encouraged to take these drugs at the same time every day, and should probably not drink grapefruit juice for one hour before and two hours after taking their medication.

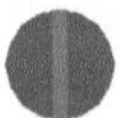

# Alpha-Blockers

The alpha-blockers prazosin (Minipress®), doxazosin (Cardura®), and terazosin (Hytrin®) are effective at reducing blood pressure, but they have not been associated with the same significant reductions in cardiovascular damage seen in studies done using other antihypertensive agents. For this reason, they are always used as additions to other antihypertensive therapy rather than as sole therapeutic agents.

## Actions and Indications

Alpha-blockers compete with norepinephrine for attachment to alpha receptor sites. Blood vessels contain the highest concentration of alpha receptors in the body. These drugs cause relaxation of the smooth muscle in both arteries and veins, thereby decreasing peripheral vascular resistance and lowering blood pressure. Because terazosin can be used as an alternative to surgery in patients with symptomatic benign prostatic hypertrophy, it can be particularly useful as a second drug in hypertensive men with concurrent BPH.

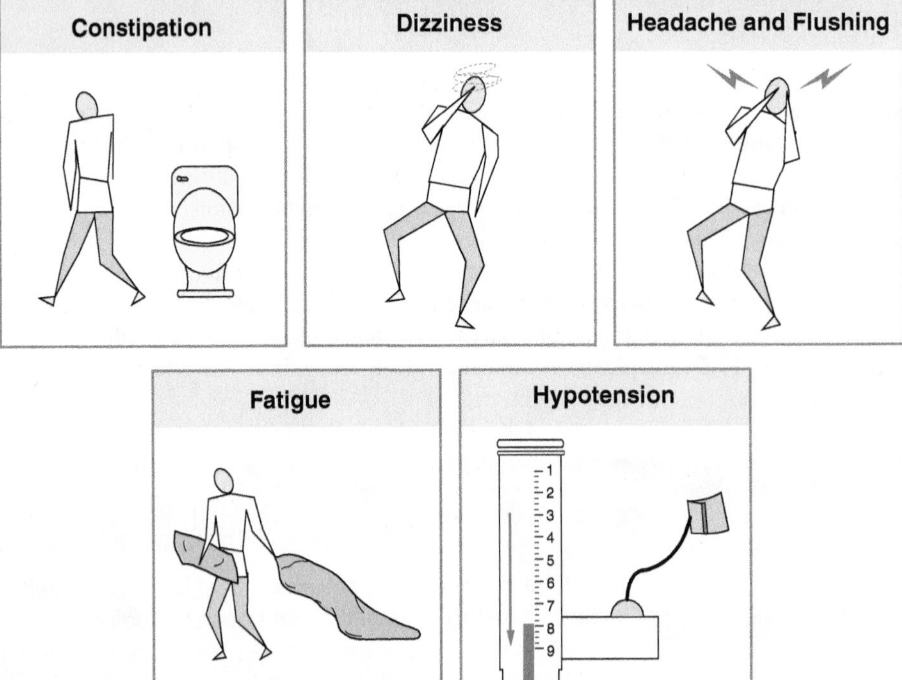


**Figure 17.5** Well-recognized adverse effects of the calcium channel blockers. (Adapted with permission from Harvey RA, Champe PC, Howland RD, et al. *Lippincott's Illustrated Reviews: Pharmacology*, 3rd edition. Baltimore: Lippincott Williams & Wilkins, 2006.)

## Administration

The alpha-blockers prazosin, terazosin, and doxazosin are available for oral use only, as either tablets or capsules. They are well absorbed orally, extensively metabolized in the liver, and excreted via the bile into the GI tract. They are available as single agents only.

These drugs should be initiated at low doses and increased gradually to avoid side effects. When alpha-blockers are added to other antihypertensives, physicians will often start patients at half the usual dose. Dosing at bedtime is recommended in order to reduce the potential for dizziness or lightheadedness. The alpha-blockers are added on to other antihypertensive therapies for the treatment of moderate hypertension. When combined with beta blockers, reflex tachycardia is minimized. They can also be used with diuretics.

## Side Effects

Reflex tachycardia, dizziness, and light-headedness early in therapy are almost universal adverse effects with these agents. These symptoms are caused by low blood pressure related to standing. Some patients may actually faint with their initial dose, and this effect is known as "first-dose syncope." Syncope can be avoided by initiating therapy at a low dose. Fluid and sodium retention can occur in some patients. The elderly are particularly sensitive to the hypotensive effects of these medications. Other side effects include headache, palpitations, and GI upset.

syncope Temporary loss of consciousness due to lack of oxygen to the brain; faint.

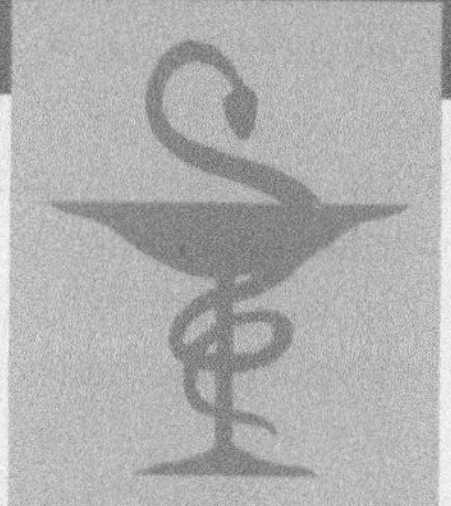

### Tips for the Technician

Because it is universally recommended that these drugs be initiated at a low dose, new prescriptions for alpha-blockers are likely to include more complex dosing regimes than is typical for most prescriptions. Technicians will need to be attentive to detail when transcribing incremental dosing instructions into the pharmacy computer system. Any time a prescription contains complex instructions, there are more opportunities for medication errors.

Patients should be warned about the possibility of low blood pressure on arising, called postural hypotension, and at any time early in therapy. First-dose syncope can occur when doses are increased or when therapy is resumed after an interruption. Patients may be more prone to postural hypotension after standing for long periods, when alcohol is consumed, or in hot weather. Accessory labels advising caution when driving should be applied to the prescription container. Patients should be advised to avoid alcoholic beverages, especially early in therapy.

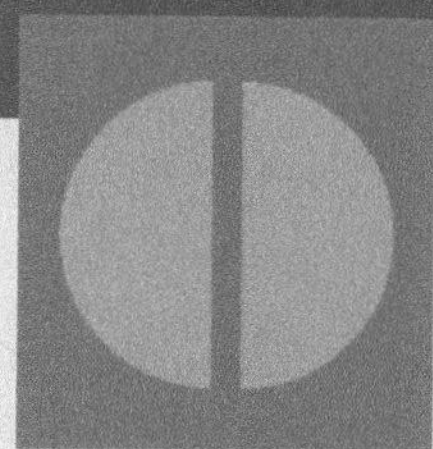

### Case 17.1

Dr. Nat Coole likes to write prescriptions for prazosin as follows: Prazosin 1 mg Q HS × 4 days, then 2 mg Q HS × 5 days, then 3 mg Q HS from day 10 onward. Using language a patient will understand, transcribe this prescription as you would on a prescription label. How might you reduce the risk of error when transcribing a complex medication order into the pharmacy computer system? How might you improve the chances of the patient administering the medication correctly?

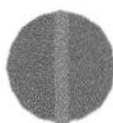

# Miscellaneous Antihypertensives

A diastolic blood pressure of >120 mm Hg is considered a hypertensive emergency and requires immediate treatment to avoid damage to the vital organs. Fortunately, improved management of chronic hypertension has reduced the number of patients who present with hypertensive crisis to less than 1%. In urgent situations, or when stage II hypertension does not respond to first-line drugs, there are several other treatment alternatives, including centrally acting alpha agonists and direct-acting vasodilators.

## Actions and Indications

The stimulation of central nervous system alpha receptors has an inhibitory effect on sympathetic outflow from the central nervous system. This inhibition results in reduced vasoconstriction, decreased peripheral vascular resistance, and reduced renin production. Although not chemically related, methyldopa (Aldomet®) and clonidine (Catapres®) are examples of centrally acting alpha agonists. These drugs are indicated for hypertension in the moderate to severe range and are recommended as adjunctive therapy, when other agents are not effective. Methyldopa is not often used because safer and more effective drugs are available.

Clonidine is useful to treat high blood pressure seen with autonomic dysfunction syndrome, which results from serious head trauma. In this condition, traumatic damage to the central nevous system results in abnormal release of catecholamines. Patients typically experience hypertension, high fevers, tachycardia, and other symptoms. Both methyldopa and clonidine can be useful in treating hypertension associated with renal failure because, unlike many other antihypertensive agents, they do not reduce renal blood flow. Clonidine is also used for several unrelated conditions, including prevention of vascular headaches and as an aid in withdrawal from opiates and nicotine.

Vasodilators act by producing relaxation of vascular smooth muscle, which decreases resistance to blood flow and, therefore, reduces blood pressure. Hydralazine (Apresoline®) is used to treat moderately severe hypertension and is almost always administered with a diuretic to prevent undesirable effects. Hydralazine monotherapy is an accepted method of controlling blood pressure in pregnancy-induced hypertension.

Minoxidil (Loniten®) directly dilates arterioles, but not veins. Minoxidil is prescribed for treatment of stage II hypertension that is refractory to other drugs. Reflex tachycardia may be severe with minoxidil and requires the concomitant use of a diuretic and a β-blocker. Additionally, minoxidil causes significant sodium and water retention that can lead to edema and congestive heart failure. This drug is available in a topical formulation to treat male pattern baldness.

Hypertensive crisis is a rare but life-threatening situation in which the diastolic blood pressure is either >150 mm Hg in an otherwise healthy person, or greater than 120 in an individual compromised by other illnesses. In the treatment of hypertensive crisis, the therapeutic goal is to reduce blood pressure as quickly as possible without causing ischemia, inadequate blood flow that results in a shortage of oxygen in the tissues. Nitroprusside (Nipride®), or sometimes nitroglycerin, labetalol, or hydralazine is administered intravenously in this situation. Nitroprusside causes prompt vasodilation. It is capable of reducing blood pressure in all patients regardless of the cause of hypertension. The drug has little effect outside the vascular system, and acts equally on all vascular smooth muscle.

ischemia Inadequate supply of oxygen to a part of the body such as the heart or brain due to obstruction of arterial blood flow.

## Administration

Clonidine is available as tablets or transdermal patches in a variety of strengths (Table 17.1). Transdermal patches are convenient for most people, and need only be changed on a weekly basis. Tablets are generally administered twice daily, and are well absorbed through the GI tract. The dose of clonidine may need to be lowered in renal failure. Rebound hypertension can occur if clonidine is abruptly discontinued.

Methyldopa is sold as tablets and as methyldopate for intravenous or intramuscular injection. Oral absorption of methyldopa is variable, and after absorption it is metabolized in the liver. Metabolites and any unchanged drug are removed via the kidneys, and doses may need to be reduced in patients with kidney disease.

Hydralazine is available for oral use and for IV or IM injection. Minoxidil is available for oral use as tablets. Both hydralazine and minoxidil oral products are rapidly and completely absorbed. Giving either drug with food is acceptable and may reduce GI upset. Both drugs are extensively metabolized. Certain populations (especially Asians or Native Americans) may metabolize hydralazine at a slower rate than other people. The dose must be reduced in these patients.

Nitroprusside is available in two different concentrations. Both must be diluted and administered intravenously. Nitroprusside is not particularly stable and solutions must be protected from light. Solutions are prepared with 5% dextrose because the drug is not compatible with saline solutions. This drug is initially dosed based on the patient's body weight and then adjusted based on the response. Nitroprusside is metabolized rapidly (half-life of minutes) and requires continuous infusion to maintain its hypotensive action.

## Side Effects

Clonidine can cause sodium and water retention and may be given with a diuretic to prevent this problem. Adverse effects are generally mild, but the drug can produce sedation and drying of the nasal mucosa. Rebound hypertension can occur following abrupt discontinuation of clonidine. The drug should be withdrawn slowly in the event of a change to the drug therapy.

The most common side effects of methyldopa are sedation and drowsiness. However, drug induced hemolytic anemia can occur and although rare, it can be very serious. Liver toxicity may occur and is more frequently seen early in therapy. The doctor will order laboratory testing to monitor the liver and watch for anemia.

The direct-acting smooth muscle relaxants, such as hydralazine and minoxidil, are not used as primary drugs to treat hypertension. They can dramatically reduce blood pressure, which results in reflex stimulation of the heart. The dramatic drop in blood pressure produced by these drugs causes increased myocardial contractility, heart rate, and oxygen consumption. In susceptible individuals, angina pectoris, myocardial infarction, or cardiac failure can result. Vasodilators increase plasma renin concentration, resulting in sodium and water retention. These undesirable side effects can be blocked by concomitant use of a diuretic and a beta-blocker.

Other adverse effects of hydralazine therapy include headache, nausea, sweating, and arrhythmia. A lupus-like syndrome can occur with high dosage, but it is reversible when the drug is discontinued. Minoxidil can cause cardiovascular effects similar to those caused by hydralazine. It is known to cause increased hair growth on the body, called hypertrichosis, and can also cause breast tenderness. Minoxidil has caused Stevens-Johnson syndrome, a sometimes life-threatening rash associated with skin sloughing.

Sodium nitroprusside exerts few adverse effects except for those of hypotension and possible cyanide toxicity. Nitroprusside metabolism results in cyanide ion production. Cyanide toxicity from the production of cyanide ions is rare and it can be effectively treated with sodium thiosulfate.

hypertrichosis Excessive hair growth.

### Tips for the Technician

It is important that patients clearly understand the importance of compliance when taking all antihypertensive medications, but following dosing regimens is especially critical with those drugs that are known to cause rebound effects with sudden discontinuation, such as clonidine, hydralazine, and minoxidil. Patients need to know that excessive weight gain could be a sign of impending heart failure and should be reported to the physician. Prescription vials should be appropriately labelled with auxiliary labels encouraging patients to follow directions exactly as written, and to continue medications unless advised by the physician to stop.

Pharmacy technicians need to be aware that hydroxyzine and hydralazine are names that look very much alike, especially when hand written, and can also sound alike. Nitroglycerin and nitroprusside injectable vials have been mistakenly substituted for each other because of proximity on pharmacy shelves and similar sounding names. Technicians should always be careful to double-check every order, but this is particularly important when there are other products with similar names. When compounding IV preparations with nitroprusside, always follow the manufacturer's advice regarding appropriate diluents, storage requirements, and protection from light.

# Review Questions

## Multiple Choice

Choose the best answer for the following questions:

1. Which of the following is a possible consequence of untreated hypertension?
   a. Kidney damage
   b. Stroke
   c. Heart attack
   d. b and c are both possible consequences
   e. a, b, and c are all possible consequences

2. Which statement is incorrect regarding the treatment of hypertension?
   a. JNC 7 recommends lifestyle changes such as quitting smoking and diet changes as the first step in treating early hypertension.
   b. There are five main drug classes used to treat hypertension.
   c. The beta antagonist drugs are the mainstay of drug therapy for hypertension and a drug from this class is usually the first drug prescribed for hypertensive patients.
   d. The goal of treatment is to prevent damage to the cardiovascular system by maintaining blood pressure below a certain acceptable level.
   e. All of these statements are incorrect regarding the treatment of hypertension

3. Which choice correctly pairs a drug class with one of its common adverse effects?
   a. Thiazide diuretics: hypokalemia
   b. Beta antagonists: tachycardia
   c. ACE inhibitors: hypokalemia
   d. Calcium channel blockers: reflex bradycardia as a result of excessive vasodilation
   e. All of the above are correct

4. What is hypertensive crisis?
   a. A person with hypertension that is going through a family emergency.

b. A life-threatening situation in which the systolic blood pressure is greater than 120 mmHg in a person with other illnesses or greater than 150 mmHg in a healthy person.

c. A life threatening situation in which the diastolic blood pressure is greater than 120 mmHg in a person with other illnesses or greater than 150 mmHg in a healthy person.

d. A severe type of hypertension for which treatment includes gradual reduction of the blood pressure over 3 to 4 months.

e. None of the above describe a hypertensive crisis.

5. Choose the correct statement regarding thiazide diuretics and their use in treating hypertension.

   a. Thiazide diuretics only lower blood pressure when the body is in a reclining position.

   b. Thiazide diuretics are often used in combination with spironolactone, a drug that helps the body eliminate even more potassium.

   c. The thiazide diuretics are not well absorbed orally and the preferred route of administration for all drugs in this class is intramuscular injection.

   d. Thiazide diuretics initially work to lower blood pressure by increasing sodium and water excretion by the kidney.

   e. All of the above are correct statements.

## True False

6. Essential hypertension is the term for the unavoidable hypertension that eventually occurs as a result of kidney disease.

   a. True

   b. False

7. Patients taking thiazide diuretics are encouraged to eat foods like bananas, avocados, and fish because they are will help replenish the body's potassium without excessive sodium intake.

   a. True

   b. False

8. It is acceptable for patients taking beta-blockers to abruptly stop taking the medication if they experience side effects such as decreased libido.

   a. True

   b. False

9. Prazosin and the other alpha-blockers are commonly used as sole therapeutic agents for the treatment of hypertension.

   a. True

   b. False

10. The direct acting vasodilators produce a dramatic drop in blood pressure that can cause chest pain, myocardial infarction, or heart failure.

    a. True

    b. False

## Matching

For questions 11 to 15, fill in each blank with the correct lettered choice below.

11. Continuing medications as prescribed is critical with some of the drugs used to treat hypertension because of the risk of development of ___________ if drugs are discontinued abruptly.
12. The number one reason for treatment failure in patients with hypertension is ___________.
13. The body maintains blood pressure within a normal range via the ___________ and the baroreceptors.
14. A patient taking ___________ for his hypertension has developed painful, swollen, and red joints, likely due to hyperuricemia, a possible adverse effect of this antihypertensive drug.
15. In a patient with asthma, diabetes, and hypertension, you would not expect a physician to prescribe ___________ as the initial choice for control of hypertension.

a. Poor choice of drug regimen by physicians
b. Hydrochlorothiazide
c. Renin-angiotensin-aldosterone system
d. Enalapril
e. Liver metabolism
f. Poor patient compliance
g. Propranolol
h. Rebound hypertension

## Short Answer

16. Why are the thiazide diuretics considered to be the cornerstone of antihypertensive drug therapy? What might be some disadvantages of these drugs?
17. If you were filling a prescription for hydrochlorothiazide and one for atenolol what auxiliary labels would you attach to each of these prescription vials?
18. One of your regular clients at the pharmacy brings in a new prescription for enalapril. Your client has recently been diagnosed with stage I hypertension. She is a 30-year-old Caucasian woman in her 3rd month of pregnancy. What do you think about the drug regimen she has been prescribed? Explain your answer, and if you feel there is a problem, how would you handle it?
19. List two side effects of hydralazine and minoxidil use.
20. Why is compliance with drug regimens such a common problem in the treatment of hypertension?

## FOR FURTHER INQUIRY

The original data that suggested hypertension was perhaps the most important risk factor for the development of heart disease and stroke came from the Framingham study. The Framingham study is an epidemiologic study begum in 1948 by what is now known as the National Heart Lung and Blood institute. Visit the Framingham study web site to learn more about the study design, as well as some of their landmark findings. Cardiac disease and stroke risk predictors are available on this web site.

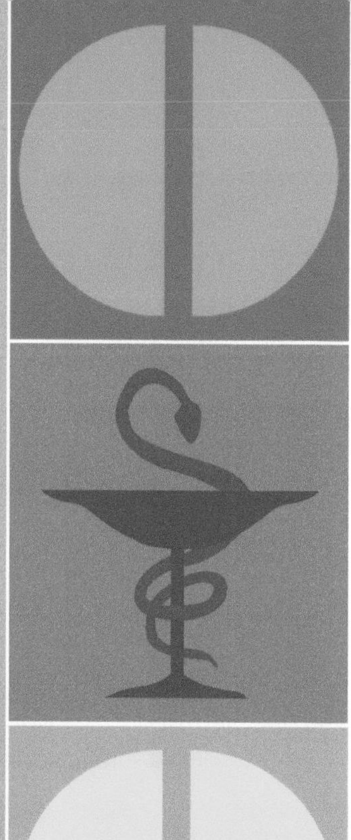

Chapter **18**

# Drugs Affecting the Blood

## KEY TERMS

- acute coronary syndrome
- angioplasty
- blood dyscrasia
- clotting cascade
- collagen
- fibrin
- fibrinogen
- hematoma
- hematopoietic
- hemostasis
- hyperlipidemia
- megaloblastic anemia
- myopathy
- peritoneum
- pernicious anemia
- pneumonitis
- polycythemia

## OBJECTIVES

After studying this chapter, the reader should be able to:

- Describe, in simple terms, the process of thrombus formation and compare the desirable role of blood clotting with the formation of an unwanted thrombus in a person with heart disease.
- List a common side effect, other than bleeding, associated with one drug from each of the following drug groups: platelet aggregation inhibitors, hirudin derivatives, vitamin K antagonists, heparin and low molecular weight heparin, and thrombolytic agents.
- Compare and contrast the roles of the nutrients iron, folic acid, and vitamin B12 with the role of epoetin alpha in the treatment of anemia.
- Explain the roles of diet and exercise as compared with drug therapy in people with elevated lipid levels at risk of developing heart disease.
- From a given list of auxiliary labels, identify those that should be affixed to a prescription vial containing an HMG-CoA reductase inhibitor.

- rhabdomyolysis
- stasis
- thrombin
- thrombosis
- thrombus
- transient ischemic attack

## DRUGS AND AGENTS COVERED IN THIS CHAPTER

### Drugs Affecting the Blood

| Platelet Aggregation Inhibitors | Anticoagulants | Thrombolytic Agents | Treatment of Bleeding |
|---|---|---|---|
| Abciximab | Dalteparin | Alteplase | Clotting Factors |
| Aspirin | Desirudin | Reteplase | Protamine sulfate |
| Clopidogrel | Enoxaparin | Streptokinase | Vitamin K |
| Dipyridamole | Heparin | | |
| Eptifibatide | Lepirudin | | |
| Ticlopidine | Warfarin | | |
| Tirofiban | | | |

| Treatment of Anemia |
|---|
| Cyanocobalamin (Vitamin B12) |
| Erythropoietin |
| Folic Acid |
| Iron |

### Lipid Lowering Agents

| HMG-CoA Reductase Inhibitors (Statins) | Fibric Acid Derivatives | Bile Acid Sequestrants | Miscellaneous Lipid lowering Agents |
|---|---|---|---|
| Atorvastatin | Fenofibrate | Colestipol | Ezetimibe |
| Fluvastatin | Gemfibrozil | Cholestyramine | Niacin |
| Lovastatin | | Colesevelam | |
| Pravastatin | | | |
| Rosuvastatin | | | |
| Simvastatin | | | |

hyperlipidemia Abnormally high fat or lipid levels in the blood.

thrombus Immature blood clot (mainly platelets) formed within a blood vessel and remaining at the site of origin.

This chapter describes drugs useful in the treatment of three different blood and blood related disorders: abnormal clotting of the blood, anemias, and hyperlipidemia (excessively high levels of any or all of the plasma lipids). Abnormal clotting of the blood can result in an unwanted clot, called a thrombus, or excessive bleeding, when clots should form but do not. Abnormal bleeding can be caused by hereditary clotting factor deficiencies, but is also a fairly common result of anticoagulant drug therapy. Correction of abnormal bleeding can include replacement of the missing factors or agents to reverse the offending drugs.

Anemias are often a result of nutritional deficiency, as in the very common iron deficiency anemia, but can also be caused by genetic anomalies that result in production of abnormal proteins, such as sickle cell anemia. Deficiency anemias are treated with vitamin and mineral supplements or by dietary changes. Although there are few treatments for inherited anemias, work on the genome and stem cells hold hope for the future.

Elevated levels of certain plasma lipids are associated with the formation of atherosclerotic plaques, which are a factor in thrombus formation and heart disease. Plasma lipids consist mostly of lipoproteins, spherical complexes of lipids and proteins. They are categorized based on their ratio of protein to fat, and are named based on their density. The goal of lipid lowering therapy is to reduce specific lipids and total cholesterol to target levels.

hemostasis Physiologic processes that arrest bleeding.

clotting cascade The series of reactions among blood clotting factors that cause clotting, or coagulation.

## Understanding Blood Coagulation

The human race would not have survived without the body's ability to stop the loss of blood after an injury to a blood vessel by clotting, or coagulating. The process of clotting and subsequent dissolution of the clot is called hemostasis. After an injury to a blood vessel, the first stage of hemostasis is blood vessel constriction, which is triggered by signalling chemicals released at the site of the injury. Next, platelets collect, or aggregate, at the site of the vascular injury and are activated by contact with the damaged tissue (**Fig. 18.1**). When they are activated, they release packets (granules) of chemical mediators that promote further aggregation and stimulate the clotting cascade, a series of reactions involving clotting factors that result in blood clotting. Thrombin, an enzyme produced after blood comes into contact with collagen (connective tissue) exposed in tissue injury, causes nearby platelets to collect. Fibrinogen, a plasma protein that acts as an adhesive, causes this loose collection of platelets to conform to the hole in the vessel wall to form a temporary plug, and thromboxane stimulates further platelet aggregation. After the platelet plug is formed, the third step in the coagulation process begins. To fortify the initial loose platelet plug, a fibrin mesh, or clot, forms to surround and stabilize the platelets. Lastly, after healing, the clot is dissolved. The clotting process involves complex interactions of 13 different clotting factors and blood components in order to produce a stable clot. **Figure 18.2** is a simplified illustration of the coagulation process. Clots formed when a sharp object cuts a vessel are life saving, but sometimes clots form inside the blood vessels, where they can cause serious damage to organs if they dislodge. A clot that adheres to a vessel wall is called a thrombus. Thrombus formation occurs most often because the walls of the arteries are damaged by the formation of fatty deposits called atherosclerotic plaque. When plaque forms within the walls of arteries it damages the wall and exposes arterial collagen. As has been described, this causes adhesion of platelets and formation of a clot or thrombus. Venous

thrombin An enzyme important in the clotting process; converts fibrinogen to fibrin.

collagen A fibrous protein of vertebrates that is a major constituent of connective tissues, such as tendon, ligament, and skin.

fibrinogen Soluble plasma protein essential to normal clotting and the precursor to fibrin.

fibrin Insoluble fibrous protein formed from fibrinogen and essential to the blood clotting process.

Resting platelet

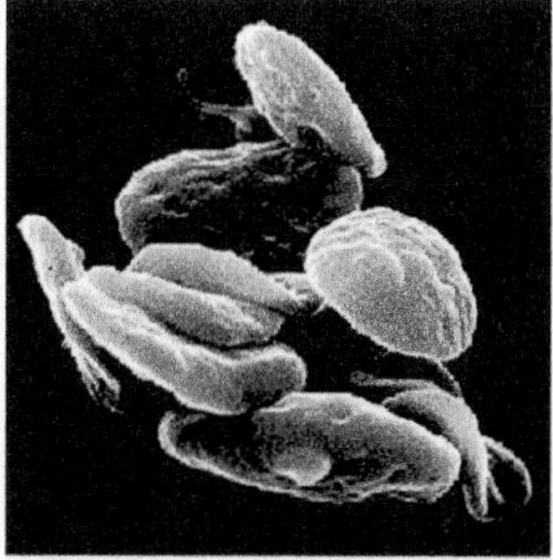

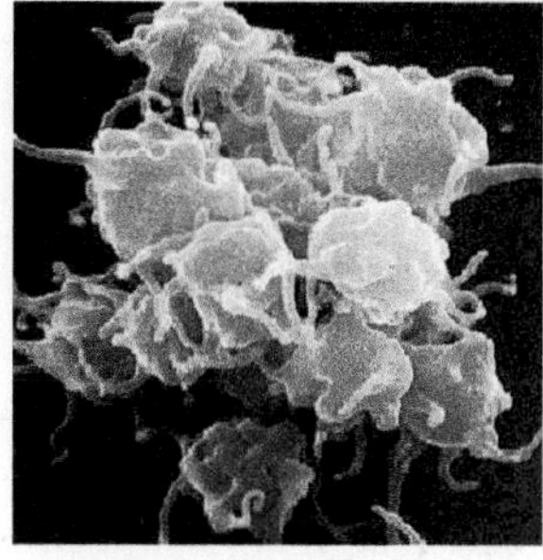

Activated platelet

**Figure 18.1** Scanning electron micrograph of resting platelets as compared with the "sticky" surface seen on activated platelets. (Reprinted with permission from Harvey RA, Champe PC, Howland RD, et al. *Lippincott's Illustrated Reviews: Pharmacology*, 3rd edition. Baltimore: Lippincott Williams & Wilkins, 2006.)

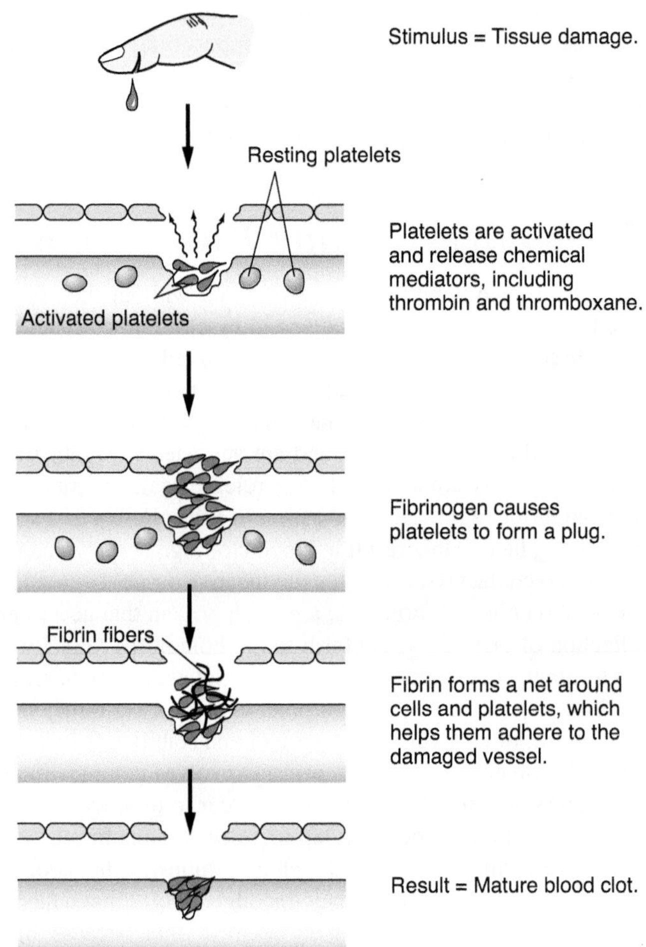
Stimulus = Tissue damage.
Resting platelets
Platelets are activated and release chemical mediators, including thrombin and thromboxane.
Activated platelets
Fibrinogen causes platelets to form a plug.
Fibrin fibers
Fibrin forms a net around cells and platelets, which helps them adhere to the damaged vessel.
Result = Mature blood clot.

**Figure 18.2** The stages involved in the formation of clots.

thrombosis Development or presence of a thrombus.

thrombosis, the formation of blood clots, occurs in people who are immobilized due to hospitalization, in people who have venous catheters, in certain heart conditions, or even from long airplane flights.

If a clot inside a blood vessel detaches from the vessel wall and floats free in the blood it is termed an embolus. The embolus moves through the bloodstream until it is trapped in a small vessel, where it will cut off the blood supply to nearby tissue. Both thrombi and emboli are dangerous, because they can occlude blood vessels and deprive tissues of oxygen and nutrients. A large embolus to the lungs, for example, will cause nearly instantaneous death.

stasis Slowing or stoppage of the normal flow of a substance, as in blood circulation.

Arterial thrombosis usually consists of a platelet-rich clot. In contrast, venous thrombosis is triggered by blood stasis (pooling) or inappropriate activation of the coagulation cascade, and results in a clot rich in fibrin. The drugs discussed in this chapter are used to prevent or treat undesirable blood clots, and include platelet aggregation inhibitors, anticoagulants, and agents that dissolve clots, called thrombolytic agents.

## Platelet Aggregation Inhibitors

Often referred to as "antiplatelet drugs," the platelet aggregation inhibitors interfere with the biochemical messages that activate platelets and stimulate platelet conglomeration. These drugs include aspirin, the thienopyridine drugs, the glycoprotein IIB/IIIA inhibitors, and dipyridamole.

## Actions and Indications

Aspirin inactivates the enzymes called cyclooxygenases (COX), found in platelets and other tissues, which are important in a number of physiologic functions, including the aggregation of platelets. Through a chemical reaction within the circulating platelets, aspirin alters the cyclooxygenase, preventing the conversion of thromboxane precursors to thromboxane. Thromboxane is an important activator of platelets and encourages their aggregation. The reaction caused by aspirin is rapid and irreversible. This means that for the approximately seven-day lifetime of a platelet exposed to aspirin, platelet aggregation is essentially prevented. Aspirin is currently used for the prevention of transient ischemic attacks (a sudden, brief loss of neurological function due to a temporary loss of oxygenation in a small area of the brain, often referred to as TIA), to reduce the risk of recurrent heart attacks, and to reduce the risk of heart attacks in people at high risk because of vessel disease. Dipyridamole is a weak platelet aggregation inhibitor that is used in combination with aspirin (Aggrenox®).

transient ischemic attack Temporary ischemia in a part of the brain caused by a brief loss of blood flow to that area, and accompanied by a reversible loss of neurological function.

The thienopyridine drugs ticlopidine (Ticlid®) and clopidogrel (Plavix®) block platelet aggregation by a mechanism different than that of aspirin, and in some studies are more effective at preventing thrombosis. These drugs prevent fibrinogen from binding to platelets, thereby blocking platelet stickiness and clumping. They are indicated for the prevention of atherosclerotic events, such as cerebrovascular accidents (CVA) or MI, in patients at risk.

There are three drugs that inhibit glycoprotein IIB/IIIA receptors by binding to this receptor complex on the platelet and preventing the platelets from releasing their granules. Abciximab (ReoPro®) is a monoclonal antibody, composed partly of human antibody fragments and partly of antibody fragments from mice. Eptifibatide (Integrelin®) is a peptide and tirofiban (Aggrastat®) is a nonpeptide that block the same part of the glycoprotein receptor. All three of these drugs are used to treat acute coronary syndrome (heart attack, or progressive angina that is thought to signify impending heart attack) and are administered during high-risk angioplasty.

acute coronary syndrome A set of signs and symptoms suggestive of sudden cardiac ischemia and including unstable angina and possibly heart attack.

Angioplasty is a procedure used to open coronary arteries. This type of procedure, which is less invasive than open-heart surgery, is called interventional cardiology. Instead of doing open-heart surgery and bypassing the clogged arteries with sections of vessels borrowed from another part of the body, cardiologists insert a catheter with a balloon tip into the clogged vessel and inflate the balloon. This opens up the artery, and once opened, a stretchy aluminum mesh tube, called a stent, is inserted to keep the vessel open. Although this procedure is much less invasive than open-heart surgery, it is not without risks. When patients are experiencing frequent angina or have recently had a heart attack, this procedure can dislodge a thrombus, causing a pulmonary embolism or stroke. Abciximab and heparin, an anticoagulant, are the drugs most often given during this procedure to prevent the risk of thrombus formation.

angioplasty Surgical reopening of a clogged blood vessel.

## Administration

Aspirin is probably the most frequently used of the platelet aggregation inhibitors. It is given orally, in low doses, for prevention of thrombotic events. Usually, an initial dose of one tablet (325 mg) is given, followed by 81 to 160 mg (one or two baby aspirin) on a daily basis. Because aspirin confers an effect for the life of the platelet, these very low doses are effective, and aspirin exerts maximal effect quickly and relatively safely. Dipyridamole and the thienopyridine drugs are also given orally. Clopidogrel is given on a once-daily basis and ticlopidine is administered twice a day. Food interferes with the absorption of ticlopidine but not of clopidogrel. Peak effect with the thienopyridine drugs occurs after three to five days. **Table 18.1** displays the drug names, formulations, and indications for these products, and the other drugs used to treat abnormal homeostasis. Abciximab is given intravenously along with heparin or aspirin during coronary interventional catheterization and angiography. After the infusion is discontinued, the antiplatelet effect persists for 24 to 48 hours. Eptifibatide and tirofiban are also used to reduce the risk of thrombotic complications from acute coronary syndrome.

**Table 18.1** Drug Names, Formulations, and Indications for the Drugs Used to Treat Abnormal Homeostasis

| Generic | Brand Name | Available as | Indications | Notes |
|---|---|---|---|---|
| **Platelet Aggregation Inhibitors** | | | | |
| Abciximab | ReoPro® | Injection | Adjunct in PCI | $$$ |
| Aspirin | Many | Tablets, EC tabs, gum, effervescent tabs, chew tabs | Prevention of MI, TIA, arthritis, aches and pain, fever | Nonprescription |
| Clopidogrel | Plavix® | Tablets | Recent MI, stroke, ACS, atherosclerotic disease | |
| Dipyridamole Aggrenox®* | Persantine® capsules | Tablets, (with aspirin) | Prevent stroke | Mainly used with aspirin |
| Eptifibatide | Integrilin® | Injection & injection conc. | ACS, adjunct in PCI | $$$ |
| Ticlopidine | Ticlid® | Tablets | Stroke prevention, if intolerant to other drugs | High-risk side effects |
| Tirofiban | Aggrastat® | Injection & injection conc. | ACS, adjunct in PCI | $$$ |
| **Anticoagulants** | | | | |
| Dalteparin | Fragmin® | Injection, PFS | Prevention of thrombosis | |
| Desirudin | Iprivask® | Powder for injection | DVT prevention | For people who cannot use heparin |
| Enoxaparin | Lovenox® | Injection, single and multidose, PFS | Prevention and treatment of thrombosis, including DVT and PE | |
| Heparin | | Injection, single and multidose, premixed IV bags | Treatment & prevention of thrombosis, embolism and coagulopathies | |
| Lepirudin | Refludan® | Powder for injection bocytopenia | Heparin-induced throm- heparin sensitive people | Off label, used for DVT in |
| Warfarin | Coumadin® | Tablets | Treatment & prevention of thrombosis, embolism | Many drug-drug & drug-food interactions |
| **Thrombolytic Agents** | | | | |
| Alteplase | Activase® | Powder for injection | Acute MI, PE or ischemic stroke, restore patency to central line | $$$ |

*(continues)*

| Generic | Brand Name | Available as | Indications | Notes |
|---|---|---|---|---|
| **Thrombolytic Agents** | | | | |
| Reteplase | Retavase® | Powder for injection | Acute MI, restore patency to central line | $$$ |
| Streptokinase | Streptase® | Powder for injection | Acute MI, PE, to restore patency to central line | |
| **Correction of bleeding** | | | | |
| Factor VIIa | NovoSeven® | Powder for injection | Bleeding in hemophilia | $$$ |
| Factor VIII | Advate®, others | Powder for injection | Bleeding in hemophilia patients | $$$ |
| Factor IX | AlphaNine®, others | Powder for injection | Bleeding in hemophilia patients | $$$ |
| Phytonadione (vitamin K) | Mephyton® Aqua-mephyton® | Tablets, injection | Vitamin K deficiency, drug-induced coagulopathy | |
| Protamine | | Injection | Reversal of heparin | |

ACS, acute coronary syndrome; DVT, deep vein thrombosis; PCI, percutaneous coronary intervention; PE, pulmonary embolism
*Aggrenox is dipyridamole with aspirin, PFS, prefilled syringe

## Side Effects

The adverse effects of greatest concern for all platelet aggregation inhibitors are related to bleeding. Aspirin, even in low doses, can cause gastrointestinal bleeding. Older patients tend to be at greater risk of GI bleeding. Especially at doses of 325 mg daily (a standard aspirin tablet) or more, patients who take aspirin run a slightly higher risk of having hemorrhagic strokes. Some patients are sensitive to aspirin, and exposure to aspirin or other nonsteroidal anti-inflammatory drugs (a family of aspirin-like drugs, such as Advil®, that are anti-inflammatory) causes bronchoconstriction in these sensitive patients. Other side effects, seen with anti-inflammatory doses of aspirin, will be discussed in Chapter 23.

An increased risk of bleeding is also seen with clopidogrel and ticlopidine, and neither these drugs, nor aspirin, should be used in patients with peptic ulcers. Physicians will usually have patients discontinue use of these drugs before surgical procedures, to reduce the risk of excessive bleeding during and after surgery. GI upset is very common with ticlopidine and less common with clopidogrel. Ticlopidine and clopidogrel have both caused a problem with the platelets called thrombotic thrombocytopenic purpura (TTP). The Food and Drug Administration requires a black box warning in the packaging for ticlopidine because of this and drug induced blood dyscrasias (abnormalities of blood components), including neutropenia and agranulocytosis. Ticlopidine has caused allergic pneumonitis (inflammation of the lungs) and kidney impairment. Because the risk of side effects related to ticlopidine use is greater than that with clopidogrel, clopidogrel is the preferred drug of the two.

Bleeding events are the most common complications of the glycoprotein IIB and IIIA inhibitors. Major bleeding can occur during interventional catheterization at the site where the catheter is threaded into the artery, or into the brain, the GI tract, or the peritoneum (the abdominal cavity). Hypotension, nausea, and fever have occurred. Because abciximab is an antibody, allergic reactions can occur.

blood dyscrasia A general term used to describe any abnormality in the blood or bone marrow's cellular components.

pneumonitis Inflammation of the lung.

peritoneum The smooth serous membrane which lines the cavity of the abdomen.

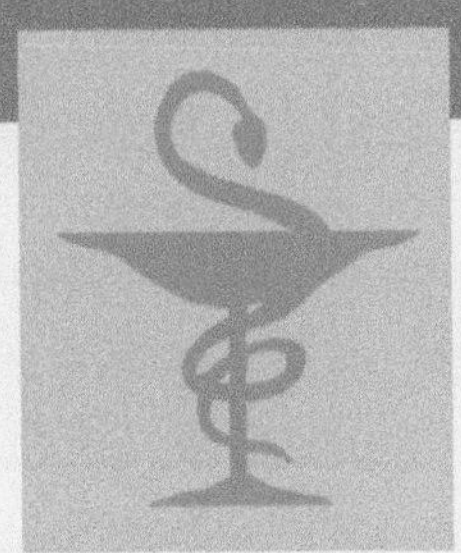

### Tips for the Technician

Aspirin should be taken with food to reduce the risk of GI irritation. Low-dose chewable aspirin tastes good and can be very dangerous to young children, so it should be kept in the original childproof container, out of the reach of young children. Patients taking any of the antiplatelet drugs should be told that it may take a little longer for bleeding to stop and that they may bruise more easily, but any excessive bleeding or bruising should be reported to the doctor. Although clopidogrel can be taken without regard to food, ticlopidine should be taken with food because food improves its absorption. People taking either of these two platelet aggregation inhibitors should avoid taking aspirin or nonsteroidal anti-inflammatory drugs. Prescription vials should be labelled with this instruction.

Abciximab and the other glycoprotein IIB/IIIA receptor inhibitors are extremely expensive drugs. Although most hospitals have purchasing contracts, the average wholesale price for abciximab is over $600 per vial. It is important to handle this product efficiently by staying within approved stock levels, rotating stock, and avoiding waste.

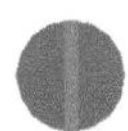

# Anticoagulants

The anticoagulants are drugs that work on a different aspect of blood coagulation than the platelet aggregation inhibitors. A number of the clotting factors in the coagulation cascade are involved with formation of fibrin, the stringy material that stabilizes the platelet plug and forms a clot. Thrombin plays a key role in coagulation, because it is required for the final steps in the generation of fibrin. The anticoagulant drugs work by interfering at different points in the production of fibrin.

Many of the anticoagulants are derived from natural sources. Heparin is a huge molecule that occurs naturally, in tiny quantities, in the mast cells of mammals. Researchers are unsure of what the role of naturally occurring heparin is, but in therapeutic doses it interferes with the action of thrombin, and as a result blocks clot formation and limits the expansion of an existing thrombus. In 1884 scientists discovered that leeches secrete a substance with anticoagulant properties that allows them to feed off of the blood of their hosts (**Fig. 18.3**). Leeches were used for centuries for the practice of bloodletting. Hirudin is the active anticoagulant compound found in the saliva of leeches, and it is a direct thrombin antagonist.

The vitamin K antagonists were discovered in the early twentieth century after cattle in North Dakota and Canada developed an unusual bleeding disorder that caused many to bleed to death. Veterinary pathologist and professor Frances Schofield linked the mystery disease to the consumption of sweet clover that had spoiled. Coumarin is present in most clovers, but when it becomes moldy, coumarin can change to dicoumarol, a potent anticoagulant. Later, other scientists isolated the chemicals responsible and eventually developed their use as rodent poisons and as anticoagulants for human use.

## Actions and Indications

The anticoagulants either inhibit the action of thrombin (heparin, low molecular weight heparins, and the hirudin derivatives) or block the synthesis of the coagulation factors (the vitamin K antagonists, such as warfarin). Until recently, heparin was the major antithrombotic drug for the treatment of deep-vein thrombosis and pulmonary embolism. Now, the low molecular weight heparins (LMWH) can be used for these conditions. Heparin or LMWH is used to prevent postoperative venous thrombosis in patients undergoing elective surgery (for example, hip replacement). Heparin and LMWH are the anticoagulants of

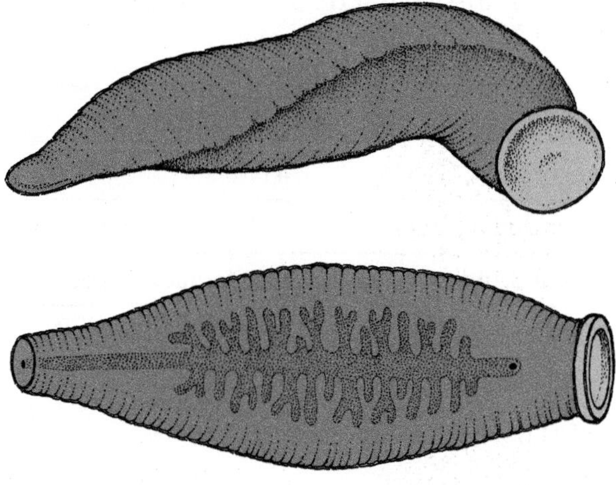

**Figure 18.3** Leeches secrete a substance with anticoagulant properties that allows them to feed off of the blood of their hosts. (Courtesy of Neil O. Hardy, Wespoint, CT)

choice for treating pregnant women because they do not cross the placenta. Heparin is given with intravenous platelet aggregation inhibitors for patients undergoing percutaneous coronary intervention, and with fibrinolytic therapy for patients with acute myocardial infarction.

Lepirudin (Refludan®) is a derivative of hirudin and is produced using recombinant DNA technology. Other, related hirudin derivatives are also available. These drugs are indicated as antithrombotic agents, but find their most important use in patients who cannot receive heparin. They are used to treat heparin induced thrombocytopenia and thrombosis, a potentially serious result of heparin therapy.

The vitamin K antagonists, or coumarin drugs, are used in patients who require long-term treatment or prevention of thrombus formation. Warfarin (Coumadin®) is the only one of these drugs available in the United States today. The clotting factors needed for coagulation reactions are synthesized in the liver. Several of these factors require the presence of vitamin K in order to be produced and become active. Warfarin treatment inhibits production and activation of these factors by blocking the action of vitamin K. Warfarin is indicated for the prevention and treatment of venous thrombosis. It is especially useful in the prevention of embolic events for people at risk, including those with atrial fibrillation or with cardiac valve replacement.

## Administration

Heparin is administered by continuous intravenous infusion for treatment of embolic events or by subcutaneous injection for prevention of embolism. Given intravenously, heparin has a speedy onset of action. This is a distinct advantage over other anticoagulants in the treatment of life-threatening embolic events. However, after initial treatment with heparin, many patients are switched to LMWH, such as enoxaparin (Lovenox®) and dalteparin (Fragmin®), because of more convenient subcutaneous administration that requires no laboratory monitoring. Because they are safer and easier to use, patients can receive treatment with the LMWH at home (**Table 18.2**). The coagulant activity of the LMWH drugs occurs about four hours after subcutaneous injection. Heparin must be given parenterally, either in a deep subcutaneous site or intravenously, because the drug does not readily cross epithelial membranes. The intramuscular route is not used for the administration of heparin type drugs because a hematoma, bleeding into the muscle, can form. Heparin is usually administered as an intravenous bolus, followed by an intravenous infusion to rapidly reach the desired degree of anticoagulation. Doses are adjusted based on laboratory tests that look at the prolongation of the time for one aspect of clotting to occur.

hematoma Localized, semisolid mass of blood that collects in a tissue or space due to a break in a vessel wall.

When long-term anticoagulation is necessary, patients who have received several days of heparin therapy will be switched over to warfarin therapy before discharge from the hos-

**Table 18.2** Comparison of Some of the Characteristics of Heparin and Low Molecular Weight Heparins (LMWHs)

| Drug Characteristic | Heparin | LMWHs |
|---|---|---|
| Intravenous half-life | 2 hours | 4 hours |
| Cost | $ (not including labs) | $$$$ (no labs required) |
| Major adverse effect | Frequent bleeding | Less frequent bleeding |
| Setting for therapy | Hospital | Hospital and outpatient |

Adapted with permission from Harvey RA, Champe PC, Howland RD, et al. *Lippincott's Illustrated Reviews: Pharmacology*, 3rd edition. Baltimore: Lippincott Williams & Wilkins, 2006.

pital. Warfarin is given orally, and can be taken by patients at home. The anticoagulation effects of warfarin can be affected by diets high in vitamin K, other drugs, and other conditions the patient may have. Because warfarin is highly protein bound and metabolized in the liver, it is prone to a number of drug interactions that will significantly affect anticoagulation. Some of the most important interacting drugs include amiodarone, sulfa antibacterial drugs, and the azole antifungal agents, but many others can also interact to a significant degree.

Warfarin therapy takes days to reach the full therapeutic effect because the response is dependent upon the disappearance of the already produced, active clotting factors in the patient's system. The dose required to achieve therapeutic anticoagulation is extremely variable between individuals and must be monitored carefully. Many factors, including the amount of vitamin K rich foods in the diet and interacting drugs, including many over-the-counter preparations, can affect warfarin dosing. For the first week of treatment, laboratory testing is usually done on a daily basis, and then weekly testing is usually required for the duration of warfarin therapy. Many hospitals and some metropolitan areas have anticoagulation programs managed by pharmacists, because effective management can be quite time consuming for physicians.

Lepirudin is administered intravenously, as are most of the other thrombin inhibitors. Desirudin (Iprivask®) is the exception, and it is given by subcutaneous injection. These drugs require dosage adjustment based on laboratory assessment, as do heparin and warfarin.

## Side Effects

Bleeding is the most common and potentially serious side effect seen with all of the anticoagulants. Monitoring of appropriate lab work is necessary to reduce the risk of unwanted bleeding with heparin, thrombin inhibitors and warfarin therapy. Lab testing is usually not necessary with the LMWH drugs, except in cases of abnormal renal function or pregnancy.

Excessive bleeding from the use of heparin is usually readily reversible by discontinuing the heparin infusion, but sometimes reversal with protamine, a heparin antagonist, is necessary. Both LMWH and heparin can induce thrombocytopenia and thrombosis, although it is less common with LMWH. HIT (heparin induced thrombocytopenia) is a kind of allergic reaction to heparin that can be life threatening, and is associated with thrombosis (see **Fig. 18.4**). Because heparin preparations are obtained from animal sources they can cause other hypersensitivity reactions. Possible reactions include chills, fever, urticaria, or anaphylactic shock.

Adverse effects associated with the hirudin derivatives include excessive bleeding and allergic reactions, including possible anaphylaxis. About half the patients receiving lepirudin develop antibodies. People self-administering desirudin should avoid taking other

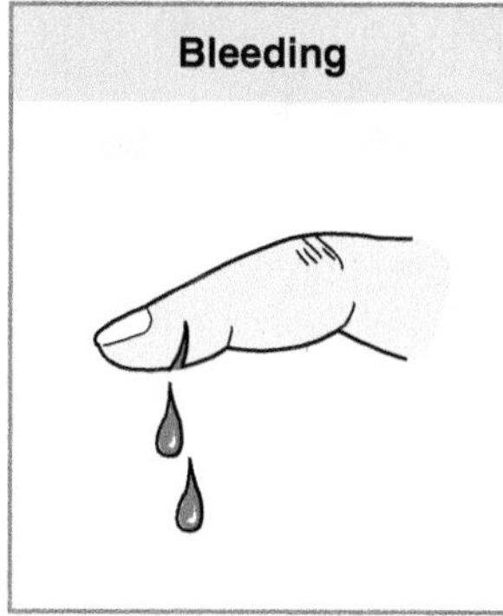

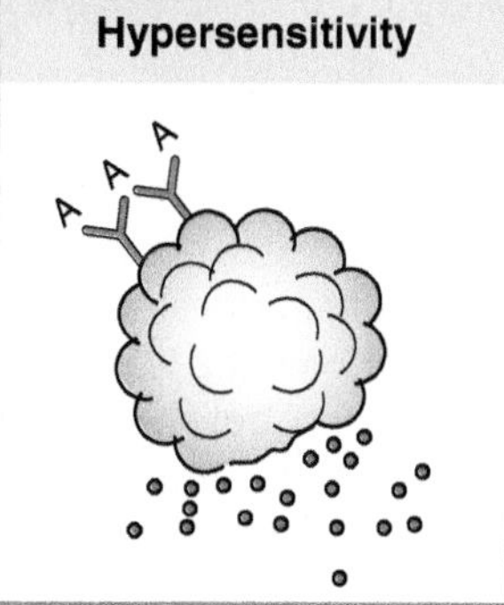

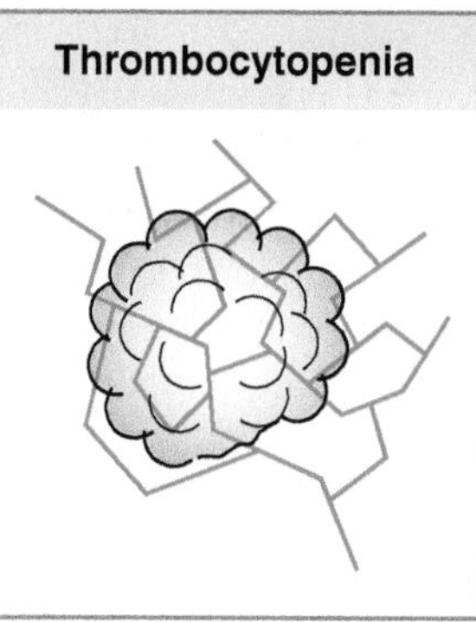


**Figure 18.4** Adverse effects of heparin and the low molecular weight heparins. Thrombocytopenia is less common with LMWH. (Adapted with permission from Harvey RA, Champe PC, Howland RD, et al. *Lippincott's Illustrated Reviews: Pharmacology,* 3rd edition. Baltimore: Lippincott Williams & Wilkins, 2006.)

drugs, such as nonsteroidal anti-inflammatory agents like ibuprofen or naproxen, that can cause bleeding and potentiate the effects of desirudin.

Although warfarin can cause diarrhea, nausea, and skin reactions, the principal untoward effect of warfarin therapy is bleeding. Maintaining laboratory values within recommended ranges reduces the risk of bleeding, but even when dosing is well controlled, bleeding can still occur. Minor bleeding, such as minor nosebleeds, or prolonged oozing after being nicked while shaving, is not usually cause for discontinuing drug treatment. Serious bleeds, such as GI bleeding or cerebral hemorrhage can occur. Since warfarin exerts its effect by antagonizing vitamin K, vitamin K can be used to reverse warfarin effects. Minor bleeding is usually treated by discontinuation of the drug and, when necessary, by administration of oral vitamin K. Severe bleeding requires larger doses of Vitamin K given intravenously.

## Tips for the Technician

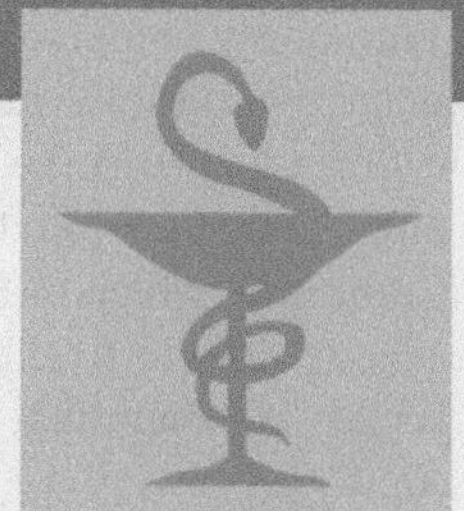

Most hospitals have premixed heparin solutions available for IV infusion so compounding isn't necessary. When it is necessary to compound a heparin intravenous solution, make sure that another technician and a pharmacist check the calculations before mixing. Heparin is incompatible with many intravenous drugs. Use a current reference, such as Trissel's *Handbook on Injectable Drugs*, to check compatibilities. Some people may self-administer low dose heparin or LMWH at home. The pharmacist should make sure they have received adequate training in sterile technique before dispensing these medications.

People taking warfarin need extensive counseling by the pharmacist to make certain they understand this medication. They need to be educated about adhering to the drug regimen, avoiding interacting drugs, and maintaining consistency in their diets. Auxiliary labels that recommend avoidance of over the counter medications except on the advice of the physician, adherence to the dosing schedule, and avoidance of alcohol should all be affixed to the prescription container. Patients should not try to make up missed doses. Pharmacy technicians can encourage patients on any long-term anticoagulant therapy to wear a medication alert bracelet or keep a drug information card in their purse or wallet.

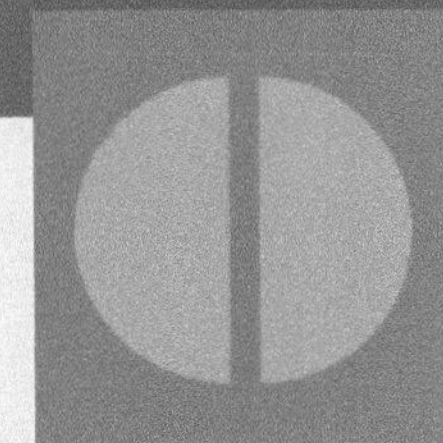

## Case 18.1

Claudia Sanger got her prescription (warfarin) for the treatment of deep vein thrombosis filled at Brown's pharmacy. The next week she returned to the counter at Brown's looking rather miserable with what appeared to be a cold. When Rosie (the pharmacy technician) asked Mrs. Sanger how she was doing with her medication, she told Rosie that the prescription was fine, but that she had a cold and a slight fever, and nothing to take for it at home. Mrs. Sanger placed several OTC items on the counter for purchase, including a combination cough and cold preparation, multiple vitamins, acetaminophen, and ibuprofen. "Are these medications okay?" asked Mrs. Sanger. Rosie tells her they are fine medicines, but the generic versions will save her money. Rosie finds the generics for her, and completes the sale. What is wrong with this scenario? How could Rosie have better served Mrs. Sanger?

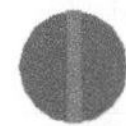

# Thrombolytic Agents

The thrombolytic agents are drugs that promote the dissolution of fibrin clots. Streptokinase, the first of these agents to be marketed and promoted for use during acute myocardial infarction, was approved for use in 1987. Use of the thrombolytic agents revolutionized the treatment of heart attack; patients who were unconscious and with a poor chance of surviving regained consciousness within minutes of the initiation of streptokinase. Since that time, more specific thrombolytic agents and new procedures continue to advance the treatment of MI. There are now six thrombolytic agents available, but the most important of these is alteplase (Activase®), sometimes referred to as tissue plasminogen activator, or TPA.

## Actions and Indications

Acute thromboembolic disease, including myocardial infarction, pulmonary embolus and certain kinds of stroke, may be treated by the administration of agents that dissolve clots. All of these agents act either directly or indirectly to break down fibrin and dissolve the clot, reopening the blood vessel. Streptokinase (Streptase®) is an enzyme that acts directly on the clot, while alteplase and reteplase (Retavasc®) activate plasminogen, which in turn causes formation of endogenous clot dissolving enzymes. Besides being used to treat embolic diseases, these drugs can also be used to open indwelling venous catheters that are blocked because of the formation of a clot at the catheter tip.

Clot dissolution and reperfusion is successful more often when therapy is started early after clot formation (within one to three hours), because clots become more resistant to dissolution as they age. In the case of the use of alteplase in strokes, the necessary diagnostic procedures to confirm the diagnosis of an embolic event, such as a CT scan, need to be available around the clock. For this reason, these effective drugs are not used for the treatment of strokes in most communities.

## Administration

All of the thrombolytic agents are administered by intravenous or intra-arterial injection in a hospital setting. Hospitals establish protocols for the use of these agents, so that unwanted effects can be minimized. Hospital pharmacies are often asked to provide these drugs in a "kit" with all the necessary ancillary drugs and diluents needed for the protocol. For example, thrombolytic therapy for acute myocardial infarction is nearly always given with aspirin as pre-treatment. Heparin infusions are given concurrently in most patients. Kits might include the thrombolytic agent and diluent, aspirin, heparin for infusion, protocols for use, and labels for the IV bags. These drugs can also be administered directly into the coronary artery, while the patient is undergoing cardiac catheterization.

## Side Effects

The thrombolytic agents do not distinguish between the fibrin of an unwanted thrombus and the fibrin of a beneficial hemostatic plug. Bleeding, therefore, is a major risk of thrombolytic therapy. For example, a previously unsuspected source of bleeding, such as a peptic ulcer, may hemorrhage following injection of a thrombolytic agent (see **Fig. 18.5**). These drugs are avoided in patients with healing wounds, pregnancy, a recent bleeding incident, or cancer. Allergic reactions can also be a problem, especially with streptokinase, which is manufactured from purified bacterial proteins.

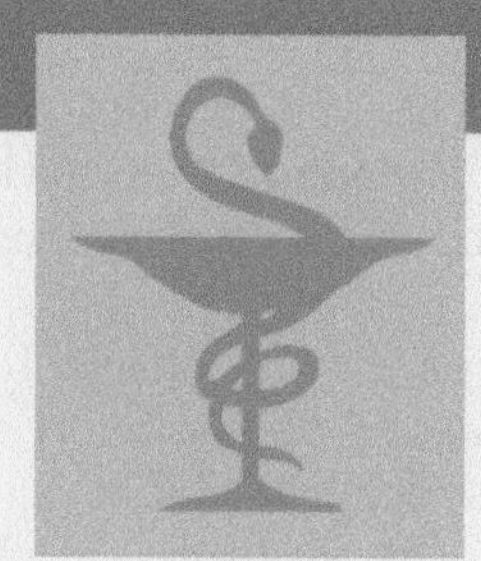

### Tips for the Technician

Reconstitution of the thrombolytic agents is normally done at the patient's bedside to avoid waste. A dose of alteplase, for example, costs more than $2,500. Hospital pharmacy technicians may be involved in preparing and supplying kits to the patient care areas. It is important for technicians to know how to access pharmacy policies and procedures, which will include directions for preparation and contents of this and other types of kits or boxes prepared by the pharmacy. Current practices for use of these drugs change frequently, and hospital-based technicians will need to continually update their education on this and other drug topics.

**A. Untreated patient**

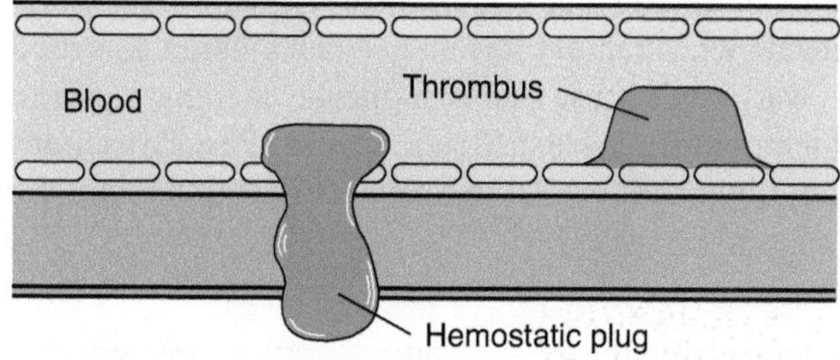


**B. Patient treated with plasminogen activator**

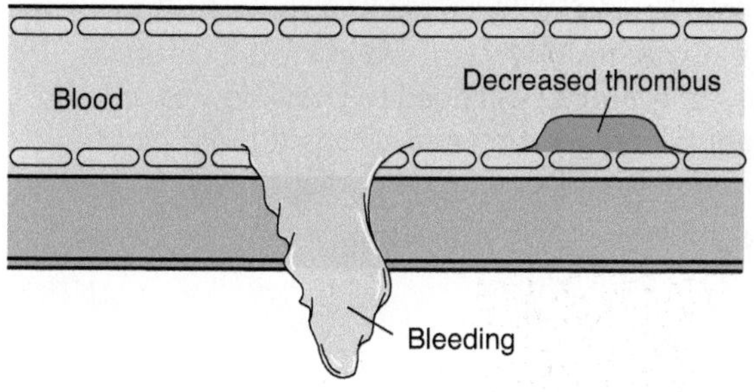


**Figure 18.5** When an unwanted thrombus is dissolved, beneficial hemostatic plugs will also be dissolved, uncovering unsuspected sources of bleeding. (Adapted with permission from Harvey RA, Champe PC, Howland RD, et al. *Lippincott's Illustrated Reviews: Pharmacology*, 3rd edition. Baltimore: Lippincott Williams & Wilkins, 2006.)

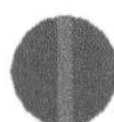

# Drugs Used for Bleeding

Bleeding problems occur most frequently as a result of drug treatment, or as a result of an inherited condition, such as hemophilia. Natural clotting factors, vitamin K, or antagonists of the anticoagulants are effective in controlling most forms of bleeding.

## Actions and Indications

Plasma coagulation factors, including recombinant factor VIIa (NovoSeven®), and factors VIII (Advate®), and IX (AlphaNine®) are indicated for bleeding episodes in patients with hemophilia. They temporarily promote hemostasis in patients who are missing these proteins essential for normal clotting. Blood transfusion is another option for treating hemophilia patients with severe hemorrhage.

Protamine sulfate antagonizes the anticoagulant effects of heparin. The positively charged protamine interacts with the negatively charged heparin molecule, forming a stable complex without anticoagulant activity. Vitamin $K_1$ (phytonadione) administration can stem bleeding problems due to the oral anticoagulants by stimulating production of clotting factors.

## Administration

Concentrated preparations of clotting factors VIII and IX are available from human donors. Factor VIIa is made using recombinant DNA technology. All of the clotting factors are administered by intravenous injection. The dose requirements depend on the extent and location of the bleeding, and the response to therapy.

Protamine is administered by slow intravenous injection to avoid side effects. It is available in solution and although it can be diluted, it does not require dilution before administration. Vitamin K can be given orally or by subcutaneous, intramuscular, or intravenous injection. The dose and route of administration of vitamin K is usually based on lab results indicating the degree of anticoagulation and the presence and amount of bleeding. The full response to vitamin K is slow, requiring about 24 hours.

## Side Effects

Use of factor replacements derived from human sources carries a small risk of transferring viral infections, such as hepatitis or HIV. Thrombosis from excessive replacement or allergic reactions can also occur.

Adverse effects of protamine administration include hypersensitivity, as well as dyspnea, flushing, bradycardia, and hypotension when rapidly injected. When vitamin K is used to reverse bleeding in patients taking warfarin, its use can complicate ongoing warfarin therapy by making dosage adjustment temporarily more difficult. Severe allergic reactions have occurred after IV administration of phytonadione, so intravenous injection is not the preferred route of administration.

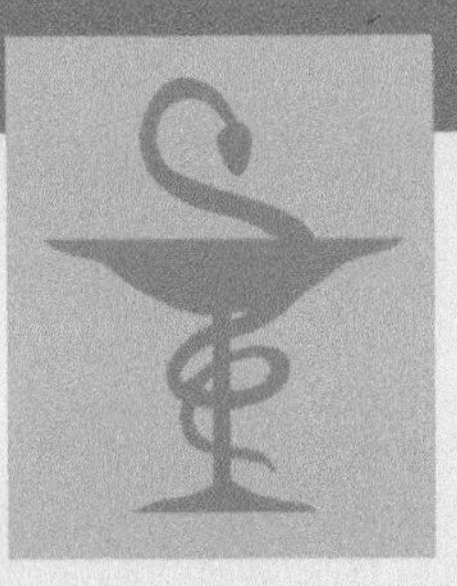

### Tips for the Technician

Protamine and vitamin K are considered antidotes, and must be kept in stock in hospital pharmacies. Clotting factors are not routinely stocked in most institutions, but technicians in pediatric hospitals, for example, will need to know how to quickly obtain them. Most clotting factors require refrigeration and reconstitution. Information on storage and reconstitution is available in the package insert for each product.

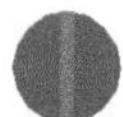 

# Drugs Used for Anemia

Anemia is defined as a below-normal plasma hemoglobin concentration resulting from too few red blood cells or abnormally low hemoglobin content in the cells. Anemia can be caused by nutritional deficiencies, chronic blood loss, low production or increased destruction of cells, and a number of other disease states. Hematopoietic agents are drugs that promote the production of red blood cells. Until recently, these were limited to the nutritional supplements iron, vitamins B12, and folic acid. With the advent of recombinant DNA technology, human hormones that stimulate production of red and white blood cells are now available. **Table 18.3** lists hematopoietic agents discussed in this chapter.

hematopoietic Relating to, or involved in, the formation of blood cells.

## Action and Indications

### Nutrients

Deficiency anemias occur because of poor diets, increased requirements during certain stages of life, poor absorption of the necessary nutrient, or drugs or disease states that affect the nutritional state or block the effects of nutrients. Iron is stored in intestinal mucosal cells until needed by the body. Iron deficiency can be caused by acute or chronic blood loss, or by insufficient intake during periods of accelerated growth in children or in menstruating or pregnant women. When iron stores are depleted, iron deficiency anemia occurs and supplementation with some form of iron is required to correct the deficiency.

Folic acid (Folvite®), or as it is sometimes called, folate deficiency may be caused by increased demand, poor absorption caused by diseases of the small intestine, or alcoholism. Treatment with drugs that antagonize the effects of folic acid (for example, methotrexate

**Table 18.3** Hematopoietic Agents, Available Formulations, and Indications for Use

| Generic Name | Brand Name | Available As | Indications | Notes |
|---|---|---|---|---|
| Cyanocobalamin (Vitamin B12) | Nascobal® | Tablets, injection, intranasal gel | Vitamin deficiency, pernicious anemia | |
| Erythropoietin | Epogen®, Procrit® | Injection | Anemia due to kidney disease, chemotherapy, or to reduce need for transfusion | Refrigerate |
| Folic Acid | Folvite® | Tablets, injection | Megaloblastic anemia, prenatal care, dietary replacement (TPN) | Low dose tabs are OTC |
| Ferrous sulfate, gluconate, and fumarate | Feratab®, Fergon®, Feostat® | Tablets, elixir, suspension, ER, chew tabs | Iron deficiency states and iron deficiency anemia | OTC |
| Iron dextran | Dexferrum® | Injection | Iron deficiency states and iron deficiency anemia | |
| Iron sucrose | Venofer® | Injection | Iron deficiency states and iron deficiency anemia | |

or trimethoprim) are another cause of folic acid deficiency. Inadequate dietary intake of folic acid during pregnancy can result in neurological abnormalities in the newborn babies, so folic acid supplementation is routinely included as part of prenatal care. Folic acid deficiency is one cause of megaloblastic anemia (abnormal immature red blood cells, called megaloblasts, are present). Vitamin B12 deficiency causes anemia that has similar red blood cell characteristics. Deficiencies of vitamin B12 can result from low dietary intake or, more commonly, from inadequate production of intrinsic factor. Specialized cells in the stomach produce intrinsic factor, and it is required for the absorption of vitamin B12. Malabsorption syndromes or gastric resection can also cause vitamin B12 deficiency. This deficiency results in pernicious anemia.

megaloblastic anemia
Anemia characterized by the presence of megaloblasts in the bloodstream; vitamin B12 and folic acid deficiencies cause this type of anemia.

pernicious anemia
Anemia marked by a decrease in number and increase in size of the red blood cell, and caused by vitamin B12 deficiency.

### Erythropoietin

Erythropoietin is a hormone produced in healthy kidneys that stimulates red cell production by the bone marrow. In chronic renal failure, production of this hormone declines and results in anemia. Human erythropoietin, called epoetin alpha (Epogen®), is manufactured using recombinant DNA technology. It is indicated in the treatment of anemia caused by end-stage renal disease, anemia associated with HIV infection, anemia resulting from cytotoxic drug therapy used in cancer, and to stimulate red blood cell production in anemic patients undergoing elective surgery.

## Administration

Iron supplements are available in a variety of formulations and for administration by both oral and parenteral routes. Ferrous sulfate is probably the most frequently administered iron salt, but ferrous gluconate and ferrous fumarate are also available without prescription for oral administration. The amount of elemental iron available for absorption differs between these three products. Ferrous fumarate contains the most (33%) and ferrous gluconate the least (12%) amount of elemental iron. Depending on the product, ferrous sulfate contains 20% to 30% elemental iron. Recommendations for iron intake are based on elemental iron.

Iron dextran (for IM or IV use) and iron sucrose (for IV administration) are used when oral iron replacement is not possible, or more rapid replacement of stores is desirable. When administered intravenously, iron products should be injected slowly, either by infusion, or by IV injection. If iron dextran is given intramuscularly, a special administration technique, called Z track, is used to prevent tissue staining.

Folic acid is a B vitamin found in low doses in most B complex tablets or capsules and also available as a single agent in low doses. The higher strength (1 mg) tablets are available by prescription only. Folate is also manufactured as a sterile solution for subcutaneous, intramuscular, or intravenous injection. It is one component of the vitamin supplementation used in parenteral nutrition.

Cyanocobalamin (Vitamin B12) is available as tablets for oral administration and as solution for subcutaneous or intramuscular injection. Oral administration is not useful when absorption is inadequate, or in pernicious anemia, where intrinsic factor is not adequately produced. Intramuscular cyanocobalamin therapy must be continued for the remainder of the life of a patient suffering from pernicious anemia.

Epoetin is administered by intravenous or subcutaneous injection. Dosing is based on the patient's diagnosis and response. Epoetin is not effective unless the patient has adequate iron stores available for the production of red blood cells. Single dose vials are preservative free and should not be reused. Epoetin must be refrigerated.

## Side Effects

Oral iron replacement therapy is often associated with GI upset and constipation. All oral iron products can cause black, tarry stools, which patients can mistake for blood in the stools. Liquid oral iron products and iron injections can stain the teeth and skin, respectively. Iron is toxic when taken in excess and iron products should be left in their original childproof containers. IV infusions of iron have been associated with severe anaphylactic reactions in some people, and are avoided when oral products can be used. Most experts recommend giving a small test dose of iron dextran at least one hour before administering the first therapeutic dose, to determine if the patient will tolerate the drug.

There are no serious side effects related to the oral intake of either folic acid or cyanocobalamin. Occasional GI upset can occur with multivitamin products, and intravenous or intramuscular administration can result in pain at the injection site.

Epoetin alpha use can cause elevations in blood pressure and edema, especially if treatment continues after hemoglobin reaches near normal. When use is continued beyond the appropriate duration, polycythemia (an excessive number of red blood cells) can result. Allergic reactions, including fever, rash, itching, and joint pain can also occur.

polycythemia An excessive number of red blood cells and amount of hemoglobin.

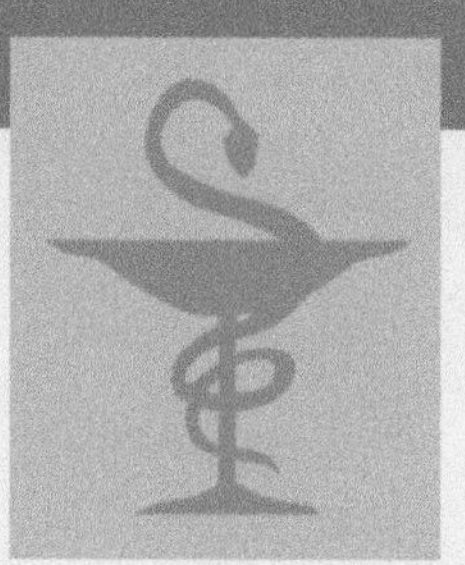

### Tips for the Technician

Warn parents about possible discoloration of the teeth when dispensing liquid vitamin supplements with iron for infants. If the medication is administered slowly, with a dropper, into the back of the cheek, the risk of tooth staining is reduced. Apply an auxiliary warning label to prescription vitamin supplements with minerals that warn of the potential for discoloration of the stools.

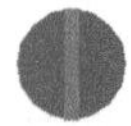

## Understanding Hyperlipidemia

There is an old proverb, "you are what you eat," that is appropriate to consider when learning about hyperlipidemia. The human body is designed to absorb nutrients and use them to synthesize all the proteins, cells, and chemical messengers needed for life. Fats are an essential part of our diets. They are converted into the steroid hormones and bile acids, and provide energy to the body. Most Americans have diets that include excessive amounts of fats and total calories, specifically dangerous fats, such as saturated and trans fats, and carbohydrates. When we eat too much of the "bad" fats, too many calories, or have a genetic inability to clear fats from the bloodstream, the body can end up depositing excess fat where it can do tremendous harm. People with chronically elevated lipid levels in the blood eventually develop atherosclerotic plaques, or fatty deposits in the arteries, that contribute to heart disease or stroke.

Hyperlipidemia is one of the most important risk factors for the development of atherosclerosis and heart disease. A 40-year-old man who does not smoke has twice the risk of having an embolic event with total cholesterol levels of 240 than the same man would if his cholesterol levels were below 200. As the leading cause of death in the United States, heart disease is responsible for more than a half million deaths every year. The cost of treating people with heart disease is more than $200 billion annually. As with cigarette smoking and hypertension, hyperlipidemia is a risk factor that can be modified. For these reasons, the treatment of elevated lipids has become a national concern and focus, and the National Cholesterol Education Program has developed treatment guidelines and goals for the prevention of heart disease (see **Fig. 18.6**). The most current of these recommendations are commonly referred to as the ATP III (Adult Treatment Panel III).

Lipid levels are increased in most people either because of an inherited inability to efficiently metabolize certain fats, or as a result of the individual's lifestyle (sedentary lifestyle and high-fat diet, for example) or both. As with the treatment of high blood pressure, the first step in treatment of elevated lipid levels is a change in diet and an increase in exercise.

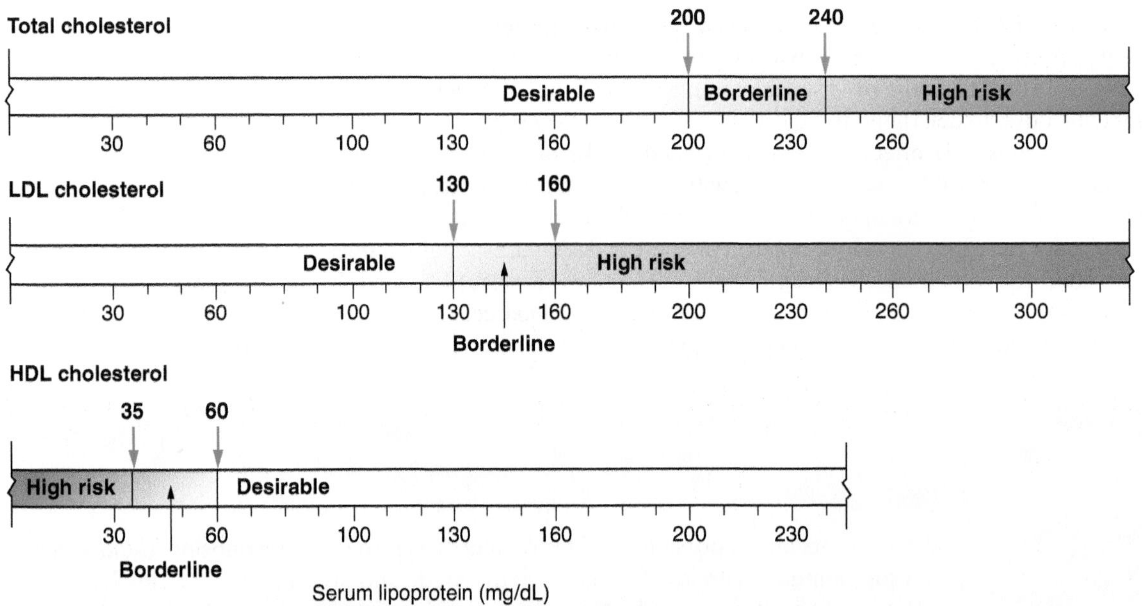


**Figure 18.6** Lipid levels for total cholesterol, LDL cholesterol, and HDL cholesterol correlated with risk. (Adapted with permission from Harvey RA, Champe PC, Howland RD, et al. *Lippincott's Illustrated Reviews: Pharmacology*, 3rd edition. Baltimore: Lippincott Williams & Wilkins, 2006.)

Fats and oils are low-density compounds as compared with other substances such as water or normal saline. A low-density liquid will float over a higher density liquid, as can be observed when mixing oil and water. Lipoproteins are spherical complexes that contain both protein and fats, and are important for transporting fats in the body. Low-density lipoprotein (LDL) and very low-density lipoprotein (VLDL) are the lipids that when elevated, are most closely associated with heart disease, and contain high concentrations of cholesterol (LDL) and triglycerides (VLDL). High-density lipoprotein (HDL) is the lipid substance that carries fats from the blood stream back to the liver for reuse, and it contains the highest percentage of proteins. An individual with high HDL levels actually has a lower risk of heart disease than the average individual. HDL is sometimes referred to as "good cholesterol" in the lay press.

Antihyperlipidemic drugs target the problem of elevated serum lipids with different mechanisms of action. Some of these agents decrease production of the lipoprotein carriers of cholesterol and triglycerides, whereas others increase the degradation of lipoprotein. Still others decrease cholesterol absorption or directly increase cholesterol removal from the body. Sometimes two lipid-lowering drugs with complementary mechanisms of action are used to increase the chance of reducing lipid levels to the target range of total cholesterol levels less than 200.

There are a number of drug classes used to treat hyperlipidemia. The HMG-CoA reductase inhibitors are a relatively new class of lipid-lowering agents commonly referred to as "statin" drugs. The fibric acid derivatives are used to reduce triglycerides, found in VLDL. Niacin and the bile acid sequestrants have been in use for many years, and ezetimibe is a new member of the lipid-lowering armamentarium.

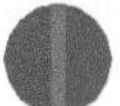

## HMG-CoA Reductase Inhibitors

This group of antihyperlipidemic agents inhibits the first enzymatic step (HMG coenzyme A reductase) in the synthesis of cholesterol. Use of these drugs prevents the formation of new plaque deposits and reduces the risk of formation of platelet thrombus. The statin drugs are the most widely prescribed antihyperlipidemic agents in the United States.

## Actions and Indications

All of the statin drugs or their metabolites are chemically similar to the precursor of cholesterol. By attaching to the enzyme HMG-CoA reductase, which is essential for cholesterol synthesis, they are able to inhibit the production of cholesterol by the liver. When levels of cholesterol within the cells fall, more LDL is removed from the bloodstream in order to synthesize cortisol and other hormones (**Fig. 18.7**). As a result, the lipid levels in the blood fall. These drugs are effective in lowering plasma cholesterol levels independent of the cause. Clinical studies have demonstrated that people at risk for heart disease who take the statin drugs do better over time than people who do not take lipid-lowering drugs.

The statin drugs are effective at lowering LDL and total cholesterol. Although they all have some effect at lowering triglycerides, only two agents, atorvastatin (Lipitor®) and simvastatin (Zocor®), have FDA-approved indications for reducing triglycerides. The FDA also gave approval to simvastatin and atorvastatin for increasing HDL, but all of the HMG-CoA reductase inhibitors have the ability to raise "good" cholesterol to a minor degree.

## Administration

The HMG-CoA reductase inhibitors are administered and absorbed orally. Most are taken once a day in the evening or at bedtime because the rate of cholesterol production increases at night. They exert their action in the liver, and are metabolized there. They are eliminated principally through the bile. Lovastatin (Mevacor®) immediate release tablets are better absorbed in the presence of food. Pravastatin (Pravachol®) and simvastatin are generally given with food to reduce GI disturbance. Refer to **Table 18.4** for a summary of the lipid-lowering agents, formulations, and indications.

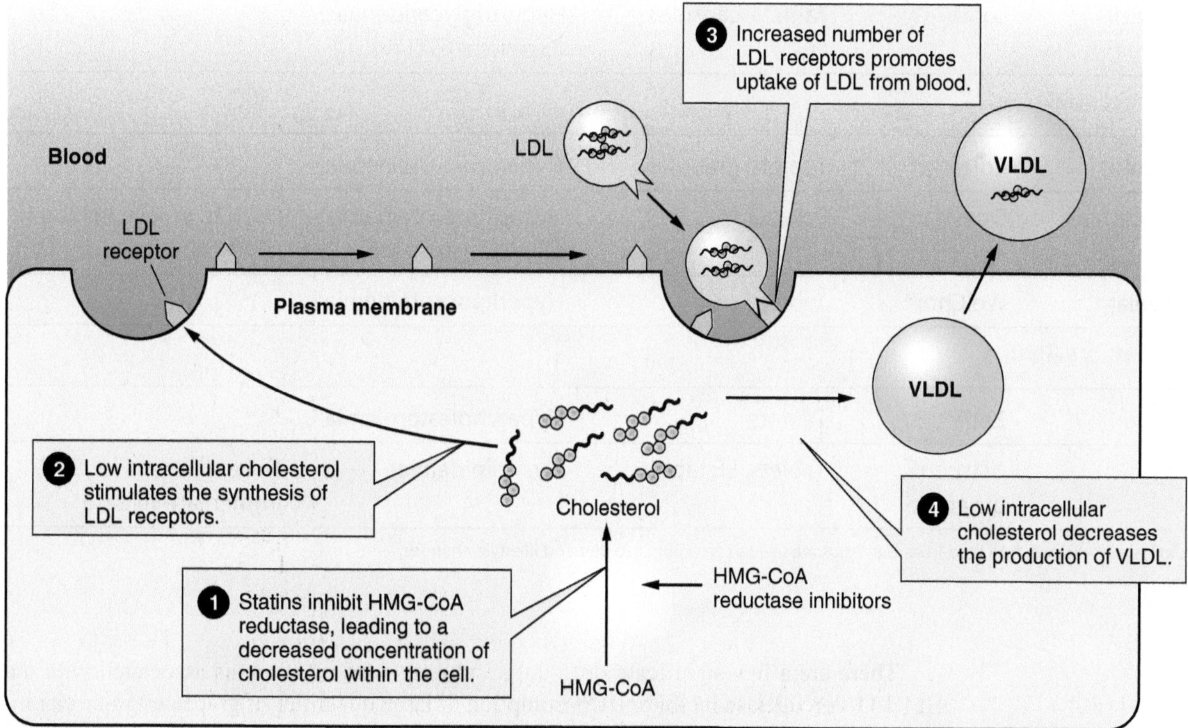


**Figure 18.7** The statin drugs reduce lipid levels in the blood by blocking the production of cholesterol in the liver. (Adapted with permission from Harvey RA, Champe PC, Howland RD, et al. *Lippincott's Illustrated Reviews: Pharmacology*, 3rd edition. Baltimore: Lippincott Williams & Wilkins, 2006.)

**Table 18.4** Summary of the Lipid-Lowering Agents, Available Formulations, and Indications

| Generic | Brand Name | Available as | Indications | Notes* |
|---|---|---|---|---|
| **HMG-CoA Reductase Inhibitors** | | | | |
| Atorvastatin | Lipitor® | Tablets | Hyperlipidemia, & to increase HDL | Statin drugs have been shown to reduce CVD risk |
| Fluvastatin | Lescol®, Lescol XL® | Capsules, ER tablets | Hyperlipidemia | |
| Lovastatin | Mevacor®, Altocor® | Tablets, ER tablets | Hyperlipidemia | * |
| Pravastatin | Pravachol® | Tablets | Hyperlipidemia | |
| Rosuvastatin | Crestor® | Tablets | Hyperlipidemia | |
| Simvastatin | Zocor® | Tablets | Hyperlipidemia, & to increase HDL | |
| **Fibric Acid Derivatives** | | | | |
| Fenofibrate | Tricor® | Tablets | Hypercholesterolemia, mixed | * |
| Gemfibrozil | Lopid® | Tablets, capsules | Hypertriglyceridemia, to reduce CVD risk | |
| **Bile Acid Sequestrants** | | | | |
| Colestipol | Colestid® | Tablets, granules | Hyperlipoproteinemia | * |
| Cholestyramine | Questran® | Powder | Hyperlipoproteinemia, biliary obstruction | Used to relieve itching in biliary obs |
| Colesevelam | WelChol® | Tablets | Hyperlipoproteinemia | |
| **Miscellaneous Agents** | | | | |
| Ezetimibe | Zetia® | Tablets | Hypercholesterolemia | * |
| Niacin | Niaspan®, others | Tablets, ER tabs | Hyperlipidemia | Dose different for ER & immediate release |

CVD, cardiovascular disease. * All lipid-lowering drugs are used as an adjunct to diet and lifestyle changes.

There are a few significant drug-drug and drug-food interactions associated with the HMG-CoA reductase inhibitors. Consumption of large quantities of grapefruit juice can increase the serum levels of simvastatin and lovastatin. The azole antifungal drugs, cyclosporine, and erythromycin increase the risk of adverse effects when given with these drugs. Niacin and gemfibrozil enhance the lipid-lowering effects of the statin drugs, but they also may increase the risk of side effects. The HMG-CoA reductase inhibitors also increase the anticoagulant effects of warfarin.

## Side Effects

The statin drugs are associated with a few minor side effects and two very important and much more serious ones. The most common side effects are heartburn and diarrhea. Central nervous system symptoms of dizziness, feelings of fatigue, and headache are also common. Rarely, some patients experience photosensitivity. The statin drugs can cause liver toxicity, and physicians will usually monitor liver function tests in order to avoid this serious side effect. These drugs are not recommended for use by patients who consume large amounts of alcohol because of the potential for liver toxicity. Rhabdomyolysis (breakdown or dissolution of muscle cells) is another rare, but very serious, side effect. Myopathy (disease of the muscle) occurs more often when the patient has renal failure or is taking interacting drugs. The destruction of muscle releases toxins into the blood stream that can cause severe kidney damage. One drug, cerivastatin, was removed from the U.S. market in 2001 because the risk of these adverse events was significantly higher than for any of the other statin drugs, and many people died from this side effect. Some consumer groups believe that rosuvastatin (Crestor®) is also excessively dangerous and have petitioned the Food and Drug Administration to review its approval. To date, the FDA has declined to do so.

rhabdomyolysis Destruction of skeletal muscle cells that is associated with the release of muscle cell contents into the circulation which causes serious metabolic disturbances.

myopathy A muscle disease.

### Tips for the Technician

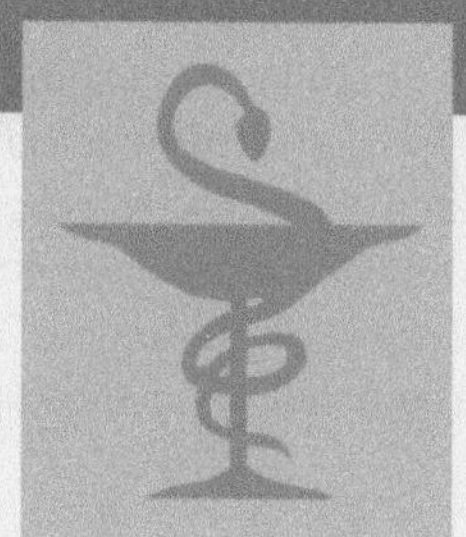

Atorvastatin, simvastatin, and pravastatin are on the list of the top 100 best-selling drugs in the United States for 2004, while fluvastatin (Lescol®) extended release and rosuvastatin are in the top 300 drugs. It is important that technicians are familiar with the use of these important drugs. All of the statin drugs should carry auxiliary warning labels advising against the consumption of alcohol. Prescription vials should also be labelled with a recommendation to take the medication with meals or a snack, to avoid large amounts of grapefruit juice, and a caution about potential drug interactions.

Because there are rare but serious side effects, patients should receive counseling from the pharmacist when they bring in a new prescription for one of the statin drugs. Patients should be familiar with side effects and be told to report any muscle pain to the physician. These drugs are contraindicated during pregnancy and in nursing mothers.

# 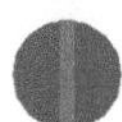 Fibric Acid Derivatives

The two fibric acid derivatives sold in the United Sates are gemfibrozil (Lopid®) and fenofibrate (TriCor®). Clofibrate, the prototype fibric acid derivative, was removed from the market because of liver toxicity.

## Actions and Indications

The fibric acid derivatives are used to treat hypertriglyceridemia. Normal triglyceride levels are less than 150 mg/dL. Treatment with one of the triglyceride drugs is not considered until use of a low-fat diet and a statin drug is maximized. People with triglyceride levels of 400 or more are treated more aggressively, possibly with the fibric acid derivatives or niacin. These drugs act on the family of genes involved in fat metabolism to stimulate production of proteins that are important in lipid breakdown. The production of VLDL in the liver is reduced and the production of HDL may be increased.

## Administration

The fibric acid derivatives are administered orally and are well absorbed after an oral dose. Fenofibrate absorption is increased in the presence of food. Gemfibrozil and fenofibrate are highly bound to albumin. As might be anticipated, they are involved in a number of drug interactions, including the potentiation of the anticoagulant effect of warfarin. Both drugs undergo metabolism in the liver and the kidneys remove metabolites. Although the VLDL levels may begin to drop within a few days, levels will continue to fall over several months.

Gemfibrozil is available in tablet form, and fenofibrate is available as tablets and capsules. Fenofibrate is administered on a once-daily basis and gemfibrozil is given twice a day. Elderly people are started on lower doses. People taking these medications should also be restricting their dietary intake of fat.

## Side Effects

Gemfibrozil is very similar to clofibrate, which was removed from the market because of liver toxicity and an apparent increased risk of death. Although no studies have been done on the newer fibric acid derivatives, there was evidence that clofibrate increased the risk of death from cancer and pancreatitis when people took it chronically. Because of this, physicians are encouraged not to leave patients on these drugs if there is not an adequate response within 2 months.

The most common adverse effects are mild gastrointestinal disturbances. Muscle pain and inflammation can occur with both drugs, and muscle weakness or tenderness should be reported to the prescriber. Patients with renal insufficiency may be at risk of developing rhabdomyolysis, especially if they are also taking one of the statin drugs. A significant number of patients will develop a change in their liver function tests, indicating an adverse effect on the liver. These tests usually return to normal once the drug is discontinued. The fibric acid derivatives increase biliary cholesterol excretion and, as a result, predispose patients to the formation of gallstones.

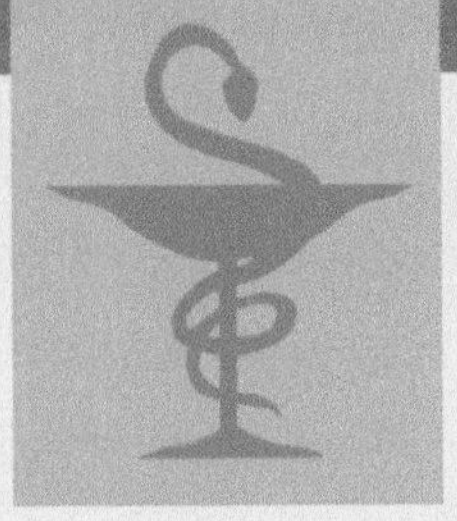

### Tips for the Technician

The manufacturer recommends that gemfibrozil be taken 30 minutes before meals, on an empty stomach, while fenofibrate is best given with meals or immediately after meals. Vials should be labelled accordingly. Patients need to be informed of potential side effects by the pharmacist during counseling, and encouraged to report any muscle pain or persistent abdominal pain. An auxiliary label warning of the potential for drug interactions should be affixed to the prescription vial.

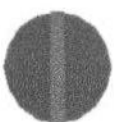

# Bile Acid Sequestrants

Cholestyramine (Questran®), colesevelam (WelChol®), and colestipol (Colestid®) are the three bile acid sequestrants presently sold in the United States. They can produce a significant reduction in LDL levels and a small increase in HDL levels. Depending on the drug used, they can be as little as one-fourth the cost of the statin drugs.

## Actions and Indications

These drugs are anion-exchange resins that bind bile acids and bile salts in the small intestine. Bile acids are synthesized from cholesterol and secreted by epithelial cells of the liver where they become part of the bile. Synthesis of bile acids is an important route for the use and elimination of cholesterol. Normally bile is delivered into the small intestine where it helps in the dissolution and absorption of dietary fats and fat-soluble vitamins. It is reabsorbed by the intestine and undergoes enterohepatic recirculation and reuse.

When the bile acid sequestrants are taken, they form an insoluble complex with the bile that is excreted in the feces. This prevents the bile acids from returning to the liver and lowers their concentration in the liver (**Fig. 18.8**). Hepatocytes must then increase conversion of cholesterol to bile acids, to replenish the supply of these compounds, which are essential components of the bile. Consequently, the intracellular cholesterol concentration decreases, and this causes increased uptake of LDL particles from the blood, causing total plasma cholesterol levels to fall. These drugs are indicated for treatment of hyperlipidemia in patients who do not respond to diet alone.

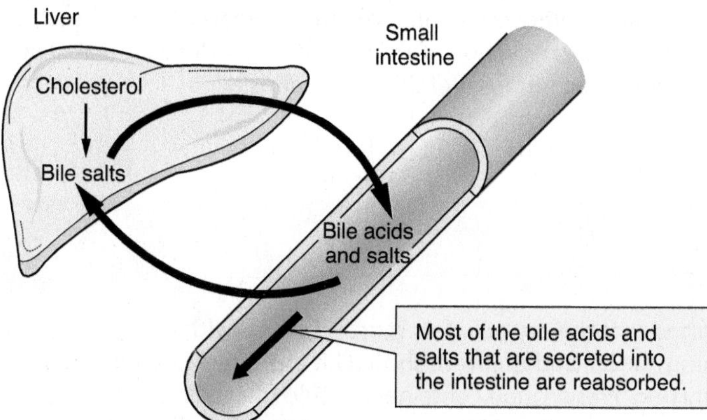


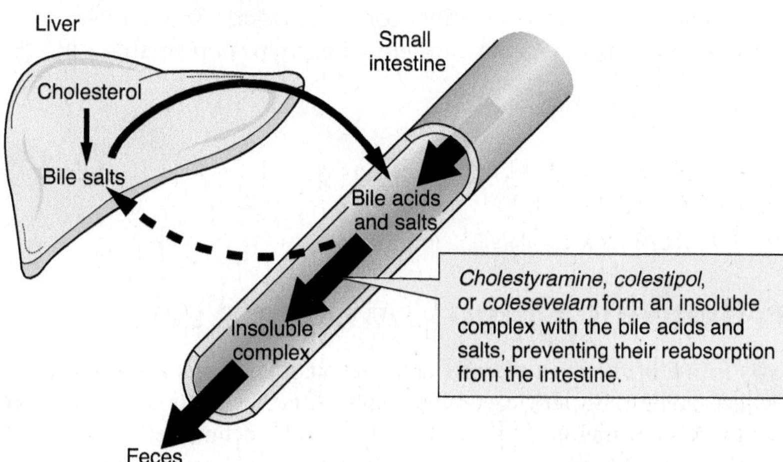


**Figure 18.8** Mechanism of action of the bile acid sequestrants. (Adapted with permission from Harvey RA, Champe PC, Howland RD, et al. *Lippincott's Illustrated Reviews: Pharmacology*, 3rd edition. Baltimore: Lippincott Williams & Wilkins, 2006.)

## Administration

Cholestyramine, colestipol, and colesevelam are taken orally. Because they are insoluble in water and are very large molecules, they are not absorbed. Instead, they are totally excreted in the feces. Cholestyramine is only available as a flavored powder that is mixed with juice or water and taken twice daily. Colestipol is available as tablets, or granules that are mixed with fluids, and given once or twice daily. Colesevelam tablets are taken once or twice daily with meals.

## Side Effects

Because these drugs work by exerting a local effect in the GI tract and are not absorbed, serious side effects are rare. Unfortunately, use of these drugs is often abandoned because of minor side effects of indigestion, gas, and constipation. Adequate fluid intake and the addition of stool softeners can reduce these unpleasant effects. The constipation, if not treated, can be serious, and these agents are not recommended for use in patients with severe chronic constipation or bowel disease.

The only other side effects occur as a result of reduced absorption of fat-soluble vitamins and folic acid. Chronic use can increase bleeding tendencies because of vitamin K malabsorption. Vitamin supplementation is recommended for patients who take these drugs chronically.

The bile acid sequestrants can significantly reduce the absorption of some drugs if they are administered concurrently. Other drugs should be taken at least an hour before or six hours after the bile acid sequestrants are administered. If bile acid sequestrants are discontinued in a patient who is taking another drug with a narrow therapeutic index, such as digoxin, there is a risk that increased absorption of the second drug will result in toxicity. Patients taking other drugs need to be informed of this potential risk.

### Tips for the Technician

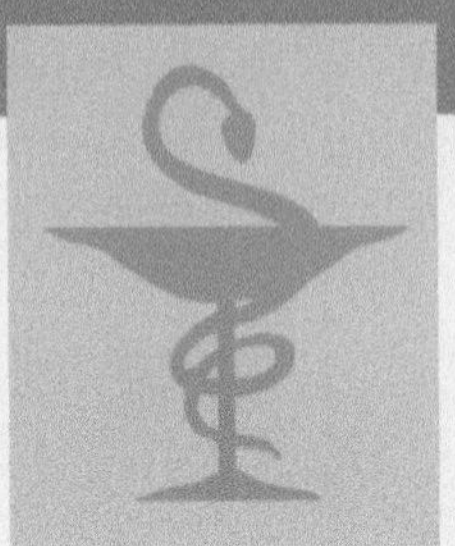

Patients should be informed that the dry powders must be mixed with non-carbonated liquids before administration, and that care should be exercised to avoid inhaling the powders when mixing. Prescription containers should be labelled with an auxiliary label instructing the patient to mix the powdered products with four or more ounces of water or juice. Prescription vials containing tablets should include instructions to swallow tablets whole; they should not be crushed. Patients should be warned by the pharmacist about the potential for constipation, and encouraged to consume plenty of liquids, fruit, and other fiber containing foods. They should also be told about the possibility of vitamin deficiency if vitamin supplements are not used.

# 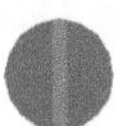 Miscellaneous Lipid-Lowering Agents

Ezetimibe (Zetia®) is one of the most recently approved antihyperlipidemic agents, and niacin (Niaspan®) is the oldest. Because ezetimibe is so new, most experts do not consider it a first-choice drug. Administration of niacin delivers a well-documented reduction in lipid levels, a significant increase in "good" cholesterol, and is the least expensive of the lipid-lowering drugs.

## Actions and Indications

In large doses, niacin inhibits the breakdown of fat in adipose tissue, which is a primary producer of circulating fatty acids. The liver normally uses circulating fatty acids for the synthesis of triglycerides. Niacin causes a decrease in the synthesis of triglycerides in the liver. Triglycerides are required for VLDL production. VLDL is used in the formation of LDL, and as a result, niacin reduces both LDL, triglyceride and total cholesterol levels. Of all the drugs used to treat hyperlipidemia, niacin is the most effective at increasing HDL, and it also reverses some of the endothelial cell dysfunction that contributes to the formation of thrombi in atherosclerosis. **Table 18.5** summarizes the effects of the antihyperlipidemic drug classes.

Ezetimibe inhibits intestinal absorption of dietary and biliary cholesterol in the small intestine, leading to a decrease in the delivery of intestinal cholesterol to the liver. This causes a reduction of hepatic cholesterol stores and an increase in clearance of cholesterol from the blood. It is selective in blocking absorption of dietary cholesterol and does not appear to prevent the absorption of fat-soluble vitamins.

## Administration

Niacin and ezetimibe are administered orally. Niacin is available in regular-release and sustained-release tablets. Generally the sustained-release formulations are better tolerated than the regular-release forms. Niacin is one of the B vitamins. When used as a vitamin supplement, niacin is administered in 50 to 100 mg doses. The dose requirement for treatment of hyperlipidemia is 1 gram or more daily. Doses for extended-release preparations are different than the dose of the immediate-release products. Two grams per day of the extended release preparations is the maximum dose. Niacin can be used in combination with statin drugs, and a product combining lovastatin and long-acting niacin is available. Niacin should be given at bedtime and the dose very gradually increased to reduce the flushing that occurs with this drug.

Unlike the bile acid sequestrants, ezetimibe is absorbed systemically and metabolized in the liver. It is excreted in the bile and through the kidneys. Lower doses may be necessary in the elderly and those with significant renal failure. It should not be used in patients with severe hepatic dysfunction. Ezetimibe tablets can be administered with or without food.

## Side Effects

Compliance has always been an issue with niacin therapy because it causes dilation of the blood vessels in the skin, or flushing. This effect is accompanied by a feeling of warmth or a burning sensation, which can be temporarily uncomfortable. Symptoms of flushing often

**Table 18.5** Characteristics of hyperepidemic drug families

| Type of Drug | Effect on LDL | Effect on HDL | Effect on Triacylglycerols |
|---|---|---|---|
| HMG-CoA reductase inhibitors (statins) | ↓↓↓↓ | ↑ | ↓↓ |
| Fibrates | ↓ | ↑↑↑ | ↓↓↓↓ |
| Niacin | ↓↓↓ | ↑ | ↓↓↓ |
| Bile acid sequestrants | ↓↓↓ | ↑ | Minimal |
| Cholesterol absorption inhibitor | ↓ | ↑ | ↓ |

HDL, high-density lipoprotein; HMG-CoA, 3-hydroxy-3-methylglutaryl–coenzyme A; LDL, low-density lipoprotein.

lessen over time. Extended-release preparations are much better tolerated, especially when taken at bedtime.

Flushing is the most common side effect, but other adverse effects include abdominal pain, nausea, and vomiting. Severe liver toxicity has occurred when patients switched from the higher doses that can be taken of the immediate-release preparations to an equivalent dose of the extended- or delayed-release products.

Ezetimibe therapy is well tolerated by most patients. The most common complaints are GI upset, abdominal pain, and diarrhea. Some patients experience muscle and joint pain. Significant elevations in liver function tests, greater than when either drug was given alone, have been seen when ezetimibe is given in conjunction with statin drugs.

## Tips for the Technician

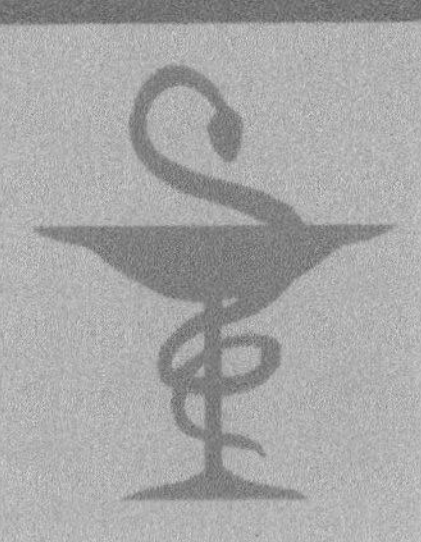

In order to help patients adhere to their niacin treatment regimens, they should be well informed of the side effects, the likelihood that the side effects will subside with time, and given tips on how to reduce the side effects. It is especially important that they take their medication at bedtime. They should avoid drinking hot beverages or alcoholic beverages when they take the niacin.

Ezetimibe can be given without regard to meals. The pharmacist should inform patients of potential side effects. Patients should be reminded of the importance of complying with the doctor's order for laboratory monitoring tests, especially if they are taking ezetimibe with a statin drug.

# Review Questions

## Multiple Choice

Choose the best answer for the following questions:

1. Which of the following best describes the process of hemostasis?
   a. Injury to vessel → platelets aggregate → platelets activated → platelet granules released → clotting factor activation → fibrin mesh is formed → healing and thrombolysis.
   b. Injury to vessel → platelets aggregate → coagulation factors activated → platelet granules released → thrombolysis.
   c. Injury to vessel → platelets aggregate → platelets activated → platelet granules released → clotting factor activation → fibrin mesh is formed.
   d. Platelets aggregate → platelets activated → platelet granules released → clotting factor activation → fibrin mesh is formed → healing and thrombolysis.
   e. None of the above are correct.

2. The platelet aggregation inhibitor ticlopidine is known to cause which of the following adverse effects?
   a. Bleeding
   b. Thrombotic thrombocytopenic purpura
   c. Asthma in aspirin sensitive individuals
   d. All of the above
   e. a and b only

3. Which of the following drugs should be taken on an empty stomach?
   a. Aspirin
   b. Heparin
   c. Streptokinase
   d. Colesevelam
   e. Gemfibrozil

4. The body requires which of the following compounds for normal production of red blood cells?
   a. Vitamin B12
   b. Iron
   c. Erythropoietin
   d. All of the above
   e. a and b only

5. Which of the following medications is able to cause dissolution of a clot, when administered intravenously?
   a. Atorvastatin
   b. Warfarin
   c. Alteplase
   d. Lepirudin
   e. Abciximab

## True/False Questions

6. Aspirin's platelet aggregation inhibiting effect disappears when the drug is no longer present in the blood stream.
   a. True
   b. False

7. Bleeding caused by excessive heparin can be rapidly reversed using vitamin K.
   a. True
   b. False

8. People with total cholesterol levels >200 should be put on diets low in saturated and trans fats and encouraged to exercise before they are put on HMG-CoA reductase inhibitor therapy.
   a. True
   b. False

9. Flushing is a common side effect of niacin, related to dilation of peripheral blood vessels.
   a. True
   b. False

10. Because of thorough screening of all new drugs by the FDA, it is safe to assume that rosuvastatin (Crestor®), the newest HMG-CoA reductase inhibitor, is safer and more effective than the older statin drugs.
    a. True
    b. False

## Matching

For questions 11 to 15, match each numbered drug to the best lettered choice below. Answer choices may be used once or not at all.

11. Warfarin
12. Desirudin
13. Cholestyramine
14. Niacin
15. Ezetimibe

a. Patient compliance with this drug can be poor because of flushing of the skin.
b. Vitamin K is an antidote to the anticoagulant effects of this drug.
c. This lipid-lowering drug binds fats in the GI tract, thereby preventing their absorption.
d. Giving protamine counteracts bleeding caused by this drug.
e. This lipid-lowering drug binds fats in the GI tract, is not absorbed, and is very inexpensive.
f. This large molecule is a thrombin inhibitor that occurs naturally, in minute amounts, in the cells of mammals.
g. This drug is a thrombin inhibitor given by subcutaneous injection, and is related to compounds found in the saliva of leeches.

## Short Answer

16. If a patient on one of the statin drugs came in complaining of feeling muscle aches and pains for the past two weeks would there be any reason for concern? Why or why not?

17. What are the advantages and disadvantages of low-dose aspirin as compared with clopidogrel for preventing thrombotic events?

18. Why are women of childbearing age and adolescents more likely to develop iron-deficiency anemia? What treatment options are available for a 21-year-old woman with iron deficiency anemia?

19. Why is it recommended that a test dose of iron dextran be given one hour before the first therapeutic dose?

20. Joe Aquafresca is on a continuous heparin infusion, receiving 1,000 units of heparin per hour. Nurse Betty calls to ask if she can inject his labetalol into the IV line where the heparin is running. Pharmacist Rich cannot come to the telephone because he is making a morphine drip. What do you tell her?

# FOR FURTHER INQUIRY

Epoetin has become a commonly, but illegally, used performance enhancing drug in sports. Find out what makes this particular agent difficult to trace, and see if you can find some cases of well-known athletes who used epoetin and got caught.

UNIT **IV**

# Drugs Affecting the Respiratory, Urinary, Gastrointestinal, and Musculoskeletal Systems

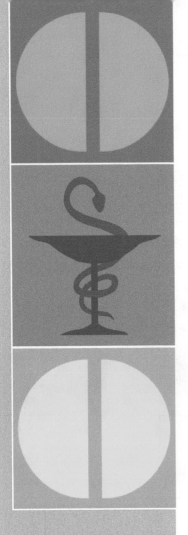

Chapter **19**

# The Anatomy and Physiology of the Respiratory, Urinary, Gastrointestinal, and Musculoskeletal Systems

*KEY TERMS*

- alimentary
- alveoli
- anal sphincter
- appendicular skeleton
- asthma
- axial skeleton
- bronchi (plural of bronchus)
- bronchiole
- bronchitis
- bursa
- cancellous bone
- cartilaginous joint
- cecum
- chronic obstructive pulmonary disease
- colon
- compact bone
- congenital
- cystitis

## OBJECTIVES

After studying this chapter, the reader should be able to:

- Describe, in simple terms, the anatomy of the respiratory system and how it interacts with the cardiovascular system in order to deliver oxygen to every cell in the body.
- List the four processes involved in urine production and identify where in the nephron each occurs.
- Trace the path of a bite of food through the digestive system and name the organs that contribute to its digestion along the way.
- Explain the relationships between muscle, bones, and joints that allow movement of the body.
- List and describe a common disease of each of the organ systems covered in this chapter.

- distal convoluted tubule
- duodenum
- emphysema
- emulsify
- epiglottis
- epiphysis
- fibrous joint
- gastrin
- glomerular filtration
- glomerulonephritis
- glomerulus
- glottis
- gout
- hematopoietic stem cell
- ileum
- insulin
- incontinent
- jejunum
- larynx
- ligament
- lithotripsy
- locomotion
- loop of Henle
- mastication
- mediastinum
- micturition
- mucosa
- muscular dystrophy
- nares
- nephron
- osteoarthritis
- osteoblast
- osteoclast
- osteomalacia
- osteomyelitis
- osteoporosis
- pepsin
- peptic ulcer
- periosteum
- peristalsis
- pharynx
- proximal convoluted tubule
- rectum
- reflux
- renal cortex
- renal medulla
- resorption
- rheumatoid arthritis
- striated
- surfactant
- synovial joint
- tendon
- thoracic cavity
- trachea
- vascular

None of the body systems function without the coordination and control of the nervous system and the power provided by the engine of life, the cardiovascular system. This chapter will describe the complementary actions and supportive functions of the respiratory, urinary, gastrointestinal, and musculoskeletal systems. Respiration, digestion, elimination, and locomotion allow for normal growth and development, not just in humans, but in all mammals. However, like the nervous system and the cardiovascular system, these organs and systems are subject to disease. In order to understand available drug therapies, students need a basic understanding of the anatomy and physiology of these systems, and some of the diseases associated with them.

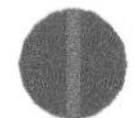

# The Respiratory System

## Anatomy of the Respiratory System

The respiratory system, whose function is to obtain oxygen from the environment, make it available for all the cells in the body, and exchange it for carbon dioxide, is a series of chambers and passageways designed to carry and hold air. The respiratory system ultimately depends on the function of the lungs, which are the key organs of respiration. The lungs are intimately connected, both anatomically and physiologically, to the heart and circulatory system. The lungs are elegantly designed to allow the exchange of oxygen for carbon dioxide, but they are dependent upon the heart and blood for delivery of the oxygen to the tissues, as described in Chapter 14. The heart rests in the space between the lungs (the mediastinum), nestled close to the left lung (see **Fig. 19.1**).

Air is pulled into the body through the nose or the mouth. The nostrils, or nares, are lined with hairs to help filter out dust and other particles. The nasal and oral cavities are lined with mucous membranes that warm and add moisture to the air before it enters the lungs. These two cavities join at the pharynx, or throat. Both air and food pass through the

mediastinum The space in the chest behind the sternum, and between the lungs.

nares Nostrils.

pharynx The anatomical area situated between the mouth and the esophagus.

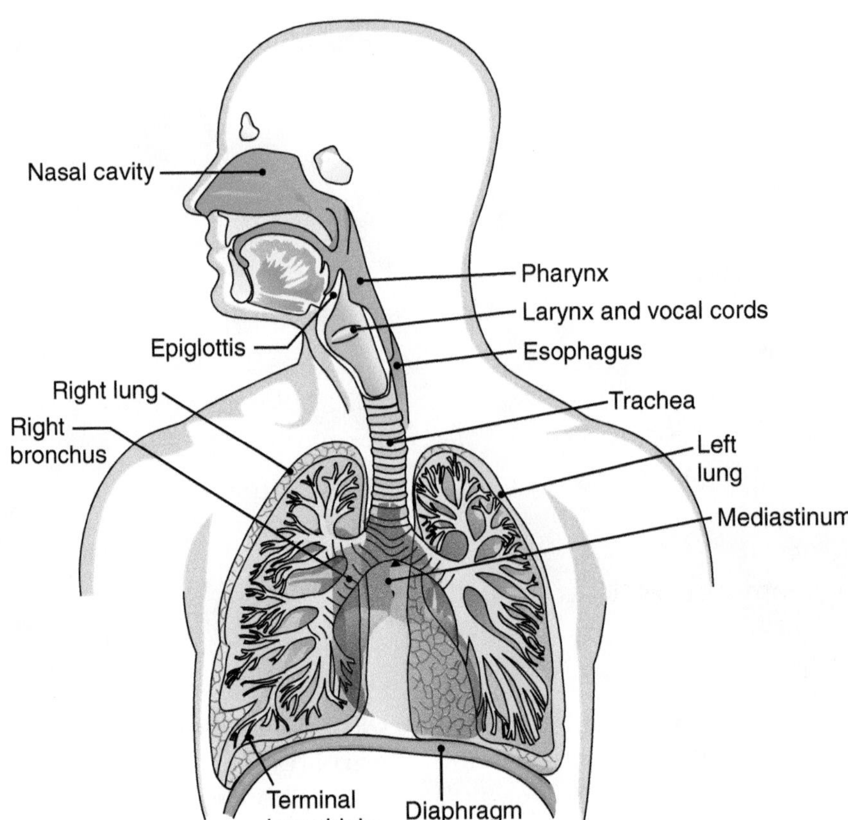


**Figure 19.1** An overview of the anatomy of the respiratory system. The shadow at the center right of the image indicates the location of the heart. (Adapted with permission from Cohen BJ. *Memmler's The Human Body in Health and Disease*, 10th edition. Baltimore: Lippincott Williams & Wilkins, 2005.)

larynx The part of the respiratory tract that is below the glottis and connected with the trachea, and contains the vocal cords.

epiglottis A cartilaginous flap that covers the glottis while swallowing food or liquids.

glottis The vocal apparatus of the larynx, including both the vocal cord tissue and the opening between the vocal cord and surrounding cartilage.

trachea The trunk of the airway that connects the larynx to the bronchi.

bronchi (plural of bronchus) The main airways that lead from the trachea to the lungs.

bronchiole One of many small, thin-walled branches off of the bronchus.

pharynx to the lower pharynx. At this point, the lower pharynx divides into the larynx, which carries air, and the esophagus, which transport food to the stomach. The larynx, commonly called the voice box, is a structure surrounded by cartilage and covered by folds of mucous membranes that separate the pharynx from the windpipe, or trachea. These membranous folds vibrate when air passes over them and are known as the vocal cords or vocal folds. The epiglottis is a small piece of cartilage that moves to cover the glottis (the space between the vocal cords) during swallowing, so that food and liquids cannot enter the trachea (**Fig. 19.2**).

The trachea is the passageway that conducts air from the larynx to the lungs. Just above the lungs the trachea divides into the right and left mainstem bronchi. The bronchi further subdivide so that a major branch of the bronchial tree feeds air to each lobe of the lungs, two on the left and three on the right. The bronchi continue to divide and branch into the smallest of passageways, called the bronchioles. The bronchi are held open with cartilage, and as they become narrower the amount of cartilage diminishes. The bronchioles do not contain cartilage, but are lined with smooth muscle under the control of the autonomic nervous system. Tiny air sacs are clustered around the end of each bronchiole. These air

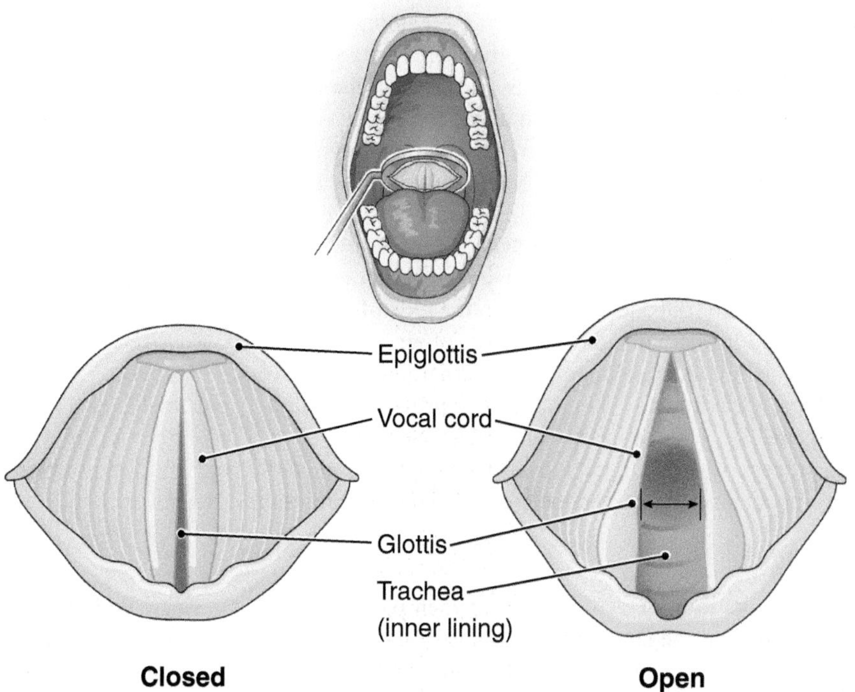


**Figure 19.2** The vocal cords in the open and closed position. (Adapted with permission from Cohen BJ. *Memmler's The Human Body in Health and Disease*, 10th edition. Baltimore: Lippincott Williams & Wilkins, 2005.)

sacs, called alveoli, expand to fill with air during inhalation and deflate during exhalation. Human lungs contain millions of alveoli, and their surface area is nearly as large as the area of a tennis court. Surfactant, secreted in the alveoli, is a slippery liquid that reduces surface tension (like liquid detergent), and prevents the alveoli from collapsing. Surfactant also aids in alveolar expansion. The walls of the alveoli are only one-cell thick and are surrounded by capillaries. It is here, through the delicate walls of the alveoli and the surrounding capillaries, that the exchange of oxygen and carbon dioxide takes place (**Fig. 19.3**).

alveoli The small thin-walled compartments of the lung that are typically arranged in saclike clusters and are the site of air exchange.

surfactant Surface-active agent; increases the emulsifying and wetting properties of a product.

## Respiratory Physiology

There are several processes involved with respiration. These processes include the expansion and filling of the lungs with air, the exchange of gases in the alveoli, the delivery of oxygen and removal of carbon dioxide to and from the tissues, and the regulation of breathing.

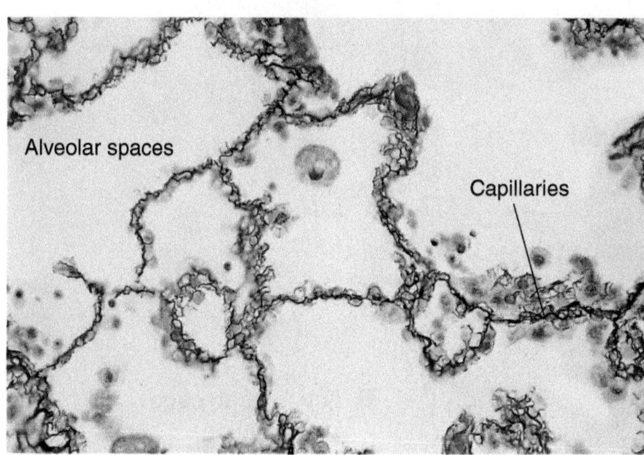


**Figure 19.3** The delicate walls of the alveoli and pulmonary capillary system are the sites of oxygen exchange in the lung. (Reprinted with permission from Mills SE. *Histology for Pathologists,* 3rd edition. Philadelphia: Lippincott Williams & Wilkins, 2007.)

## Ventilation

Ventilation is the exchange that occurs during breathing between air in the lungs and the air in the environment. During inhalation, the diaphragm and the external intercostal muscles contract. The external intercostal muscles attach at the underside of the rib above and run diagonally between the ribs to attach at the top of the rib below. When these muscles contract, the ribs are lifted up and out. When the diaphragm contracts it pushes down on the abdominal organs located below it. As a result of these two actions, the volume of the thoracic cavity, which is the space that contains the lungs, expands (**Fig. 19.4**).

thoracic cavity Division of the body cavity that lies above the diaphragm; the chest, which contains the heart and lungs.

With the expansion of the thoracic cavity, the pressure inside the lungs is less than the outside (ambient) air pressure. This negative pressure gradient causes air to flow from the area of higher pressure (outside the lungs) to the area of lower pressure (inside the lungs). The alveoli expand to accommodate the influx of air.

During exhalation the diaphragm and external intercostals relax. This reduces the volume of the thoracic cavity and creates a positive pressure gradient in relationship to the ambient air pressure. The change in pressure causes air to move out of the lungs. In order for the ongoing process of ventilation to occur, the lung tissue must inflate, the muscles of ventilation must function normally, and the bronchi and bronchioles must remain unobstructed.

## Gas Exchange

Gas exchange occurs in the alveoli, where oxygen passes through the single cell layer of alveolar epithelium and the single cell layer of the capillary basement membrane to reach the blood stream. The air we inhale from the atmosphere contains about 21% oxygen, or a partial pressure of about 159 mmHg (millimeters of mercury), but once it is mixed with residual air in the lungs it contains about 100 mmHg of oxygen.

The deoxygenated blood returning to the lungs contains about 40 mmHg of oxygen, whereas fully oxygenated arterial blood leaving the lungs contains an oxygen pressure of about 98 mmHg. Exchange of oxygen from the lungs to the bloodstream occurs because of

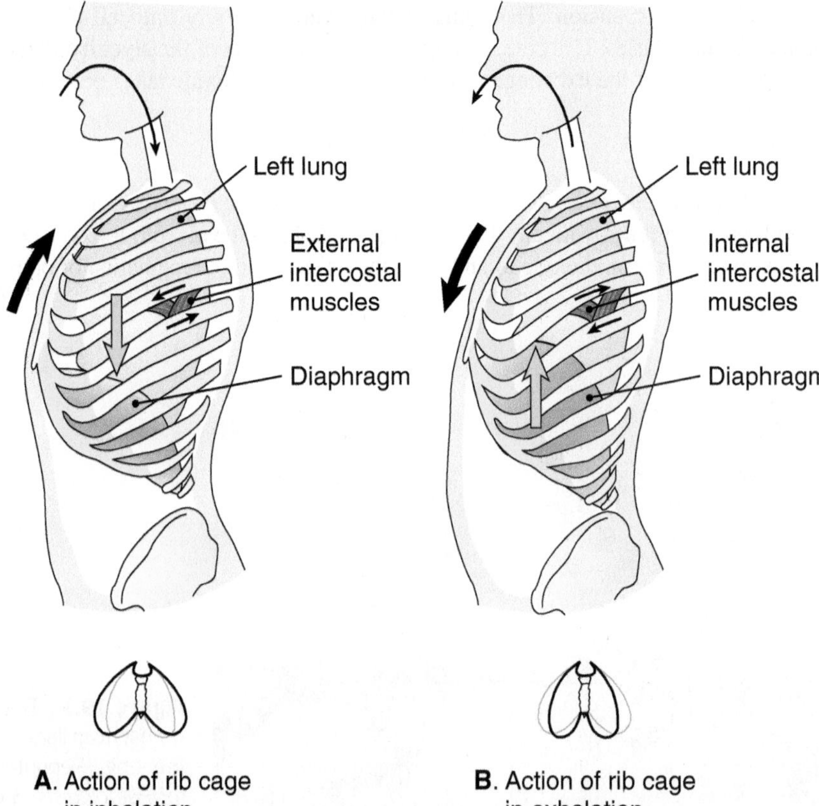


**Figure 19.4** During inhalation (A), the diaphragm and the external intercostal muscles contract, allowing the lungs to expand. During exhalation (B), internal intercostal muscles and diaphragm push air out. (Adapted with permission from Cohen BJ. *Memmler's The Human Body in Health and Disease*, 10th edition. Baltimore: Lippincott Williams & Wilkins, 2005.)

diffusion, the movement of a substance from an area where it is in a higher concentration to an area of lower concentration (**Fig. 19.5**). However, if not for the presence of hemoglobin in red blood cells, the ability of the blood to hold oxygen would be minimal. This is because the blood would only be able to carry the small amount of oxygen that could dissolve into it. Fortunately, humans and other mammalian blood cells contain hemoglobin. In humans, this iron-containing protein reversibly attaches to and carries oxygen, which increases the oxygen carrying capacity of blood about 70-fold. When hemoglobin levels are low, as in iron deficiency anemia, oxygen carrying capacity of the blood is reduced.

Most tissues have an oxygen concentration of about 40 mmHg, so when oxygenated blood reaches tissues, the process of diffusion begins again. Here in the tissues, oxygen is released from hemoglobin where it passes through capillary basement membranes into cells. The cells contain a higher concentration of carbon dioxide, produced during cellular metabolism, than does the blood. Carbon dioxide, therefore, diffuses from cells into the blood. Some carbon dioxide attaches to hemoglobin but the majority is converted to bicarbonate ion, which dissolves in the plasma and is carried back to the lungs. In the lungs, it is converted back to a gas, and is exchanged for oxygen in the process of ventilation.

### Regulation of Breathing

Regulation of breathing is complex and is controlled by the respiratory center in the brain stem, input from the autonomic nervous system, and feedback from receptors that register the concentrations of oxygen and carbon dioxide in the blood. Although we can consciously increase or decrease our rate of breathing, the control of ventilation is ultimately, and very fortunately, under involuntary control.

Rising levels of carbon dioxide are the single greatest stimulus to breathing. For example, during periods of increased metabolism such as vigorous exercise, carbon dioxide production increases as a result of vastly increased energy and oxygen consumption. Rising levels of carbon dioxide trigger a response in the central nervous system. To meet the increased oxygen requirements of tissues, the respiratory rate must increase. A higher respiratory rate increases the supply of oxygen to the bloodstream, but the heart also must beat harder and faster to get the blood to the tissues. Once the metabolic rate of the muscles returns to normal, carbon dioxide production falls and the heart and respiratory rates return to their resting levels.

## Diseases of the Respiratory System

Disorders of the respiratory system include diseases affecting any part of the system from the nasal cavity and sinuses to the lungs. Because many infectious agents and allergens are airborne, respiratory infections and allergies are common. People who are exposed to airborne environmental contaminants, such as tobacco smoke or the components of smog, run

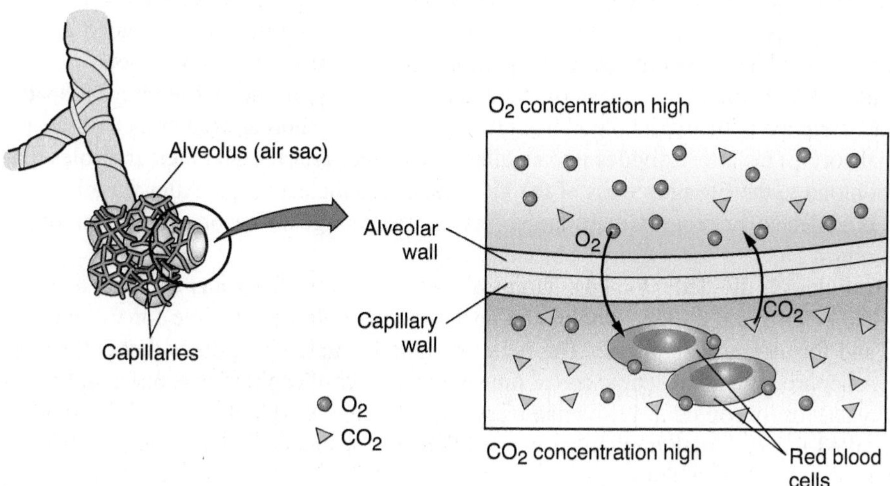


**Figure 19.5** Oxygen and carbon dioxide exchange across the alveoli and capillary membranes, down the concentration gradients.

asthma A lung disorder with recurring episodes of airway constriction and symptoms of labored breathing accompanied by wheezing and coughing.

bronchitis Acute or chronic inflammation of the bronchi, often due to infection.

emphysema A lung disease usually due to smoking, in which distention and reduced elasticity of alveoli causes air accumulation and impaired air exchange.

chronic obstructive pulmonary disease Progressive, irreversible pulmonary diseases, emphysema or chronic bronchitis, related to smoking and characterized by difficulty breathing and a chronic cough.

renal cortex The outer part of the kidney, which contains the glomerulus and parts of the tubules.

renal medulla The center portion of the kidneys where the urine collecting system is located.

nephron Single excretory unit of the kidney, where blood is filtered and urine formed.

glomerulus An intertwined mass of capillaries that is situated at the origin of each nephron through which the blood is filtered.

proximal convoluted tubule The portion of the vertebrate nephron that lies between the glomerulus and the loop of Henle.

a higher risk of developing virtually all respiratory disorders. Individuals who live in agricultural areas may have a higher risk of allergic rhinitis and asthma.

Asthma is a condition that occurs because the airways react to allergens, exercise, or other triggering factors by constricting and preventing the efficient exhalation of air. Exposure to irritants or other triggers leads to inflammation and the presence of white blood cells in the airways. Mast cells, a type of white blood cell containing histamine and other chemical mediators, are present in abnormally high numbers in the bronchi of asthmatic patients. When activated mast cells release these mediators, they cause edema, mucus production, and bronchoconstriction (constriction of the airways). Asthma is characterized by reversible airway obstruction and is not generally a progressive condition. Although deaths due to asthma are not common, they have been on the rise sine the 1980s.

Bronchitis is inflammation of one or both of the bronchi, usually because of infection. Chronic bronchitis is a result of chronic inflammation and infection that occurs in response to long-term exposure to environmental contaminants, such as cigarette smoke. In chronic bronchitis, the airways are inflamed and excessive secretions are produced. People who suffer chronic bronchitis have a much higher risk of developing emphysema. Emphysema causes a gradual loss of elasticity of the alveoli, making the efficient exchange of oxygen more and more difficult. Chronic bronchitis and emphysema are sometimes grouped together under the name chronic obstructive pulmonary disease (COPD).

Much less common than asthma or COPD, cystic fibrosis (CF) is a genetic disease that affects the cells that produce mucus, both in the GI and respiratory tracts. CF is characterized by the production of thick and sticky mucus. CF patients cannot clear mucus from the lungs and it causes frequent infections and damage to the respiratory tract, as well as malabsorption and other problems in the GI tract. A generation ago children with CF did not often live past their twenties. Newer, more consistent treatments have extended the life expectancy of CF patients into the thirties and forties. The genetic error that causes CF has been identified, and ongoing genetic research raises hopes for a cure in the not too distant future.

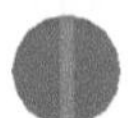

# The Urinary System

The urinary system is made up of two kidneys, two ureters connecting the kidneys to the bladder, the urinary bladder, and the urethra. The kidneys do the main work of the urinary system: elimination of waste products and fluid and electrolyte regulation.

## Anatomy of the Urinary System

The kidneys are at the back of the upper abdomen, just under the last rib. The left kidney is slightly higher than the right because of the presence of the liver on the right side (refer to **Fig. 19.6**). The kidneys are approximately 4 inches long, 2 inches wide, and about 1 inch thick. They are encapsulated in a fibrous sac and a layer of adipose tissue intended to protect them. The kidneys lie outside of the peritoneum, the thin, shiny membranous sac that surrounds most of the other organs of the abdominal cavity, in the retroperitoneal space. They are supplied with arterial blood from the renal artery, a short arterial branch of the abdominal aorta. This artery divides into smaller and smaller arteries, and then arterioles that present blood to the filtration units of the kidneys, called the nephrons. After filtration, the blood is collected in progressively larger vessels that merge to become the renal veins, which return blood to the inferior vena cava.

The kidney is divided into two anatomical areas, the renal cortex and the renal medulla (**Fig. 19.7**). The renal cortex contains the nephrons, the units responsible for filtration of blood and formation of the urine. The renal medulla is made up of ducts that collect the urine. A nephron is a microscopic coiled tube with a cluster of capillaries at one end, known as a glomerulus (or sometimes Bowman's capsule). The tiny tube that leaves each glomerulus is called the proximal convoluted tubule. This tubule makes a hairpin turn in what is

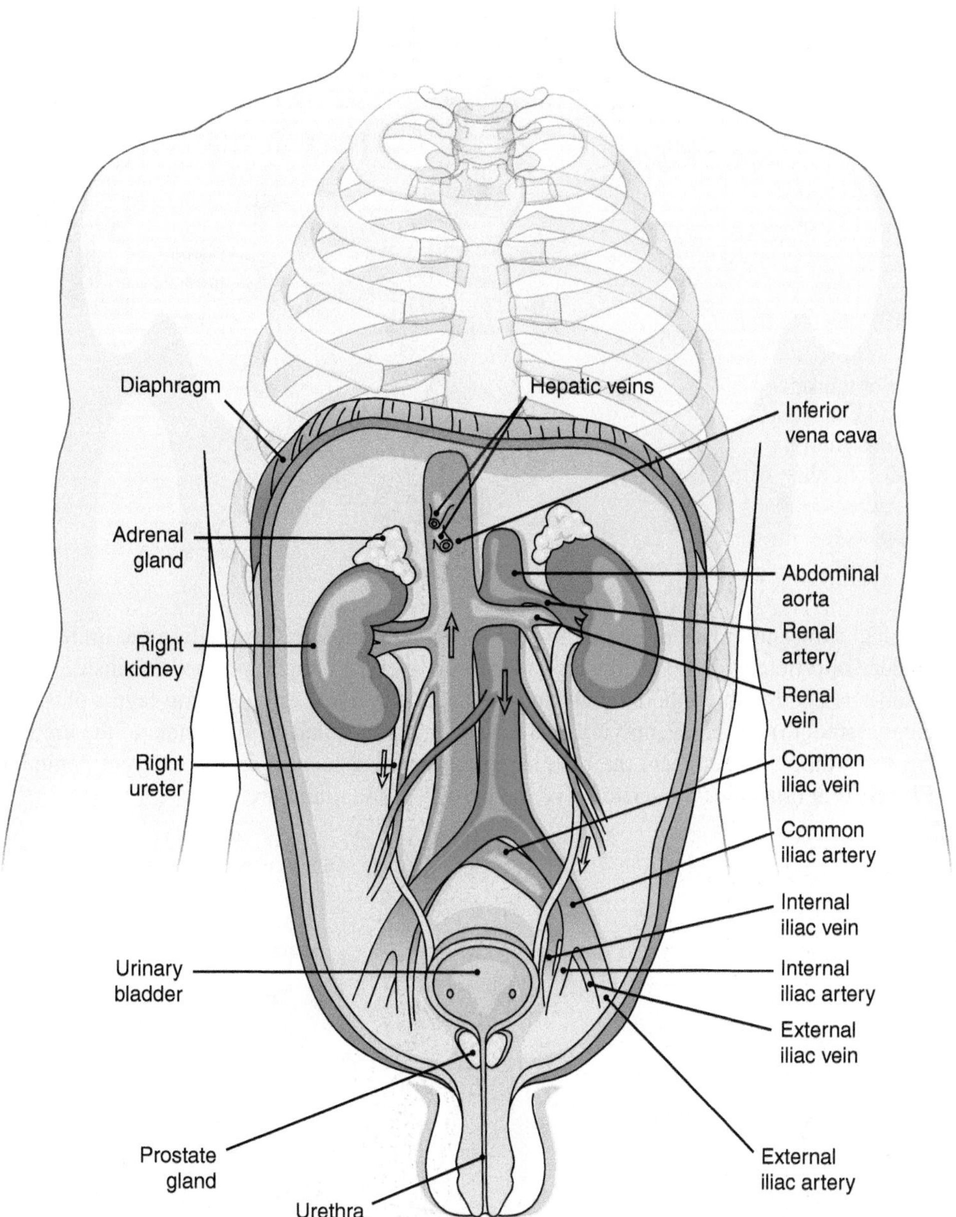


**Figure 19.6** The male urinary system, including major vessels. (Reprinted with permission from Cohen BJ. *Memmler's The Human Body in Health and Disease*, 10th edition. Baltimore: Lippincott Williams & Wilkins, 2005.)

loop of Henle The U-shaped portion of the renal tubule in vertebrates; begins at the proximal convoluted tubule and ends in the distal convoluted tubule.

distal convoluted tubule Winding portion of the nephron between the loop of Henle and the nonsecretory part of the nephron; important in the concentration of urine.

known as the Loop of Henle, which then travels back towards the glomerulus as the distal convoluted tubule (see **Fig. 19.8**). The kidneys contain more than a million nephrons each. If they all could be uncoiled and laid end to end they would extend about 75 miles. This system of microscopic tubules empties into a system of collecting ducts that join together and eventually empties into the ureters.

The ureters are long (10 + inches, depending on body size) thin tubes that extend from the kidneys down to the urinary bladder. They enter the bladder at an angle and run through the smooth muscle of the bladder, such that when the bladder is full, pressure on the ureters prevents backflow of urine. Urine moves down the ureters through a combination of grav-

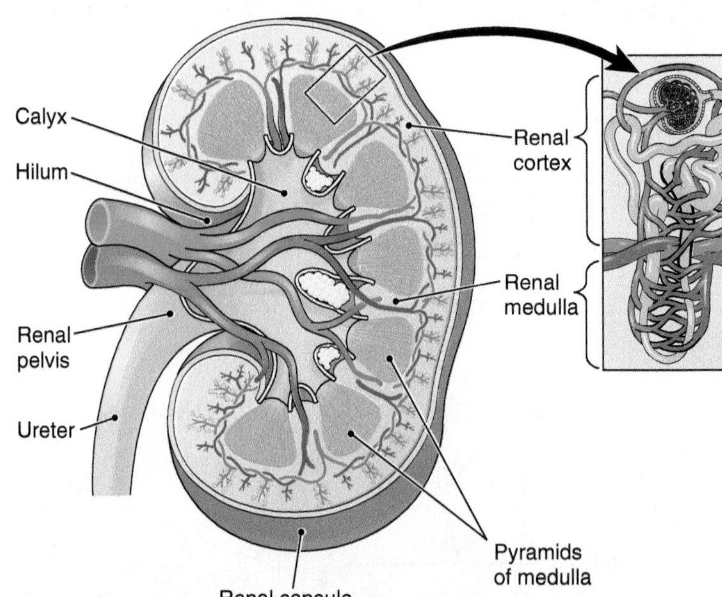


**Figure 19.7** A cross-sectional view of the kidney showing the cortex, medulla, calyx, and blood supply. The inset shows the anatomical design of the nephron. (Adapted with permission from Cohen BJ. *Memmler's The Human Body in Health and Disease*, 10th edition. Baltimore: Lippincott Williams & Wilkins, 2005.)

itational flow and muscular contraction of the smooth muscle surrounding the ureter. The bladder is a stretchy, balloon-like reservoir for temporarily holding urine. The inside of the bladder is lined with epithelial cells and the outside is made up of several layers of involuntary (smooth) muscle. Emptying of the bladder is controlled by sphincters of the urethra, the short tube that connects the bladder to the opening located in the external genitalia. **Figure 19.9** illustrates the anatomy of the ureters, bladder and urethra.

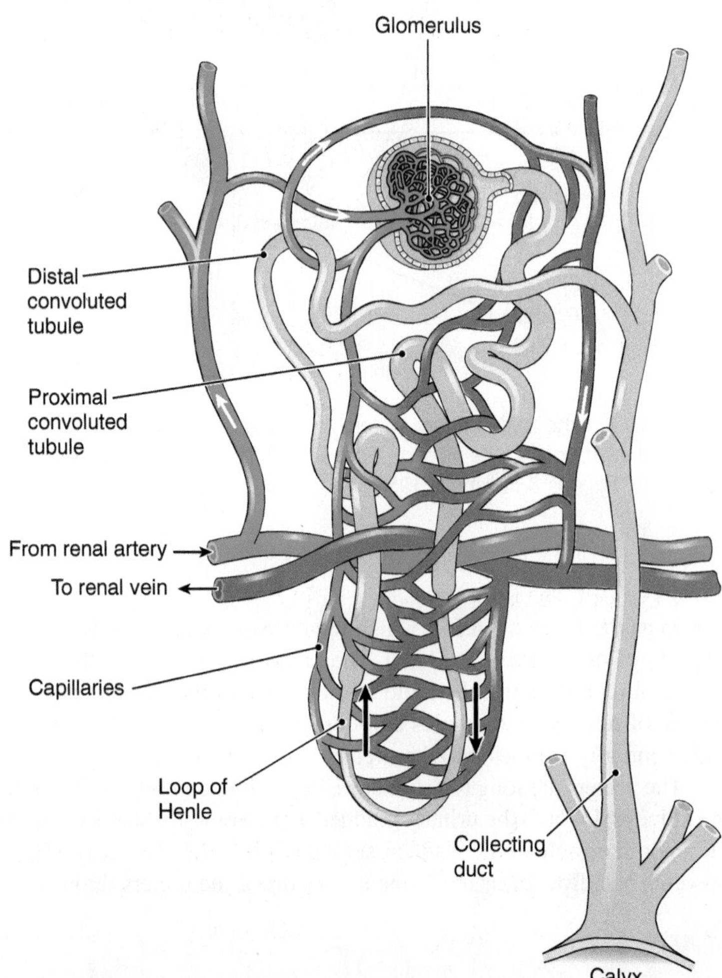


**Figure 19.8** The nephron. (Adapted with permission from Cohen BJ. *Memmler's The Human Body in Health and Disease*, 10th edition. Baltimore: Lippincott Williams & Wilkins, 2005.)

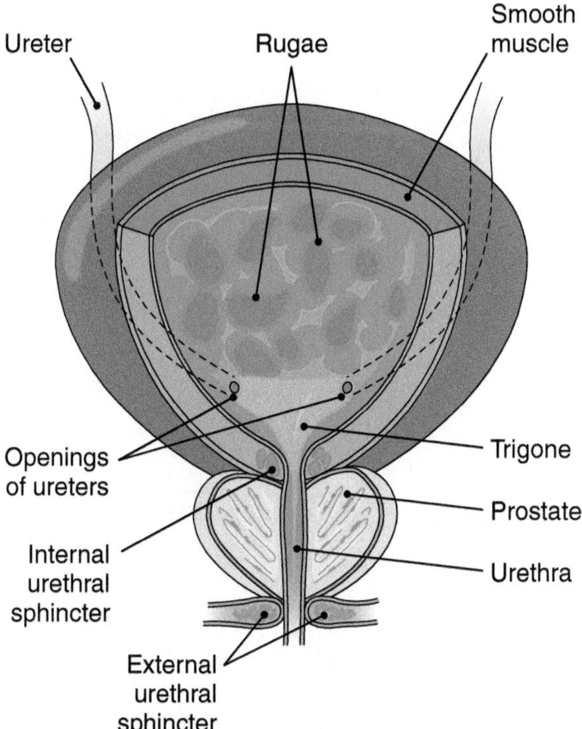


**Figure 19.9** The anatomical structure of the ureters, bladder, and urethra. (Reprinted with permission from Cohen BJ. *Memmler's The Human Body in Health and Disease*, 10th edition. Baltimore: Lippincott Williams & Wilkins, 2005.)

## Urinary System Physiology

The kidneys regulate water, electrolyte, and acid-base balance through mechanisms involved with the production of urine. They eliminate many of the byproducts associated with both cellular metabolism and metabolized drugs as well as other toxins processed in the liver. One of these byproducts is a nitrogenous compound called urea. The liver converts ammonia, a toxic byproduct of the synthesis of proteins, to urea, a much less toxic compound that is then removed by the kidneys. Levels of urea in the blood are one indication of how well the kidneys are functioning.

### Formation of Urine

The formation of urine is a highly complex process of filtration, diffusion, active transport and osmosis. Whereas diffusion involves movement of a substance (solute) across a semi-permeable membrane to balance its concentration, osmosis involves the movement of water or other solvent across a concentration gradient. Osmosis occurs because the membrane is permeable to water or another solvent, but the solute cannot pass. The interweaving of the capillaries and tubules of the nephron make possible the back and forth exchanges of fluid and permeable solutes between the bloodstream and the collecting system that is necessary for the formation of the urine. The following description of urine production is graphically represented in **Figure 19.10**.

Blood enters each glomerulus through an incoming (afferent) arteriole and leaves through a smaller outgoing (efferent) arteriole. Because the diameter of the outgoing vessel is smaller, blood pressure increases against the walls of the capillaries of the glomerulus. The increased pressure due to the smaller outgoing vessel forces fluid, salts, and small molecules, including sodium, potassium, amino acids, and glucose, through the walls of the capillaries in a process referred to as filtration. Since it occurs in the glomerulus, this process is called glomerular filtration. In the healthy adult with normal renal function, the kidneys filter about 125 ml of blood every minute, or 180 L every day. The normal blood volume in an adult is about 5 L. This means, on average, our entire blood volume is being filtered more than 30 times a day!

glomerular filtration
Filtration of the blood through the tuft of capillaries at the origin of the nephron in the kidney.

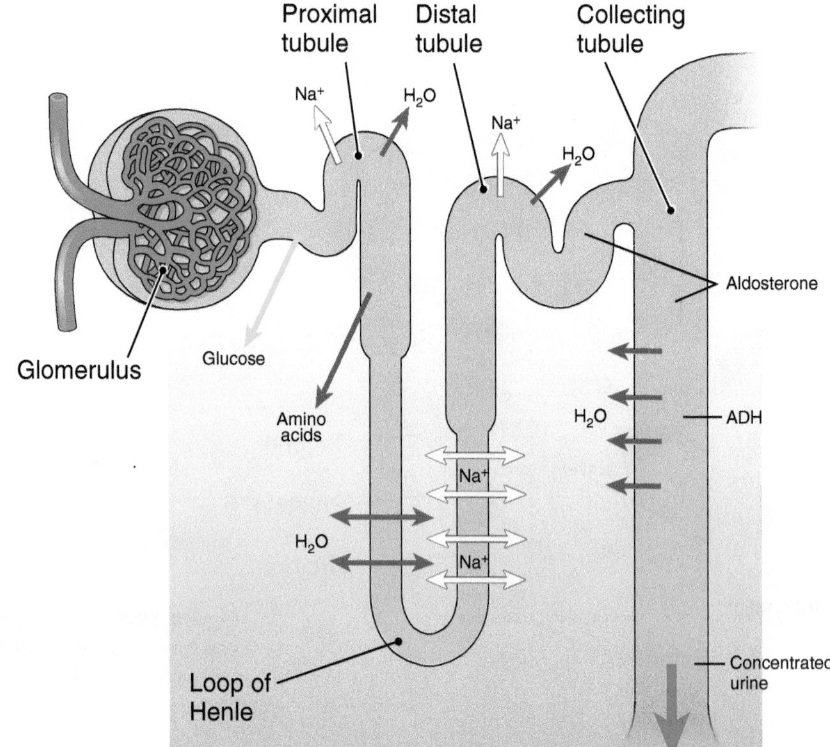


**Figure 19.10** The concentration of urine is accomplished through diffusion and osmosis that is possible because of changes in permeability in the tubules and the actions of hormones. (Adapted with permission from Cohen BJ. *Memmler's The Human Body in Health and Disease*, 10th edition. Baltimore: Lippincott Williams & Wilkins, 2005.)

The solution forced through the capillary walls is called the filtrate, and is a dilute solution similar to interstitial fluid. Although the kidneys form about 160 L of filtrate each day, we only produce about 1.5 L of urine daily. This is because most of the fluid in the filtrate is reabsorbed back into the bloodstream. Because the fluid in the tubules is so dilute, water passes from the proximal tubule back into the adjacent capillaries by osmosis. In the Loop of Henle, the walls of the tubules become less permeable to water. Here electrolytes are actively transported out of the tubule, causing the fluid inside to be more dilute, and the fluid surrounding the tubules to be more concentrated with sodium and other electrolytes. The actions of aldosterone and antidiuretic hormone modulate the reabsorption of water and sodium. The distal tubule and collecting duct are permeable to water, and because the outside fluid is "salty" as a result of active transport, water flows out of these sections of the tubule by osmosis. It is here that the final concentration of the urine occurs.

Besides the filtration and reabsorption processes, the tubule is the site of active transport of several compounds. Sodium is actively transported out of the tubule, into interstitial fluids, which helps to concentrate the urine because water follows it out. Glucose, amino acids, phosphate and other salts are also actively transported out early in the urine formation process. Potassium and hydrogen is excreted into the fluid in the distal tubules and collecting tubules. It is the excretion of hydrogen ions into the urine that allows the kidneys to adjust blood pH.

## Urination

micturition Urination.

incontinent Unable to voluntarily retain urine or feces.

The emptying of the bladder is called urination or micturition. Urination is under both voluntary and involuntary control. This is important because removal of waste must occur, whether a person is able to consciously control urination or not. An individual who cannot control urination is referred to as being incontinent. When the bladder is full, stretch receptors send nerve impulses to an area in the spinal cord responsible for bladder control. Reflex motor impulses return to the bladder causing the smooth muscle to contract. If both the internal and external urethral sphincter muscles relax, urination ensues. Muscular control of the external sphincter, which can develop late in some children, allows for voluntary control of urination.

### Homeostatic Functions of the Kidney

The kidneys, along with the closely aligned adrenal glands, are the organs that regulate fluid and electrolyte homeostasis and to a significant degree, the pH of the blood. The pH, or acidity of the blood, is normally maintained between 7.3 and 7.4. If the blood pH becomes too acidic (lower pH), the kidneys excrete more hydrogen ions into the urine, and fewer hydrogen ions are excreted if the blood becomes too alkaline (higher pH). Similarly, if presented with excessive serum concentrations of potassium, calcium, or other components of blood, the kidneys step up removal of those compounds. Reclamation of these same components is increased when levels are low.

The kidneys regulate blood pressure through the secretion of renin. Aldosterone, produced by the adrenal glands, and antidiuretic hormone (ADH), produced by the pituitary gland, work in the nephron to maintain adequate blood volume. Although not often thought of in this way, the kidneys are endocrine glands, responsible for the production of erythropoietin and calcitriol. Erythropoietin stimulates the bone marrow to produce red blood cells. Calcitriol is the active form of vitamin D and is important in the maintenance and repair of bone tissue.

## Diseases Related to the Urinary System

There are a variety of diseases responsible for altering the function of the urinary system both directly and indirectly, but the most serious of these affect the function of the kidneys themselves. The two most common causes of kidney failure are diabetes and hypertension. High blood pressure can damage the tiny capillaries in the glomerulus so that normal filtration cannot occur. Diabetes is an impairment of glucose utilization. When glucose is not removed from the bloodstream, excess sugar is presented to the nephron for removal from the filtrate. If the concentration of sugar exceeds the ability of the active transport system to remove it, the sugar damages the nephron. This damage is called diabetic nephropathy and can eventually cause complete renal failure.

Dehydration, advancing age, and the long-term use of certain medications can also impair kidney function. Edema, electrolyte imbalance, and anemia are common results of renal failure. Acute renal failure can usually be treated with fluids and medications, but may require dialysis, or the removal of waste products with an artificial filtration machine. Chronic renal failure is treated with dialysis and when possible, kidney transplantation.

Pyelonephritis is caused by an infection of the kidney. When infections are not adequately treated they can become chronic inflammatory conditions that lead to a deterioration in kidney function over time. Some urinary system diseases are congenital, or inherited, abnormalities. These would include anatomical abnormalities and polycystic kidney disease.

congenital Existing at birth; usually referring to conditions acquired during development of the fetus, regardless of their cause, i.e., congenital herpes.

Autoimmune and other diseases can cause inflammation of the glomerulus, referred to as glomerulonephritis. One of the most frightening causes of glomerulonephritis is systemic lupus erythematosus, commonly referred to simply as lupus. As the name implies, lupus is a systemic disease and can affect many organ systems in the body. There is no cure for lupus and when the inflammatory processes are not well controlled it can cause permanent damage to kidneys, lungs, and central nervous system.

glomerulonephritis Inflammation of the capillary tuft in the nephron of the kidneys.

Kidney stones, or calculi, are formed when substances like calcium and uric acid occur in higher concentrations than normal in the filtrate. This may be coupled with lower than normal water concentrations. As a result, solutes precipitate out and form crystals, which can grow into stones the size of a grain of sand to stones large enough to fill the renal pelvis (**Fig. 19.11**). The movement of a kidney stone down into the ureter causes excruciating pain, called renal colic, and is often the first sign that stone formation has occurred. A stone in a ureter can cause obstruction, and if it does not pass naturally, has to be removed. Calculi that do not pass naturally are either treated with lithotripsy or are surgically re-

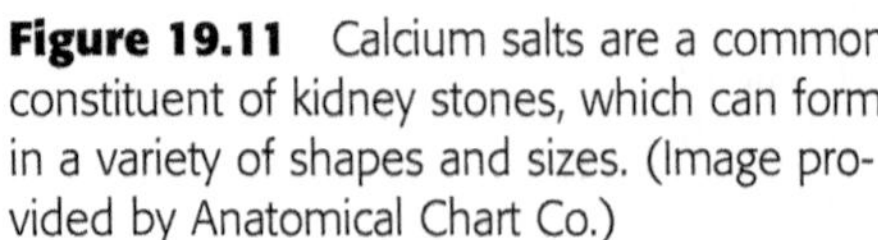

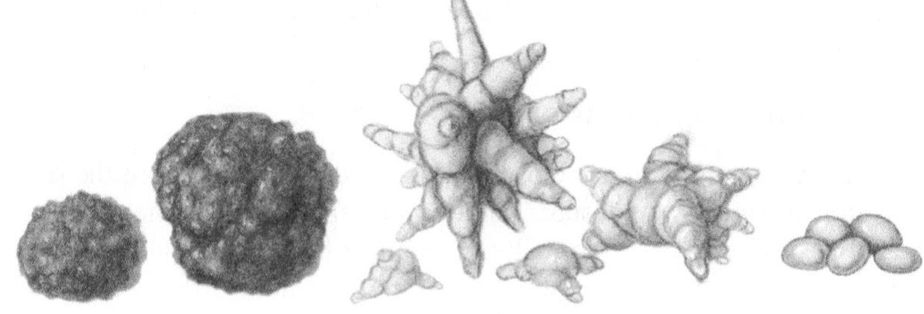

**Figure 19.11** Calcium salts are a common constituent of kidney stones, which can form in a variety of shapes and sizes. (Image provided by Anatomical Chart Co.)

lithotripsy A procedure that uses sound waves to break up kidney stones into pieces small enough to be easily eliminated.

cystitis Inflammation of the urinary bladder (often caused by infection).

moved. Lithotripsy is a procedure that uses high-energy waves, precisely targeted at the stone, to break it up into tiny pieces that can pass without surgery.

The most common disease of the bladder is infection, known as cystitis, or bladder infections. Bladder infections are ten times more common in women, where the urethra is very short and in close proximity to the anus. Urinary catheterization, diabetes, and incomplete emptying of the bladder because of physical anomaly or partial obstruction increase the risk of cystitis.

Bladder obstruction can be caused by benign prostatic hypertrophy in men. Benign prostatic hypertrophy is an enlargement of the prostate that is not due to a malignancy and is common in aging men. An enlarged prostate puts pressure on the urethra, which causes partial obstruction and inability to empty the bladder completely. When the bladder does not empty completely this can lead to infection, and if untreated, kidney damage from the backflow of urine. Men with this condition commonly complain of frequent urge to urinate with minimal urine flow.

Urinary incontinence is a common condition in older women, and is sometimes associated with menopause. Stress incontinence occurs as a result of a weakened bladder sphincter muscle, and involves loss of a small amount of urine when laughing, sneezing, or lifting puts pressure on the bladder. Urge incontinence results from the inability to control bladder contractions once the urge to urinate is perceived.

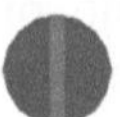

## The Gastrointestinal System

The gastrointestinal, or digestive, system is responsible for the intake and digestion of the raw materials needed for life, and elimination of the remaining waste. Every body system needs a constant supply of nutrients and water for normal growth, development, and maintenance, and this is supplied through the GI tract. The gastrointestinal system is actually several structures and organs, which contribute, in serial fashion, to the processes of digestion (**Fig. 19.12**).

Possibly the best way to envision the anatomy and understand the physiologic processes of the GI tract is to follow a bite of food from your plate, to your mouth, through digestion and elimination. Imagine your favorite meal, sitting irresistibly in front of you. Seeing it is enough to make your mouth water. The fragrance of a juicy, perfectly barbecued steak or perhaps fresh spaghetti and sauce with lots of garlic wafts up to your nose and starts the flow of saliva and digestive juices. In fact, you may notice that just reading about a meal is enough to make saliva flow. Your food begins its digestive journey as soon as the first bite reaches your mouth.

### The Oral Cavity, Esophagus, and Stomach

mastication Chewing with the teeth.

The mouth, or oral cavity, is the first structure in the gastrointestinal system. The oral cavity is designed for the intake of food and liquids. The teeth provide for the initial breakdown of food through chewing, or mastication. The tongue is a muscular structure that is

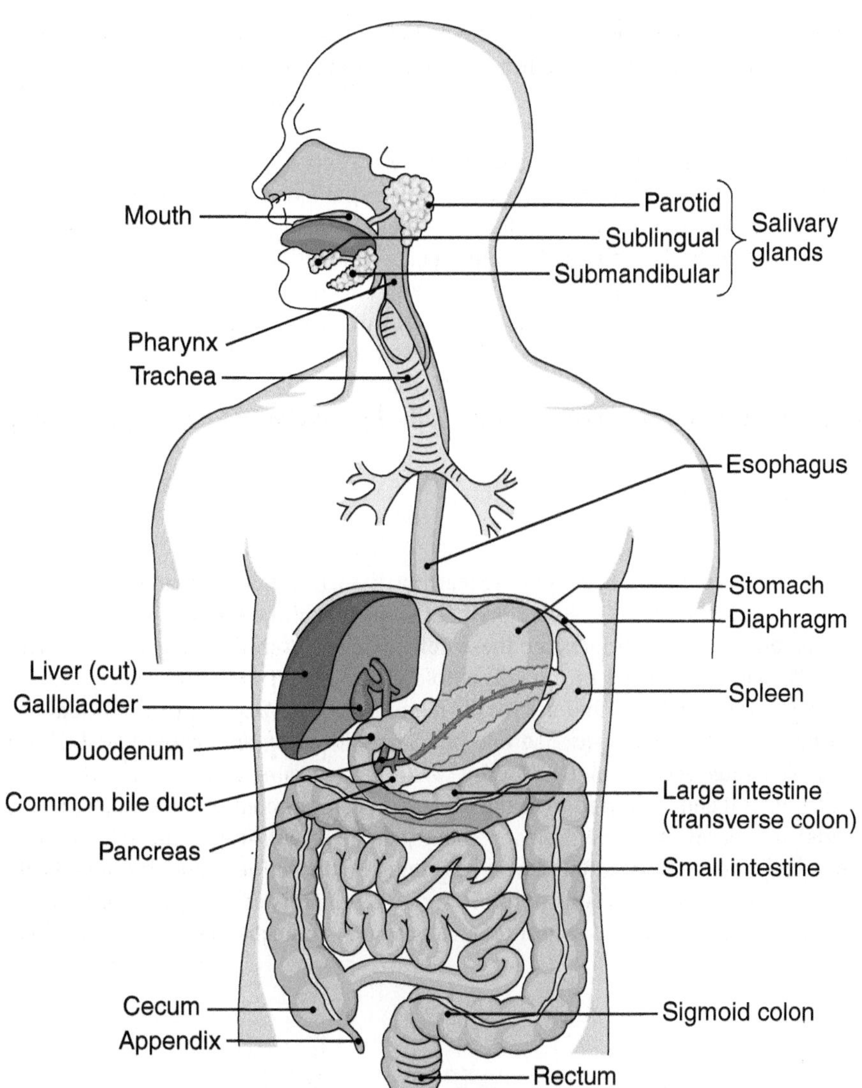


**Figure 19.12** The gastrointestinal system. (Reprinted with permission from Cohen BJ. *Memmler's The Human Body in Health and Disease*, 10th edition. Baltimore: Lippincott Williams & Wilkins, 2005.)

covered with tiny sensory organs called taste buds. In response to the stimulation of the taste and smell of food, salivary glands located under the structure of the tongue and on the sides of the mouth secrete saliva. That first bite of your favorite meal is in contact with amylase, an enzyme in the saliva that digests carbohydrates before you even swallow. Once the bite is appropriately chewed and mixed with saliva, your tongue helps push it to the pharynx, where it is swallowed.

During the involuntary action of swallowing, the soft palate and epiglottis protect the integrity of the trachea from contamination with food, and the food and liquid moves into the esophagus. The esophagus is a tube-like structure surrounded by smooth muscle, and lined with mucus producing epithelial cells. Food moves down the approximately 10-inch length of the esophagus through a muscle action called peristalsis. Peristalsis is a series of wave-like muscle contractions that is responsible for the GI motility that propels food from the esophagus onward through the length of the alimentary canal. Mucus production helps lubricate its passage until it reaches the end of the esophagus and the lower esophageal sphincter, a muscular ring that relaxes to admit food into the stomach.

peristalsis Waves of involuntary contraction passing along the walls of the GI tract responsible for the movement of food to the intestines and waste through the intestines.

alimentary Concerned with, or relating to, nourishment or the organs of digestion.

Food collects and is temporarily held for further digestion in the stomach. The stomach is a J-shaped organ on the left side of the upper portion of the abdominal cavity. It is made up of three layers of smooth muscle and is lined with special secretory cells. Most of these secretory cells produce mucus that protects the lining of the stomach, while others produce digestive acid and enzymes. When empty, the stomach collapses into folds, but it can stretch to hold as much as two liters (approximately the volume of a half-gallon container of milk or ice cream).

gastrin A peptide hormone that is secreted by the gastric mucosa; contributes to the secretion of gastric acid.

pepsin An enzyme that in an acid medium digests most proteins.

The presence of food causes the stomach to secrete gastrin, a hormone that along with histamine and acetylcholine causes the parietal cells in the stomach lining to secrete hydrochloric acid. Pepsin, an enzyme that digests protein, is also produced in the stomach. While in the stomach, food is churned through peristaltic action and mixes with the hydrochloric acid and pepsin for further digestion. The sphincter between the stomach and the duodenum relaxes about every twenty minutes. After twenty minutes in the stomach, your dinner, which is now an acidic mass of partly digested food, begins to move through the pyloric sphincter. About every fifteen to twenty minutes (called the stomach emptying time), the stomach releases another bolus of partially digested food to the small intestine.

mucosa A mucous membrane.

## The Small Intestine, the Liver, the Gall Bladder, and the Pancreas

duodenum The first and shortest part of the small intestine that extends from the pylorus to the jejunum.

jejunum The section of the small intestine that connects the duodenum to the ileum.

ileum The last segment of the small intestine.

The small intestine is so named because of its narrow diameter. It is about an inch in diameter and is about ten feet long in the living body. Like the rest of the GI tract, it is lined with epithelial cells, but in the small intestine these cells extend out in tiny fingers called villi (**Fig. 19.13**). The cellular surface of the villi is folded into even smaller protrusions called microvilli. The presence of villi and microvilli increases the surface area for nutrient absorption in the small intestine more than one hundred fold, to an area about the size of a tennis court. The majority of food and drug absorption occurs in the small intestine. Beneath the epithelial cells, referred to as the mucosa, a layer of connective tissue contains blood vessels and nerves. The capillaries in this tissue layer will carry nutrients away as they are absorbed, and the nerves found here help regulate the action of the smooth muscle layer below. The smooth muscle is responsible for ongoing peristalsis. The sections of the small intestine are named the duodenum (connects to the stomach), the jejunum, and the ileum.

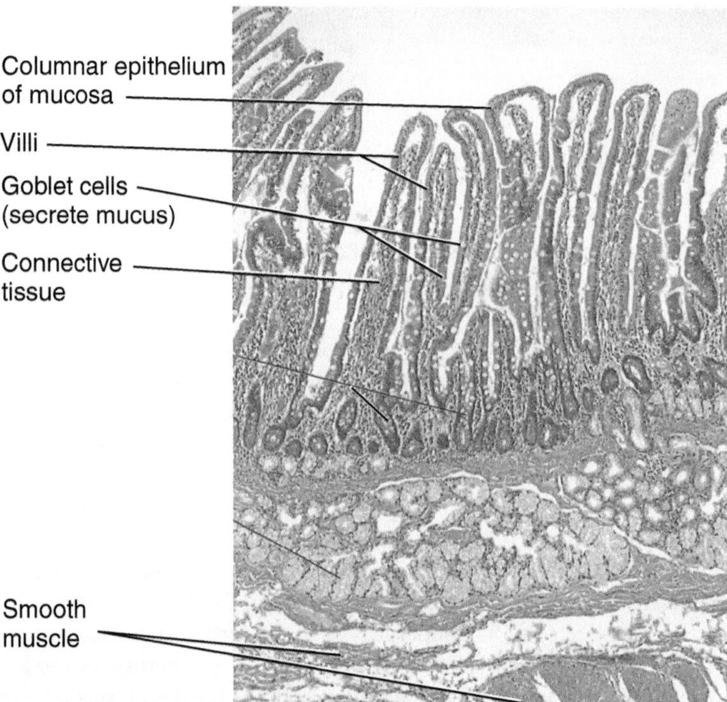


**Figure 19.13** An electron micrograph of the small intestine in cross section. (Micrograph reprinted with permission from Cormack, DH. *Essential Histology*, 2nd edition. Philadelphia: Lippincott Williams & Wilkins, 2001.)

Once in the small intestine, your dinner is subjected to further digestion by enzymes secreted by specialized secretory cells in the intestinal mucosa. Both the liver and the pancreas contribute to the processes of digestion at this point. The liver is a highly vascular (rich in blood supply) organ tucked underneath the rib cage on the right side of the abdomen. The functions of this remarkable organ are diverse and include synthesis of proteins, cholesterol, bile and other compounds, storage of glucose, iron, and some vitamins, and removal and detoxification of many byproducts of metabolism and drugs. Bile produced by the liver moves down to the gallbladder where it is stored until needed for digestion. When the gall bladder contracts it sends bile down the common bile duct into the small intestine. Bile emulsifies (reduces the size of the fat particles and distributes them evenly through the food mass) the fats in your dinner so they can be more easily absorbed.

vascular Relating to blood vessels or indicating an area is well suppled with vessels.

emulsify To disperse in an emulsion or convert immiscible liquids into an emulsion.

The pancreas is a gland that is crucial to the digestion of food and the utilization of carbohydrates. Not only does it produce enzymes that digest fats, proteins, and carbohydrates, it also secretes insulin, the hormone responsible for normal utilization of carbohydrates. The enzymes produced here move out of the pancreas through the pancreatic duct. This duct connects to the common bile duct very near where it joins the small intestine (see **Fig. 19.14**). With the action of these enzymes, your dinner is now broken down into particles that are absorbable. Fats are converted into fatty acids and glycerol, proteins into amino acids, and carbohydrates are converted to starch and then sugars. Most of these nutrients, as well as vitamins, minerals and most drugs will be absorbed through the villi in the small intestine, where they will pass into the capillaries and be carried into the enterohepatic circulation. The nonabsorbable remains of your dinner now pass into the large intestine.

insulin Peptide hormone secreted by the pancreas that regulates blood sugar levels.

cecum Pouch-like section of the intestine (off of which the appendix extends) that connects the ileum to the colon.

colon Also known as the large intestine, the colon extends from the cecum to the rectum.

## The Large Intestine

The large intestine is larger in diameter (2.5 inches), but shorter in length at about 5 feet, than the small intestine. Although the large intestine absorbs water and to a small degree, some remaining nutrients and drugs, no further digestion occurs here. The bacteria of the large intestine produce vitamin K, which is absorbed here. The large intestine is named by anatomic subdivisions. The cecum connects the small intestine to the colon, and the colon, further divided into ascending, transverse, and descending regions, connects to the rectum. The large intestine continues the movement of the residual portion of your dinner through peristaltic action. Once most of the nutrients and water have been absorbed, the remaining solid waste (feces) arrives at the rectum, where the pressure it exerts stimulates elimination through the anal sphincter.

rectum The last portion of the colon, which connects the colon to the anus.

anal sphincter The musculature surrounding and able to close the anus.

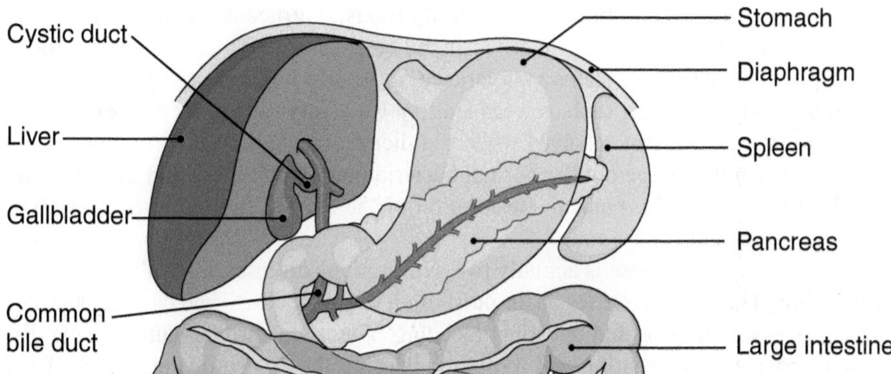


**Figure 19.14** The pancreas, liver, and gall bladder, the accessory organs of digestion. (Adapted with permission from Cohen BJ. *Memmler's The Human Body in Health and Disease*, 10th edition. Baltimore: Lippincott Williams & Wilkins, 2005.)

## Diseases of the Gastrointestinal System

Disorders of the digestive system can occur anywhere along the alimentary canal from the oral cavity, where poor dental care or oral lesions can affect chewing and swallowing, to the rectum and anus, where constipation and hemorrhoids are common complaints. Diseases can be caused by a number of factors, including chemical, mechanical, and inflammatory problems.

### Indigestion and Ulcers

reflux A backward flow.

The most common gastrointestinal complaints for which people request drug therapy begin in the esophagus and stomach, where an excess production of gastric acid can cause heartburn and indigestion. Heartburn, named because of a burning sensation in the upper abdomen, is usually caused by reflux (backflow) of stomach acid into the esophagus. Chronic reflux is called gastroesophageal reflux disease, or GERD. Some medications, excessive coffee and alcohol consumption, certain foods, and more serious conditions such as GI ulceration can cause similar symptoms of irritation and the sensation of discomfort or pain in the stomach. Most people will refer to this as indigestion, but it is important to realize that this sensation can also be a sign of a serious illness.

peptic ulcer An ulcer in the mucous membrane of the wall of the stomach or duodenum.

The condition of ulceration of the mucosa in either the stomach or duodenum is referred to as peptic ulcers. Peptic ulcers can be associated with a number of causative factors, including stress, smoking, or drug therapy with aspirin or other drugs. Most people with recurrent ulcers are found to have *Helicobacter pylori* infections of the GI tract. *H. pylori* infection causes an inflammatory response in the GI mucosa that is responsible for eventual ulceration.

### Diseases of the Intestines

Although, strictly speaking, diarrhea, gas, and constipation are not diseases, they are the most common intestinal complaints. Diarrhea is a symptom characterized by frequent, watery bowel movements, and constipation is characterized by infrequent, hard bowel movements. Both complaints can be related to very serious disorders, but are more often associated with short-term conditions. Gas is produced by bacteria in the intestine and is normally a result of consumption of particular food types. Typically, this complaint is short lived and easily treated.

Diarrhea can be a symptom of infection, malabsorption syndromes, medication use, or diet. Food poisoning, serious infections such as cholera or typhoid, or simple viral infections can all begin with initial symptoms of diarrhea. However, where most viral infections resolve in 24 hours, the diarrhea caused by cholera can cause such severe dehydration and electrolyte imbalances that some patients with this illness may require hospitalization within 24 hours.

When the intestinal tract is shortened through surgery, or patients have a genetic predisposition or other inability to break down certain foods, diarrhea can result. Causes can include celiac disease, which is an inherited inability to absorb gluten-containing foods (wheat, barley or other grains), lactose intolerance, or gastric bypass surgery. People who overeat foods with lots of fiber, such as fresh fruit, or eat a very fatty meal may experience a similar form of diarrhea that resolves when the diet returns to normal. Antibiotics can cause diarrhea when they wipe out the normal bacteria that inhabit the colon and allow an overgrowth of an unwanted organism. Restoration of the normal flora is often enough to restore bowel movements to normal.

Inflammatory bowel disease is actually two autoimmune diseases, Crohn's disease and ulcerative colitis. These two diseases occur most often in young adults and cause symptoms of pain, diarrhea, weight loss, and intestinal bleeding. These are chronic, autoimmune diseases associated with exacerbation and remissions during the course of the illness. If not well controlled, they can lead to life-threatening complications.

Constipation is often a result of inadequate fluid intake, sedentary lifestyle, or inadequate intake of dietary fiber. Severe constipation can be a symptom of intestinal obstruction, either from a tumor or sometimes from a foreign body. Other causes of constipation can include medication use, pregnancy, and advancing age.

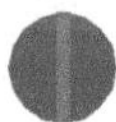

# The Musculoskeletal System

The skeleton and attached muscles provide the framework and support for the body. Bones protect the internal organs, work with the muscles to allow locomotion (movement) and strength, manufacture blood cells, and act as a storage depot for calcium and phosphorus. Muscles provide movement, body alignment and balance, and warmth through metabolism of glucose.

locomotion Movement or the ability to move from place to place.

## The Bones

The human skeleton is made up of 206 bones that are of four main types; long bones, short bones, irregular bones, and flat bones (see **Fig. 19.15**). The bones of the arms and legs are long bones, and they serve as levers to allow for the most efficient use of the attached muscles. Short bones are found in the wrists and ankles, and as the name implies, are short.

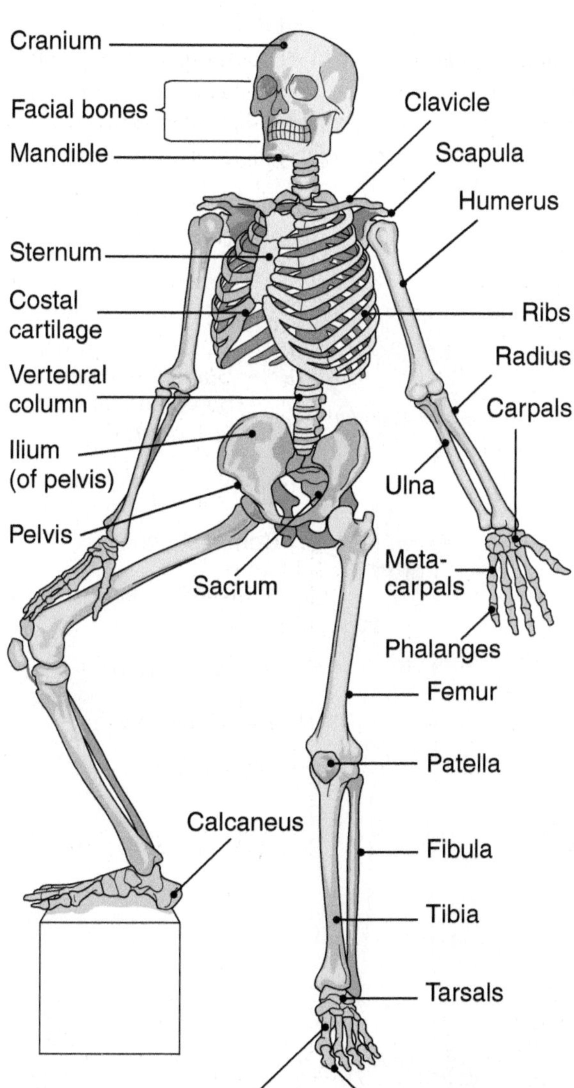


**Figure 19.15** The human skeleton, with the axial skeleton shown in yellow and appendicular skeleton in blue. (Reprinted with permission from Cohen BJ. *Memmler's The Human Body in Health and Disease*, 10th edition. Baltimore: Lippincott Williams & Wilkins, 2005.)

Small bones are essential to make up these complex joint structures, which allow for movement in many directions. Flat bones have a large surface for the attachment of large muscles and the protection of internal organs. These include the bones of the shoulder and pelvic girdles, the ribs, and the skull. The irregular bones have unique shapes appropriate to their function. Vertebral bones, which surround and protect the spinal chord, are an example of this type of bone. The skeleton is described in terms of two divisions. The axial skeleton is the central framework, and includes the skull, vertebrae, ribs, the sternum, and sacrum. The appendicular skeleton is made up of the bones of the extremities.

axial skeleton The articulated bones of the head and trunk.

appendicular skeleton The bones that make up the shoulder girdle, the pelvis, and the upper and lower extremities.

Bone is an organ and is made up of living tissue, with its own blood supply and enervation. There are two types of bone tissue. Cancellous bone, spongy and vascular, is found at the end of the long bones and at the center of other bones. Cancellous bone forms in a matrix that looks something like a honeycomb. Compact bone is denser and provides the hard outer portions of all bones. It forms in rings around a central canal that contains the blood supply. The spongy ends of the long bones are called the epiphysis and are the site of bone lengthening during growth and development (**Fig. 19.16**). The outside of the bone is covered with a fibrous layer of connective tissue called the periosteum.

cancellous bone Bone that has a lattice-like structure.

## Physiological Processes

All bones undergo constant repair and resorption, or breakdown. Together these processes are called remodeling. Cells called osteoclasts remove bone and osteoblasts lay down new bone. Remodeling is regulated by vitamin D, calcitonin, which is a hormone produced by the thyroid gland in humans, and parathyroid hormone, from the parathyroid gland. Calcitonin inhibits bone removal by osteoclasts and promotes bone formation by osteoblasts and uptake of calcium from the circulation. Parathyroid hormone stimulates bone

compact bone Noncancellous; made up of layers of bone formed around a central canal.

epiphysis The part of the long bone where growth occurs; growth plate.

periosteum Tough, fibrous connective tissue that surrounds bones except the joint surfaces.

resorption The loss of substance, for example bone mass, through normal or disease processes.

osteoclast A cell associated with bone resorption or breakdown.

osteoblast Cell that gives rise to bone.

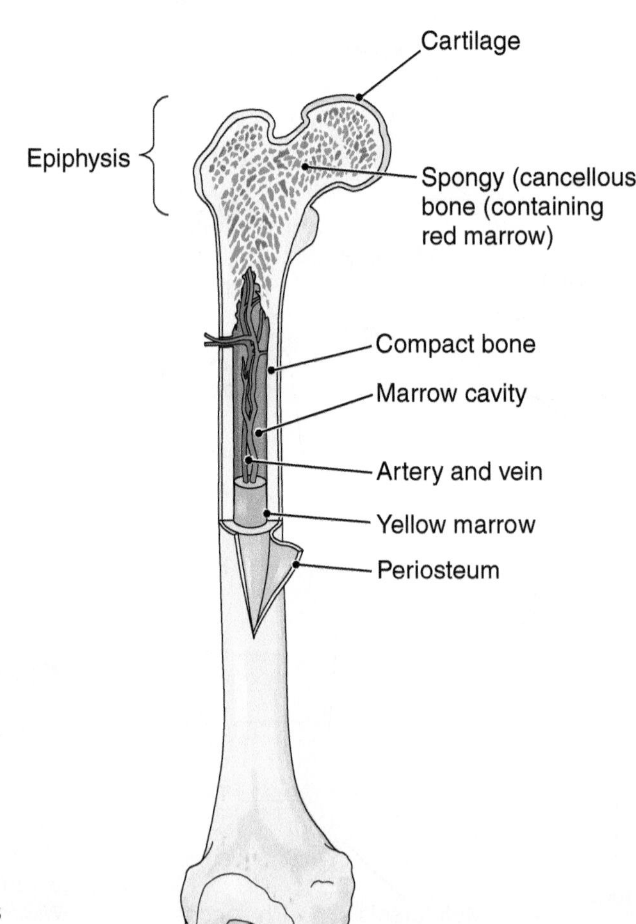


**Figure 19.16** The anatomical structure of a long bone. (Adapted with permission from Cohen BJ. *Memmler's The Human Body in Health and Disease*, 10th edition. Baltimore: Lippincott Williams & Wilkins, 2005.)

resorption and calcium and phosphorus release into the circulation. Vitamin D stimulates calcium absorption from the intestinal tract, helps to maintain a normal relationship between calcium and phosphorus levels, and promotes bone mineralization.

Bone marrow is the tissue that forms the center of large bones. Bone marrow is categorized as two types, red and yellow marrow. Yellow marrow contains blood vessels and nerves, but is composed mostly of fat. During times of great demand, yellow marrow can be converted to red marrow. Red marrow is the site of formation of blood cells. Blood cells are formed from hematopoietic stem cells. These stem cells differentiate and give rise to all three classes of blood cells: leukocytes, erythrocytes, and thrombocytes. In adults, the sites that produce the most blood cells include the pelvic and shoulder girdles, the ribs, and the vertebrae. The bone marrow produces billions of red blood cells every day. Old red blood cells are removed at the same rate by the spleen.

hematopoietic stem cell Cell that gives rise to distinct daughter cells, including a cell that will reproduce and differentiate into mature blood cells.

## The Joints

Joints are areas where two or more bones articulate, or join. There are three main types of joints, classified based on the materials which connect the bones. These include immobile fibrous joints, like the connections between the bones of the skull, and cartilaginous joints, which allow for minimal movement, such as those between the vertebrae. Synovial joints are very mobile, contain a joint space, and are lubricated with synovial fluid. In these joints, a thin layer of cartilage covers the ends of the bones. Some joints also contain small, fluid-filled sacs called bursae, which help cushion the joint at points of stress (see **Fig. 19.17**).

Synovial joints occur in six different mechanical arrangements, including ball and socket joints, gliding joints, and hinge joints. The hip is an example of a ball and socket joint and allows for rotational movement. A number of gliding joints are found in the wrist, and the elbow contains a hinge joint, similar to a door hinge. The mechanical configuration of the joint defines the kind of movement possible. Synovial joints are held together and supported by ligaments, a type of connective tissue.

fibrous joint Union of two bones with fibrous tissue resulting in a joint that is nearly immobile; examples include joints between the bones of the skull.

cartilaginous joint A joint in which the bony surfaces of the two juxtaposed bones are united with cartilage; for example, the vertebral joints.

synovial joint Mobile joint that is lined with synovial membrane and contains synovial fluid.

bursa Singular of bursae, a small sack between tendon and bone that contains a synovial fluid; facilitates smooth movement of joints.

ligament Tough band of fibrous tissue that connects and supports the bones in a joint or supports or maintains the position of some organs.

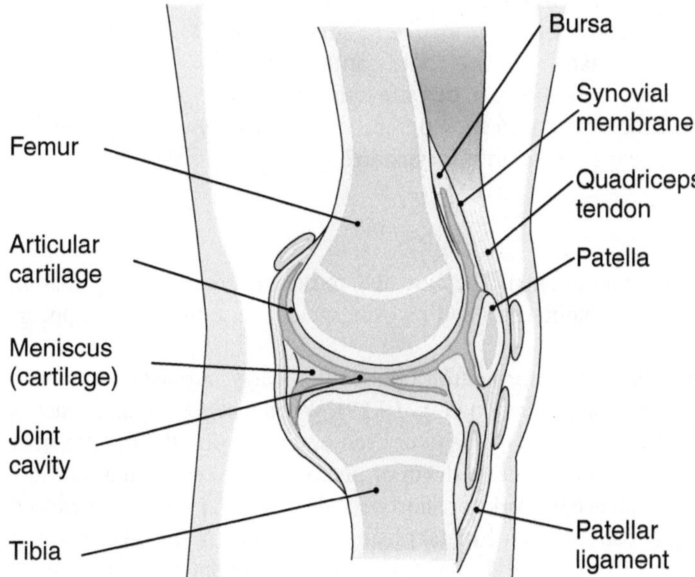


**Figure 19.17** Diagram of a synovial joint (the knee) showing the relationship of connective tissues to the bones. (Reprinted with permission from Cohen BJ. *Memmler's The Human Body in Health and Disease*, 10th edition. Baltimore: Lippincott Williams & Wilkins, 2005.)

## Muscles

striated Marked by parallel lines or grooves; as in striated muscle.

There are three types of muscle in the human body. The smooth muscle of blood vessels and bronchioles is under involuntary control. Although cardiac muscle is striated (striped), and is structurally more similar to skeletal muscles, it is also under involuntary control (**Fig. 19.18**). Skeletal muscle is under voluntary control, is attached to bones, and through contraction and relaxation allows for coordinated movement of the body. The skeletal muscles make up about forty percent of the total body weight in the normal adult of average weight and fitness.

### Muscle Function

tendon Strong, fibrous connective tissue that joins muscle to bone so that muscle can initiate movement at joints.

Muscles are made up of individual muscle fibers, bundled together by fibrous connective tissue. Multiple bundles are then bound together in a connective tissue sheath. These connective tissue layers join together to form the tendon. Muscle cells are themselves long and cylindrical and contain many nuclei. Skeletal muscle cells are excitable, meaning that they can transmit electrical current along the cell membranes. Muscle fibers are also contractile, meaning that they can shorten and thicken. They are able to do this because of alternating layers of two different kinds of protein, actin and myosin, which cause the striped appearance of skeletal muscle.

#### Case 19.1

Just out of graduate school, Minnie Montaine moved to a small California town and got a job working for the local newspaper as a reporter. In her spare time, Minnie played tennis and golf. She walked to work every day, and prided herself on being physically fit. When the newspaper looked for staff volunteers for a backpacking trek on the John Muir Trail in honor of its 90th anniversary, Minnie was one of the first to volunteer. Unlike the other hikers, she had never been backpacking before, but was confident in her fitness level. Rather than doing any further fitness preparation, she spent most of her prep time finding the right equipment, learning the history of the trail, and studying maps, so that she could write about her journey intelligently. Two days before the trip, she learned that the first day of hiking was twelve miles, and the last two miles included an altitude climb of 2,000 feet. Undaunted, Minnie pulled on her 38-pound backpack, and set out with the group on the trail two days later. Although the scenery was glorious, by the eighth mile (at 9,500 feet), Minnie was feeling very winded. By the eleventh mile, she developed cramps in her calf muscles, and had to sit down and get a friend to massage them. She made it to the camp late that afternoon, put up her tent, and climbed into her sleeping bag. The next morning she awoke so sore she didn't know if she could make it out of bed, and wasn't sure she could continue. Her trail mates told her that moving would make her feel better, but she had a hard time believing that! Why do you think Minnie developed such painful muscles? Why was an otherwise fit young woman so unexpectedly unfit for hiking?

Recall from Chapter 4 that the motor neuron (nerves that carry impulses to muscle) joins the muscle at the neuromuscular junction (**Fig. 19.19**). When a nerve impulse reaches the muscle, the layers of actin and myosin slide over each other, causing the muscle fiber to shorten. This motion requires energy, in the form of glucose and oxygen, and the flow of calcium ions. Although muscles can work for short periods of time at levels that exceed the supply of oxygen and glucose (anaerobic metabolism), this results in the production of lactic acid. It is the build-up of lactic acid during anaerobic metabolism that causes mus-

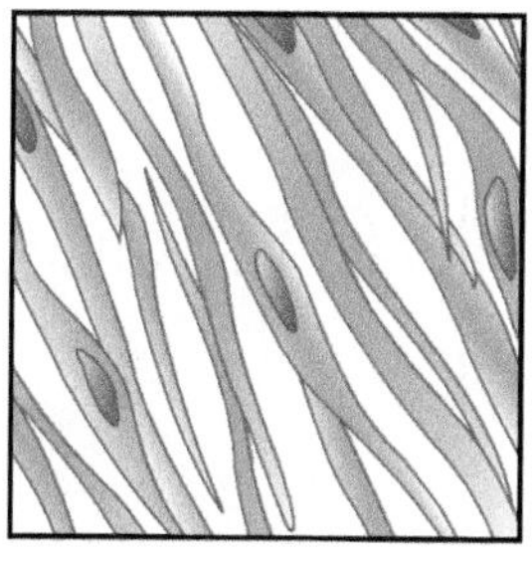


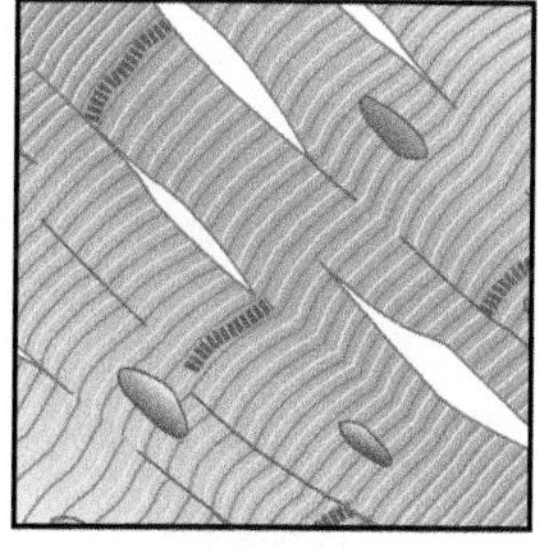


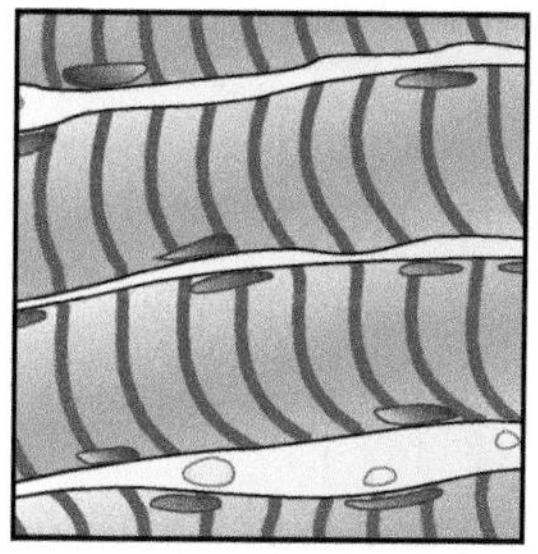


**Figure 19.18** The three types of muscle in the human body. Smooth muscle and cardiac muscle are under involuntary nervous control, while skeletal muscle is under voluntary control. (Adapted with permission from Cohen BJ. *Memmler's The Human Body in Health and Disease*, 10th edition. Baltimore: Lippincott Williams & Wilkins, 2005.)

cles to fatigue. Regular exercise and training stimulates capillary formation, and increases the ability to store and process energy.

There are more than 600 separate muscles, but they function in groups to elicit movement. For instance, the muscles of the head work as a group to provide chewing motions and facial expression. Muscles responsible for movement of synovial joints usually function in opposing pairs. When one muscle contracts, the opposing muscle must relax. Motion of the forearm illustrates this point. When the biceps brachii contracts, the opposing triceps brachii must relax, as seen in **Figure 19.20**.

Muscles generally attach to bone at two or more points. The tendon is a strong, cord-like bundle of connective tissue that connects the muscle to the periosteum of the bone. Attachment occurs at a stable point of the skeleton at one end, called the origin, and a movable point at the other end, called the insertion. When the muscle flexes it shortens, pulling on both points. Through motion of the joint, the bone at the insertion site is moved in the direction of the bone where the origin of the muscle is located.

The use of different muscles working together allow for very complex and coordinated body movements. Through exercise and repetitive practice, human beings are able to become highly proficient and fluid in the use of their muscles. Our ability to move is as diverse as our interests. Whether a football player, ballerina, or surgeon, our musculoskeletal systems provide the potential for us to move in nearly every way imaginable.

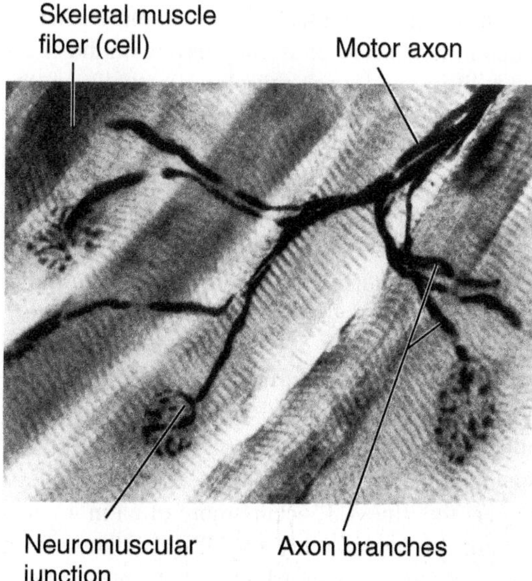


**Figure 19.19** An electron micrograph of a motor axon, muscle fibers, and the neuromuscular junction, where nerve impulses are translated into muscle contraction. (Reprinted with permission from Cormack DH. *Essential Histology*, 2nd edition. Philadelphia: Lippincott Williams & Wilkins, 2001.)

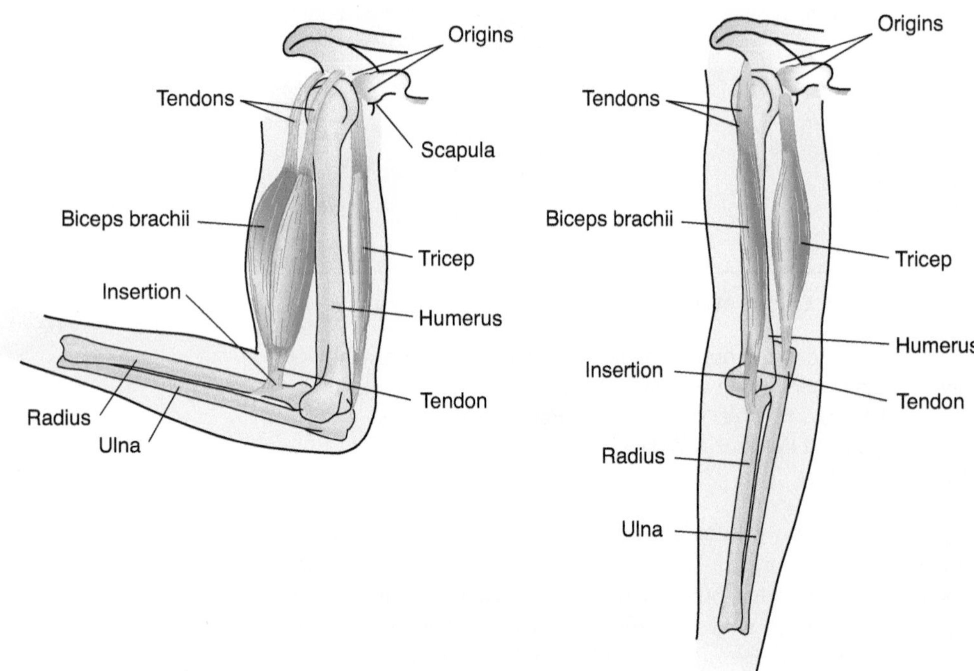


**Figure 19.20** Muscle opposition; when the biceps contracts, the triceps must stretch. (Adapted with permission from Cohen BJ. *Memmler's The Human Body in Health and Disease*, 10th edition. Baltimore: Lippincott Williams & Wilkins, 2005.)

## Disorders of the Musculoskeletal System

The most common disorders of the musculoskeletal system are related to wear and tear, improper use, and lack of fitness. Repetitive motion can cause injury to joints, muscles, and underlying tissues. Tendonitis, bursitis, and rupture of ligaments can be a result of sports- or work-related injuries.

Muscles are designed to protect underlying structures and support bones and joints. When muscles are not fit they provide less effective protection. For example, back pain can occur when an individual puts too much strain on the vertebrae. This occurs more often in individuals who do not have strong abdominal muscles. The constant pressure on the intervertebral cartilage and tissues from improper lifting and weak muscles eventually causes damage, which results in compression of the spinal nerve in that space, causing severe, and often debilitating pain.

osteoarthritis Degenerative arthritis that usually begins during middle or old age, marked by pain, swelling, and stiffness.

Osteoarthritis is a degenerative joint disease caused by a lifetime of use of the joints. Obesity and weak muscles exacerbate osteoarthritis. It occurs most often in weight-bearing joints, such as the hips, knees, and vertebral columns, but can also occur in hands and wrists. In osteoarthritis the joint lining and cartilage deteriorate, causing pain in the joints with movement.

rheumatoid arthritis Chronic, inflammatory, autoimmune disease marked by pain and inflammation of the joints leading to eventual joint destruction.

Another disease, rheumatoid arthritis, is a much more serious condition. Rheumatoid arthritis is an autoimmune disorder that is a result of an abnormal immune response to joints and sometimes other tissues. Antibody complexes attach to tissues in the joints, causing pain, inflammation, and, if uncontrolled, deformities and loss of function (see **Fig. 19.21**). Family members of people with rheumatoid arthritis have a higher risk of developing the disease, but no one knows what triggers the illness. It occurs more often in women than men and usually begins in middle age, but can begin at any age. The childhood form of the disease is called juvenile rheumatoid arthritis and can afflict babies and toddlers.

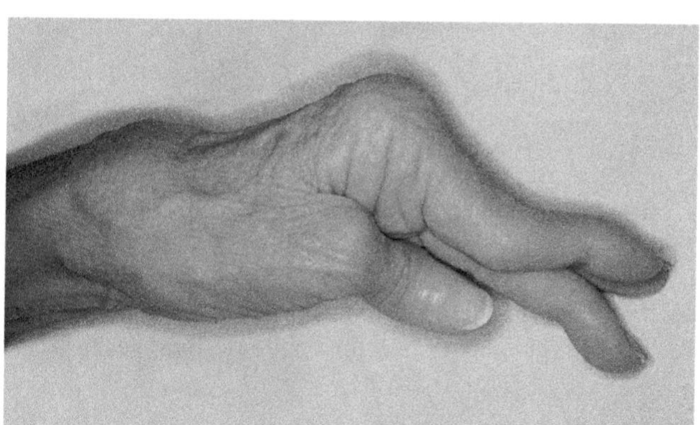

**Figure 19.21** The joint deformities of the hand typically seen in a patient with rheumatoid arthritis can cause pain and limitations of movement and strength. (Reprinted with permission from Strickland JW, Graham TJ. *Master Techniques in Orthopaedic Surgery: The Hand*, 2nd Edition. Philadelphia: Lippincott Williams & Wilkins, 2005.)

Like rheumatoid arthritis, other autoimmune disorders, such as systemic lupus erythematosus, psoriatic arthritis, and the inflammatory bowel diseases have unknown causes, and can cause joint pain. In each of these diseases the body loses some of its ability to recognize itself, and develops inflammatory processes that damages its own tissue. Rheumatoid arthritis is the most common of the autoimmune diseases and is the only one to cause widespread destruction of joints.

Gout is a metabolic disease that affects the joints and is caused by overproduction or reduced elimination of uric acid. Deposits of uric acid crystals can form in the cartilage and other connective tissues of the joints. An acute attack of gouty arthritis usually occurs in a single joint and causes severe pain and inflammation of the joint. Gouty arthritis usually occurs in joints of the lower extremities, such as knees, toes, and ankles. Uric acid can deposit in the kidneys, where the crystals can cause damage. Gout occurs more frequently in men.

gout Metabolic disease marked by painful inflammation, deposits of uric acid crystals in the joints, and an excessive level of uric acid in the blood.

Osteoporosis is a metabolic disease of the bones, where there is an increase in bone breakdown without a commensurate deposition of new bone. Bones become weak and break easily. Although everyone loses some bone density with age, people with osteoporosis have a dramatic loss of bone mineralization. This disease is most common in post-menopausal women, but can also occur in younger women and in men. Lack of weight-bearing exercise, immobility, and nutritional deficiencies can contribute to osteoporosis.

osteoporosis Bone disease, mainly of older women, that causes a decrease in bone mass and in more porous and brittle bones that can lead to fracture.

Osteomalacia, or rickets, is a softening of bone due to lack of calcification. This is most often due to vitamin D deficiency in the diet, but can also be seen when vitamin D is not converted to the active form because of liver disease, or when absorption of calcium is impaired.

osteomalacia Softening of the bones in adults that is analogous to rickets in the young.

Infection of the bone is called osteomyelitis. This usually occurs when there is both a break in the skin that causes an infection of the soft tissues, and an underlying chronic illness, such as diabetes, that weakens the immune defenses. Osteomyelitis can result from systemic infections such as tuberculosis, or from use of dirty needles by drug abusers.

osteomyelitis Inflammation of the bone usually caused by infection of bacterial origin.

The muscular dystrophies are a group of genetic muscle disorders that are characterized by progressive weakness and degeneration of skeletal muscle. The most serious of these, Duchenne muscular dystrophy, occurs mainly in boys, usually before the age of five. By the age of 20, most of these patients require a ventilator to breath. The genes causing this defect have been identified, and there is important research being done, but at present no cure for these diseases.

muscular dystrophy One of a group of hereditary diseases characterized by progressive degeneration of muscles.

# Review Questions

## Multiple Choice

Choose the best answer for the following questions:

1. Circle the answer that best describes the pathway of oxygen processed by the respiratory system.
   a. Air is drawn in through the nasopharynx, passes into the esophagus, through the bronchioles to the alveoli where oxygen passes through capillaries to enter the bloodstream.
   b. Air is drawn in through the nasopharynx, passes through the trachea to the airways, into the alveoli where oxygen passes through capillaries to enter the bloodstream. In tissues, oxygen is exchanged for carbon dioxide, which is then returned to the lungs and blown out.
   c. Air is drawn in through the nares to the mediastinum where it is exchanged across the alveoli. In tissues, oxygen is exchanged for carbon dioxide, which is then returned to the lungs and blown out.
   d. Air is drawn in through the nasopharynx, passes into the trachea, through the airways to the alveoli. Oxygen is exchanged for carbon dioxide in the aorta and $CO^2$ is removed from the bloodstream.
   e. Air is drawn in through the nasopharynx, passes into the esophagus, through the bronchioles to the alveoli where oxygen passes through capillaries to the bloodstream. Oxygen is exchanged for carbon dioxide in the aorta and $CO^2$ is removed from the bloodstream.

2. Of the following statements, which one does not describe one of the processes involved with respiration?
   a. A negative pressure gradient causes air to flow from the area of higher pressure outside the lungs to the area of lower pressure inside the lungs.
   b. Surfactant, a slippery liquid that reduces surface tension, prevents the alveoli from collapsing and also aids in their expansion.
   c. Stem cells differentiate and give rise to all three classes of blood cells; leukocytes, erythrocytes, and thrombocytes.
   d. Hemoglobin in red blood cells attaches to and carries oxygen.
   e. All of the above processes are involved with respiration.

3. Identify the statement about renal anatomy and physiology that is not correct.
   a. The urinary system is made up of two kidneys, two ureters connecting the kidneys to the bladder, the urinary bladder, and the urethra.
   b. The nephron is a microscopic unit in the kidney responsible for the filtration of blood and the formation of urine.
   c. The kidneys regulate water, electrolyte, and pH balance through mechanisms involved with the production of urine.
   d. In respiration, carbon dioxide is inhaled and exchanged with oxygen carried from the tissues via the blood.
   e. Dehydration, advancing age, and the long-term use of some drugs can cause impairment of kidney function.

4. Which of the following is a common complaint related to the gastrointestinal tract?
   a. Diarrhea
   b. Gout

c. Hypercholesterolemia
d. Inflammatory bowel disease
e. All of the above

5. What essential function does the musculoskeletal system perform?
   a. The skeleton and muscles provide the framework and support for the body.
   b. The skeleton anchors and works with the muscles to provide for locomotion and strength.
   c. Bones act as a storage depot for calcium and phosphorus.
   d. The skeleton manufactures blood cells and muscles produce body heat.
   e. All of the above are true.

## True/False

6. Osteoporosis is a metabolic disease of the bones characterized by bone weakness where bones break easily.
   a. True
   b. False

7. The most common disease of the bladder is urinary retention due to benign prostatic hypertrophy.
   a. True
   b. False

8. Asthma occurs when airways that are hypersensitive to allergens, exercise, or other stimulants constrict and prevent the efficient exhalation of air.
   a. True
   b. False

9. The pancreas is a gland that is crucial to the digestion of carbohydrates and the utilization of protein.
   a. True
   b. False

10. Rheumatoid arthritis is different from osteoarthritis because it is an autoimmune condition that results in inflammation and destruction of joints.
    a. True
    b. False

## Matching

For numbers 11 to 15, match the word or phrase with the correct lettered choice from the list below. Choices will not be used more than once and may not be used at all.

11. Tendon
12. Ligament
13. Synovial joint
14. Cartilaginous joint
15. Osteoblast

a. A mobile joint, with a joint space that is lubricated with fluid
b. Connective tissue that attaches muscle to bone
c. Cell that differentiates to give rise to all three classes of blood cells
d. Cell responsible for forming new bone
e. Connective tissue that holds and supports synovial joints
f. A joint that allows minimal movement
g. Cell responsible for breakdown of bone

### Short Answer

16. Describe peristalsis, the action that propels food through the gastrointestinal tract.

17. What are some common causes of heartburn and indigestion? Why should chronic heartburn or indigestion not be ignored?

18. Compare diffusion and osmosis and describe their roles in the production of urine.

19. Describe how muscles, bones, and joints function to allow movement.

20. List a common disease associated with each of the organ systems discussed in this chapter.

## FOR FURTHER INQUIRY

Use the Internet to learn more about one of the body systems discussed in this chapter. Try a search on Google using the terms "anatomy," "physiology," and "activities" to locate some interesting and educational activities to further your interest.

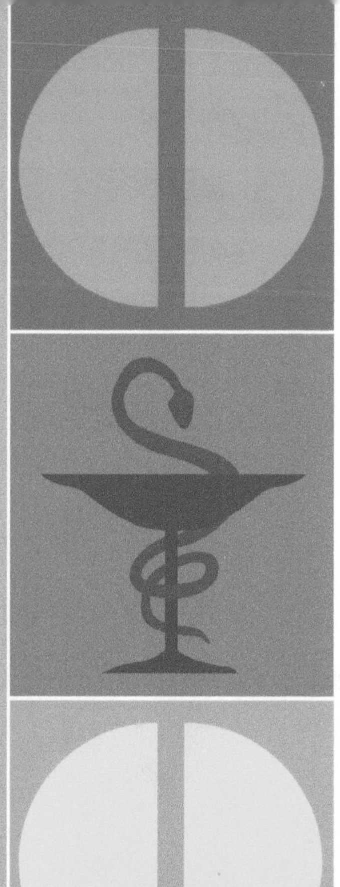

Chapter **20**

# Drugs Affecting the Respiratory System

## KEY TERMS

- apnea
- atopic dermatitis
- cytokine
- metered dose inhaler
- nebulizer
- pruritus
- rhinitis

## OBJECTIVES

After studying this chapter, the reader should be able to:

- Compare and contrast the causes, pathology, characteristics of the patients, and goals of treatment of chronic obstructive pulmonary disease and asthma.
- Describe or, if model devices are available, demonstrate the appropriate use and care of metered dose inhalers and spacers.
- List the brand and generic names of three inhaled corticosteroids, and explain why inhalation is the preferred route of administration for corticosteroids in the treatment of asthma.
- Identify the role in chronic obstructive pulmonary disease, if any, of the long-acting beta agonists, ipratropium, aminophylline, and the leukotriene inhibitors.
- Explain the role of antihistamines in the treatment of allergic rhinitis. Describe two major differences between first- and second-generation antihistamines, and list three possible side effects of the antihistamine drugs.

## DRUGS COVERED IN THIS CHAPTER*

### Long-Term Asthma and COPD Control Medications

| Bronchodilators | Respiratory Corticosteroids | Alternative Pulmonary Anti-Inflammatory Drugs |
|---|---|---|
| Albuterol | Beclomethasone | Cromolyn |
| Epinephrine | Budesonide | Nedocromil |
| Formoterol | Flunisolide | Montelukast |
| Metaproterenol | Fluticasone | Zafirlukast |
| Pirbuterol | Triamcinolone | Zileuton |
| Salmeterol | | |
| Terbutaline | | |
| Ipratropium | | |
| Tiotropium | | |

### Drugs for Migraines

| Methylxanthine Derivatives | Antihistamines |
|---|---|
| Aminophylline | Azelastine |
| Theophylline | Cetirizine |
| | Chlorpheniramine Maleate |
| | Cyproheptadine |
| | Diphenhydramine |
| | Fexofenadine |
| | Hydroxyzine |
| | Loratadine |
| | Promethazine |

### Cough Suppressants, Expectorants, and Decongestants

Codeine
Hydrocodone
Dextromethorphan
Guaifenesin
Pseudoephedrine
Oxymetazoline

Asthma, chronic obstructive pulmonary disease (COPD), and allergic rhinitis are increasingly common diseases of the respiratory tract. Known environmental factors contribute to the occurrence of these diseases. We inhale particles from the air, such as pollen, tobacco smoke, toxins, or smog, on a chronic basis with deleterious consequences for our delicate respiratory tissues. These foreign particles stimulate an immune response, which over time can cause permanent damage. Although the distribution and pathology of these diseases differ, they share some common characteristics and treatments.

Asthma is a chronic disease associated with abnormal reactivity of the bronchioles to triggers. It affects twenty million people in the United States, many of them children. More than 5,000 people in the Unites States die every year from asthma, and nearly two million asthma related emergency room visits occur annually. Asthma is the most common chronic illness in children. COPD affects approximately thirty million people in the United States, and is the fourth most common cause of death. Most people who develop this disease are smokers or people who have worked in close contact with environmental toxins. As it progresses, COPD can become profoundly disabling because the airways and lungs become less flexible and less able to exchange air.

Allergic rhinitis is an extremely common condition, affecting approximately twenty percent of the population. Popularly known as "hay fever," allergic rhinitis is caused by reactions to airborne allergens, such as pollen or molds, and is typically seasonal in nature. Unlike allergic rhinitis, most upper respiratory infections are self-limited and are treated symptomatically. Medications used to treat congestion and cough associated with allergic conditions are often the same drugs used to treat the symptoms of viral infections of the upper respiratory tract ("colds"). For that reason, cold medicines will be covered in this chapter.

Drugs used for respiratory disorders are members of numerous drug classes, including sympathomimetic agents, antihistamines, corticosteroids and other modulators of immune response, mucolytic agents and expectorants, and cough suppressants, among others.

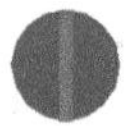

## Drugs Used to Treat Asthma and Chronic Obstructive Pulmonary Disease

Asthma is characterized by episodes of acute, reversible bronchoconstriction that cause shortness of breath, cough, chest tightness, wheezing, and rapid respiration (**Fig. 20.1**). A variety of factors, such as exposure to dust mites, pollen, or cigarette smoke, and exercise, can trigger asthma. Asthma is a disease of exacerbation and remission, and the goals of treatment are to both relieve symptoms associated with acute attacks and prevent the recurrence of asthmatic attacks.

Chronic obstructive pulmonary disease (chronic bronchitis and emphysema) results in irreversible airway constriction and loss of elasticity in the airways and lungs. Whereas asthma is often thought of as a disease of childhood, COPD is a condition found in middle aged and elderly people. Many of the same drugs used to treat asthma are used to treat the disorders of COPD. The goals of COPD therapy are to increase airflow, alleviate symptoms, and decrease exacerbations of the disease. COPD is a progressive disease that eventually leads to death. Since 90% of COPD cases are related to smoking, the best way to prevent the disease is to not smoke.

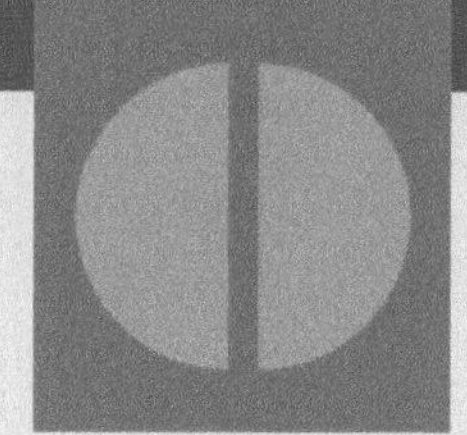

### Case 20.1

Mrs. Marla Burroughs is a 35-year-old woman you know as a frequent customer at the local Nice & Neighborly Pharmacy. She comes in for her inhaler and antibiotics for chronic bronchitis. On this particular day she looks very worried and asks for your help. Marla says that today her doctor told her that if she doesn't quit smoking she will be on a ventilator by the time she is 50 years old! What assistance can you give her?

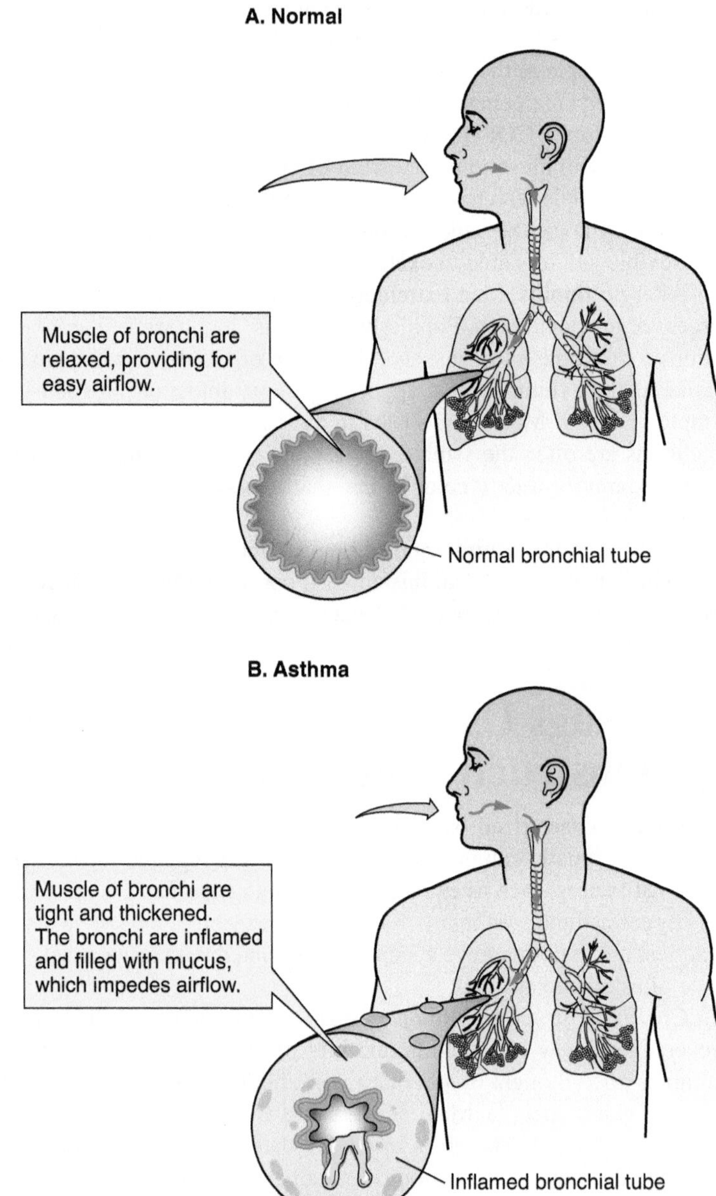


**Figure 20.1** The function of a normal airway (A) and the effects of asthma on an airway (B). (Adapted with permission from Harvey RA, Champe PC, Howland RD, et al. *Lippincott's Illustrated Reviews: Pharmacology,* 3rd edition. Baltimore: Lippincott Williams & Wilkins, 2006.)

Inflammation of the bronchioles plays an important role in the etiology of both asthma and COPD. Removing triggering factors from the environment, when possible, can help prevent exacerbations of asthma. Many of the long-term, disease modifying treatments for asthma are designed to modify the body's reactions to the triggering agents that cause the inflammation, thereby allowing normal activity and exercise. In COPD, smoking cessation is of utmost importance. Other important measures include treatment of infections and the judicious use of theophylline and oral corticosteroids when necessary. Drugs used to treat these disease fall into two broad categories: those used to treat acute exacerbations and those used to prevent further exacerbations or deterioration over time.

## Bronchodilators

Selective $\beta_2$-agonists are the drugs of choice for the treatment of mild asthma and provide the foundation of treatment for asthma and COPD of any severity. Beta agonists have no anti-inflammatory effects, but are potent bronchodilators. Therefore, they are effective to treat acute bronchoconstriction, but do not prevent attacks. Ipratropium (Atrovent®) and tiotropium (Spiriva®) are used for treatment and prevention of bronchospasm in COPD.

## Actions and Indications

Beta$_2$-agonists selectively relax the smooth muscle that surrounds the bronchioles. They combat acute bronchoconstriction and provide symptomatic relief of wheezing and chest tightness. When symptoms of asthma occur once or twice a week, the use of a fast-acting $\beta_2$ agonist, such as albuterol (Proventil®), is the treatment of choice. No daily preventative medication is needed in these patients. When a patient has more severe forms of asthma, the fast acting $\beta_2$ agonists are considered the best agents for reversal of acute attacks. Because they are used to treat acute asthma attacks, the short-acting beta-agonists are sometimes referred to as "rescue" agents.

In persistent asthma, treatment with long acting $\beta_2$-agonists, such as formoterol (Foradil®) and salmeterol (with fluticasone as Advair®), can sometimes be beneficial. These two drugs are chemical analogs of albuterol but they have a greater affinity for the receptor, which accounts for their longer duration of action. They are not a substitute for drugs that prevent acute exacerbations of asthma, such as the inhaled corticosteroids. Long-acting $\beta_2$ agonists are prescribed only for administration at regular intervals for maintenance therapy, not for treatment of acute symptoms.

Treatment of COPD includes bronchodilation with beta-agonists as well as the anticholinergic bronchodilators, ipratropium, and tiotropium. By antagonizing the effects of acetylcholine, these drugs allow the bronchioles to dilate. They are as effective as the beta-agonists in COPD, but play a minor role in the treatment of asthma. Short-acting and long-acting beta$_2$-agonists and the inhaled anticholinergics produce bronchodilation, relieve symptoms, and improve the quality of life of COPD patients on a temporary basis. No available drugs are able to prevent the progressive loss of pulmonary function in people with these diseases.

## Administration

Drugs used to treat pulmonary diseases can be delivered to the respiratory tissues by systemic administration or by direct, local administration via inhalation. When drugs are given by mouth or by injection, they reach the bloodstream, or systemic circulation, where they can cause effects throughout the body. When it is possible, inhalation is the preferred route of administration for treating airway disease, because the drug is delivered directly to the airways, resulting in less systemic absorption and therefore fewer systemic side effects. The beta-agonists are available in a variety of formulations for inhalation and a few for systemic administration. **Table 20.1** lists the products available for treatment of asthma and COPD.

The short-acting beta$_2$-agonists albuterol and pirbuterol (Maxair®) can be inhaled every six hours as maintenance therapy. They are also used as rescue agents, given more often for short periods of time during acute exacerbations. These drugs are available in a device called a metered dose inhaler (MDI), which includes a small, pressurized canister containing the drug and a mouthpiece for administration (**Fig. 20.2**). A set dose of the drug is delivered every time the patient presses down on the canister to actuate it, or cause it to spray. Effective use of an inhaler requires coordination of breathing with actuation of the device. Inhalers are not recommended for children until they are capable of coordinating the use of the inhaler with some adult support. Even when the MDI is used properly, only about ten percent of an inhaled dose gets into the bronchioles. Spacing devices (refer to **Fig. 20.3**) will improve the efficiency of metered dose inhaler usage in young children and can reduce some unpleasant side effects of the use of inhalers in all ages.

metered dose inhaler A device for delivering measured doses of aerosolized medication to the airways.

Some beta-agonists are also available for inhalation with a nebulizer. This device uses a small compressor pump to convert the drug solution into a mist that the patient inhales through a mouthpiece (**Fig. 20.4**). Albuterol, levalbuterol (Xopenex®), terbutaline (Brethine®), and others are available for use with nebulizers. Even though this method of delivery is more effective than metered dose inhaler administration, much of the drug is still lost to the environment.

nebulizer A device used to convert a sterile medication solution into an extremely fine spray for inhalation into the lungs.

Although systemic administration is associated with more side effects, a number of beta-agonists are available for oral or subcutaneous administration. Albuterol and terbu-

**Table 20.1** A Comparison of the Names, Indications, and Formulations of Drugs Used to Treat Respiratory Conditions Discussed in This Chapter

| Generic | Brand Name | Available as | Indications | Notes |
|---|---|---|---|---|
| **Bronchodilators** | | | | |
| Albuterol | Proventil®, Ventolin® | Tablets, MDI, ER tabs, syrup, soln for nebulizer | Tx and prevention of bronchospasm | Adults and children |
| Epinephrine | Adrenalin®, microNefrin®, Primatene® | Injection, solution for nebulizer, MDI, topical solution | Inhalation & injection, tx of bronchospasm, topical—for nasal congestion | Emergencies, all ages; inhaler not for children |
| Formoterol | Foradil® | Inhalation powder | Prevention of broncho-spasm | Adults and children ≥12 |
| Levalbuterol | Xopenex® | Solution for nebulizer | Tx and prevention of bronchospasm | Enantiomer of albuterol |
| Metaproterenol | Alupent® | Aerosol, solution for inhalation | Tx of bronchospasm | |
| Pirbuterol | Maxair® | MDI | Tx and prevention of bronchospasm | Adults and children ≥12 |
| Salmeterol (and fluticasone) | Advair® | Powder for inhalation | Prevention of broncho-spasm | Children ≥4 years |
| Terbutaline | Brethine® | Tablets, injection | Tx and prevention of bronchospasm | Adults and children ≥12 |
| Ipratropium | Atrovent® | MDI, solution for inhalation | Prevention of broncho-spasm, COPD | Adults; nasal for adults and children ≥12 |
| Tiotropium | Spiriva® | Powder for inhalation | Prevention of broncho-spasm, COPD | |
| **Respiratory Corticosteroids** | | | | |
| Beclomethasone | QVAR®, Beconase AQ® | MDI, 40 and 80 µg/ inhalation, nasal aerosol | Preventative treatment of asthma, prevent and treat allergic rhinitis | Adults and children* |
| Budesonide | Pulmicort®, Rhinocort® | Powder and susp. For inhalation, nasal spray, and nasal inhaler | Preventative treatment of asthma, prevent and treat allergic rhinitis | Adults and children |
| Flunisolide | AeroBid®, Nasalide® | MDI, nasal spray | Preventative treatment of asthma, prevent and treat allergic rhinitis | Adults and children |
| Fluticasone | Flovent®, Flonase® | MDI, powder for inhala-tion, nasal spray | Preventative treatment of asthma, prevent and treat allergic rhinitis | Adults and children |
| Triamcinolone | Azmacort®, Nasacort® | MDI, nasal spray | Preventative treatment of asthma, prevent and treat allergic rhinitis | Adults and children |

*(continues)*

| Generic | Brand Name | Available as | Indications | Notes |
|---|---|---|---|---|
| **Mast Cell Stabilizers** | | | | |
| Cromolyn | Intal®, NasalCrom® | MDI, nasal spray, solution for inhalation | Preventative treatment of asthma, prevent and treat allergic rhinitis | Adults and children ≥2 |
| Nedocromil | Tilade® | | Prevention of asthma, maintenance treatment | Adults and children |
| **Leukotriene Inhibitors** | | | | |
| Montelukast | Singulair® | Tablets, chewable tabs, granules | Prevention of asthma, maintenance treatment tx of allergic rhinitis | Asthma – Adults and children ≥1 |
| Zafirlukast | Accolate® | Tablets | Prevention of asthma, maintenance treatment | Adults and children ≥5 |
| Zileuton | Zyflo® | Tablets | Prevention of asthma, maintenance treatment | Adults and children ≥12 |
| **Methylxanthine derivatives** | | | | |
| Aminophylline | | Tablets, oral liquid, suppositories, injection | Relief or prevention of bronchospasm of COPD, asthma | |
| Theophylline | Theolair®, Theo24®, others | Tablets, capsule, ER tabs and caps, syrup, elixir | Relief or prevention of bronchospasm of COPD, asthma | |
| **Antihistamines** | | | | |
| Azelastine | Astelin® | Nasal Spray | Symptomatic tx of allergic rhinitis | Adults and children ≥5 |
| Cetirizine | Zyrtec® | Tablets, chew tabs, syrup | Symptomatic tx of allergic rhinitis, chronic urticaria | Adults and children ≥2 |
| Chlorpheniramine Maleate | Chlor-Trimeton® | Tablets, chew tabs, ER tabs & caps, syrup | Symptomatic tx of allergic rhinitis | Adults and children ≥6 |
| Cyproheptadine | | Tablets, syrup | Hypersensitivity reactions | Adults and children ≥2 |
| Diphenhydramine | Benadryl® | Capsules, tablets, chew tabs, elixir, syrup, injection | Hypersensitivity reactions, motion sickness, cough | Gold standard tx for allergic reactions |
| Fexofenadine | Allegra® | Tablets and capsules | Symptomatic tx of allergic rhinitis, chronic urticaria | Adults and children ≥6 |

*(continues)*

**Table 20.1** A Comparison of the Names, Indications, and Formulations of Drugs Used to Treat Respiratory Conditions Discussed in This Chapter *(continued)*

| Generic | Brand Name | Available as | Indications | Notes |
|---|---|---|---|---|
| **Antihistamines (continued)** | | | | |
| Hydroxyzine | Vistaril®, Atarax® | Tablets, capsules, syrup, suspension, and injection antiemetic (injection only) | Atopic or contact dermatitis, sedative, | Hydroxyzin HCL and hydroxyzine pamoate |
| Loratadine | Claritin® | Tablets, orally disintegrating tabs, syrup | Symptomatic tx of allergic rhinitis | Adults and children ≥2 |
| **Cough suppressants, Expectorants, Decongestants** | | | | |
| Dextromethorphan | Delsym®, others | Gelcaps, lozenges, liquid, suspension | Temporary relief of cough | Age 2 and up |
| Guaifenesin | Robitussin®, others | Liquid, tablets, ER tabs, capsules | Expectorant | Age 2 and up |
| Oxymetazoline | Afrin® | Spray | Decongestant, temporary use | Age 6 and up |
| Phenylephrine | Neo-Synephrine®, Entex LA, ER® | Nasal spray & drops, tablets (OTC), injection, ophthalmic (Rx) | Nasal congestion, hypotension, some forms of glaucoma | |
| Pseudoephedrine | Sudafed® | Tablets, capsules, ER tabs, liquid, drops | Decongestant, for short-term use | Age 2 and up. Found behind the Rx counter |

COPD, chronic obstructive pulmonary disease; ER, extended release; MDL, metered dose inhaler; Tx, treatment.

taline are available as tablets, and albuterol as syrup for oral administration. Metaproterenol (Alupent®), a nonspecific beta-agonist, is supplied as tablets and syrup, in addition to products for inhalation. Terbutaline and epinephrine (Adrenaline®) are both available for subcutaneous injection. Salmeterol and formoterol have a long duration of action, providing bronchodilation for at least twelve hours. They are inhaled with a device that delivers the drug as a dry powder. Ipratropium is available in a number of formulations for inhalation, including a solution for use with a nebulizer and in a metered dose inhaler. It is combined with albuterol in MDI form and as a nebulizer solution. Tiotropium is only sold as a dry powder inhaler.

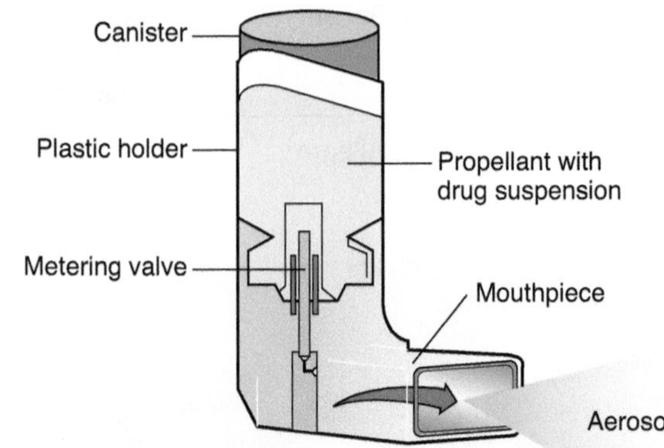


**Figure 20.2** Metered dose inhalers are made up of two detachable parts: the canister containing the drug and a mouthpiece with a device that regulates the dose.

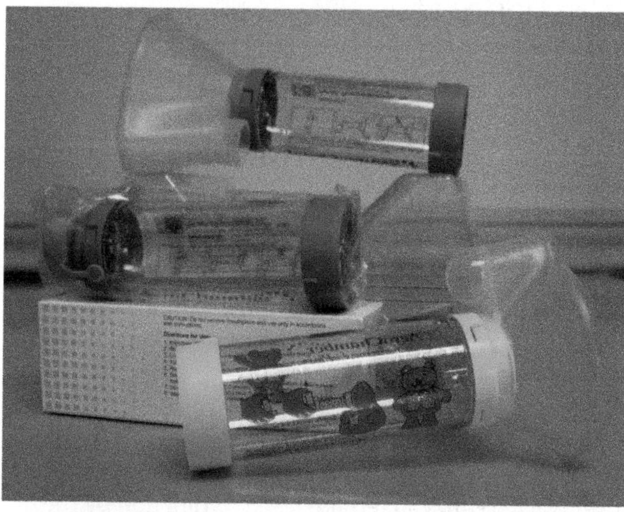

**Figure 20.3** Spacers are marketed in a variety of styles for use with metered dose inhalers. The spacers in the front and back are made for children and cover the nose and mouth.

## Side Effects

Selective $\beta_2$-agonists used repeatedly or in high doses can have deleterious cardiac effects. Fatal arrhythmias have occurred in asthma patients using salmeterol along with frequent use of short acting beta agonist inhalers. Beta-agonists can produce adverse CNS effects that include anxiety, fear, tension headache, and tremor. Feelings of jitteriness and an increased heart rate are fairly common, even with selective beta-agonists.

As you recall, drugs are made up of two mirror-image molecules of identical structure called enantiomers. Even though they are chemically identical, one of these enantiomers is always more active at the receptor than the other. Some pharmaceutical companies remove the less active enantiomer, and claim to have a better, safer product. Although promoted as causing fewer side effects, levalbuterol (Xopenex®), the L-enantiomer of albuterol, has not been shown to be safer or more effective than albuterol in controlled clinical trials. Levalbuterol costs the pharmacy and the patient about six times as much as albuterol.

Dry mouth is a fairly common complaint associated with the use of both ipratropium and tiotropium. Tiotropium can occasionally cause urinary retention and constipation, both typical consequences of anticholinergic use. These adverse effects occur less frequently than they do with systemic administration of anticholinergic drugs.

Use of the dry powder inhalers is associated with throat irritation and coughing. The drugs inhaled using metered dose inhalers leave a bad taste in the mouth and can also be

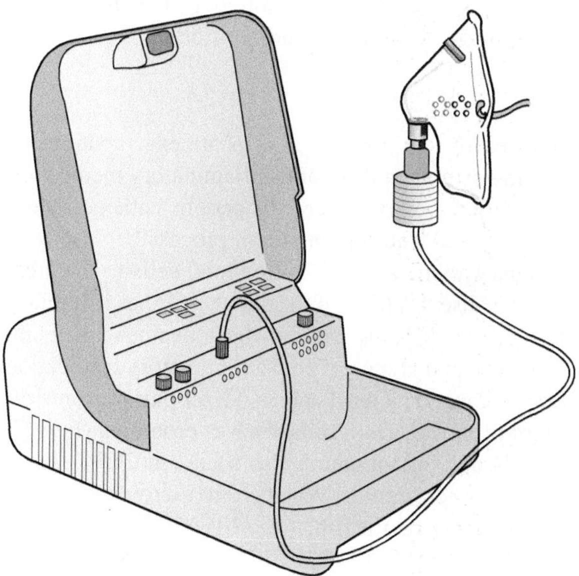

**Figure 20.4** A nebulizer aerosolizes bronchodilators to deliver them more effectively than an MDI.

irritating. By using a spacer with the MDI, the large particles of drug that cause the bad taste and irritation drop to the bottom of the spacer to prevent these issues. Spacers cannot be used with dry powder inhalers.

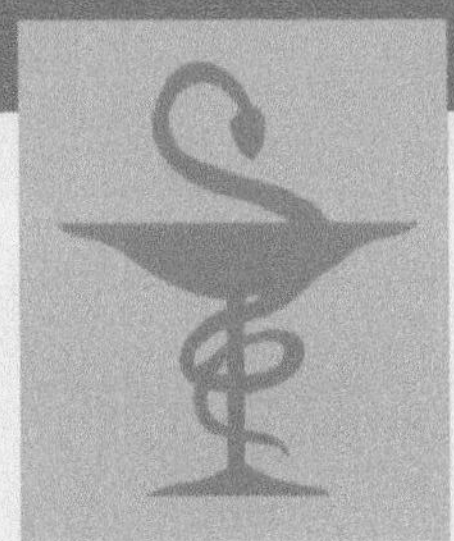

## Tips for the Technician

Technicians can play a very important supportive role in guiding patients with respiratory diseases. Most retail pharmacies sell air purifiers, spacers to be used with inhalers, and nebulizers. Technicians should become familiar with this equipment and its use in order to provide customers with sound information about the various devices available.

Metered dose inhalers must be shaken before use and a shake well sticker should be applied. Dry powder inhaler devices do not need to be shaken. Dry powder inhalers are activated when the user breathes in, and require less coordination by the user. Unlike MDIs, these devices deliver the medication in different ways. Some devices need to be reloaded by the patient before each dose, while others contain a preset number of doses. Each of these devices has a unique system for loading and activation.

Patient instructions are included with all inhalers. Encourage inexperienced patients to look them over while still in the pharmacy so the pharmacist can answer any questions they might have. When patients routinely use more than one inhaler, it is important that they use their beta agonist inhaler first, and wait a few minutes before using other inhalers. When multiple "puffs" of the same medication are ordered, patients should wait one minute between inhalations. This allows the bronchioles to open up, so that subsequent medication is delivered lower into the airways, where it will be the most effective.

## Respiratory Corticosteroids

Glucocorticoids are endogenous hormones synthesized from cholesterol by the adrenal glands. In humans, the most important of these hormones is cortisol. Cortisol is important in the body's response to stress; it increases the levels of glucose in the blood and suppresses some aspects of the immune response, among other actions. Synthetic derivatives of cortisol are used pharmacologically for their anti-inflammatory effects in a variety of diseases. Unit V, and especially Chapter 27, will cover the physiology of the steroid hormones in more detail. This discussion is limited to the inhaled corticosteroids.

### Actions and Indications

The respiratory corticosteroids are indicated for the prevention of acute exacerbations of asthma. In the stepwise approach to treating asthma, a daily anti-inflammatory medication is added when wheezing and other symptoms are persistent. In people with persistent asthma symptoms, chronic inflammation occurs. The inflammation process begins when endogenous chemicals activate the immune system and call white blood cells to the area. These cells release other chemicals, which cause swelling of tissues and further irritability of the bronchi. An inhaled corticosteroid, which helps prevent the movement of white blood cells to the bronchioles, is generally the first choice of anti-inflammatory medication for adults with asthma. In young children, however, a mast cell stabilizer that prevents release of histamine and other inflammatory chemicals from cells, such as cromolyn (Intal®) or nedocromil (Tilade®), is preferred. Although inflammation also occurs in COPD, these patients are generally less responsive to the corticosteroids. When corticosteroids are found to be useful, the inhaled route is preferred over systemic use.

The inhaled corticosteroids inhibit many of the cells involved with inflammation in the bronchi and bronchioles. The numbers of these cells found in the airways are reduced after treatment with corticosteroids for a month or more. In addition, the corticosteroids reduce airway edema and make the airways less sensitive to the triggers that induce bronchoconstriction. The peak effects of the corticosteroids take several weeks to develop. Absorption of the drug from respiratory tissue is low. Inhaled corticosteroids are not effective in the treatment of acute asthma attacks. When sprayed into the nasal cavity, the corticosteroids are also effective in treating allergic rhinitis via similar mechanisms of action. The desired clinical effects of reduced congestion, itching, and improvement of other symptoms occur within a few hours to days.

## Administration

Although the corticosteroids are used systemically for short periods and may be given intravenously when people with asthma are hospitalized, inhalation is the preferred route of administration for maintenance and prevention of acute asthma attacks. Oral and intravenous use of the corticosteroids will be discussed in Chapter 27. When a patient experiences seasonal asthma exacerbations, inhaled corticosteroids can be started several weeks before and continued through the time period where the client is most at risk of an acute attack, for example, through the springtime. The drug dose can be minimized, or the drug discontinued altogether, after the risk period is past. In asthma, the goal is to use the lowest corticosteroid dose possible to maintain the patient in a symptom free state.

Besides being available in a surprising array of products for oral inhalation, respiratory corticosteroids are available as nasal sprays for use in allergic rhinitis. Along with the standard MDI, inhalation devices for use in asthma include dry powder inhalers in a variety of strengths. Fluticasone (Flovent®) and beclomethasone (QVAR®) MDIs are formulated in different dosage strengths per use. Fluticasone is also marketed in a dry powder for inhalation in multiple dosage strengths. Budesonide (Pulmocort®) is marketed in both a dry powder inhaler format and in a formulation for inhalation via nebulizer. Nasal sprays are metered dose pumps used by removing the protective clip and cap, and pressing down on the device (**Fig. 20.5**).

## Side Effects

The advantage of inhaling the corticosteroids is that very little is absorbed into the blood stream. Serious side effects are seen with long-term systemic corticosteroid use, but are

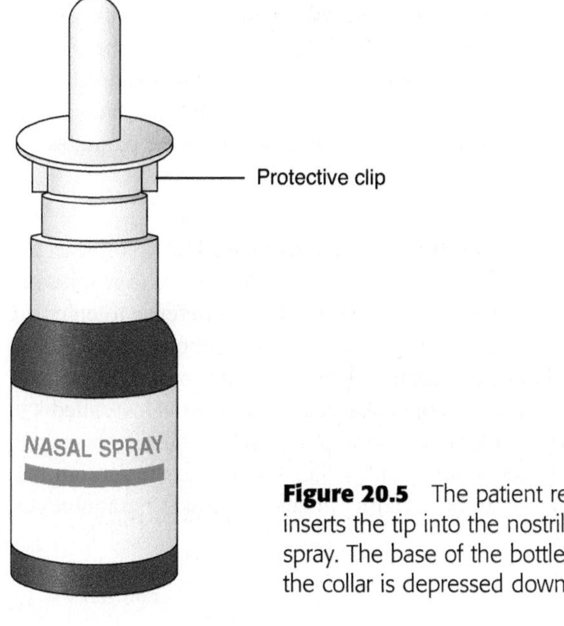


**Figure 20.5** The patient removes the protective clip and cap and inserts the tip into the nostril to use the metered dose pump nasal spray. The base of the bottle is supported with the thumb while the collar is depressed downward the index and middle fingers.

much less likely and less severe when the same medications are inhaled. In some patients, long-term use of inhaled corticosteroids at maximal doses can cause minor suppression of the production of cortisol by the body. There is some evidence that long-term inhaled corticosteroid use can cause delayed growth in young children. In clinical studies, this difference in growth is quite small. Inhaled corticosteroids are associated with the more common side effects of cough, throat irritation, and oral candidiasis. Oral candidiasis, or thrush, is a yeast infection of the mouth that can be quite painful, but is easily treated. Local side effects are reduced when patients use a spacer with their inhalers. Rinsing the mouth after use of the inhaler reduces the likelihood of oral candidiasis.

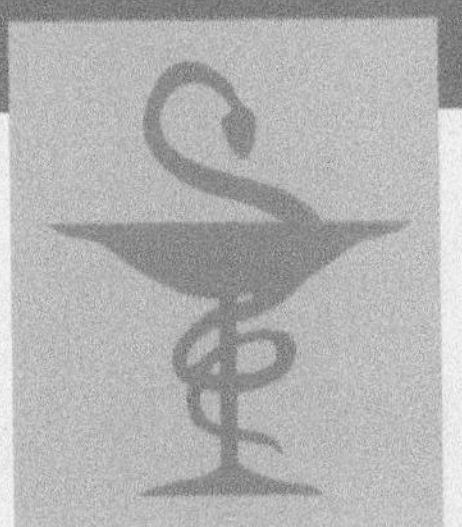

### Tips for the Technician

Technicians need to use special caution when dispensing inhalers that are available in different strengths. It is important to read the package label every time you remove one from the shelf because packages are often deceptively similar in appearance. Before dispensing, apply a "shake well" label to all metered dose inhalers. Dry powder inhaler devices are not shaken before use. Other auxiliary patient instruction labels pertinent to use of a metered dose inhaler include instructions to rinse the mouth after using the inhaler and clean the mouthpiece after each use.

Packages do come with patient package inserts for reference, but the pharmacist should make certain that patients or parents understand the techniques used for administration of these products before they leave the pharmacy. Patients should be advised to use their bronchodilator inhaler first and wait several minutes before administering their corticosteroid inhaler. This allows the airways to open, so that particles of the second drug are deposited further down in the airways for better drug effect. The patient should be instructed that rinsing the mouth after drug administration helps to prevent mouth infections. It is very important that people understand that the inhaled corticosteroids are not effective to treat acute asthma exacerbations.

## Alternative Pulmonary Anti-Inflammatory Drugs

Although the corticosteroids are the most effective pulmonary anti-inflammatory agents, there are alternative medications for long-term prevention of asthma that can be used in place of the steroids, or added on to a regimen of beta agonists and inhaled steroids. The mast cell stabilizers, cromolyn and nedocromil, are first-line drugs, while the leukotriene modifiers may allow reduction of the dose of inhaled corticosteroids in some patients.

### Actions and Indications

Several lines of defense protect the human body from foreign invaders. The first line of defense includes physical barriers like the skin, or the mucous produced in the respiratory tract. When a foreign organism or substance penetrates the first line of defense to enter the body, white blood cells recognize the invader, and begin the antigen-antibody response that results in inflammation. First white blood cells designed to engulf the invading material (granulocytes) are drawn to the location by endogenous chemical substances called cytokines. Many different types of cells can release cytokines early in the immune response. Other white blood cells called lymphocytes produce antibodies specific to the foreign material. Antibodies and enzymes combine with the invading material, allowing granulocytes to surround and remove it more easily.

cytokine Small proteins secreted by cells that are involved with cell to cell communication and regulation, especially of the immune system.

Mast cells, a type of white blood cell, play a key role in the body's defense against invading bacteria, viruses, and other proteins the body recognizes as "foreign." When activated during the immune response, mast cells release granules containing chemicals such as histamine and leukotrienes that attract more white blood cells, cause edema, and promote the inflammatory response. Allergies and the irritability of the airways seen in asthma occur because of an exaggerated immune response to triggering agents or events that should be recognized by the immune system as relatively harmless.

Cromolyn and nedocromil inhibit the release of histamine, leukotrienes, and other inflammatory chemicals by the mast cells and other granulocytes. They are as effective as low-dose inhaled steroids, but less effective than mid or high dose steroids in asthma. Mast cell stabilizers are indicated in the long-term management of asthma and can be used before potential exposure to exercise, cold air, or allergens to prevent acute attacks. Cromolyn is also indicated for the treatment of allergic rhinitis and has been used off-label for the treatment of chronic urticaria (hives).

Leukotrienes are potent mediators of inflammation that cause contraction of the smooth muscle, increase local edema, increase mucus secretion, and attract and activate inflammatory cells in the airways of patients with asthma. There are three drugs that inhibit the actions of the leukotrienes: montelukast (Singular®), zafirlukast (Accolate®), and zileuton (Zyflo®). Montelukast and zafirlukast are indicated for the prevention and chronic treatment of asthma. Montelukast can be used to treat asthma in children as young as 1 year of age. Zileuton is indicated for the symptomatic treatment of asthma, but is rarely used because of a greater risk of side effects than the other two drugs. These drugs are less effective than the corticosteroids and the mast cell stabilizers, and are second-line drugs in the treatment of asthma.

## Administration

Cromolyn and nedocromil are administered via inhalation in asthma. Cromolyn is available in a solution for use with a nebulizer and in a metered dose inhaler. It is sold over the counter in a metered nasal spray for use in allergic rhinitis. Nedocromil is marketed as a metered dose inhaler only.

The leukotriene inhibitors are administered orally and are well absorbed. This makes administration easier, but also results in a greater risk of systemic side effects. All of the leukotriene inhibitors are metabolized by the liver and are subject to drug interactions with other drugs metabolized by the same enzyme systems (cytochrome P-450 and others). All three products are manufactured in tablet form. In addition, montelukast is available as chewable tablets for children, and as granules that can be mixed into soft foods for younger children. Zafirlukast should be taken on an empty stomach because the presence of food reduces the absorption of the drug.

## Side Effects

The mast cell stabilizers, cromolyn and nedocromil, are not absorbed from the respiratory tract. Medication that lands in the mouth and is swallowed is absorbed in miniscule amounts from the GI tract. Because of this lack of systemic absorption, there are no systemic side effects clearly attributable to either drug. Their use is associated with throat irritation, dry mouth, cough, and an unpleasant taste in the mouth (especially nedocromil). Occasionally patients may experience wheezing or cough with these inhalers. Using a beta-agonist, if prescribed, before the mast cell stabilizing drug can reduce the risk of bronchospasm.

The leukotriene inhibitors are fairly well tolerated by most patients. The most common side effects include headache and GI upset, but they can also cause hepatotoxicity, eosinophilia, and joint and muscle pain, in rare instances. Hepatotoxicity occurs more frequently with zileuton use than with the other two drugs. Zileuton and zafirlukast have also been associated with reduced white blood cell counts.

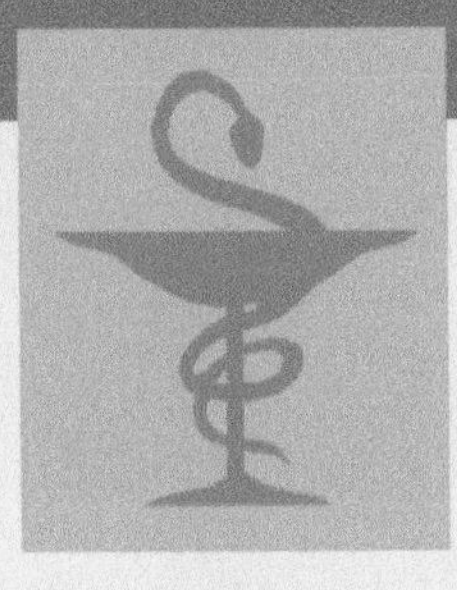

## Tips for the Technician

Patients should be instructed that these drugs are used to prevent asthmatic attacks, not to treat acute bronchospasm. It is important for patients to take their medication as directed, even when they are symptom free. Technicians will label metered dose inhalers with auxiliary "shake well" labels, and zafirlukast with an auxiliary label instructing the patient to take the drug on an empty stomach. Pharmacists should educate patients about the risk of drug interactions and side effects with the leukotriene inhibitors.

## Methylxanthine Derivatives

One of the most famous Americans to suffer from asthma was Theodore Roosevelt, our twenty-sixth president. He was born in 1858 and grew up in New York City, where coal burning was the major source of heat and energy, and a tremendous source of air pollution. Although the traditional asthma treatments of the day were not purified and delivered via inhaler, we now know their use was pharmacologically rational. Teddy was given cigarettes made of plants that contained potent anticholinergic agents to smoke and very strong coffee to drink. Coffee, tea, and chocolate all contain methylxanthine (or xanthine) derivatives known to possess stimulant, diuretic, and bronchodilatory effects. Theophylline (Theolair® and many others) and the related drug aminophylline are the methylxanthine derivatives most often used for COPD, and sometimes asthma.

### Actions and Indications

Use of theophylline and aminophylline for asthma, COPD, and as a respiratory stimulant in neonates has waxed and waned over the last fifty years. In therapeutic doses, these drugs cause bronchodilation and exert some minimal anti-inflammatory effect in the airways. They increase heart rate and contractility, cause CNS stimulation, and vasodilation. They are indicated for the treatment of COPD, after the use of anticholinergic and beta-agonist drugs. They can be used for the treatment of asthma, but are generally relegated to use in patients whose asthma is difficult to control, and where other alternatives have failed. Occasionally they are used to treat apnea (intermittent cessation of breathing) in neonates, however, caffeine is considered a safer alternative and is much more frequently used for this condition.

apnea Temporary cessation of breathing.

### Administration

Theophylline and various salts or derivative of theophylline, are available in a variety of products for oral, injectable, and rectal administration. The most convenient and widely used of the products are extended-release tablets and capsules that may be given once or twice daily. Theophylline must be administered every six hours when immediate-release products are used. When intravenous administration is desired, aminophylline is the preferred drug.

The methylxanthine derivatives undergo metabolism in the liver and the metabolites are excreted in the urine. Elimination of these drugs is extremely variable from patient to patient and serum levels are monitored in order to void toxicity. Drug dosing for these agents is based on the total amount of theophylline. Products cannot be interchanged without dosage adjustment because they contain different amounts of theophylline. Several drug interactions have an important bearing on serum levels of theophylline. People who smoke eliminate these drugs much more rapidly than nonsmokers, and are likely to require higher theophylline doses. A number of drugs increase theophylline levels, including two important infection-fighting drug classes that are frequently used to treat respiratory infections. The macrolide antibiotics (erythromycin, clarithromycin and azithromycin) and the quinolones (ciprofloxacin and many other drugs) are likely drug choices for treating bronchitis. When these drugs are taken with the theophylline derivatives they cause significant elevations in theophylline serum levels.

### Side Effects

The use of theophylline and related drugs is waning because in spite of the ability to monitor serum levels, they are difficult to dose, individuals handle the drugs differently, and the toxic dose is fairly close to the therapeutic dose (narrow therapeutic index). Therapeutic effects and side effects are closely correlated to serum levels. At serum levels in the therapeutic range or slightly above, side effects can include headache, irritability, and nausea and vomiting. At higher serum concentrations, central nervous system stimulation can lead to seizures, hypotension (related to vasodilation) becomes problematic, and cardiac arrhythmias can occur.

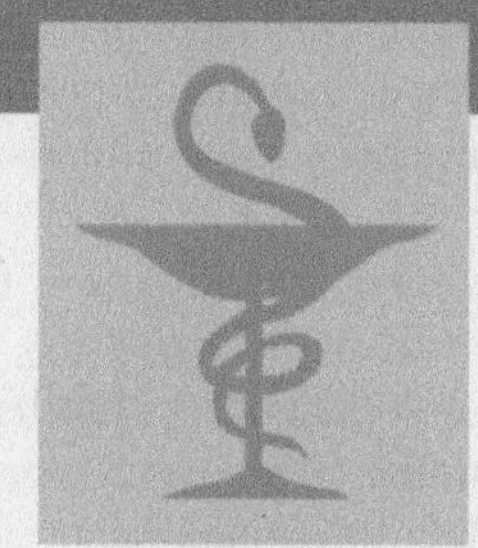

#### Tips for the Technician

All clients should receive consultation from the pharmacist when treatment with theophylline or related drugs is initiated. It is important that patients or their families understand the potential side effects and drug interactions and the importance of following their physician's orders for serum level monitoring.

The hospital-based technician will need to be aware of dosing differences between theophylline products. Products cannot be freely interchanged without verifying product equivalence with the pharmacist. For example, 100 mg of an aminophylline product contains only 80 mg theophylline. Hospital-based pharmacy technicians should be aware that many drugs and additives are incompatible with aminophylline intravenous solutions.

## Drugs Used to Treat Allergic Rhinitis, Coughs, and Colds

Rhinitis is inflammation of the mucous membranes of the nose. This inflammation may be caused by allergies or infection and is typically accompanied by nasal discharge, sneezing, and congestion. Allergic rhinitis, or hay fever, is usually seasonal, and often accompanied by itchy, irritated eyes. Treatment includes antihistamines, decongestants, and intranasal application of corticosteroids or cromolyn to combat inflammation. Preventative measures, such as air filters that remove allergens from the environment, can be quite useful.

rhinitis Inflammation of the mucous membrane of the nose.

The rhinitis that accompanies viral upper respiratory infections is self limited and treated symptomatically with decongestants or combination products designed to treat multiple cold symptoms. Coughing is a natural response to airway irritation and aids the process of clearing foreign material. However, coughs can be symptomatic of asthma, bronchitis, or simple viral infections. The medications for cough covered in this chapter are for the symptomatic treatment of coughs accompanying simple upper respiratory infections.

### Antihistamines

Most lay people think of histamine only as the cause of food allergies, skin reactions, and hay fever, and the seasonal misery associated with it. Antihistamines are likely to be found in the medicine cabinets of most Americans. However, histamine is an important biogenic amine involved in cell signalling, and research over the past thirty years has demonstrated that it mediates normal physiologic functions in the brain and the stomach, as well as being involved with allergic reactions and the immune response. Like all chemicals involved with cellular communication, histamine works by interacting with receptors. Scientists have so far identified three types of histamine receptors and research in this area continues. The $H_1$ receptor is activated in allergic reactions, activation of $H_2$ receptors in the parietal cells of the stomach cause acid secretions, and stimulation of the $H_3$ receptors found in the central and peripheral nervous system tissue appears to modulate the release of other neurotransmitters.

## Actions and Indications

The antihistamines can be subdivided into classifications based on chemical structure, but for the purpose of this discussion they will be considered one pharmacologic class with two "generations." All antihistamines are reversible antagonists at the $H_1$ receptor, and they prevent the typical effect of histamine stimulation at this receptor, including sneezing and runny nose associated with allergic rhinitis. First-generation antihistamines are nonselective and can activate $H_1$ receptors found in the central nervous system, which accounts for their reputation as "sedating" antihistamines. The second-generation, "nonsedating" antihistamines are selective for peripheral $H_1$ receptors. Antihistamines do nothing to prevent the release of histamine, and they do not reverse the effects of histamine once it binds to receptors and the inflammatory process begins.

pruritus Itching.

atopic dermatitis An inflammatory skin condition, characterized by dry skin, itchy, scaly rash, and often associated with allergies.

As a group, the antihistamines are indicated for allergic reactions, including in some cases the treatment of hives, and the pruritus (itching) associated with atopic dermatitis, an allergic skin condition commonly referred to as eczema. Several first-generations antihistamines, including the phenothiazine-like drugs and diphenhydramine (Benadryl®), have strong anticholinergic effects. These anticholinergic effects explain the antinauseant and the drying effects of antihistamines. Because of their drying effect on secretions, antihistamines are generally not recommended for routine use in either asthma or eczema. If mucous becomes thick, it becomes more difficult for the natural removal processes in the lungs to clear it out. These drugs are often found in cough and cold preparations (for drying nasal secretions), are useful as sedatives, and are effective for prevention of motion sickness. Diphenhydramine is used in hospitals for treating allergic reactions to medications and dystonia caused by antipsychotic agents or the antiemetic phenothiazines. In spite of its significant sedating effects, diphenhydramine remains the standard antihistamine to which other drugs are compared.

## Administration

Antihistamines for the treatment of allergic rhinitis are administered orally and are well absorbed. Most of the first-generation antihistamines require administration every 6 hours, so a number of extended-release products are available. The second-generation antihistamine fexofenadine (Allegra®) is given every 12 hours, while cetirizine (Zyrtec®) and loratadine (Claritin®) only require once-daily dosing. Because of the variety of indications for use, the antihistamines are available in an assortment of formulations for oral, injectable, rectal, and topical administration. Refer to Table 20.1 for a comparison of the names, uses, and available formulations of drugs described in this chapter.

As is typical of all drug products, indications for use influence the available product formats. In other words, an antihistamine indicated for use in vomiting is likely to be manufactured as a solution for injection and as suppositories for rectal administration, since oral administration in a nauseated patient is not particularly successful. Promethazine (Phenergan®), a drug classified as both an antihistamine and a phenothiazine, is available for injection and as a suppository for treatment of nausea and vomiting, and as tablets and liquids for use in the treatment of allergies and upper respiratory symptoms. Diphenhydramine, which is available in solution for injection and in nearly every conceivable kind of oral preparation, is also sold as a cream or combined with calamine lotion for hypersensitivity reactions of the skin. With the exception of azelastine nasal spray (Astelin®), the second-generation, nonsedating antihistamines are administered orally.

Among these, cetirizine and loratadine are available in oral formulations appropriate for use in children.

## Side Effects

The most common side effect of the nonspecific antihistamines is sedation. The sedating effects of these drugs can be additive with other CNS depressant medications. Promethazine, diphenhydramine, and hydroxyzine (Atarax® and Vistaril®) are the most sedating of the first-generation agents. When these three drugs are administered intravenously, side affects such as dizziness, hypotension, and sedation can be profound. Of the second-generation antihistamines, cetirizine is the most likely to cause drowsiness, although it is minimal. Lower antihistamine doses are recommended for elderly patients, who are more likely to become oversedated, confused, dizzy, or hypotensive. Children can exhibit a paradoxical response to antihistamines and become excitable and wakeful instead of being sedated.

Because of the anticholinergic effects, these drugs can cause urinary retention, especially in men with benign prostatic hypertrophy. Promethazine and hydroxyzine can cause dyskinesias because of their chemical relationship to the phenothiazines. These are more likely in the elderly and in newborn infants of mothers who are given these medications. The antihistamines should not be used in pregnancy because of the possibility of fetal malformations when used early in pregnancy and the risk of toxic effects in the neonate when used late in pregnancy.

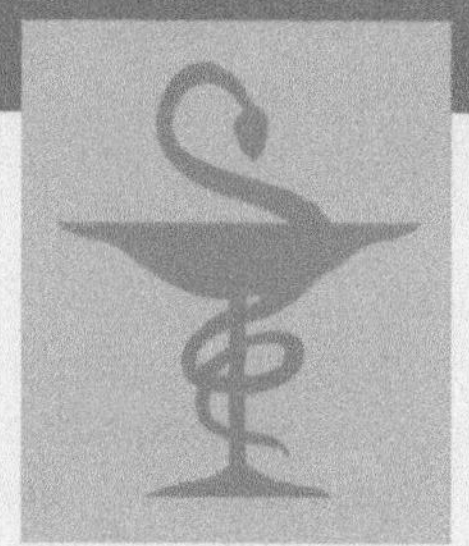

### Tips for the Technician

Many antihistamines are available without prescription. Technicians should urge patients to read the package labelling for warnings and contraindications (conditions that preclude the use of a drug). Any prescription antihistamine or combination antihistamine product should be labelled with auxiliary labels that warn of potential sedation and discourage the consumption of alcoholic beverages. Extended-release products should not be crushed. Hydroxyzine is manufactured as the hydrochloride and pamoate salts. Verify which product is ordered before dispensing. Promethazine suppositories are stored in the refrigerator and should be labelled accordingly.

# Cough Suppressants, Decongestants, and Expectorants

Americans have more than one billion colds every year. Colds are the most common form of infection, and the most common reason for children to miss school. Drug manufacturers sell an enormous number of products for the treatment of cold symptoms, even though colds go away on their own in a few days anyway. However, when patients are so uncomfortable with cold symptoms that they cannot sleep, decongestants, cough suppressants, and expectorants can be useful. These drugs are indicated for the short-term treatment of symptoms accompanying colds and other upper respiratory infections.

## Actions and Indications

Alpha-adrenergic agonists constrict small vessels in the nasal mucosa and reduce congestion and airway resistance. Pseudoephedrine (Sudafed®), phenylephrine (neo-Synephrine®), oxymetazoline (Afrin®), and others are alpha-agonists useful as nasal decongestants. These products are used for short-term reversal of nasal congestion.

Throat irritation caused by viral infection and postnasal drip stimulates the cough centers in the CNS. The opiate cough suppressants, including codeine, decrease the sensitivity of these cough centers. The antitussive actions occur at doses lower than those required for analgesia (refer to Chapter 9 for additional information). Dextromethorphan (Delsym®), a synthetic derivative of morphine, suppresses the response of the cough center by the same mechanism. It has no analgesic or addictive potential and is less constipating than codeine.

An expectorant is a drug that promotes the removal of sputum from the lungs. Guaifenesin (Robitussin®, others), the most frequently used expectorant, works by increasing the production of mucous and decreasing the viscosity of mucous, thereby leading to greater ease in expelling it from the airways. Use of iodinated glycerol does not consistently prove effective in studies and at this time is rarely used. Some experts believe that drinking adequate fluids and using a room air humidifier provides results equal to or superior to the use of an expectorant. Successful treatment with guaifenesin requires use of effective doses and consumption of plenty of fluids.

## Administration

Many nasal decongestant products are designed for local use in the nose, either as nasal sprays or drops. Most nasal decongestant products are available without a prescription. Pseudoephedrine is perhaps the most universally used orally administered decongestant. It is available in a variety of formulations, including regular-release tablets and capsules, chewable tablets, extended-release tablets, pediatric liquid in two concentrations and infant drops in a higher concentration formula.

Dextromethorphan is available alone and in many combination products for colds. It is a nonprescription drug that is taken by mouth. The combination of dextromethorphan with guaifenesin in cough preparations is common. Like dextromethorphan, guaifenesin is administered orally and is available without prescription in most strengths and formulations. It is available as a single drug entity formulated in tablets, capsules, and liquids, as well as being combined with a variety of other drugs for relief of cold symptoms.

## Side Effects

When administered as an aerosol, nasal decongestants work quickly and cause few systemic side effects. However, they should be used no longer than several days, because rebound nasal congestion occurs on discontinuation after more prolonged use. Oral administration of decongestants can elevate blood pressure, especially in hypertensive clients. People with glaucoma and cardiac disease, and patients taking MAO inhibitors should avoid using systemic decongestants.

Adverse effects related to use of dextromethorphan and guaifenesin are uncommon in normal doses. Nausea and vomiting may occur with either drug. Patients taking monamine oxidase inhibitors, including selegiline, cannot use dextromethorphan. There are no significant drug interactions with guaifenesin. Both dextromethorphan and pseudoephedrine carry some risk of abuse. Dextromethorphan can cause hallucinations when taken in extremely high doses, and pseudoephedrine can be converted to the stimulant methamphetamine. By federal law, pseudoephedrine-containing products are now stored behind the prescription counter. Individuals who purchase them must show identification, and pharmacies must keep records of purchaser's identification.

### Tips for the Technician

Any prescription for a narcotic antitussive should be properly labelled with auxiliary warning instructions. Patients should be cautioned that they could experience drowsiness when taking these products and should avoid operating complex machinery. In addition, attach a label to the container that directs the patient to avoid the consumption of alcoholic beverages.

Many products used for the common cold are available without prescription. Although consumers may seek the advice of a technician regarding these products, it is important to refer questions requiring clinical judgement to the pharmacist. Even though drugs are sold over the counter, they can interact with prescription medications and may not be indicated for use by some people because of their underlying disease states. This is the case with the orally administered alpha adrenergic agonists pseudoephedrine and phenylephrine (Entex® LA and others). Consumers should be encouraged to read and follow all of the package instructions for use of any over the counter drug, especially if they have never used the product before.

# Review Questions

## Multiple Choice

Choose the best answer for the following questions:

1. Which of the following statements about asthma is true?
   a. Asthma is the most common chronic disease in children.
   b. More than 5,000 people die of asthma every year in the United States.
   c. Nearly two million asthma related emergency room visits occur annually in the United States.
   d. Beta-agonist inhalers are the foundation of treatment of acute asthma.
   e. All of the above are true.

2. Which of the following is the most common cause of COPD in the United States?
   a. Childhood asthma
   b. Working for many years in an occupation that requires you to live at a high altitude
   c. Smoking
   d. Industrial exposure
   e. Living in a smoggy environment

3. What is the goal of asthma treatment?
   a. Prevent asthma attacks
   b. Keep asthma from altering the lifestyle of the family or patient
   c. Relieve symptoms associated with the disease
   d. a and c
   e. b and c

4. Of the following medication combinations, which is most likely to be used for the treatment of COPD?
   a. Albuterol MDI and budesonide MDI
   b. Albuterol and ipratropium MDI, plus an oral corticosteroid
   c. Albuterol and Advair® inhalers-plus montelukast tablets
   d. Albuterol and cromolyn MDI
   e. A short-acting beta-agonist alone

5. The pharmacy technician will apply which of the following auxiliary instruction to a Flovent® MDI?
   a. Shake well
   b. Rinse mouth after each use
   c. Clean mouthpiece after each use
   d. All of the above should be applied
   e. None of the above should be applied

## True/False

6. Theophylline is a first-line drug in the treatment of asthma because it is effective, easy to use, and is relatively free of side effects.
   a. True
   b. False

7. Spacers are used with metered dose inhalers mainly to reduce the unpleasant taste of the medications.
   a. True
   b. False

8. The most common side effect of orally administered antihistamines of both generations is drowsiness, but drowsiness is less significant with second-generation antihistamines.
   a. True
   b. False

9. An expectorant is a drug that promotes the removal of sputum from the lungs.
   a. True
   b. False

10. Decongestants cause blood vessels to dilate so that the patient can breathe through them more easily.
    a. True
    b. False

## Matching

For numbers 11 to 15, match the drug name with the correct pharmacologic class from the list below. Choices will not be used more than once and may not be used at all.

| | |
|---|---|
| 11. Oxymetazoline | a. Second-generation antihistamine |
| | b. Expectorant |
| 12. Aminophylline | c. Decongestant |
| | d. Methylxanthine derivative |
| 13. Atrovent® | e. Respiratory corticosteroid |
| 14. Zyrtec® | f. First-generation antihistamine |
| 15. Benadryl® | g. Bronchodilator |

## Short Answer

16. Explain why it is more desirable to administer corticosteroids by inhalation rather than by mouth.

17. Why should patients who use a short-acting beta-agonist MDI along with another, anti-inflammatory MDI, such as cromolyn or a corticosteroid, administer the short-acting beta-agonist first?

18. Patients with moderate asthma are usually treated with a beta-agonist, such as albuterol, and another drug such as the inhaled corticosteroids or mast cell stabilizers. What is the difference in how these drugs act, and what are their roles in asthma treatment?

19. What is the most important preventative measure a person can take to prevent COPD?

20. Which people should avoid taking nasal decongestants?

## FOR FURTHER INQUIRY

Besides being considered more mature, sophisticated, and appealing to the opposite sex, nonsmokers also reap multiple health benefits. Learn more interesting facts about the damaging effects of tobacco use and how to quit smoking by searching on the Internet or by visiting one of the web sites listed here. Recommended sites include the following: www.cdc.gov/tobacco/index.htm, www.anti-smoking.org, and www.smokefree.gov.

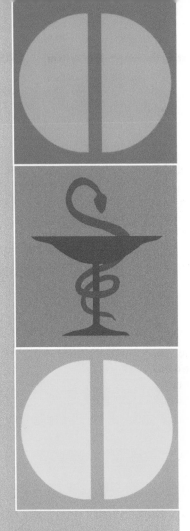

Chapter **21**

# Diuretics and Other Drugs Affecting the Urinary System

## OBJECTIVES

After studying this chapter, the reader should be able to:

- List four classes of diuretics and describe their mechanism of action, including where in the nephron they exert their effect.
- Describe two common side effects seen with the loop diuretics and thiazide diuretics and explain how the side effects relate to the mechanism of action of the drugs.
- Explain what precautions a pregnant pharmacy technician should take when filling prescriptions for androgen inhibitors and why there is a concern.
- List three side effects common to the urinary tract antispasmodics.
- Define "erectile dysfunction" and identify two drugs used to treat this condition by their generic names.

*KEY TERMS*

- erectile dysfunction
- hirsutism
- oxotoxic

## DRUGS COVERED IN THIS CHAPTER*

### Diuretics

| Loop Diuretics | Thiazide Diuretics | Potassium-Sparing Diuretics | Miscellaneous Diuretics |
|---|---|---|---|
| Bumetanide | Chlorothiazide | Amiloride | Acetazolamide |
| Ethacrynic Acid | Chlorthalidone | Spironolactone | Mannitol |
| Furosemide | Hydrochlorothiazide | Triamterene | |
| Torsemide | Metolazone | | |

### Drugs for BPH

| Androgen Inhibitors | Alpha-Blockers |
|---|---|
| Dutasteride | Tamsulosin |
| Finasteride | Terazosin |

### Urinary Tract Antispasmodic and Analgesic Agents

Oxybutynin
Tolterodine
Trospium
Phenazopyridine

### Drugs for Erectile Dysfunction

Sildenafil
Tadalafil
Vardenafil

** Medications covered in this chapter exert effects on the urinary tract.*

Pathology in the urinary system occur as a result of aging, illnesses that affect the kidneys and urinary tract, such as diabetes or hypertension, and damage caused by drugs, infection, or other sources of injury. Renal failure is the most serious problem, but more common complaints include urinary tract infections, benign prostatic hypertrophy (BPH), urinary incontinence, and erectile dysfunction in men. This chapter will focus on drugs that act on the urinary system, including the diuretics and the drugs used to treat BPH, urinary incontinence, and erectile dysfunction. A discussion of antibiotics and urinary antiseptics used to treat bladder and other urinary tract infections can be found in Chapters 29 and 30.

# Diuretics

Drugs that increase the production and flow of urine are called diuretics. The efficacy of the different classes of diuretics varies and is dependent upon the site and mechanism of their action. Further discussion of the thiazide diuretics can be found in Chapter 17.

## Actions and Indications

The major clinical uses of diuretics are in managing disorders involving abnormal fluid retention (for example in heart failure) or in treating hypertension. Diuretics may be useful to control edema and hypertension in chronic renal failure, and are sometimes indicated in acute renal failure. Diuretics must be used judiciously in renal failure because dehydration can be the cause of, or exacerbate, acute or chronic renal failure.

Diuretics exert their action by reducing the reabsorption of sodium and chloride in the tubules of the kidney. As a result, the excretion of both fluids and electrolytes increases. The potential for fluid removal is dependant upon the site of diuretic action, and diuretics are often classified accordingly (**Fig. 21.1**). Drugs that act upon the loop of Henle are the most effective at mobilizing fluid and sodium and are called loop diuretics. Compared to all other classes of diuretics, these drugs produce copious amounts of urine. Furosemide (Lasix®) was the ninth most frequently dispensed drug in the United States in 2004. Use of furosemide and bumetanide (Bumex®), an equally effective loop diuretic, is quite common in hospitals.

The thiazide and thiazide-like diuretics act mainly in the distal tubule to decrease the reabsorption of sodium. They exert a minor effect in the proximal tubule. After the loop diuretics, the thiazide-type diuretics are the next most effective class. The thiazides reduce the excretion of calcium in the urine, an effect that is useful in people who form calcium oxalate kidney stones. This diuretic class is useful in the treatment of diabetes insipidus, a disease characterized by the voluminous production of dilute urine, which is caused by defects in the production or action of antidiuretic hormone. In diabetes insipidus, the thiazide diuretics exert the seemingly paradoxical effect of reducing urine volume.

Potassium-sparing diuretics act in the collecting tubule to inhibit sodium reabsorption and potassium excretion. The major use of the potassium-sparing drugs is in the treatment of hypertension, where they are most often combined with a thiazide diuretic (Dyazide®, Maxzide®). The potassium-sparing diuretics are less effective at producing diuresis than the thiazides and more effective than the carbonic anhydrase inhibitor, acetazolamide (Diamox®). Spironolactone is a direct aldosterone antagonist and is useful in conditions where there is an excess of aldosterone, such as in heart failure.

Acetazolamide is a weak diuretic that works by inhibiting the reabsorption of bicarbonate ions in the proximal convoluted tubule. As a result, urine pH increases and retention of hydrogen ions causes mild metabolic acidosis (reduction of the pH of the blood). This drug loses its diuretic effect after a few days of therapy and is more often used for its other pharmacologic effects. It lowers intraocular pressure in glaucoma by inhibiting carbonic anhydrase in the eye. Backpackers or hikers who experience nausea, headache, and shortness of breath associated with rapid ascent to altitudes of 10,000 feet or higher can take acetazolamide for five days in advance of a hike to prevent acute mountain sickness.

Mannitol is an example of a simple, hydrophilic chemical substance that, when filtered by the glomerulus, causes diuresis. This is due to its ability to carry water with it, by osmosis, into the forming urine. The word osmosis describes the movement of water (solvent) across a semipermeable membrane. This movement of solvent occurs when a nonpenetrable solute, in this case mannitol, is concentrated on one side of the membrane. The movement of the solvent tends to balance the concentration of the solute. In the kidneys, if the substance that is filtered subsequently undergoes little or no reabsorption, there will be an increase in urine output. Diuretics with this mechanism of action are called osmotic diuretics. Osmotic diuretics increase water excretion rather than increasing sodium excretion, so they are not useful for treating conditions where sodium retention occurs. They are a mainstay of treatment for patients with increased intracranial pressure or acute renal failure due to shock, drug toxicities, and trauma.

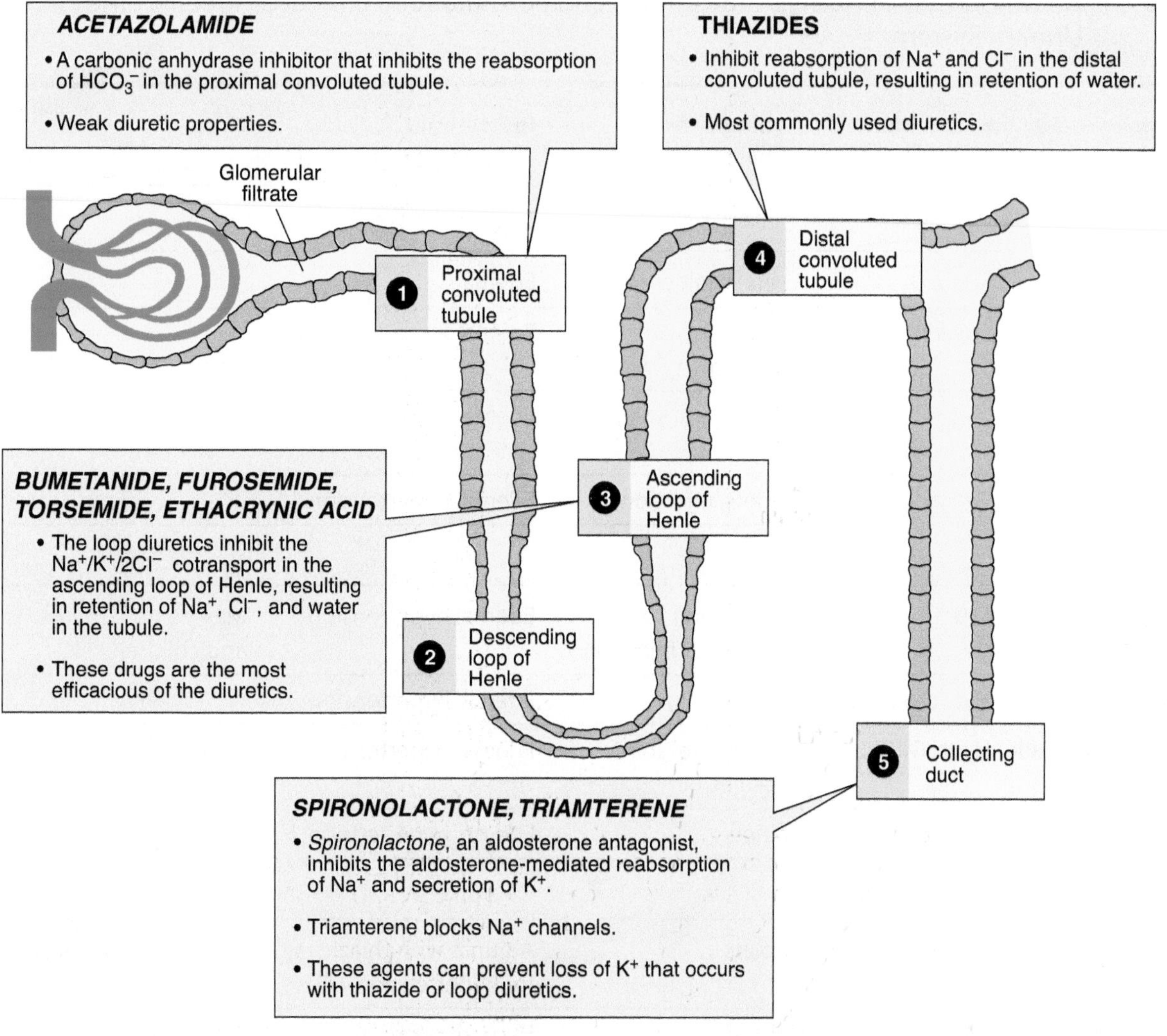


**Figure 21.1** The sites of diuretic action in the renal tubule. (Adapted with permission from Harvey RA, Champe PC, Howland RD, et al. *Lippincott's Illustrated Reviews: Pharmacology*, 3rd edition. Baltimore: Lippincott Williams & Wilkins, 2006.)

## Analogy

Most little kids, at one time or another, have done the backyard experiment of putting salt on a snail. When you salt a snail, the salt immediately draws all the water out of the snail's body and it shrivels up and dies. Mannitol works to draw water into the urine much like the salt works to draw water out of a snail. The high concentration of solute (the salt and the mannitol) draws fluid across the concentration gradient in order to even out the concentration of solute.

## Administration

All of the loop diuretics are adequately absorbed orally, and are available in a variety of formulations for oral use (see **Table 21.1**). In addition, these drugs can be administered by direct intravenous injection. Furosemide and bumetanide can be given by intramuscular injection.

**Table 21.1** A Comparison of Names, Indications, and Formulations of Drugs Affecting the Urinary System

| Generic | Brand Name | Available as | Indications | Notes |
|---|---|---|---|---|
| **Loop Diuretics** | | | | |
| Bumetanide | Bumex® | Tablets, injection | Edema | |
| Ethacrynic Acid | Edecrin® | Tablets, powder for injection | Edema | |
| Furosemide | Lasix® | Tablets, oral soln, injection | Edema, hypertension, HF | |
| Torsemide | Demadex® | Tablets, injection | Edema, hypertension | |
| **Thiazide Diuretics** | | | | |
| Chlorothiazide | Diuril® | Tablets, oral susp, powder for injection | Edema, hypertension | May be used in infants and children |
| Chlorthalidone | Hygroton® | Tablets | Edema, hypertension | |
| Hydrochlorothiazide | HydroDIURIL® | Tablets, oral soln, capsules | Edema, hypertension | Used in infants and children |
| Metolazone | Zaroxolyn® | Tablets | Edema, hypertension, HF | |
| **Potassium-Sparing Diuretics** | | | | |
| Amiloride | Midamor® | Tablets | Adjunct with thiazides for hypertension, HF | Give with food |
| Spironolactone | Aldactone® | Tablets | Hypertension, HF, edema, primary hyper-aldosteronism | Aldosterone antagonist properties |
| Triamterene | Dyrenium®, Dyazide®, Maxzide® | Capsules | Edema | Dyazide®, Maxzide® include hydrochloro-thiazide |
| **Other Diuretics** | | | | |
| Acetazolamide | Diamox® | Tablets, ER caps, injection | Glaucoma, mountain sickness, edema, some forms of epilepsy | |
| Mannitol | Osmitrol® | Vials and bottles for IV infusion | Acute renal failure, cerebral edema, glaucoma, overdoses | Concenrated solutions may crystalize |
| **Alpha-Blockers** | | | | |
| Tamsulosin | Flomax® | Capsules | BPH | |
| Terazosin | Hytrin® | Capsules | BPH, Hypertension | |

BPH, benign prostatic hypertrophy; ER, extended release; HF, heart failure.

*(continues)*

| Generic | Brand Name | Available as | Indications | Notes |
|---|---|---|---|---|
| **Androgen Inhibitors** | | | | |
| Dutasteride | Avodart® | Tablets | BPH, | |
| Finasteride | Proscar®, Propecia® | Tablets | BPH, male pattern baldness | |
| **Urinary Tract Antispasmodic and Analgesic** | | | | |
| Oxybutynin | Ditropan® | Tablets, ER tabs, soln, transdermal | Overactive Bladder | |
| Tolterodine | Detrol® | Tablets, ER caps | Overactive Bladder | |
| Trospium | Sanctura® | Tablets | Overactive Bladder | |
| Phenazopyridine | Pyridium® | Tablets | Bladder analgesic | |
| **PDE 5 Inhibitors** | | | | |
| Sildenafil | Viagra® | Tablets | Erectile Dysfunction | |
| Tadalafil | Cialis® | Tablets | Erectile Dysfunction | |
| Vardenafil | Levitra® | Tablets | Erectile Dysfunction | |

The thiazide diuretics are well absorbed through the GI tract, can be taken without regard to food, and are available in a variety of products. Only chlorothiazide is available for injection, where it is more likely to be administered to pediatric patients than adults. The potassium-sparing diuretics and acetazolamide are administered orally. Absorption of amiloride is poor and it should be administered with food to maximize absorption. The other potassium-sparing diuretics can be given without regard to meals.

Mannitol, an osmotic diuretic, must be administered by slow intravenous injection or by intravenous infusion. Mannitol solutions are available in 5%, 10%, 15%, and 20% concentrations in larger volumes ready for infusion, and in 25% concentration, in 50 mL vials. Mannitol in concentrations greater than 15% is prone to crystallization at cool room temperatures. The solution can be used after warming in a warm water bath or other warming device.

## Side Effects

Side effects are more common with administration of the loop diuretics because they cause the greatest diuresis. By increasing the volume of urine, and the excretion of sodium, potassium, and other electrolytes, the loop diuretics alter the concentration of electrolytes in the blood. To varying degrees, the thiazide diuretics cause similar changes in electrolytes and blood volume. Hypokalemia, or reduced blood levels of potassium, is the most problematic of the likely electrolyte changes. Low potassium levels can result in weakness, muscle cramping, delirium, and arrhythmias. Hypokalemia is especially dangerous in patients who take digoxin because it increases the risk of digoxin toxicity. Other electrolytes, including magnesium and calcium, can also be depleted. Dehydration can occur, and in some individuals (especially the elderly or those who have other illnesses) can undermine renal function or cause acute renal failure. In some cases, volume depletion results in hypotension.

Uric acid retention can occur as a result of treatment with furosemide, ethacrynic acid, or the thiazide diuretics. In the kidneys, the diuretics compete with uric acid for secretion. Elevated uric acid levels increase the risk of acute gouty attacks, especially in patients with this disease. Other metabolic effects, including altered glucose metabolism, can occur with the loop diuretics and the thiazide diuretics. Altered glucose metabolism can impact the treatment of diabetes.

The loop diuretics can cause hearing impairment, especially when administered by rapid intravenous injection, if given in large doses, or when given in conjunction with other drugs toxic to the ears. The damage to hearing can be permanent if treatment with the ototoxic drug continues. Ethacrynic acid is the most likely of the loop diuretics to cause deafness.

ototoxic Toxic to the nerves and other anatomical structures involved in hearing.

While hypokalemia is associated with use of the thiazide and loop diuretics, hyperkalemia is a side effect of the potassium-sparing diuretics. Elevated potassium levels can occur as a result of kidney failure, and the potassium-sparing diuretics are contraindicated in people with chronic renal failure. Amiloride has a more pronounced effect on potassium retention in some patients, but it is the least commonly used drug of this class. The potassium-sparing diuretics interact with other drugs that elevate potassium levels, including the ACE inhibitors, potassium supplements, and also with salt substitutes, which contain high levels of potassium.

The loop and thiazide diuretics can cause nausea and vomiting. These diuretics are sulfa-containing compounds, with the potential to cause allergic reactions in sulfa sensitive patients. Rarely, the thiazides and loop diuretics can suppress the production of blood cells in the bone marrow, and cause other sulfa-related side effects.

Besides antagonizing the effects of aldosterone, spironolactone has weak antiandrogen activity. As a result, some men taking the drug may experience adverse sexual side effects, including inability to maintain an erection and gynecomastia, or breast enlargement and tenderness. Women who take this drug may experience changes in their menstrual cycles. Because of the antiandrogen activity, spironolactone has been used to treat women with hirsutism, or excessive body hair.

hirsutism Excessive hair growth, especially male patterned hair distribution in women.

Acetazolamide is another sulfa-containing compound and sulfa type side effects such as allergic reactions and bone marrow suppression can occur with it as well. As is true with all diuretics, fluid and electrolyte abnormalities can occur. Because this drug is a mild diuretic, these abnormalities are mild. Mannitol can also cause fluid and electrolyte abnormalities. Physicians exercise caution when administering this drug to patients with compromised cardiovascular systems, because it can temporarily increase the load on the heart.

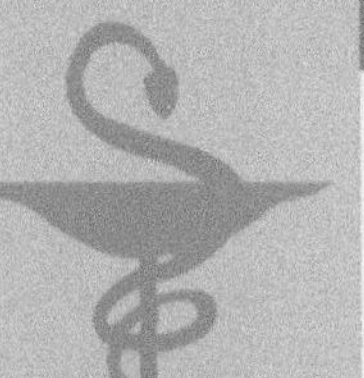

## Tips for the Technician

Bumetanide, torsemide (Demadex®), furosemide, the thiazide diuretics, and acetazolamide are all sulfonamide derivatives, and can cause allergic reactions in patients who are allergic to sulfa drugs. Therefore, complete and accurate patient profiles are necessary to prevent unnecessary risk of exposure. As sulfa derivatives, these drugs can predispose patients to photosensitivity, and prescription vials should be labelled with the appropriate auxiliary warning label.

The loop and the thiazide diuretics may be taken with food or milk to prevent nausea or GI upset. Because of the effects on uric acid and glucose metabolism, patients with gout or diabetes should be forewarned about the possibility that they may require changes in their treatment while taking the loop or thiazide diuretics. All patients on diuretics should be warned about the possibility of dizziness on arising. Getting up slowly can prevent this problem.

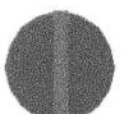

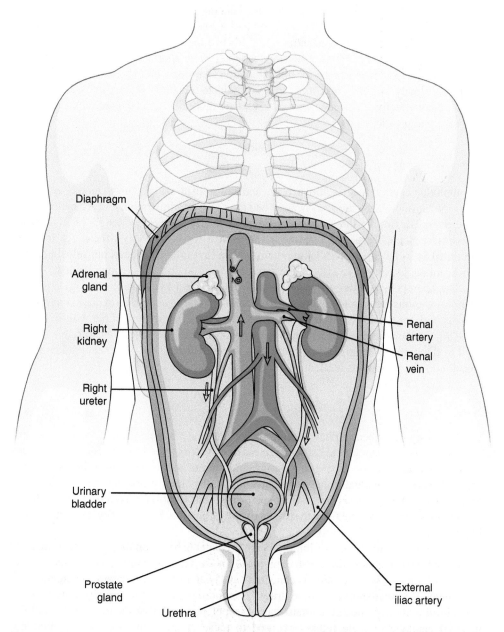

## Drugs for Treatment of Prostate Disease

The prostate gland wraps around the urethra in men (see **Fig. 21.2**). Situated under the bladder, the primary function of the prostate is to add seminal fluid to the sperm before it is ejaculated. As a man ages, the prostate gland enlarges and puts pressure on the urethra. Sometimes this enlargement is malignant, but more commonly it is benign. Recent advancements in the study of BPH have shown that symptoms are caused not only by mechanical pressure, but also by neurologic changes in the bladder and prostate. In the past, the standard treatment for BPH was surgical resection of the gland. Now pharmacologic treatments are used initially and are effective in a significant number of patients. Drug treatments include alpha-adrenergic antagonists and androgen inhibitors.

Diaphragm
Adrenal gland
Right kidney
Right ureter
Urinary bladder
Prostate gland
Urethra
Renal artery
Renal vein
External iliac artery

**Figure 21.2** Anatomy of the male reproductive system. (Adapted with permission from Cohen BJ. *Memmler's The Human Body in Health and Disease*, 10th edition. Baltimore: Lippincott Williams & Wilkins, 2005.)

## Actions and Indication

The alpha-antagonists are used as an alternative to surgery in patients with symptomatic BPH. Blockade of α-receptors decreases tone in smooth muscle, thereby causing relaxation of the bladder neck and the smooth muscle of the prostate, and improvement in urine outflow. Two nonspecific alpha-blockers, terazosin (Hytrin®) and doxazosin (Cardura®), are indicated for treatment of hypertension and are used for BPH. Although alpha-antagonists are not first-line drugs in the treatment of hypertension, they are a useful option in men who have both disorders. Tamsulosin (Flomax®) is an alpha-antagonist that specifically blocks alpha-receptors in the prostate gland. It is indicated for the treatment of BPH, but not for hypertension. All alpha-antagonists cause rapid improvement in urine outflow and the effect is not dependent on the degree of prostate enlargement.

The other class of drugs used to treat BPH is the 5α-reductase inhibitors, or the androgen inhibitors. These drugs block the enzyme that converts testosterone to the more potent dihydrotestosterone (DHT), a hormone that plays a role in the enlargement of the prostate. These drugs also reduce the concentration of DHT in the scalp, thereby reducing hair loss in male pattern baldness. Finasteride (Proscar®) is FDA approved for treatment of male pattern baldness and is marketed for this indication as Propecia®. The androgen inhibitors work very slowly, and may take three to six months to reduce prostate size by 20%. These drugs are not effective in all men with BPH and are more likely to be effective in men with very enlarged prostates.

## Administration

The alpha-blockers terazosin, doxazosin, and tamsulosin are given by mouth, as either tablets or capsules. They are readily absorbed after oral administration and are metabolized in the liver. The dose of these drugs should be gradually increased when initiated to avoid hypotensive side effects. If the dosing is interrupted for several days, the drugs must be reinitiated as if the patient was taking them for the first time. Although tamsulosin has no significant antihypertensive effects, the same approach to dosing is recommended.

The androgen inhibitors, finasteride and dutasteride (Avodart®), are well absorbed after oral administration and are metabolized in the liver. No alteration in dose is needed in patients with renal failure, but these drugs are used with caution in people with liver failure. They can be administered without regard to meals. Because results are variable and related to duration of therapy, a minimum of six months treatment is recommended before abandoning the therapy as ineffective.

## Side Effects

As previously described, alpha-blocking drugs can cause hypotension, occasionally with blood pressures low enough to cause dizziness or even loss of consciousness. This problem is especially apparent on arising and during initiation of the medication. It is for this reason that doses are gradually increased early in therapy. Less problematic undesirable effects include GI upset, nasal congestion, and drowsiness. Caution is exercised when administering these drugs to patients with serious liver dysfunction, because they are metabolized in the liver.

Side effects of the androgen inhibitors are predictable based on their pharmacologic effects. Men who take these drugs can experience reduced libido or impotence. Although not indicated for use in women, serious concerns have been raised with regard to potential risk to pregnant women exposed to these drugs. The androgen inhibitors are absorbed through the skin. Based on studies in animals, there is a potential risk that the development of the external genitalia of male fetuses exposed to these drugs in utero could be inhibited. Women of childbearing age who are or could become pregnant are cautioned not to come in contact with tablets, tablet dust, or leaky capsules.

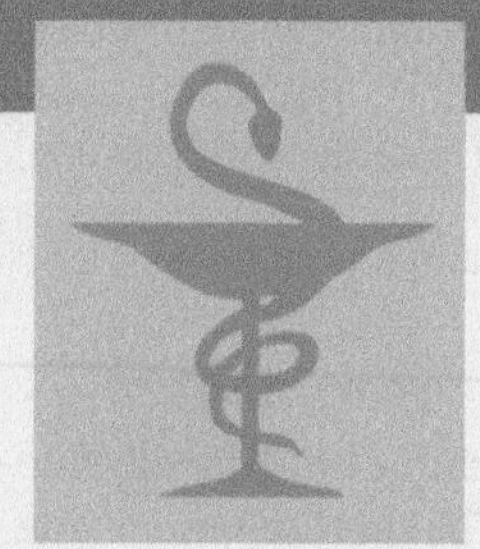

**Tips for the Technician**

Clients should be warned by the pharmacist about the possibility of low blood pressure on arising, dizziness, and drowsiness, especially early in therapy with the alpha-blockers. Patients may be more prone to postural hypotension after standing for long periods, when alcohol is consumed, or in hot weather. Auxiliary labels advising caution when driving or consuming alcohol should be applied to the prescriptions.

Female pharmacy technicians who are pregnant need to exercise caution when filling prescriptions for either finasteride or dutasteride. Reasonable precautions include: wear gloves, avoid handling broken or crushed tablets, do not use automated counting machines, and use good handwashing techniques after handling the medication. Delegating the responsibility of handling these medications to a male or non-pregnant coworker is another option. Thorough cleaning of equipment used in dispensing these drugs is important in order to prevent contamination of subsequently handled drugs. Men taking these medications should be warned of the potential risk posed to pregnant women in their homes caused by handling broken tablets, tablet dust, or leaky capsules.

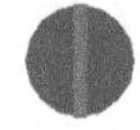

# Urinary Tract Antispasmodics and Analgesics

Urinary incontinence is a problem that affects a surprising number of older individuals, especially women. Although approximately one third of women over the age of 65 experience some form of incontinence, only half of these will ever mention the problem to their physicians. As our population ages and the market for treatments of what can be an embarrassing problem increases, pharmaceutical companies will undoubtedly continue to develop new antispasmodic drug treatments.

## Actions and Indications

The urinary antispasmodics are anticholinergic drugs indicated for the treatment of urge incontinence, or what is commonly termed overactive bladder. Urge incontinence is characterized by the sudden and uncontrollable need to urinate. People with urge incontinence feel the need to urinate frequently during the day and may wake up multiple times in the night to urinate. This is different from stress incontinence, which is characterized by incontinence episodes with sneezing, coughing, or strenuous exercise. Drug therapy is not indicated for the treatment of stress incontinence. The urinary antispasmodics work by inhibiting bladder contractions. Pelvic floor strengthening exercises are an effective nonpharmacologic means to increase bladder control in both types of incontinence.

The urinary tract analgesic phenazopyridine (Pyridium®) is useful in the early treatment of cystitis or for treatment of bladder pain caused by trauma. It has no antibacterial or other action on the bladder and therefore does not treat underlying causes of bladder pain. Phenazopyridine is a dye that is excreted into the urine. It has a topical analgesic effect conferred by an unknown mechanism.

## Administration

Urinary tract antispasmodics are available for oral administration in immediate release and sustained-release preparations. Tolterodine in the long-acting formulation (Detrol® LA) is administered once daily, whereas the regular release formulation is given twice a day. Oxybutynin (Ditropan®) is manufactured as syrup for oral use and transdermal patch. Transdermal oxybutynin patches are applied topically, twice weekly. Phenazopyridine is administered orally, usually for the first two days of treatment of a urinary tract infection, to reduce pain and urgency.

## Side Effects

The urinary antispasmodic agents are anticholinergics and as might be anticipated, side effects are similar to those seen with other anticholinergic drugs. The most common side effects are dry mouth, constipation, headache, and dizziness. Other reported anticholinergic side effects include dry eyes, urinary retention, and blurred vision. Because sweating can be inhibited by these medicines, some individuals may become more sensitive to heat, and extreme heat should be avoided.

Phenazopyridine administration is usually not accompanied by significant side effects because the duration of use is limited. Some people may experience GI upset, headache, or rash. In cases where the dose or duration is excessive, or the drug is used in people with poor renal function, hemolytic anemia can develop. This form of anemia is uncommon, but when it does occur it is often related to an adverse reaction to a drug the patient is receiving.

### Tips for the Technician

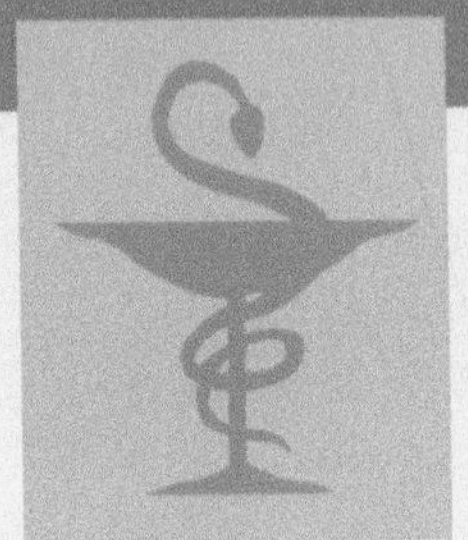

The urinary antispasmodics can cause drowsiness or dizziness that could impair patients' ability to operate complex machinery. Consumption of alcoholic beverages can intensify this effect. The pharmacist should caution clients regarding these and other typical anticholinergic side effects. Auxiliary labels warning of the possibility of drowsiness that is made worse by alcohol consumption should be affixed to the prescription vials. Trospium (Sanctura®) is taken on an empty stomach and should be labelled accordingly.

Phenazopyridine is one of several drugs that can alter the color of urine. It causes a dark, reddish-orange discoloration that patients may confuse with blood if they are not warned of this effect. Phenazopyridine should be taken after meals to avoid GI upset. Prescription containers need to be labelled appropriately.

# Drugs Used to Treat Erectile Dysfunction

erectile dysfunction
Routine inability to maintain an erection sufficient for sexual intercourse.

Erectile dysfunction (ED) is a form of impotence and is defined as the consistent inability to sustain an erection sufficient for sexual intercourse. Until the approval of the phosphodiesterase inhibitor sildenafil (Viagra®) in 1998 there were no safe, effective, orally administered drugs to treat this syndrome. Presumably because of a new willingness to discuss the condition, and the availability of new treatments, the number of men who requested help for ED from their physicians tripled from 1985 to 1999. Tadalafil (Cialis®) and vardenafil (Levitra®) are the latest phosphodiesterase inhibitors approved for the treatment of ED.

## Actions and Indications

In most men, erectile dysfunction is a result of injury to the nerves or impairment of blood flow to the penis. Diseases such as diabetes, injury such as spinal cord injury, and side effects of drugs can all result in erectile dysfunction. Smoking and lifestyle choices that cause vascular disease are other possible causes of ED. In order for an erection to occur, nerve impulses travel from the brain down the spinal cord to the penis, allowing the influx of arterial blood where it is temporarily trapped due to compression of veins responsible for outflow (see **Fig. 21.3**). The influx of blood is dependent upon smooth muscle relaxation in the corpus cavernosum, which is mediated by the chemical cyclic guanosine monophosphate (GMP), a nucleotide that plays many important roles in the body.

By inhibiting phosphodiesterase type 5 (PDE5 inhibitors), the enzyme responsible for the destruction of cyclic GMP in the penis, these drugs allow levels of cyclic GMP to increase. The resultant smooth muscle relaxation allows the influx of arterial blood needed to cause an erection. The PDE5 inhibitors have no effect in the absence of sexual stimulation, which is required in order to trigger the production of cyclic GMP. The phosphodiesterase inhibitors are indicated only for the treatment of erectile dysfunction. There is no sound clinical evidence that they are effective in the treatment of female sexual dysfunction.

## Administration

All three PDE5 inhibitors are administered orally. Sildenafil and vardenafil absorption is reduced or delayed by high-fat meals, so it makes sense for consumers to take them on an empty stomach. The elderly and people with severe renal or hepatic failure require lower doses of the drugs. The usual recommendation is that the drugs be taken an hour before anticipated sexual activity. Sildenafil and vardenafil can be taken as long as four hours in advance, while the manufacturers of tadalafil claim that it can be taken as far as 36 hours in advance of sexual activity. No more than one dose per day is recommended.

## Side Effects

Although these drugs are fairly specific for inhibition of PDE 5, they affect other phosphodiesterases to a lesser degree. As a result, smooth muscle relaxation and other pharmacologic activity is not entirely restricted to the genitourinary tract. Because vasodilation can be more widespread, there is a risk that a significant drop in blood pressure can occur when these drugs are taken. This effective is additive to the actions of other vasodilating drugs, such as the alpha-adrenergic blocking agents, nitroglycerin, or other nitrates, and can be very dangerous. The combination of vasodilators with the ED drugs is absolutely con-

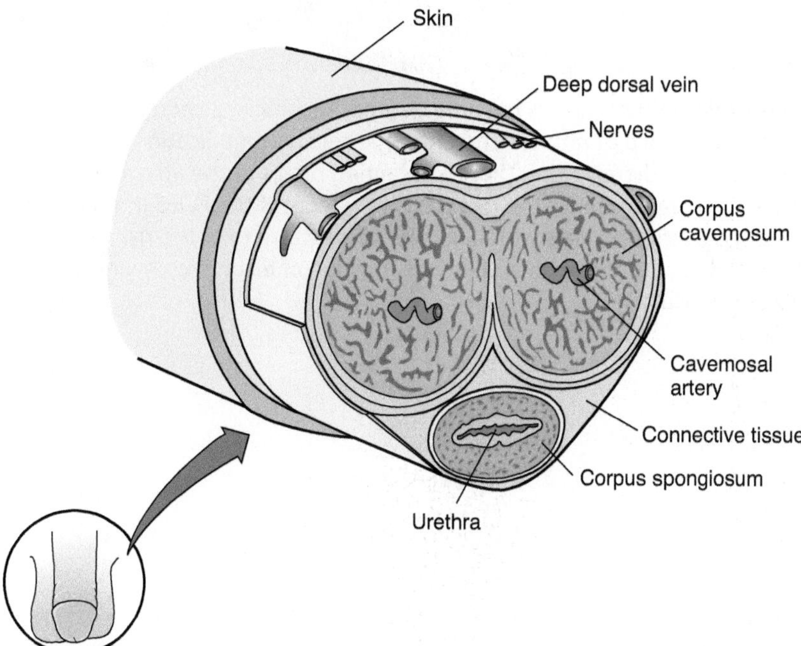


**Figure 21.3** A cross section of the penis, showing blood supply and anatomical structures. (Source: Miller TA. Diagnostic Evaluation of Erectile Dysfunction. *Am Fam Physician.* 2000 Jan 1;61(1):95–104,109–10; Cohen BJ. *Memmler's The Human Body in Health and Disease*, 10th edition. Baltimore: Lippincott Williams & Wilkins, 2005.)

traindicated. Hypotension, nasal congestion, and flushing can also occur as a result of vasodilation. Headache is a fairly common side effect of these drugs, but may not be a result of vasodilation. Chest pain, myocardial infarction, and cardiac arrhythmias may result when people with serious underlying heart conditions take PDE5 inhibitors. Priapism, a painful and persistent erection, can occur. Patients should report a painful and persistent erection to the physician.

## Case 21.1

In the movie *Something's Gotta Give*, the character played by Jack Nicholson experiences a mild heart attack while at his young and beautiful girlfriend's beach house. When he is wheeled into the emergency room, the doctor, played by Keanu Reeves, starts an IV in order to give him a nitroglycerin infusion. Dr. Keanu questions Nicholson repeatedly about whether he takes Viagra®. With his girlfriend and her mother at his side, of course Nicholson denies using the drug. When Keanu tells Nicholson he could die with the combination of Viagra and nitroglycerin, the film moves to a close shot of Nicholson's face as he turns to yank the IV out of his own arm. He has to admit that he did take a Viagra tablet. Although the movie scene is hilarious, this drug combination is no laughing matter! What role do you think the communication skills of the health care worker play in a situation like this? What factors might make it easier for a man who takes ED medications to discuss potential problems with the health care professional?

Through the inhibition of cyclic GMP, the PDE5 inhibitors can also affect the retinal response to light. Blurred vision, eye pain, and altered perception of color have been reported with all three drugs. More recently, reports of a sudden loss of vision that can either resolve or become permanent prompted the FDA to warn health care providers of this risk. Loss of vision occurs because of a disruption in the blood supply to the optic nerve. It is not yet known whether this is due to a direct effect of the drugs, underlying disease, or a combination of the two.

## Tips for the Technician

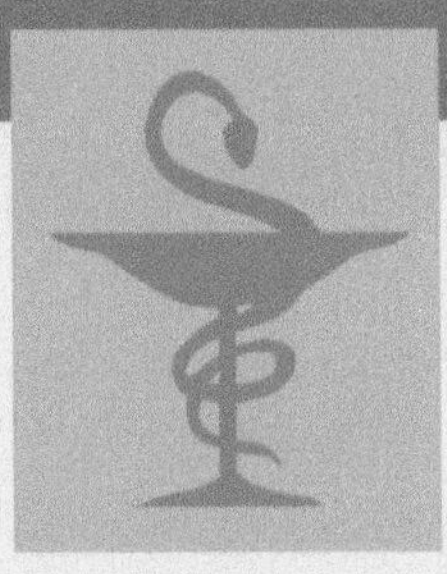

Many drugs interact with these agents to some degree. Technicians should be especially mindful of the presence of nitrates and antihypertensives medications on the patient's profile and immediately bring these interacting drugs to the attention of the pharmacist. Alcohol can increase the hypotensive effects of the PDE5 inhibitors. Appropriately label prescription vials with auxiliary labels warning of the risk of drug interactions and cautioning against the consumption of alcoholic beverages while taking these medications.

# Review Questions

## Multiple Choice

Choose the best answer for the following questions:

1. Which of the following drugs is not a loop diuretic?
   a. Spironolactone
   b. Furosemide
   c. Bumetanide
   d. Torsemide
   e. Ethacrynic acid

2. Circle the letter that corresponds to a common side effect seen with both the loop and thiazide diuretics.
   a. Hypertension
   b. Hearing loss
   c. Electrolyte abnormalities
   d. All of the above are common
   e. None of the above is common

3. Which drug(s) should not be used at the same time as sildenafil, tadalafil, or vardenafil?
   a. Furosemide or hydrochlorothiazide
   b. Phenazopyridine
   c. Vitamin C or Vitamin E
   d. Lactulose or milk of magnesia
   e. Nitroglycerin or terazosin

4. Which of the following side effects are typical of the urinary antispasmodics?
   a. Dry mouth
   b. Constipation
   c. Blurred vision
   d. All of the above
   e. None of the above

5. Treatment for benign prostatic hypertrophy include all of the following except
   a. Terazosin
   b. Imipramine
   c. Surgical resection of the prostate
   d. Doxazosin
   e. Drug treatment with 5a-reductase inhibitors

## True/False

6. Phenazopyridine is a urinary tract analgesic that frequently turns the urine blue-green.
   a. True
   b. False

7. Diuretics that act upon the loop of Henle are the most effective at mobilizing fluid and sodium and are called loop diuretics.
   a. True
   b. False

8. Erectile dysfunction is a form of impotence caused by a consistent and sustained disinterest in having sexual intercourse, which is treated with phosphodiesterase type 5 inhibitors.
   a. True
   b. False

9. The urinary antispasmodics are anticholinergic drugs indicated for the treatment of urge incontinence, or what is commonly termed overactive bladder.
   a. True
   b. False

10. Backpackers or hikers who experience nausea, headache, and shortness of breath associated with rapid climbs can take acetazolamide in advance of a hike to prevent acute mountain sickness.
    a. True
    b. False

## Matching

For numbers 11 to 15, match the drug name with the correct statement pertaining to instructions, side effects, or warnings from the list below. Choices will not be used more than once and may not be used at all.

11. Tolterodine
12. Vardenafil
13. Mannitol
14. Phenazopyridine
15. Tamsulosin

a. Shake well before using
b. Avoid taking with nitrates or other vasodilators
c. Dry mouth and blurred vision can occur
d. Check for crystallization before dispensing
e. Shake well before use
f. May cause discoloration of urine
g. Dizziness on arising can occur

## Short Answer

16. What precautions should a pregnant pharmacy technician take when dispensing finasteride?

17. What auxiliary labels would be applied to a prescription of an alpha-adrenergic blocking agent?

18. What are the most likely reasons a patient will receive a prescription for a diuretic?

19. List two possible side effects caused by spironolactone.

20. What are the most likely side effects observed with the use of thiazide and loop diuretics? How do these relate to the action of the drugs?

## FOR FURTHER INQUIRY

Organ transplantation plays an important, sometimes life-saving role in treatment for people with severe renal failure. Investigate the indications for kidney transplantation, the sources of kidneys, and the exclusion criteria for potential transplant recipients. Learn about the drugs that organ recipients must take to prevent organ rejection.

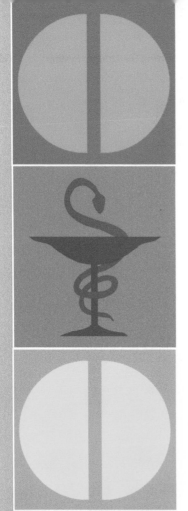

Chapter **22**

# Treatment of Gastrointestinal Disorders

## OBJECTIVES

After studying this chapter, the reader should be able to:

- List three factors that contribute to the development of peptic ulcer disease.
- Compare and contrast the actions of the $H_2$ receptor antagonists and the actions of the proton pump inhibitors on the production of gastric acid.
- Explain the three physiologic processes that result in nausea and vomiting. Describe two factors that can trigger these mechanism and two antiemetic drugs that work by inhibiting the same mechanisms.
- Name two antidiarrheal medications and list a common side effect for each.
- Describe the mechanism of action of a stimulant laxative and a bulk laxative and name an example of each. Explain how stool softeners differ from laxatives.

*KEY TERMS*

- dyspepsia
- emesis
- emetogenic
- flatulence
- ileus

## DRUGS COVERED IN THIS CHAPTER

### Drugs for Peptic Ulcers and Reflux Disease

| $H_2$ Receptor Antagonists | Proton Pump Inhibitors | Miscellaneous Drugs | Antacids |
|---|---|---|---|
| Cimetidine | Lansoprazole | Misoprostol | Magnesium & Aluminum Hydroxides |
| Famotidine | Omeprazole | Sucralfate | Calcium Carbonate |
| Nizatidine | Esomeprazole | | |
| Ranitidine | Pantoprazole | | |
| | Rabeprazole | | |

### Drugs for Nausea and Vomiting

| Antihistamines and Phenothiazines | $5HT_3$ Receptor Blockers | Miscellaneous Antiemetics |
|---|---|---|
| Dimenhydrinate | Dolasetron | Dronabinol |
| Meclizine | Granisetron | Scopolamine |
| Prochlorperazine | Ondansetron | Metoclopramide |
| Promethazine | | Traditional remedies |
| Thiethylperazine | | |
| Trimethobenzamide | | |

### Drugs for Bowel Disorders

| Antidiarrheals and Antiflatulents | Aminosalicylates | Laxatives |
|---|---|---|
| Activated attapulgite | Sulfasalazine | Bisacodyl |
| Bismuth Subsalicylate | Mesalamine | Bulk laxatives (methylcellulose, psyllium) |
| Diphenoxylate/Atropine | | Docusate |
| Kaolin/Pectin | | Glycerin Suppositories |
| Loperamide | | Lactulose |
| Simethicone | | Magnesium salts |
| | | Polyethylene Glycol |
| | | Senna |

This chapter describes drug classes used to treat some common and a few less common medical conditions involving the gastrointestinal tract. These diseases include peptic ulcer disease, acid reflux, including gastroesophageal reflux disease (GERD), nausea and vomiting, including chemotherapy related emesis, inflammatory bowel disease, diarrhea, constipation, and indigestion. Some of the drug classes used to treat these conditions are described in other chapters. Their descriptions here will be abbreviated, and the reader is referred back to other chapters for more complete details.

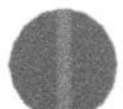

# Drugs Used for Reflux and Ulcer Disease

dyspepsia Stomach discomfort following meals; indigestion.

gastritis Inflammation of the mucous membrane of the stomach.

Acid reflux and peptic ulcers are just two of many possible causes of dyspepsia, chronic or recurrent discomfort centered in the upper abdomen. Gastritis caused by foods, beverages, or medications (spicy or greasy foods, coffee and alcoholic beverages, nonsteroidal anti-inflammatory drugs), pancreatitis, gall bladder disease, and abdominal cancers are all possible causes of chronic abdominal pain. The drugs discussed here may have application for disorders other than peptic ulcer disease and reflux disease; these will be noted accordingly.

Peptic ulcers are erosions in the lining of the stomach or duodenum (**Fig. 22.1**). Normally the epithelial layers of the stomach and intestines are covered by a layer of mucus to protect tissues below from the corroding effects of digestive enzymes and stomach acid. In peptic ulcer disease there is a malfunction of the production of this mucus layer. There can be a number of causes for the malfunction, including infection with *Helicobacter pylori*, use of nonsteroidal anti-inflammatory drugs, excessive alcohol consumption, smoking, and the severe physical stress accompanying serious illness and hospitalization.

The most common cause of GI ulceration is infection with *H. pylori* (**Fig. 22.2**). This organism is also strongly associated with later development of stomach cancers. When *H. pylori* infection is confirmed, its eradication dramatically reduces the risk of ulcer recurrence. Eradication of the organism requires treatment with multiple antibiotics, usually for two weeks. Typically, the antibiotic regimen includes clarithromycin (Biaxin®) and metronidazole (Flagyl®), and sometimes amoxicillin or tetracycline in various combinations. In addition to antibiotics, proton pump inhibitors or $H_2$ receptor antagonists are used to control the production of acid and protect the mucosal lining.

## Histamine$_2$ Receptor Antagonists

In the 1960s, pharmacologists knew that histamine caused increased secretion of gastric acid from parietal cells of the stomach, but they also knew traditional antihistamines did nothing to block this effect. The presence of a second kind of histamine receptor was unknown at the time. By manipulating the antihistamine molecules and then testing the resulting compounds to see if they could block acid secretion, pharmacologists eventually came

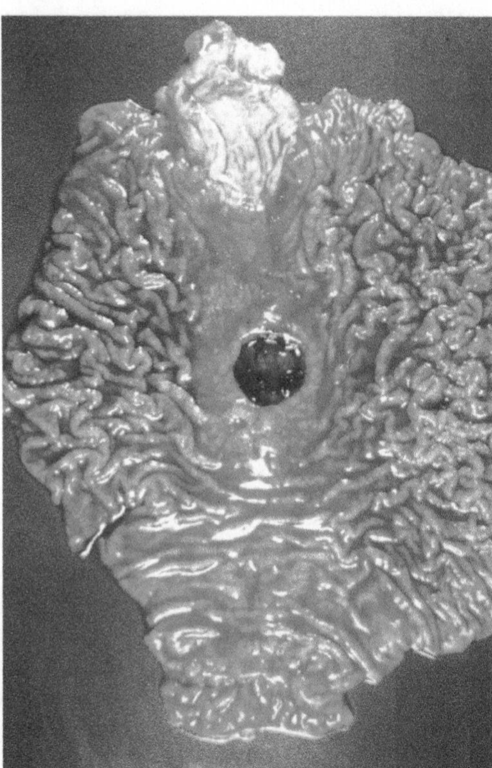

**Figure 22.1** A photograph showing the damaged mucosal tissue in peptic ulcer disease. (Reprinted with permission from Rubin E and Farber JL. *Pathology*, 3rd edition. Philadelphia: Lippincott Williams & Wilkins, 1999.)

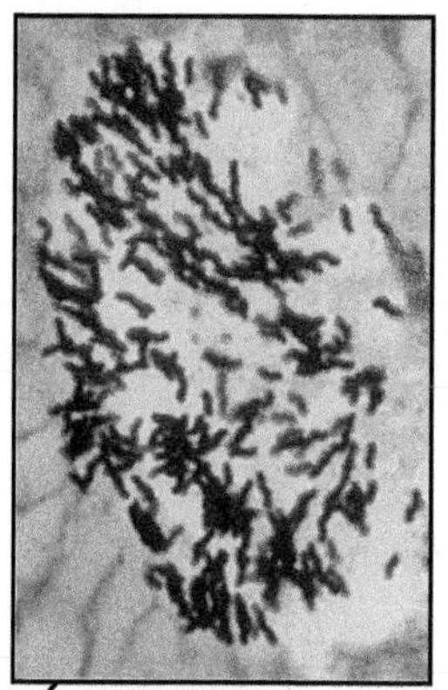

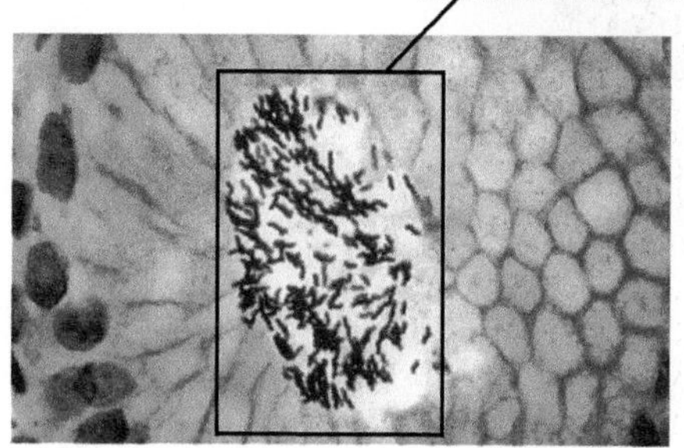

**Figure 22.2** *H. pylori* infection in gastric mucosal tissue. (Adapted with permission from Harvey RA, Champe PC, Howland RD, et al. *Lippincott's Illustrated Reviews: Pharmacology*, 3rd edition. Baltimore: Lippincott Williams & Wilkins, 2006.)

up with a precursor to cimetidine that had some effect at blocking histamine induced acid secretion. Further study of molecular structure and action at what scientists then believed was a second histamine receptor eventually led to the production and approval of cimetidine, the first $H_2$ receptor antagonist and the prototype of the class.

## Actions and Indications

The histamine$_2$ receptor antagonists, cimetidine (Tagamet®), famotidine (Pepcid®), ranitidine (Zantac®), and nizatidine (Axid®), compete with histamine to bind at receptors in the parietal cells in the stomach (**Fig. 22.3**). When bound to the receptors, gastric acid secretion is dramatically reduced. In people who have not been treated with acid suppressing drugs, there are a number of stimulants to acid production, including meals, caffeine, and the production by the pancreas of insulin. Treatment with an $H_2$ receptor antagonist blocks the production of acid even in the presence of these stimulants. In their prescription strengths, these drugs are indicated for the treatment of peptic ulcers, GERD, and erosive esophagitis. All of the $H_2$ receptor antagonists are available in lower strengths for the treatment of heartburn and acid indigestion.

When ulcers are not treated early enough, they can penetrate through the outer layers of the epithelium down to more vascular tissues. At that point ulcers may begin to bleed and in severe cases they can perforate. Bleeding ulcers can be a life-threatening condition, and treatment is aimed at stopping the bleeding. Cimetidine, ranitidine, and famotidine are used for the treatment of bleeding ulcers and for the prevention of stress ulcers. These drugs are also indicated in hypersecretory syndromes, where an abnormally large amount of acid secretion occurs in the stomach.

## Administration

The $H_2$ receptor antagonists are well absorbed and administered orally for four to eight weeks in the treatment of peptic ulcers. The dose and frequency of administration depends on the disease being treated. Hypersecretory conditions require more frequent dosing, but peptic ulcers can generally be treated using once or twice daily dosing. The concurrent use of antacids can reduce the absorption of cimetidine and ranitidine, so doses of these drugs should be staggered.

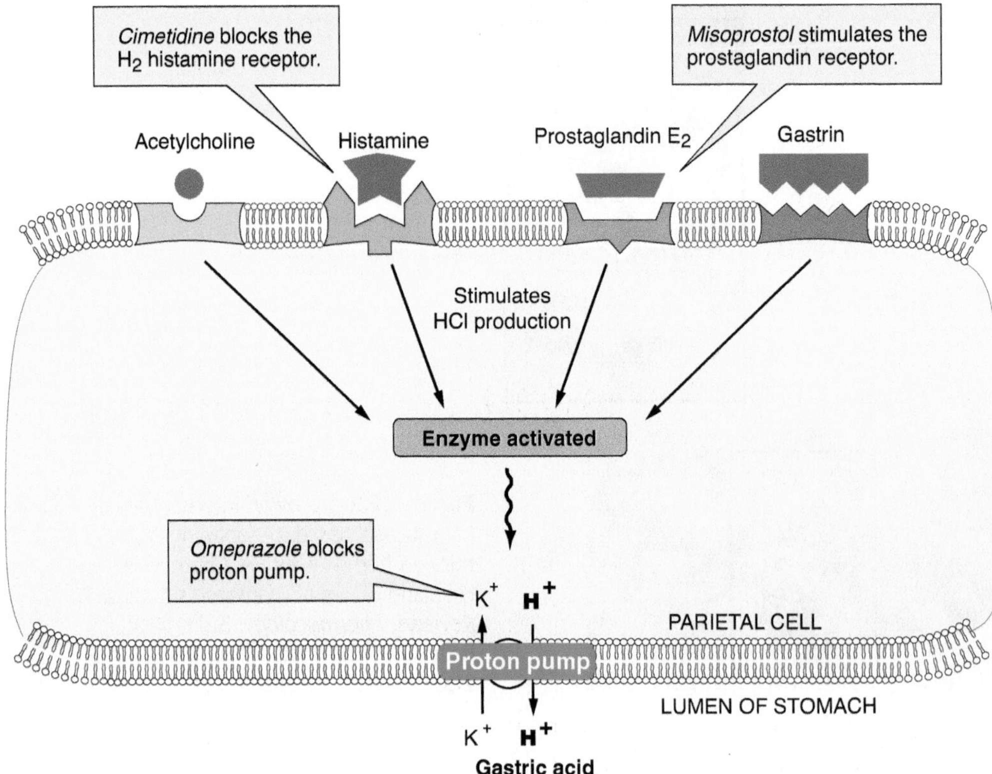


**Figure 22.3** Mechanisms of action of some drug classes used to treat peptic ulcer and acid reflux disease. (Adapted with permission from Harvey RA, Champe PC, Howland RD, et al. *Lippincott's Illustrated Reviews: Pharmacology*, 3rd edition. Baltimore: Lippincott Williams & Wilkins, 2006.)

Pediatric patients can safely take either ranitidine or famotidine. As a result, these two drugs are available in quite a variety of formulations for oral administration. Besides tablets, there are oral liquids and chewable, effervescent, and orally disintegrating tablets. **Table 22.1** shows the brand and generic names and formulations of drugs discussed in this chapter.

To prevent ulceration in seriously ill, hospitalized patients, or when patients cannot take their medication orally, cimetidine, famotidine, and ranitidine can be administered parenterally. They are most commonly given by continuous infusion for prevention of stress ulcers, but can be given by intermittent intravenous infusion. Cimetidine and famotidine can be given by IV push over two minutes or more. All three can also be administered intramuscularly.

## Side Effects

As a class, the $H_2$ receptor antagonists are considered quite safe. However, not long after cimetidine was approved, reports of altered mental states, including confusion, agitation, hallucinations and disorientation came to the attention of the FDA. These CNS effects occurred most often in patients with renal insufficiency or in the elderly, who may also have compromised renal function. As a result, doses of $H_2$ receptor antagonists are reduced in people with renal failure. Cimetidine is less often used than other $H_2$ receptor antagonists because of an increased risk of drug interactions and side effects observed with its use. To a lesser degree, ranitidine can be involved with drug interactions. Important drug interactions can occur when digoxin, several antiarrhythmic agents, warfarin, and a number of anticonvulsants are given with cimetidine. Nizatidine can cause changes in liver function tests, indicating possible damage to the liver, but these abnormalities are reversible when the medication is discontinued. Typical side effects observed with the use of the $H_2$ receptor antagonists are headache and dizziness.

**Table 22.1** A Comparison of Generic Names, Brand Names, Indications, and Available Formulations of Drugs Used for Upper GI Diseases Discussed in This Chapter

| Generic | Brand Name | Available as | Indications | Notes |
|---|---|---|---|---|
| **$H_2$ Receptor Antagonists** | | | | |
| Cimetidine | Tagamet® | Ulcers, GERD, hyper-secretory states, GI bleed, heartburn | Tablets, liquid, injection | |
| Famotidine Complete® | Pepcid®, Pepcid | Ulcers, GERD, hyper-secretory states, GI bleed, heartburn | Tablets, gel caps, chew tabs, injection, powder for susp. | Pepcid Complete includes antacid |
| Nizatidine | Axid® | Ulcers, GERD, heartburn | Tablets, capsules | |
| Ranitidine | Zantac® | Ulcers, GERD, hyper-secretory states, GI bleed, heartburn | Tablets, syrup, inj. effervescent tabs | |
| **Proton Pump Inhibitors** | | | | |
| Lansoprazole | Prevacid® | Ulcers, GERD, hyper-secretory states, erosive esophagitis | Capsules, granules for susp, disintegrating tabs, powder for injection | Oral products are ER to protect from acid |
| Omeprazole | Prilosec® | Ulcers, GERD, hyper-secretory states, erosive esophagitis | ER capsules and tablets, powder for oral suspension | |
| Esomeprazole | Nexium® | Same | ER capsules | S isomer of omeprazole |
| Pantoprazole | Protonix® | GERD, erosive esophagitis, hyper-secretory states | ER tabs and powder for injection | |
| Rabeprazole | Aciphex® | Ulcers, GERD, hyper-secretory states, erosive esophagitis | ER tablets | |
| **Miscellaneous Drugs** | | | | |
| Misoprostol | Cytotec® | Prevent NSAID ulcers, cervical ripening and labor induction | Tablets | |
| Sucralfate | Carafate® | Peptic ulcer disease, treatment of NSAID GI side effects | Tablets and suspension | |
| **Antacids** | | | | |
| Calcium Carbonate | Tums®, Dicarbosil® | Calcium replacement, gastric hyperacidity | Chew tabs, suspension, gum | |

*(continues)*

**Table 22.1** A Comparison of Generic Names, Brand Names, Indications, and Available Formulations of Drugs Used for Upper GI Diseases Discussed in This Chapter *(continued)*

| Generic | Brand Name | Available as | Indications | Notes |
|---|---|---|---|---|
| **Antacids** | | | | |
| Aluminum Hydroxide | Amphojel® | Reduce phosphate absorption, gastric hyperacidity | Tablets, capsules, and suspension | Maalox & Mylanta combine Al and Mg hydroxide |
| Magnesium Hydroxide | Milk of magnesia | Laxative, gastric hyper-acidity | Chew tabs and suspension | |
| Magaldrate | Riopan® | Gastric hyperacidity | Suspension | |

ER, extended release; GERD, gastroesophageal reflux disease; NSAID, nonsteroidal anti-inflammatory drugs.

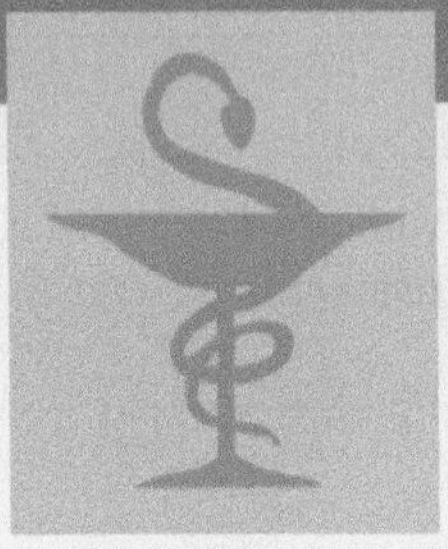

**Tips for the Technician**

$H_2$ receptor antagonists can be administered orally without regard to food. Clients who take nonprescription products should be encouraged to report ongoing GI symptoms to their physicians. Technicians will need to appropriately label cimetidine and ranitidine prescription vials with auxiliary labels warning of drug interactions. While no special storage conditions are required for most of these products, famotidine injection should be refrigerated. Once famotidine granules for suspension are mixed, they are stable for 30 days only, and should be labelled with a 30-day expiration date.

## Proton Pump Inhibitors

The proton pump inhibitors (PPIs) were investigated in the 1980s and most reached the market in the 1990s. Experience has shown them to be more effective at reducing acid secretion in the stomach and equally as safe as the $H_2$ receptor antagonists. Four of the five PPIs were in the top 20 most prescribed drugs in the United States in 2004.

### Actions and Indications

The proton pump inhibitors are so named because they block the final step in the production of stomach acid, the release of hydrogen ions into gastric fluids. All of theses drugs are prodrugs (inactive compounds), and are activated once they are absorbed into the blood stream. From there, the drugs are picked up and concentrated in the parietal cells. In the parietal cells they irreversibly bind to the active cellular proton pumps, and prevent the release of hydrogen ions, $H^+$. At peak effectiveness they reduce gastric acid production by 90% or more. They are metabolized in the liver and are cleared from the bloodstream fairly rapidly. However, the effects on the proton pump continue after the drug is out of the body.

All of the proton pump inhibitors are very similar and are equally effective. They are superior in effectiveness to the $H_2$ receptor antagonists for suppressing acid production and healing peptic ulcers. For this reason, they are the preferred drugs for treating GERD, peptic ulcers, and hypersecretory conditions. Clinical studies have shown that PPIs reduce the risk of bleeding from an ulcer caused by aspirin and other nonsteroidal anti-inflammatory agents (NSAIDS). When combined with antibiotics, PPIs are successful at eradicating ulcers caused by *H. pylori*.

Esomeprazole (Nexium®) is the active, S-enantiomer fraction of omeprazole (Prilosec®). As presented in Chapter 1, AstraZeneca Pharmaceuticals marketed esomeprazole in order to hold on to the huge income brought into the company by omeprazole after its patent expired. Esomeprazole is, for our purposes, the same drug as omeprazole, and offers no advantages in effectiveness, duration of action, or side effect profile.

## Administration

The proton pump inhibitors are given orally, and in the case of pantoprazole (Protonix®), intravenously. These drugs are acid labile, and enteric coating protects the tablets and contents of capsules. Food delays the absorption of the PPIs and reduces the availability of esomeprazole. Therefore, if tolerated, these drugs should be administered an hour before meals or two hours after. Lansoprazole (Prevacid®) and omeprazole are available as products for suspension. Omeprazole suspension is sold in 20-mg packets, to be mixed by the patient and used immediately after mixing. It must be taken on an empty stomach. Lansoprazole granules for suspension are enteric coated. They, too, are packaged in unit of use envelopes and mixed immediately before administration.

Because of their mechanism of action (irreversible binding to the acid pumps), the PPIs are effective when given once daily. However, some prescribers prefer to give them twice daily, especially in treatment of hypersecretory conditions and in the treatment of active ulcer disease.

## Side Effects

Side effects are infrequent, and occur in only about five out of every one hundred patients treated. The most common are gastrointestinal side effects, including nausea, diarrhea, and abdominal pain. Dizziness and headache are typical of the adverse central nervous system effects caused by this class. Rarely, skin reactions, gynecomastia, and elevated liver enzymes can occur. Omeprazole is known to interact with several drugs, sometimes significantly. Of note are interactions between omeprazole and carbamazepine or phenytoin. In both cases, the drug levels of the anticonvulsants can increase significantly.

Prolonged therapy with agents that suppress gastric acid, such as the PPIs and $H_2$ receptor antagonists, may result in reduced absorption of vitamin $B_{12}$, because acid is required for its absorption. Some scientists have hypothesized that the PPIs may predispose patients to certain forms of gastric cancers because the lower acid levels may allow bacteria to grow in the stomach. To date, no such relationship is proven.

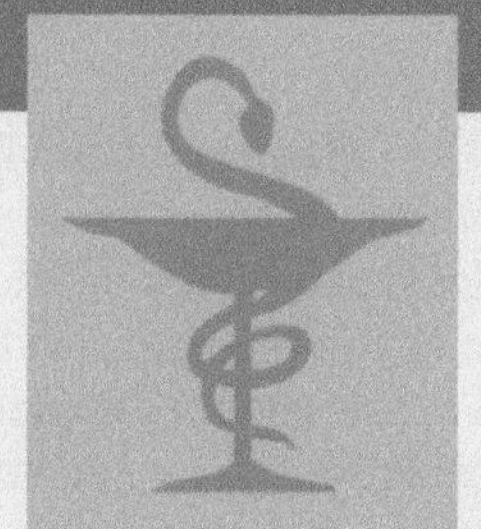

### Tips for the Technician

Because dizziness can occur, auxiliary labels cautioning patients about driving should be affixed to prescription vials. Esomeprazole must be taken on an empty stomach and should be labelled as such. For the other PPIs, administration before meals is preferred, but pantoprazole can be taken without regard to food. Proton pump inhibitor tablets and capsules cannot be crushed because the drug will be broken down by stomach acid. However, the omeprazole and lansoprazole capsules can be opened up and mixed into applesauce and swallowed. The granules should not be chewed. Likewise, lansoprazole disintegrating tablets are not chewable tablets. The tablet is placed on the tongue to disintegrate, and then swallowed with water. Technicians should affix the appropriate auxiliary labels to prescription bottles, and make sure the pharmacist instructs patients in the appropriate use of these medications.

# Miscellaneous Drugs for Peptic Ulcer Disease

Although they have very different mechanisms of action, both misoprostol (Cytotec®) and sucralfate (Carafate®) have a mucosal protective action on the stomach lining. They are not routinely used to treat peptic ulcer disease, but are useful in specific situations. Misoprostol and sucralfate are not chemically related.

## Actions and Indications

Prostaglandin E2, produced by the gastric mucosa, inhibits secretion of stomach acid and stimulates secretion of mucus and bicarbonate. Misoprostol, an analog of prostaglandin, mimics these actions. The nonsteroidal anti-inflammatory drugs (NSAIDs) are prostaglandin synthesis inhibitors. Inhibition of prostaglandin synthesis is responsible for the anti-inflammatory effects of this drug class, since prostaglandins are important mediators of inflammation. Unfortunately, inhibition of prostaglandin synthesis also reduces the natural mechanisms that protect the stomach lining from ulceration. Misoprostol has a greater affinity for prostaglandin receptors in the stomach than do the NSAIDs, which allows it to exert its protective effect.

Misoprostol is approved for prevention of gastric ulcers induced by NSAIDs. Because it is a prostaglandin, misoprostol causes uterine contractions, and is used off label with mifepristone to terminate an unwanted pregnancy, early in the pregnancy. It can also be used vaginally to induce labor.

Sucralfate is a complex of sucrose, aluminum, and sulfate used to protect and hasten healing of the stomach lining. The protective effects of sucralfate are due to local action at the site of ulceration. When the drug reaches the stomach it is activated by stomach acid and forms a sticky, pasty substance that binds to the damaged gastric mucosa. This substance buffers stomach acid and protects the ulcerated tissue from acid and digestive enzymes. The complex formed between the drug and the tissue is fairly stable and remains in place for up to six hours after a dose, allowing tissues to heal. Sucralfate is indicated in the treatment of peptic ulcer disease. It is used off-label to protect the gastric mucosa in patients who take NSAIDs, to prevent stress ulcers in hospitalized patients, and for treatment of stomatitis in cancer patients.

## Administration

Both misoprostol and sucralfate are administered orally. Misoprostol is available as tablets in two dosage strengths and is taken with meals. It is rapidly absorbed and subsequently converted to the active drug form in the liver. The kidneys are responsible for the elimination of the active metabolite.

Sucralfate is marketed as tablets and in a suspension form. Absorption of sucralfate is minimal; at least 95% of each dose remains in the GI tract. This medication should be administered on an empty stomach, at least one hour before meals. Treatment for more than eight weeks is not recommended.

## Side Effects

The most common adverse effects associated with misoprostol are diarrhea, abdominal pain, nausea, and vomiting. GI complaints are usually self-limiting, but can be severe enough to cause discontinuation of the drug. Diarrhea is dose related and occurs in fifteen to forty percent of patients. These side effects are a result of the action of prostaglandins on the smooth muscle of the GI tract. A much more serious result of this pharmacologic effect occurs when misoprostol is given to a pregnant woman. Misoprostol causes contraction of the smooth muscle of the uterus and can result in premature labor, damage to the muscle wall of the uterus, and fetal death. When given to women of childbearing age, misoprostol can cause menstrual cramps and other menstrual disorders. Normally misoprostol is not administered to women of childbearing age unless the benefit outweighs the potential risk if the patient were to become pregnant while taking the medication.

Because sucralfate is not significantly absorbed, all consistently reported side effects relate to effects in the gastrointestinal tract. Most common of these is constipation, but nausea, dry mouth, stomach upset, and flatulence can also occur. Sucralfate contains aluminum, small amounts of which are absorbed. Normally, there is no problem eliminating these small quantities of aluminum, but in rare cases people with renal failure may develop aluminum toxicity.

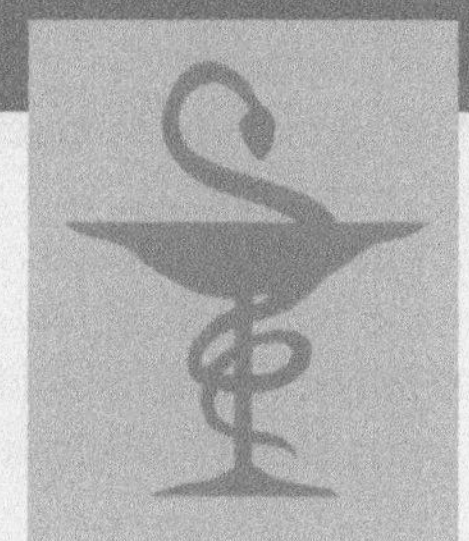

## Tips for the Technician

It is very important that patients purchasing misoprostol for the first time receive careful counselling by the pharmacist. All patients need to understand that a pregnant woman who takes this medication could have a miscarriage, and for this reason, the medication should not be shared with other people. Auxiliary labels warning against use during pregnancy are available, and are recommended for use on misoprostol prescription vials. This medication is better tolerated when given after meals. Attach an auxiliary label to the vial that instructs patients to take the medication with food. The drug names mifepristone and misoprostol are examples of drug names that look and sound similar. Special caution is warranted when dealing with drugs with look alike, sound alike counterparts.

Sucralfate is taken on an empty stomach, one hour before meals. To help remind patients of the appropriate administration times, the pharmacy technician should label prescription vials "take one hour before meals, on an empty stomach." The pharmacist will alert clients to the possibility of constipation caused by sucralfate.

# Antacids

Antacids were the first drugs routinely and effectively used for the treatment of indigestion, peptic ulcer disease, and acid reflux disease. The first mention of the use of calcium carbonate for indigestion dates back 5,000 years. Ancient peoples probably used ground shells and coral, which are made of calcium carbonate, for relief of dyspepsia. Much later, the English pharmacist Charles Henry Phillips concocted a suspension of magnesium hydroxide for use as a laxative or antacid. He patented it in 1873, and named it Phillips Milk of Magnesia, a product still in use today. Until the development of the $H_2$ receptor antagonists, antacid therapy was the cornerstone of treatment for peptic ulcer disease.

## Actions and Indications

Antacids are weak bases that react with gastric acid to form water and a salt, thereby reducing gastric acidity. Because the digestive enzyme, pepsin, is inactivated at a pH greater than four, antacids also reduce its activity. In addition, there is some evidence that they stimulate the synthesis of prostaglandin in the stomach. They are sold without a prescription for use in treatment of heartburn and indigestion. Antacids can promote healing in peptic ulcer disease, and are used for symptomatic relief in reflux disease and gastritis.

Antacid products vary widely in their chemical composition. Commonly used antacids are salts of aluminum, magnesium, and calcium. Examples include aluminum hydroxide, magnesium hydroxide, and calcium carbonate. Magaldrate is a distinct chemical entity made up of aluminum and magnesium hydroxide. Aluminum hydroxide is administered in patients with chronic renal failure to reduce excessive phosphorus levels by binding phosphorus in the GI tract. Magnesium oxide is used as a magnesium supplement.

The acid-neutralizing ability of an antacid depends on composition, and to some degree on how long it stays in contact with gastric acid. Acid neutralizing capacity must be balanced with risk of side effects when choosing an antacid. Antacids that are well absorbed usually carry greater potential for causing side effects. Before the ready availability of low-cost antacids in every drug and grocery store, baking soda (sodium bicarbonate), was frequently used as an antacid. Although quite effective, sodium bicarbonate is absorbed systemically and can cause abnormalities in the pH of the bloodstream. Repeated use of baking soda as an antacid, therefore, is not recommended. Calcium carbonate has a high degree of acid neutralizing capacity and is fairly well absorbed, an advantage in people who need a source of calcium.

## Administration

Antacids are taken by mouth. They are available in an assortment of combinations, package sizes, and formulations, including liquids, chewable tablets, and gum. When antacids are administered as liquids, they disperse more rapidly, take effect more quickly, and are more effective than chewable tablets. They are not as convenient as chewable tablets, however. If chewable tablets are used, they should be thoroughly chewed before swallowing, and followed with a glass of water. Although some of the antacid compounds are available as capsules or tablets, those formulations are used for indications other than GI distress or treatment of ulcer disease, such as mineral replacement therapy.

## Side Effects

Although considered safe enough to be sold for self-treatment, antacids can cause unwanted effects, especially if they are used excessively or by patients who have other health conditions. Magnesium salts act as laxatives, and magnesium-containing antacids can cause loose stools or diarrhea in some people. Some magnesium is absorbed from these products, and when patients with kidney disease use magnesium-containing antacids chronically, they can develop magnesium toxicity.

While magnesium can cause diarrhea, aluminum hydroxide can be constipating. The binding of phosphate by aluminum-containing antacids can lead to loss of this essential mineral, and eventually, to low phosphate levels. Sodium bicarbonate can cause belching and flatulence, in addition to the potential for causing abnormally alkaline blood pH when taken repeatedly. All antacid products can cause dose-related rebound production of gastric acid. This is usually not a significant concern because most patients who take these drugs routinely are also taking some type of acid suppressant.

The sodium content of some antacids can be significant, and is listed on most package labeling. Sodium content is of concern to some patients with hypertension or congestive heart failure who need to control their intake of sodium. There are several antacids, such as calcium carbonate, that are "low-sodium" products.

Antacids, some of which look similar to each other (see **Fig. 22.4**), are involved with a number of important drug interactions. They can alter the absorption of other drugs by affecting their dissolution and solubility. They can alter the removal of some drugs by changing the pH of the urine. Antacids can bind to some drugs in the GI tract to form an insoluble compound, thereby significantly reducing the bioavailability of the other drug.

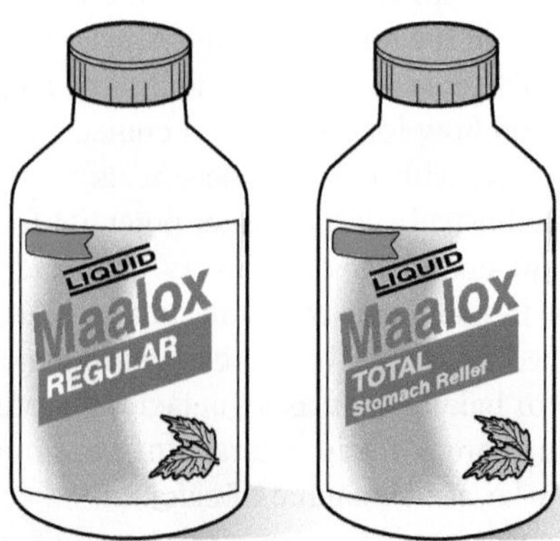


**Figure 22.4** Brand name extension can cause confusion among consumers as exemplified by similar-looking labels on Maalox Regular and Maalox Total Stomach Relief.

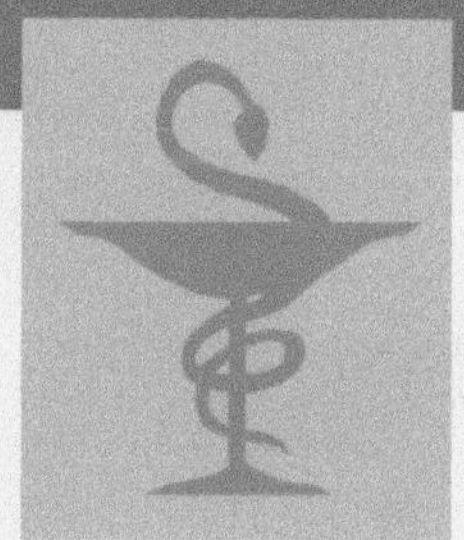

## Tips for the Technician

Because most antacid products are sold without prescriptions, technicians play an important role in directing customers to the desired products, and referring those who might need additional information to the pharmacist. In retail pharmacies, the technician is often the first person a client approaches with questions about nonprescription items. It is important for technicians to be good listeners, and know how to ask customers questions that will elicit important information. Sometimes this role requires technicians to be sensitive to inquiries that reveal the presence of underlying issues that should be referred to the pharmacist. The motivated pharmacy technician student will not underestimate the importance of developing good listening and communications skills, and a thorough knowledge of available products as part of becoming a valuable member of the pharmacy team.

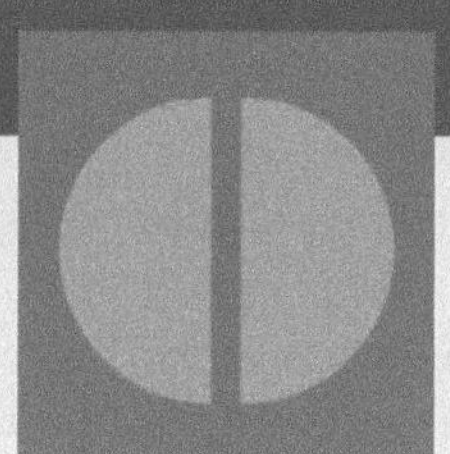

## Case 22.1

Ivana Sauermilch, CPT, is working the night shift at the local 24-hour pharmacy. At four in the morning, Perry Stalles, who appears to have been drinking, carries a bottle of Maalox® Total Stomach Relief to her at the cash register. "May I help you?" Ivana asks. Perry says he has been celebrating his 21st birthday with friends and asked the cab driver to stop at the pharmacy so he could get an antacid. He wants to know if Maalox® is a good antacid, because he thinks he is going to need one. What is Maalox® Total Stomach Relief? How do you think Ivana should advise the young man?

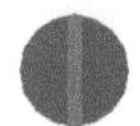

# Drugs for Nausea and Vomiting

Strictly speaking, a discussion of antiemetic drugs belongs with a discussion of drugs that affect the central nervous system. Triggering factors cause the symptom of nausea, and the response by the gastrointestinal tract called emesis, or vomiting, by stimulating the vomiting center in the brain. In order to prescribe the correct medication, the prescriber needs to know the underlying cause of the nausea and vomiting (refer to **Figure 22.5**).

emesis Vomiting.

There are three major pathways that trigger nausea and subsequent vomiting. The chemoreceptor trigger zone (CTZ), located in an area of the brain that is not protected from the systemic circulation, responds directly to chemical stimuli in the blood or cerebrospinal fluid, and causes the release of dopamine and serotonin, and subsequent activation of the vomiting center. Stimulation of the CTZ is responsible for most drug-induced vomiting. Irritation in the GI tract (from bacteria or toxins, for instance) also causes release of dopamine and serotonin. Lastly, the vestibular center (involved with balance) releases histamine and acetylcholine when stimulated, as in motion sickness. Input from any one of these three pathways triggers the vomiting center in the medulla, which directly mediates nausea and vomiting. Treatment of nausea and vomiting involves use of medications designed to counteract the effects of dopamine and serotonin in the GI tract and CTZ, and histamine and acetylcholine in the vestibular system.

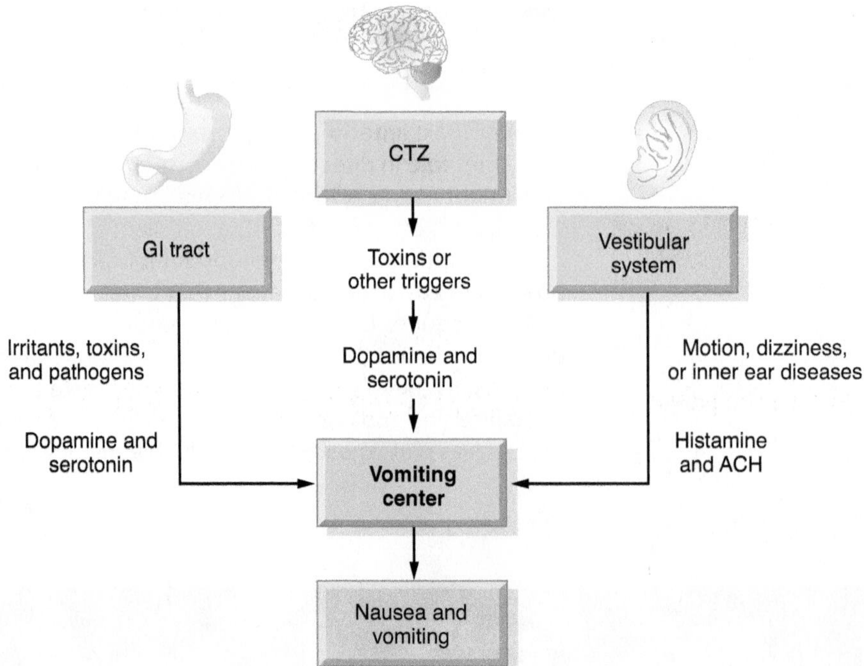


**Figure 22.5** The physiologic mechanisms underlying nausea and vomiting.

## Antihistamines and Phenothiazines

Although chemically related, members of these classes have different antiemetic mechanisms, and therefore different uses. Neither of these drug classes is recommended for routine treatment of the nausea and vomiting associated with pregnancy.

### Actions and Indications

The phenothiazine-type antiemetics, including promethazine (Phenergan®), prochlorperazine (Compazine®), and thiethylperazine (Torecan®) have potent antidopaminergic activity and effectively reduce nausea and vomiting caused by activation of the chemoreceptor trigger zone. As such, they are useful in the treatment of drug-induced vomiting (postoperative nausea and chemotherapy induced nausea) as well as vomiting caused by viral infections. They are not effective for the nausea and vomiting associated with motion sickness. Although promethazine is a potent antidopaminergic agent, it also exerts strong antihistaminic action and is approved for treatment of motion sickness. It is less often used for this however, because it is highly sedating.

The antihistamines exert their antiemetic effect through anticholinergic action, and are therefore much less effective at treating vomiting due to stimulation of the CTZ. They are effective in preventing nausea due to motion sickness and are effective at treating nausea caused by local irritation of the gastrointestinal tract. Meclizine (Antivert®) is used to treat vertigo and nausea associated with disorders of the inner ear, such as Ménière's Disease. Trimethobenzamide (Tigan®) is a weak antihistaminic drug with limited antinauseant effect. Unlike other antihistamines, it does not prevent nausea due to local GI irritation, but rather seems to work at the CTZ.

### Administration

While all of the antihistamine and phenothiazine antiemetics can be administered orally, several are manufactured for intramuscular or rectal administration. Promethazine and prochlorperazine can be given intravenously, but this route is not encouraged. Too rapid IV administration can result in severe hypotension. When patients are actively vomiting, rectal administration is the only feasible route for use of an antiemetic at home. Promethazine and prochlorperazine are available as rectal suppositories in a number of different strengths. Trimethobenzamide can be administered by mouth, by intramuscular injection, or rectally. For a description of available products by generic and brand names, refer to **Table 22.2**. In the treatment of drug induced vomiting, pretreatment with one of the antidopaminergic agents can be helpful.

### Side Effects

As discussed in Chapters 12, the phenothiazines are known to cause abnormal muscle movements. Although these effects are more likely to occur with chronic use of the phenothiazines, one particular form of abnormality, torticollis, can occur after a single dose. This involuntary contraction of neck and back muscles and twisting of the neck is usually successfully reversed with diphenhydramine (Benadryl®). Other side effects, such as hypotension, restlessness, and induction of seizures can also occur. Giving higher doses of the phenothiazines improves antiemetic activity, but side effects are dose limiting. Although it is not classified as a phenothiazine, trimethobenzamide can also cause atypical movements and can induce seizures.

With short-term use the most common side effect of both the phenothiazine and antihistamine drugs with short-term use is sedation. Both drug classes can cause anticholinergic side effects, such as dry mouth, but these symptoms are more likely to occur with use of antihistamines.

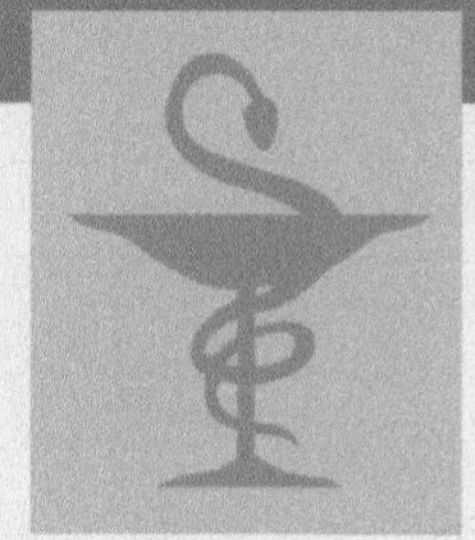

### Tips for the Technician

All antihistamine and phenothiazine prescription containers should be labelled with auxiliary warnings about the risk of sedation. Adult patients should be specifically warned about the dangers of driving while being treated with these highly sedating medications. When the prescription is intended for a child, the pharmacist may need to provide instruction on the proper administration of suppositories.

Medical personnel, including pharmacy technicians, may develop contact dermatitis from repeated skin contact with phenothiazines. Contact with injectable or liquid products is obviously of greater concern than contact with tablets or capsules. Thorough handwashing after any skin contact with these drugs may reduce the chance of developing dermatitis.

## 5-hydroxytriptamine$_3$ Receptor Blockers

Prevention and control of nausea and vomiting are paramount to successful cancer chemotherapy. People that suffer from nausea and vomiting after chemotherapy may develop electrolyte abnormalities, have chronic loss of appetite, develop nutritional deficiencies, and in some cases become so discouraged that they decide to forego potentially lifesaving chemotherapy treatment. The 5-hydroxytriptamine$_3$ ($5HT_3$) receptor antagonists are some of the most effective agents at preventing chemotherapy-induced nausea and vomiting (CINV). Refer to **Figure 22.6** for a comparison of antiemetic efficacy in CINV.

### Actions and Indications

The $5HT_3$ receptor antagonists selectively block one type of serotonin receptor located in both the GI tract and in the CTZ. The result of this action is a decrease in the stimulation, from the CTZ and the GI tract, of the vomiting center. Because of their ability to block input from both of these sites, these drugs are considered first-line treatment for chemotherapy induced nausea and vomiting. These drugs are fairly selective, and exert limited effects on other serotonin receptors in the heart and blood vessels.

**Table 22.2** A Comparison of Antiemetic Drug names, Indications, and Formulations

| Generic Name | Brand Name | Available as | Indications | Notes |
|---|---|---|---|---|
| **Antihistamines** | | | | |
| Dimenhydrinate | Dramamine® | Tablets, chew tabs, liquid, injection | Treatment of N&V, vertigo of motion sickness | Rx & OTC |
| Meclizine | Antivert® | Tablets, capsules, chew tabs | Treatment of N&V, vertigo of motion sickness, vestibular diseases | Rx & OTC |
| Trimethobenzamide | Tigan® | Capsules, injection suppositories | Relief of N&V | |
| **Phenothiazines** | | | | |
| Prochlorperazine | Compazine® | Tablets, ER caps, suppositories, injection, syrup | Control of severe N&V | Children >2 years |
| Promethazine | Phenergan® | Tablets, injection, suppositories, syrup | Postop N&V, motion sickness. Also used to prevent CINV | Children >2 years |
| Thiethylperazine | Torecan® | Injection | Relief of N&V | Not used in children |
| **$5HT_3$ Receptor Blockers** | | | | |
| Dolasetron | Anzemet® | Tablet, injection | Prevent CINV, prevent postop N&V, treat postop N&V | |
| Granisetron | Kytril® | Tablet, oral solution, injection | Prevent CINV, prevent N&V assoc. with radiation | |
| Ondansetron | Zofran® | Tablet, oral solution, injection, orally disintegrating tab | Prevent CINV, prevent postop N&V, prevent N&V assoc. with radiation | |
| **Miscellaneous Antiemetic Agents** | | | | |
| Dronabinol | Marinol® | Capsules | Prevent CINV, treat anorexia in AIDS patients | Not used in children |
| Metoclopramide | Reglan® | Tablets, syrup, injection | Diabetic gastroparesis, prevent CINV, prevent postop N&V, tx of GERD | ↑ risk of side effects in children |
| Vitamin $B_6$ | | Tablets, capsules, injection | Recommended for morning sickness | |
| Phosphorated Carbohydrate Soln | Emetrol® | Oral solution | Recommended for morning sickness, N&V in children | |
| Cola syrup | | Syrup | N&V in children | |
| Ginger | | | Recommended for morning sickness | |

CINV, chemotherapy induced nausea and vomiting; ER, extended release; N&V, nausea and vomiting.

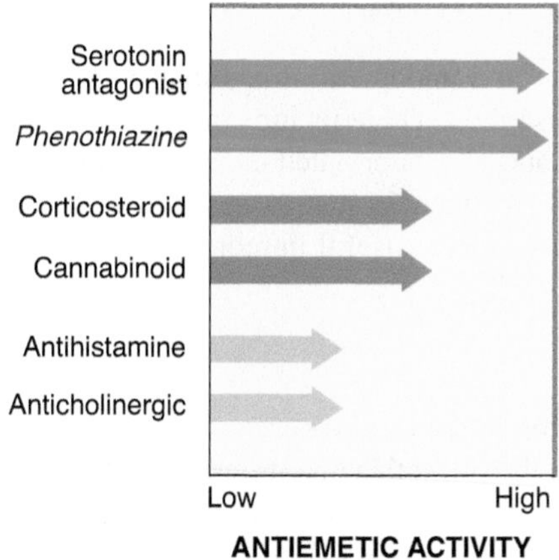


**Figure 22.6** Relative efficacy of various antiemetic drugs in the treatment of the nausea and vomiting associated with chemotherapy. (Adapted with permission from Harvey RA, Champe PC, Howland RD, et al. *Lippincott's Illustrated Reviews: Pharmacology*, 3rd edition. Baltimore: Lippincott Williams & Wilkins, 2006.)

## Administration

All of the most frequently used $5HT_3$ receptor blockers can be administered by the oral route or by intravenous injection. Ondansetron (Zofran®) solution for injection must be diluted before administration. It is available premixed, for intravenous piggyback administration. Both ondansetron and granisetron (Kytril®) are available in oral solutions, especially helpful for use in children. Ondansetron is manufactured as an orally disintegrating tablet.

When used for the prevention of CINV, these drugs are administered as a single dose, thirty minutes to an hour before the start of chemotherapy. Most cancer treatment facilities combine the $5HT_3$ receptor blockers with other drugs to maximize control of nausea and vomiting, especially when highly emetogenic (likely to produce vomiting) chemotherapy regimens are used. They are often administered with a corticosteroid such as dexamethasone, and sometimes a second antiemetic drug such as promethazine or metoclopramide. Chemotherapy patients develop anticipatory vomiting, meaning that the thought, sight, or smell of the drugs is enough to trigger vomiting. In patients who have anticipatory vomiting, pretreatment with an antianxiety drug and use of biofeedback techniques can be helpful. Antiemetic medications are sometimes continued for a day or two after chemotherapy, but the high cost of these medications may prevent patients from being able to continue beyond the day the chemotherapy is administered.

emetogenic Causes vomiting; usually in reference to a drug side effect.

## Side Effects

Most side effects caused by $5HT_3$ receptor antagonists are related to their actions in the GI tract and central nervous system. Headache is the most common side effect and is caused by all three drugs. Other central nervous system effects, such as dizziness and fatigue, can occur. In the gastrointestinal tract, ondansetron and granisetron are commonly associated with constipation, while dolasetron is more likely to cause diarrhea. Cardiovascular changes, including arrhythmia and hypotension can occur with dolasetron. Patients with underlying cardiovascular problems are given this medication with caution. Serious allergic reactions are possible, but uncommon.

### Tips for the Technician

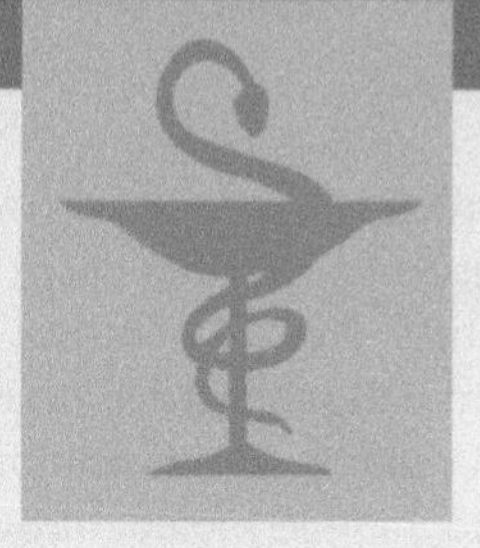

Because these medications are fairly safe and taken on a short-term basis only, few special instructions are required. Formulas for extemporaneously compounded rectal suppositories and solutions are available for some of these medications. Technicians may be asked to compound these products. Remember that all extemporaneously compounded products should be appropriately labelled with expiration date, lot number, and any special storage instructions.

## Miscellaneous Antiemetic Drugs

There are a number of miscellaneous antinauseant and antiemetic drugs that do not fit neatly into the pharmacologic categories already described. These include metoclopramide (Reglan®), dronabinol (Marinol®), scopolamine, and phosphorylated carbohydrate solution (Emetrol®), an older medication long used for treatment of nausea in young children and pregnant women. Scopolamine, an anticholinergic agent useful in motion sickness, is discussed in Chapter 5.

### Actions and Indications

Metoclopramide is a dopamine antagonist with action in the central nervous system and in the GI tract. Although it is chemically unrelated to the phenothiazine drugs, its antiemetic action is similar. In addition, metoclopramide increases GI motility through an unknown mechanism. This effect makes it useful in conditions where stasis (lack of movement) results in nausea, indigestion, and constipation. Metoclopramide is indicated in the prevention of chemotherapy induced and postoperative nausea and vomiting for treatment of diabetic gastroparesis (poor gastric motility can occur as a result of diabetes), and symptomatic gastroesophageal reflux disease.

Dronabinol is chemically identical to tetrahydrocannabinol, the principal psychoactive ingredient found in *Cannabis sativa*, and exerts the same effects in the central nervous system as marijuana. These include euphoria, appetite stimulation, altered perception of reality, and a reduction in cognitive ability and memory, among other actions. The mechanisms of the antiemetic and appetite stimulant effects are unknown. Dronabinol appears to be moderately effective in preventing CINV in studies done to date. It is indicated for use in chemotherapy patients who do not respond adequately to conventional therapy. It is also indicated for the treatment of loss of appetite in AIDS patients.

A number of other remedies can be used to treat nausea, including vitamin $B_6$ or ginger for the nausea of pregnancy, and cola syrup or phosphorylated carbohydrate solution (Emetrol®) for viral infections in children too young to be treated with antiemetics. Phosphorylated carbohydrate solution is thought to act directly on the GI tract to reduce smooth muscle contraction. Although shown to be effective in some small studies, the mechanisms of action of vitamin $B_6$ and ginger in nausea associated with pregnancy are unknown.

### Administration

Metoclopramide is usually administered thirty minutes before chemotherapy by intravenous infusion, and then repeated for several doses for prevention of CINV. For other indications, the oral route is usually preferred. This medication should be taken before meals. Higher doses are used for the prevention of chemotherapy-induced nausea and vomiting than for other indications.

Dronabinol is available only as gelatin capsules for oral administration. Dosage varies depending on tolerance to the drug and the condition for which it is being used. In the treatment of CINV the drug is given one or more hours before chemotherapy and then repeated at regular intervals afterward for several doses.

Vitamin $B_6$, phosphorylated carbohydrate solution, cola syrup, and ginger are orally administered. Phosphorylated carbohydrate solution should be taken undiluted, and without water or liquid immediately thereafter. Vitamin $B_6$, phosphorylated carbohydrate solution, and cola syrup are available without prescription.

### Side Effects

The usefulness of both dronabinol and metoclopramide are limited by side effects. As a dopamine antagonist that enters the CNS, metoclopramide might be expected to cause extrapyramidal symptoms or Parkinson-like symptoms, and it does. These symptoms are more common when high doses are administered and are more common in children or young adults who receive the drug. They can be reversed or prevented by administration of diphenhydramine. More common side effects seen with metoclopramide include drowsiness, fatigue and restlessness, and diarrhea due to increased GI motility. Although 20% to

30% of patients experience side effects, they are usually mild and transient at lower doses. At higher doses, the rate of side effects is higher and they may be significant enough to cause discontinuation of therapy.

Dronabinol causes increased sympathetic activity in the central nervous system. The resultant central nervous system effects, such as euphoria and other mood changes, altered perception of reality, inability to concentrate, and poor memory, are more consistently seen in patients taking higher doses. However, some patients developed psychotic episodes while taking low to average doses of the drug. Dronabinol can affect the cardiovascular system. Effects on blood pressure vary, but some people experience a drop in blood pressure on standing, which may result in dizziness or light-headedness. Dronabinol can cause elevated heart rate in some patients, especially those receiving higher doses.

Because of complex central nervous system effects and potential cardiovascular effects, this drug should be used cautiously in people with high blood pressure and heart disease, avoided completely in patients with psychiatric disorders, and used at lower doses in the elderly. It should not be given to children. The drug is highly fat soluble and effects may linger for days. People taking this medication must not drive or try to engage in any activity requiring judgement or coordination.

Vitamin $B_6$, phosphorylated carbohydrate solution, cola syrup, and ginger are not associated with any serious side effects when used as directed. Vitamin $B_6$ is water soluble, and does not build up in the body even at higher than necessary doses. Cola syrup and phosphorylated carbohydrate solution both contain sugar, and should be avoided in diabetic patients. Vomiting can be a very serious condition, especially in young children, where it can quickly lead to dehydration and serious electrolyte imbalances. The danger of self-treatment of any condition is in waiting too long to see a physician when an illness is more serious than it first appears.

## Tips for the Technician

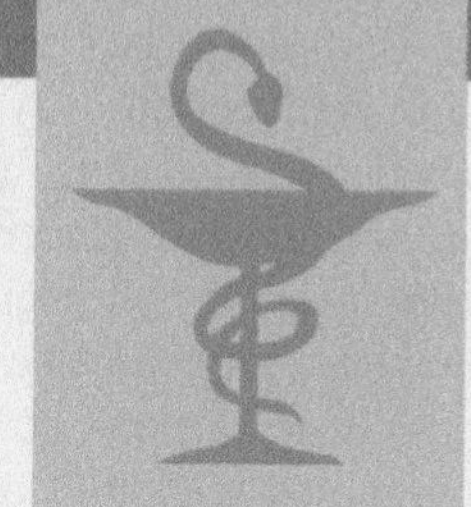

Users of metoclopramide should be counseled regarding potential side effects, including the possibility of involuntary movements, drowsiness, or light-headedness. Patients should notify their physicians if they experience involuntary movements. Pharmacy technicians need to make certain that appropriate warnings are given to the patient about the dangers of driving if they feel tired or light headed. The appropriate cautionary labels should be affixed to the prescription vial.

Dronabinol is a CIII controlled substance and as such, access to the drug must be monitored and the drug must be inventoried. One or more trustworthy members of the pharmacy staff, often including a technician, will be responsible for controlled substance inventories on a regular basis. Hospitals, and most retail pharmacies store controlled substances in specially locked cabinets, so that they are easier to monitor. This particular drug also requires special storage for stability reasons. The soft gelatin capsules must be stored in a tightly sealed container, between 46° and 59° F. Unless the pharmacy has a temperature-controlled cool storage area, this means the drug must be refrigerated.

Patients taking this drug must not drive, and the manufacturer recommends they stay in the company of a responsible adult. Patients should be warned that this drug has an additive effect with other psychoactive medications, and consumption of alcohol, other CNS depressants, or stimulants should be avoided. When dronabinol is taken with drugs that increase heart rate, such as tricyclic antidepressants, bronchodilators, or other sympathomimetics, an additive effect on heart rate can occur. Appropriately label prescription vials with auxiliary labels indicating the drug should be stored in the refrigerator, alcohol and other drugs should be avoided, and patients should not drive while taking this medication.

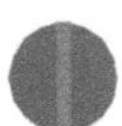

# Drugs for Bowel Disorders

ileus Obstruction of the bowel or intestine usually due to failure of peristalsis.

The initial symptoms of most bowel disorders are diarrhea (frequent loose or watery bowel movements) or constipation (hard, infrequent bowel movements). These symptoms can be related to a variety of serious diseases, but are far more likely to be related to less serious causes. Diarrhea can be caused by viral infections, changes in diet, or stress. More serious causes include bacterial infection or the inflammatory bowel diseases, such as Crohn's disease or ulcerative colitis. Constipation is usually caused by a diet low in fiber and a sedentary lifestyle. However, it can be a symptom of irritable bowel syndrome or ileus, a potentially life-threatening paralysis of the bowel. In this chapter, drugs to treat the symptoms of diarrhea and constipation are discussed. Treatment of the inflammatory bowel diseases, which are autoimmune in nature, involves some of the same drugs used to treat rheumatoid arthritis. Most of these will be covered in the next chapter. The aminosalicylates, however, exert local antiinflammatory effects on the GI tract, and will be discussed here.

## Antidiarrheals and Antiflatulents

Irritation of the GI tract caused by the presence of unabsorbable substances, toxins, or pathological organisms increases the motility of the intestines and may cause inflammation. Inflammation and increased peristaltic movement can cause fluids to be secreted into the gut or inadequately reabsorbed. The result of either or both mechanisms is diarrhea. Commonly used antidiarrheal drugs include antimotility agents, adsorbents, and anti-inflammatory agents.

### Actions and Indications

Two analogues of the opioid meperidine, diphenoxylate and loperamide (Imodium®), are widely used to control diarrhea. They interact with opiate receptors in the GI tract to slow peristaltic movement, thereby allowing for reabsorption of fluids. Both drugs lack analgesic activity and CNS effects at the doses used to treat diarrhea, but at higher doses typical opioid effects begin to occur with diphenoxylate. Atropine is added to discourage the abuse of this drug. Lomotil®, the product containing diphenoxylate and atropine, is a controlled substance indicated for use as an antidiarrheal in the treatment of acute, nonspecific diarrhea. Loperamide has a mechanism of action similar to diphenoxylate, but it is less well absorbed and therefore carries less risk of abuse. It is indicated for use in acute, nonspecific diarrhea. Loperamide is not a controlled substance and can be purchased without a prescription but is recommended for short-term use only.

Adsorbent agents, such as kaolin-pectin suspension (Kapectolin®), activated attapulgite (Parepectolin®), and bismuth subsalicylate (Pepto Bismol®), are widely used to control diarrhea. These agents act by adsorbing intestinal toxins or microorganisms, and by protecting the intestinal mucosa from irritation. Kaolin and attapulgite are highly refined clays, and pectin is a polysaccharide demulcent and thickener derived from fruit.

In addition to its adsorptive actions, bismuth subsalicylate decreases fluid secretion into the bowel. This effect is probably due to the action of salicylate, which is released when the compound dissociates in the GI tract. Bismuth subsalicylate is indicated for treatment of nausea and control of diarrhea. It is used with some success in the prevention of traveler's diarrhea when taken four times daily, for up to two weeks, during periods of high-risk travel.

flatulence The presence of gas or air in the GI tract to the degree that distention and discomfort occur.

Flatulence, or gas, can result from swallowing air, drinking carbonated beverages, or eating foods that are partially digested by gas-forming bacteria in the GI tract. In most situations gas passes through the GI tract in the same way that feces do. In some cases, however, large volumes of flatus are produced or retained and become quite painful. Simethicone (Mylicon®) is a surface-active agent that disperses excess flatus and prevents formation of gas pockets. It is available without prescription and has been used to treat gas symptoms, and colic in infants.

## Administration

The antidiarrheals are taken by mouth. They are available in a variety of formulations, as seen in **Table 22.3**. None of the antidiarrheal products should be given to children under three years of age except when prescribed by a physician. Antidiarrheals are administered after each loose bowel movement, up to a maximum number of doses each day. Clients purchasing antidiarrheals for self-treatment should be urged to read the instructions and adhere to the maximum dosage recommendations.

Simethicone is also administered orally. It is available as capsules, tablets, chewable tablets, and drops appropriate for use in infants or children. The drops are a suspension and must be shaken before using. Simethicone and antacid combinations are typically found in preparations for indigestion, such as Mylanta®.

## Side Effects

The most important unwanted effect of most antidiarrheals is constipation, which can become severe. It can occur as a result of using any of the antidiarrheals discussed here, but is more likely after use of the antiperistaltic agents, diphenoxylate with atropine or loperamide. Drowsiness or dizziness can occur in some patients taking these agents. Dry mouth can also occur. Neither diphenoxylate with atropine or loperamide should be used to treat the severe diarrhea caused by toxigenic bacteria associated with food poisoning or contaminated water, including *Salmonella, E. coli*, or *Shigella*. The use of either drug can prolong or aggravate diarrhea caused by these infections.

The adsorbent antidiarrheals are known to interact with some drugs to prevent or delay their absorption. The risk of an interaction of any importance can be avoided by appropriate spacing between doses of the antidiarrheals and other drugs. Bismuth subsalicylate, an ingredient found in a number of non-prescription antidiarrheals, might cause discoloration of the tongue and stools, an effect that is alarming to uninformed patients. People who are allergic to aspirin should not take this medication.

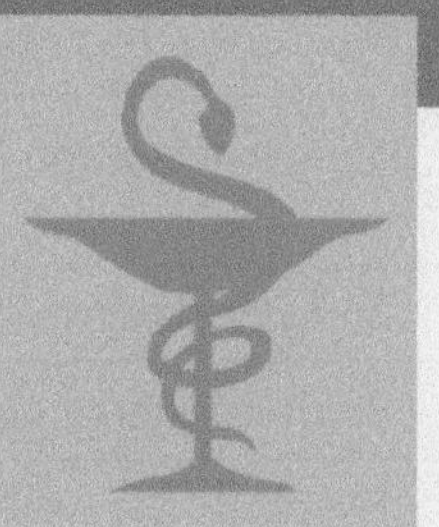

### Tips for the Technician

Diphenoxylate with atropine is a controlled substance, and technicians need to follow all applicable state and federal regulations regarding storage, dispensing, and record keeping. Patients receiving diphenoxylate with atropine or loperamide should be warned of the potential for these drugs to cause drowsiness, and the prescription vials appropriately labelled. Clients purchasing over the counter antidiarrheal agents should be encouraged to read and follow label directions carefully. The technician should direct them to the pharmacist if they have any concerns about the use of these medications.

# The Aminosalicylates

The aminosalicylates are a group of drugs that share a common active metabolite, mesalamine, also known as 5-aminosalicylic acid. These drugs are used in autoimmune conditions that affect the large intestine. They were the first drugs capable of inducing and maintaining remission in these diseases.

## Actions and Indications

The first aminosalicylate to be used for inflammatory bowel disease was sulfasalazine (Azulfidine®). This drug is cleaved within the bowel to mesalamine and sulfapyridine. Although the exact mechanism of action of this and related drugs is not completely understood, mesalamine is thought to have local antiinflammatory activity in the intestine. Sulfapyridine

**Table 22.3** A Comparison of Names, Indications, and Formulations of Drugs Used to Treat Conditions of the Lower GI Tract

| Generic | Brand Name | Available as | Indications | Notes |
|---|---|---|---|---|
| **Antidiarrheals** | | | | |
| Activated attapulgite | Parepectolin® | Liquid, tablets | Treatment of diarrhea | |
| Bismuth Subsalicylate | Pepto Bismol® | Suspension, tablets | Treatment of diarrhea, to prevent traveler's diarrhea | May discolor tongue, stools |
| Diphenoxylate | Lomotil® | Tablets, liquid | Management of non-specific diarrhea | Combined with atropine |
| Kaolin/Pectin | Kapectolin® | Suspension | Treatment of diarrhea | |
| Loperamide | Imodium® | Tablets, capsules, liquid | Management of non-specific diarrhea | |
| **Antiflatulent** | | | | |
| Simethicone | Mylicon® | Tablets, capsules, drops, chew tabs | Relief of symptoms caused by excess gas | Has been used for colic |
| **Aminosalicylates** | | | | |
| Sulfasalazine | Azulfidine® | Tablets, EC tabs | Ulcerative colitis, RA, juvenile RA | |
| Mesalamine | Asacol®, Pentasa® | ER tabs and caps, suppositories | Chronic inflammatory bowel disease | |
| **Laxatives** | | | | |
| Bisacodyl | Dulcolax® | Suppositories, EC tablets, tablets | Constipation | Stimulant laxative |
| Cascara Sagrada | | Tablets, liquid | Constipation | Stimulant laxative |
| Docusate | Colace® | Capsules, tablets, syrup | Prevention of constipation | Stool softener |
| Glycerin | Sani-Supp® | Suppositories, liquid | Constipation, can be used in children | Hyperosmotic laxative |
| Lactulose | Cephulac®, Enulose® | Solution, crystals for reconstitution | Constipation, hepatic encephalopathy | Hyperosmotic laxative |
| Magnesium salts | Magnesium citrate, Epsom salts, MOM | Liquid, granules, suspension | Constipation | Saline laxative |
| Methylcellulose | | Powder, tablets | Constipation | Bulk laxative |
| Polyethylene Glycol + electrolytes | GoLYTELY® | Powder for oral solution | Bowel evacuation | |
| Psyllium | Metamucil® | Powder, granules, wafers | Constipation, irritable bowel syndrome | Bulk laxative |
| Senna | Senokot® | Tablets, granules, liquid | Constipation | Stimulant laxative |

EC, enteric coated; ER, extended release; MOM, milk of magnesia; RA, rheumatoid arthritis.

has antibacterial activity and may alter immune response in some way. Sulfasalazine is indicated for the treatment of ulcerative colitis, rheumatoid arthritis, and juvenile rheumatoid arthritis. It is used off-label for the treatment of certain patients with Crohn's disease, ankylosing spondylitis, and psoriatic arthritis. Mesalamine (Asacol®) and other drugs that are metabolized to mesalamine are indicated for the treatment of ulcerative colitis.

### Administration

The aminosalicylates are administered orally or rectally. Mesalamine is manufactured as extended release tablets, capsules, and rectal suppositories. Sulfasalazine is available as tablets and enteric-coated tablets. The goal of an extended-release formulation is to deliver the active metabolite to the lower GI tract, and to avoid the GI irritation that some people experience.

### Side Effects

There is a risk of allergic reaction associated with taking sulfasalazine and other aminosalicylates that contain sulfonamide components. Patients who develop symptoms of an allergic reaction should discontinue the medication and contact their physician. The most common side effects observed with the use of the aminosalicylates are headache, nausea or loss of appetite, and abdominal pain. Less frequent, but more serious side effects include liver and kidney toxicity and drug-induced anemias.

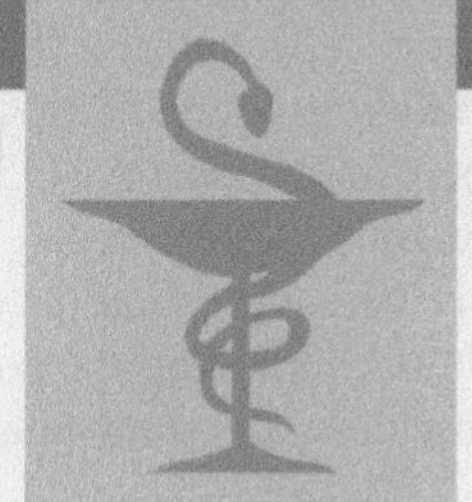

#### Tips for the Technician

It is important for the pharmacist to counsel all patients receiving one of the aminosalicylates for the first time. Patients need to know the symptoms of allergic reactions as well as symptoms that might indicate the development of a drug-induced anemia. Sulfasalazine produces dark yellow discoloration of the urine in most people. Technicians can warn patients of this by attaching the appropriate auxiliary label to the prescription vial. Enteric-coated or extended-release tablets and capsules should be swallowed whole. Uncoated sulfasalazine tablets leave dusty residue on equipment surfaces. These should be cleaned before using the equipment again for other prescriptions so that the dust does not contaminate another patient's medication.

## Laxatives

Laxatives are used to relieve constipation, defined as infrequent or difficult bowel movements, or in some cases to prepare the bowel for diagnostic procedures. The need for laxatives is usually related to a change in normal routines (such as travel), lack of exercise, a diet that is low in fiber, or inadequate fluid intake. Although occasional laxative use is safe, people who require more frequent use of laxatives will benefit from increasing their fluid intake, the amount of fiber in the diet, and regular exercise.

### Actions and Indications

The laxatives are classified based on their mechanisms of action as stimulants, bulk forming, saline, and hyperosmotic laxatives. They work by increasing peristaltic movement in the GI tract. Stimulant laxatives directly irritate or stimulate nerve or mucosal tissues in the GI tract. Saline laxatives are nonabsorbable salts that attract water into the stool, thus increasing the volume inside the GI tract. Bulk-forming laxatives also increase the volume of the stool, but they accomplish this with nonabsorbable fiber that retains water. When the volume of the stool increases, peristalsis is stimulated. Hyperosmotic laxatives and suppositories draw water into the bowel or rectum through osmosis. The nonabsorbable solute draws water across the concentration gradient, where it is retained in the bowel, increasing the volume of stools and stimulating peristalsis.

Laxatives are indicated for the occasional treatment of constipation or for evacuation of the bowel before examinations or diagnostic procedures. Fiber laxatives are sometimes used to regulate bowel habits in people with irritable bowel syndrome. Lactulose (Cephulac®) is used as a laxative, but also in the treatment of hepatic encephalopathy to increase the elimination of ammonia.

Stool softeners work by a different mechanism and are not, strictly speaking, laxatives. They facilitate the mixing of fats and water into the stool, making it softer. Stool softeners are used to prevent constipation, prevent straining with bowel movements, and to ease bowel movements when stools are hard and painful to pass.

## Administration

The majority of laxatives are taken orally, but a number are formulated for rectal administration as a suppository or an enema. Saline laxatives include milk of magnesia and magnesium citrate solution, and both are given orally. The stimulant laxatives cascara sagrada and senna compounds (Senokot®) are available for oral use, singly and in combination with other laxatives and stool softeners. Bisacodyl (Dulcolax®) is a stimulant laxative that is available as tablets, rectal suppositories, and enema.

The bulk forming laxatives are sold in a variety of preparations for oral use. Preparations include tablets, granules and powder for dilution in juice or water, capsules, and even wafers. The uncoated tablets can be difficult to swallow and should be taken with plenty of fluids. Lactulose solution is taken by mouth. Glycerin suppositories (Sani-Supp®), another hyperosmotic laxative, are manufactured in formulations for pediatric and adult rectal administration. Both lactulose and glycerin are hyperosmotic laxatives. The most commonly used stool softener, docusate, is sold as tablets, capsules, and syrup.

Products used for bowel preparation are usually given orally, although some physicians also use enemas. Many of these products are prescription items, including the polyethylene glycol and electrolyte solution, GoLYTELY®. Most other laxatives are available without prescription.

## Side Effects

Chronic use of laxatives, especially stimulants, is very detrimental and may result in laxative dependence. Diarrhea, cramping, and fluid and electrolyte imbalance can occur in sensitive patients or when laxatives are used inappropriately. Individuals with undiagnosed severe abdominal pain, vomiting, or other symptoms that may indicate appendicitis should not use laxatives, and should contact their physician immediately. Use of lactulose can cause gas, belching, and abdominal discomfort. Esophageal or intestinal obstruction has occurred in people taking bulk-forming laxatives without adequate intake of fluids.

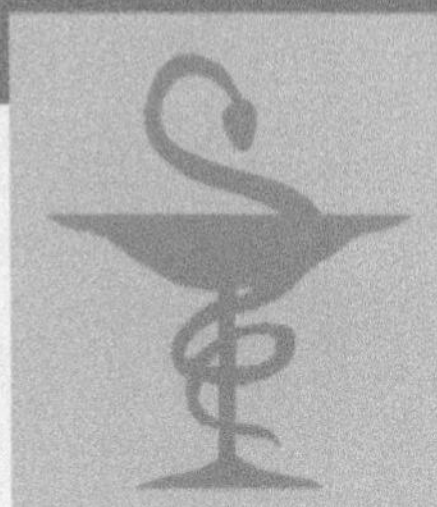

### Tips for the Technician

Technicians may have an opportunity to interact with people looking for nonprescription laxatives. If the technician discovers that a client is using laxatives frequently or routinely, refer the client to the pharmacist, who can present the dangers of laxative abuse. The pharmacist or technician can remind patients with constipation to be sure to include plenty of water, fresh fruit, and fiber in the diet. Cascara sagrada and senna can cause reddish, brown, or black discoloration of the urine. Although they are flavored, the taste of magnesium citrate solutions improves with refrigeration. In hospital pharmacies, the technician can arrange to have some magnesium citrate stock refrigerated and ready to use.

# Review Questions

## Multiple Choice

Choose the best answer for the following questions:

1. Which of the following is not a factor that can contribute to the development of peptic ulcers?
   a. Smoking
   b. Eating spicy food
   c. Alcohol consumption
   d. Use of nonsteroidal anti-inflammatory drugs
   e. Infection with *H. pylori*

2. Circle the letter corresponding to the $H_2$ receptor antagonist most often involved with drug interactions.
   a. Famotidine
   b. Ranitidine
   c. Cimetidine
   d. Nizatidine
   e. None of the above

3. Sucralfate works by
   a. Reducing acid production by blocking $H_2$ receptors in gastric parietal cells
   b. Forming a sticky paste that adheres to the surface of damaged mucosa
   c. Increasing prostaglandin mediated mucus production
   d. Inhibiting thee excretion of hydrogen ions
   e. Neutralizing stomach acid

4. Which of the following pairs of antiemetics work by antagonizing the effects off dopamine?
   a. Metoclopramide and promethazine
   b. Diphenhydramine and Emetrol®
   c. Meclizine and prochlorperazine
   d. All of the above
   e. None of the above

5. Milk of magnesia is considered a
   a. Bulk-forming laxative
   b. Stool softener
   c. Hyperosmotic laxative
   d. Stimulant laxative
   e. Saline laxative

## True/False

6. Calcium carbonate is an effective antacid that is also useful as a calcium supplement.
   a. True
   b. False

7. $H_2$ receptor antagonists are the drugs of choice for the treatment of peptic ulcer disease because they are safer and more effective than the proton pump inhibitors.
   a. True
   b. False

8. Diphenoxylate and loperamide are derivatives of the opioids, but loperamide is poorly absorbed and is available without prescription.
   a. True
   b. False

9. Sulfasalazine is used to treat ulcerative colitis as well as some other autoimmune diseases, such as rheumatoid arthritis.
   a. True
   b. False

10. The most common side effects of the antihistamine antiemetics is torticollis.
   a. True
   b. False

## Matching

For numbers 11 to 15, match the condition with the correct lettered choice of a drug used to treat or prevent it from the list below. Choices will not be used more than once and may not be used at all.

| | |
|---|---|
| 11. Chemotherapy-induced nausea and vomiting | a. Ondansetron |
| 12. Traveler's diarrhea | b. Misoprostol |
| 13. Seasickness | c. Dimenhydrinate |
| 14. NSAID induced ulcers | d. Milk of Magnesia |
| 15. Nausea of pregnancy | e. Vitamin $B_6$ |
| | f. Pepto Bismol® |
| | g. Lactulose |

## Short Answer

16. In what situations is dronabinol useful, and what limits its usefulness?

17. List two advantages and two disadvantages of the proton pump inhibitors in the treatment of peptic ulcer disease or acid reflux disease.

18. How do the adsorbent antidiarrheal agents work?

19. How do bulk laxatives differ from stool softeners? Give an example of each.

20. Explain the antiemetic action of the $5HT_3$ antagonists. Give the brand name and indication for use of two of these drugs.

# FOR FURTHER INQUIRY

Irritable bowel syndrome is a functional disorder (meaning there is a problem with some normal function without any physical abnormality) of the bowel that occurs fairly commonly in the Unites States. Investigate the cause of this syndrome, drug treatment, and other methods that can help control this disorder, or research another GI disorder that interests you.

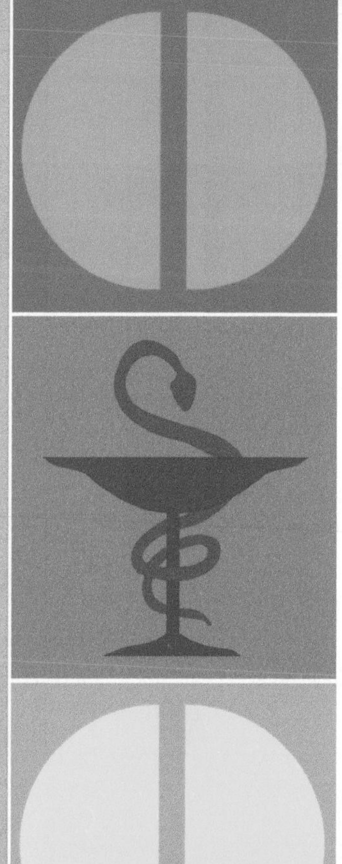

Chapter **23**

# Drugs Used to Treat Musculoskeletal Disorders

## KEY TERMS

- arthritis
- aseptic technique
- biologicals
- dysmenorrhea
- pyrogen
- teratogenic
- tinnitus
- tophi
- intrathecal
- uricosuric

## OBJECTIVES

After studying this chapter, the reader should be able to:

- Describe the mechanism of action of the nonsteroidal anti-inflammatory drugs, their three major therapeutic effects, and the most common side effect associated with their use.
- Define the term "disease-modifying antirheumatic drug," describe why these agents are used, and list three drugs that are considered to be part of this group.
- List the brand and generic names of one drug used for each of the following conditions: rheumatoid arthritis, gout, and osteoporosis. Name an auxiliary label the pharmacy technician will apply to prescriptions for each drug listed.
- Compare and contrast the actions of acetaminophen with the actions of aspirin or other nonsteroidal anti-inflammatory drugs. Explain why consumers need to be aware of the acetaminophen content of medications.
- Describe two differences and two similarities between the skeletal muscle relaxants cyclobenzaprine and baclofen.

## DRUGS COVERED IN THIS CHAPTER

### Nonsteroidal Anti-inflammatory Drugs

| Salicylates | Propionic Acid Derivatives | Acetic Aid Derivatives | Enolic Acid Derivatives | COX-2 Inhibitors |
|---|---|---|---|---|
| Asprin | Fenoprofen | Diclofenac | Piroxicam | Celecoxib |
| Choline salicylate | Ibuprofen | Etodolac | | |
| Diflunisal | Ketoprofen | Ketorolac | | |
| | Naproxen | Nabumetone | | |
| | | Sulindac | | |

### Disease-Modifying Antirheumatic Drugs

| TNF Inhibitors | Other DMARDs |
|---|---|
| Adalimumab | Gold salts |
| Etanercept | Hydroxychloroquine |
| Infliximab | Leflunomide |
| | Minocycline |
| | Methotrexate |
| | Sulfasalazine |

### Drugs for Gout / Drug Treatment for Osteoporosis

| Drugs for Gout | Drug Treatment for Osteoporosis: Bisphosphonates | Drug Treatment for Osteoporosis: Miscellaneous Drugs for Osteoporosis |
|---|---|---|
| Allopurinol | Alendronate | Calcitonin |
| Colchicine | Etidronate | Raloxifene |
| Probenecid | Ibandronate | |
| | Pamidronate | |
| | Risedronate | |

### Drugs for Mild Pain / Skeletal Muscle Relaxants

| Drugs for Mild Pain | Skeletal Muscle Relaxants |
|---|---|
| Acetominephen | Baclofen |
| | Carisoprodol |
| | Cyclobenzaprine |
| | Dantrolene |
| | Diazepam |
| | Metaxalone |
| | Tizanidine |

Because we humans spend a great deal of time in motion, both at work and at play, our musculoskeletal systems are the origin of many complaints. Musculoskeletal disorders often arise from overuse or misuse of the muscles, bones, joints, and connective tissues. Most people experience muscle strain, broken bones, or back pain at some time in their lives. If not, they know someone who has. Beyond these common complaints, however, is a realm of chronic and debilitating disorders of bones, joints, and muscles that are estimated to cost American society $65 billion dollars annually in lost productivity, disability, and health care.

People are often surprised to learn that there are more than 100 different forms of joint, muscle, and connective tissue diseases. These include osteoporosis, autoimmune disorders such as rheumatoid arthritis, and many other forms of arthritis, or inflammation of the joints. Some form of arthritis affects nearly one of every six Americans at some time in their lives. People tend to think of arthritis as a disease of the elderly, but sadly, children as young as six months of age can develop a form of arthritis called juvenile rheumatoid arthritis. This chapter will cover drugs used to treat musculoskeletal disorders, including sprains and strains, osteoarthritis, the autoimmune diseases, and osteoporosis.

arthritis Inflammation of the joints caused by infection, trauma, and metabolic or other causes.

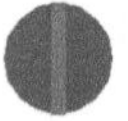

# Nonsteroidal Anti-inflammatory Drugs

Hippocrates and the ancient Romans left records of the use of willow bark to relieve pain and fever. The bark and leaves of the willow tree contain salicin, which was converted to salicylic acid and widely used for pain and fever in the early nineteenth century. A French chemist originally synthesized and reported the discovery of a crude form of acetylsalicylic acid in the late nineteenth century. Ultimately, Felix Hoffman, who was said to be searching for a drug to relieve his father's arthritis pain, came across the earlier research and developed a more refined process to make acetylsalicylic acid. He worked for Bayer Company and convinced them to manufacture the drug, which they patented as Aspirin®.

Shortly after World War I, Bayer Corporation lost their patent on the name, and aspirin became a common name used worldwide. Aspirin is the oldest and most commonly used nonsteroidal anti-inflammatory drug (NSAID) and is the drug to which all other anti-inflammatory agents are compared. As the name implies, the nonsteroidal anti-inflammatory drugs are not related to the anti-inflammatory corticosteroids. Although some sources make a distinction between the salicylates (aspirin-like drugs) and NSAIDs, aspirin will be considered the prototype of the NSAIDs in this text.

## Actions and Indications

Inflammation is a normal, protective response to tissue injury. It is the body's defensive effort to inactivate or destroy invading organisms, remove irritants, and set the stage for tissue repair. Inflammation is triggered when cytokines signal white blood cells that tissue injury has occurred or foreign substances have been detected. When this complex process begins, cells are mobilized, enzymes released, and antibody activated, with the result of tissue edema, inflammation, and the beginning of the healing process. When healing is complete, the inflammatory process usually subsides. However, sometimes the inflammation reactions are inappropriate and create tissue injury, as seen in asthma or rheumatoid arthritis. In these situations, drugs with anti-inflammatory or immunosuppressive properties may be required to control the immune response and prevent tissue damage.

The cytokines, or chemical mediators, released at the initiation of the inflammation process vary with the type of inflammatory process. They include histamine, leukotriene, bradykinin, thromboxane, prostaglandins, and many, many others. All of the NSAIDs act by inhibiting the synthesis of prostaglandins. They work by blocking the action of two enzymes that are crucial to the formation of prostaglandins, cyclooxygenase-1 and 2. Referred to as COX-1 or COX-2, these enzymes are responsible for prostaglandin synthesis in different areas. COX-1 regulates prostaglandin synthesis responsible for some normal cellular processes, such as production of protective mucus in the stomach, platelet aggregation, and kidney function. COX-2 regulates production of prostaglandins at the sites of injury, but this enzyme is also found in normal brain, kidney and bone tissue, where its role is still not completely understood.

The NSAIDs inhibit COX-1 and COX-2 to varying degrees (see **Fig. 23.1**). In the past decade, pharmaceutical companies produced three drugs that were COX-2 specific, thinking they would offer a greater degree of safety because of fewer GI side effects. The COX-2 inhibitors have about equal anti-inflammatory effects and are less likely to cause GI side effects. However, two of the three drugs have been removed from the market because of unwanted effects on the heart and kidneys. Celecoxib (Celebrex®) is the only remaining COX-2 specific inhibitor.

The COX-2 inhibitors are unique among the NSAIDs in that they provide no protective effect against platelet aggregation, a response due to inhibition of COX-1. Aspirin is also unique in that it irreversibly confers the antiplatelet aggregation effect used for prevention of myocardial infarction. Other NSAIDs inhibit platelet aggregation, but the effect only lasts as long as the drug is present in the bloodstream.

The NSAIDs, including aspirin, have three major therapeutic actions. They are anti-inflammatory, analgesic, and antipyretic, meaning they reduce inflammation, pain, and fever. Because aspirin and the NSAIDs inhibit cyclooxygenase activity, they impede the synthesis of prostaglandins and reduce inflammation in which prostaglandins act as mediators. One of the prostaglandins is thought to sensitize nerve endings to the action of bradykinin, histamine, and other chemical mediators responsible for causing pain. Thus, by decreasing prostaglandin synthesis, aspirin and other NSAIDs repress the sensation of pain.

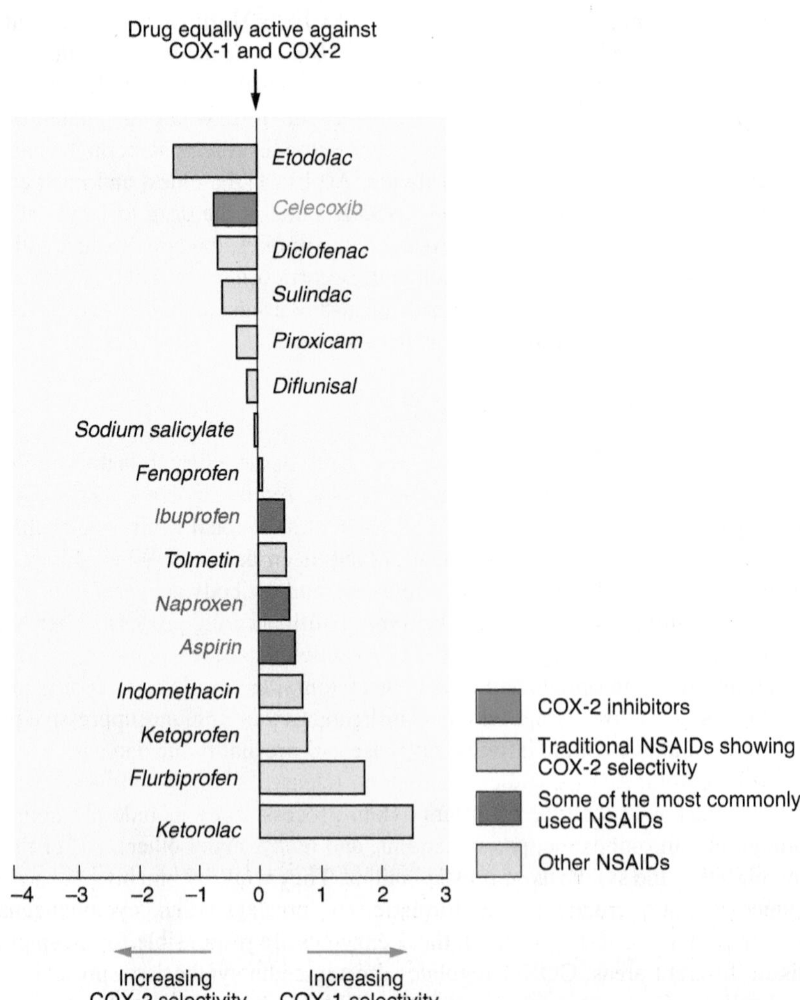


**Figure 23.1** Relative COX-1 and COX-2 inhibition by selected NSAIDs. (Adapted with permission from Harvey RA, Champe PC, Howland RD, et al. *Lippincott's Illustrated Reviews: Pharmacology*, 3rd edition. Baltimore: Lippincott Williams & Wilkins, 2006.)

Acetaminophen, which has no effect on prostaglandins, has no anti-inflammatory effects, and is less effective at relieving pain associated with swelling or inflammation (see **Fig. 23.2**). NSAIDs are used for the management of mild to moderate pain and are more effective than the opiates at relieving pain in which inflammation is involved. Combinations of opioids and NSAIDs are more effective than either alone.

Fever occurs when the thermoregulatory center in the brain is reset. This up regulation can be caused by prostaglandins produced when a fever-inducing agent (pyrogen) is released from activated white cells. The salicylates lower body temperature in patients with fever by blocking prostaglandin synthesis. Aspirin resets the "thermostat" toward normal, and body temperature of febrile patients decreases by the usual mechanisms of peripheral vasodilation and sweating. Aspirin has no effect on normal body temperature.

pyrogen A substance that, when in the bloodstream, causes fever.

## Analogy

The thermoregulatory center in the brain is a little like a thermostat. In healthy states, most people's "thermostat" is set to keep the body at about 98.6°F when measured orally. The body makes adjustments to cool or heat itself through sweating or flushing when excessively warm, or shivering and vasoconstriction when cold. The presence of pyrogens (fever producers) causes the body's "thermostat" to reset at a level higher than usual. This is an adaptive response that helps the body kill invading microorganisms, and explains why you shiver with a fever even though you are warmer than usual.

The NSAIDs are indicated for use in many arthritic diseases. They are frequently used for treatment of mild to moderate pain associated with soft tissue injury, such as athletic injuries or dental procedures. Indomethacin (Indocin®), an acetic acid derivative NSAID, can be used to correct a cardiac anomaly seen in some premature infants called patent ductus arteriosis. The ductus arteriosus is an opening in the fetal heart that allows blood to bypass the baby's lungs before birth. When it fails to close after birth, it can cause problems in the newborn. Both indomethacin and its close relative sulindac (Clinoril®) are indicated

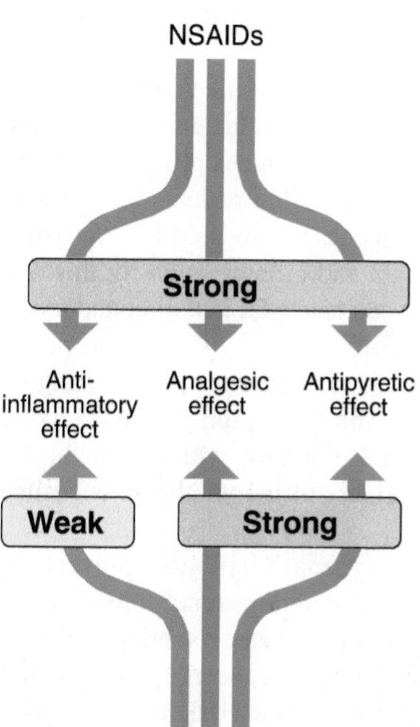


**Figure 23.2** The comparative actions of NSAIDs and acetaminophen. (Adapted with permission from Harvey RA, Champe PC, Howland RD, et al. *Lippincott's Illustrated Reviews: Pharmacology*, 3rd edition. Baltimore: Lippincott Williams & Wilkins, 2006.)

for the treatment of gouty arthritis. Ketorolac (Toradol®), another acetic acid derivative, is used for the short-term relief of postoperative or other acute pain. The recommendation for the maximum duration of ketorolac treatment is five days.

The propionic acid derivatives ibuprofen (Motrin®, Advil®), naproxen (Naprosyn®, Aleve®), fenoprofen (Nalfon®), and ketoprofen (Orudis®) are some of the most widely used NSAIDs. They are indicated for treatment of rheumatoid and osteoarthritis, as well as being used for pain relief. Ibuprofen and naproxen in nonprescription strengths are used for the reduction of fever, and are the most popular drugs in prescription strength for the treatment of arthritis. This group of drugs is also indicated for the treatment of dysmenorrhea, painful menstrual periods

dysmenorrhea Painful menstruation.

## Administration

The effects of the NSAIDs, including the salicylates, are dose related. The antipyretic and analgesic effects occur at low doses, whereas anti-inflammatory effects require higher doses. This is especially important when considering the use of aspirin. The pharmacokinetics of aspirin is dose dependent. When higher doses are administered, the time for the drug to be removed is longer, so the drug is likely to accumulate, and serum salicylate levels must be monitored. Because the use of high dose aspirin is complicated by the requirement for laboratory monitoring, the newer NSAIDs are nearly always used instead of aspirin for treatment of arthritis and other inflammatory processes.

All of the nonsteroidal anti-inflammatory drugs, including the salicylates, are well absorbed orally, and nearly all are exclusively orally administered. There are a few exceptions, including aspirin and indomethacin, which are both available as rectal suppositories. Ketorolac is available for intramuscular or intravenous injection, as well as in tablet form. Several NSAIDs are available in formulations for administration to children or adults who have difficulty swallowing. Choline salicylate (Arthropan®) is an aspirin-like drug sold as a liquid. Aspirin is also sold as a chewable, low dose tablet, and indomethacin is available as a suspension. The use of ibuprofen in children has increased dramatically over the past decade, and manufacturers provide a number of child-friendly formulations. These include infant drops, oral suspension, and chewable tablets in two strengths. **Table 23.1** lists the generic and brand names, indications, and available formulations of the drugs for arthritis and gout discussed in this chapter.

## Side Effects

The most common adverse effects of the NSAIDs are related to the GI tract and range from dyspepsia to formation of bleeding ulcers. Epigastric distress can be related to local effects, but GI ulceration is a result of depression of prostaglandin related mucus production in the GI tract. A microscopic amount of GI bleeding is almost universal in patients treated with salicylates. The propionic acid derivatives are less likely to cause serious GI bleeding than aspirin and gained wide acceptance in the treatment of pain and inflammation for this reason. Although promoted as safe to the GI tract, celecoxib can cause GI irritation and ulceration but at a lower rate than other NSAIDs (see **Fig. 23.3**).

tinnitus The sensation of noise, such as ringing or buzzing, in the ear.

Side effects involving the central nervous system, such as headache, tinnitus (ringing or roaring in the ears), and dizziness are well documented. These symptoms are most likely to occur at anti-inflammatory doses. CNS symptoms are most common with indomethacin. Despite being a potent anti-inflammatory agent, the usefulness of indomethacin is limited because of the high rate of CNS and GI side effects.

All of the NSAIDs can affect renal function. Cyclooxygenase inhibitors prevent the synthesis of prostaglandins that are responsible for maintaining renal blood flow. Decreased synthesis of prostaglandins can result in sodium and water retention and may cause edema in some patients. Celecoxib has been noted to cause exacerbation of hypertension as well as fluid retention, and is associated with at least as much risk to kidney function as the other NSAIDs. The elderly appear to be especially prone to the toxic effects of NSAIDS on the kidney and to developing GI ulceration.

**Table 23.1** The Generic and Brand Names, Indications, and Available Formulations of the Drugs for Arthritis and Gout Discussed in This Chapter

| Generic | Brand Name | Available as | Indications | Notes |
|---|---|---|---|---|
| **NSAIDs** | | | | |
| Aspirin | Bufferin®, St. Joseph's®, Bayer®, others | Tablets, chew tabs, effervescent tabs, suppositories, gum | Pain, fever, RA, prevent MI, osteoarthritis, inflammation | Avoid use in children with viral infections |
| Choline salicylate | Arthropan® | Liquid | RA, osteoarthritis, inflammation | |
| Diflunisal | Dolobid® | Tablets | Treatment of pain, RA, osteoarthritis | |
| Celecoxib | Celebrex® | Capsules | Osteoarthritis and RA | |
| Diclofenac | Voltaren® | Tablets, ER tabs | Osteoarthritis and RA, ankylosing spondylitis, dysmenorrhea | |
| Etodolac | Lodine® | Tablets, ER tabs, capsules | Treatment of pain, RA, osteoarthritis | Immediate release only for pain |
| Fenoprofen | Nalfon® | Capsules, tablets | Treatment of pain, RA, osteoarthritis | |
| Ibuprofen | Motrin®, Advil®, others | Tablets, capsules, chew tabs, drops, suspension | Pain, fever, RA, osteo-arthritis, inflammation | OTC and Rx |
| Indomethacin | Indocin® | Capsules, ER caps, suspension, injection | Osteoarthritis, RA, gouty arthritis, patent ductus arteriosus | |
| Ketoprofen | Orudis® | Tablets, capsules, ER caps | Osteoarthritis, RA, primary dysmenorrhea, pain | OTC and Rx |
| Ketorolac | Toradol® | Injection, tablets | Acute pain, moderate to severe | Max use 5 days |
| Meloxicam | Mobic® | Tablets | Osteoarthritis | |
| Nabumetone | Relafen® | Tablets | Treatment of pain, RA, osteoarthritis | |
| Naproxen | Naprosyn®, Aleve® | Tablets, ER tabs, suspension | Pain, fever, RA, osteoarthritis, inflammation, ankylosing spondylitis | OTC and Rx |
| Piroxicam | Feldene® | Capsules | Osteoarthritis, RA | |
| Sulindac | Clinoril® | Tablets | Osteoarthritis, RA, gout, inflammation, ankylosing spondylitis | |

*(continues)*

**Table 23.1** The Generic and Brand Names, Indications, and Available Formulations of the Drugs for Arthritis and Gout Discussed in This Chapter *(continued)*

| Generic | Brand Name | Available as | Indications | Notes |
|---|---|---|---|---|
| **DMARDs** | | | | |
| Adalimumab | Humira® | Injection | RA | Refrigerate |
| Etanercept | Enbrel® | Injection | Ankylosing spondylitis, JRA, RA, psoriatic arthritis | Refrigerate |
| Infliximab | Remicade® | Injection | Crohn's disease, RA, *JRA, ankylosing spondylitis, psoriatic arthritis | Refrigerate |
| Gold sodium thiomalate | Myochrysine Aurolate® | Injection | RA | |
| Hydroxy-chloroquine | Plaquenil® | Tablets | Systemic lupus, malaria, RA | |
| Leflunomide | Arava® | Tablets | RA, *psoriatic arthritis | |
| Methotrexate | Trexall® | Tablets, injection | RA, JRA, psoriasis, cancers | |
| Minocycline | Minocin® | Capsules | *Early RA | |
| Sulfasalazine | Azulfidine® | Tablets, EC tabs | Ulcerative colitis, RA, *JRA, ankylosing spondylitis, Crohn's disease, psoriatic arthritis | |
| **Drugs for Gout** | | | | |
| Allopurinol | Zyloprim® | Tablets, injection | Gout, hyperuricemia of malignancy, some kidney stones | Injection not for gout |
| Colchicine | | Tablets, injection | Acute gout | |
| Probenecid | | Tablets | Gout, hyperuricemia | |
| **Other Analgesics** | | | | |
| Acetaminophen | Tylenol® | Tablets, capsules, ER tabs, caps, chew tabs, elixir, suppositories, drops | Analgesic, antipyretic, OA | OTC, max dose = 4 g/day in adults |

*off-label use

EC, enteric coated; ER, extended-release; JRA, juvenile rheumatoid arthritis; MI, myocardial infarction; OA, osteoarthritis; RA, rheumatoid arthritis.

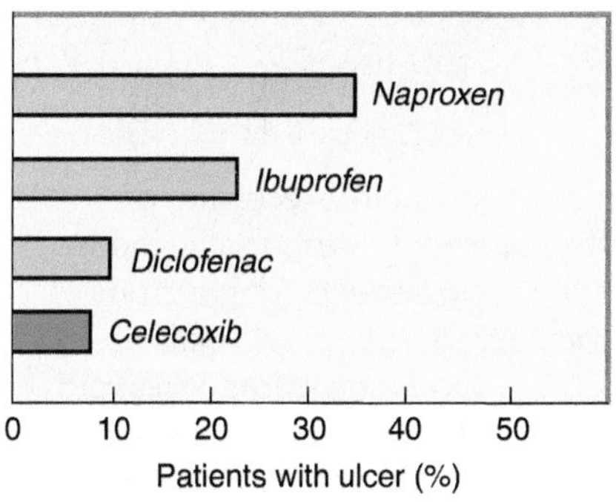


**Figure 23.3** The relative risk of developing GI ulceration from some commonly used NSAIDs. (Adapted with permission from Harvey RA, Champe PC, Howland RD, et al. *Lippincott's Illustrated Reviews: Pharmacology*, 3rd edition. Baltimore: Lippincott Williams & Wilkins, 2006.)

Before the advent of child safety caps, aspirin overdose was a fairly common cause of pediatric emergency room visits. Baby aspirin, which tastes good, was in nearly every household with children and was a likely target for childhood ingestion. Children are particularly prone to salicylate intoxication, which can be mild or severe. The mild form is called salicylism, and is characterized by nausea, vomiting, hyperventilation, headache, confusion, dizziness, and tinnitus. When large doses of salicylate are taken, severe salicylate intoxication can result in hallucinations, convulsions, coma, respiratory and metabolic acidosis, and death from respiratory failure (**Fig. 23.4**).

Although aspirin is one of the best fever-reducers available without a prescription, it is infrequently recommended for use in children. Aspirin is no longer recommended for children or adolescents with fever because its use in certain cases is associated with an increased risk of developing Reye's syndrome. Reye's syndrome is a very rare and sometimes fatal illness that usually develops in children after they have influenza or chickenpox. While the connection with aspirin use is still controversial, the FDA and other groups recommend avoidance of aspirin in children with fevers related to viruses. Since most parents are not qualified to determine whether or not a child has a viral illness, its use is routinely avoided.

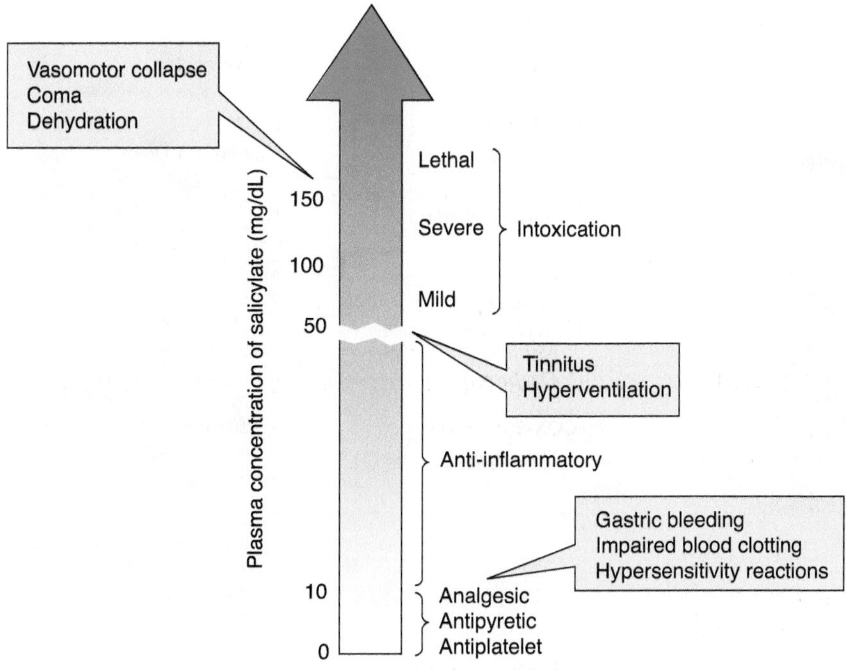


**Figure 23.4** The effects of aspirin are dose related, and high doses can result in very dangerous toxic effects. (Adapted with permission from Harvey RA, Champe PC, Howland RD, et al. *Lippincott's Illustrated Reviews: Pharmacology*, 3rd edition. Baltimore: Lippincott Williams & Wilkins, 2006.)

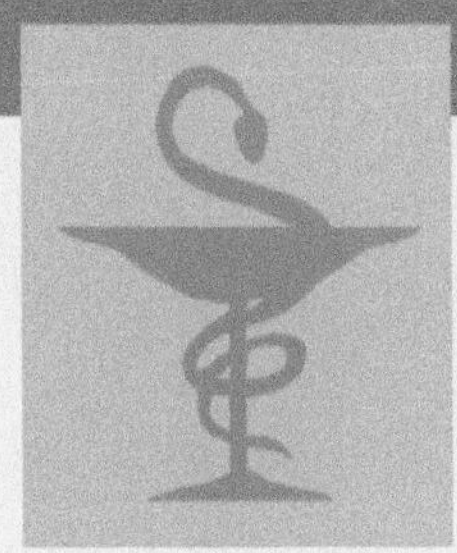

## Tips for the Technician

Although it is a good idea for the pharmacist to counsel all patients receiving prescription NSAIDs regarding potential side effects, this education is especially important for elderly clients, who are more likely to experience side effects. These drugs must be taken with food to protect the stomach from local irritation, and vials should be labelled with the appropriate auxiliary. Clients should be warned to avoid taking the medications at the same time as other GI irritants, such as alcoholic beverages. The NSAIDs interact with warfarin to increase the risk of bleeding. Patients receiving warfarin need to be warned against buying nonprescription pain relievers without checking first with the physician or pharmacist. **Figure 23.5** summarizes some advantages and disadvantages of the NSAIDs.

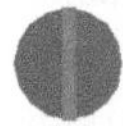

# Disease-Modifying Antirheumatic Drugs

Aspirin and the other nonsteroidal anti-inflammatory drugs remained the mainstay of the treatment of arthritis for many years. They treat pain and reduce swelling, allowing people afflicted with these diseases to continue most daily activities. Unlike the corticosteroids, there are no exceptional long-term consequences of their use. However, the NSAIDs do not prevent damage to joints or other tissues. The disease-modifying antirheumatic drugs

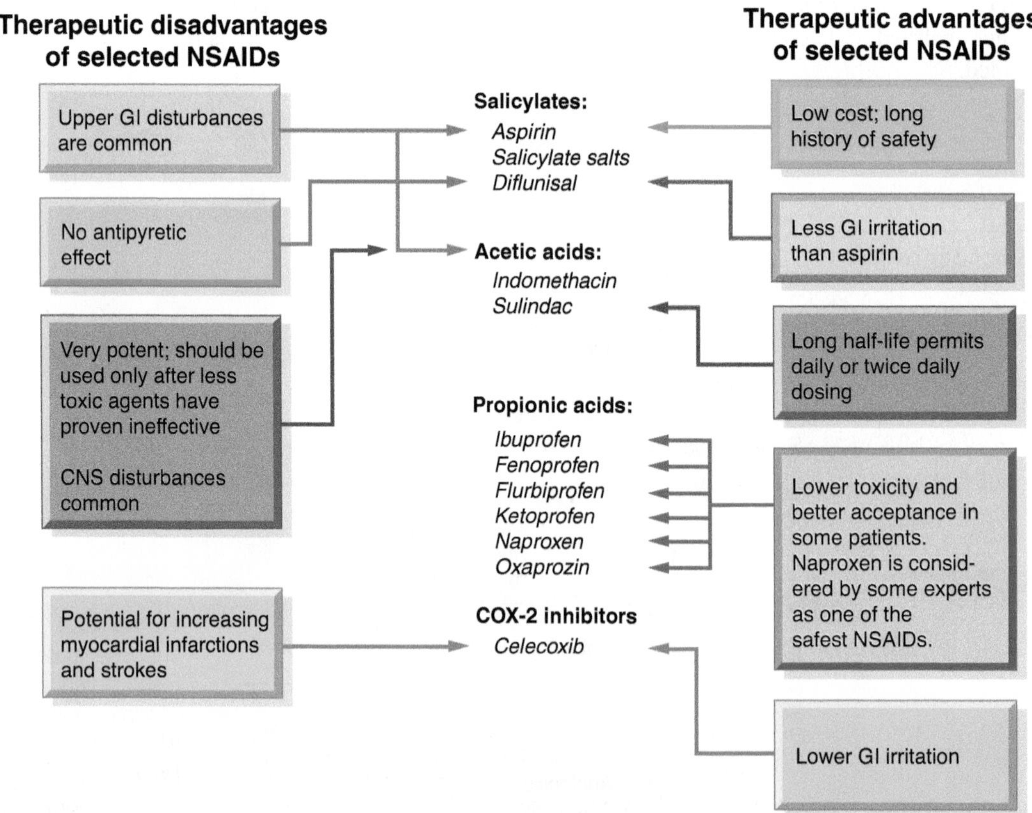


**Figure 23.5** A summary of advantages and disadvantages of the NSAIDs. (Adapted with permission from Harvey RA, Champe PC, Howland RD, et al. *Lippincott's Illustrated Reviews: Pharmacology*, 3rd edition. Baltimore: Lippincott Williams & Wilkins, 2006.)

(DMARDs) are a group of unrelated drugs that have the potential to reduce or prevent joint damage in rheumatoid arthritis, and organ damage in other autoimmune disease. Most of these drugs are used primarily to slow the course of the disease in autoimmune disorders, but some have other roles, which are covered in other chapters.

## The TNF Inhibitors

Cells in the body are able to adapt and change partly because they can receive and send chemical signals. It is chemical signalling that directs muscle cells to flex, nerves to sense pain, and white blood cells to react to invasions by bacteria or other invasions. Chemical signals include neurotransmitters, hormones, and the many mediators of inflammation already mentioned. The chemicals that mediate many forms of cell-to-cell communications are cytokines, and they include tumor necrosis factor.

### Actions and Indications

Tumor necrosis factor, or TNF, plays a central role in the inflammatory processes associated with rheumatoid arthritis and other autoimmune diseases. TNF "recruits" inflammatory cells to the joints or other affected tissues, where they release enzymes and other chemicals that cause damage. Three drugs, adalimumab (Humira®), etanercept (Enbrel®), and infliximab (Remicade®), specifically target the role of TNF in autoimmune diseases. The TNF inhibitors are bioengineered antibodies that bind to and inactivate TNF. Although relatively new drugs, they are already used widely to stop the destruction of joints and other tissues. Unlike many DMARDs they begin to relieve symptoms fairly quickly, often after the first dose. They are indicated for the treatment of rheumatoid arthritis, ankylosing spondylitis, juvenile rheumatoid arthritis, and infliximab is used for Crohn's disease. Most of these agents are used off-label for psoriatic arthritis.

### Administration

Antibodies, vaccines, and other products referred to as biologicals (treatments derived from the immune response of living organisms) are rarely orally administered, because gastric acid and enzymes break them down. The TNF inhibitors are antibodies, and they must be given by injection. Infliximab (Remicade®) is given intravenously, and therefore requires a visit to the doctor's office on an every eight-week basis during maintenance therapy, and more often at the initiation of therapy. The intravenous infusion runs in over two hours. Adalimumab (Humira®) and etanercept (Enbrel®) are given subcutaneously and can be self-administered by the patient.

biologicals Antibodies, vaccines, cultures, or other products made from living organisms and used to treat or prevent disease.

### Side Effects

It is not surprising that the most common side effects to the TNF inhibitors are allergic in nature, since all three drugs are proteins. Infliximab infusions may be accompanied by shortness of breath, rash, and headache. Subcutaneous injection of the other two products is associated with skin reactions at the injection site, including hives. Both of these products sting when injected.

Other reactions of a more serious nature are also known to occur. A few patients have new onset or exacerbations of neurological disorders such as seizures or multiple sclerosis while taking these medications. The exact nature of the relationship of the neurological diseases to the drugs is unclear, and this adverse effect is rare. Other serious reactions are predictable based on the pharmacologic actions of these drugs. Because TNF inhibitors impact the immune response, they can impair the ability of the body to fight infections. They pose a serious risk to people with chronic infectious diseases such as tuberculosis or valley fever (coccidioidomycosis). Infections acquired before or during treatment can become fatal when the host's immune system is suppressed with a TNF inhibitor. Infections at the site of injection can occur, and are related to poor aseptic technique (method used to maintain sterility of products or equipment).

Our immune system plays a role in removing our own cells when they become abnormal. Cancerous cells develop tumor antigens that the body recognizes and normally re-

aseptic technique Methods used by pharmacists and technicians to maintain the sterility of sterile products during compounding.

moves before tumors become established. There is concern that over the long-term these drugs may predispose the users to cancers because part of the response to malignant cells is suppressed. Since they have been in widespread use for less than a decade, it remains to be seen whether or not this theoretical risk becomes a problem.

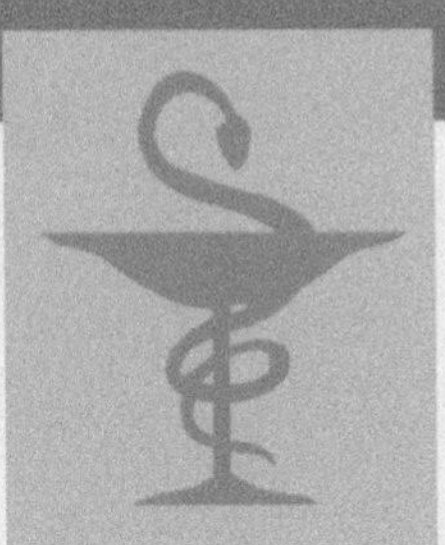

## Tips for the Technician

All biological products have short shelf lives and usually require refrigeration. Such is the case with the TNF inhibitors, which must be stored under refrigeration. Once prescriptions are filled, they will be returned to the refrigerator to await pick-up by the patient. Be sure to attach a label directing the patient to store the drug in the refrigerator at home. These drugs are some of the most expensive made, with one-month's treatment costing more than a thousand dollars. It is essential they not be wasted because of improper storage.

Patients need thorough training on how to prepare and inject these solutions using aseptic technique. This information and training is provided in the physicians office, but be prepared to refer patients to the pharmacist if they have questions regarding injection technique. Although the packages contain patient instructions and an alcohol wipe for each injection, it might be helpful for patients to purchase extra alcohol wipes to have at home.

## Other DMARDs

The first written description of what we know as the rheumatic diseases was written in 123 AD. It is not surprising that the treatment of these disorders has undergone many transformations over the centuries. What might be surprising is that some relatives of a few early antiarthritic remedies are still used. The use of willow bark, which contains salicylates, was already mentioned. In the late seventeenth century there are records of the use of the bark of another plant, the Cinchona tree, found in the Andes Mountains of South America, for arthritis. Cinchona bark contains the antimalarial drug quinine. Although we still do not know how it works, hydroxychloroquine (Plaquenil®) is an important disease-modifying agent in the battle against the rheumatic diseases. Other traditional arthritis remedies included placing a gold coin in an afflicted joint. Gold sodium thiomalate (Myochrysine®) was one of the first very effective disease modifying agents of the twentieth century and is sometimes still used today.

For most of the last half of the twentieth century, the treatment of rheumatoid arthritis and other autoimmune diseases was conservative, with NSAIDs, rest, and the occasional use of corticosteroids playing the most important roles. Now a more aggressive approach is taken in the hopes that treatment can delay the onset of destruction of joints and other tissues. In addition to rest, strengthening exercises, and anti-inflammatory agents, the current standard of care is to start therapy with disease-modifying antirheumatic drugs early in the disease.

### Actions and Indications

All of the disease-modifying agents appear to work by modulating the immune response to the patient's own tissues. Although they share some pharmacologic affects, the DMARDs are not chemically related. Unlike the TNF inhibitors, these drugs take weeks to months to achieve their peak effects. They are anti-inflammatory, but do not have specific analgesic properties.

Methotrexate (Trexall®) is used alone or in combination with other DMARDs. It is the mainstay of modern treatment for severe rheumatoid or psoriatic arthritis. Response to methotrexate occurs sooner than is usual for other slow-acting agents; relief often begins within 3 to 6 weeks of starting treatment. It is a cytotoxic drug also used for cancer chemotherapy and suppresses the immune system through its toxicity to white blood cells. This may or may not be the mechanism of action in the treatment of arthritis. It is indicated for the treatment of rheumatoid and juvenile rheumatoid arthritis, as well as psoriasis and psoriatic arthritis.

Leflunomide (Arava®) is thought to work by reducing the development of autoimmune lymphocytes. Leflunomide can be used alone as an alternative to methotrexate, or as an addition to methotrexate in combination therapy. It is approved for the treatment of rheumatoid arthritis, where it not only reduces pain and inflammation associated with the disease but also appears to slow the progression of structural damage.

The mechanism of action of hydroxychloroquine in the treatment of patients with rheumatoid arthritis and systemic lupus erythematosus is unknown. However, it is effective in most cases for the treatment of these diseases, particularly mild to moderate disease. Hydroxychloroquine is often combined with other agents, such as sulfasalazine, for additional benefit. Sulfasalazine was already discussed for its use in the treatment of the inflammatory bowel diseases (Chapter 22). This drug is an effective DMARD approved for use in rheumatoid and juvenile rheumatoid arthritis, and is used off label for psoriatic arthritis and ankylosing spondylitis. The mechanism of action of sulfasalazine is incompletely understood, but the drug and its metabolites have an affinity for connective tissue and demonstrate anti-inflammatory effects in animals.

Gold salts are effective in the treatment of rheumatoid arthritis, especially when given intramuscularly. The mechanism of action is unknown. Until the 1980s intramuscular gold salts were the most often used DMARD agents. Now, there are many drugs with better safety records that are used first. Auranofin is an oral gold product. It is easier to use, but is much less effective than gold sodium thiomalate.

Minocycline (Minocin®), a tetracycline antibiotic. When it is given soon after the diagnosis of rheumatoid arthritis is made, it appears to reduce the severity of the disease on a permanent basis. Many experts believe that some form of infection causes the abnormal immune response in autoimmune diseases, but no organism has ever been identified. Whether minocycline works because of its antibiotic effect or for another reason is not known.

## Administration

Gold sodium thiomalate is given by intramuscular injection on a weekly basis. With the exception of the TNF inhibitors and gold sodium thiomalate, all the other DMARDs are orally administered and well absorbed. Dosing regimens vary widely, but most drugs are administered once daily. Sulfasalazine is given twice daily, and hydroxychloroquine and minocycline are given once or twice daily. Methotrexate is administered on a once-weekly basis for treatment of the autoimmune diseases. This is a very important distinction to make; misprinting the label so that patients take this drug daily can and has resulted in death.

## Side Effects

Many of the DMARDs have serious side effects, so they require careful monitoring by the physician. The DMARDs are not used frivolously and the benefit of preventing permanent tissue damage must outweigh the risks associated with their use. Because of side effects, gold injections are rarely used today, in spite of their effectiveness. Gold causes mouth sores, rash, diarrhea, and a metallic taste in the mouth in up to about one third of all patients. Although less common, a significant numbers of patients will develop drug induced anemias, kidney, or liver damage.

Methotrexate frequently causes mouth ulcers, nausea and loss of appetite, and abdominal discomfort. It can cause liver damage, and people taking the drug should limit their intake, or avoid, alcohol altogether. Some people develop a serious lung condition in reaction to methotrexate therapy. Since methotrexate works by blocking the body's use of folic acid, patients can minimize side effects by taking a vitamin that contains folic acid on a daily basis. This folate antagonism causes methotrexate to be teratogenic (causes the formation of abnormalities in a fetus) and an abortifacient. It should not be administered to women who are or may become pregnant. Women who wish to become pregnant should stop the methotrexate at least three months in advance.

teratogenic Causing or tending to cause fetal malformations.

Leflunomide, which inhibits cellular metabolism by blocking the use of a different nutrient, causes adverse effects very similar to those caused by methotrexate. Like methotrexate, leflunomide is teratogenic. Men or women who either want to father a child or become pregnant must use a special detoxification protocol to rid the body of the drug before proceeding with pregnancy plans.

The most common reactions to treatment with hydroxychloroquine and sulfasalazine are nausea and GI disturbances. Both drugs can cause hemolytic anemia in people with an inherited enzyme deficiency called G6PD deficiency. Hydroxychloroquine can cause retinal damage, but this effect is dose related and can be prevented by using low dose therapy and checking the eyes at regular intervals. Sulfasalazine may cause allergic reactions because it is a sulfonamide. More serious effects include hepatitis and bone marrow suppression, but these are rare and generally occur early in therapy.

Minocycline is relatively safe, but has minor side effects in common with the tetracycline antibiotics. GI upset is the most likely side effect of minocycline. Diarrhea and fungal overgrowth can occur because the normal balance of bacteria in the GI tract is disturbed. However, because minocycline is completely absorbed this is usually not a significant problem. Minocycline can cause skin rashes, photosensitivity, and alterations in pigmentation of the skin. Rarely minocycline can cause kidney and liver toxicity.

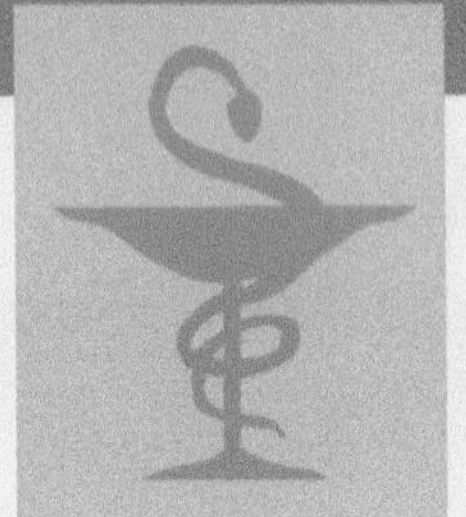

### Tips for the Technician

Because the use of these drugs requires extensive monitoring and careful adherence to administration schedules, the pharmacist should counsel all people with new prescriptions for the DMARD drugs. Special attention should be paid to the interpretation of prescription directions. Methotrexate is never administered on a daily basis. In the treatment of the autoimmune disorders, it is always given once weekly. Warn patients of the dangers to the fetus of taking either leflunomide or methotrexate while pregnant by attaching the appropriate auxiliary label to the prescription vial. Patients should be cautioned to avoid alcohol consumption while taking these products too. Technicians should take care to avoid unnecessary exposure to tablet dust when dispensing methotrexate, leflunomide, or any cytotoxic medications and follow established standards for personal protection.

Auxiliary labels warning patients to avoid excessive sun exposure should be attached to prescription vials of minocycline and sulfasalazine. Sulfasalazine should be taken with plenty of water, and minocycline should be taken on an empty stomach, if possible. Because calcium and other minerals bind the tetracyclines to reduce their absorption, patients should be directed to avoid milk or other dairy products and antacids for an hour before and two hours after each minocycline dose.

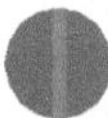

## Drugs for the Treatment of Gout

Gout is a form of arthritis that is caused by abnormal metabolism of uric acid. Like many of the arthritic disorders, it is a systemic disease that can cause problems in other areas besides the joints. Uric acid levels are elevated in gout, either from overproduction or impaired elimination. When uric acid crystals are deposited in joints, they cause inflammation and excruciating pain (see **Fig. 23.6**). Uric acid can deposit in the kidneys to create stones or deposit in soft tissues to form tophi. The goal of therapy is to reduce the frequency of painful acute gout attacks and prevent further uric acid deposition in the tissues.

tophi Uric acid crystals deposited in tissues, characteristic of gout.

Genetic predispositions, medications, and diet can increase the risk of developing acute gout. Consumption of alcoholic beverages and excess consumption of foods rich in purines, such as organ meats, red meat, and certain shellfish are avoided in patients with gout. Gouty arthritis is the most common form of inflammatory joint disease in men older

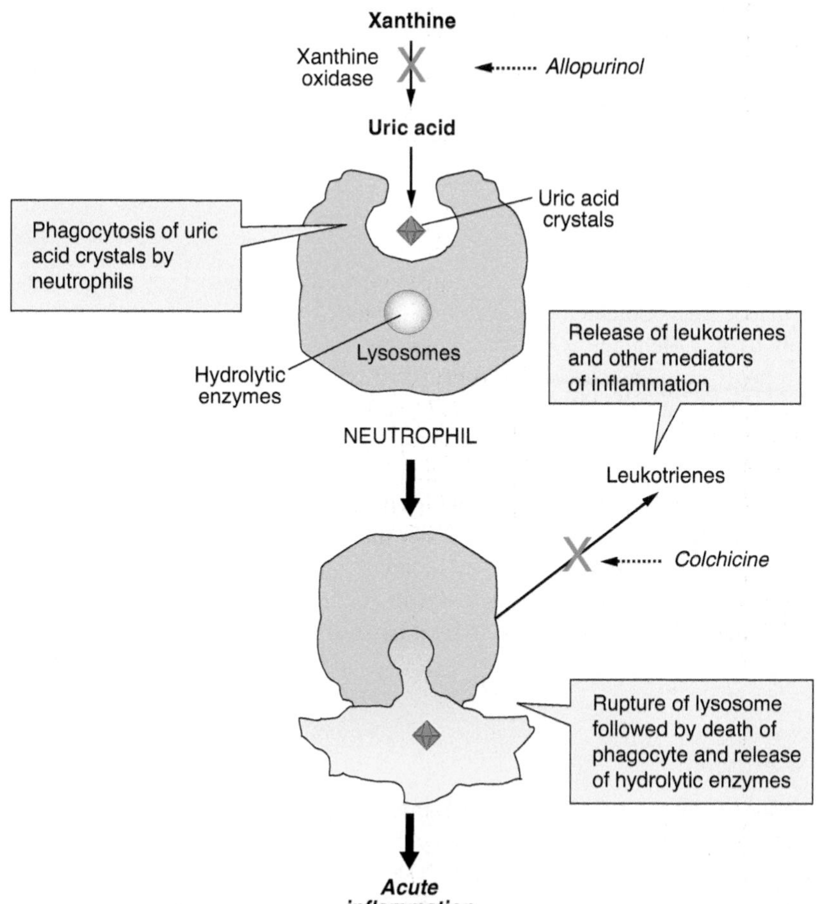


**Figure 23.6** The role of uric acid and the actions of allopurinol and colchicines. (Adapted with permission from Harvey RA, Champe PC, Howland RD, et al. *Lippincott's Illustrated Reviews: Pharmacology*, 3rd edition. Baltimore: Lippincott Williams & Wilkins, 2006.)

than 40 years. The drugs of choice for treatment of an acute gouty attacks are the NSAIDs, which are started at maximum doses as soon as possible after the onset of an attack and tapered off afterwards. Colchicine is another agent that can be used in acute gout.

Drugs that will prevent recurrences of gout are as important as treatment for acute attacks. After the first gouty attack subsides, laboratory testing is done to determine whether the patient overproduces uric acid or has impaired elimination of uric acid. If there is reduced elimination, a uricosuric drug will be prescribed. A uricosuric agent promotes elimination of uric acid. Probenecid is the most frequently used uricosuric agent. Allopurinol (Zyloprim®) is the only drug available to reduce the formation of uric acid.

uricosuric An agent that promotes, or relates to, the excretion of uric acid.

## Actions and Indications

Colchicine is the oldest known medication for gout. It is derived from the roots of the herb *Colchicum autumnale*. Colchicine is a highly effective treatment when it is started at the onset of an attack. The mechanism of action of colchicine is not completely clear, however pharmacologists believe that colchicine interrupts the inflammatory response by inhibiting the uptake of uric acid crystals by white blood cells. Colchicine is indicated for the treatment of acute gout.

Probenecid works in the tubules of the kidneys, where it competes with uric acid for reabsorption. This competition results in increased elimination of uric acid through the urine. When probenecid is given with the penicillin antibiotics, the same competition for reabsorption occurs, and the penicillin is preferentially reabsorbed. As a result, the effects of the antibiotic are prolonged. Probenecid is sometimes given with penicillin for this very purpose. Probenecid is indicated for the treatment of hyperuricemia associated with gout, and as an adjuvant to treatment with penicillins and cephalosporin antibiotics in order to increase serum levels of the antibiotics and prolong their effects.

Allopurinol inhibits the enzyme responsible for converting the precursors of uric acid to uric acid. This makes allopurinol useful when a high rate of cell breakdown causes a dangerous elevation in uric acid levels, as can sometimes be seen during cancer chemotherapy when cytotoxic drugs are used. Allopurinol is indicated for prevention of gouty attacks in those patients who over produce uric acid, and as an adjunct to cancer chemotherapy.

## Administration

Colchicine, probenecid, and allopurinol are administered orally for gout. They are well absorbed through the GI tract. Colchicine is available for intravenous injection, but this formulation is rarely used. Colchicine is dosed based on individual needs, but is often given every one to two hours until an acute attack subsides or until side effects prevent continuation. Patients cannot repeat this procedure for at least 3 days.

Probenecid and allopurinol are given on a routine basis for gout prevention. Probenecid is given twice daily and allopurinol can be administered once daily. Probenecid is a sulfonamide and should not be used in patients with sulfa allergy. Both drugs are better tolerated when taken with food or milk. Adequate water intake must be maintained with both drugs to prevent formation of kidney stones. The recommended daily fluid intake with probenecid is six to eight full glasses of water daily, and with allopurinol is 10 to 12 glasses of water daily. Allopurinol injection is used to treat hyperuricemia associated with cancer chemotherapy.

## Side Effects

Colchicine is no longer the first choice in the treatment of acute gout because of the high rate of side effects. About 80% of patients who take this drug will experience gastrointestinal side effects of diarrhea, nausea, and vomiting. The drug inhibits cell division and can temporarily interfere with sperm production in men, and can cause drug-induced anemias. Toxicity is increased in people with kidney or liver failure and in the elderly.

When probenecid therapy is started, there is an increased amount of uric acid moving from tissues through the kidneys. This can precipitate an acute gouty attack and cause formation of kidney stones. Other common side effects of probenecid therapy include rash and gastrointestinal problems. Side effects from allopurinol can include rashes, GI upset, headache, and kidney toxicity. The most serious adverse effect is a severe hypersensitivity syndrome. In this rare reaction bone marrow suppression, liver toxicity, and renal failure is life threatening.

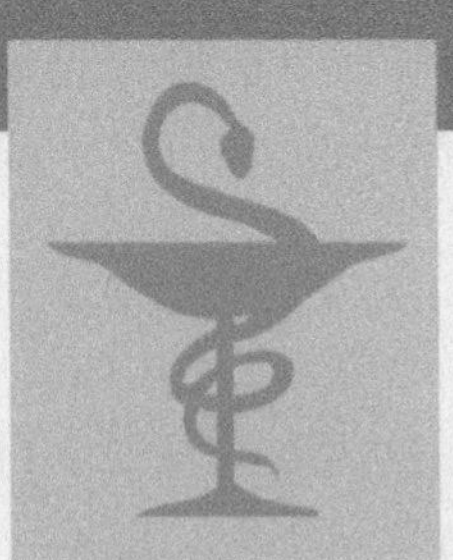

### Tips for the Technician

Whenever clients receive prescription medication like allopurinol or colchicine, which has the potential to cause drug-induced anemias, they should be educated about the symptoms that might indicate the presence of this side effect. This is information the pharmacist should provide during the patient consultation. Allopurinol can cause drowsiness. Be certain patients are warned of this effect by attaching an auxiliary warning label to the prescription container. Auxiliary labels should be affixed to both allopurinol and probenecid prescriptions instructing the patient to take them with plenty of water. Both drugs should be administered with food. Probenecid cannot be taken with the salicylates because they counteract its effect.

Colchicine is highly toxic to children, and like all medications, it should be kept out of their reach. Colchicine should be discontinued at the first signs of GI upset or as soon as the acute attack subsides. This drug should be protected from light exposure and kept in the amber prescription vial.

# 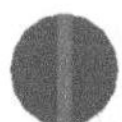 Drug Treatment for Osteoporosis

Osteoporosis is a condition of bone fragility caused by progressive loss of bone mass seen with advancing age. It is more common in postmenopausal women, but can also occur in older men and younger women. Bone fractures occur more often in people with osteoporosis and are a major cause of disability among the elderly. Of the approximately 25 million American women who have osteoporosis, about eight million have had a fracture. Inadequate calcium and vitamin D intake during adolescence and early adulthood, sedentary lifestyle and tobacco use contribute to bone loss. Treatment and prevention measures include adequate intake of calcium and vitamin D, weight-bearing exercise, and smoking cessation (see **Table 23.2**). Estrogen hormone replacement may be indicated in some women (see Chapter 27) to encourage maintenance of bone density. The goals of osteoporosis therapy are to prevent the problem of osteoporosis-related fractures.

## Bisphosphonates

The bisphosphonates are analogs of the mineral pyrophosphate, and include etidronate (Didronel®), risedronate (Actonel®), alendronate (Fosamax®), pamidronate (Aredia®), ibandronate (Boniva®), and others. They comprise an important drug group used for the treatment of disorders of bone remodeling. Bone remodeling is the ongoing process of breakdown of bone by cells called osteoclasts, and repair by cells called osteoblasts. In osteoporosis, the osteoclasts are more active than osteoblasts, resulting in a rapid loss of bone density (**Fig. 23.7**).

### Actions and Indications

The bisphosphonates work by penetrating the bone and binding at sites where bone loss is actively proceeding. They inhibit the actions of the osteoclasts at these sites. They also seem to inhibit the growth of new osteoclasts, and increase the rate of cell death of the old osteoclasts. The actions of the bisphosphonates are specifically targeted at osteoclasts. They do not interfere with the growth or actions of osteoblasts, which are, in the meantime, laying down new bone. The net result is a gradual increase in bone density. The gain in bone density is maintained for as long as the drug is taken (up to 10 years in clinical trials), but gradual bone loss begins again after discontinuation. The bisphosphonates are indicated for the treatment of osteoporosis and Paget's disease, as well as for treatment of metastatic bone cancers. In addition, alendronate and risedronate have been approved for the prevention of osteoporosis. The injectable bisphosphonates can be used to treat hypercalcemia when calcium levels are high enough to cause symptoms in the patient.

**Table 23.2** Strategies for Prevention and Treatment of Osteoporosis

| |
|---|
| Calcium-rich diet and/or calcium supplements, with adequate vitamin D intake |
| Quit smoking |
| Avoid excess alcohol and caffeine intake |
| Regular weight-bearing exercise |
| Regular screening of bone density |
| Avoid use of medications that can reduce bone density whenever possible (corticosteroids) |
| Treatment with bisphosphonates, estrogens, and selective estrogen-receptor modulators |

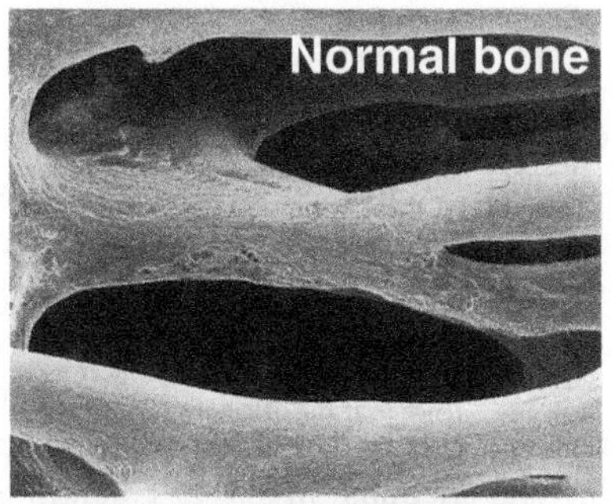


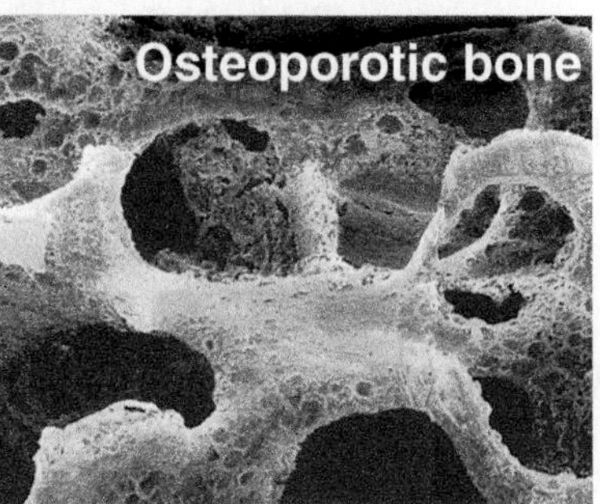


**Figure 23.7** Changes in bone density seen in osteoporosis. (Reprinted with permission from Harvey RA, Champe PC, Howland RD, et al. *Lippincott's Illustrated Reviews: Pharmacology*, 3rd edition. Baltimore: Lippincott Williams & Wilkins, 2006.)

## Administration

The bisphosphonates are administered by mouth in the treatment or prevention of osteoporosis. Alendronate, the first oral bisphosphonate, was originally given as a 10-mg dose on a once-daily basis. More recent studies show that it can be given just as successfully on a weekly basis. Several tablet strengths are now available, because different doses are used in treatment and prevention, and daily or weekly dosing. Risedronate comes in two strengths only, one for daily and one for weekly dosing, for both prevention and treatment of osteoporosis. The newest bisphosphonate, ibandronate, is orally administered in different strengths for daily or monthly use, but the same dose is used for both treatment and prevention of osteoporosis. A new injectable form is now available for IV administration on an every-3-month basis.

Etidronate and pamidronate are used for Paget's disease of the bone and for hypercalcemia due to malignancy. Etidronate is available in both tablets and solution for intravenous infusion, while pamidronate is available in products for intravenous infusion only. When these drugs are used to treat hypercalcemia, the dose is based on the serum calcium levels.

Even though most of the bisphosphonates are administered orally, their absorption is poor; less than 10% of a given dose is absorbed. Refer to **Table 23.3** for a comparison of the products available for the treatment of osteoporosis. Food significantly interferes with absorption, so the drugs are taken fasting, with eight ounces of water, 30 minutes to 1 hour before eating breakfast. Patients must sit upright for at least half an hour to avoid side effects.

## Side Effects

Oral bisphosphonates cause a number of side effects that are generally minor but can become serious. The most common side effects are gastrointestinal and include irritation and pain in the esophagus and stomach, diarrhea, nausea and vomiting. Esophageal pain can be a precursor to more serious esophageal ulcerations and bleeding. Patients who stay upright for at least 30 minutes after taking the dose are less likely to develop serious esophageal problems.

All of these drugs can cause a drop in blood levels of calcium as calcium is moved into bone. Most patients will take calcium supplements in addition to the bisphosphonate prescription. They should not be taken at the same time because the calcium can interfere with the absorption of the bisphosphonates.

**Table 23.3** Drugs for Treatment of Osteoporosis and Other Bone Conditions

| Generic | Brand Name | Available as | Indications | Notes |
|---|---|---|---|---|
| **Bisphosphonates*** | | | | |
| Alendronate | Fosamax® | Tablets, oral solution | Osteoporosis treatment and prevention, Paget's disease | |
| Etidronate | Didronel® | Tablets, injection | Hypercalcemia of malignancy (HCM), Paget's disease | Oral for Paget's Disease |
| Ibandronate | Boniva® | Tablets, injection | Postmenopausal osteoporosis treatment and prevention | |
| Pamidronate | Aredia® | Powder for inj., injection | HCM, Paget's disease | Refrigerate after mixing |
| Risedronate | Actonel® | Tablets | Osteoporosis treatment and prevention, Paget's disease | |
| **Other Drugs for Osteoporosis** | | | | |
| Calcitonin | Miacalcin® | Nasal spray, injection | Postmenopausal osteoporosis, Paget's Disease, hypercalcemia | Refrigerate |
| Raloxifene | Evista® | Tablets | Osteoporosis treatment and prevention | For postmenopausal women only |

Inj, injection; HCM, hypercalcemia of malignancy.
*Oral bisphosphonates must be given with a full glass of water, on an empty stomach, in an upright position.

Rarely these drugs can cause inflammation and irritation of the eye. Although irritation is generally not serious, rare severe inflammation has occurred during treatment with pamidronate. This problem resolves when the bisphosphonate is discontinued.

## Tips for the Technician

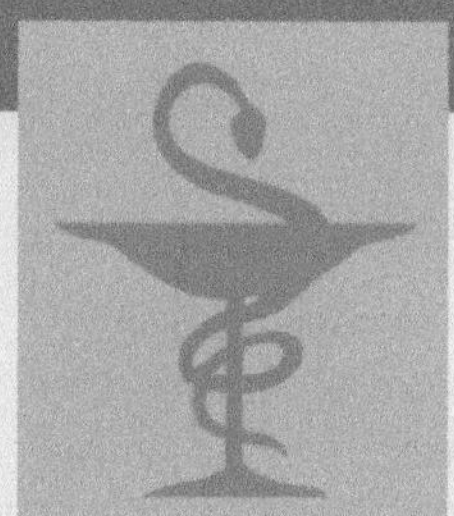

Because the bisphosphonates require specific administration techniques, the pharmacist should counsel patients when they first receive the medication. Patients should be instructed to report esophageal irritation or pain and eye irritation to the physician. Prescription vials are labelled with auxiliary instructions to take the medication with a full eight-ounce glass of water, and on an empty stomach. The oral bisphosphonates come in strengths that are appropriate for daily, weekly, and in one instance, monthly dosing. This means that tablet strengths vary 7- to 30-fold. The technician needs to use great care when selecting the medication from the shelf to fill a prescription. Always double-check the name and strength of every product before removing it from the shelf to fill a prescription. An error could be quite serious.

## Miscellaneous Drugs for Osteoporosis

### Actions and Indications

Calcitonin and raloxifene are two additional drugs that are used for the treatment of osteoporosis. Both drugs are useful in treating patients who should not use estrogen replacement and do not tolerate the bisphosphonates. Calcitonin is a hormone that reduces bone breakdown by inhibiting osteoclast function. It is often given to women who develop fractures from their osteoporosis because it is thought to exert an analgesic effect. For reasons that are poorly understood, the increases in bone mass seen with calcitonin only continue for a few years. Resistance to its effects eventually develops. Calcitonin is approved for the treatment of Paget's disease of the bone and hypercalcemia.

Raloxifene is a unique compound that binds to estrogen receptors but only activates selective receptors. While it exerts an estrogenic effect on bone by reducing bone resorption, it blocks estrogen receptors in the uterus or the breast. It has a beneficial, estrogen-like effect on total cholesterol levels. Raloxifene is FDA approved for the prevention and treatment of osteoporosis.

### Administration

Calcitonin is available for subcutaneous or intramuscular injection or as an intranasal spray. When the parenteral product is used, it is given every other day. The nasal spray is used in alternating nostrils, one spray daily. Both products must be stored in the refrigerator. Like most drugs for osteoporosis, patients should take calcium and vitamin D while receiving calcitonin.

Raloxifene is taken orally, where it is quickly absorbed. It undergoes extensive first-pass metabolism in the liver, so that only a small amount gets into the systemic circulation. It can be given without regard to meals. Both ampicillin and cholestyramine significantly reduce the absorption of raloxifene, so these combinations are avoided.

### Side Effects

Women who take raloxifene have an increased risk of blood clot formation, similar to that seen with the use of estrogen. For this reason, the product is not recommended for women who are immobile. Because of its anti-estrogen actions, the most common side effects are hot flashes and vaginal dryness and irritation. Raloxifene is only used to treat osteoporosis in postmenopausal women. Raloxifene has the potential to interact with warfarin and NSAIDs, with the possibility of increased side effects of either drug.

Calcitonin is fairly well tolerated. The most common side effects include nasal irritation and rhinitis with use of the nasal product. Use of the injectable product is associated with nausea with or without vomiting, especially early in therapy, and injection site reactions. Allergic reactions may occur with either product.

### Tips for the Technician

Both formulations of calcitonin require special storage conditions. Prescription labeling should include directions to the patient to keep the products in the refrigerator. After the first use, the nasal spray can be left at room temperature (no higher than 77°F) for 30 days, but then any leftover medication must be discarded. In most pharmacies, the pharmacist or technician will assemble the nasal spray pump before dispensing the product. Instructions on how to use the spray are included in the package and are intended for the patient.

Patients should be taking calcium and vitamin D while on raloxifene and other osteoporosis treatments. A patient package insert is dispensed with each prescription. Attach an auxiliary label warning patients that there are drug interactions with this drug. Clients should speak to the pharmacist to find out about problematic drug combinations.

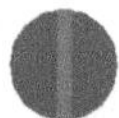

# Acetaminophen

After caffeine and alcohol, acetaminophen is the most commonly used drug in the United States. About one in five adults take this medication every week. However, recent information indicates that when this drug is taken routinely at the maximum recommended doses, it is not as safe as consumers believe.

## Actions and Indications

Acetaminophen is a nonprescription analgesic and antipyretic agent (Tylenol®) without anti-inflammatory properties. It inhibits prostaglandin synthesis in the CNS, but has no significant effect on cyclo-oxygenase in peripheral tissues.It does not affect platelet adhesion and provides no protective antithrombotic effect for people with heart disease.

Acetaminophen is a suitable substitute for the analgesic and antipyretic effects of aspirin for patients with gastric complaints, for patients at risk of bleeding, or for those who do not require the anti-inflammatory action of aspirin. Acetaminophen is the analgesic/antipyretic of choice for children with viral infections or chicken pox.

## Administration

Acetaminophen is administered either orally or rectally and is rapidly absorbed. Oral absorption is reduced and delayed by the presence of food. It is advisable to take the medication on an empty stomach. Total acetaminophen dose in adults should not exceed 4 grams daily, and at this maximum dose should not continue for more than a few days. Acetaminophen is contained in many different products, a fact of which most people are unaware. It is important for consumers to be aware of the presence of acetaminophen in their medications and the maximum dose recommendations, because chronic excessive use of acetaminophen is very dangerous.

## Side Effects

With normal therapeutic doses and occasional use, acetaminophen is virtually free of any significant adverse effects. Skin rash and minor allergic reactions occur infrequently. With large doses of acetaminophen given chronically, however, very serious and potentially life-threatening liver and kidney toxicity can occur. The risk of liver damage is magnified if other drugs that are toxic to the liver, such as alcohol, are also consumed. Acute overdoses of acetaminophen frequently result in hepatic necrosis (cell death) and a prolonged death. Unfortunately, most people are unaware of the dangerous nature of chronic acetaminophen usage or acetaminophen overdose.

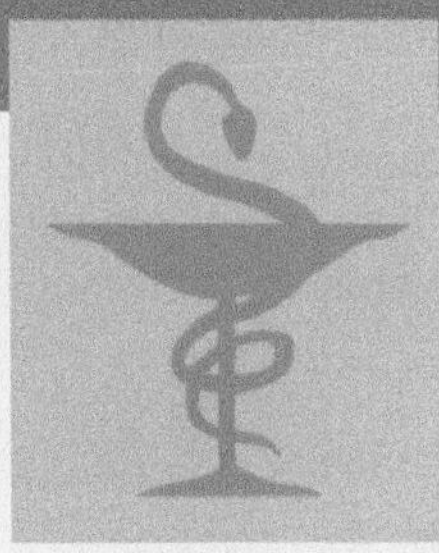

## Tips for the Technician

In retail pharmacies, people receiving prescription products containing acetaminophen should be warned to limit their intake of other acetaminophen-containing products. Parents buying children's acetaminophen formulations should be encouraged to check with the pharmacist about appropriate doses. In hospitals, pharmacies often have systems for monitoring patient intake of acetaminophen from various medicines, and a warning system for the nurses administering medications. Pharmacy technicians may be involved with collecting data on drug utilization (for example total daily use of acetaminophen) for review by pharmacists.

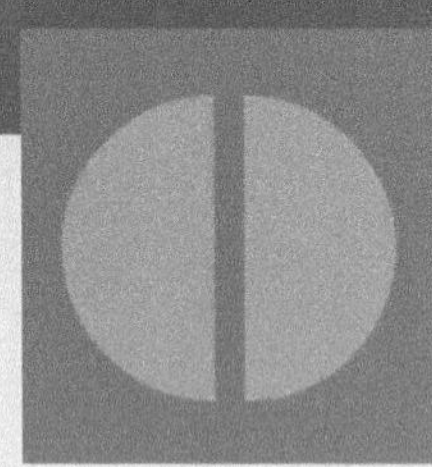

## Case 23.1

Ruby Olay is the mother of 5 young children and a frequent customer of the pharmacy where Henry Hicks is the technician. Ruby comes to the pharmacy just about the time that the staff is ready to close the store. She states that her 2-year-old daughter Rosie has a high fever. She says there are acetaminophen drops and liquid at home and wants Henry to tell her how much she can give. She also purchases a combination cold medication for Rosie. How should Henry advise her?

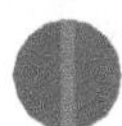

# Skeletal Muscle Relaxants

Unlike the neuromuscular blocking agents, the skeletal muscle relaxants (sometimes called spasmolytics) discussed in this chapter do not impair the ability to use all of the muscles. With the exception of dantrolene, these agents exert their effects on the central nervous system. This group of drugs is not chemically related.

## Actions and Indications

The skeletal muscle relaxants discussed in this chapter are used to treat muscle spasm and spasticity. Not all muscle relaxants are useful in all conditions. Centrally acting compounds such as carisoprodol (Soma®), cyclobenzaprine (Flexeril®), or metaxalone (Skelaxin®) are usually used to treat muscle spasm that can occur as a result of trauma or injury. For example, one of these drugs might be used to treat back injury or muscle spasms after an automobile accident. Although their precise mechanisms of action are incompletely described, they are thought to work through general depression of the central nervous system.

Baclofen (Lioresal®), dantrolene (Dantrium®), tizanidine (Zanaflex®), and diazepam (Valium®) are used for the spasticity that can accompany cerebral palsy or neuromuscular disorders such as multiple sclerosis. These drugs are much more effective than the other skeletal muscle relaxants. Their spasmolytic mechanisms of action vary. Diazepam enhances the inhibitory effects of the CNS inhibitory neurotransmitter, gamma-aminobutyric acid (GABA). Researchers believe this effect occurs in both spinal nerves and in the brainstem. Baclofen is an analog of GABA and its effects are also likely to be related to the actions of GABA. Tizanidine is a centrally acting alpha adrenergic agonist similar to clonidine, but without significant antihypertensive effects. It decreases spasticity presumably by inhibiting nerve transmission to muscles. Dantrolene exerts action directly on muscle tissue to reduce contractility. It also causes central nervous system depression, which may contribute to the muscle relaxant effect.

## Administration

The muscle relaxants presented in this chapter can be taken by mouth and are well absorbed when orally administered. Refer to **Table 23.4** for a listing of available products. Tizanidine is generally not used for extended periods of time, but rather for acute treatment of spasticity. Dantrolene injection is used for the treatment of malignant hyperthermia only (refer to Chapter 7). Diazepam is available for intravenous administration, but is less likely to be administered in this way for muscle spasms or spasticity related to cerebral palsy or muscle trauma. Diazepam is the drug of choice in treating tetanic spasms and seizures due to *Clostridium tetani* infections (tetanus), a syndrome that is rarely seen because of the availability of tetanus immunization.

Baclofen is available as tablets for oral use, but also in a formulation for intrathecal injection. Drugs administered by this route are injected directly into the cerebrospinal fluid surrounding the spinal cord. Baclofen is administered via a small pump that is implanted under the skin in the abdominal region. A catheter is inserted into the intrathecal space of the spine, then tunneled under the skin and connected to the pump. The drug is delivered in this way to provide chronic control of spasticity in patients who do not tolerate oral administration. Trained personnel must refill the pump.

intrathecal Within or introduced into the space between the organs of the CNS and the sheath that surrounds them.

## Side Effects

Centrally acting compounds such as carisoprodol, cyclobenzaprine, metaxalone, diazepam, and others cause side effects related to central nervous system depression. The most common of these include drowsiness, dizziness, and ataxia. Carisoprodol sometimes causes GI upset and can be taken with food to reduce that effect. Because of its CNS depressant effects, carisoprodol abuse has occurred in some patients.

**Table 23.4** Drugs Used for Treatment of Muscle Spasm and Spasticity

| Generic | Brand Name | Available as | Indications | Notes |
|---|---|---|---|---|
| Baclofen | Lioresal® | Tablets, intrathecal injection, orally disintegrating tablets | Spasticity due to MS, spinal cord injuries | |
| Carisoprodol | Soma® | Tablets | Acute musculoskeletal pain, muscle spasm | |
| Cyclobenzaprine | Flexeril® | Tablets | Acute musculoskeletal pain, muscle spasm | |
| Dantrolene | Dantrium® | Capsules, injection | Spasticity due to MS, spinal cord injuries | Injection for malignant hyperthermia only |
| Diazepam | Valium® | Tablets, injection, oral soln, oral concentrate | Spasticity associated with cerebral palsy, spinal cord injury | |
| Metaxalone | Skelaxin® | Tablets | Acute musculoskeletal pain, muscle spasm | |
| Tizanidine | Zanaflex® | Tablets | Acute and chronic treatment of spasticity | Mainly short-term use |

MS, multiple sclerosis; soln, solution.

Cyclobenzaprine is related to the tricyclic antidepressants, and like the tricyclics, can cause dry mouth, constipation, hypotension, and arrhythmia. Like the tricyclics, cyclobenzaprine should not be administered to patients receiving MAO inhibitors. Cyclobenzaprine can accentuate problems of urinary retention in men with BPH. Besides drowsiness and dizziness, cyclobenzaprine can cause mental confusion.

The side effects most frequently observed with oral administration of baclofen include drowsiness, dizziness, headache, confusion, nausea, and hypotension. Rarely, oral baclofen can cause seizures. Risks associated with intrathecal use are related to implantation of the infusion device as well as administration of the drug itself and include the same effects as for oral use, as well as risk of infection, increased risk of seizures, and a syndrome that resembles malignant hyperthermia, which can occur when intrathecal baclofen is abruptly discontinued.

Tizanidine causes drowsiness, dizziness, and hypotension fairly frequently. These side effects are sometimes severe enough that patients cannot continue taking the medication. Because side effects can be significant and are dose related, the dose of this drug is gradually increased to improve patient tolerance. Besides the more common side effects, this drug can cause liver injury and hallucinations.

Dantrolene also has the potential to cause hepatotoxicity, which is sometimes fatal. Along with the typical side effects of drowsiness, dizziness, weakness, and diarrhea, dantrolene can significantly increase the risk of seizures. Neither tizanidine nor dantrolene is used for routine muscle strains or spasm, but should be reserved, because of the risk of serious side effects, for muscle spasticity due to multiple sclerosis or other neuromuscular disorders.

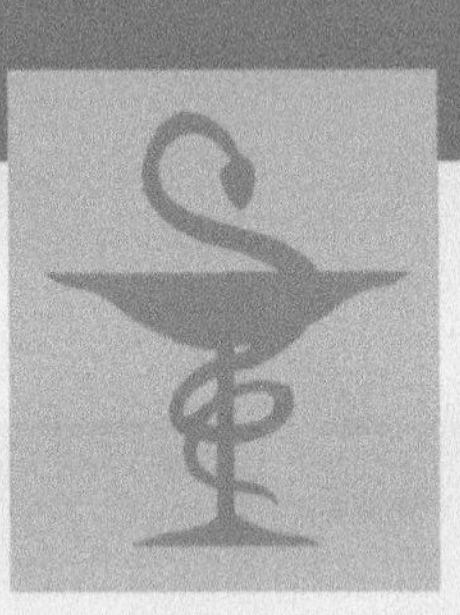

## Tips for the Technician

These medications cause drowsiness or dizziness and prescription containers should uniformly be labelled with auxiliary labels cautioning patients about driving or operating complex machinery while taking them. In all cases, patients should avoid alcoholic beverages and other CNS depressants while taking these medications. Label prescription vials appropriately. The pharmacist should counsel patients taking tizanidine and baclofen about the risk of drug-related toxicity.

# Review Questions

## Multiple Choice

Choose the best answer for the following questions:

1. How do the centrally acting skeletal muscle relaxants and dantrolene differ from the neuromuscular blocking agents?
   a. The skeletal muscle relaxants can be orally administered.
   b. Patients retain the ability to use their muscles while taking the skeletal muscle relaxants.
   c. The skeletal muscle relaxants can be administered to outpatients.
   d. Only experienced professionals should administer neuromuscular blockers and only with resuscitation equipment readily available.
   e. All of the above are true.

2. Which of the following statements regarding the NSAIDs is not true?
   a. Aspirin and the salicylates are not considered NSAIDs because their actions are completely different.
   b. The NSAIDs are antipyretic, analgesic, and in adequate doses, anti-inflammatory.
   c. The most common side effect experienced with use of NSAIDs is GI irritation.
   d. NSAIDs can cause GI bleeding.
   e. Several NSAIDs are available without prescription.

3. Which of the following factors are not known to increase the risk of osteoporosis?
   a. Menopause
   b. Immobility
   c. Low calcium intake, especially during adolescence
   d. Puberty
   e. Smoking

4. Which of the following drugs or groups are not considered disease modifying antirheumatic drugs?
   a. Remicade®, Enbrel®, and Humira®
   b. Aspirin, naproxen, and ibuprofen
   c. Hydroxychloroquine and sulfasalazine
   d. Methotrexate and leflunomide
   e. Minocycline

5. Select the letter corresponding to the true statement regarding the oral administration of the bisphosphonates.
   a. They are administered on an empty stomach, at least 30 minutes before the first meal of the day.
   b. Patients should take these drugs with a full glass of water.
   c. After taking the medication patients must stay in the upright position for 30 minutes.
   d. Oral absorption is very poor.
   e. All of the above are true.

## True/False

6. The maximum dose of acetaminophen in normal adults is 4 grams per day.
   a. True
   b. False

7. Patients who take skeletal muscle relaxants should be more concerned about excitation and insomnia than drowsiness or dizziness while taking these medications.
   a. True
   b. False

8. Allopurinol and probenecid are indicated for the treatment of acute gouty arthritis attacks.
   a. True
   b. False

9. Many of the DMARDs have serious side effects, but their careful use in RA and other autoimmune conditions can prevent permanent damage to joints and other tissues.
   a. True
   b. False

10. Aspirin can interfere with the uricosuric effect of probenecid.
    a. True
    b. False

## Matching

For numbers 11 to 15, match the drug name with the correct lettered indication for its use from the list below. Choices will not be used more than once and may not be used at all.

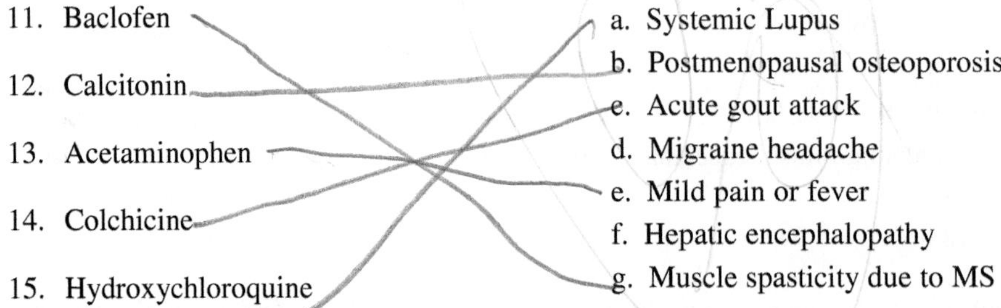

11. Baclofen
12. Calcitonin
13. Acetaminophen
14. Colchicine
15. Hydroxychloroquine

a. Systemic Lupus
b. Postmenopausal osteoporosis
c. Acute gout attack
d. Migraine headache
e. Mild pain or fever
f. Hepatic encephalopathy
g. Muscle spasticity due to MS

## Short Answer

16. What are some of the risks of taking methotrexate? What do technicians need to remember about the dosing of methotrexate in rheumatoid arthritis to avoid a life-threatening mistake?

17. Not all nonsteroidal anti-inflammatory drugs have the same indications. List three nonsteroidal anti-inflammatory drugs by brand and generic name and their unique indications.

18. What special handling and labelling is required when dispensing the TNF inhibitors?

19. Why is it important to understand drugs like the NSAIDs and other agents used to treat arthritis?

20. Explain the differences and similarities between cyclobenzaprine, carisoprodol, and metaxalone versus baclofen and dantrolene.

# FOR FURTHER INQUIRY

Some experts still do not agree that there is good evidence that use of salicylates during a febrile illness caused by influenza or chicken pox increases a child's risk of developing Reye's syndrome. In a small group or individually, read about Reye's syndrome and the research done in the 1980s that connected the use of salicylates to this often-fatal illness. In Australia, where the syndrome was first described, discussion of the initial research continues. Visit www.tga.gov.au/npmeds/aspirin_reye.htm, and other web sites to learn more about this interesting controversy in medicine.

UNIT V

# Drugs Affecting the Endocrine System

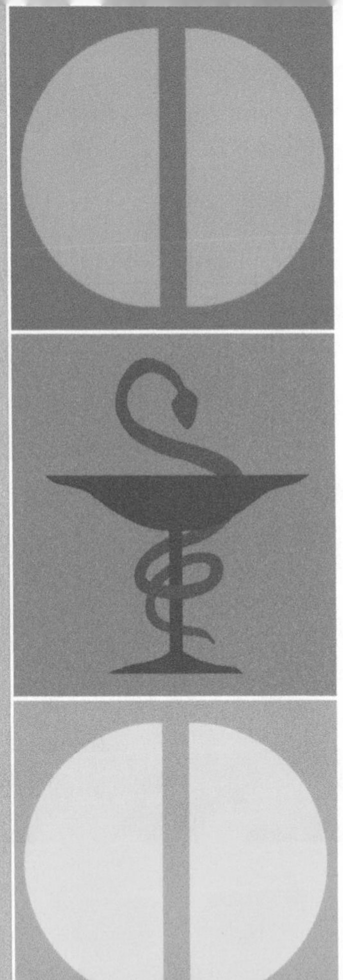

Chapter **24**

# Anatomy and Physiology of the Endocrine System

## KEY TERMS

- androgen
- anterior
- autocrine
- endocrine
- exocrine
- glucocorticoids
- hormone
- hydrophobic
- mineralocorticoid
- paracrine
- posterior
- steroid
- zygote

## OBJECTIVES

After studying this chapter, the reader should be able to:

- Compare and contrast the cell signaling actions of neurotransmitters (paracrine) with the actions of hormones (endocrine).
- Define the term hormone, and compare the two general chemical types of hormones and how they interact with receptors.
- Describe negative feedback mechanisms, through which most hormone secretion is controlled.
- List five hormones described in this chapter and explain the effects of each on the body.
- Describe the typical symptoms of one of the deficiency syndromes presented in this chapter.

A fully formed adult human being begins as a mass of rapidly dividing, undifferentiated cells. Undifferentiated cells all look alike. They contain the necessary genetic material to either become a whole person or a particular group of cells, but at this point they are indistinguishable from one another. After a certain number of divisions the cells begin to organize and different cell patterns occur. What happens to cause this change? This is a question that scientists are still grappling with, but the evidence indicates that communication from genetic material within the cell and interactions between cells play a role in causing these changes. The transfer of chemical messages from one cell to another and from proteins within cells causes the biochemical changes that allow for differentiation and growth over the next 40 weeks that, if all goes well, results in a healthy infant.

These amazing processes, and the continuing growth and development that occur after birth, are a result of cell signaling. Our cells are endowed with the ability to send and receive signals that allow adaptation to the cellular environment and provide for changes in the organism as a whole. Autocrine communication occurs when cells produce a protein or other substance to which they themselves respond.

autocrine Of or related to self-signalling; secretion of a substance by cells that affects only members of the same cell type.

The nervous system uses signaling through electrical impulses and neurotransmitters to control heart rate, respiration, and muscle movement. Messages move from one nerve cell to the next along a string of cells. Some cells release histamine, prostaglandins, thromboxane, and other mediators that call nearby cells to respond. This cell-to-cell communication is called paracrine signaling, and it results in a nearly immediate response when the released compounds attach to receptors on nearby cells.

paracrine Substance secreted by a cell that acts on nearby cells.

Endocrine signaling occurs when endocrine glands send signals to distant cell systems by releasing chemicals into the blood stream. Endocrine signaling causes changes in cellular metabolism that can be carried out over hours, weeks, and years. These naturally occurring chemicals are called hormones. Hormones and the glands that release them make up the endocrine system. They are responsible for slow signaling that controls utilization of nutrients in the biochemical processes that provide energy and maintain and repair tissue (cellular metabolism). In other words, the endocrine system controls the normal growth and development processes required for life, health, and reproduction. These three types of communication interact to ensure a normal physiologic state while allowing for growth and change.

endocrine Pertaining to glands or their secretions that are distributed in the body by way of the bloodstream.

hormone An endogenous substance, secreted into the bloodstream, which causes a specific response in target cells, usually located at a distant site.

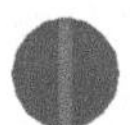

# Hormones

Unlike neurotransmitters and cytokines, hormones signal tissues at a distance. Endocrine tissues produce hormones and release them into the bloodstream, which in turn carries them to the target tissues. Hormones may affect a wide variety of target tissues or very specific tissues. Target tissue cells contain hormone specific receptors either on their surfaces or inside the cells to which hormones attach and cause a response.

Hormones fall into two general chemical types: those derived from amino acids and those derived from cholesterol. Hormones derived from amino acids are hydrophilic, often large, and for the most part are either proteins or peptides (lower molecular weight chains of amino acids from which proteins are made). Because these substances are hydrophilic, they interact with receptors on the outside of the cell. The binding of the hormone to the receptor causes a response inside the cell that alters cellular metabolism. Insulin and thyroxine are examples of this type of hormone.

Other hormones are derived from cholesterol and are hydrophobic (not readily mixing with water) and fat-soluble. These hormones penetrate cells and interact with receptors inside. The hormone-receptor complexes interact directly with genetic material within cells to alter cellular metabolism and production of proteins. These hormones are referred to as steroid hormones (derived from cholesterol), and include the sex hormones.

hydrophobic Resistant to absorption of water or lack of affinity for water.

steroid A group of compounds that contain a 17-carbon ring system; includes some hormones and sterols.

## Regulation of Hormones

There are innumerable biochemical processes necessary to maintain homeostasis, or stability, of normal functions in the human body. These processes are adjusted through feedback of information to the controlling tissue that subsequently causes an up or down regulation of a function in the target tissue. This type of control mechanism is called a negative feedback mechanism. It is different from a positive feedback mechanism, which stimulates increasing up-regulation of a process. In any type of feedback mechanism the last step of a series of changes comes back to control the first step.

Most hormones are regulated through a negative feedback mechanism, but some, such as oxytocin, operate with a positive feedback mechanism. In a negative feedback control system, information about a hormone or its effect is returned to the controlling tissues. If the information indicates low levels or activity of the hormone, the gland increases hormone secretion until feedback returns indicating that levels are normal. At that point, hormone production will be turned down.

### Analogy

There are a number of analogies that can be used to describe a negative feedback system. Probably the one most often used is the analogy of the thermostat. A thermostat senses temperature much like the pancreas senses the presence of glucose. When the temperature is too high, the air conditioner switches on. When the temperature falls to the level set on the thermostat, the air conditioner turns off. In this analogy, elevated temperatures correlate to elevated glucose levels. When glucose levels are too high, the pancreas "turns on" insulin production until glucose concentration falls to the preset level. At that point, insulin secretion is turned off until glucose levels rise again.

A simple explanation of how the pancreas controls insulin production might clarify this point. Insulin is required for cells in the body to utilize their most important energy source, glucose. When blood glucose levels are elevated, for example after a meal, the pancreas picks up this information and secretes insulin into the blood stream. Insulin circulates out to the tissues and interacts with receptors on cell surfaces, which results in movement of glucose from the bloodstream into the tissues. Movement into tissues causes the concentration of the glucose in the blood to fall. The new, lower blood glucose levels circulate back through the pancreas where they register and cause a reduction in insulin release down to basal levels, where it will stay until the next snack or meal (**Fig. 24.1**).

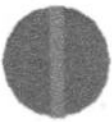

## Endocrine System

The endocrine system is made up of glands and other tissues that synthesize and secrete hormones. These glands are located throughout the body, from the pituitary gland directly below the brain, to the sex organs. By regulating hormone production, the endocrine glands coordinate our metabolism, normal growth and development, sexual maturation, and reproduction. **Figure 24.2** shows the location of the glands of the endocrine system.

### The Pituitary Gland

The pituitary gland is the size of a large pea and lies directly below the brain, at about the level of the bridge of the nose and halfway between the front and the back of the skull. The pituitary gland secretes hormones that modulate the activity of other glands in the endocrine system. Hormones that control the release of other hormones can be recognized by the suffix -tropin, meaning to act on. An example is adrenocorticotropin, which is secreted by the pituitary and acts on the adrenal glands to cause the secretion of cortisol. The activ-

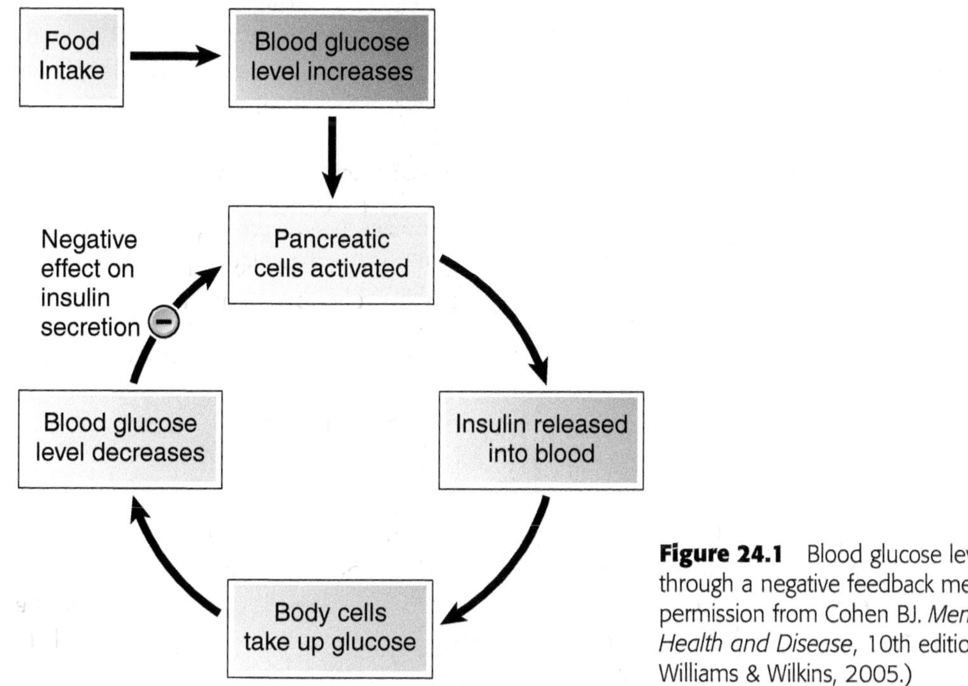


**Figure 24.1** Blood glucose levels regulate insulin release through a negative feedback mechanism. (Reprinted with permission from Cohen BJ. *Memmler's The Human Body in Health and Disease*, 10th edition. Baltimore: Lippincott Williams & Wilkins, 2005.)

ity of the pituitary is in turn controlled by the hypothalamus, a part of the brain directly above the pituitary.

The hypothalamus is physically connected to the pituitary by the infundibulum, a tissue bridge through which blood vessels and nerves carry information. The pituitary releases hormones to the systemic circulation only when it is signaled by the hypothalamus. The hy-

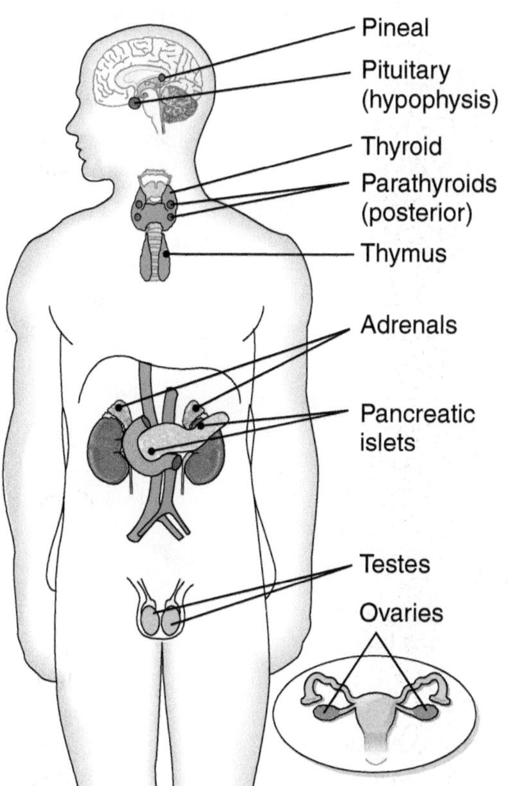


**Figure 24.2** Glands of the endocrine system . (Adapted with permission from Cohen BJ. *Memmler's The Human Body in Health and Disease*, 10th edition. Baltimore: Lippincott Williams & Wilkins, 2005.)

pothalamus uses nerve signaling and compounds called releasing hormones to stimulate this hormone release. For example, when gonadotropin-releasing hormone (GnRH) is sent to the pituitary, it releases the gonadotropins, follicle stimulating hormone (FSH) and leuteinizing hormone (LH), which initiate puberty and sexual maturation and control many normal reproductive functions.

anterior Located or situated toward the front of the body.

posterior Situated at or toward the back part of the body.

The pituitary gland is divided into two lobes, the anterior (front) and posterior (back) pituitary. The anterior lobe produces seven hormones that affect other glands or tissues in the body. The posterior pituitary releases three hormones that are produced in the hypothalamus and delivered to the pituitary. **Figure 24.3** illustrates the anatomy of the hypothalamic-pituitary axis and the hormones secreted by the pituitary. The tissues that each hormone affects and the names of the hormone secreted are displayed. **Table 24.1** lists the most important hormones, the gland that secretes them, and describes the actions of the hormones.

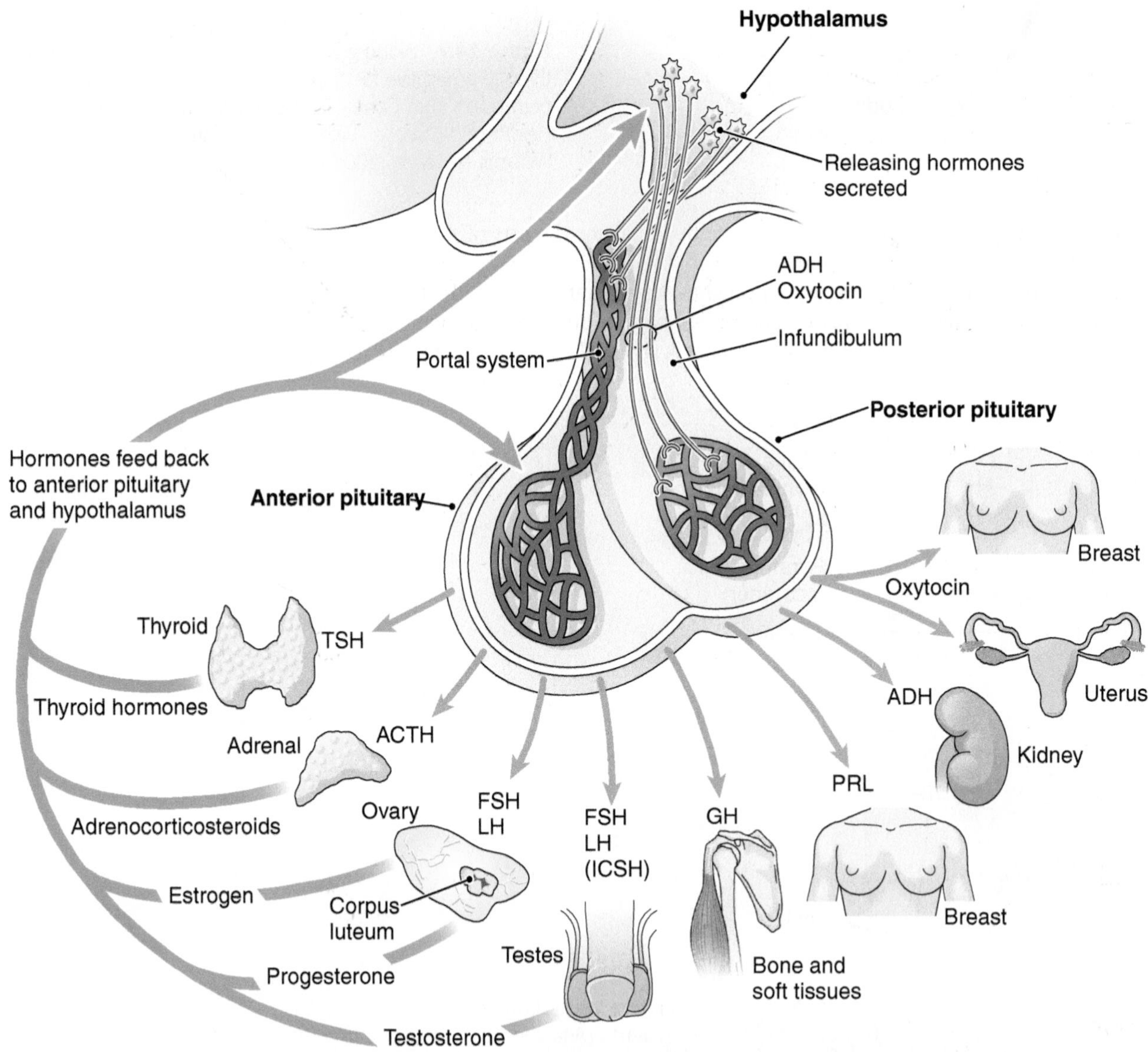


**Figure 24.3** The hypothalamus, pituitary gland, hormones, and target tissues. (Adapted with permission from Cohen BJ. *Memmler's The Human Body in Health and Disease*, 10th edition. Baltimore: Lippincott Williams & Wilkins, 2005.)

**Table 24.1** A Summary of the Major Hormones, Their Sources and Target Tissues, and Their Actions

| Gland Name | Major Hormones | Target Tissues | Action |
|---|---|---|---|
| Posterior Pituitary | Antidiuretic Hormone (ADH) | Kidney | Promotes reabsorption of water (↓ elimination of water) |
| | Oxytocin | Uterus and breasts | Contraction of uterus and milk let-down reflex |
| Anterior Pituitary | Growth Hormone (somatotropin) | All body tissues | Stimulates protein synthesis, causes growth in adolescence |
| | Thyroid stimulating Hormone (TSH or thyrotropin) | Thyroid gland | Stimulates the thyroid gland to produce thyroid hormone |
| | Adrenocorticotropic Hormone (ACTH) | Adrenal glands | Stimulates production of steroid hormones, especially in stress |
| | Prolactin | Breasts | Stimulates milk production |
| | Follicle Stimulating Hormone (FSH) | Ovaries and testes | Stimulates the development of germ cells (ova and spermatozoa) |
| | Leuteinizing Hormone | Corpus luteum and gonads | Causes ovulation in females, secretion of sex hormones in both |
| | Melanocyte Stimulating Hormone | Melanocytes | Production of melanin in skin, also affects appetite and libido |
| Thyroid Gland | Thyroxine (T4), Triiodothyronine (T3) | Tissues throughout the body | Normal growth and development, metabolism |
| | Calcitonin | Bone | Opposes bone loss, increases calcium deposition in bone |
| Adrenal Glands | Epinephrine, norepinephrine | Heart, bronchioles, blood vessels, eyes, other tissues | "Fight or flight"—↑ HR, BP, dilates pupils, ↑ blood flow to muscles, dilates bronchioles |
| | Cortisol | Tissues throughout the body, liver | ↑ Glucose levels, suppress inflammation |
| | Aldosterone | Kidneys, sweat glands | ↑ Sodium reabsorption, reduces sodium loss through sweat, causes fluid retention |
| Pancreas | Insulin | Skeletal muscle, fat, hypothalamus, liver, others | ↓ Blood sugar by ↑ utilization, ↑ storage of glucose as glycogen in liver, as fat in fat cells |
| | Glucagon | Liver | ↑ Blood sugar, releases glucose from glycogen stores in liver |
| Ovaries | Estrogen | Tissues throughout the body, breasts, uterus | Secondary female sex characteristics, preparation of uterus for pregnancy, many others |
| Ovaries | Progesterone | Tissues throughout the body, uterus | Supports implantation of fertilized ovum |
| Testes | Testosterone | Tissues throughout the body, testes | Secondary male sex characteristics, spermatogenesis, many others |
| Thymus | Thymosin | Lymphocytes, lymphatic tissue | Maturation of lymphocytes |
| Pineal Gland | Melatonin | Brain, unknown | Wake-sleep cycles, puberty onset |

## The Thyroid and Parathyroid Glands

The thyroid gland is located in the neck, near the top of the trachea. In humans the gland has a butterfly shape, with one lobe on either side of the trachea and a tissue bridge called the isthmus (**Fig. 24.4**). The thyroid gland is critically important for normal growth and development from infancy. An infant whose thyroid gland does not develop will suffer from a lack of both physical and intellectual growth unless thyroid hormone is replaced, a syndrome called cretinism. For this reason the law requires that all neonates be checked for the presence of adequate thyroid hormone at birth. Hypothyroidism is more common in adults, and results in weight gain, sensitivity to cold, feeling sluggish and other symptoms.

Excessive thyroid production can also occur. The result of excessive thyroid activity is called hyperthyroidism and can be due to an enlarged thyroid gland, inflammation of the thyroid, tumors of the thyroid, and other causes. Hyperthyroidism, or thyrotoxicosis, can cause an increased level of activity and anxiety, weight loss, rapid pulse, sweating, and tremors. In the most severe form it can cause a life-threatening hypermetabolic state known as thyroid storm.

The thyroid gland produces peptide hormones, including two kinds of thyroid hormone, thyroxine and triiodothyronine, and calcitonin. Both thyroid hormones contain iodine, a nutrient required for thyroid health. Thyroxine is produced in the largest quantities and is the hormone found in the highest concentrations in the bloodstream. Once in tissues, thyroxine is converted to the more active triiodothyronine.

Calcitonin plays an important role in calcium metabolism and bone health. Calcitonin causes calcium to leave the bloodstream and deposit in the bones. Its effects are balanced by parathyroid hormone, released from the parathyroid glands. The parathyroid glands are four small pieces of tissue embedded in or attached to the thyroid gland. Parathyroid hormone promotes calcium movement from the bones to the bloodstream. Parathyroid and calcitonin production and release is controlled through a negative feedback mechanism based on blood levels of calcium. Along with the active form of vitamin D, these hormones regulate calcium absorption from the GI tract, calcium blood levels, calcification of bone, and calcium conservation in the kidneys.

glucocorticoids A group of corticosteroids that affect carbohydrate metabolism, especially by increasing blood sugar, and that have pronounced anti-inflammatory activity.

mineralocorticoid Any of a group of corticosteroids that primarily regulate fluid and electrolyte balance.

## The Adrenal Glands

The adrenal glands are small glands located at the top of the kidneys. They are made up of two layers of tissue and each layer secretes different hormones. The adrenals play a critical role in helping the body to function during times of physical or other severe stress. The adrenal medulla produces epinephrine and norepinephrine, which, because they are released into the bloodstream, can be considered as hormones. The adrenal cortex secretes glucocorticoids and mineralocorticoids, which are steroid hormones. Norepinephrine and epinephrine raise heart rate, direct blood to the muscles, dilate the eyes, and raise blood sugar levels, all in response to what the brain perceives as danger. These effects are known as the fight or flight response, and are discussed in Chapter 4.

Glucocorticoids are also released in response to stress. They raise the concentration of sugars and other nutrients in the bloodstream. In addition, they suppress the inflammatory

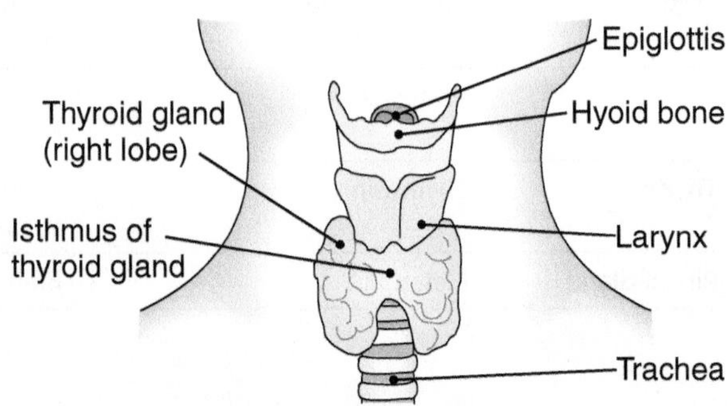


**Figure 24.4** The thyroid gland is shown in relation to other structures. (Adapted with permission from Cohen BJ. *Memmler's The Human Body in Health and Disease*, 10th edition. Baltimore: Lippincott Williams & Wilkins, 2005.)

response. Cortisol is the most important endogenous glucocorticoid. Mineralocorticoids regulate electrolyte balance, help regulate the concentration of urine and fluid balance, and are required for life. Aldosterone is the principal steroid with mineralocorticoid activity.

Unusually low adrenal function due to suppression from taking corticosteroids, or for other reasons, gives rise to a condition called Addison's disease. In this syndrome, the patient experiences increasing weakness and fatigue, loss of appetite, weight loss, fluid and electrolyte imbalances, and an inability to respond to physical stresses. If not corrected, this syndrome can lead to death. Excessive secretion of cortisol, or chronic drug treatment with steroids, results in Cushing syndrome. This condition is associated with a moon-shaped face, fat pads on the back ("buffalo hump"), fluid retention and weight gain, bone weakening, diabetes, easy bruising, fragile skin, and hirsutism.

## The Pancreas

The pancreas is both an endocrine and an exocrine gland (a gland that secretes substances into a duct, like the salivary glands). It secretes digestive enzymes into the pancreatic duct, and insulin into the blood stream. The islets of Langerhans are the insulin secreting cells within the pancreas (see **Fig. 24.5**). Insulin acts on muscle and other tissues to increase the utilization of glucose. Glucagon, which is also secreted by the islets of Langerhans, raises blood sugar by acting on the liver to increase the breakdown of glycogen, a form of stored energy, to glucose. Both glucagon and insulin are peptide hormones. Together these two hormones modulate the levels of glucose in the blood and play an important role in normal utilization of energy for growth and health.

exocrine Secreting outwardly, usually via a duct, for example salivary glands.

Diabetes mellitus, the most common of all endocrine illnesses, occurs because of a complete lack of insulin production in type I diabetes. In type II diabetes, there is a relative lack of insulin as compared with need. This disease is associated with obesity and resistance within tissues to the effect of insulin. Type II diabetes is linked to high cholesterol levels, high blood pressure, and heart disease in what is referred to as metabolic syndrome. Unfortunately, the rise in national rates of obesity is associated with an increasing occurrence rate of type II diabetes, which now is even occurring in children. Type II diabetes is completely preventable. It is prevented by eating a healthy diet that includes protein, healthy fats, and complex carbohydrates instead of simple sugars, and by exercising regularly.

Early symptoms of diabetes can include excessive thirst, frequent urination, exaggerated hunger, lack of energy, and more frequent infections. Poorly controlled type I and type II diabetes eventually will result in damage to many organ systems, including the cardiovascular system, the eyes, and the kidneys.

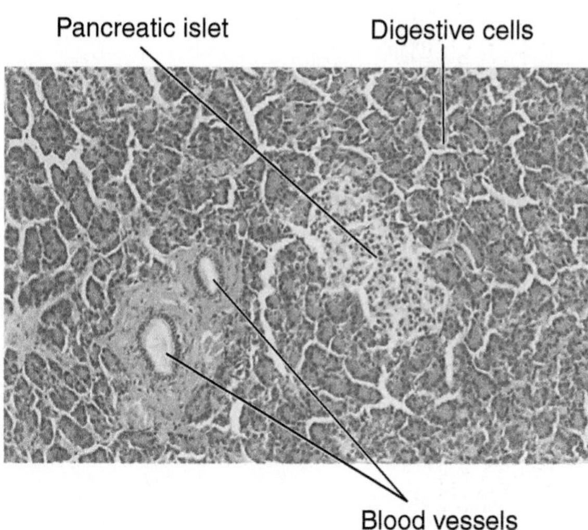


**Figure 24.5** A microscopic view of pancreatic tissue, showing islet cells and exocrine cells of the pancreas. (Reprinted with permission from Cohen BJ. *Memmler's The Human Body in Health and Disease*, 10th edition. Baltimore: Lippincott Williams & Wilkins, 2005.)

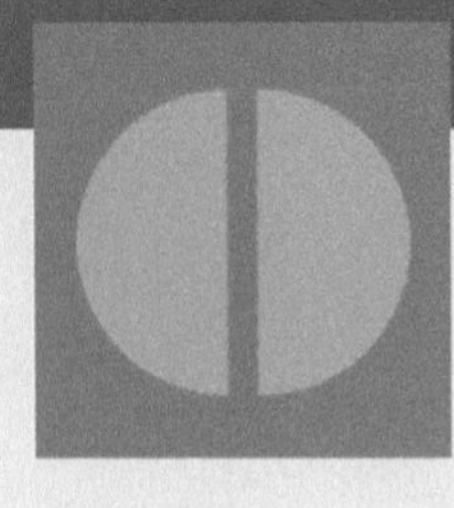

## Case 24.1

Dexter Rose is an unfortunate youngster who was allowed to eat sugary snacks and junk food beginning when he was 18 months old. Dexter is now 15 years old and at 5 feet 7 inches, he weighs 210 pounds. Because he was always overweight and kids made fun of him, he never wanted to participate in sports. His favorite pastime is watching sports on television. He began to feel extra tired and experienced blurred vision recently, and his parents noticed he was always getting sick. He finds that he needs to use the restroom frequently and is often thirsty. Now his pediatrician tells his parents that he has type II diabetes, and must give himself insulin. What lifestyle changes can help Dexter to return to health?

## The Ovaries and Testes

The ovaries in the female and the testes in the male are responsible for producing ova and spermatozoa, the germ cells needed for sexual reproduction. In addition, they are the main source of female and male sex hormones. The testes produce testosterone, the hormone responsible for the secondary sex characteristics of males, including greater muscle mass, facial hair, and the characteristic body structure (broad shoulders and narrow hips) of men. Male hormones are known as androgenic steroid hormones. The testes are under the control of the pituitary gland. Leuteinizing hormone (LH) stimulates the testes to produce testosterone. Follicle stimulating hormone (FSH), along with testosterone, promotes the production of spermatozoa.

androgen A general term referring to male sex hormones.

The ovaries secrete estrogen and progesterone. Estrogen is responsible for the development of the secondary sex characteristics of women, and the development of the mammary glands (breasts). Female sex hormones follow a monthly cycle and are under the regulation of the pituitary gland. In the mature female, an ovum will ripen each month under the influence of FSH. The follicle that contains the ripening ovum secretes estrogen, which thickens the lining of the uterus in preparation for pregnancy. The elevated estrogen levels in the blood feed back to the pituitary gland, which responds by increasing leuteinizing hormone. LH causes rupture of the follicle and release of the ovum into the fallopian tube, a process called ovulation. The ruptured follicle is called the corpus luteum, and it secretes some estrogen and large amounts of progesterone. If fertilization occurs, the zygote (fertilized egg) implants into the wall of uterus. Progesterone levels remain high to sustain the pregnancy. If fertilization does not occur, hormone levels fall and menstruation occurs, starting the cycle all over again.

zygote A single cell formed from the union of the male and female germ cells at fertilization, and capable of developing into an embryo.

## The Thymus and the Pineal Glands

The thymus is a two-lobed gland located in the upper portion of the chest cavity, on either side of the trachea. It is closely tied to the immune system, and is intimately involved with the maturation and health of that system. The thymus is larger and more active in infancy through young adulthood than in old age. During development, lymphocytes gravitate to the thymus and mature there. These lymphocytes are called T (for thymus) cells. T cells play an important roll in identifying and reacting to substances recognized as "foreign." T cells are supposed to develop self-tolerance, but when that fails, autoimmune responses occur. Thymosin is a peptide hormone secreted by the thymus and involved with maturation of the lymphocytes into T cells.

The pineal gland is a tiny gland located above and posterior to the pituitary. It produces the peptide hormone melatonin. Secretion of this hormone occurs during the hours of darkness. The retina, which detects light, directly signals the pineal gland to stimulate secretion of melatonin as light wanes. The pineal gland is large in children and begins to shrink at puberty. Melatonin levels influence wake-sleep cycles and appear to affect the onset of puberty.

### Other Hormones

Other tissues besides glands can also secrete hormones. The prostaglandins, although originally found in the prostate, are secreted by most tissues and affect a bewildering number of cell types. Some of these actions have already been described. The kidneys secrete erythropoietin, the hormone that stimulates the bone marrow to produce red blood cells. The placenta produces hormones that help to maintain a pregnancy and prepare the breasts for milk production. The GI tract produces numerous substances that act both as true hormones, released into the blood stream, and through paracrine signaling. Included in these substances is gastrin, produced by the stomach, which stimulates production of gastric acid and pepsin. Researchers are identifying more and more substances that contribute to homeostasis through local and distant cell signaling.

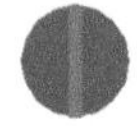

## Hormones and Treatment of Endocrine Disorders

The diseases of the endocrine system are related to excessive production of a hormone (hyperfunctioning gland) or underproduction of hormones (hypofunctioning gland). One example already discussed is that of hypo- or hyperthyroidism. More recently, researchers have discovered that resistance to hormones can contribute to diseases that appear to be caused by hypofunctioning glands. In type II diabetes, resistance to insulin complicates treatment for many patients.

When diseases related to hypofunction or hyperfunction occur, they are treated with replacement hormones, or drugs that mimic or antagonize the effects of a hormone. When hormone resistance occurs, drugs that alter the response of target tissues may be used. However, hormones are not used exclusively to treat disease due to hyperfunctioning or hypofunctioning glands. They can be used to intentionally interfere with usual feedback mechanisms or cell-to-cell communication in order to control some body function. For example, female hormones are used to manipulate ovulation and prevent pregnancy. We use steroid hormones to control excessive inflammation associated with allergic reactions or asthma. Growth hormone is used to increase the stature of very small children.

In the past, hormones were simply extracted from animal tissues. Since human and animal forms of hormones are not identical, these extracts could result in allergic reactions, production of antibodies to the substances, or incomplete responses. The use of hormone extracts presented difficulties with purification and quantification of the drug. Now many human hormones can be exactly replicated through recombinant DNA technology, by splicing the gene responsible for production of the hormone into a rapidly replicating organism, such as a bacterium. The organisms with the new gene rapidly reproduce and the offspring carry the new gene. The bacteria become mass producers of the human hormone, which is harvested and purified. Other hormones or related drugs are synthesized in the laboratory and provide a response similar to the actual hormone. In the next several chapters, the wide variety of hormones and related drugs for the treatment of endocrine and related conditions will be discussed. These drugs are important; at least six different antidiabetic agents, two drugs for thyroid insufficiency, and numerous female sex hormones appear on the top 200 drugs sold for 2006.

# Review Questions

## Multiple Choice

Choose the best answer for the following questions:

1. Cell to cell communication involving chemical signaling is known as?
   a. Long-distance signaling
   b. Advanced cell communication
   c. Apoptosis
   d. Paracrine signaling
   e. Endocrine signaling

2. Long-distance signaling between cell systems is carried out when endocrine glands release what?
   a. Neurotransmitters
   b. Chemotactic factors
   c. Hormones
   d. Biogenic amines
   e. All of the above

3. When the accumulation of substance A slows the production of substance A, this is known as?
   a. Negative feedback
   b. The mechanism by which oxytocin synthesis is controlled in the body
   c. Positive feedback
   d. Circular feedback
   e. None of the above

4. Which of the following exerts direct control over the function of the pituitary gland?
   a. Infundibulum
   b. Glucose levels in the bloodstream
   c. Adrenal glands
   d. Hypothalamus
   e. Releasing hormones

5. Which of the following is true about the adrenal glands?
   a. They are responsible for production of glucocorticoids and mineralocorticoids.
   b. They play an important role in the response to stress.
   c. The adrenal glands sit on top of the kidneys.
   d. Administration of corticosteroids can cause adrenal suppression.
   e. All of the above are correct.

## True/False

6. Steroid hormones are not considered to be true hormones because they are derived from cholesterol.
   a. True
   b. False

7. Hypothyroidism beginning in adulthood causes the same symptoms and outcome as hypothyroidism beginning in infancy.
   a. True
   b. False

8. Many hormones, such as insulin and calcitonin, are made of chains of amino acids called peptides.
   a. True
   b. False

9. Most endocrine diseases are caused by a malfunctioning endocrine gland that fails to produce normal levels of the hormone in the body.
   a. True
   b. False

10. Thymosin is a hormone that is secreted by the pancreas and controls blood levels of glucose.
    a. True
    b. False

## Matching

For numbers 11 to 15, match the word or phrase with the correct lettered choice from the adjacent list. Choices will not be used more than once and may not be used at all.

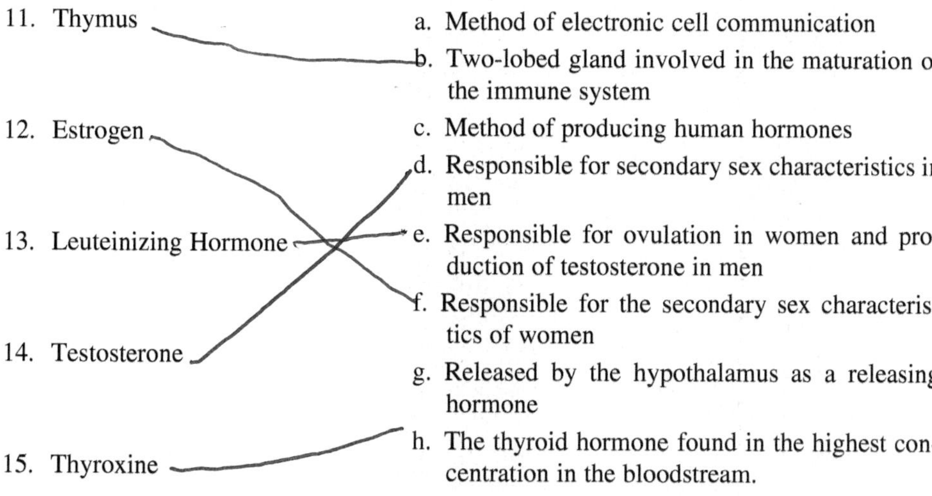

11. Thymus
12. Estrogen
13. Leuteinizing Hormone
14. Testosterone
15. Thyroxine

a. Method of electronic cell communication
b. Two-lobed gland involved in the maturation of the immune system
c. Method of producing human hormones
d. Responsible for secondary sex characteristics in men
e. Responsible for ovulation in women and production of testosterone in men
f. Responsible for the secondary sex characteristics of women
g. Released by the hypothalamus as a releasing hormone
h. The thyroid hormone found in the highest concentration in the bloodstream.

## Short Answer

16. Explain why a lack of insulin is detrimental to health, and describe the mechanism of insulin function in the body.

17. List at least three of the basic functions in the body that the endocrine system coordinates.

18. Explain the difference between steroid and peptide hormones and how their chemical differences affect their action in cell signaling.

19. Explain the negative feedback response common in the endocrine system. A diagram may be used.

20. Explain what causes the release of gonadotropins and what effects they have in males and females.

## FOR FURTHER INQUIRY

Investigate the role of the thymus gland and thymosin in the development of immunity or the pineal gland and melatonin in sleep-wake cycles. How does aging affect the function of the thymus gland? What is the relationship between sunlight, melatonin production, and mood?

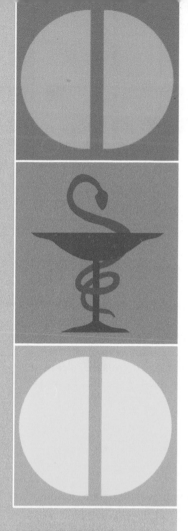

Chapter **25**

# Hypothalamic, Pituitary, and Thyroid Hormones

## KEY TERMS

- acromegaly
- depot injection
- diurnal
- exophthalmos
- goiter
- hyperthyroidism
- hypothyroidism
- idiopathic

## OBJECTIVES

After studying this chapter, the reader should be able to:

- Describe the relationship between the actions of the hypothalamus and the pituitary gland in the control of hormone release by other glands.
- List three aspects of somatropin or somatrem use with which patients must be familiar before leaving the pharmacy with a new prescription.
- Compare and contrast the posterior pituitary hormones vasopressin and oxytocin.
- Identify the three treatment options available to a person suffering from hyperthyroidism.
- Explain why levothyroxine is the preferred drug for use in the treatment of hypothyroidism.

## DRUGS COVERED IN THIS CHAPTER

| Hypothalamic and Pituitary Hormones | | Drugs Affecting the Thyroid Gland |
|---|---|---|
| Corticotropin | Somatropin (human growth hormone) | Iodide salts |
| Cosyntropin | Vasopressin | Levothyroxine |
| Desmopressin | | Liothyronine |
| Octreotide (somatostatin) | | Methimazole |
| Oxytocin | | Propylthiouracil |
| Somatrem | | Thyroid hormone, desiccated |

The nervous and endocrine systems monitor and adjust all of the important functions of the human body. Hormone release is principally modulated by the pituitary gland, but it is in turn controlled by the part of the brain called the hypothalamus. "Releasing" or "inhibiting" hormones are produced in the hypothalamus and sent to the pituitary to direct the release of pituitary hormones. Each hypothalamic regulatory hormone controls the release of a specific hormone from the anterior pituitary. The hormones secreted by the hypothalamus and the pituitary glands are peptides or proteins.

# Hormones of the Hypothalamus and Pituitary

Although a number of hypothalamic and pituitary hormone preparations are currently available, their use is mainly limited to diagnostic tests or treating specific hormonal deficiencies or excesses.

## Adrenocorticotropic Hormone

diurnal Having a daily cycle or occurring during the daytime.

Adrenocorticotropic hormone (ACTH) is cyclically released from the anterior portion of the pituitary gland. Its release follows a diurnal rhythm, meaning that it follows a daily cycle and is released at about the same time every day. The highest concentration of ACTH occurs early in the morning and the lowest in the evening.

### Actions and Indications

ACTH acts on the adrenal glands by interacting with receptors on the cell surfaces. The activated receptors switch on proteins inside the cell that in turn cause synthesis (from cholesterol) and release of cortisol. See **Figure 25.1**. Because many synthetic corticosteroids are readily available for oral use, ACTH is no longer used to treat patients with low levels of cortisol. It is easier and safer to simply replace the adrenal hormones with hydrocortisone and an aldosterone substitute, when necessary. ACTH is indicated for exacerbation of multiple sclerosis. This form of treatment is not common, because injectable corticosteroids work more directly and are easier to use. The most important role for ACTH is as a diagnostic tool for differentiating between primary adrenal insufficiency known as Addison disease and caused by adrenal atrophy, and secondary adrenal insufficiency caused by the inadequate secretion of ACTH by the pituitary.

### Administration

Like all hormones of the anterior and posterior pituitary, ACTH is a peptide hormone. As such it cannot be administered orally, because it is susceptible to destruction by pepsin and other enzymes that digest proteins in the GI tract. Two formulations of ACTH are available (see **Table 25.1** for product information on all the drugs presented in this chapter). Corticotropin is an extract from the anterior pituitaries of domestic animals and cosyntropin is a synthetic segment of human ACTH. Corticotropin is administered intramuscularly or subcutaneously, while cosyntropin is administered intramuscularly or intravenously.

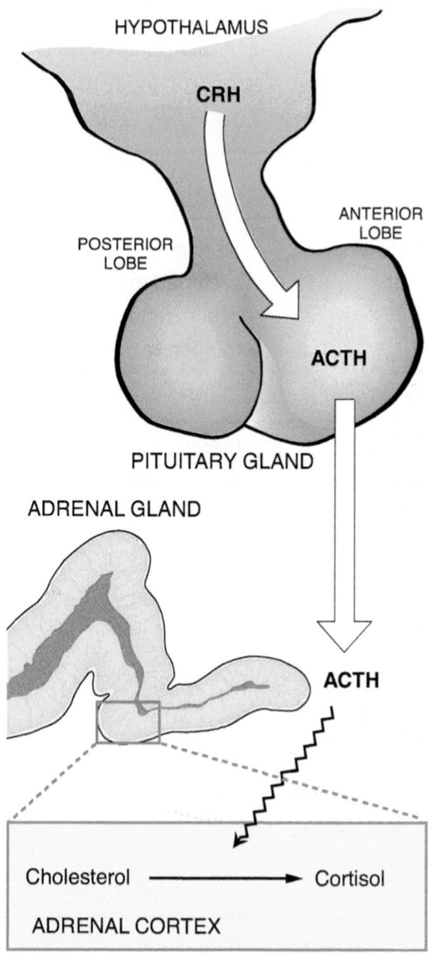


**Figure 25.1** The actions of the pituitary on the adrenal gland. (Adapted with permission from Harvey RA, Champe PC, Howland RD, et al. *Lippincott's Illustrated Reviews: Pharmacology*, 3rd edition. Baltimore: Lippincott Williams & Wilkins, 2006.)

Both forms of ACTH are used for diagnosis of adrenal gland function. The drug is injected and the response is monitored by checking plasma cortisol levels. In the patient with normal adrenal function, plasma cortisol levels will increase appropriately.

## Side Effects

Adrenocorticotropic hormone has few side effects when used one time for diagnostic purposes. The animal extracted form, corticotropin, is associated with allergic reactions, including the possibility of anaphylaxis. When used more frequently, corticotropin can cause fluid retention that leads to hypertension, heart failure, or increased intracranial pressure. Muscle weakness, hypokalemia, hyperglycemia, pancreatitis, GI bleeding, and an impaired immune response can become problematic. After prolonged use, this drug will suppress the body's production of ACTH and glucocorticoids. Abrupt withdrawal of the drug without replacement glucocorticoids can result in very serious illness, or even death.

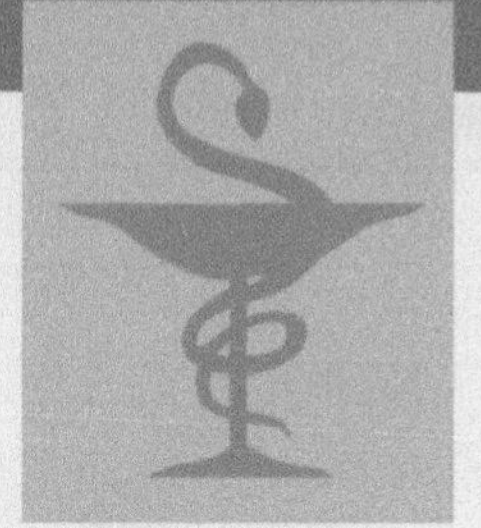

### Tips for the Technician

Reconstituted corticotropin and ACTH gel is kept refrigerated. Patients should be warned that the injections are painful. When the drug is brought to room temperature beforehand, injection is less uncomfortable. Patients taking the drug for ACTH deficiency must be warned not to abruptly discontinue this medication, because adequate adrenocortical steroids are necessary for life.

**Table 25.1** Product Names, Formulation, and Indications for Pituitary and Thyroid Hormones

| Generic | Brand Name | Available as | Indications | Notes |
|---|---|---|---|---|
| **Hypothalamic and Pituitary Hormones** | | | | |
| Corticotropin | Acthar® Gel | Repository Injection | Diagnostic testing, inflammatory diseases | Steroid replacement preferred to use of corticotropin, refrigerate |
| Cosyntropin | Cortrosyn® | Powder for injection | Diagnostic testing | |
| Desmopressin | DDAVP®, Stimate® | Tablets, nasal solution, injection | Diabetes insipidus, pre-op to prevent bleeding in patients with hemophilia | Refrigerate nasal soln and injection |
| Octreotide (somatostatin) | Sandostatin® | Injection, depot injection | Acromegaly, carcinoid tumors, VIPomas | Refrigerate<br>Room temp ok x 30 days |
| Oxytocin | Pitocin®, others | Injection | Initiation, improvement of contractions, control post-partum bleeding | Check labelling for storage |
| Somatropin (human growth hormone) | Genotropin®, Nutropin®, Serostim®, others | Powder for injection, injection | Growth failure, growth hormone deficiency, AIDS wasting (Serostim® only) | Refrigerate |
| Somatrem | Protropin® | Powder for injection | Treatment of growth failure | Refrigerate |
| Vasopressin | Pitressin® | Injection | Diabetes Insipidus, abdominal distention, esophageal varices | |
| **Thyroid Hormones** | | | | |
| Levothyroxine | Synthroid®, Levoxyl®, others | Tablets, powder for injection | Hypothyroidism, treatment of goiter | |
| Liothyronine | Cytomel®, Triostat® | Tablets, injection | Hypothyroidism, treatment of goiter | |
| Thyroid, desiccated | Armour Thyroid® | Tablets | Hypothyroidism, treatment of goiter | Less consistent than levothyroxine |
| **Antithyroid Drugs** | | | | |
| Iodide salts | Lugol's Solution | Solution | Thyrotoxicosis, preparation for surgery, radiation emergency | Short-term effectiveness |
| Methimazole | Tapazole® | Tablets | Hyperthyroidism | |
| Propylthiouracil | | Tablets | Hyperthyroidism | |

## Growth Hormone and Somatostatin

Growth hormone (GH), or somatotropin, is a peptide hormone secreted by the anterior pituitary gland. Its release and synthesis is controlled by growth hormone releasing hormone (GHRH), a compound produced by the hypothalamus. Another hormone, somatostatin, inhibits the release of growth hormone and indirectly affects the thyroid gland. The presence of growth hormone feeds back to regulate the release of GHRH. Like many hormones, the release of GH follows a cyclic pattern of release, with highest levels of release occurring during deep sleep.

### Actions and Indications

Growth hormone influences a wide variety of biochemical processes. By stimulating protein synthesis, muscle and bone growth are promoted. This is one of many hormones that are important in the regulation of glucose levels and utilization of fat. Although GH exerts many physiologic effects directly on target tissues, some are mediated through insulin-like growth factors I and II, which are secreted by the liver and other tissues in response to GH signaling.

Somatropin, the generic name of human growth hormone of recombinant DNA origin, is used in the treatment of growth hormone deficiency in children. It is indicated for growth failure in children that occurs for other reasons, such as chronic renal insufficiency. This drug can be used to prevent muscle wasting and weight loss seen in patients with AIDS. The use of growth hormone for short stature in normal children is controversial and problematic. Most health professionals feel that use of growth hormone to increase height in otherwise normal children is an unjustified and potentially risky use of limited medical resources for essentially cosmetic reasons. Studies indicate that the average child will only gain an additional one to two inches in height with growth hormone treatment. This use is supposed to be reserved for the shortest two to three percent of children. Somatrem is another recombinant DNA growth hormone that is therapeutically equivalent to somatropin, but varies from human growth hormone because of an additional amino acid.

#### Case 25.1

Trula Short has two children, a boy who is 10 years old and a girl, 13. She is a friend of Brian O'Neil, who is the technician in her local pharmacy. Trula calls Brian one day to tell him how distressed her son is because of his height. She says he is the shortest kid in class and gets picked on all the time. She is 5′2″ and her husband Riley Short is 5′6″. She wants to know if Brian knows of a drug that can be used to make her son taller. If you were Brian, what would you tell her? Investigate the use of growth hormone for short stature in the library or on reliable Internet sources to formulate an answer.

Although somatostatin (growth hormone inhibiting hormone) is released from the hypothalamus, it is also found in cells throughout the body. It not only inhibits the release of GH, but also of insulin, glucagon, and gastrin. Octreotide is a synthetic analog of somatostatin available for use in the treatment of acromegaly, a condition caused by excessive production of growth hormone that results in enlarged facial features, skull, and bones of the extremities (**Fig. 25.2**). When this condition begins in childhood, it can result in what is referred to as gigantism, Octreotide is also useful in the treatment of some gastrointestinal tumors, such as carcinoid tumors, that produce hormones and cause a syndrome of profuse diarrhea and flushing.

acromegaly A disorder that is caused by chronic overproduction of growth hormone by the pituitary gland, similar to gigantism.

### Administration

As peptide hormones, somatropin, somatrem, and octreotide are administered only by injection. Somatropin and somatrem are available as sterile powder that must be reconstituted before IM or subcutaneous injection. Octreotide is available as an immediate-release injection and in a long-acting formulation intended to remain at the sight of injection where it slowly and consistently releases the medication, referred to as a depot injection. The depot

depot injection Formulation that uses a vehicle designed to remain in "storage" at the site of injection so that absorption and drug action occurs over a prolonged period.

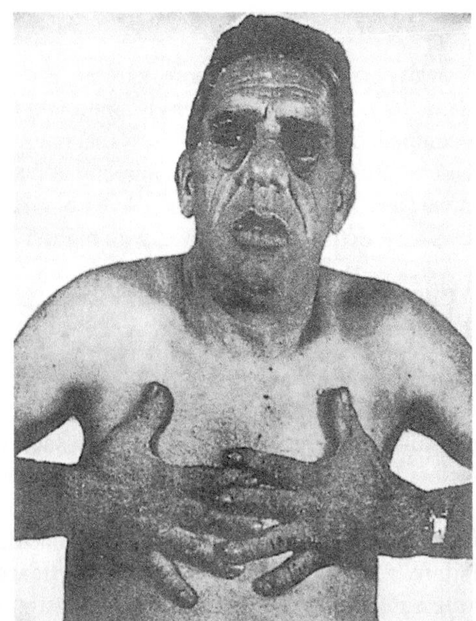

**Figure 25.2** Acromegaly, a condition caused by excessive production of growth hormone, is characterized by enlarged facial features, skull, and bones of the extremities. (Reprinted with permission from Porth CM. *Pathophysiology Concepts in Altered Health States*, 6th edition. Philadelphia: Lippincott Williams & Wilkins, 2002.)

formulation is administered every 4 weeks intramuscularly and the regular injection is dosed twice daily, subcutaneously or intravenously. All of these drug products should be stored in the pharmacy under refrigeration. However, octreotide injection is stable for 14 days at room temperature.

## Side Effects

Side effects of somatropin and somatrem are generally mild and uncommon. Headache, weakness, and edema can occur. Metabolic side effects, including hyperglycemia and hypothyroidism, can occur. Development of persistent antibodies to the drug occur in up to 40% of patients treated with somatrem, while only about 2% of patients receiving somatropin develop antibodies. Recall that somatrem contains an extra amino acid, while somatropin is identical to human growth hormone.

In patients who receive somatostatin (octreotide), adverse effects occur with some frequency. People with acromegaly are at a greater risk of experiencing side effects. Gastrointestinal effects are most common, and include abdominal discomfort, diarrhea, and nausea. Slow heart rate and other arrhythmias can occur. Headache, dizziness, fatigue, and injection site pain are not unusual.

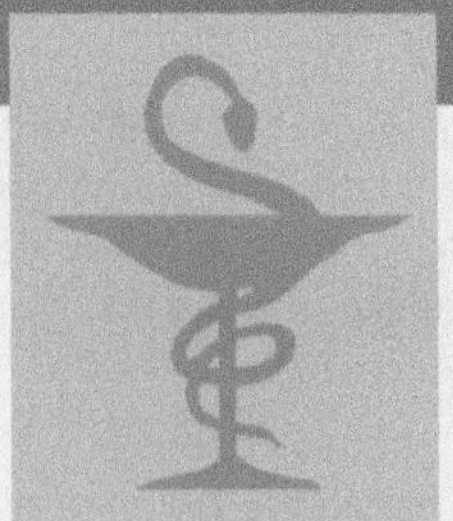

### Tips for the Technician

The prescribing physician will have educated most new patients with prescriptions for somatropin or somatrem on product reconstitution and injection techniques. Technicians should verify that clients feel comfortable with mixing and injecting the drug, and if not refer them to the pharmacist. Clients may require additional materials, such as alcohol wipes, which most pharmacies sell. Growth hormone products must be stored in the refrigerator and are stable under refrigeration for 14 days after reconstitution. To prevent unintentional waste of these costly medications, verify that prescriptions are appropriately labelled with storage instructions and that patients understand the requirement for refrigeration before and after reconstitution.

People receiving octreotide will probably use the immediate-release injection at first, until the prescriber can determine what the patient response to the drug will be. If the initial treatment is successful, patients will be switched to the long-acting form of octreotide. The long-acting formulation must be given IM into the gluteal muscle, and will therefore require that someone other than the patient administer the medication. It is important for the pharmacist to verify that the person administering the drug is appropriately trained. Patients may choose to leave octreotide out of the refrigerator in a cool place, as long as they will use the product within 14 days.

## Vasopressin and Oxytocin

The posterior pituitary is responsible for the secretion of vasopressin (Pitressin®) and oxytocin (Pitocin®). Vasopressin, or antidiuretic hormone (ADH), helps maintain the total body water content at around 60% of the body mass in adults. Oxytocin plays a crucial role in the birth process and production of milk in women, and a less well-defined role in bonding, social relationships, and sexual activity in both men and women. Both of these hormones are peptide hormones made up of nine amino acids and they differ by only two amino acids.

### Actions and Indications

The posterior pituitary hormone vasopressin exerts its most significant affect on the renal tubules, where it promotes the reabsorption of water, and therefore, the concentration of the urine. In addition, vasopressin exerts an affect on the smooth muscle of blood vessels and other tissues, especially in higher concentrations, where it causes constriction. It is available as a purified posterior pituitary extract, assigned the generic name vasopressin, and as the synthetic equivalent, desmopressin (DDAVP®). Both drugs are indicated to stop or prevent bleeding in very specific circumstances, such as in an unusual condition of the upper GI tract called esophageal varices. They are sometimes used to prevent bleeding in people with hemophilia who are undergoing medical or surgical procedures. The most important application of vasopressin or desmopressin is in the treatment of diabetes insipidus.

Diabetes insipidus (DI) is characterized by the production of voluminous amounts of very dilute urine and is unrelated to diabetes mellitus. People with diabetes insipidus urinate very frequently and are constantly thirsty. This problem can result in electrolyte abnormalities, bed-wetting, and dehydration. DI is caused either by a lack of production of ADH or by a lack of sensitivity of the kidneys to ADH. The most common form of DI, often referred to as neurogenic DI, is treated with vasopressin.

Although chemically similar to vasopressin, oxytocin has different pharmacologic effects. It exerts a direct and selective action on the smooth muscle of the uterus and the breast. Oxytocin causes constriction of the smooth muscle in blood vessels, but it has significantly less of this effect than vasopressin. In the uterus, it causes uterine contractions. The strength of the contractions is related to the sensitivity of the uterus to the hormone. As the pregnancy nears term, the number of oxytocin receptors in the uterine muscle increases, causing the uterus to be more sensitive to oxytocin release. Although a number of factors, including the pressure of the fetus on the cervix, sex hormones, and the presence of prostaglandins, contribute to the preparation of the uterus for birth, it is oxytocin release that provides the tremendous impetus necessary to deliver the infant.

In a woman who is pregnant, prolactin prepares the breast and initiates the production of milk. After giving birth, infant suckling at the breast initiates the further release of oxytocin. It stimulates contraction of smooth muscle in the breast causing milk letdown, or ejection. The oxytocin released by the suckling infant plays a role in maternal behavior and bonding and causes post-partum contraction of the uterus, which controls bleeding.

Oxytocin is indicated for use in the initiation of labor when it is advisable for medical reasons, or for improving the quality of contractions when labor is not progressing. It is also used for the initiation of labor when an aborted pregnancy is inevitable (when the fetus dies) or to help empty the uterus after an incomplete abortion. It can be administered after birth to reduce the risk of postpartum bleeding, and to aid in milk letdown.

## Administration

Both desmopressin and vasopressin are peptide hormones and therefore are destroyed in the GI tract if they are orally administered. Although desmopressin is very poorly absorbed, there is an oral formulation of the drug. Its use requires initiation at a low dose and titration upward until an adequate therapeutic effect is attained. The absorption and bioavailability of the nasal solution of desmopressin is much better than the tablets, and the nasal pump spray is easy to use. Both desmopressin and vasopressin are available in a sterile solution for injection. Vasopressin is given intramuscularly or subcutaneously and desmopressin is given subcutaneously or by direct intravenous injection. Oxytocin is also destroyed by enzymes in the GI tract and is given by intravenous infusion to induce labor and by intramuscular or intravenous injection after delivery to control postpartum bleeding.

## Side Effects

Because of its potent effect on water balance, action on blood vessels, and requirement for carefully individualized dosing, use of vasopressin carries some associated risk. High doses can result in excessive water retention, water intoxication, and seizures. The vasoconstrictive effects may result in chest pain, or even cardiac arrest in patients with heart disease. Although these side effects can occur with the nasal formulations, they are more likely to occur when the drug is given by injection. Nasal formulations are more commonly associated with GI upset, irritation of the nose and eyes, headache, and facial flushing.

When oxytocin is administered properly, toxicity is uncommon. However, when administered in excessive doses, contractions can be so powerful as to cause uterine spasm, rupture of the uterus, and damage to the fetus. Although the antidiuretic and pressor activities of oxytocin are very much lower than those of vasopressin, oxytocin can cause maternal hypertension, arrhythmias, and water intoxication.

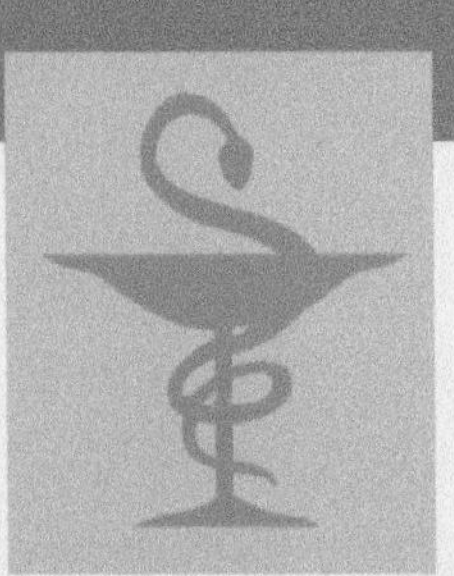

### Tips for the Technician

Only hospital-based technicians are likely to handle oxytocin, injectable vasopressin, and injectable desmopressin. Storage recommendations for these drugs differ from product to product. Oxytocin should be stored in the refrigerator unless it is used quickly. This product can only be stored at room temperature for 30 days. Vasopressin injection can be stored at room temperature. The two injectable products, Pitocin® and Pitressin®, have names that look and sound alike. Technicians need to be extra cautious when interpreting orders for these drugs.

Desmopressin injection and nasal formulations must be refrigerated. Be sure a label instructing the client to store the product in the refrigerator is affixed to the prescription. The desmopressin nasal products come with patient instructions, which must be included with the prescription. Refer patients to the pharmacist if they are unsure of administration techniques.

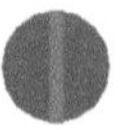

# The Thyroid Gland, Hormones, and Related Drugs

Although it is quite small, the thyroid gland plays an important role in maintaining human health. Every aspect of metabolism is regulated by the thyroid gland, whose hormones stimulate protein synthesis, increase the levels of glucose available for energy consumption by tissues, and through production of calcitonin, encourage bone growth. Parathyroid hormone, produced by the embedded parathyroid glands, contributes to healthy bone and calcium metabolism.

The thyroid gland is in turn regulated by the hypothalamus and pituitary. In the normal person, when the hypothalamus signals the pituitary (with thyrotropin releasing hormone or TRH), the pituitary releases TSH, or thyroid stimulating hormone. TSH acts in the thyroid gland to stimulate production and release of the thyroid hormones, triiodothyronine ($T_3$) and thyroxine ($T_4$). When thyroid levels are in the normal range, their presence feeds back to the hypothalamus, which in turn reduces TRH, TSH, and thyroid hormone production. In patients with thyroid disease, one of these steps is abnormal.

Diseases of the thyroid gland can be divided into four broad categories: overproduction and underproduction of thyroid hormone and benign enlargement and malignant tumors of the thyroid gland. Underproduction of thyroid hormone, or hypothyroidism, is fairly common and can have many possible causes. These include the autoimmune disorder Hashimoto's thyroiditis, surgery or radioactive iodine therapy for hyperthyroidism that results in too little remaining functional tissue, and idiopathic (without a known cause) hypothyroidism. The thyroid gland requires iodine in order to produce thyroid hormone. In most industrialized nations, iodine is added to table salt to prevent hypothyroidism and the benign enlargement of the thyroid gland, called goiter, which is caused by iodine deficiency. Hypothyroidism can also occur because the pituitary gland is not functioning normally.

Hyperthyroidism is the overproduction of thyroid. Hyperthyroidism can be caused by a malfunction of the pituitary gland, hormone-secreting tumors of the thyroid gland, or benign enlargement of the thyroid gland. Graves' disease, an autoimmune disease that causes stimulation of the thyroid gland, is the most common cause of hyperthyroidism. In severe forms it can be associated with exophthalmos, or bulging of the eyes.

Once a diagnosis of thyroid disease is made, there are a number of pharmacologic and nonpharmacologic treatment options for physicians to chose. The usual treatment for hypothyroidism is thyroid replacement therapy, either using thyroid extract or synthetic replacement hormones. The most common treatment of hyperthyroidism is use of radioactive iodine, a substance that when taken orally makes its way to the thyroid where it causes the gland to shrink. Although surgery is an option, it is performed less frequently today than in the past. Antithyroid drugs and sometimes iodide solutions are used to suppress thyroid function before surgery, and antithyroid drugs can also be used as primary therapy.

hypothyroidism Deficient activity of the thyroid gland that results in a lowered metabolic rate and associated symptoms.

idiopathic Arising spontaneously with no known cause.

goiter Enlargement of the thyroid gland that can result from insufficient iodine intake.

hyperthyroidism Excessive activity of the thyroid gland that results in signs of increased metabolic rate, an enlarged thyroid gland, and other symptoms.

exophthalmos Abnormal protrusion of the eyeball.

## Actions and Indications

Thyroid hormones and thyroid extract are approved for treatment of hypothyroidism, goiter, and some forms of thyroid cancer. Some prescribers use these agents to treat obesity, a practice that is both ineffective and dangerous. Levothyroxine, the most active enantiomer of thyroxine, is the drug of choice when thyroid replacement is needed because of its longer duration of action, consistent potency, and reasonable cost. Although levothyroxine contains only $T_4$, it is readily metabolized to $T_3$ in the body, which parallels the conversion of endogenous thyroxin to triiodothyronine.

Thyroid USP, an extract of desiccated porcine thyroid glands, is rarely prescribed today because of inconsistent potency between and within brands. Liothyronine ($T_3$ or triiodothyronine) is another thyroid hormone indicated for the treatment of hypothyroidism. It acts more rapidly and disappears more quickly than thyroxine, a possible advantage in some situations, but it is also more expensive. Use of liothyronine results in laboratory findings that indicate low $T_4$ levels, a result which may be confusing to practitioners.

Propylthiouracil (PTU) and methimazole are drugs used to suppress the production of thyroid hormone. They do not block the activity of thyroid hormone on peripheral tissues, nor do they inhibit the release of thyroid hormone that is stored in the thyroid gland. PTU inhibits the conversion from thyroxine ($T_4$) to the active hormone, triiodothyronine ($T_3$). These antithyroid drugs are indicated for the treatment of hyperthyroidism, and when given for 6 months or more, they can induce remission in Grave's disease. They are also used to prepare patients for surgery or treatment with radioactive iodine. By pretreating with antithyroid drugs there is reduced risk of thyroid storm. Thyroid storm is a life-threatening hypermetabolic state brought on by the rapid release of excess thyroid hormone into the blood stream, a situation that can occur as a result of surgery.

Although small amounts of the mineral iodine is essential for normal synthesis of thyroid hormone, high doses of iodine can inhibit the synthesis and release of thyroid hormone and reduce the vascularity of the gland. For this reason, potassium iodide combined with iodine (strong iodine solution or Lugol's solution) can be used for preparation of the thyroid gland before surgery. Iodine suppression of the thyroid is only effective for a short period of time. After a few weeks, the thyroid gland ceases to respond to the effects of the therapy. Iodine is used to protect the thyroid gland during emergencies where exposure to radioactivity would damage it, such as in the event of a nuclear power plant disaster.

## Administration

All thyroid hormones are effective when administered by the oral route, although absorption can be variable. Because the bioavailability of different brands of levothyroxine varies, patients are encouraged to stay with one brand of drug. Patients should take levothyroxine on an empty stomach to improve its absorption. Liothyronine is more completely absorbed than levothyroxine. A number of drugs and foods can affect the absorption of thyroid hormones. It is recommended that patients separate the administration of iron, antacids, bile acid sequestrants (cholestyramine and others), sucralfate, and simethicone from their thyroid dose by at least four hours.

Besides oral preparations, levothyroxine and liothyronine are available for parenteral use. Liothyronine is given by intravenous injection, while levothyroxine can be administered by IM or IV injection. Liothyronine injection must be stored under refrigeration. Parenteral administration of thyroid hormone is used in coma related to myxedema, a life-threatening state that results from uncorrected hypothyroidism. It is also used when people with hypothyroidism are unable to take their medications orally.

The antithyroid drugs are available for oral administration only. Several doses of PTU are required per day, but methimazole can usually be given once or twice daily. These drugs are slow to reach peak effect, because stored thyroid hormone must be depleted first. Iodide treatment is given orally, three times a day. It begins to act quickly and for this reason can be used to treat thyroid storm, or to prevent damage from radioactive exposure.

## Side Effects

The side effects of treatment with thyroid hormone are usually related to excessive doses, and are similar to the symptoms of hyperthyroidism. Doses are adjusted based on response and laboratory testing to avoid toxic doses. Signs of excessive dose can include rapid heart rate, palpitations, cardiac arrhythmia, elevated blood pressure, tremors, nervousness, weight loss, nausea and vomiting, heat intolerance, and hair loss. Allergic reactions to thyroid extract can occur. Drug interactions are reported for several drugs. As noted above, a number of drugs can adversely affect absorption of thyroid hormones. In addition, thyroid hormone replacement can alter the dose requirements of insulin or other antidiabetic drugs, warfarin, and digoxin.

The side effects of the antithyroid drugs are less predictable than those related to thyroid hormone replacement. The most serious side effects seen with the antithyroid drugs are agranulocytosis and other blood abnormalities, vasculitis, and liver toxicity. More commonly, they can cause GI upset, skin rashes, and signs of hypothyroidism including mental depression, cold intolerance, hair loss, and edema. Iodine administration causes local irritation to the mouth and GI tract, a metallic taste in the mouth, burning of the mouth and gums, and gastric pain. It is poisonous in excessive doses, and must be kept out of the reach of children.

## Tips for the Technician

When pharmacies purchase thyroid extract and levothyroxine it is appropriate to purchase a single brand with a good record of consistent bioavailability. Decisions regarding the brand purchased ought not to be made based on price alone. It is the expected standard that prescriptions for these drugs will be filled with the same brand of drug from month to month unless a change is unavoidable.

Patients need to be instructed by the pharmacist to notify the physician if symptoms of thyroid toxicity occur. They need to be informed that thyroid therapy is taken for life, except in rare cases. Technicians should affix auxiliary labels to the prescription vial that instruct the patient to take levothyroxine on an empty stomach, avoid interacting drugs, and continue taking the medication unless otherwise directed by the physician.

For best results, it is desirable for patients to take PTU or methimazole in equally divided doses. The pharmacist should alert patients to the symptoms associated with agranulocytosis.

The taste of strong iodine solution, or Lugol's solution, can be improved by diluting it in juice or water. It is a good idea for the technician to label this product with instructions to keep it out of the reach of children.

# Review Questions

## Multiple Choice

Choose the best answer for the following questions:

1. The patient or their responsible family member should be comfortable with which of the following aspects of the use of somatropin or somatrem before leaving the pharmacy?
   a. Injection techniques
   b. Sterile reconstitution
   c. Storage requirements
   d. Possible side effects
   e. All of the above

2. Indicate the choice that correctly identifies the accepted uses of oxytocin.
   a. Induction of labor when medically necessary and improvement in the quality of labor.
   b. Prevention of milk production and release in nonnursing mothers.
   c. Reduction of the risk of postpartum bleeding and stimulation of milk letdown.
   d. a and c.
   e. b and c.

3. Which of the following is incorrect regarding the superiority of levothyroxine over other thyroid hormone products for treatment of hypothyroidism?
   a. Levothyroxine has a longer duration of action.
   b. Levothyroxine potency is more predictable than that of thyroid extract.
   c. Levothyroxine absorption is superior to other products.
   d. Levothyroxine is less expensive than liothyronine.
   e. None of the above is incorrect.

4. Vasopressin or desmopressin are used for what indications, below?
   a. Treatment of diabetes insipidus
   b. Prevention or treatment of bleeding in limited circumstances
   c. Induction of labor
   d. a and b
   e. All of the above

5. For which of the following products is ongoing refrigeration required?
   a. DDAVP®
   b. Sandostatin®
   c. Levothyroxine injection
   d. Cytomel®
   e. Lugol's solution

## True/False

6. Oral administration of most peptide hormones is unsuccessful because the enzyme pepsin destroys them.
   a. True
   b. False

7. The posterior pituitary hormones vasopressin and oxytocin differ by only two amino acids and share a small degree of overlap in pharmacologic activity.
   a. True
   b. False

8. Thyroid hormones help people with normal thyroid activity safely lose weight by increasing their metabolic rates.
   a. True
   b. False

9. Pitocin® and Sandostatin® can be stored for a short time in the refrigerator, but it is preferable to store them at room temperature.
   a. True
   b. False

10. The hormones secreted by the hypothalamus and the pituitary glands are peptides or proteins.
    a. True
    b. False

## Matching

For numbers 11 to 15, match the drug name with the correct lettered choice indicating the available formulation from the list below. Choices will not be used more than once and may not be used at all.

11. Corticotropin
12. Propylthiouracil
13. Somatrem
14. Iodide salts
15. Oxytocin

a. Tablets
b. Capsules
c. Injection
d. Solution
e. Repository injection
f. Powder for injection

## Short Answer

16. What are some similarities and some differences between oxytocin and vasopressin?
17. List the possible treatment options for a person with hyperthyroidism.
18. If a client is getting a prescription filled for growth hormone for the first time, what does he or she need to know about its use?
19. Why is levothyroxine generally considered superior to liothyronine or thyroid extract in the treatment of hypothyroidism?
20. When are iodide solutions used in the treatment of thyroid problems, and how do they work?

# FOR FURTHER INQUIRY

During a nuclear event, radioactive iodine can be released into the air. As part of emergency preparedness, the CDC and FDA have developed guidelines for protecting the thyroid gland during such an event. Use the Internet or your school library to investigate the use of potassium iodide to protect the thyroid gland in the event of radiation emergencies.

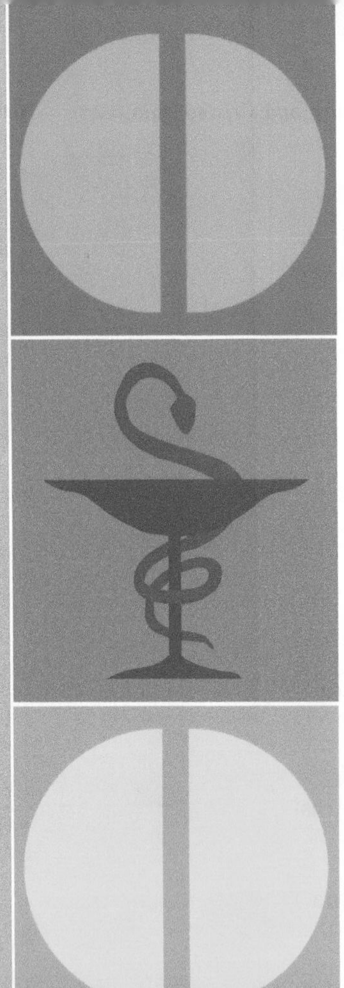

## Chapter 26

# Insulin and Other Drugs for Diabetes

### KEY TERMS

- hypoglycemic agent
- lipodystrophy
- polydipsia
- polyphagia
- postprandial
- secretagogue
- Type 1 diabetes
- Type 2 diabetes

## OBJECTIVES

After studying this chapter, the reader should be able to:

- Compare and contrast diabetes type 1 and type 2, and state the goals of treatment of diabetes.
- Describe the three classic symptoms characteristic of diabetes that are directly or indirectly caused by the inability of tissues to utilize glucose.
- Explain the differences between short, rapid, intermediate, and long-acting insulin, and describe how each is administered.
- Describe the mechanisms of action of the insulin secretagogues, insulin sensitizers, and the glucose absorption inhibitors, and list an example in each drug category.
- List the common symptoms of hypoglycemia, and explain the actions of glucagon and when it would be used.

## DRUGS COVERED IN THIS CHAPTER

| Insulin Preparations | Other GI Hormones |
|---|---|
| Aspart insulin | Exenatide |
| Glargine insulin | Glucagon |
| Glulisine insulin | |
| Lente (Insulin zinc) | |
| Lispro insulin | |
| NPH insulin suspension | |
| Regular | |
| Ultralente (Extended insulin zinc) | |

### Oral Antidiabetic Agents

| **Insulin Sensitizers** | **Inhibitors of Glucose Absorption** | **Insulin Secretagogues** |
|---|---|---|
| Metformin | Acarbose | Glipizide |
| Pioglitazone | Miglitol | Glimepiride |
| Rosiglitazone | | Glyburide |
| | | Nateglinide |
| | | Repaglinide |
| | | Tolbutamide |
| | | Tolazamide |

Diabetes mellitus was probably recognized as early as 1500 BC, when a disease involving production of copious urine was described in the Ebers papyrus. Although the first known use of the word "diabetes" occurred in Greece in the late second century BC, legend has it that it was a Roman physician who noticed flying insects circulating around the urine of a diabetic patient. He tasted the urine, found it to be as sweet as honey, and added the descriptive Latin term "mellitus" to the name. For the next thousand years, physicians used the taste of urine to diagnose diabetes, and described it as a "melting down of the flesh into urine," thinking that the cause of the disease was a malfunction of the kidneys.

Progress in understanding the cause and finding a treatment for diabetes was very slow. An entry in *The New American Cyclopaedia* published in 1859 gave this description of diabetes:

> The large excretion of urine begins to attract attention, and the patient complains that despite his excessive appetite he grows thinner and weaker; the mouth is pasty, the skin dry and hard, the bowels constipated . . . vision often becomes dim, the gums are spongy, . . . the memory and intellect fail . . . ( Ripley G. *The New American Cyclopaedia*. D. Appleton and Company, New York, 1859: page 438.)

In their search for understanding, physicians of the late 1800s realized that eliminating starches and sugar from the diet of diabetics could slow the progress of the disease. Exercise was recognized as helpful, and children with diabetes were encouraged to exercise when possible. In 1869 the young German medical student Paul Langerhans identified two types of tissue in the pancreas, one that secreted digestive enzymes and another type, "islands" embedded within the pancreas, whose function was not understood. Later research concluded that this tissue was the source of insulin, and it was named the "islets of Langerhans" in honor of Paul Langerhans' discovery.

Scientists soon discovered that they could cause diabetes in dogs by removing the pancreas. The name insulin (Latin for islands) was coined for the unidentified pancreatic substance, produced by the normal islets of Langerhans, which was now understood to be missing in the diabetic patient. There was a frantic search to extract and purify this mysterious pancreatic hormone in the early 1900s. Children that developed diabetes rarely survived into adulthood, and their parents, some of them wealthy, were ready to try any remedy possible (**Fig. 26.1**). Canadian physicians Frederick Banting, Charles Best, James Collip, and John Macleod are credited with the isolation and purification of insulin, and Banting and Professor Macleod were awarded the Nobel Prize for this important discovery. Soon afterwards, Eli Lilly Company bought the right to manufacture insulin. For the first time, the availability of the purified and effective hormone provided hope for people with diabetes.

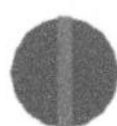

## Understanding Diabetes

Diabetes is a complex metabolic disorder related to a complete or relative lack of insulin. Insulin and other pancreatic hormones regulate the utilization of glucose by the tissues. When insulin levels are inadequate, glucose is not utilized and elevated levels of glucose in the blood (hyperglycemia) result. It is elevated glucose levels that directly cause two of the common presenting symptoms of diabetes, polyuria and polydipsia. Polyuria, or the passage of excessive volumes of urine, occurs because there is so much sugar in the blood the kidneys cannot prevent it from spilling into the urine. When that happens, water follows by osmosis. Patients who lose excessive amounts of water through the urine experience chronic, excessive thirst, or polydipsia. When insulin is completely absent, the tissues cannot utilize glucose and therefore they starve, even though dietary intake of calories is adequate. This accounts for the wasting away of the body described in early accounts of diabetes, in spite of polyphagia (great appetite and consumption of food), the third of the classic signs of diabetes. The high levels of blood glucose are the main cause of the many complications of diabetes. Drugs that reduce blood glucose levels are called hypoglycemic agents.

polydipsia Excessive or abnormal thirst.

polyphagia Excessive or abnormal hunger.

hypoglycemic agent Drug used to reduce blood glucose levels.

Type 1 diabetes Form of diabetes that usually develops during childhood or adolescence and is characterized by a lack of insulin secretion requiring replacement.

Type 2 diabetes Diabetes often seen in obese adults, characterized by impaired insulin utilization and inadequate compensation of insulin production; initially diet, exercise, and oral antidiabetic agents are used for treatment.

We now describe diabetes as falling into two major classifications. Type 1 diabetes, sometimes referred to as insulin dependent diabetes, is most likely to be diagnosed in children and young adults, and is the result of a complete lack of insulin production. In type 1 diabetes, the cells that produce insulin are destroyed, probably through an autoimmune process. Type 1 diabetes makes up about 10% of all cases of diabetes. Type 2 diabetes, by far the most common form, occurs because of insulin resistance in the tissues and an inability of the insulin producing cells in the pancreas to increase production of insulin enough to compensate for this resistance. Type 2 diabetes is sometimes called noninsulin-dependent diabetes, because other, oral medications are usually effective in its treatment. Although this is typically a disease of overweight adults, more and more children are developing this

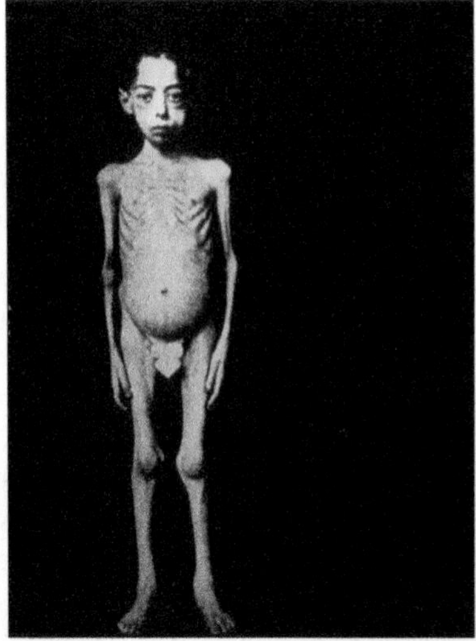
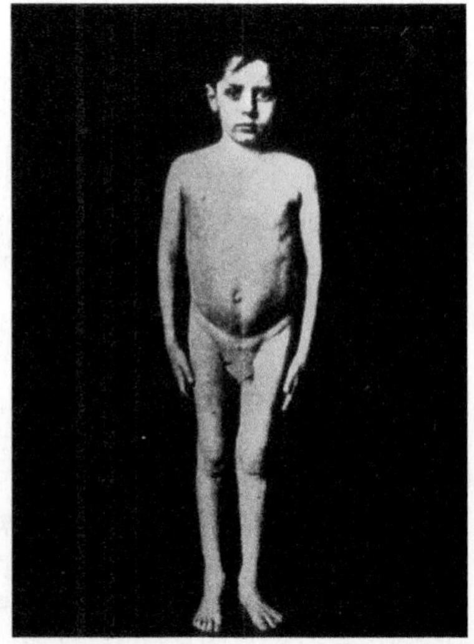

**Figure 26.1** Historic photograph of a child with diabetes before and after receiving newly discovered insulin. (Image is from the National Library of Medicine (http://wwwihm.nlm.nih.gov/). Original photographs are from the World Health Organization (WHO).

disease because of a nearly epidemic increase in obesity of childhood. Refer to **Table 26.1** for a comparison of the two types of diabetes.

## An Overview of the Treatment of Diabetes

The goal of the treatment of diabetes is to normalize blood sugars in order to prevent the many serious, long-term complications of the disease. The blood glucose level of a normal person who has not been fasting is in the range of the low to mid 100s (reported as mg glucose/dl blood). In the past, diabetic patients with blood glucose levels in the low 200s were considered to be within the acceptable range. Currently, more intensive treatment is considered the standard of care, and the goal is to keep glucose levels below 200 mg/dl at all times. Although the risk of hypoglycemia is increased with intensive treatment, long-term complications are dramatically reduced.

Long-term complications of poorly controlled diabetes include kidney failure, blindness, nerve damage that can cause pain in the limbs, GI complications, impotence, and, finally, vessel disease. Diabetic vascular complications can include hypertension and cardiovascular disease. Poor circulation results in sores on the feet and legs that can become chronically infected, and sometimes will lead to amputation. (See **Fig. 26.2** for some of the long-term complications of diabetes.) Diet and exercise continue to play a key role in controlling blood sugar levels. Although drug treatment of diabetes has advanced dramatically, the patient who consumes an appropriate diet, exercises regularly, and is educated about the disease will always have a better outcome than one who does not.

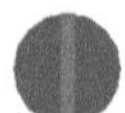

# Insulin

Insulin is a hormone consisting of two peptide chains. Its secretion in a healthy person is triggered by high blood glucose. Insulin release can be stimulated, amplified, or inhibited by the presence of the amino acids leucine and arginine, the hormone glucagon, the actions of the sympathetic nervous system, and other hormones through complex interactions. Insulin remains the only effective treatment for type 1 diabetes, and is an important agent

**Table 26.1** A Comparison of the Common Features of Type 1 and Type 2 Diabetes.

| | Type 1 (Insulin-Dependent Diabetes) | Type 2 (Noninsulin-Dependent Diabetes) |
|---|---|---|
| Age of onset | Usually during childhood or puberty | Frequently over age 35 |
| Nutritional status at time of onset | Frequently undernourished | Obesity usually present |
| Prevalence | 10 to 20 percent of diagnosed diabetics | 80 to 90 percent of diagnosed diabetics |
| Genetic predisposition | Moderate | Very strong |
| Defect or deficiency | β cells are destroyed, eliminating the production of insulin | Inability of β cells to produce appropriate quantities of insulin; insulin resistance; other defects |

(Reprinted with permission from Harvey RA, Champe PC, Howland RD. *Lippincott's Illustrated Reviews: Pharmacology*, 3rd edition. Baltimore: Lippincott Williams & Wilkins, 2006.)

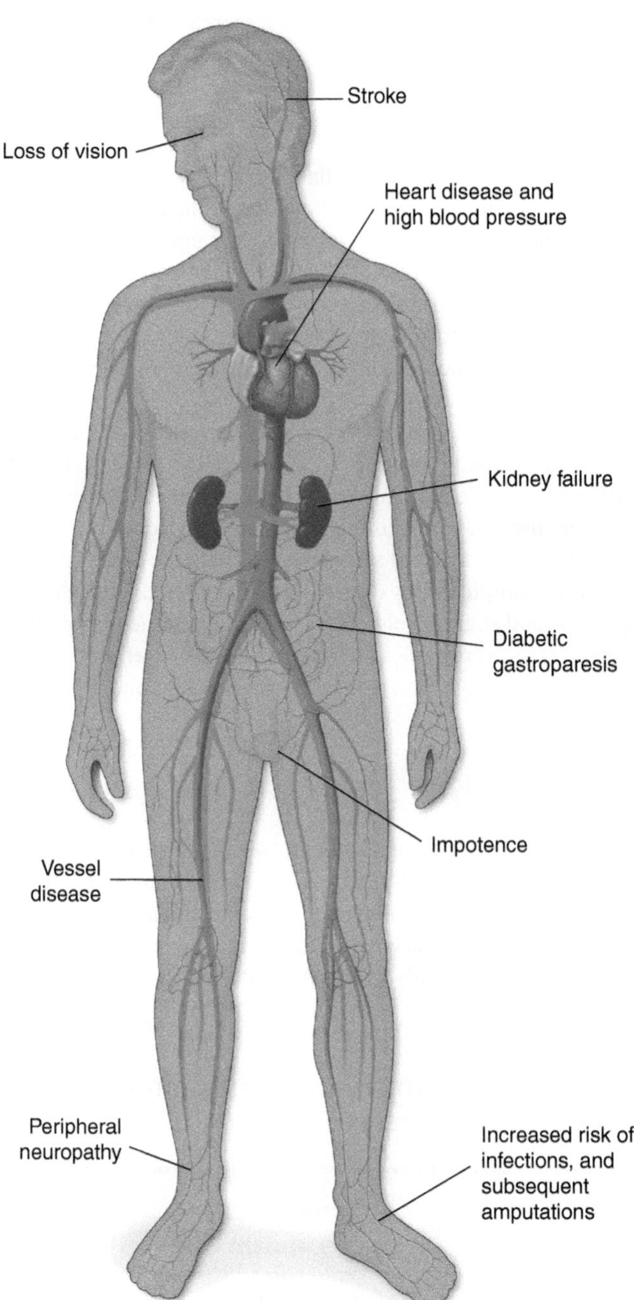


**Figure 26.2** Poorly controlled blood sugars are more likely to lead to long-term complications of diabetes. (Reprinted with permission from Premkumar K. *The Massage Connection: Anatomy and Physiology*. Baltimore: Lippincott Williams & Wilkins 2004.)

in type 2 patients who are poorly controlled in the early stages of disease or because of illness or other stressors.

Although insulin became available in the 1920s, it was derived from animal sources until recently. Human insulin and porcine insulin are closely related, but the availability of human insulin in 1983 reduced the occurrence of antibody production and reduced the dose requirements for most patients. Human insulin is synthesized, using recombinant DNA technology, by bacteria or yeast that are altered to contain the human gene responsible for insulin production.

## Actions and Indications

Human insulin is used as hormone replacement in people with Type 1 diabetes and can be used in patients with Type 2 diabetes when the disease is inadequately controlled by diet and exercise alone. Insulin increases glucose transport into cells, thereby reducing blood glucose levels. It encourages the formation of glycogen, a compound that is made from glucose and stored in the liver for later use. Insulin encourages the formation of protein in muscle cells and inhibits the breakdown of fat.

Modifications of human insulin have produced a variety of insulin preparations with different onsets and durations of action. Preparations are classified accordingly, and are usually referred to as rapid- or short-acting, intermediate-acting, and long-acting (see **Fig. 26.3**). Regular insulin is a short-acting insulin solution. It quickly lowers blood sugar and is safe for use during pregnancy. Lispro (Humalog®), aspart (NovoLog®), and glulisine (Apidra®) insulin are classified as rapid-acting because of their very rapid onset and very short duration of action. Intermediate- and long-acting insulin analogs include isophane (NPH), insulin zinc suspension (lente), insulin glargine (Lantus®), and extended insulin zinc suspension (ultra lente). Onset and duration vary due to the size and composition of the insulin crystals, as well as the amino acid sequences of the polypeptides. The less soluble an insulin preparation is, the longer its duration of action. Dose, injection site, blood supply, temperature, and physical activity can also affect the duration of action of the various preparations. A list of the most important insulin preparation, oral antidiabetic agents and other hormones, their indications, and available dosage forms is shown in **Table 26.2**.

## Administration

Because it is a peptide hormone, digestive enzymes destroy insulin administered by the oral route. Insulin is therefore administered by injection, most often subcutaneous injection. When elevated glucose levels constitute an urgent medical situation, rapid or short acting insulin (regular insulin and lispro insulin are suitable) will be given by intravenous injection or continuous infusion. Only insulin in solution can be administered intravenously. Insulin suspensions are given by subcutaneous injection.

Physicians use insulin preparations with different pharmacokinetic properties in order to improve diabetic control and patient compliance. For example, a patient may use a low dose of long-acting insulin for basal glucose control, and rapid-acting insulin dosed according to blood glucose levels at mealtimes. Rapid-acting insulin analogs are administered to mimic the mealtime release of insulin. In order to successfully use these flexible insulin

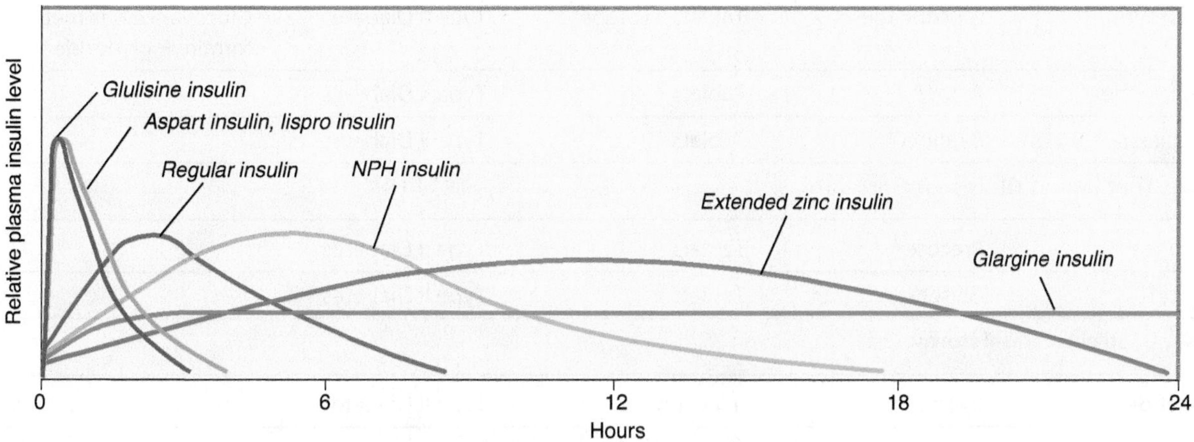


**Figure 26.3** Graph shows the onset and duration of action of several human insulin analogs. (Adapted with permission from Harvey RA, Champe PC, Howland RD. *Lippincott's Illustrated Reviews: Pharmacology*, 3rd edition. Baltimore: Lippincott Williams & Wilkins, 2006.)

**Table 26.2** The Most Important Insulin Preparation, Oral Antidiabetic Agents, and Other Hormones, Their Indications and Available Dosage Forms

| Generic | Brand Name | Available as | Indications | Notes |
|---|---|---|---|---|
| **Insulins** | | | | |
| Aspart | NovoLog® | Injection | Diabetes | Rapid acting |
| Glargine | Lantus® | Injection | Diabetes | Long acting |
| Glulisine | Apidra® | Injection | Diabetes | Rapid acting |
| Lente | Humulin L® | Injection | Diabetes | Intermediate acting |
| Lispro | Humalog® | Injection | Diabetes | Rapid acting |
| NPH | Humulin N® | Injection | Diabetes | Intermediate acting |
| Regular | Humulin R®, Novolin R Pen® | Injection, cartridge | Diabetes | May be given IV Short acting |
| Ultralente | Humulin U® | Injection | Diabetes | Long acting |
| NPH + Regular | Humulin 70/30, Humulin 50/50 | Injection | Diabetes | Premixed in set ration |
| **Insulin Secretagogues** | | | | |
| Glipizide | Glucotrol®, Glucotrol XL® | Tablets and ER tabs | Type II Diabetes | |
| Glimepiride | Amaryl® | Tablets | Type II Diabetes | |
| Glyburide | DiaBeta®, Micronase® | Tablets, micronized tabs | Type II Diabetes | Glynase®, PresTab® are micronized tablets |
| Nateglinide | Starlix® | Tablets | Type II Diabetes | Take right before meals |
| Repaglinide | Prandin® | Tablets | Type II Diabetes | Take right before meals |
| Tolbutamide | Orinase® | Tablets | Type II Diabetes | |
| **Insulin Sensitizers** | | | | |
| Metformin | Glucophage® | Tablets, ER Tabs | Type II Diabetes | Glucovance® is metformin + glyburide |
| Pioglitazone | Actos® | Tablets | Type II Diabetes | |
| Rosiglitazone | Avandia® | Tablets | Type II Diabetes | |
| **Drugs That Inhibit Glucose Absorption** | | | | |
| Acarbose | Precose® | Tablets | Type II Diabetes | |
| Miglitol | Glyset® | Tablets | Type II Diabetes | |
| **Other Gastrointestinal Hormones** | | | | |
| Exenatide | Byetta® | Injection | Type II Diabetes | |
| Glucagon | GlucaGen® | Powder for Injection | Severe Hypoglycemia | |

ER tabs, extended-release tablets.

dosing regimens, the patient must use a blood glucose testing machine on a regular (3 to 4 times daily or more) basis. Most pharmacies sell blood glucose testing equipment. **Figure 26.4** illustrates two of the numerous possible insulin dosing regimes.

Insulin pumps are sometimes used to continuously deliver insulin to patients with type 1 diabetes. The insulin will be administered through a venous catheter that remains in place. While the pump is connected, insulin is delivered in small amounts by continuous infusion to meet the basal insulin requirement of the patient. The blood sugar is tested throughout the day and extra insulin doses can be given when needed. An additional insulin dose, if needed, is calculated and programmed into the pump, which then delivers a bolus of insulin.

A variety of premixed combinations of human insulin, such as 70% NPH insulin plus 30% regular insulin, or 50% combinations of each of these, are also available. These are sometimes ordered by physicians to simplify the insulin regimen for patients who have a difficult time managing a more complex insulin regimen.

For many years pharmaceutical companies have looked for alternate methods of insulin administration in order to make its use easier and less painful. Insulin can be injected using an insulin pen, a prefilled injection device that allows the patient to dial in a dose and inject it accurately without drawing up the insulin. The pen is easy to use and only requires that a new needle be attached each time, and that the pen be primed with insulin before the first injection. Early in 2006, Pfizer Corporation received FDA approval for the first noninvasive insulin. Exubera® is an inhaled, short-acting insulin that is aimed at providing mealtime coverage for type 1 diabetics, thereby reducing the need for injections to one or possibly two injections daily. The inhaler device is less compact than a metered dose inhaler and more complicated to use. It is not yet approved for use in children. Research continues to find other effective insulin delivery systems, such as an insulin transdermal patch or sublingual spray.

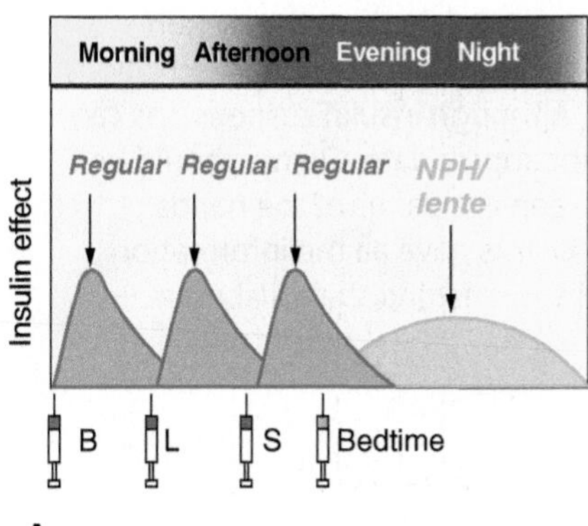


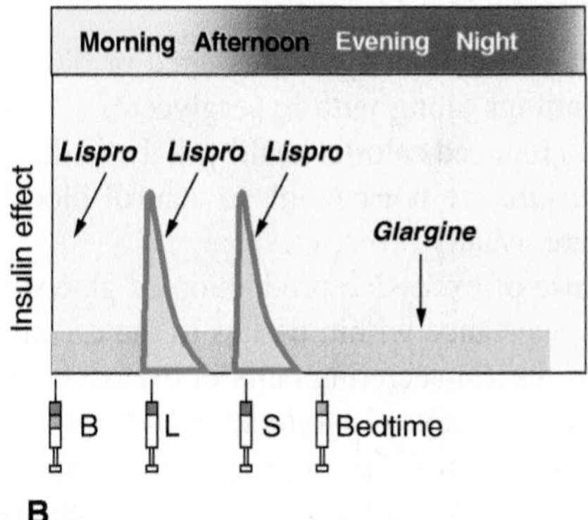


**Figure 26.4** Two of the numerous possible insulin dosing regimens (B, breakfast; L, lunch; S, supper). (Adapted with permission from Harvey RA, Champe PC, Howland RD, et al. *Lippincott's Illustrated Reviews: Pharmacology*, 3rd edition. Baltimore: Lippincott Williams & Wilkins, 2006.)

## Side Effects

The most serious and common adverse effect associated with use of any insulin is hypoglycemia, or low blood sugar. People with diabetes often do not produce adequate amounts of glucagon, epinephrine, and cortisol, the naturally occurring compounds that normally provide an effective defense against hypoglycemia. Severe hypoglycemia can be quite dangerous and result in coma, seizures, and death if not corrected. Patients with diabetes are taught to recognize its signs, such as feeling weak, dizzy, or confused (**Fig. 26.5**) and reverse it immediately with orange juice or another source of rapidly absorbed sugar. Other insulin side effects include pain at the injection site, hypersensitivity reactions, and lipodystrophy, an uneven distribution of fat tissues that occurs because of frequent injections at the same site.

lipodystrophy
Abnormality of fat metabolism especially involving loss of fat from or deposition of fat in tissue.

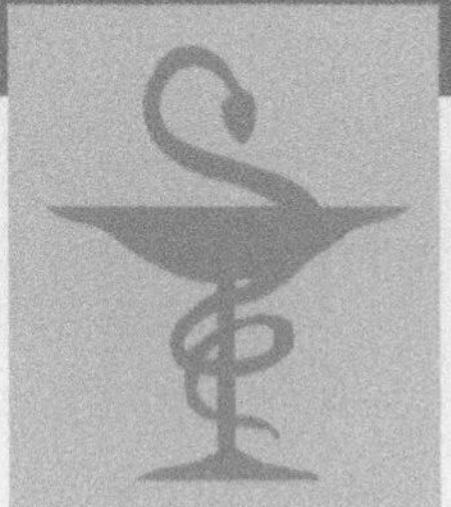

### Tips for the Technician

Diabetes can be a complex disease that requires intensive monitoring. Technicians can help patients by staying informed and knowledgeable about the equipment and devices stocked in their own pharmacies. Encourage diabetic patients to wear a medical identification bracelet, or carry information that identifies them as being diabetic, at all times. If the patient uses insulin, he or she should always carry adequate supplies for monitoring and administering the drug, know the signs of hypoglycemia, and carry candy or sugar packets to take in the event of hypoglycemia.

Insulin should always be stored in the refrigerator while in the pharmacy, but can be stored at cool room temperature once it is opened. Room temperature insulin is less painful to inject. Insulin must be protected from temperature extremes and cannot be frozen. Depending on the manufacturer, insulin vials are discarded 28 or 30 days after opening. In order to discard them at the appropriate time, the person opening the vial should label it with the date opened. Verify that insulin prescriptions are properly labelled regarding storage conditions. Although insulin suspensions can be labelled with "shake well," vigorous shaking is not appropriate. Clients should be taught to disperse particles by rolling the vials between the palms of the hands. Technicians play an important role in assuring that clients have all the information and equipment they need in order to be successful at managing their diabetes.

# Oral Antidiabetic Agents

People with type 2 diabetes are almost always overweight, usually middle-aged or older, and are likely to have other abnormal metabolic findings along with hyperglycemia. The first and most important treatment for this disease is a reduced calorie, healthy diabetic diet, and adequate exercise. For some people, these measure are not enough to control blood sugar. In these patients, oral hypoglycemic agents are usually effective.

Hyperglycemia occurs in type 2 diabetes because of excessive production of glucose (usually related to excessive calorie consumption), resistance within tissues to the effects of insulin, and inadequate secretion of insulin from insulin-secreting cells in the islets of Langerhans, called beta cells. Most of the available drugs employed to treat this disease increase production of insulin, reduce insulin resistance, or otherwise improve the effectiveness of endogenous insulin. A few drugs directly alter glucose absorption or metabolism, sometimes through a variety of mechanisms.

**Symptoms Caused by Hypoglycemia**

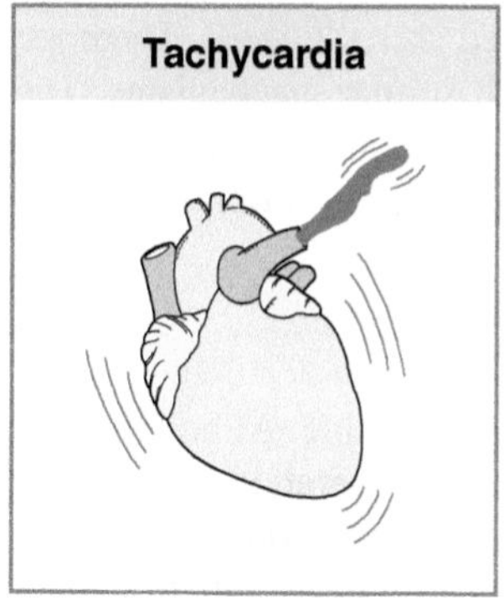


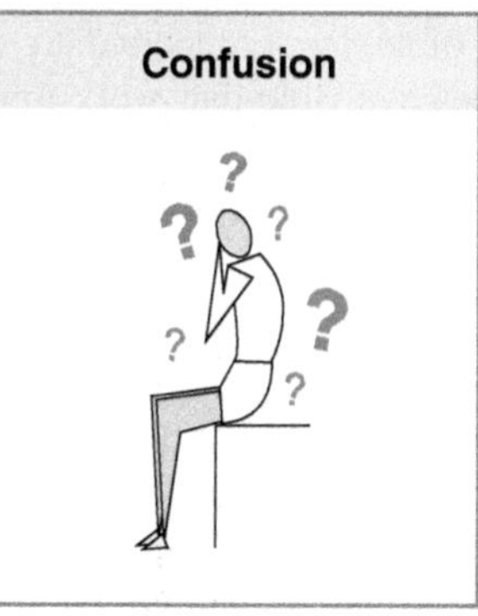


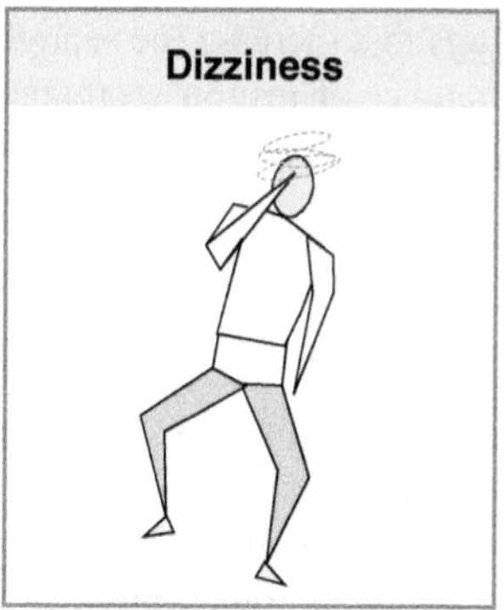


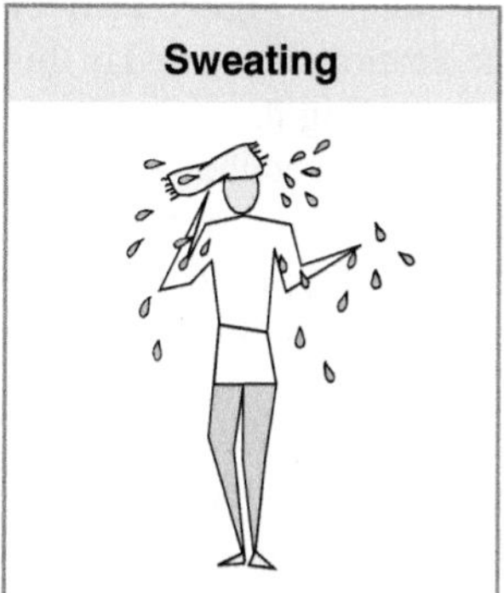


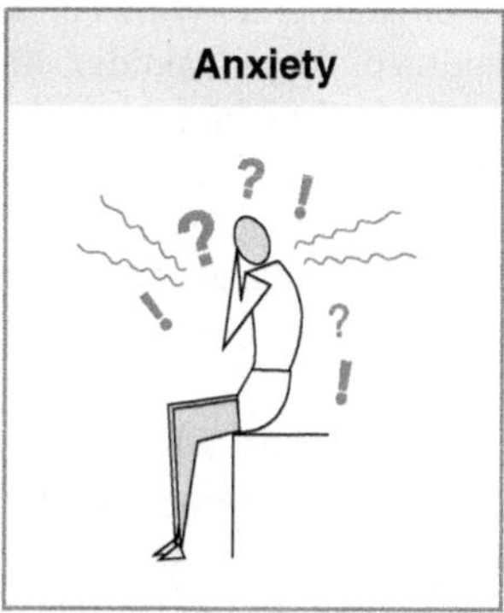


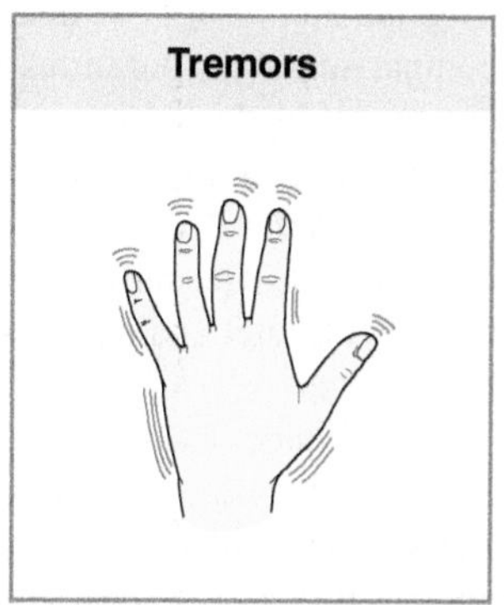


**Symptoms Caused by Hyperglycemia**

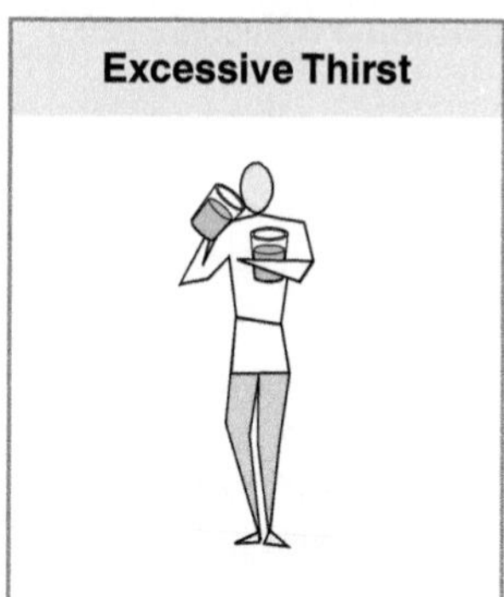


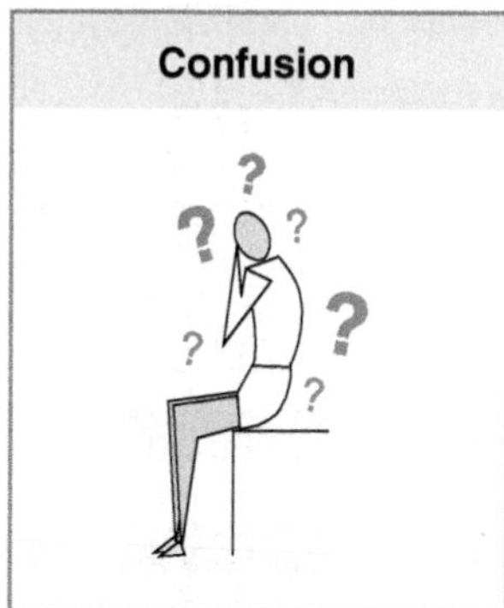


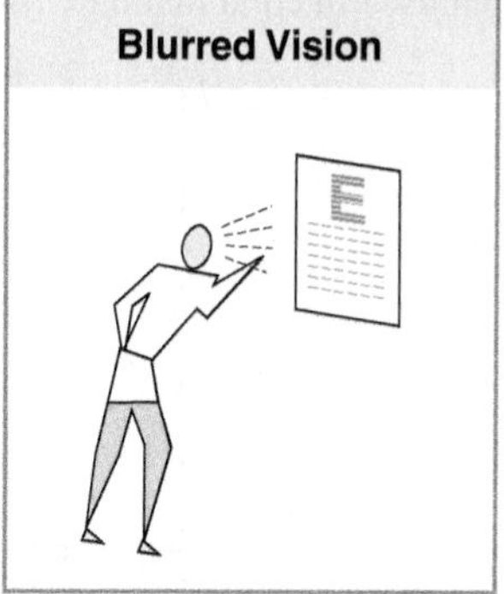


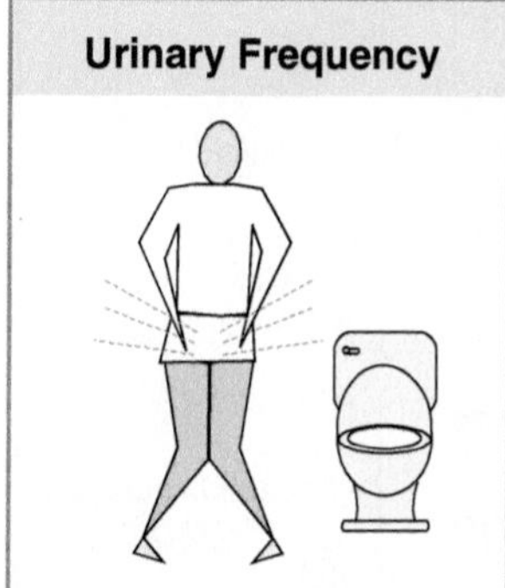


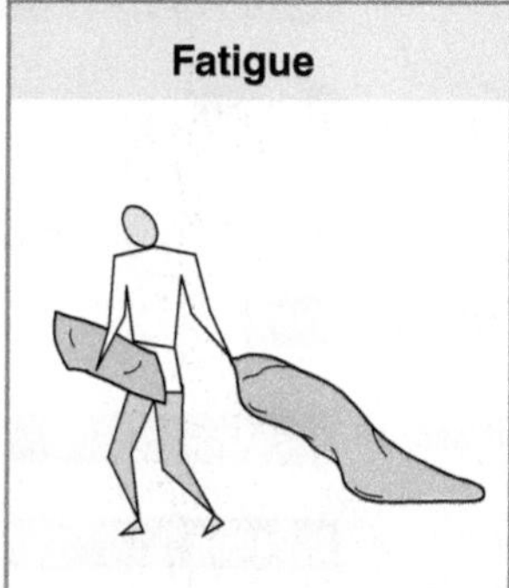


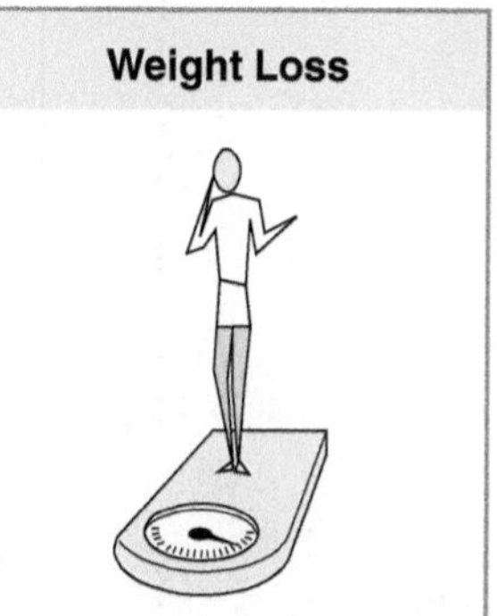


**Figure 26.5** The symptoms of hypoglycemia compared to the symptoms of hyperglycemia. (Adapted with permission from Harvey RA, Champe PC, Howland RD, et al. *Lippincott's Illustrated Reviews: Pharmacology*, 3rd edition. Baltimore: Lippincott Williams & Wilkins, 2006.)

## Drugs That Increase Insulin Secretion

secretagogue Substance that stimulates secretion.

Drugs that increase the secretion of another compound are called secretagogues. There are a number of insulin secretagogues available that work through similar mechanisms. The first drugs developed, the sulfonylureas, are related to other sulfonamide compounds. Two newer agents, repaglinide (Prandin®) and nateglinide (Starlix®), are nonsulfonylurea secretagogues referred to as meglitinides.

### Actions and Indications

The sulfonylurea drugs were the first oral hypoglycemic agents available. Although there are still some first generation sulfonylurea drugs used, the second-generation derivatives, glyburide (DiaBeta®, Micronase®), glipizide (Glucotrol®), and glimepiride (Amaryl®) are far more commonly prescribed. First-generation sulfonylureas drugs differ from second-generation drugs because of their shorter durations of action. Refer to **Figure 26.6** for a comparison of the durations of action of the oral antidiabetic medications discussed in this chapter. All of the sulfonylurea hypoglycemic agents work by increasing the secretion of insulin from functional beta cells in the islets of Langerhans. After prolonged therapy, these drugs may reduce production of glucose by the liver and increase sensitivity of target tissues to insulin. The sulfonylurea drugs are indicated for the treatment of type 2 diabetes, as an adjunct to diet and exercise. They can be given in combination with other oral antidiabetic agents.

Repaglinide and nateglinide are not sulfonylurea drugs, but they have similar actions. Like the sulfonylureas, their action is dependent upon functioning insulin producing pancreatic cells. They increase the release of insulin in much the same way as the sulfonylurea drugs. However, in contrast to the sulfonylureas, the meglitinides have a rapid onset and short duration of action, and are used to regulate postprandial (after meals) hyperglycemia. They are indicated as an adjunct to diet and exercise for the treatment of type 2 diabetes, and are often used in combination with another oral antidiabetic agent, metformin (Glucophage®).

postprandial Occurring after a meal.

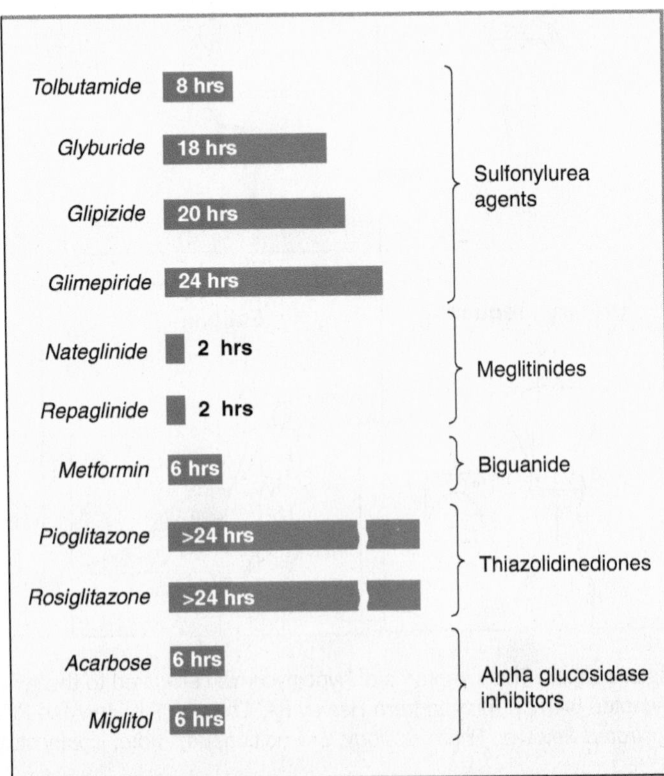


**Figure 26.6** A comparison of the durations of action of some of the oral antidiabetic drugs. (Adapted with permission from Harvey RA, Champe PC, Howland RD, et al. *Lippincott's Illustrated Reviews: Pharmacology*, 3rd edition. Baltimore: Lippincott Williams & Wilkins, 2006.)

## Administration

All of the insulin secretagogues are administered by mouth. Glimepiride, glipizide, and the older sulfonylureas are rapidly and completely absorbed after oral administration. Absorption of standard glyburide tablets is adequate, but is significantly less than the absorption of the micronized tablets (Glynase®, PresTab®). People who are switched to the micronized tablets will require a lower dose of the drug than the regular tablets. For this reason, the two types of tablets cannot be interchanged.

Although they are sometimes given twice daily, glimepiride, glipizide, and glyburide can be given once daily because of their extended duration of action. They are generally given with breakfast, but glipizide is given 30 minutes before eating for best effect. The more frequent dosing required for use of first generation sulfonylurea drugs, including tolazamide (Tolinase®) and tolbutamide (Orinase®), can result in poor patient compliance. Repaglinide and nateglinide are administered within the 30-minute period before each meal. Food delays but does not reduce the absorption of nateglinide. Both drugs are rapidly and completely absorbed when taken on an empty stomach, as recommended.

## Side Effects

The most important side effect seen with the oral insulin secretagogues is hypoglycemia. The risk of hypoglycemia appears to be less with use of nateglinide and repaglinide than the sulfonylureas. The sulfonylurea agents can cause allergic reactions in patients allergic to other sulfonamide drugs. Other adverse reactions typical of the sulfonamides are also possible, including skin rashes, and drug-induced anemias. The sulfonylureas are associated with mild GI upset. Weight gain can result from taking sulfonylurea drugs, nateglinide, or repaglinide. Delayed excretion of glyburide and glimepiride may cause hypoglycemia in people with kidney failure. All of these drugs are avoided in people with liver failure because they are metabolized in the liver and have the potential for drug accumulation.

A number of potentially important drug interactions can occur with both the sulfonylureas and nateglinide and repaglinide. Corticosteroids, thyroid hormone, thiazide diuretics, sympathomimetic drugs, and estrogens are known to increase glucose levels in some people. Other drugs, such as warfarin, the NSAIDs, and some beta-blockers may increase the effect of the sulfonylureas and meglitinides. The combination of the lipid-lowering drug gemfibrozil and repaglinide can cause severe hypoglycemia. Excessive consumption of alcohol causes poor glucose control through addition of extra calories and alteration of glucose metabolism, and should be avoided.

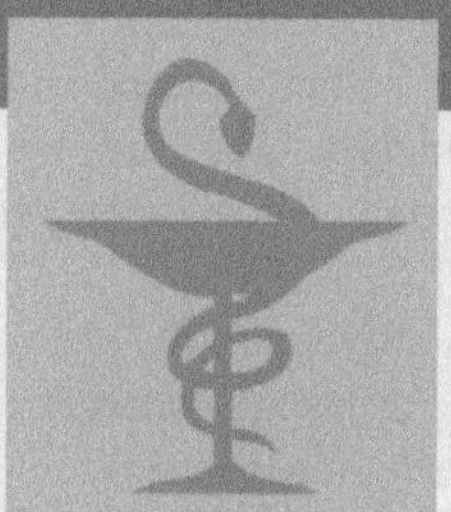

### Tips for the Technician

A good pharmacy technician always checks the patient profile for allergies before filling any new prescription. When technicians receive new prescriptions for sulfonylurea drugs, they need to verify that the patient is not allergic to sulfonamide derivatives before proceeding. The pharmacist must be made aware if the patient is sulfa allergic.

Prescription labelling should include warnings regarding the consumption of alcoholic beverages and potential for drug interactions. Patients must be advised not to discontinue these medications except on the order of the physician. It is important that all patients be aware of the symptoms of hypoglycemia, and report hypoglycemic episodes to the doctor. The pharmacist should warn people taking meglitinides to only take these drugs before a meal. If they skip a meal, they should also skip the dose of medication.

## Insulin Sensitizers

Two classes of oral hypoglycemic drugs work by improving the efficiency of insulin. The biguanides, which in the United States include only metformin, and the thiazolidinediones (TZD), which include pioglitazone (Actos®) and rosiglitazone (Avandia®), are considered insulin sensitizers. These drugs lower blood sugar by improving the response to insulin in target cells.

### Actions and Indications

Metformin increases the sensitivity of cells to insulin. As a result, target cells, such as skeletal muscle, are better able to take up and use glucose. Like the sulfonylureas, metformin requires some insulin to be present in order to act, but unlike the sulfonylureas, it does not promote insulin secretion. Metformin reduces the production of glucose from glycogen breakdown by the liver. Excess glucose produced by the liver is the major source of high blood sugar in type 2 diabetes. Metformin also slows intestinal absorption of sugars.

A very important property of this drug is its ability to cause a modest reduction in total cholesterol levels after routine use for 4 or more weeks. Weight loss occurs in some patients because metformin can reduce appetite, an advantage in type 2 diabetes. Metformin is the only oral hypoglycemic agent proven to decrease cardiovascular mortality in diabetic patients, and for this reason, many experts recommend its use early in treatment. It is indicated for treatment of type 2 diabetes, alone or in combination with one of the other oral agents or insulin.

The TZDs also increase the sensitivity of tissues to the action of insulin, but by a different mechanism of action. Pioglitazone and rosiglitazone trigger the synthesis of proteins that are needed for effective insulin action. Both drugs significantly reduce glucose levels and improve the sensitivity of tissues to available insulin, but they do not increase insulin production. In addition, pioglitazone reduces triglyceride levels and increases HDL, "good cholesterol" levels. Both drugs reduce hepatic production of glucose. Peak effects of the TZDs may not be achieved for several weeks.

The TZDs are used in conjunction with diet and exercise for type 2 diabetes. Rosiglitazone is indicated for use alone or in combination with metformin or the sulfonylurea drugs when a single drug, along with diet and exercise, provides inadequate control. Pioglitazone is used alone, with metformin, the sulfonylureas, or insulin for the treatment of type 2 diabetes.

### Administration

Metformin is absorbed orally, but absorption is incomplete. When taken with a meal, the food delays and further reduces the absorption of the drug. However, metformin is usually taken with meals in order to prevent the GI upset that can occur. It is usually administered twice a day, but may be administered three times a day. Both immediate-release and delayed-release metformin tablets are available. Metformin is not metabolized, and it is excreted via the kidneys. For this reason it is generally not recommended for use in people with renal failure.

Pioglitazone and rosiglitazone are rapidly and well absorbed after oral administration. Pioglitazone absorption is slowed when it is given with meals. These drugs are metabolized in the liver and then removed by the kidneys. No dosage adjustment is required in renal impairment. Because the hypoglycemic effect caused by the TZDs is indirect and not dependent upon the presence of the drug in the bloodstream, they are effective when taken once a day.

### Side Effects

The insulin sensitizers do not promote the secretion of insulin, and they do not cause hypoglycemia when they are used alone. When these drugs are combined with other oral antidiabetic drugs, the risk of hypoglycemia can increase. The side effects typical of the insulin sensitizers are very different from the other oral hypoglycemic agents. **Figure 26.7**

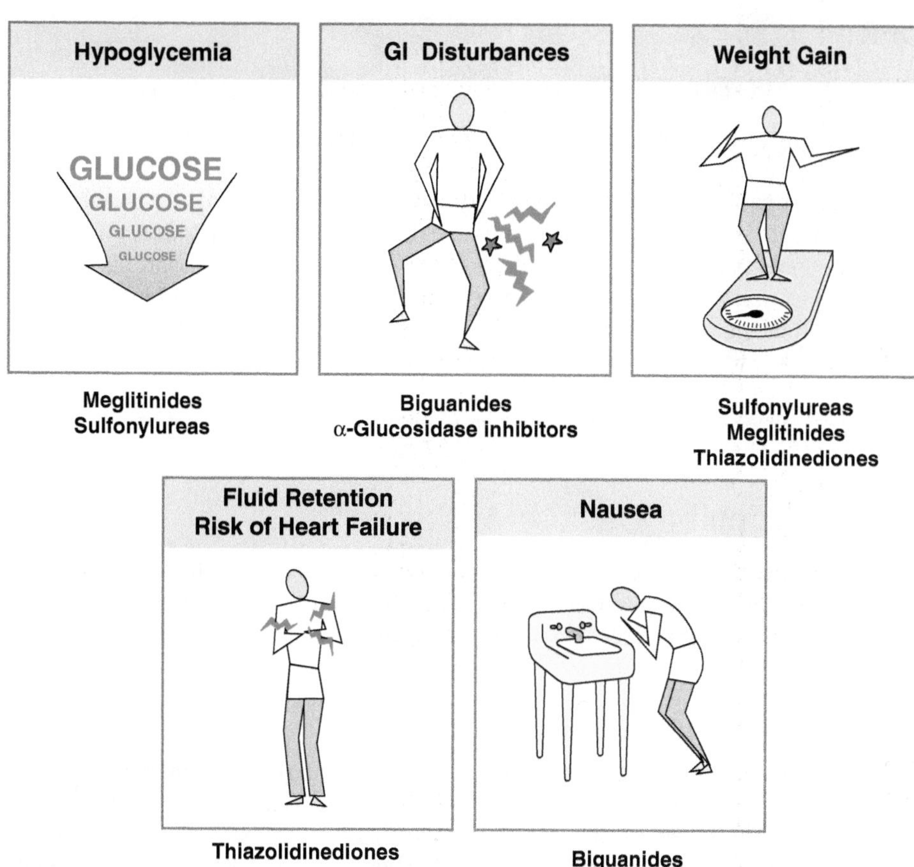


**Figure 26.7** Troubling adverse effects seen with the oral antidiabetic agents discussed in this chapter. (Adapted with permission from Harvey RA, Champe PC, Howland RD, et al. *Lippincott's Illustrated Reviews: Pharmacology*, 3rd edition. Baltimore: Lippincott Williams & Wilkins, 2006.)

illustrates the side effects that are representative of each class of the oral antidiabetic agents. Metformin typically causes GI upset, including nausea, diarrhea, loss of appetite, and an unpleasant taste in the mouth. Although it is very rare, metformin use can predispose patients with kidney, liver, or heart failure to lactic acidosis, a potentially life-threatening build-up of lactic acid in the body. Drug interactions include an increase in the effects of metformin by cimetidine, furosemide, nifedipine, and other agents. Drug classes that interfere with glucose metabolism, such as corticosteroids or sex hormones, can alter the effectiveness of all of the antidiabetic agents.

Troglitazone, the first TZD, was approved in 1997. Within months, reports of liver toxicity began to appear, and 3 years after its approval it was removed from the market because of the risk of serious or fatal liver toxicity. By the time it was removed, pioglitazone and rosiglitazone were available for sale. Use of these drugs has not been associated with the same risk of liver damage. Although hepatotoxicity is extremely rare with the thiazolidinediones on the market today, the FDA recommends they not be used in people with liver disease or elevated liver enzymes. The TZDs are associated with weight gain, sometimes significant, and fluid retention. Fluid retention is worse when the drugs are combined with insulin, and can become serious enough to cause heart failure.

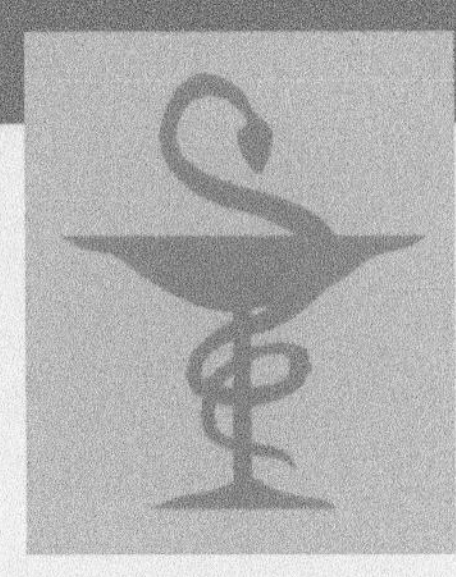

## Tips for the Technician

As with other oral antidiabetic agents, prescription labelling should include warnings regarding the consumption of alcoholic beverages. Prescriptions for metformin extended-release tablets should be labelled "do not crush." The pharmacist should verify that patients taking metformin are aware of the signs of lactic acidosis, and that those patients taking a TZD know to report rapid weight gain and shortness of breath to their physician. Patients taking other antidiabetic agents in combination with metformin or the thiazolidinediones should be made aware of the symptoms of hypoglycemia and report hypoglycemic episodes to the doctor.

# Drugs That Inhibit Glucose Absorption

Acarbose (Precose®) and miglitol (Glyset®) are two drugs that work to reduce carbohydrate absorption through similar mechanisms. They are classified as alpha-glucosidase inhibitors. They are less likely to be used than other agents because of their annoying GI side effects.

## Actions and Indications

Both acarbose and miglitol reduce and delay the absorption of glucose from the GI tract by competing with dietary carbohydrates to bind with alpha glucosidase. Alpha glucosidase is the enzyme found in the intestinal lining that breaks down the carbohydrates consumed in the diet. The action of this enzyme converts carbohydrates into glucose and other simple sugars so that they can be absorbed into the blood stream. Acarbose also inhibits pancreatic amylase, which is responsible for the breakdown of starch into sugars. As a consequence of taking these medications, the increase of blood glucose that occurs after meals is blunted. Unlike the other oral hypoglycemic agents, these drugs do not stimulate insulin release, nor do they increase insulin action in target tissues. Both drugs are indicated for use as an adjunct to diet and exercise in the treatment of type 2 diabetes. Each is also indicated for use in conjunction with insulin, or metformin (acarbose), or the sulfonylureas (miglitol).

## Administration

The alpha glucosidase inhibitors are available as tablets for oral administration. They are taken with the first bite of each meal. The absorption of acarbose is negligible, but miglitol is completely or partly absorbed, depending on the dose. Although miglitol is absorbed, it has no systemic action.

## Side Effects

When dietary carbohydrates are not absorbed, they remain in the GI tract and are digested by resident bacteria. Bacteria release carbon dioxide when they metabolize sugars, and the result is an increase of gas formation. Unabsorbed sugars draw fluid into the intestine through osmosis and can cause diarrhea. As might be anticipated, the major side effects of these drugs are flatulence, diarrhea, and abdominal cramping. People with inflammatory bowel disease, colonic ulceration, malabsorption syndromes, or other chronic bowel disorders that might deteriorate because of these effects are not good candidates for treatment with alpha glucosidase inhibitors.

It is possible that the absorption of digoxin, propranolol, and ranitidine can be reduced because of diarrhea caused by the alpha glucosidase inhibitors. Intestinal absorbants, such as activated charcoal and digestive enzymes, will reduce the effectiveness of these drugs when taken concurrently. As previously noted, a number of drugs can alter glucose metabolism. The corticosteroids, thyroid hormones, some diuretics, sympathomimetic drugs, estrogens, NSAIDs, and some beta-blockers can potentially affect glucose levels, and therefore can affect the control of blood sugar in patients taking acarbose and miglitol.

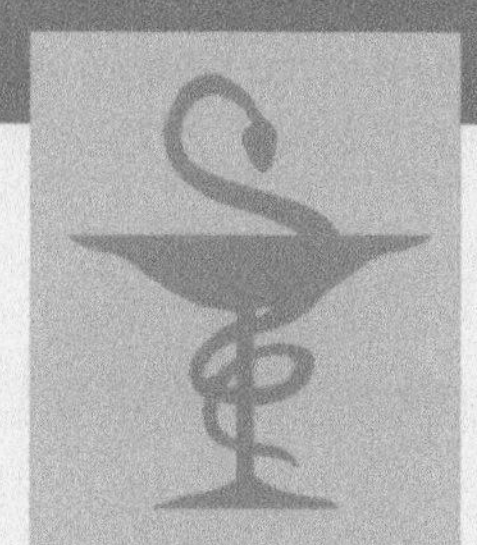

**Tips for the Technician**

Patient education plays an important role in the treatment of diabetes, and although technicians do not legally participate in the actual patient education process, they can encourage patients to utilize available education resources. As with other oral hypoglycemic agents, clients taking acarbose or miglitol should be encouraged to follow a diabetic diet, get adequate exercise, and recognize the symptoms of hyper- and hypoglycemia. They should be made aware of the GI side effects and reminded that these effects often subside with time.

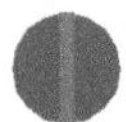

# Other Gastrointestinal Hormones

Researchers are constantly discovering and identifying new compounds that play a role in regulating body functions. Incretin hormones are two such hormones, produced by the gastrointestinal tract in response to food intake. These hormones, glucose-dependent insulinotropic peptide, or GIP, and glucagon like peptide-1, or GLIP-1, appear to play an important role in the production and efficiency of insulin. They are chemically similar to glucagon, another gastrointestinal hormone involved with carbohydrate homeostasis. Glucagon is important in balancing the effects of insulin on blood glucose levels.

## Incretin Analogs

When food is taken into the GI tract, insulin is secreted. If an equal amount of carbohydrate is given intravenously, the amount of insulin secretion is less. This effect is referred to as the "incretin effect," and is apparently impaired in type 2 diabetes. This effect underscores the important role of gastrointestinal hormones in the digestion and absorption of nutrients. A number of incretin analogs are under investigation for the treatment of type 2 diabetes. The FDA approved one, exenatide (Byetta®), in April of 2005.

### Actions and Indications

Exenatide, derived from the venom of the Gila monster, is the first of the incretin analogs to be FDA approved. By interacting with the GLIP-1 receptor, it increases insulin secretion, slows gastric emptying time, decreases hunger and thus food intake, and reduces glucagon secretion. Exenatide promotes beta cell regeneration, reduces programmed cell death of insulin-producing beta cells in the pancreas, and increases the sensitivity of tissues to insulin. Consequently, weight gain, hyperglycemia, and loss of beta cells are reduced. Exenatide is indicated for use in type 2 diabetes, for those people who do not achieve adequate glucose control with diet, exercise, and other medications.

### Administration

Because exenatide is a peptide hormone, it cannot be administered orally. It is injected subcutaneously twice a day, before breakfast and the evening meal. It is supplied in multidose, prefilled injector pens. These must be stored in the refrigerator and cannot be frozen. Patients must carefully change the hypodermic needle before each injection.

### Side Effects

The most common reported side effect with the use of exenatide is nausea. The nausea is dose related, and likely to dissipate over time. Hypoglycemia can occur, especially when exenatide is being used with a sulfonylurea agent. Other reported side effects include vomiting, headache, and excessive sweating. Obviously, the inconvenience and discomfort of twice daily injections are another drawback to use of this drug. Exenatide has not been available for long enough to be certain there will be no long-term consequences associated with its use.

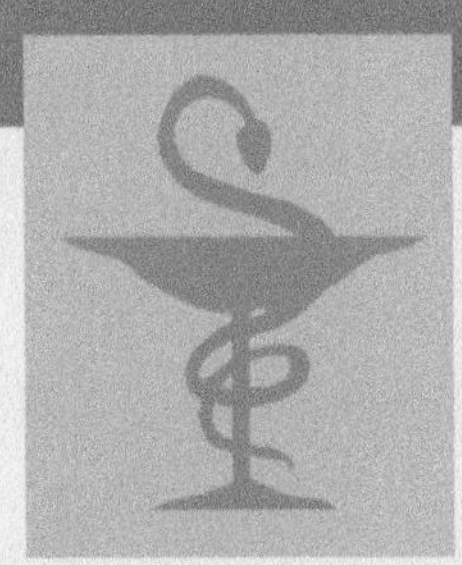

#### Tips for the Technician

Exenatide pens deliver a pre-measured dose of the drug. They are available in 5μ per dose and 10μ per dose strengths. Technicians need to carefully choose the appropriate strength device when filling prescriptions. This drug is expensive and must be stored under refrigeration to avoid waste. Each prescription must be dispensed with the patient package insert, which instructs users on how to use the device. Be sure that patients understand the instructions, and that the package is clearly labelled "refrigerate" before the prescription is dispensed.

## Glucagon

Glucagon is synthesized in the alpha cells of the islets of Langerhans and is usually thought of as the hormone that opposes the action of insulin. Whereas insulin is secreted when glucose levels rise, glucagon is released when glucose levels fall. The balance between these two hormones is largely responsible for the maintenance of blood sugar levels in the normal range.

### Actions and Indications

Glucagon acts principally on the liver where it stimulates the conversion of glycogen into glucose and also encourages the synthesis of glucose from other energy sources such as fat or protein. The release of glucagon occurs in response to hypoglycemia or stress, and is suppressed after a meal. Hypoglycemia is a common and potentially dangerous complication of the use of insulin. The preferred way to treat insulin-induced hypoglycemia (insulin reactions) is by administering high sugar foods. However, when hypoglycemia is severe, patients may lose consciousness, and food should never be administered to an unconscious person.

Glucagon products are synthesized using recombinant DNA technology and are identical to human glucagon. Glucagon is indicated for the reversal of severe hypoglycemia and is available in emergency kits for this purpose. It is also used as a diagnostic aid for certain procedures.

### Administration

Glucagon is another of the many peptide hormones that is ineffective when administered by mouth. Reconstituted glucagon powder for injection can be administered intravenously, intramuscularly, or subcutaneously. For emergency treatment of hypoglycemia by a friend or family member, the injection is given subcutaneously.

### Side Effects

Glucagon can cause nausea and vomiting, so the patient is always turned to the side before glucagon is injected to avoid the possibility of choking. Diabetic patients can also lose consciousness when their blood sugar is excessively high. Glucagon will obviously not correct hyperglycemia. Family members should seek help immediately when glucagon is used, especially if the patient does not regain consciousness within a few minutes. As soon as a hypoglycemic patient becomes alert, he or she should eat. Glucagon effects are short lived and hypoglycemia can recur when the effect of glucagon disappears.

## Tips for the Technician

Most retail pharmacies carry glucagon emergency kits, and technicians need to become familiar with them. Both Eli Lilly and Novo Nordisk manufacture glucagon emergency kits that are fairly easy to use. Before it is necessary to use the kit, family members are strongly advised to practice giving diabetic patients their insulin injections so that they feel comfortable giving an injection in case of an emergency. Prior to reconstitution, glucagon and glucagon kits are stored at room temperature. Type 1 diabetics should have a glucagon emergency kit available for use by family members at all times.

## Case 26.1

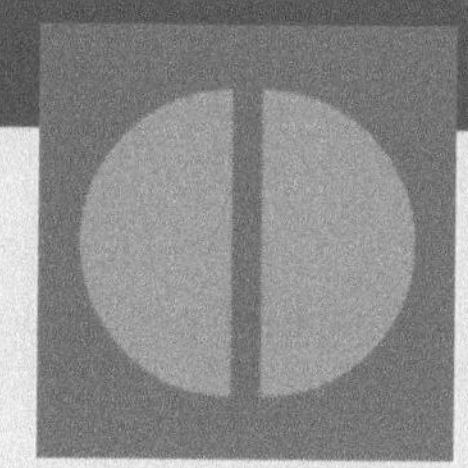

Brigitta Sweet is the parent of a recently diagnosed 10-year-old diabetic child. Her son is an avid soccer player, and his diabetes is fairly well controlled. At his last appointment, the endocrinologist told Brigitta's son it was good for him to get out and get the exercise that soccer provides. She cautioned Brigitta that her son's insulin requirements would go down when he exercised strenuously, and recommended that she purchase a glucagon kit. That day Brigitta purchased the kit. Saturday after his first game, she walked into her son's room to find him unarousable on his bedroom floor. She frantically opened the glucagon kit and found that she needed to reconstitute the powder, draw the medicine up into the syringe, remove the air bubbles, and then inject the drug, a process she had never attempted. She knows she cannot give her son candy or sugar when he is unconscious, yet she is afraid of giving him the injection because she has no idea what she is doing. Meanwhile, she fears that her son's life hangs in the balance.

# Review Questions

## Multiple Choice

Choose the best answer for the following questions:

1. Type 1 diabetes is different from type 2 diabetes in all of the following ways except?
   a. Patients with type 2 diabetes have a relative lack of insulin, while people with type 1 diabetes completely lack insulin.
   b. Type 1 diabetes usually begins in childhood or young adulthood whereas type 2 diabetes usually begins in adulthood.
   c. The goals of treatment are different for type 1 and type 2 diabetes.
   d. Oral antidiabetic agents are usually effective in type 2 diabetes, but not type 1 diabetes.
   e. Type 1 diabetes is probably caused by autoimmune destruction of the islets of Langerhans, while type 2 diabetes is closely related to obesity and diet.

2. Which of the following is not one of the classic symptoms or findings of diabetes?
   a. Polyphobia
   b. Polydipsia
   c. Hyperglycemia
   d. Polyphagia
   e. Polyuria

3. Of the following, which statement is correct regarding the islets of Langerhans?
   a. Islets of Langerhans are a vacation hot spot off the coast of the Netherlands.
   b. They are islets of tissue in the pancreas, discovered by Paul Langerhans, which produce glucagon and insulin.
   c. They are islands of tissue in the liver, discovered by Paul Langerhans, which produce insulin.
   d. The beta cells in the islets produce glucagon and the alphas cell produce insulin.
   e. The islet cells multiply in type 1 diabetes, causing an excess of insulin.

4. Which of the following drug classes are used to treat type 2 diabetes?
   a. Sulfonylurea drugs
   b. Insulin sensitizers such as metformin
   c. Alpha glucosidase inhibitors
   d. Insulin
   e. All of the above

5. Select the problem, listed below, that is not a potential consequence of poorly controlled diabetes.
   a. Poor circulation in the feet and legs
   b. Kidney failure
   c. Blindness
   d. Hypothyroidism
   e. Damage to nerves

## True/False

6. Diabetes is a complex metabolic disorder, characterized by hyperglycemia related to a complete or relative lack of insulin, which can result in damage to the kidneys, eyes, heart, blood vessels, and nervous system.
   a. True
   b. False

7. Exubera® is an inhaled, long-acting insulin that is aimed at providing all day basal control of glucose with one inhalation in the morning.
   a. True
   b. False

8. Canadian physicians Frederick Banting, Charles Best, James Collip, and John Macleod are credited with the isolation and purification of insulin.
   a. True
   b. False

9. Insulin secretagogues, such as glyburide or glimepiride, work by increasing the secretion of insulin from remaining functional $\beta$ cells.
   a. True
   b. False

10. Metformin rarely causes GI upset, and can increase appetite, resulting in a potential for further weight gain in diabetics who take it.
    a. True
    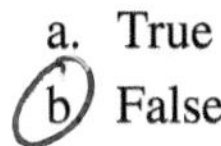
    b. False

## Matching

For numbers 11 to 15, match the drug description with the correct lettered choice from the list below. Choices will not be used more than once and may not be used at all.

11. Short-acting insulin that can be given IV
12. Rapid-acting insulin that is used for glucose control at meals
13. Long-acting insulin that is used for basal insulin requirements
14. Rapid-acting insulin secretagogue for postprandial increase in blood sugar
15. Short-acting inhaled insulin

a. Nateglinide
b. Insulin glargine
c. NPH insulin
d. Regular insulin
e. Metformin
f. Lispro insulin
g. Exubera®

## Short Answer

16. What is the purpose of having rapid-, short-, medium-, and long-acting insulin analogs, and when might each be used? What kind of insulin can be administered by intravenous injection?
17. Why is it important for diabetics to know the difference in the symptoms of hyperglycemia and hypoglycemia?
18. What auxiliary labels should a technician place on a prescription for NPH insulin?
19. What are some of the drug classes that can negatively affect glucose blood levels, and thereby complicate treatment of diabetes?
20. Explain the goal of treatment of diabetes, and two important steps that people with type 1 and type 2 diabetes can take to achieve that goal.

# FOR FURTHER INQUIRY

Find out about alternative insulin formulations or new approaches to insulin administration that are undergoing research and development. You can investigate on the Internet or call Eli Lilly or Novo Nordisk. Pharmaceutical company contact information is available in the most commonly used drug reference books.

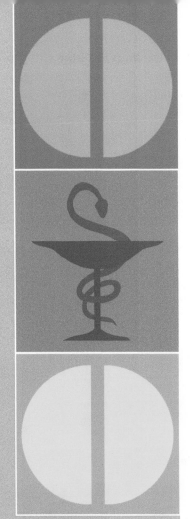

Chapter **27**

# The Steroid Hormones

*KEY TERMS*

- amenorrhea
- anabolic
- carcinogenic
- catabolism
- endometriosis
- precocious puberty
- spermatogenesis

## OBJECTIVES

After studying this chapter, the reader should be able to:

- Explain why it is dangerous for patients to abruptly discontinue the use of long-term corticosteroid treatment, and describe one measure that pharmacy technicians can take to prevent this from happening.
- List three indications for use of corticosteroids and four potential adverse effects from long-term use of high dose (greater than the physiologic production) of corticosteroids.
- Compare and contrast four different forms of hormonal contraceptives, and describe their appropriate use, advantages, and disadvantages.
- List the appropriate auxiliary labels and written information that should be included on oral hormone prescriptions.
- Describe the inappropriate use of anabolic steroids, the risks to the user, and the legal step that was taken by the DEA to reduce this inappropriate use.

## DRUGS COVERED IN THIS CHAPTER

### Corticosteroids

Betamethasone
Dexamethasone
Fludrocortisone
Hydrocortisone
Methylprednisolone
Prednisolone
Prednisone
Triamcinolone

### Sex Hormones

**Estrogens**
Conjugated estrogens
Estradiol
Estrone
Ethinyl Estradiol

**Progestins**
Medroxyprogesterone
Megestrol
Norelgestromin
Norethindrone
Norgestrel
Carboprost
Dinoprostone
Mifepristone

**Androgens and Anabolic Steroids**
Danazol
Methyltestosterone
Nandrolone
Oxandrolone
Testosterone

### Uterine Active Agents

Carbopost
Dinoprostone
Mifepristone

Steroid hormones are a family of important hormones derived from cholesterol. Steroids are so named because they possess four fused rings in their chemical structure that are typical of this class of chemicals. Steroids can be subdivided into several different categories, each of which plays a different role in the body. Of these categories, the androgens, estrogens, and progestins are frequently grouped together as sex hormones, and the glucocorticoids and mineralocorticoids as adrenocorticotropic hormones. Different tissues in the body secrete steroid hormones. The cortex of the adrenal glands secretes adrenocorticotropic hormones and precursors to androgens, while the male and female gonads are the primary sites of sex hormone synthesis. The adrenal glands are a minor source of androgens in men, but a major source of androgens in women.

The steroid hormones play critical roles in maintaining homeostasis during periods of physical stress and in normal growth, development, and reproduction. Cortisol is the most abundant endogenous glucocorticoid. In times of physical or mental stress, the hypothalamus signals the pituitary to secrete adrenocorticotropic hormone, which in turn signals the adrenals to secrete cortisol (**Fig. 27.1**). There are cortisol receptors in every type of cell where it exerts a variety of physiologic effects. The term glucocorticoid is derived from the increase in blood sugar that occurs as a result of the release of cortisol. However, the best known of the physiologic effects of glucocorticoids is the suppression of the immune response. The use of synthetic glucocorticoids for their anti-inflammatory effect is one of the most important applications of these drugs.

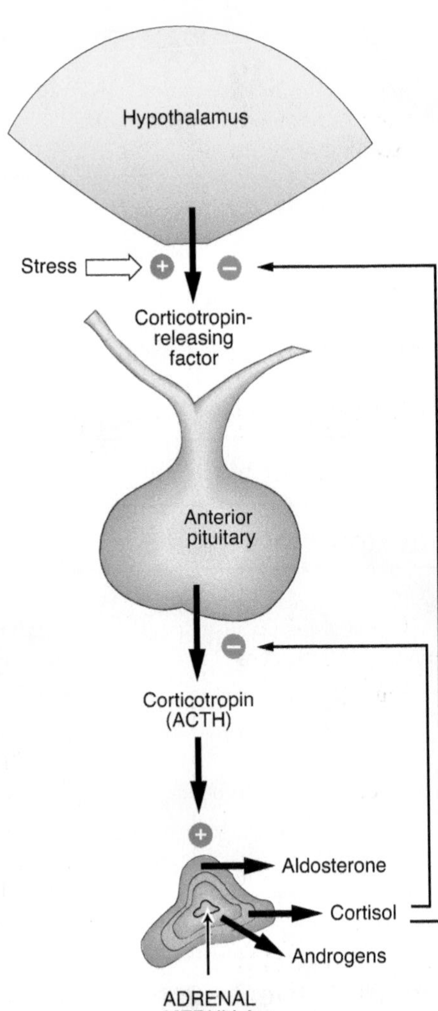


**Figure 27.1** The synthesis and secretion of endogenous steroid hormones by the adrenal glands is regulated by feedback mechanisms and is affected by outside factors like physiologic stress or intake of steroid medications. (Adapted with permission from Harvey RA, Champe PC, Howland RD, et al. *Lippincott's Illustrated Reviews: Pharmacology*, 3rd edition. Baltimore: Lippincott Williams & Wilkins, 2006.)

The principal mineralocorticoid secreted by the adrenals is aldosterone. The name mineralocorticoid is derived from the critical role of aldosterone in maintaining the levels of minerals, especially sodium, in the blood. This effect and the effect of maintaining adequate blood volume is essential for life. The kidneys are the most important sites of mineralocorticoid activity, where the hormone promotes the reabsorption of sodium. Aldosterone also targets sweat glands to reduce the loss of sodium in perspiration, and taste buds to heighten the sensation of saltiness in order to encourage salt intake.

The sex hormones testosterone, estrogen, and progesterone are produced in the testes and ovary, respectively. These hormones are required for normal physical maturation and secondary sex characteristics in men and women, and for sexual reproduction. There are many therapeutic uses for synthetic sex hormones, including use as contraceptive agents, for hormone replacement therapy, and in the management of osteoporosis. A number of hormone antagonists are used in cancer chemotherapy and will be discussed in Chapter 33.

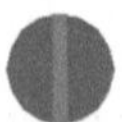

## Adrenocorticotropic Hormones

Cortisol was first isolated and identified in the 1930s. Scientists understood its potential for use as an anti-inflammatory agent, and the battle was on within several pharmaceutical companies for developing an inexpensive way to synthesize it. Upjohn pharmaceuticals eventually developed hydrocortisone (Cortef®, Solu-Cortef®, many others), the synthetic equivalent of cortisol, which was anticipated to be a tremendous asset in the treatment of inflammatory conditions. Later, prednisone (Sterapred®), methylprednisolone (Medrol®, Solu-Medrol®), and dexamethasone (Decadron®) were added to the range of available corticosteroids.

## Actions and Indications

The glucocorticoids increase the production of glucose and increase blood glucose levels. By raising glucose levels, glucocorticoids provide the body with the energy it requires to combat stress caused by trauma, fright, infection, blood loss, or debilitating disease. These hormones cause a decrease in circulating lymphocytes and macrophages, two types of blood cells, by redistributing them out of the blood stream to the lymphatic system. This effect compromises the body's ability to fight infections, but is useful in some forms of leukemia where too many white blood cells reach the blood stream. In contrast to the effect on white blood cells, glucocorticoids increase the blood levels of hemoglobin, red blood cells, and platelets.

The most important pharmacologic effect of the glucocorticoids is their ability to dramatically reduce inflammation and to suppress immunity. There are many, complex mechanisms that contribute to the anti-inflammatory effects of the steroids. Glucocorticoids switch off the genes responsible for the synthesis of leukotrienes, prostaglandins, and inflammatory enzymes, among other important mediators of inflammation. Glucocorticoids inhibit the release of histamine from mast cells, and as previously mentioned, reduce the numbers of circulating lymphocytes and macrophages

The glucocorticoids synthesized for medicinal use are often referred to as corticosteroids, and include the original hydrocortisone, prednisone, methylprednisolone, triamcinolone (Aristocort®, Kenalog®), and the longer-acting dexamethasone, among others. These drugs have a tremendous number of uses and are available in an impressive array of formulations appropriate for the indication. For example, hydrocortisone is available for intravenous injection in treatment of asthma or other severe inflammatory conditions, adrenal insufficiency, or shock, in a long-acting injectable form for injection into inflamed tissues or joints, in topical preparations for allergic reactions or itching, and rectal formulations for inflammatory bowel disease, among others. Refer to **Table 27.1** for a

**Table 27.1** A Comparison of Commonly Used Corticosteroids, Their Brand Names, Indications, and Available Formulations

| Generic | Brand Name | Available as | Indications | Notes |
|---|---|---|---|---|
| Betamethasone plain, acetate & Na phosphate | Celestone®, Celestone Soluspan® | Syrup, injection, LA injection | Inflammation, joint & soft tissue injection | Acetate (Soluspan) = LA |
| Dexamethasone plain, acetate & Na phosphate | Decadron®, Dexasone LA ® | Tablets, injection, LA injection | Allergies, diagnostic, joint & soft tissue injections | Acetate = LA |
| Fludrocortisone | Florinef® | Tablets | Replacement, salt-losing syndromes | |
| Hydrocortisone, HC acetate | Cortef®, Solu-Cortef® | Tablets, injection, cream, ointment, lotion, others | Replacement, inflammation, topical | |
| Methylprednisolone plain, acetate & Na succinate | Medrol®, Depo-Medrol®, Solu-Medrol® | Inflammation, joint & soft tissue injection | Tablets, injection, LA injection | Acetate (Depo-Medrol®) is LA |
| Prednisolone Na Phosphate | Pediapred®, Orapred® | Liquid, injection | MS, soft tissue inflammation | Often used in pediatrics |
| Prednisone | Orasone® | Tablets, oral solution, syrup | Replacement, inflammation | |
| Triamcinolone, acetonide | Aristocort®, Kenalog® | Tablets, syrup, injection | Inflammation, joint & soft tissue injection | Acetonide is LA |

LA, Long acting.

comparison of some of the more frequently used products. The corticosteroids are indicated for replacement therapy when there is insufficient production by the adrenal glands, for diseases associated with inflammation (acute illnesses such as asthma or systemic lupus erythematosus), when the immune response is excessive (such as allergic skin conditions), and as an adjunct to or component of cancer chemotherapy.

The mineralocorticoids help to control the body's water volume and concentration of electrolytes, especially sodium and potassium. Aldosterone acts on kidney tubules and collecting ducts, causing reabsorption of sodium, bicarbonate, and water, and plays a key role in creating more concentrated urine. Although synthetic corticosteroids have varying glucocorticoid and mineralocorticoid properties (see **Fig. 27.2**), one drug, fludrocortisone, exerts strong mineralocorticoid activity. Fludrocortisone is used exclusively in adrenal insufficiency and in syndromes where patients have difficulty maintaining adequate sodium levels.

## Administration

Corticosteroids are available in nearly every kind of formulation imaginable. There are products for oral, intravenous, intramuscular, topical, and rectal administration, to name but a few. There are numerous corticosteroid products suitable for instillation into the eyes and ears, including several combinations of cortisteroids and antibiotics. Hydrocortisone cream, ointment, lotion, spray, and other formulations are available without a prescription for itching or irritation due to insect bites, eczema, and other causes. More potent topical corticosteroids are available by prescription only. Long acting injectable products can be injected into inflamed joints, providing a more localized effect, or into muscle for a sustained systemic effect.

When they are orally administered, corticosteroids are well absorbed. They are metabolized in the liver and the metabolites removed by the kidneys. Because systemic adminis-

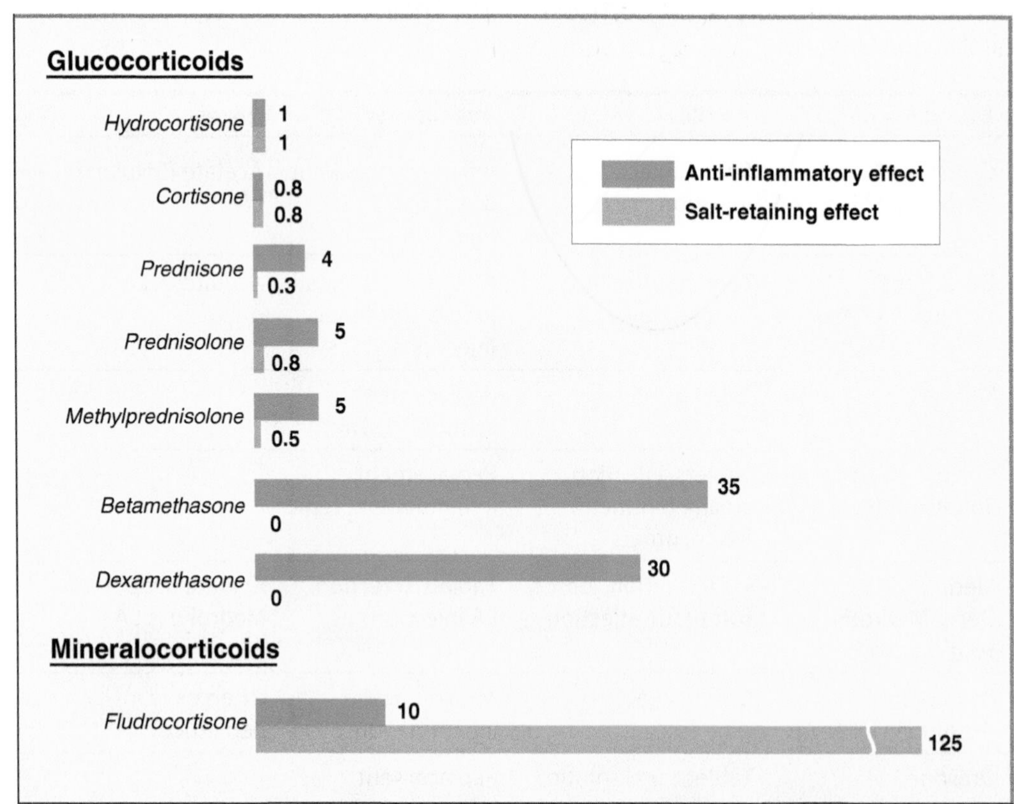


**Figure 27.2** The relative anti-inflammatory and sodium retaining effects of some commonly used corticosteroid drugs. (Adapted with permission from Harvey RA, Champe PC, Howland RD, et al. *Lippincott's Illustrated Reviews: Pharmacology*, 3rd edition. Baltimore: Lippincott Williams & Wilkins, 2006.)

tration of corticosteroids can suppress the body's production of cortisol, most physicians use short courses of corticosteroids whenever possible. When short courses of treatment are not possible, doses may have to be tapered down before discontinuation to allow the adrenal glands to recover normal function. This process can result in complicated and potentially confusing prescription directions, but tapering is a necessity. Less adrenal suppression occurs when corticosteroids are given once a day, in the morning, or on an every-other day schedule.

## Side Effects

Adverse systemic effects of the corticosteroids are directly related to the dose administered and the duration of use of the drugs. Because the corticosteroids exert effects on nearly every tissue, side effects can be quite wide-ranging and very serious. It is sometimes difficult for people who take these medications systemically to accept the serious nature of potential side effects, possibly because most people feel so much better while they are taking a corticosteroid. This sense of well being conferred by use of corticosteroids is sometimes referred to as corticosteroid euphoria.

One of the most important adverse effects of the systemic use of these medications is suppression of the normal function of the adrenal glands, and consequently, altering their interaction with the pituitary gland and the hypothalamus. When corticosteroids are used locally, adrenal suppression is less likely, but can still occur in some situations. For example, infants and young children are much more likely to absorb potent topical steroids through the skin than adults. Suppression of the adrenal glands occurs when doses that exceed normal physiologic steroid production are given for 2 or more weeks.

Long-term corticosteroid use can cause diabetes, osteoporosis, retention of fluid and sodium, delayed wound healing, skin fragility, and increased susceptibility to infection. Fluid retention and electrolyte imbalance can be especially profound with fludrocortisone, which should only be used when sodium retention is desired. Other less common corticosteroid side effects, also related to dose or duration of therapy, include psychoses, hypertension, peptic ulcer disease, and cataract formation.

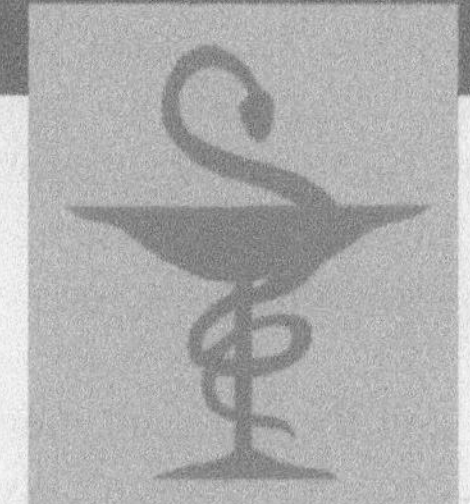

### Tips for the Technician

One of the biggest challenges technicians will face when working with the corticosteroids is keeping the formulations straight. Consider the drug triamcinolone, which is available in multiple formulations and strengths. It is manufactured for oral use as tablets and syrup. Injectable triamcinolone is available as triamcinolone acetonide (the most commonly used form), triamcinolone diacetate, and triamcinolone hexacetonide, and each of these is manufactured in more than one concentration. Finally, triamcinolone acetonide is available in a metered dose inhaler, nasal spray, and topically, as cream, lotion, ointment, and paste, in several strengths and sizes! Fortunately, most pharmacies do not carry every possible formulation, but it makes sense for technicians to become familiar with the appropriate route of administration and use of the products on hand. It is important to remember that as a general rule (one or two exceptions exist), suspensions are never given intravenously. Special caution should be used when dispensing prednisone and prednisolone, two look-alike and sound-alike products that are always close to each other on the shelf.

Label oral corticosteroid prescriptions with an auxiliary warning instructing patients not to discontinue taking the medications except on the advice of their physician. When oral preparations are prescribed, technicians should apply an auxiliary label directing patients to take the medication with meals. Make certain that topical preparations are labelled for "external use only," and apply "shake well" labels to all corticosteroids suspensions and inhaled preparations.

# Sex Hormones

The sex hormones are essential for normal sexual maturation, sex characteristics, and reproduction. Although male and female hormones are present in both men and women, it is the amount of circulating hormone that differs between the sexes. There are three endogenous (originating within the body) estrogen hormones. The ovaries synthesize estradiol, the most potent, while estrone and estriol are produced in the adrenal glands and the liver of men and women. Progesterone, the natural progestin, is produced in response to luteinizing hormone secretion (LH). In females, the corpus luteum and the placenta secrete LH, and in males, the testes secrete it. It is also synthesized by the adrenal cortex in both sexes. The androgens are a group of steroids that have anabolic effects (they promote the growth of tissues) and masculinizing effects in both males and females. Testosterone, the most important androgen, is synthesized in the testes, and in smaller amounts, by cells in the ovary of the female and the adrenal glands. Other androgens secreted by the testes are 5-alpha-dihydrotestosterone (DHT), androstenedione, and small amounts of dehydroepiandrosterone (DHEA).

anabolic The aspect of metabolism concerned with molecular synthesis and tissue building.

## Estrogens and Progestins

Estrogens and progestins have been available for use in a number of applications since the late 1930s. Some of their uses are controversial, and some downright dangerous. Diethylstilbestrol (DES), a synthetic estrogen touted in the 1940s and 50s as a drug that could prevent miscarriages, is now known to be teratogenic, a drug that promotes the development of birth defects, and carcinogenic, an agent that promotes the development of cancer. Mothers, and their daughters who were exposed to this drug in utero, have an increased risk of developing a variety of different types of cancer. More recently, the use of estrogens and progestins for treatment of the symptoms of menopause has become controversial because of safety concerns.

carcinogenic Substance that may produce or promote cancer.

### Actions and Indications

After being synthesized by the ovaries, estrogens are released into the bloodstream and act by binding to estrogen receptors in the target tissues of the breast, uterus, and bone, among others (**Fig. 27.3**). Estrogens promote the maturation and maintenance of the female reproductive system, and promote the development of the secondary sex characteristics in adolescent girls. They cause metabolic effects, including retention of fluids and deposition of calcium in bone. When estrogens are taken therapeutically they mimic the actions of endogenous estrogen. They can suppress ovulation, improve bone mineralization, and suppress some types of cancer.

The corpus luteum, the adrenal glands, the testes in males, and the placenta (during pregnancy) synthesize endogenous progesterone. Progesterone reduces the contractility of the uterus, works with estrogen to prepare the lining of the uterus for pregnancy, promotes fat deposition, and prepares the breasts for lactation. Progesterone plays a key role in maintaining pregnancy when it occurs, and when it does not, progesterone is responsible for initiating menstruation.

Estrogens are indicated for the prevention of postmenopausal osteoporosis, and alone or in combination with progesterone for the treatment of the symptoms of menopause. Estrogens are sometimes indicated in the treatment of certain carcinomas of the breast in selected postmenopausal women and some men, and in the treatment of hormone sensitive cancers of the prostate. Vaginal estrogen is indicated in the treatment of vaginal dryness and irritation associated with menopause. Estrogens are used in combination with progestins as contraceptive agents.

amenorrhea The abnormal absence of menstruation.

endometriosis Presence and growth of endometrial tissue outside the uterus that can result in severe pain with the menses and infertility.

Progestins are used to treat amenorrhea (lack of menstruation) and dysfunctional uterine bleeding. The synthetic progestin norethindrone is used in oral contraceptives and can be used to treat endometriosis, a condition where the tissue that lines the uterus gets into the pelvic cavity to cause discomfort, and in severe cases, infertility. Progestins can also be

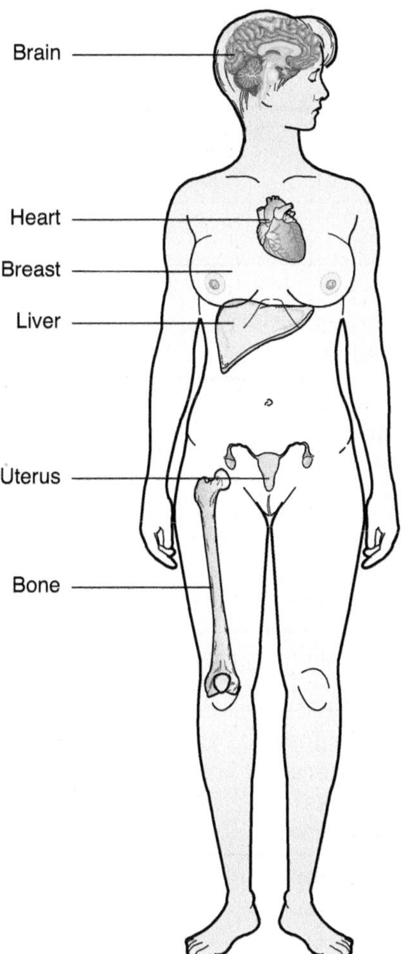


**Figure 27.3** The tissues targeted by estrogens.

used as an adjunct to treatment of certain forms of cancer. They are used alone, or in combination with estrogens, as contraceptive agents. Medroxyprogesterone acetate (Depo-Provera®) is used in treatment of certain cancers and as a contraceptive. Megestrol (Megace®) is used as an appetite stimulant. They are also combined with estrogen for the treatment of the symptoms of menopause. Natural progesterone (Prometrium®) as well as synthetic agents are used for this indication.

## Administration

Estradiol (Delestrogen®, Estrace®, Vivelle®, others), the most potent of the endogenous forms of estrogen, is the most commonly prescribed for relief of symptoms of menopause, and for prevention of postmenopausal osteoporosis. Products containing estrone and conjugated estrogens (Premarin®, the name and product are derived from pregnant mares' urine) are also available. Ethinyl estradiol is the form of estradiol typically used in combination contraceptives. **Table 27.2** displays the most commonly used sex hormone products, their brand names, formulations, and indications.

Estrogens prescribed for therapeutic use are well absorbed through the GI tract, skin, and mucous membranes. Various products are designed for use as transdermal patches, for oral administration, injection, topical, and vaginal administration. When naturally occurring estrogens are administered orally, they undergo first-pass metabolism in the liver, significantly reducing the amount that reaches the blood stream. Topical or transdermal estrogen does not undergo immediate metabolism, and as a result doses are lower when topical application is used. The synthetic estrogens, ethinyl estradiol and mestranol, are well absorbed orally, and are longer acting than natural estrogens.

**Table 27.2** A Comparison of Some Commonly Prescribed Sex Hormone Products and Contraceptives, Including Brand Name, Indications, and Formulations

| Generic | Brand Name | Available as | Indications | Notes |
|---|---|---|---|---|
| **Estrogens** | | | | |
| Conjugated Estrogens | Premarin®, Prempro® | Tablets, injection, vaginal | Menopause sx, prevent osteoporosis, injection: abnormal bleeding | Prempro® contains progestin |
| Estradiol | Estrace®, Vivelle®, Delestrogen®, Climara®, others | Tablets, LA injection, topical, transdermal, vaginal | Hypogonadism, menopause sx, adjunct in some cancers, prevent osteoporosis | |
| Estrone (Esterified Estrogens) | Menest® | Tablets | Hypogonadism, menopause sx, adjunct in some cancers, prevent osteoporosis | |
| **Progestins** | | | | |
| Medroxyprogesterone acetate | Depo Provera®, Provera® | Tablets, injection | Endometrial hyperplasia, amenorrhea, abnormal uterine bleeding, injection: contraception | Depo Provera® long-acting contraceptive |
| Megestrol | Megace® | Tablets, suspension | Palliative treatment in some cancers, appetite stimulant | |
| Progesterone | Prometrium®, etc | Capsules, injection, vaginal gel | Endometrial hyperplasia, amenorrhea, infertility due to progesterone deficiency | |
| **Contraceptives** | | | | |
| Combination Contraceptives | | | | |
| Ethinyl estradiol + Ethynodiol | Demulen®, Zovia® | Tablets | Oral Contraceptive | Oral contraceptives come in many dose combinations. |
| Ethinyl estradiol + Norethindrone | Norinyl®, Ovcon®, Ortho-Novum, Loestrin® | Tablets | Oral Contraceptive | Biphasic and triphasic types are designed to mimic the normal cycle. |
| Ethinyl estradiol + Norgestrel | Ovral®, Lo Ovral® | Tablets | Oral Contraceptive | |
| Ethinyl estradiol + Levonorgestrel | Alesse®, Triphasil®, Trivora® | Tablets | Oral Contraceptive | |
| Ethinyl estradiol + Norgestimate | Ortho Tricyclen® | Tablets | Oral Contraceptive | |
| Norelgestromin + Ethinyl Estradiol | Ortho Evra® | Transdermal Patch | Contraceptive | |

*(continues)*

| Generic | Brand Name | Available as | Indications | Notes |
|---|---|---|---|---|
| **Progestin Only Contraceptives** | | | | |
| Norethindrone | Ortho-Micronor®, NorQD®, others | Tablets | Oral contraceptive | |
| Norgestrel | Ovrette® | Tablets | Oral contraceptive | |
| **Emergency Contraceptives** | | | | |
| Levonorgestrel | Plan B® | Tablets | Emergency contraception | 1st dose within 72 hours of unprotected sex |
| Levonorgestrel + Ethinyl Estradiol | Preven® | Tablets | Emergency contraception | |
| **Androgens and Anabolic steroids** | | | | |
| Danazol | Danocrine® | Endometriosis, fibrocystic breast disease | Capsules | |
| Methyltestosterone | Methitest®, Virilon®, Android® | Hypogonadism, delayed puberty, metastatic breast cancer | Tablets, buccal tabs, capsules, injection | All androgens and anabolic steroids are CIII controlled substances |
| Nandrolone | Deca-Durabolin® | Treatment of anemia | LA injection | |
| Oxandrolone | Oxandrin® | Appetite stimulant, to promote weight gain | Tablets | |
| Testosterone | AndroGel®, Depo-Testosterone®, Delatestryl®, others | Hypogonadism, delayed puberty, metastatic breast cancer | Topical gel, LA injection, buccal tabs | |

LA, long- acting; SX, symptoms.

Like estrogens, progestins are well absorbed orally and undergo first-pass metabolism. They can be administered parenterally, and some synthetic progestins are available as transdermal patches for contraception. Long-acting medroxyprogesterone is administered by deep IM injection every three months in the doctor's office as a contraceptive agent. When administered in this way, it inhibits ovulation and menstruation and is suggested for women who have trouble following oral contraceptive regimens. Transdermal contraceptive patches offer the advantage of being applied once a week, but some users complain that patches can come off. Besides transdermal and injected contraceptives, a number of intrauterine devices and vaginal rings impregnated with hormones are available as contraceptive agents. Intrauterine devices are implanted in the doctor's office, but patients insert the vaginal rings themselves. Patient package inserts are included with all hormones that instruct patients about the appropriate use of the drugs.

Many combination oral contraceptive agents are designed to mimic the normal hormonal cycle and contain different ingredients over the course of the month. Most oral contraceptives (28 day packages) include seven tablets with no hormones for use on the last 7 days of the month. These tablets are included as place markers to aid patient compliance. In some oral contraceptives these seven tablets contain an iron replacement and in others they are inert. A woman who misses a single tablet during the first 21 days can simply take the tablet when the missed dose is discovered, or she can double up the dose on the next night. If she misses two doses or more, she should contact her pharmacist or physician to determine how to adjust her schedule. Another form of contraception should be used for at least the next week and preferably through the remainder of her cycle. Of course, missing tablets from the last 7 days of the cycle will not increase the risk of pregnancy.

Emergency contraceptives are higher doses of levonorgestrel (Plan B®), or levonorgestrel plus ethinyl estradiol (Preven®), the same hormones found in some oral contraceptives. These medications, sometimes referred to as the "morning after pill," are taken in two oral doses to prevent pregnancy after unprotected sexual intercourse. They should be administered as soon as possible, and no later than 72 hours after unprotected sex. The second dose is taken 12 hours after the first dose.

## Side Effects

The risks of estrogen therapy, whether taken as hormone replacement or for contraception, are well known and are a frequent topic in the news media (**Fig. 27.4**). The side effects are related to the dose taken and the duration of therapy. Low-dose estrogen therapy, when combined with progestin, is associated with a low risk of side effects, especially when taken for less than 5 years. The risk of side effects accumulates beyond that time.

When taken without progestin, estrogen increases the risk of uterine and cervical cancers in women who still have a uterus. Estrogens and progestins increase the risk of blood clots, high blood pressure, and may adversely affect the cardiovascular system in other ways. Postmenopausal women who take estrogen or estrogen plus progesterone may have a higher risk of developing breast cancer.

Both progestins and estrogens can cause mood swings, changes in libido, headache, nausea, and vomiting. Use of emergency contraceptives is associated with a fairly significant risk of nausea and vomiting, but is otherwise quite safe. Both hormone classes can cause breast tenderness. Neither estrogens nor progestins should be taken during pregnancy

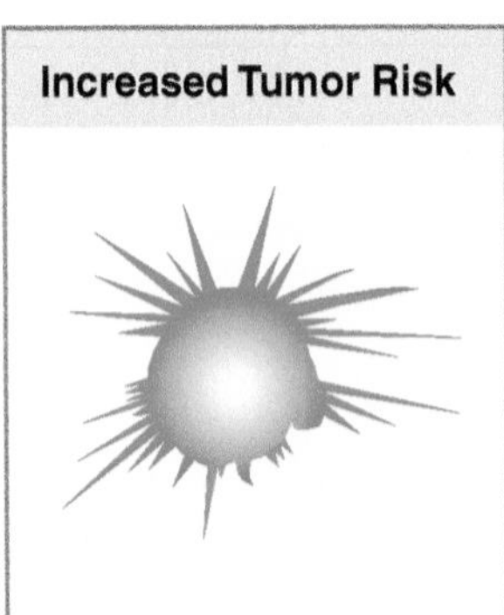

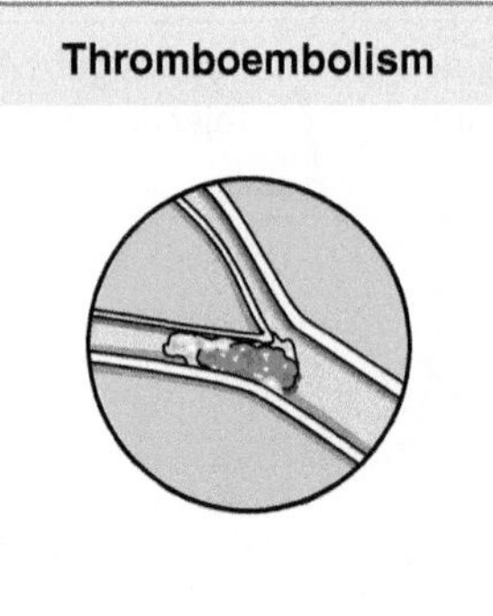

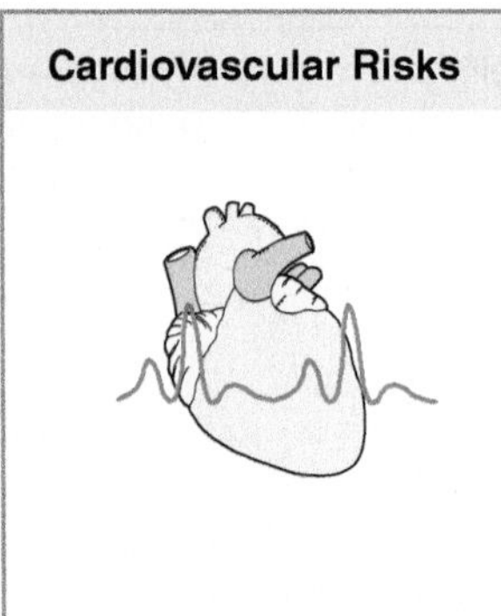

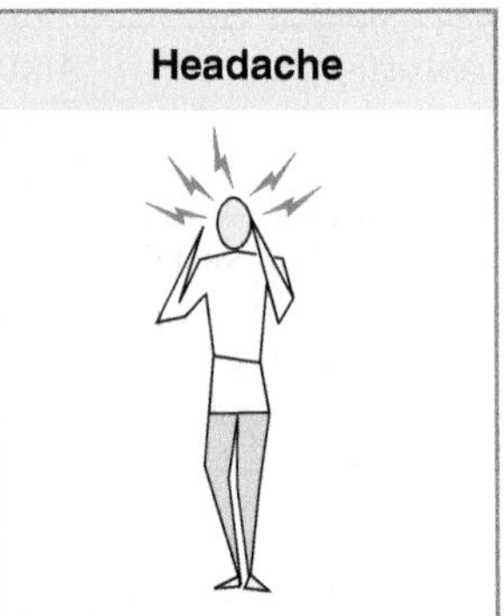

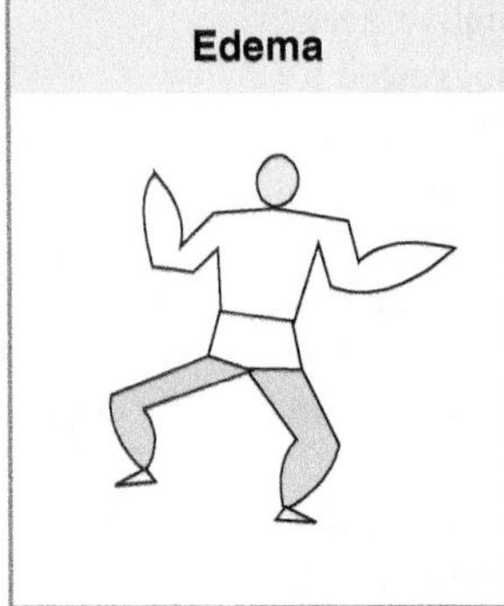

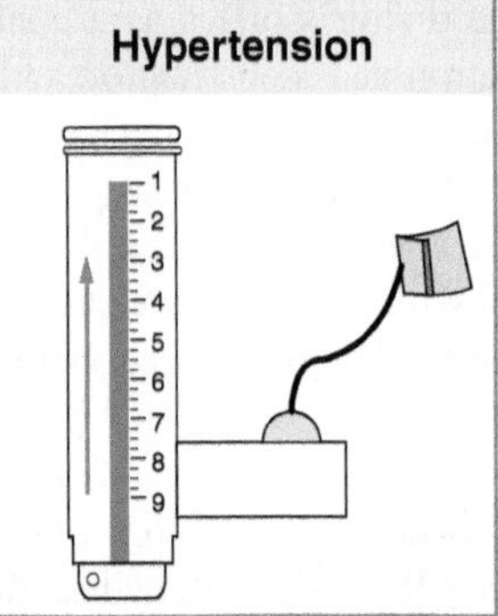

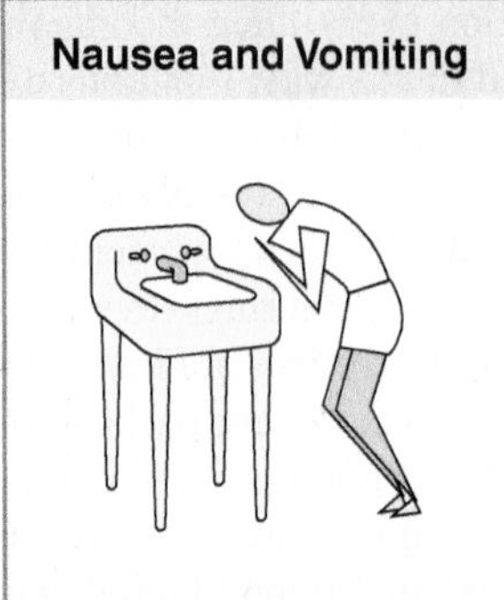


**Figure 27.4** Adverse effects associated with estrogen therapy. (Adapted with permission from Harvey RA, Champe PC, Howland RD, et al. *Lippincott's Illustrated Reviews: Pharmacology*, 3rd edition. Baltimore: Lippincott Williams & Wilkins, 2006.)

because they can cause abnormalities of the genitals in the infant. The risks associated with use of contraceptive hormones increase with the age of the woman, and the cardiovascular risks are higher still in women who smoke. It is important to note that although there are risks associated with hormonal contraceptives, they are significantly less than the risks associated with pregnancy. The hormonal contraceptives, when used according to directions, are very effective forms of contraception, and therefore the benefit of their use outweigh the risks in the vast majority of sexually active women. Relative to other easy-to-use preventative measures, oral contraceptives are the most effective (**Fig. 27.5**). Only sterilization and surgically implanted hormone devices are more effective.

Progestin-only contraceptives can cause acne, mood disturbances, spotting, and weight gain. Women who use injectable medroxyprogesterone acetate as a contraceptive have the same risks from use of this agent as those who take oral progestins. In addition, they may have prolonged infertility, menstrual irregularities, and ongoing weight gain with continued use. Weight gain can be significant, and may be problematic in women with type II diabetes.

### Tips for the Technician

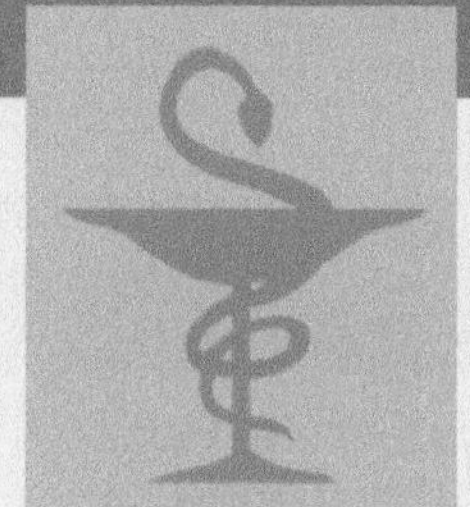

All estrogen and progestin products come with a patient package insert. It is the responsibility of the pharmacy staff members to provide this information to patients. The pharmacist should counsel women receiving hormone prescriptions for the first time regarding the risks of use. All patients should be informed that no hormonal contraceptive protects the user from sexually transmitted diseases.

Patients may ask technicians for advice on missed contraceptive doses, information about side effects, or about the availability of emergency contraceptives. It is important for technicians to know to refer these questions to the pharmacist. Pharmacists are allowed to dispense emergency contraceptives without a prescription in some cases. Emergency contraceptives are readily available from most family planning clinics. Although emergency contraceptives are not abortifacients, some pharmacies choose not to carry these products, and some pharmacists may refuse to dispense them based upon their personal religious beliefs. Because of inconsistent ability to access these medications, many states are enacting legislation to assure that patients can obtain them when they are needed. Be sure that you are familiar with emergency contraception laws in your state.

An auxiliary label to instruct patients that hormones may be taken with food to lessen the risk of GI upset should be attached to oral contraceptive and hormone replacement prescriptions. Warning labels that discourage smoking while taking contraceptive or other hormones, and that instruct the user to discontinue the drug in the event of pregnancy are also appropriate. An auxiliary label that instructs users to apply patches to clean, dry skin, and to rotate patch placement sites should be affixed to prescriptions for hormone replacement or birth control patches. Women who take oral contraceptives should be warned that some drugs could interact with and possibly reduce the effectiveness of oral contraceptives. Commonly prescribed drugs that may reduce contraceptive effectiveness include some antibiotics, anticonvulsants, and benzodiazepine sedative hypnotic agents.

## Uterine Active Agents

Three drugs are available in the United States that can terminate a pregnancy. Their use is controversial, and complicated by the legal requirements placed on doctors who want to prescribe them.

| Contraceptive method | Relative failure rate* |
|---|---|
| Vasectomy (male sterilization) | 0.02 |
| Tubal ligation (female sterilization) | 0.13 |
| *Norgestrel* implants | < 0.2 |
| Estrogen/progestin oral contraceptives | 0.25 |
| Progestin-only oral contraceptives | 1.2 |
| Intrauterine device (IUD) | 1.4 |
| Diaphragm | 1.9 |
| Condom | 3.6 |
| Withdrawal | 6.7 |
| Spermicide | 11.9 |
| Rhythm | 15.5 |

*Number of pregnancies per 100 hundred women using the method for 1 year

**Figure 27.5** Relative risk of failure for commonly used forms of contraception. Failure rates represent the number of pregnancies in 100 women who use the method for 1 year. (Adapted with permission from Harvey RA, Champe PC, Howland RD, et al *Lippincott's Illustrated Reviews: Pharmacology*, 3rd edition. Baltimore: Lippincott Williams & Wilkins, 2006.)

## Case 27.1

Emergency contraception products Plan B® and Preven® are used for prevention of pregnancy after unprotected sex, including sexual assault. Professional pharmacy organizations, such as APhA and ASHP, believe that pharmacy staff members have a right to refuse to fill a prescription because of religious beliefs, as long as patients are referred to a pharmacy where the medication is available and can be filled within the required time frame for use.

Consider the following case that occurred in a chain pharmacy in Texas. In Texas, as in most states, pharmacists are not required to fill legal prescriptions if they object to filling them on religious or ethical grounds. In this case, reported to have occurred in February of 2004, a pharmacist refused to dispense emergency contraceptives to a rape victim because he felt that to do so would be immoral. Two other pharmacists on duty also refused to fill the prescription. Later that evening, and without a referral, the woman found a pharmacist that filled the prescription. The managers of the first chain store eventually fired all three of the pharmacists who refused to fill the prescription for violating the patient's right to receive service. As a result of the ongoing controversy over filling these prescriptions, many states have enacted legislation allowing "conscience clauses" for pharmacy employees, while still protecting patients' rights to obtain care. Late in 2006, the FDA approved one version of these drugs, Plan B®, to be sold without a prescription to women 18 years of age or older.

## Actions and Indications

Mifepristone (also known as RU 486 and Mifeprex®) is a progestin antagonist used to terminate a pregnancy during the first 7 weeks. Administration of this drug early in pregnancy results in abortion of the fetus due to the interference with progesterone in 85% of women. Dinoprostone and carboprost are prostaglandins that effectively terminate pregnancies from the twelfth to the twentieth week. Dinoprostone is also used to stimulate uterine contractions in the case of intrauterine fetal death. They stimulate the pregnant uterus to contract in the same way that endogenous prostaglandins stimulate labor at full term.

### Administration

Mifepristone is rapidly and completely absorbed after oral administration. The woman takes three tablets by mouth, which must be administered in a doctor's office, clinic, or hospital. She is sent home after she takes the medication, but returns to the office on day three and day 14 to verify that the abortion is complete. Dinoprostone and carboprost are administered vaginally or intramuscularly, respectively.

### Side Effects

Use of mifepristone or the prostaglandins may result in incomplete abortion and a risk of subsequent bleeding. This risk is fairly high with the prostaglandins, but only about 5% with mifepristone. However, incomplete abortion may require surgical intervention, or result in bleeding that requires the use of transfusions.

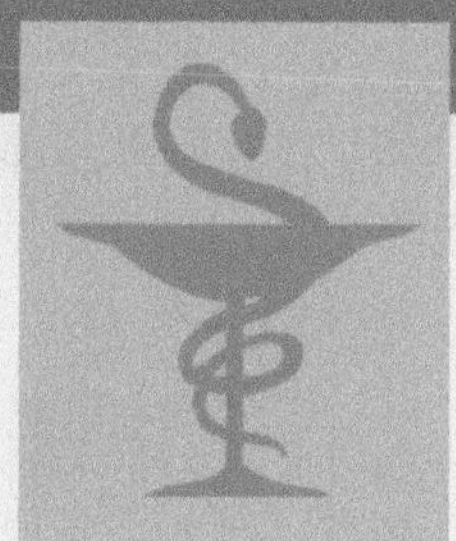

**Tips for the Technician**

Mifepristone is not distributed through pharmacies so technicians will not handle this drug. The prostaglandins are used in hospitals only. Carboprost injection is stored in the refrigerator and dinoprostone vaginal suppositories are stored in the freezer.

## Androgens and Anabolic Steroids

All endogenous androgenic steroid hormones have anabolic activity, and all anabolic steroids have some masculinizing characteristics. However, the hormones synthesized for use as anabolic agents are less masculinizing than the androgens, and are therefore considered part of a different therapeutic class.

### Actions and Indications

Endogenous testosterone promotes maturation of the male sex organs and the development of secondary sex characteristics, such as facial hair and the lower pitched voice associated with maturation in adolescent boys (**Fig. 27.6**). Both male and female fetuses have testosterone and estrogen receptors in the brain, and it is felt that the higher levels of either estrogen or testosterone shape the brains of the developing fetus and encourage what we recognize as typical personality characteristics associated with the sexes. Native testosterone also encourages spermatogenesis (the formation of spermatozoa), growth of the long bones, and muscle development in males. Androgen replacement is indicated for use in the absence of adequate natural testosterone. This can occur as a result of injury to the pituitary gland from tumors or trauma, or injury to the testicles from toxic substances such as chemotherapy or alcohol abuse.

spermatogenesis The process of male gamete formation.

Like the androgens, endogenous anabolic steroids promote muscle and other body tissue building processes in conjunction with adequate protein and calorie consumption. These drugs are indicated for treatment of certain forms of anemia, and for control of metastatic breast cancer in some women. Oxandrolone (Oxandrin®) is used to promote weight gain in patients who are losing weight because of chronic illness, after extensive surgery, or for other reasons are in a catabolic state (a destructive metabolic state where tissues are consumed as energy sources).

catabolism Destructive metabolism whereby complex materials are broken down into waste products and energy.

Anabolic steroids are sometimes illegally obtained and used by athletes as performance enhancing drugs. In an effort to curb this inappropriate and dangerous use, the Drug Enforcement Administration has categorized all androgenic and anabolic steroids as controlled substances. Not only is this use dangerous (see side effects), there is growing evi-

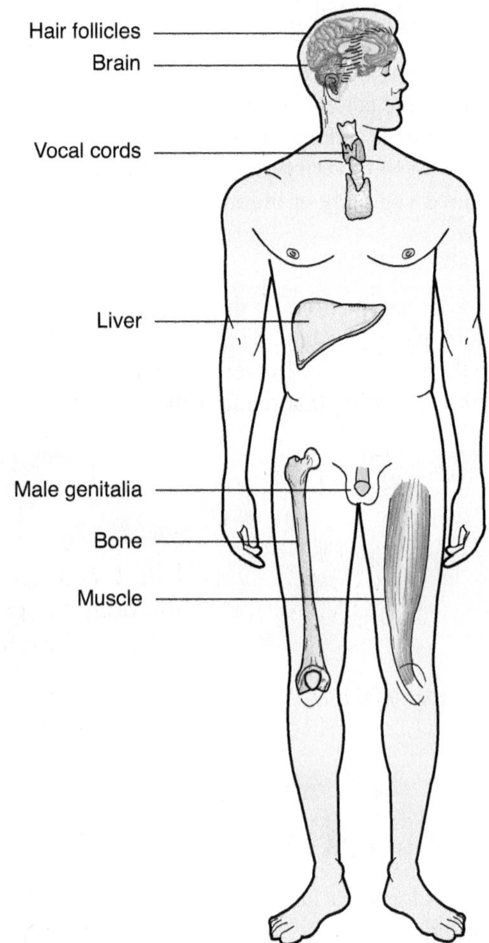


**Figure 27.6** The tissues targeted by testosterone and the anabolic steroids.

dence that it is questionably effective. While anabolic steroids are known to increase muscle mass, evidence suggests that the new muscle tissue may be structurally flawed. Weight gain is at least partially due to retention of sodium and water. Furthermore these drugs do not improve agility or endurance, and no study has ever demonstrated that they improve overall performance.

Danazol (Danocrine®) is an androgen used for the treatment of severe endometriosis, fibrocystic breast disease, and off-label for precocious puberty (early puberty) in girls. The androgenic effects of this drug are relatively weak and its most important action is to suppress the production of FSH and LH in the pituitary.

precocious puberty
Unexpectedly early onset of puberty that can be due to a disease process in the glands that secrete sex hormones.

## Administration

Testosterone is not effective when it is taken by mouth because of first pass metabolism in the liver. Testosterone is effective when it is absorbed through the mucous membranes of the mouth, and a product that adheres to the gum to utilize buccal absorption is available. Other testosterone products include a gel (AndroGel®) that is applied topically to the shoulders, upper arms, or abdomen, a testosterone transdermal patch (Androderm®), long-acting testosterone injection (Depo-Testosterone®), and implantable testosterone pellets. Methyltestosterone (Methitest®), a synthetic androgen, can be taken as buccal tablets or orally, and danazol is taken orally. The anabolic steroid oxandrolone is taken orally and nandrolone (Deca-Durabolin®) is a long-acting injectable product administered by deep intramuscular injection.

### Side Effects

When women take androgens for cancer or endometriosis, masculinization can occur. Acne, growth of facial hair, deepening of the voice, male pattern baldness, and excessive muscle development are possible. Similar cosmetic and physical changes can occur or be accentuated in men. Menstrual irregularities can occur in women. Because of possible effects on the genitalia or masculinization of a female fetus, pregnant women should not use androgens or anabolic steroids.

Because use of androgenic steroids suppresses the natural production of testosterone in males, use of androgens or anabolic steroids can cause impotence, decreased sperm count and subsequent infertility, and gynecomastia. They can also stimulate excessive growth of the prostate. Androgens increase total cholesterol levels, and lower levels of HDL, the "good" cholesterol. By causing these changes and increasing sodium and fluid retention, they increase the risk for premature coronary heart disease.

In addition to the possible side effects already listed, use of anabolic steroids by young athletes can cause premature closing of the epiphysis of the long bones, which stunts growth and interrupts development. Long-term use and high doses are required to maintain increased muscle mass in the athletes who abuse these drugs. This kind of misuse can result in reduction of testicular size, often-fatal liver damage, increased aggression, psychotic episodes, and an addiction syndrome.

## Review Questions

### Multiple Choice

Choose the best answer for the following questions:

1. When technicians fill prescriptions for prednisone tablets, which of the following should be considered?
   a. Prednisone and prednisolone look and sound alike, but they are not the same drug.
   b. A warning label advising patients not to abruptly discontinue the medication should be affixed to the prescription vial for corticosteroids that are prescribed for chronic use.
   c. A patient package insert should always be sent home with the patient.
   d. a and b are correct.
   e. None of the above is true.

2. Circle the letter corresponding to the incorrect statement about use of the contraceptive hormones.
   a. Contraceptive hormones protect the users against sexually transmitted diseases.
   b. Long acting medroxyprogesterone can cause significant weight gain.
   c. When used according to directions, oral contraceptives are among the most effective forms of contraception.
   d. Contraceptive hormones can be taken orally, given by IM injection, or applied as a transdermal patch.
   e. Contraceptive hormones increase the risk of blood clots.

3. Which of the following is not an appropriate use of corticosteroids?
   a. Treatment of acute inflammatory illnesses such as systemic lupus erythematosus
   b. Inhaled, for the prevention of asthmatic attacks
   c. Chronic oral use for the treatment of diabetes
   d. Applied topically for treatment of minor skin irritations
   e. Replacement therapy in adrenal insufficiency

4. Which of the following are adverse consequences that young athletes who abuse androgens might incur?
   a. Anabolic steroid induced rage, dependence, or psychosis
   b. Life-threatening liver damage
   c. Increased cardiovascular risks
   d. Arrest for abuse of a controlled substance
   e. All of the above

5. Indicate the auxiliary label that is inappropriate to apply to a prescription for oral contraceptives.
   a. Do not take this drug if you become pregnant
   b. May cause drowsiness
   c. Smoking should be avoided while taking this medication
   d. Certain medications may alter the effectiveness of birth control pills
   e. May take with food to lessen the chance of stomach upset

## True/False

6. Technicians should carefully transcribe directions for tapering the dose of corticosteroids to minimize the chance of patient administration errors that could result in an adverse drug reaction.
   a. True
   b. False

7. The cardiovascular risks associated with use of contraceptive hormones (blood clots, heart attacks) decrease with the age of the woman, but are higher in women who smoke.
   a. True
   b. False

8. Pharmacy staff members who are ethically opposed to abortion have the right to refuse to fill prescriptions for emergency contraceptives without referring the client to another pharmacy where she can get the prescription filled.
   a. True
   b. False

9. Fludrocortisone, the corticosteroid with the greatest mineralocorticoid activity, should only be used when fluid and sodium retention is desired.
   a. True
   b. False

10. Danazol, a drug with mild androgenic properties, is used to treat endometriosis, an often painful condition where the tissue that lines the uterus get into the pelvic cavity.
    a. True
    b. False

## Matching

For numbers 11 to 15, match the drug name with the appropriate use or indication from the list below. Choices will not be used more than once and may not be used at all.

11. Dexamethasone acetate
12. Megestrol
13. Methylprednisolone sodium succinate
14. Hydrocortisone 1% cream
15. Norgestrel

a. Intra-articular injections into an acutely inflamed joint
b. Intravenous infusion for acute lupus nephritis
c. Treatment of elevated intracranial pressure
d. Appetite stimulant
e. Contraception
f. Self treatment of minor skin irritation or itching

## Short Answer

16. Why should patients be warned not to abruptly discontinue corticosteroids after taking them for 2 weeks or more? What can technicians do to help make sure abrupt discontinuation does not occur?
17. List four adverse effects that can occur as a result of chronic administration of corticosteroids.
18. Compare the advantages and disadvantages of medroxyprogesterone injections as a contraceptive agent to oral contraceptives or contraceptive patches.
19. Name the mineralocorticoid produced in the adrenals and explain its role.
20. Why are anabolic steroids used as performance enhancing drugs and why is the use inappropriate?

## FOR FURTHER INQUIRY

Questions regarding the wisdom of the use of hormone replacement therapy for the treatment of the symptoms of menopause are as yet unanswered. Although some physicians suggest that low doses of estrogen and progesterone are safe, there are some women that should probably not receive these medications. Investigate some of the alternative, natural, or herbal treatments suggested for the symptoms of menopause. Do you believe there is adequate evidence to suggest they are safe and effective?

UNIT VI

# Antimicrobials

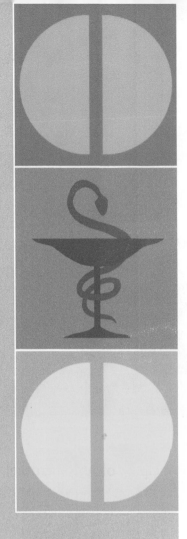

Chapter **28**

# The Immune System, Infectious Disease, and the Principles of Antimicrobial Therapy

## OBJECTIVES

After studying this chapter, the reader should be able to:

- Explain how adaptations may improve the ability of micro-organisms to survive and reproduce.
- List four tissues that play an important role in the defense of the human body against infection and state whether these tissues provide a nonspecific or specific form of defense.
- Compare and contrast the roles of B and T lymphocytes in the immune system.
- Describe how misuse of antibiotics can encourage the development of antibiotic resistant organisms.
- Define the following terms: pathogen, infectious disease, communicable disease, virulence, and immunity.

*KEY TERMS*

- antibody
- broad spectrum
- communicable
- culture
- immunity
- infectious disease
- lymph
- lymphocyte
- macrophage
- micro-organism
- normal flora
- parasite
- pathogenic
- phagocyte
- resistance
- vector
- virulent
- zoonosis

Micro-organisms fill a very important ecological niche in the biosphere. They add to the fertility of soil, provide food for marine creatures, break down organic matter, and can even detoxify inorganic compounds. If it were not for the ability of microbes to degrade dead plants and animals, we would be up to our elbows in debris. It is the presence of micro-organisms that supports the existence of all life on earth. Although it may not be pleasant to imagine, every human body, even one that is kept meticulously clean, is covered with micro-organisms. The microscopic organisms that reside in or on our bodies include bacteria, fungi, and even tiny members of the spider family called mites.

Most of these organisms are harmless, and many provide helpful services to the body. For instance, the GI tract is filled with numerous species of bacteria that aid in digestive processes, manufacture vitamin K, and maintain a balance in the GI tract that helps to hold harmful bacteria at bay. Of all the microbes that live on the surface of our skin or in the GI tract, bacteria make the greatest contribution. These resident microbes are frequently referred to as normal flora.

While most micro-organisms are not harmful, the body is under constant attack from pathogenic (disease-causing) micro-organisms. Pathogens cause infectious diseases that range from mild colds to lethal epidemics that wipe out hundreds of thousands of people in a matter of months. Thankfully, the body is endowed with a network of defenses, called the immune system, which keeps most infectious agents out.

normal flora Micro-organisms expected to be present on body surfaces or in the intestines and that under normal circumstances do not cause disease.

pathogenic Capable of causing disease.

infectious disease Disease caused by the presence and growth of pathogenic micro-organisms.

communicable Capable of being transmitted from person to person or between animals of other species; especially disease.

vector An organism, such as an insect, that transmits a pathogen from one source to another.

zoonosis An infectious disease that can pass from animals to humans under natural conditions.

## 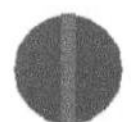 Infectious Diseases

An infectious disease is an illness caused by the entrance into the body of pathogenic organisms, such as bacteria, viruses, fungi, or parasites, which multiply there (**Fig. 28.1**). Most infectious diseases are also communicable, or contagious, meaning that they can be passed on to other people through personal contact, contact with body fluids or discharge, or via a vector (carrier). Many people think only blood-sucking insects that take blood from a sick individual and move on to bite a healthy person qualify as vectors. In truth, insects are the most important vectors (especially mosquitos, ticks, and fleas), but birds, rodents, pets, and food animals can also carry diseases. If infectious diseases cause illness in animals, and move from animal populations to cause disease in humans, then the diseases are referred to as zoonotic infections. Infections with this capacity include some forms of influenza, West Nile virus, and parasites, among others.

Some infections are mild and easy for the body to fight off, while others are devastating. The outcome of an infection depends on two major factors; the ability of the patient to fight off the infection, and the disease-producing characteristics of the infecting organism.

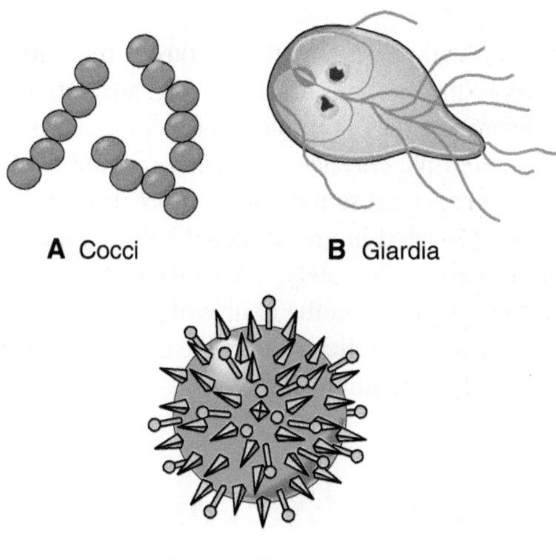


**Figure 28.1** Representations of Streptococcus bacteria **(A)**, Giardia intestinalis, a parasite **(B)**, and the virus that causes influenza **(C)**. Note that streptococcus are 0.6 to 1 micrometers, giardia is 10 to 20 micrometers in length, and influenza viruses are 0.08 to 0.12 micrometers. (A and B: reprinted with permission from McConnell TH. *The Nature of Disease*. Baltimore: Lippincott Williams & Wilkins, 2007; C: LifeART image © 2007 Lippincott Williams & Wilkins. All rights reserved.)

virulent A markedly pathogenic organism, able to rapidly overcome the body's defense mechanisms.

micro-organism A microscopic organism.

Disease producing organisms that rapidly overcome the defenses of the host's body are said to be highly virulent.

Micro-organisms (organisms that cannot be seen with the naked eye) expend all of their energy to fulfill one purpose: to reproduce. While it may seem odd to think of micro-organisms as having behavior, they readily adapt to obstacles that impede their survival and reproduction. The most well-adapted microbes live in an intimate relationship with another organism without causing death. Organisms that are not lethal to the host have an opportunity to reproduce and infect other hosts. Pathogens that quickly kill their host are less likely to survive themselves, and are less well adapted to spread to other hosts. Compare the adaptations of the HIV virus, which causes AIDS, and the Ebola virus. HIV is a disease that does not appear for months to years after the patient is infected, and during this time, HIV can spread to others. Even after 25 years of research on the disease, HIV-AIDS continues as a worldwide epidemic. On the other hand, Ebola is a disease that kills its victim within 7 days. Clearly, the Ebola virus is much less well adapted than the HIV virus.

## Case 28.1

Since the sole purpose of any micro-organism is survival and reproduction, it makes sense that an organism that rapidly kills its host will not be a microbial "high achiever." Take, for example, the Ebola-Zaire virus. At the beginning of the last large outbreak in Zaire, a charcoal worker arrived at a local hospital with the typical Ebola symptoms of rapid onset of a high fever and diarrhea. The charcoal worker died when internal bleeding, vomiting of blood, and shock developed within a week of the onset of his disease. This organism is spread through contact with body fluids, which victims produce profusely, not through inhaled droplets. In this case, and in most Ebola epidemics, secondary cases occur in hospital workers, who do their jobs without the benefit of modern protective equipment. A laboratory technician was the next person infected, followed by physicians and nurses who were caring for him. Once the infection was identified, proper protective equipment, and isolation controlled the outbreak.

Ebola has been known to wipe out entire villages, because it kills 80% to 100% of its victims after a period of about a week. Partly because of the rapidity with which the disease kills, the high death rate, and the low likelihood of long-distance travel by people who live in the area where it is found, and partly due to its limited ability to spread by means other than contact with body fluids, Ebola-Zaire has never caused an epidemic outside of the African continent.

Micro-organisms reproduce so quickly they can undergo many generations of reproduction in a matter of days. Because of this rapid reproductive rate, mutations and adaptations, some successful and some not, can make significant changes in a microbial population in a matter of weeks. Successful adaptations (those that improve the chances of microbial survival) might make the organisms less lethal, more contagious, or cause them to be more resistant to antimicrobial medications. Antimicrobial resistance (covered in greater detail below) gravely impacts our ability to successfully treat infectious diseases. Ultimately, the question of whether or not the person with an infectious disease survives depends on the ability of that person to fight off the infection. The harmless microbes that live unnoticed on the skin of someone healthy can cause death in the individual with an inadequate immune system.

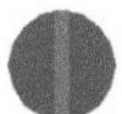

## Understanding the Immune System

Human beings benefit from many layers of defense against foreign invaders, whether something as minor as a splinter, or something as potentially deadly as cholera (see **Table**

**28.1**). Our first, and arguably, most important line of defense is our skin. Healthy and intact skin forms a barrier that most micro-organisms cannot breach. The constant production of tears, nasal, and respiratory secretions that contain enzymes, and even the secretion of stomach acid provide another layer of protection. Tiny hairs that move mucus and trapped micro-organisms up and out of the airways protect the respiratory tract. Our normal flora fill up most of the available ecological space where a pathogen could take hold, and these microbes protect their space by secreting proteins or enzymes that inhibit many potential invaders. These defense mechanisms are innate and nonspecific, but we have other, highly specific defense mechanisms that are mediated through the immune system.

The immune system is made up of organs, including the spleen and the bone marrow, a specialized circulatory system called the lymphatic system, and highly specialized defensive white blood cells (**Fig. 28.2**). The lymphatic system is a network of vessels that carries fluid called lymph. Lymph arises from the interstitial fluid, which passes out of capil-

lymph Clear fluid similar to plasma that passes from the blood, to intercellular spaces of body tissue, into the lymphatic vessels and contains lymphocytes.

## Analogy

Imagine an area of Yellowstone National Park that is high in the mountains, far from human interference. In remote areas, animals occupy territories or niches. This is similar to the territory occupied by normal flora in the GI tract. Wolves, for example, live in harmonious groups and roam across an area that is theirs. They mark their territory with urine, so that other wolves from outside the group will stay away. If something happens to the family group, so that they become sick or are killed, a new group of wolves, or a different predator species will move into their space. In the case of gaps in the normal flora of the GI tract, the new group is often pathogenic.

**Table 28.1** The Specific and Nonspecific Defenses That Protect Humans From Disease

| Nonspecific defenses | Actions |
|---|---|
| Skin | Provides a mechanical barrier against penetration of micro-organisms |
| Secretions | Enzymes and pH of secretions are antibacterial |
| Respiratory tract mucus and ciliated cells | The "ciliary elevator" moves mucus and micro-organisms out of the respiratory tract |
| Normal Flora | Fills available niches so that pathogens cannot colonize |
| Lymphatic System | Lymph circulates through lymph nodes and spleen where it is filtered; white blood cells accumulate here |
| **Specific Defenses** | |
| Lymphocytes | Lymphocytes produce antibody, coordinate the immune response, and destroy cells that have consumed micro-organisms |
| Antibody | Highly specific proteins attach to "foreign" material and identify it for destruction |
| Macrophages | Cells in the lymphatic system and other tissues designed to consume micro-organisms |

phagocyte A cell capable of engulfing and destroying foreign material, such as bacteria.

macrophage A phagocytic cell that arises from the bone marrow and moves out to tissues where it functions in the destruction of foreign antigens and stimulates other immune system cells.

lymphocyte White blood cells, differentiated in the lymphatic tissue; B and T lymphocytes are responsible for the production of antibody and other aspects of immunity.

antibody A protein that is produced by B lymphocytes, after sensitization by an antigen, to act specifically against the antigen in an immune response; also called immunoglobulin.

laries and bathes the cells of the body. Most of the interstitial fluid eventually circulates directly back into the capillaries, but some does not. This small portion passes into lymphatic capillaries, which progressively increase in size to become lymphatic vessels. Lymph only flows in one direction, so lymphatic vessels, like veins, contain valves to help move the fluid forward. Eventually, the lymphatic system drains its fluid back into the right and left subclavian veins. Along the way, lymph moves through tiny tissue sacs called lymph nodes. There are hundreds of lymph nodes in the body, but they are mainly concentrated in the groin, abdomen, armpits, and neck.

The inner walls of the lymph nodes are lined with one type of phagocyte (cells that engulf and destroy foreign particles, bacteria, or other invaders), called macrophages (**Fig. 28.3**). Macrophages remove foreign material that enters the lymphatic system. The number and activity of these cells increases when the body is combating an infection, and as a result, lymph nodes often become enlarged and noticeable by the patient. The enlarged lymph nodes are commonly referred to as "swollen glands."

The lymph nodes contain many of the specialized white blood cells called lymphocytes. While all white blood cells play a role in the body's defenses, it is the lymphocytes that, when mature, may produce antibody (proteins involved in the immune response), or play other important roles in the destruction of microbes. Like all blood cells, lymphocytes are born in the bone marrow. The majority of them move to the thymus gland, where they mature into T cells (T for thymus). The lymphocytes that stay in the bone marrow to mature are called B cells. Once mature, the B cells moves into the circulation and the lymphatic system. When B cells are activated they produce antibody, proteins that attach to foreign particles or diseased cells to mark them for destruction.

T cells serve in two important capacities in the immune processes. Helper T cells coordinate the response of other immune cells. They signal B cells when it is time to produce antibody, activate the other class of T cells, and call phagocytic cells to the scene. The other T

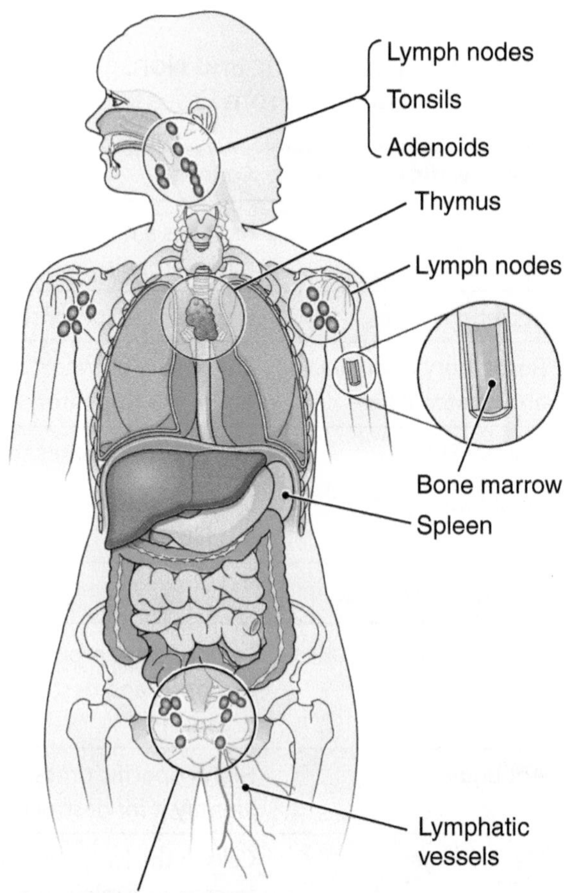


**Figure 28.2** Tissues and organs of the immune system, illustrated here, are an important part of providing protection against invading micro-organisms. (Adapted with permission from McConnell TH. *The Nature of Disease*. Baltimore: Lippincott Williams & Wilkins, 2007.)

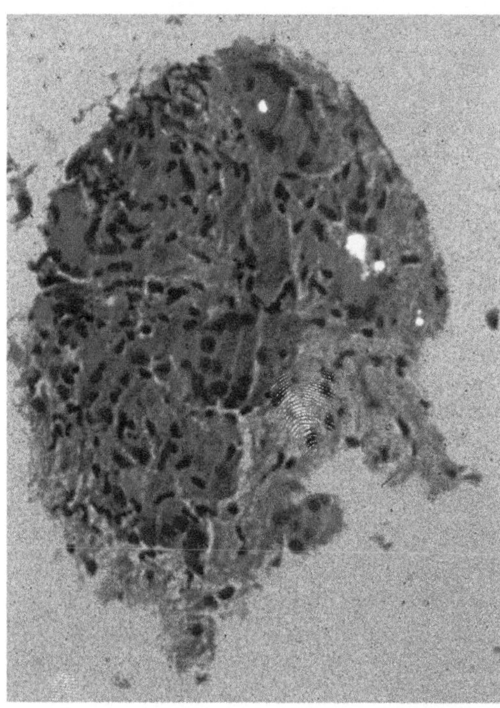

**Figure 28.3** Photomicrograph of a macrophage, an important immune system cell that engulfs foreign particles. (Reprinted with permission from Cagle PT. *Color Atlas and Text of Pulmonary Pathology*. Philadelphia: Lippincott Williams & Wilkins, 2005.)

cells, when activated by the helper T cells, become what are known as killer T cells. Killer T cells destroy diseased cells that contain foreign particles. For example, killer T cells will destroy cells that contain viruses to keep the virus from replicating inside of the cell.

The lymphatic fluid eventually passes through the spleen, located in the upper left side of the abdomen, before returning to the blood stream. The spleen has two major functions. The best known of these is as a filter for the blood. The spleen is highly vascular, and as the rich supply of blood feeds through, aging red blood cells and platelets are removed and recycled. The spleen also stores red blood cells and can produce them during times of stress. The second major role of the spleen is as an organ of the immune system. Lymphatic tissue makes up a significant portion of the spleen, and it functions in a way similar to that of lymph nodes. Blood and lymph are filtered, and foreign particles or organisms removed. The spleen holds a large supply of lymphocytes, which become active during infectious processes. Like the lymph nodes, the spleen can become enlarged when the body is fighting infection.

After fighting off an infection, lymphocytes retain "memory" of the organisms they encountered, which results in immunity, or protection from reinfection with the same organism. For example, if a person has chickenpox while in grade school and then is exposed again in adulthood, he or she will not get sick again. The kind of immunity conferred by having an infection is called natural active immunity, and is life-long. Immunity that develops as a result of immunization or vaccination is also active immunity, but is considered artificial and generally does not last nearly as long as natural immunity. The protection conferred by T cells, B cells, and antibodies they produce is highly specific to a particular foreign particle. The body never develops complete immunity to organisms that can rapidly change their make-up (like cold viruses) because the antibodies produced for the old infection won't match the new virus. For the same reason, it is impossible to create a successful vaccine to prevent the common cold.

immunity Ability of the body to resist an infectious disease; classified as active, passive, natural, or acquired.

People survive colds, infected scrapes, or the chicken pox all the time without using antimicrobials, so we know the body can combat infection without the help of medications. Most people are not aware that even with the best medications, the body cannot survive infection without a functional immune system. People who are elderly, or very young, or are being treated with cancer chemotherapy or corticosteroids, are more likely to die of a serious infection because their immune systems are less capable of fighting it. When antimicrobial effectiveness is compromised because of misuse, successful treatment of at-risk patients is even more difficult.

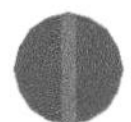

# Principles of Antimicrobial Therapy

The development of immunizations and use of antibiotics revolutionized health care in a way that no other new treatments have accomplished since. It is estimated by some experts that since the discovery of penicillin alone, more than 200 million lives have been saved. However, indiscriminate use of antibiotics can cost lives. While physicians and pharmacists work together to make appropriate medication selections, technicians will be better equipped to support good patient care if they understand the basic principles of antimicrobial use.

## The Germ Theory of Disease

For centuries, infectious diseases could not be appropriately prevented or treated because physicians were not aware of their cause. After the microscope was developed in the late seventeenth century by Anton Van Leeuwenhoek, he went on to discover the presence of microorganisms in pond water. However, it was not until the late nineteenth century that Louis Pasteur and others proved that microbes were the cause of infectious diseases. Besides developing pasteurization, a process that prevents the spoilage of milk and other beverages, Pasteur's research went a long way to convince physicians and surgeons that sterilizing instruments, washing hands, and cleaning surgery rooms could save lives.

Louis Pasteur's work went beyond pasteurization to expand Edward Jenner's concept of vaccination. Jenner theorized and then demonstrated that infections with weakened organisms could confer immunity in people exposed to more virulent forms of a disease. Late in his career, Pasteur developed the first rabies and anthrax vaccines and opened doors to the development of many other immunizations.

From Pasteur's work, Joseph Lister derived the concept of antisepsis. When he incorporated the use of antiseptics and clean instruments into hospital practices, rates of infection and death fell dramatically. Paul Ehrlich postulated that compounds could be created that would specifically target pathogenic organisms without harming people. The work of these and other scientific giants led directly to the development and use of antibiotics and other antimicrobial compounds.

## Appropriate Use of Antimicrobials

resistance The failure of an infection or other disease to respond to treatment.

Use of antimicrobials has unquestionably saved millions of lives, and yet inappropriate use of these drugs encourages the development of adaptations in microbes that allows them to survive in the presence of drugs intended to kill them. When an antibiotic is ineffective at either killing or inhibiting the growth of bacteria, the bacteria are said to be resistant. Some bacteria are inherently resistant to specific antimicrobials, while others develop resistance. The use of many antimicrobials is permanently compromised because of microbial resistance. In order to avoid development of resistance, prescribers must know the identity of the infecting organism and its susceptibility to available drugs.

### Identification of the Organism

Physicians can usually determine whether bacteria, viruses, fungi, or parasites cause an infection based on the symptoms the patient exhibits and the history of their illness. Doctors will ask about symptoms of fever, rash, GI upset, or respiratory symptoms, and will consider travel, food consumption, and exposure to individuals who are sick when they make a diagnosis. Since they see many patients every day, they are likely to have a good idea of what is "going around."

culture To grow in a laboratory; especially bacteria in infectious diseases.

Once a likely cause is determined, physicians must identify a specific organism before any antimicrobial medications are prescribed. Bacteria and fungi can be cultured, or grown in the laboratory, and then identified by laboratory technicians. Organisms are grown in petri dishes on specific nutrients called growth medium (**Fig. 28.4**) Once grown in culture,

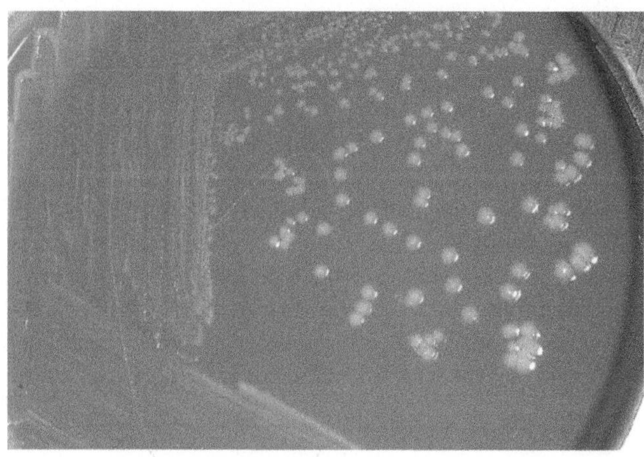

**Figure 28.4** A photograph of bacterial colonies cultured on growth medium. In order to identify the organisms, a laboratory technician examines the colonies, stains the organisms, and studies them under the microscope. (Reprinted with permission from McClatchey KD. *Clinical Laboratory Medicine*, 2nd edition. Philadelphia: Lippincott Williams & Wilkins, 2002.)

they are inspected for characteristic features, stained, and examined under the microscope. Gram stain is a violet-colored stain taken up by certain bacteria, and Gram staining is one tool used by laboratory technicians to identify organisms (**Fig. 28.5**).

Identification of viruses requires the patient's blood be tested for the level of antibodies to specific viruses. When identifying parasites, the laboratory technician usually looks for the parasite, ova, or other signs of a parasitic infection in the sample. Most parasites are identified using stool, blood, or sputum samples. Rarely tissue samples must be used. Exact identification of the infecting organism is essential, because drugs are quite specific. In other words, antibiotics cannot be used to kill viruses, and antiviral drugs will not kill bacteria. Furthermore, drugs are specific for particular types of organisms within any one class of microbes. After the infecting organism is identified by its genus and species, its sensitivity to available medications is tested.

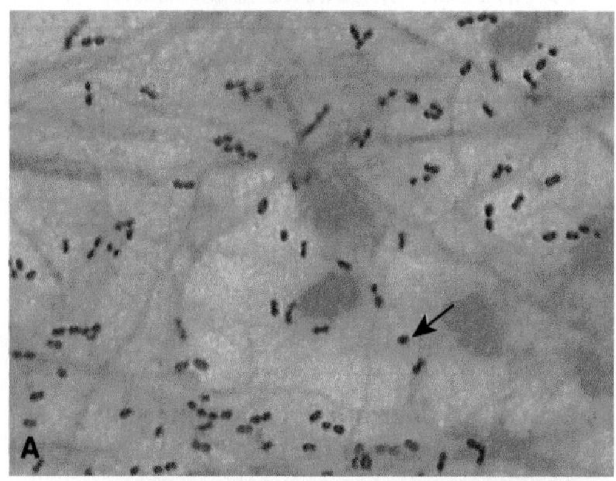


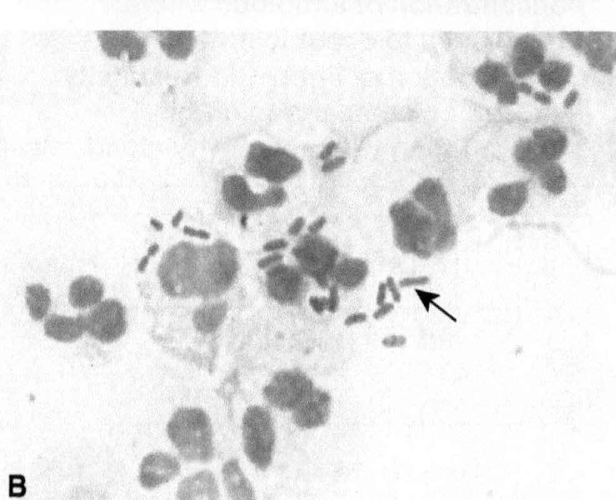


**Figure 28.5** Gram-positive organisms, such as the Anthrax bacillus **(A)**, pick up Gram stain and appear purple. Gram negative organisms appear pink **(B)**. (A: reprinted with permission from Tasman W and Jaeger E. *The Willis Eye Hospital Atlas of Clinical Ophthalmology*, 2nd edition. Philadelphia: Lippincott Williams & Wilkins, 2001; B: reprinted with permission from Koneman EW, Allen SD, Janda WM, et al. *Color Atlas and Textbook of Diagnostic Microbiology* (4th and 5th editions). Philadelphia: Lippincott, 1992, 1997.)

## Sensitivity Testing

Once bacteria and fungi are cultured, the cultures are tested for sensitivity to antimicrobial agents. This is an essential step to find a drug that will effectively treat an infection. This is accomplished by exposing the organisms, which are mixed with growth medium in a test tube, to several standard concentrations of the antimicrobial drug being tested (**Fig. 28.6**). After 24 hours in a temperature-controlled environment, the test tubes are checked for bacterial growth. Simply stated, if there are no signs of bacterial growth in the test tubes that correspond to less than usual concentrations of the drug in the blood, then the organism is considered to be sensitive to the antimicrobial. If the bacteria grow in spite of the presence of normal concentrations of the drug, it is considered to be resistant to the antimicrobial. Precise standards for determining sensitivity are set by the Clinical Laboratory Standards Institute.

Fortunately, sensitivity testing for antiviral medications is rarely needed because the majority of viral infections resolve without treatment. For people with infections that require treatment, sensitivity testing similar to that used with bacterial or fungal infections is not an option. Drug selection is usually based on information regarding treatment success or failure in the local area. The genotypes of viruses can be tested and checked for genetic evidence of mutations that confer resistance, a practice recommended by the CDC for AIDS patients. More often, viral resistance is identified when, in spite of treatment, patients do not improve.

parasite An organism that must get nutrition and shelter from another organism in order to survive.

Parasites are organisms that live with, in, or on another organism in order to survive. Luckily, with the exception of Giardia and pinworms, parasitic infections are rare in the United States and Canada. Because these infections are uncommon, most physicians are unfamiliar with appropriate drug treatment. Prescribers normally depend on recommendations from the Center for Disease

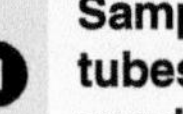

1
Samples of bacteria are placed into tubes containing growth medium and varying concentrations of antibiotic.


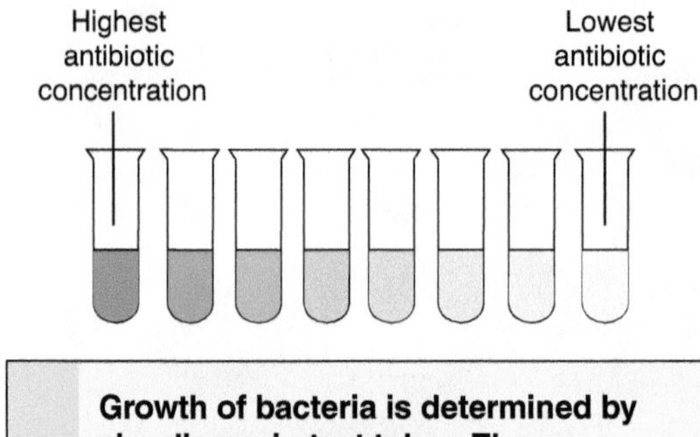

Highest antibiotic concentration
Lowest antibiotic concentration
2
Growth of bacteria is determined by cloudiness in test tubes. The concentration of antibiotic where growth fails to occur is noted. Determination of antibiotic sensitivity is based on comparison of this concentration with sensitivity standards.


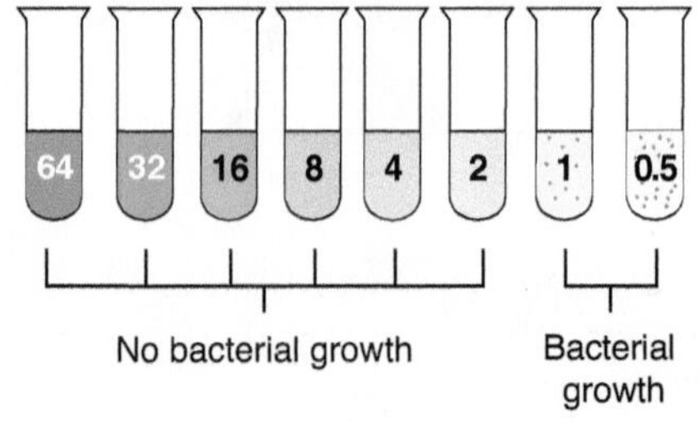


**Figure 28.6** One process used to determine bacterial sensitivity in the laboratory. (Adapted with permission from Harvey RA, Champe PC, Howland RD, et al. Lippincott's Illustrated Reviews: *Pharmacology*, 3rd edition. Baltimore: Lippincott Williams & Wilkins, 2006.)

Control and Prevention (CDC) in Atlanta, Georgia, or other experts when they need to make appropriate drug selections for parasitic infections.

### Resistance

Bacteria are said to be resistant to an antibiotic if an effective therapeutic dose of the antibiotic does not prevent their growth. Antibiotics may be effective against a broad range or a narrow range of organisms, while they are ineffective against others. For example, gram-negative organisms are inherently resistant to penicillin. Microbial species that are normally responsive to a particular drug may develop resistance, either through selection of resistant individuals (a kind of survival of the fittest), by acquiring a gene for resistance from other organisms, or through spontaneous mutations.

When antibiotics are not dosed appropriately, or the person taking the medication is not compliant with the instruction, the hardiest organisms may survive to reproduce again. This is a form of natural selection with the end result of loss of antibiotic effectiveness. When spontaneous mutations occur, they may or may not be an advantage to the organism. However, if the cell survives the mutation, it will be passed on to future generations. Most mutations have little or no effect on the organism, but some may produce antibiotic resistant strains of an organism. Often, the genes for antibiotic resistance are contained in packets of genetic material called plasmids. Plasmids can move between organisms and enter other organism types, thereby transferring resistance characteristics from one group of bacteria to another, and even from one genus of bacteria to another.

The spread and increase of bacterial resistance is of grave concern to experts because it critically restricts our ability to treat some of the most virulent bacteria and viruses. Overuse and misuse of antimicrobials are two factors that encourage the development of resistance. Studies have demonstrated that antibiotic resistance declines when antibiotic use is either limited, or when antibiotics are prescribed and used correctly. This is another reason that it is so important for pharmacy staff members to teach and encourage patients to use their medications properly.

## The Perfect Antimicrobial

If pharmaceutical chemists could create the perfect antimicrobial, what kind of characteristics would they look for? Although pharmaceutical companies are constantly touting the advantages of broad-spectrum antibiotics (those that kill or slow the growth of a wide range of bacteria), most infectious disease experts agree that the ideal antimicrobial is specific and targeted to one group of organisms. By using antimicrobials with a narrow spectrum, fewer bacteria are being exposed to the effects of the antibiotics, and pressure toward resistance is reduced. Broad-spectrum antibiotics are less desirable because they kill harmless or helpful bacteria, thereby creating an opening for the invasion of a pathogen.

broad spectrum A term used to describe an antibiotic that is effective against a wide range of microorganisms.

The perfect antimicrobial would kill the microbe, not simply slow its growth, and it would exert this effect by targeting some aspect of the microbial growth and reproduction that is dissimilar to mammalian functions. When drugs work through mechanisms that are unique to microbes, side effects brought on by disruption of host cells are reduced. Ideally, this drug would penetrate to the site of the infection without disturbing the normal flora of the intestinal tract, and without requiring intravenous or intramuscular injection. The perfect antimicrobial should also be reasonably priced.

When all of these characteristics are considered together, it is little wonder there is no perfect antimicrobial. It is fair to question whether such a drug could ever exist. Certainly at this point, our best antimicrobials are the ones floating through our own bloodstreams. Our white blood cells and antibodies are specific, go precisely where they are needed, only attack foreign invaders, and are free. It may be that in the future, the perfect antimicrobials will be the ones that spur on our own defenses. In the meantime, our best hope is to use the good antimicrobials we have sparingly and correctly, because safe, effective, affordable new antimicrobials are very hard to find.

# Review Questions

## Multiple Choice

Choose the bast answer to the following questions:

1. Circle the statement below that is not true about the ways micro-organisms help the body.
   a. They aid the digestive process.
   b. They produce vitamin K.
   c. They provide food for killer T cells.
   d. They help prevent the invasion of pathogens.
   e. All of the above are false.

2. Significant changes can occur in bacterial populations in relatively short time periods because of which of the following?
   a. Many generations of bacterial reproduction occur in a short period of time.
   b. Mutations occur frequently and are always beneficial.
   c. Mutations occur rarely and are never beneficial.
   d. Appropriate use of antibiotics encourages change.
   e. The effect of gamma rays from the sun encourage mutations.

3. One of the important functions of the spleen is?
   a. Produces stomach acid and digestive enzymes
   b. Exchanges oxygen for carbon dioxide in respiration
   c. Controls the blood pH
   d. Filters blood to remove aging cells
   e. Filters blood to remove toxins and impurities

4. Microbes that were once killed by a specific antibiotic but are no longer affected by it are said to have developed what?
   a. Resistance
   b. Super powers
   c. Beta lactamase
   d. An impenetrable cell membrane
   e. None of the above

5. In some cases, plasmids are known to transfer resistance from one organism to another. What does a plasmid contain that allows this to occur?
   a. Enzymes used to combat antimicrobials
   b. Genetic material coding for resistance
   c. A virus
   d. Organelles from the bacteria
   e. Nothing, it is not known if they do play a part in resistance

## True/False

6. The spread of microbial resistance is not very important because we can always develop new antibiotics.
   a. True
   b. False

7. A communicable disease can be passed from one person to another.
   a. True
   b. False

8. Our first and possibly most important line of defense against pathogens is our own white blood cells.
   a. True
   b. False

9. Natural active immunity comes from getting immunized with vaccines.
   a. True
   b. False

10. Parasitic infection is a major health problem in North America.
    a. True
    b. False

## Matching

For questions 11 to 15 match the definition or description to the correct word or phrase from the list below. Choices will be used once or not at all.

11. A "package" of genetic material transferred from one organism to another.
12. Pathogenic organism
13. The lymph nodes are most concentrated here
14. T cells mature in this gland
15. Identified in the lab by culturing

A. An organism that causes disease in its host
B. Plasmids
C. Groin, abdomen, armpits, and neck
D. Thymus
E. Bone marrow
F. Legs, head, feet, and back
G. Bacteria or Fungi

## Short Answer

16. Explain two ways that an individual can develop immunity to an infection caused by a virus.

17. Explain two ways that resistance can occur due to inappropriate use of antibiotics.

18. Explain the basics of how a normally functioning lymphatic system helps to fight infections.

19. Explain why the usefulness of some antimicrobials is permanently compromised.

20. How are organisms tested for resistance to a certain antimicrobial agents?

# FOR FURTHER INQUIRY

If the world of microbiology interests you, consider reading one of the many fascinating nonfiction works about science and the battle against infection. Although there are many titles available, the following are entertaining and well reviewed. *The Hot Zone: A Terrifying True Story* by Richard Preston, is a highly entertaining, if somewhat exaggerated account of the Ebola Virus that reads like a thriller. *Scourge: The Once and Future Threat of Smallpox* by Jonathan B. Tucker, is interesting both from a scientific and political perspective, and *The Great Influenza*, by John M. Barry, is pertinent, frightening, and critically acclaimed.

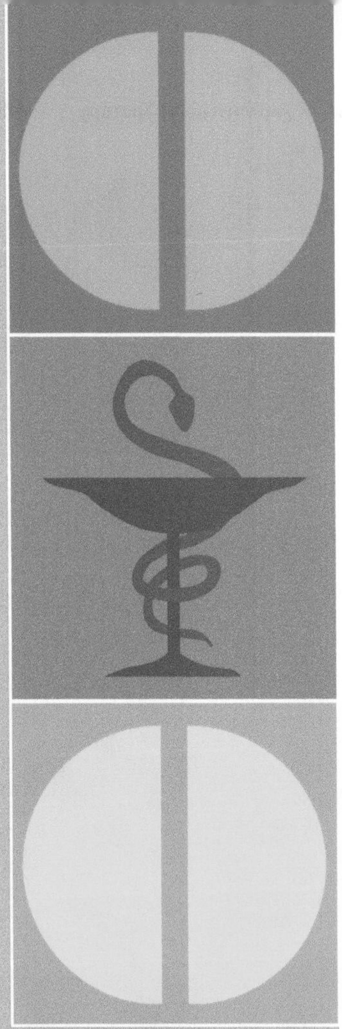

## KEY TERMS

- antibacterial
- antibiotic
- bacteriocidal
- bacteriostatic
- buffer
- cyanosis
- hyponatremia
- idiosyncratic
- intravenous piggy-back
- nephritis
- otitis media
- phlebitis
- ribosome
- sepsis
- synergistic effect

Chapter **29**

# Antibiotics: Cell Wall and Protein Synthesis Inhibitors

## OBJECTIVES

After studying this chapter, the reader should be able to:

- Define the following terms: antibiotic, antibacterial, bacteriocidal, bacteriostatic, nosocomial, community acquired.
- List the name of a commonly used drug, two potential side effects, and the route(s) of administration for the extended spectrum penicillins, antistaphylococcal penicillins, antipseudomonal penicillins, and first-, second-, and third-generation cephalosporins.
- Explain why the use of highly effective antibiotics such as meropenem, imipenem, and vancomycin should be restricted to only the most seriously ill patients with difficult to treat infections.
- Compare and contrast the aminoglycoside antibiotics with the third-generation cephalosporins, including mechanisms of action, uses, routes of administration, and side effects.
- List an antibiotic from each of the following classes or groups discussed in the chapter, an indication for its use, and the auxiliary labelling that should accompany a prescription filled in a retail practice setting: tetracycline, macrolide, and "other protein synthesis inhibitors."

## DRUGS COVERED IN THIS CHAPTER

### Antibiotics That Inhibit Bacterial Cell Walls

**β-Lactam Antibiotics**

**Penicillins**

***Natural***

Penicillin G
Penicillin V

***Extended Spectrum***

Amoxicillin
Ampicillin

***Antistaphylococcal***

Dicloxacillin
Methicillin
Nafcillin
Oxacillin

***Antipseudomonal***

Carbenicillin
Piperacillin
Ticarcillin

**Cephalosporins**

***1st Generation***

Cefadroxil
Cephazolin
Cephalexin
Cephradine

***2nd Generation***

Cefaclor
Cefotetan
Cefoxitin
Cefprozil
Cefuroxime

***3rd Generation***

Cefdinir
Cefoperazone
Cefotaxime
Ceftazidime
Ceftizoxime
Ceftibuten
Ceftriaxone

***4th Generation***

Cefepime

**Carbapenems**

Ertapenem
Imipenem/Cilastatin
Meropenem

**Monobactams**

Azactam

**β-Lactamase Inhibitors**

Clavulanic Acid
Sulbactam
Tazobactam

**Other Cell Wall Inhibitors**

Bacitracin
Vancomycin

### Antibiotics That Inhibit Protein Synthesis

**Tetracyclines**

Demeclocycline
Doxycycline
Minocycline
Tetracycline

**Aminoglycosides**

Amikacin
Gentamicin
Neomycin
Streptomycin
Tobramycin

**Macrolides**

Azithromycin
Clarithromycin
Erythromycin

**Other Protein Synthesis Inhibitors**

Chloramphenicol
Clindamycin
Linezolid
Quinupristin/Dalfopristin

By the early 1900s the idea that microbes caused infectious disease was well established. But while more and more physicians were focusing on cleanliness and sterility, infections were still the number one cause of death around the world. The research chemist Paul Ehrlich promoted the idea that it should be possible to invent a compound that would kill a specific micro-organism without causing undue harm to the body, what he referred to as chemotherapy. Biochemical and medical researchers were avidly hunting for compounds that would serve as "magic bullets," drugs that would target specific organisms without harming patients.

Alexander Fleming was one of those researchers. He earned his degree in medicine in 1906 and was keenly interested in the defense mechanisms of the human body. When World War I erupted, he served in the British Army's medical corps, where he was discouraged by the inability to treat wound infections, which often resulted in death. After the war, he went back to his research. One day in 1928 he left a culture dish smeared with a common skin dwelling bacteria called staphylococcus on the counter and then left on a holiday. On his return he discovered the petri dish was covered with bacteria, except for a wide ring of clear space around a mold growth that contaminated the dish. In a moment of insight, instead of tossing the ruined culture plate in with the other glassware that needed washing, Fleming decided to investigate further. He correctly believed that the mold was producing a substance that inhibited the growth of the surrounding bacteria. The mold was identified as Penicillium notatum, and he named the unidentified compound it secreted penicillin. It took 12 years and a team of Oxford researchers to finally isolate the drug penicillin, but Fleming's discovery changed health care forever. Besides saving millions of lives, his discovery gave momentum to the developing pharmaceutical industry and its search for other lifesaving drugs.

Also as a result of Fleming's discovery, a new word was added to the scientific lexicon: antibiotic. Antibiotics are defined as chemical substances produced by micro-organisms that inhibit the growth of other microorganisms. Now the word is often used interchangeably with the term antibacterial, any drug used to kill or suppress the growth of bacteria.

antibiotic A drug produced by or derived from a micro-organism and able to kill or inhibit the growth and reproduction of another micro-organism.

antibacterial Intended to kill or prevent the growth or reproduction of bacteria.

Most of the medications discussed in the first half of Chapter 29 are antibiotics that are chemically related to penicillin and work through similar mechanisms of action. These include the penicillins, cephalosporins, and a few others. The second half of the chapter covers drugs that, although chemically unrelated to each other, are loosely related through their mechanisms of action.

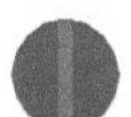

## Cell Wall Inhibitors

Drugs that inhibit cell wall formation are only effective against certain micro-organisms, and only those that have a cell wall. In order to treat infections appropriately, the causative bacteria must be correctly identified. The shape of bacteria is an important clue in identification of the organism. **Figure 29.1** illustrates the shapes of some common bacterial pathogens. Bacteria can also be neatly divided into two general types based on biochemical differences in their cell walls, another aid to identification. Staining the organisms with Gram's stain makes differentiation of cell wall types possible. Gram-positive organisms have a cell wall that absorbs the stain, and gram-negative organisms do not. Nearly all bacteria have one of these cell wall types, with the exception of Mycoplasma species, which have no cell walls, and Mycobacterium species, which have a different type of cell wall.

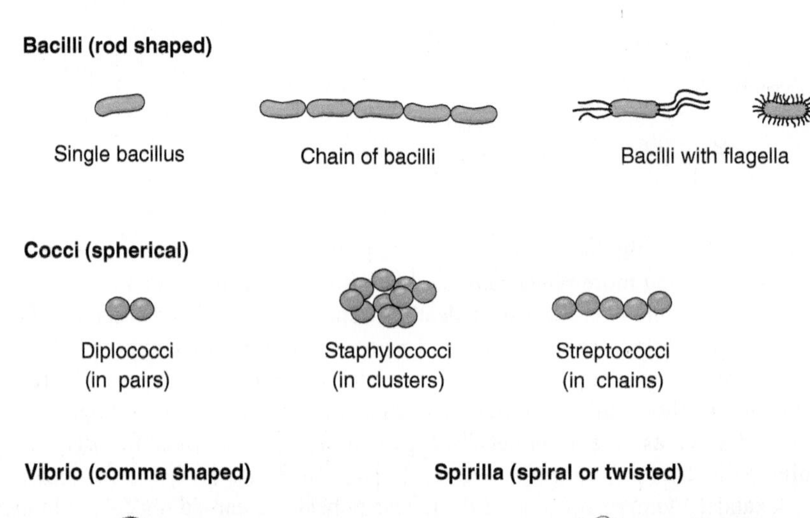


**Figure 29.1** Common shapes and arrangements of some important bacteria. (Adapted with permission from McConnell TH. *The Nature of Disease.* Baltimore: Lippincott Williams & Wilkins, 2007)

# Beta-Lactam Antibiotics

Drugs that are chemically related to penicillin are called β-lactam antibiotics, for the lactam ring contained in their chemical structure. These include the naturally occurring penicillin and cephalosporin antibiotics and their many synthetic cousins. Members of the β-lactam antibiotic group differ from one another because of their spectrum of activity, stability to stomach acid, and susceptibility to degradation by enzymes that some bacteria synthesize.

## Actions and Indications

The β-lactam antibiotics are among the most widely used antibiotics, but increased resistance limits their use in some cases. These drugs interfere with bacterial cell wall synthesis. The cell wall is a layered structure surrounding the organism that protects it from changes in osmotic pressure and provides support and shape (**Fig. 29.2**). Without their cell wall, bacteria cannot survive. While most bacteria require cell walls to survive, mammals and most other animals do not have these structures. This is important, because antibiotics that work by preventing bacteria from forming cell walls affect an area of bacterial metabolism that has no bearing on human metabolism. As a result, these antibiotics are some of our safest drugs.

Cell wall inhibitors are bacteriocidal, meaning they kill bacteria. The β-lactam antibiotics are most effective when bacteria are rapidly reproducing because this is the time when cell walls are formed. They are ineffective against organisms that lack a cell wall, such as protozoa, fungi, mycobacterium (cause of tuberculosis and leprosy), and viruses.

bacteriocidal Capable of killing bacteria.

Penicillins, cephalosporins, and related drugs bind to specific proteins (penicillin-binding proteins) in the cell wall in order to act. Some organisms are resistant to these antibiotics because they have fewer of the bindings sites. Others are resistant because their cell walls are less penetrable and the drugs must cross through the cell wall in order to take effect. In general the cell walls of gram-negative organisms are more difficult to penetrate, making these organisms more likely to be resistant to the β-lactam antibiotics.

The β-lactam antibiotics are indicated for the treatment of infection caused by susceptible organisms. When the organism identification is not final, physicians will prescribe a medication based on their knowledge of the infection site and the organisms most likely to cause infections there, patient specific information, and an understanding of the usual spectrum of activity of the drugs. This is referred to as empiric therapy. Because of their safety, β-lactam antibiotics are frequently chosen for empiric therapy.

Certain antibiotics are considered drugs of choice for specific infections. For example, penicillin G (Pfizerpen®) and penicillin VK (Veetids®) are naturally occurring penicillins that are mainly effective against gram-positive organisms, such as streptococcus. Penicillin VK is the drug of choice for the treatment of strep throat, caused by streptococcus bacteria. Penicillin G is the drug of choice for pneumococcal pneumonia, syphilis, and meningitis caused by *Neisseria meningitidis* (**Fig. 29.3**). Neisseria species are gram-negative cocci that are also responsible for causing gonorrhea.

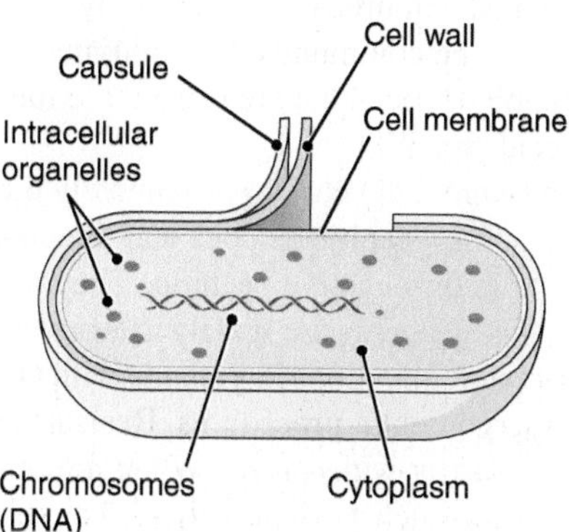


**Figure 29.2** An example of a cell wall, the membrane that surrounds and protects most bacteria. (Adapted with permission from McConnell TH. *The Nature of Disease*. Baltimore: Lippincott Williams & Wilkins, 2007)

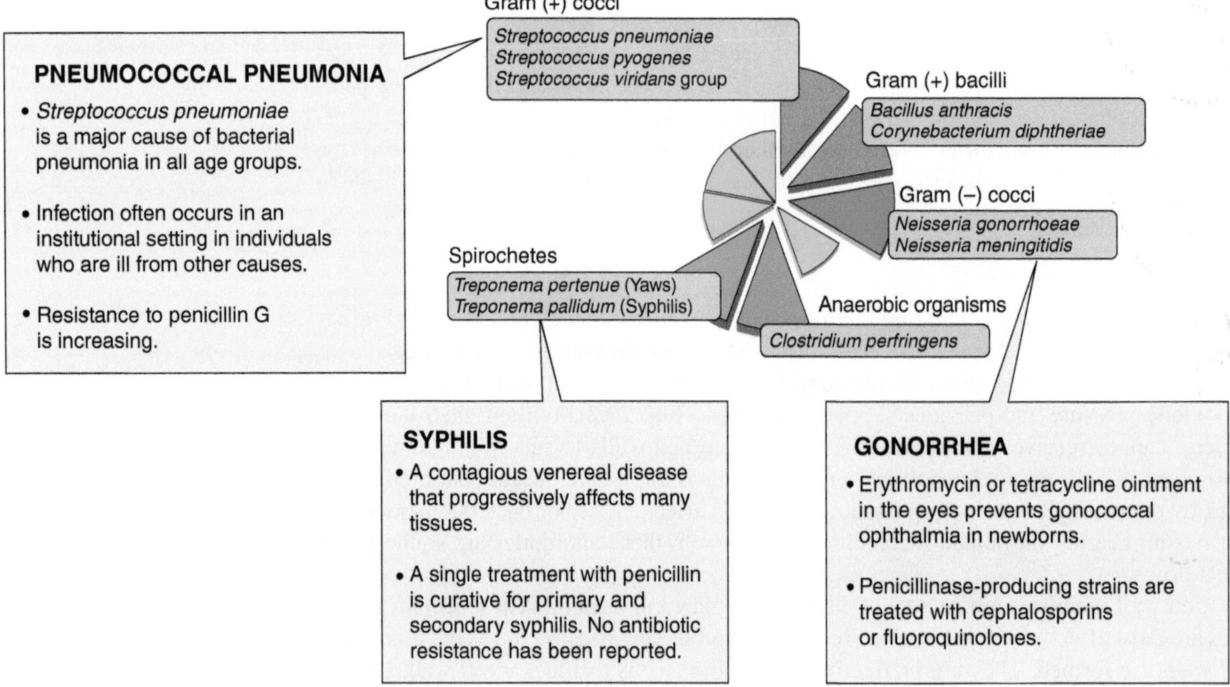

Gram (+) cocci
Streptococcus pneumoniae
Streptococcus pyogenes
Streptococcus viridans group
Gram (+) bacilli
Bacillus anthracis
Corynebacterium diphtheriae
Gram (–) cocci
Neisseria gonorrhoeae
Neisseria meningitidis
Spirochetes
Treponema pertenue (Yaws)
Treponema pallidum (Syphilis)
Anaerobic organisms
Clostridium perfringens
PNEUMOCOCCAL PNEUMONIA
• Streptococcus pneumoniae is a major cause of bacterial pneumonia in all age groups.
• Infection often occurs in an institutional setting in individuals who are ill from other causes.
• Resistance to penicillin G is increasing.
SYPHILIS
• A contagious venereal disease that progressively affects many tissues.
• A single treatment with penicillin is curative for primary and secondary syphilis. No antibiotic resistance has been reported.
GONORRHEA
• Erythromycin or tetracycline ointment in the eyes prevents gonococcal ophthalmia in newborns.
• Penicillinase-producing strains are treated with cephalosporins or fluoroquinolones.


**Figure 29.3** Some therapeutic applications of penicillin G. (Adapted with permission from Harvey RA, Champe PC, Howland RD, et al. Lippincott's Illustrated Reviews: *Pharmacology*, 3rd edition. Baltimore: Lippincott Williams & Wilkins, 2006.)

There are many other forms of penicillin besides penicillin G and penicillin VK. The other members of the penicillin family can be categorized as either antistaphylococcal, extended spectrum, or antipseudomonal penicillins. Penicillins are considered antistaphylococcal when they are resistant to the action of the enzyme penicillinase, produced by staphylococci. Drugs in this group include methicillin, the prototype, nafcillin (Unipen®), and dicloxacillin (Dynapen®). Methicillin is no longer available because it causes more serious side effects than the other drugs in the group. Use of the antistaphylococcal penicillins is limited to the treatment of infections caused by sensitive staphylococci.

Some staphylococcus species are part of the normal flora of the skin. Although *Staphylococcus aureus* is often found on the skin or nasal mucosa of healthy people, it can also be responsible for serious infections. *S. aureus* can cause infections as minor as localized skin infections or food poisoning, to more serious soft tissue infections (for example cellulitis), to life-threatening conditions such as pneumonia, endocarditis, or sepsis (a disease complex caused by overwhelming infection carried throughout the body by the blood stream). Previously a serious cause of nosocomial (hospital acquired) infections only, methicillin-resistant *staphylococcus aureus* (MRSA) now can be community acquired, meaning infections can be contracted outside of hospitals. Staphylococci that are resistant to methicillin are also resistant to the other anti-staphylococcal penicillins.

sepsis An infection of the bloodstream and the systemic response it causes.

Although ampicillin (Principen®) and amoxicillin (Amoxil®) have approximately the same effect as penicillin on gram-positive organisms such as staphylococcus and streptococcus, they are somewhat more effective against some gram-negative bacteria. They are therefore referred to as extended-spectrum penicillins. These agents are widely used in the treatment of respiratory infections, and by dentists to prevent infections in patients with abnormal heart valves or prosthetic joints who are to undergo dental procedures. Resistance to these antibiotics because of inactivation by penicillinase is widespread. When amoxicillin or ampicillin is combined with a β-lactamase inhibitor, such as clavulanic acid or sulbactam, they are protected from degradation, which extends their antimicrobial spectrum.

Carbenicillin (Geocillin®), ticarcillin (Ticar®), and piperacillin (Pipracil®) are called antipseudomonal penicillins because of their activity against Pseudomonas aeruginosa, a gram-negative bacillus that causes very serious nosocomial and sometimes community acquired infections. These antibiotics are effective against many other gram-negative bacilli as well. Combination of ticarcillin with clavulanic acid: (Timentin®) and piperacillin with tazobactam (Zosyn®) protects the drugs against penicillinase and broadly extends the antimicrobial spectrum of these antibiotics. These added compounds do not have intrinsic antibiotic activity and are never used alone.

The cephalosporins are β-lactam antibiotics that are closely related both structurally and functionally to the penicillins. Cephalosporins, like penicillins, block cell wall synthesis. In general, they are more impervious than the penicillins to destruction by β-lactamase, but they are subject to the same bacterial resistance mechanisms. Cephalosporins are classified as first, second, third, or fourth generation, based largely on the susceptibility of bacteria to their action. They are some of the most frequently used antibiotics and are prescribed for a variety of types of infections (**Fig. 29.4**). Experts believe that the overuse of

**First-generation cephalosporins**

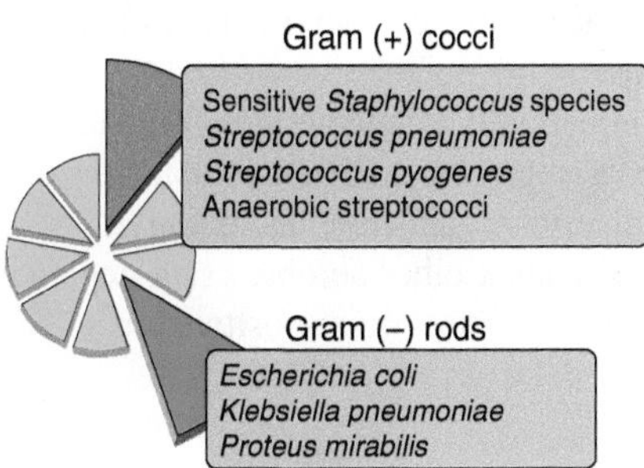


**Second-generation cephalosporins**

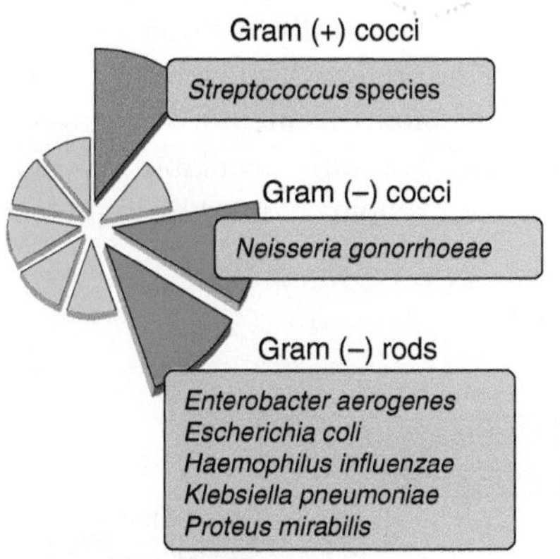


**Third-generation cephalosporins**

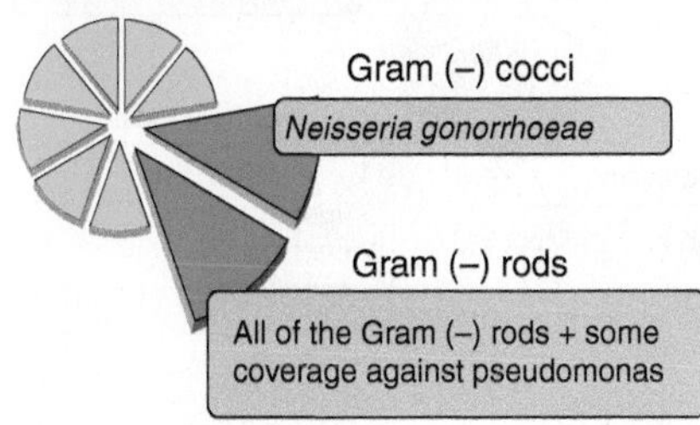


**Figure 29.4** Summary of the sensitivities of organisms to the cephalosporin antibiotics. (Adapted with permission from Harvey RA, Champe PC, Howland RD, et al. *Lippincott's Illustrated Reviews: Pharmacology*, 3rd edition. Baltimore: Lippincott Williams & Wilkins, 2006.)

broad-spectrum cephalosporins (such as the third-generation drugs) contributes significantly to the development of resistance in bacteria, including methicillin resistance.

Cephalosporins designated as "first-generation," for example cefazolin (Ancef®) and cephalexin (Keflex®), are effective against approximately the same organisms as penicillin G. Second-generation cephalosporins, such as cefuroxime (Ceftin®), display greater activity against a few additional gram-negative organisms, but activity against gram-positive organisms is weaker. Third-generation cephalosporins have even further enhanced activity against gram-negative organisms, including most enteric organisms. Ceftriaxone (Rocephin®) or cefotaxime (Claforan®) are often used in the treatment of meningitis because they reach effective concentrations in the cerebrospinal fluid. Cefepime (Maxipime®), classified as a fourth-generation cephalosporin, has a wide spectrum of antibacterial activity against gram-positive and gram-negative organisms including pseudomonas.

The carbapenems, imipenem (Primaxin®), meropenem (Merrem®), and ertapenem (Invanz®), are chemically related to penicillin. Imipenem must be given with cilastatin to protect it from degradation by bacterial enzymes. Imipenem and meropenem have a very broad spectrum of activity against both gram-negative and gram-positive microbes, including aerobic and anaerobic organisms (**Fig. 29.5**). Many experts regard imipenem and meropenem as two of the most reliable agents available to treat difficult infections, and they are generally reserved for the treatment of seriously ill people in order to discourage development of resistance. While it is also considered a broad spectrum antibiotic, ertapenem is not as effective in killing Pseudomonas and Acinetobacter species, two organisms that can cause serious infections usually acquired in hospitals.

Aztreonam (Azactam®), which is the only commercially available monobactam, has antimicrobial activity directed primarily against the large gram-negative rods that are associated with intestinal infections (gram-negative enteric organisms), including *E. coli*, Salmonella, and Shigella, among others. It also acts against other aerobic gram-negative rods, including *Pseudonomas aeruginosa*. It lacks activity against gram-positive organisms and anaerobes. Aztreonam is resistant to the action of β-lactamase enzymes.

## Administration

Most of the penicillins are subject to some degree of degradation in the acidic environment of the stomach. Drugs that are broken down by stomach acid are considered to be acid labile. Instability in the presence of acid is an important reason why some of the β-lactam drugs can only be given by injection. Penicillin G used to be given orally, but because penicillin VK is much more stable in the presence of acid, it is the preferred, and the only available oral natural penicillin for treatment of susceptible infections. Penicillin VK, amoxicillin, and amoxicillin combined with clavulanic acid are only available as oral preparations. Oral penicillins are normally taken on an empty stomach in order to protect them from stomach acid.

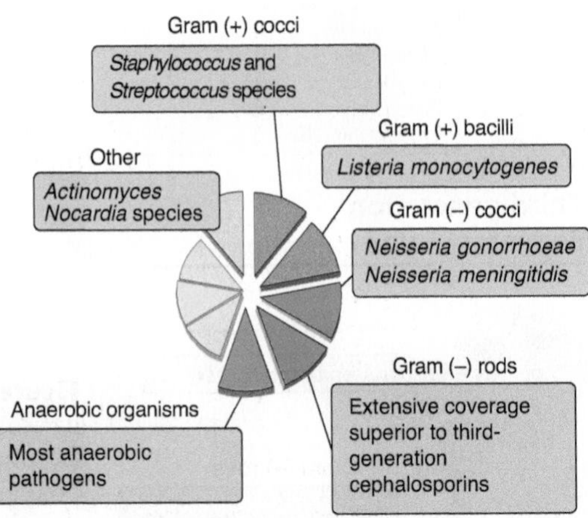


**Figure 29.5** The range of antimicrobial activity makes imipenem and meropenem especially useful for difficult to treat infections. (Adapted with permission from Harvey RA, Champe PC, Howland RD, et al. *Lippincott's Illustrated Reviews: Pharmacology*, 3rd edition. Baltimore: Lippincott Williams & Wilkins, 2006.)

Another factor that determines the choice of route of administration is the seriousness of the infection. Penicillin G is given intravenously for life-threatening infections, such as meningitis. Procaine penicillin G (Wycillin®) and benzathine penicillin G (Bicillin®) are long acting formulations given intramuscularly. They are slowly absorbed into the circulation and persist at low levels over a long time period, making them useful in the treatment of syphilis or when patient compliance is an issue. Ticarcillin, piperacillin, and the combinations of ampicillin with sulbactam (Unasyn®), ticarcillin with clavulanic acid, and piperacillin with tazobactam must be administered by intravenous or intramuscular injection.

Many of the cephalosporins are poorly absorbed after oral administration, too. First-generation drugs cefadroxil (Duricef®), cephradine (Velosef®), and cephalexin, second-generation agents cefaclor (Ceclor®) and cefprozil (Cefzil®), and third-generation drugs cefdinir (Omnicef®) are the only cephalosporins that are available in oral preparations. Of all the cephalosporins, only the third-generation drugs cross into the central nervous system in adequate amounts to treat infections there.

The carbapenems cannot be administered by mouth. Imipenem and meropenem are administered IV, and penetrate well into body tissues and fluids. Aztreonam can be administered either intravenously or intramuscularly, but not orally. **Table 29.1** lists the most important cell wall inhibitors by drug class, with brand names, formulations, and indications for use.

## Side Effects

Penicillins and cephalosporins are among the safest of all drugs. However, side effects can still occur. Allergic reactions are the most important adverse effects of the penicillins. Because they are closely related compounds, the cephalosporins should be used with caution in individuals who are allergic to penicillins. Approximately 10% of people with true penicillin allergy will also be allergic to cephalosporins. Patients who have had an anaphylactic response to penicillins should not receive cephalosporins. About 5% of people who take penicillin will experience some kind of allergic reaction, ranging from a rash to marked swelling of the lips and tongue, and anaphylaxis.

**Table 29.1** Names, Indications, and Formulations of Antibiotics That Inhibit Bacterial Cell Wall Synthesis

| Generic | Brand Name | Available as | Indications | Notes |
|---|---|---|---|---|
| **Natural Penicillins** | | | | |
| Penicillin G Aqueous | Pfizerpen® | Powder for injection, premixed IVPB bags | Meningitis, pneumonia caused by sensitive organisms | Store premixed bags in freezer, reconstituted soln in refrigerator |
| Penicillin G Benzathine | Bicillin L-A® | Sterile susp for IM injection in prefilled syringe | Syphilis, URI* caused by sensitive strep | Refrigerate, look-alike, sound-alike names |
| Penicillin G Procaine | Wycillin® | Sterile susp for IM injection in prefilled syringe | Bacteria sensitive to prolonged, low penicillin levels, syphilis | Refrigerate, look-alike, sound-alike names |
| Penicillin VK | V-Cillin K®, Veetids® | Tablets, powder for oral solution | Infections due to susceptible strep and pneumococci | Refrigerate solution |

(continues)

**Table 29.1** Names, Indications, and Formulations of Antibiotics That Inhibit Bacterial Cell Wall Synthesis *(continued)*

| Generic | Brand Name | Available as | Indications | Notes |
|---|---|---|---|---|
| **Extended-Spectrum Penicillins** | | | | |
| Amoxicillin | Amoxil®, Trimox® | Capsules, powder for oral suspension, chew tabs, tabs for oral suspension | UTI, URI caused by susceptible organisms | Look-alike, sound-alike names. Shake well, refrigerate oral suspension |
| Ampicillin | Principen® | Capsules, powder for oral suspension, powder for injection | Systemic, skin abdominal, & GU infections due to sensitive bacteria | Short IV stability in D5%/W. Look-alike, sound-alike names. Shake well, refrigerate oral suspension |
| **Antistaphylococcal Penicillins** | | | | |
| Dicloxacillin | Dynapen® | Capsules, powder for oral suspension | Infections due to susceptible staphylococci | Shake well, refrigerate oral suspension |
| Nafcillin | Unipen®, Nafcil® | Capsules, tablets, powder for injection, IVPB premix | Serious infections due to susceptible staphylococci | IVPB premixes stored frozen |
| Oxacillin | Bactocill® | Capsules, powder for oral solution, powder for injection, IVPB premix | Serious infections due to susceptible staphylococci | Refrigerate oral solution, IVPB premixes stored frozen |
| **Antipseudomonal Penicillins** | | | | |
| Carbenicillin | Geocillin® | Tablets | UTI, prostatitis due to sensitive bacteria | Not effective for systemic infections |
| Piperacillin | Pipracil® | Powder for injection, ADD-vantage vials | Serious infections due to sensitive bacteria | Refrigerate after reconstitution |
| Ticarcillin | Ticar® | Powder for injection | Serious infections due to sensitive bacteria | Refrigerate after reconstitution |
| **Penicillin Combinations** | | | | |
| Pen G Procaine + Benzathine | Bicillin C-R® | Sterile susp for IM injection in prefilled syringe | Some strep infections | Refrigerate. Look-alike, sound-alike names |
| Amoxicillin + Clavulanate | Augmentin®, Augmentin XR® | Tablets, chew tabs, powder for oral suspension, ER tabs | URI, UTI, OM, other infections due to sensitive bacteria | Dose based on amoxicillin component. Shake well, Refrigerate oral suspension |
| Ampicillin + Sulbactam | Unasyn® | Powder for Injection | Serious infections due to sensitive bacteria | Refrigerate after reconstitution |
| Piperacillin + Tazobactam | Zosyn® | Powder for injection, ADD-vantage vials, IVPB premix | Serious infections due to sensitive bacteria | IVPB premixes stored frozen |

*(continues)*

| Generic | Brand Name | Available as | Indications | Notes |
|---|---|---|---|---|
| **Penicillin Combinations** | | | | |
| Ticarcillin + Clavulanate | Timentin® | Powder for injection, ADD-vantage vials, IVPB premixes | Serious infections due to sensitive bacteria | Refrigerate after reconstitution, IVPB premixes stored frozen |
| **1st-Generation Cephalosporins** | | | | |
| Cefadroxil | Duricef® | Capsules, tablets, powder for suspension | UTI, strep throat, skin infections due to sensitive bacteria | Shake well, refrigerate oral suspension |
| Cephazolin | Ancef® | Powder for injection, ADD-vantage vials, IVPB premix | Serious infections due to sensitive bacteria | Refrigerate after reconstitution, IVPB premixes stored frozen |
| Cephalexin | Keflex® | Capsules, tablets, powder for susp. | Infections due to sensitive bacteria | Shake well, refrigerate oral suspension |
| Cephradine | Velosef® | Capsules, powder for suspension | URI, UTI, OM & skin infections due to sensitive bacteria | Shake well, refrigerate oral suspension |
| **2nd-Generation Cephalosporins** | | | | |
| Cefaclor | Ceclor® | Capsules, ER tabs, powder for suspension | URI, UTI, OM, & pneumonia due to sensitive bacteria | Shake well, refrigerate oral suspension |
| Cefotetan | Cefotan® | Powder for injection, ADD-vantage vials, IVPB premix | Serious infections due to sensitive bacteria | Refrigerate after reconstitution, IVPB premixes stored frozen |
| Cefoxitin | Mefoxin® | Powder for injection, IVPB premix | Serious infections due to sensitive bacteria | Refrigerate after reconstitution, IVPB premixes stored frozen |
| Cefprozil | Cefzil® | Tablets, powder for oral suspension | URI, OM, tonsillitis due to sensitive bacteria | Shake well, refrigerate oral suspension |
| Cefuroxime | Ceftin®, Zinacef® | Tablets, powder for oral suspension, powder for injection, IVPB premix | URI, OM, UTI, GU, other serious infections due to sensitive bacteria | Shake well, store susp in or out of refrigerator refrigerate IV after mixing, IVPB premixes stored frozen |
| **3rd-Generation Cephalosporins** | | | | |
| Cefdinir | Omnicef® | Capsules, powder for oral suspension | Pneumonia, URI due to sensitive bacteria | Shake well, store oral suspension at room temp |
| Cefoperazone | Cefobid® | Powder for injection and IVPB premixes | Serious infections due to sensitive bacteria | Refrigerate after reconstitution, IVPB premixes stored frozen |
| Cefotaxime | Claforan® | Powder for injection and IVPB premixes | Serious infections due to sensitive bacteria | Refrigerate after reconstitution, IVPB premixes stored frozen |

*(continues)*

**Table 29.1** Names, Indications, and Formulations of Antibiotics That Inhibit Bacterial Cell Wall Synthesis *(continued)*

| Generic | Brand Name | Available as | Indications | Notes |
|---|---|---|---|---|
| **3rd-Generation Cephalosporins** | | | | |
| Ceftazidime | Fortaz®, Tazicef®, others | Powder for injection, ADD-vantage vials, IVPB premixes | Serious infections due to sensitive bacteria | Refrigerate after reconstitution, IVPB premixes stored frozen |
| Ceftizoxime | Cefizox® | Powder for injection IVPB premixes | Serious infections including STDs due to sensitive bacteria | Refrigerate after reconstitution, IVPB premixes stored frozen |
| Ceftibuten | Cedax® | Capsules, powder for oral suspension | URI, OM, tonsillitis due to sensitive bacteria | Shake well, refrigerate oral suspension |
| Ceftriaxone | Rocephin® | Powder for injection, ADD-vantage vials, IVPB premixes | Serious infections including STDs due to sensitive bacteria | Refrigerate after reconstitution, IVPB premixes stored frozen |
| **4th-Generation Cephalosporin** | | | | |
| Cefepime | Maxipime® | Powder for injection, ADD-vantage vials | Serious infections, especially pseudomonas | Refrigerate after reconstitution |
| **Carbapenems and Monobactams** | | | | |
| Ertapenem | Invanz® | Powder for injection | Serious infections when other drugs ineffective | Less effective than other monobactams. Refrigerate solutions |
| Imipenem/Cilastatin | Primaxin® | Powder for injection, ADD-vantage vials | Serious infections when other drugs ineffective | Refrigerate after reconstitution |
| Meropenem | Merrem® | Powder for injection | Serious infections when other drugs ineffective | Refrigerate after reconstitution |
| Aztreonam | Azactam® | Powder for injection, IVPB premixes | Serious infections when other drugs ineffective | Refrigerate after reconstitution, IVPB premixes stored frozen |
| **Other Cell Wall Inhibitors** | | | | |
| Bacitracin | | Ointment, eye ointment, powder for injection | Topical-superficial infections, limited systemic use | |
| Vancomycin | Vancocin® | Staphylococcal infections, especially MRSA, PO for *Clostridium difficile* | Powder for injection, ADD-vantage vials, capsules, powder for oral solution | Refrigerate IV and solution after reconstitution |

ER, extended release; GU, genitourinary; IVPB, intravenous piggyback; MRSA, methicillin resistant staph aureus; OM, otitis media; PO, by mouth; STD, sexually transmitted disease; strep, streptococci; URI, upper respiratory infection; UTI, urinary tract infection.

Diarrhea is a fairly common side effect of antibiotic use that is caused by disruption of the normal balance of intestinal micro-organisms. It occurs to a greater extent with antibiotics that are incompletely absorbed after oral administration, or that have an extended antibacterial spectrum. All of the drugs mentioned in this chapter have the potential to cause diarrhea, sometimes severe.

Many medications and some infections have the potential to cause inflammation in the kidneys called acute interstitial nephritis. Although all penicillins have the potential to cause this condition, methicillin was much more likely to do so. This trait is the main reason methicillin use declined and it was removed from the market. Another side effect common to the class is irritation to nerve tissue, which is important in certain situations. Penicillin drugs can provoke seizures if very high blood levels are reached. This is unlikely to occur unless excessively high doses are administered intravenously, high doses are infused rapidly, or the patient has renal failure. Likewise, high levels of imipenem are associated with seizures, but meropenem is less likely to cause them. Epileptic patients are particularly at risk for this side effect of the penicillins and carbapenems. Lastly, the antipseudomonal penicillins, and more importantly, cefamandole, cefoperazone, and cefotetan can predispose at-risk patients, such as those receiving anticoagulants, to bleeding.

interstitial nephritis Inflammation of the renal tubules and glomerulus; often a reaction to a medication.

## Tips for the Technician

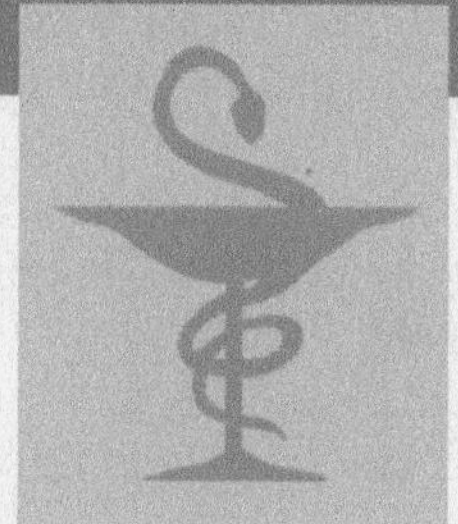

Oral penicillins and cephalosporins are often prescribed for use in children, and are usually available in granules or powders for suspension. These products are mixed in the pharmacy, immediately prior to dispensing. Nearly all must be stored in the refrigerator and are stable for 14 days after mixing. Cefdinir and cefuroxime suspensions are only good for 10 days under refrigeration. Cephradine is stable for 7 days out of the refrigerator, but 14 days under refrigeration. Refrigeration generally improves the taste and is recommended when available. Suspensions of all kinds are always labelled with "shake well" instructions. In addition, antibiotic suspensions should be labelled with refrigeration instructions when necessary, and instructions to finish all the medication unless otherwise directed by the doctor. Even though not all penicillins are equally acid labile, oral penicillins are routinely labelled with instructions to take the medication on an empty stomach. Oral cephalosporins can usually be taken with food.

Injectable penicillins and cephalosporins arrive in the pharmacy as dry powders for reconstitution unless they are premixed intravenous piggybacks. **Intravenous piggybacks (IVPB), sometimes referred to as mini bags, are small sterile IV bags that can be "piggybacked" onto the IV line attached to a large volume parenteral. Use of these bags allows for more expedient administration of IV drugs than administration by slow IV injection, because they can be given without constant supervision by nursing staff.** Premixed piggyback penicillins and cephalosporins are delivered and stored frozen, and then thawed before use. If they are not used once thawed, they can usually be returned to the refrigerator and kept for 2 or more days, depending on the drug. Before reconstitution of dry powders for injection, penicillin and cephalosporin products are stored on the shelf. After reconstitution, most injectable penicillins and cephalosporins are good for several days if stored in the refrigerator. However, the stability of ampicillin is quite variable, depending on the diluent. Stability data is available in the package insert or in an intravenous admixture reference.

intravenous piggyback A small-volume, single-dose, sterile preparation used to administer medications into an IV line at specific times.

## Other Cell Wall Inhibitors

Other cell wall inhibitors include vancomycin and bacitracin. Vancomycin (Vancocin®) is increasingly important because of its effectiveness against drug-resistant MRSA and enterococci. Although bacitracin (Baciguent®) was once more widely used, its use is generally restricted to topical application because of its potential for toxicity.

## Actions and Indications

Vancomycin inhibits synthesis of components of the bacterial cell wall. It weakens the cell wall and damages the underlying cell membrane, eventually killing the bacteria. Vancomycin is primarily effective against gram-positive organisms and is usually reserved for organisms resistant to others antibiotics, such as MRSA and enterococcus, and for severe infections, such as endocarditis. Vancomycin can also be used for enterocolitis associated with antibiotic use. Bacitracin works by inhibiting bacterial cell wall synthesis, and is active against a wide variety of gram-positive organisms.

## Administration

Vancomycin and bacitracin are both large molecules that are not absorbed orally. They can be administered orally, however, to treat colitis caused by overgrowth of *Clostridium difficile*, associated with antibiotic use. Bacitracin is less likely to be used for this indication than vancomycin, and vancomycin is less frequently used than another antimicrobial, metronidazole. Vancomycin is given intravenously for systemic infections, and its dose must be adjusted in patients with impaired renal function. Hospital pharmacists often adjust doses for physicians based on serum drug levels and knowledge of patient-specific parameters, such as height, weight, and renal function.

Bacitracin is far more likely to be applied topically than by any other route. It is available without prescription, alone and in combination with other antibiotics, for use on minor cuts and scrapes. The ophthalmic ointment is sold by prescription only.

## Side Effects

As compared with most of the other cell wall inhibitors, systemic administration of bacitracin is unacceptably risky. Along with overgrowth of nonsusceptible bacteria, use of injectable bacitracin is associated with renal failure, hearing loss, allergic reactions, tightness in the chest, and low blood pressure. Some hearing loss can even occur after prolonged topical use over large areas.

Although not as toxic as bacitracin, vancomycin shares some of these adverse effects. Vancomycin can cause hearing loss, especially if it is administered with other ototoxic drugs, or when drug levels are excessive for prolonged periods. Similarly, kidney damage from vancomycin use can occur with excessive vancomycin levels or when vancomycin is used while the patient is taking other nephrotoxic drugs. When vancomycin is administered too rapidly, a syndrome of flushing, reddened skin, itching, and in severe cases, fever and chills can occur. This is commonly referred to as "red man's syndrome" and occurs because of vancomycin induced histamine release. It is not considered a true allergic reaction, because when the infusion is slowed, patients who have experienced this reaction can usually continue treatment. Vancomycin can cause true allergic reactions, however. It is often associated with pain at the injection site.

### Tips for the Technician

Only hospital-based technicians are likely to handle vancomycin for injection. Although it is available in 500-mg and 1-g vials, technicians will most often have to work with odd doses and calculate the appropriate vancomycin volumes to add to piggyback bags. Be sure to have calculations checked before compounding and dilute the sterile powder according to manufacturers recommendations. When doses of 500 mg or 1 g are prescribed, Add-Vantage® system vials are available. Add-vantage® and similar systems are designed for ease of preparation, a lower risk of contamination during preparation, and reduced waste. These piggyback systems are closed to room air or touch contamination, and are easily reconstituted by nurses immediately before administration.

Every 500 mg of vancomycin should be diluted with at least 100 mL of appropriate IVPB fluid before administration. Appropriate dilution reduces the risk of pain at the site of administration. When technicians are finished with compounding operations, it is important to label any partial vials with the drug concentration, the date of reconstitution and the initials of the compounding technician before refrigeration, so that remaining drug can safely be used later.

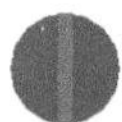

# Protein Synthesis Inhibitors

A number of antibiotics exert their antimicrobial effects by targeting the bacterial ribosome. All cells contain ribosomes, which are small cellular organelles responsible for synthesizing proteins based on instructions within nucleic acids. Bacterial ribosomes differ somewhat from their mammalian counterparts, but share many similarities. Although these antibiotics usually spare the host cells, they are associated with greater risks of toxicity than the antibiotics that block cell wall synthesis.

ribosome Granular organelles found in the cytoplasm of cells and responsible for protein synthesis.

## Tetracyclines

The tetracyclines are a group of closely related compounds that, as the name implies, contains four rings in their chemical structure. Additions to the ring structures are responsible for variation in their pharmacokinetics, and small differences within the class.

### Actions and Indications

The tetracyclines pass through the cell walls of susceptible organisms, where the drug binds reversibly to the bacterial ribosome. By blocking access to the nucleic acid where protein synthesis occurs, cell wall formation is inhibited. The tetracyclines are broad-spectrum antibiotics, and are effective against gram-positive and gram-negative bacteria, as well as several types of atypical bacteria (mycoplasma, rickettsia, and chlamydia), and even some nonbacterial microbes such as protozoa. The tetracyclines are considered bacteriostatic drugs because they inhibit the growth and reproduction of bacteria without killing them. When bacterial replication is controlled, the immune system is able to manage the destruction of the infecting organisms. This drug class is ineffective against viruses and fungi. The tetracyclines are the drugs of choice for a few exotic infectious diseases, including Lyme disease, plague, and cholera (refer to **Fig. 29.6**), and are also used for more mundane infections like sinus infections or acne.

bacteriostatic Capable of inhibiting the growth and replication of bacteria.

The most frequently used tetracyclines include tetracycline (Sumycin®), minocycline (Minocin®), and doxycycline (Vibramycin®). Tetracycline is used in low doses for the treatment of acne. The CDC recommends doxycycline to prevent malaria when travellers visit countries where chloroquine resistant forms of malaria occur. Minocycline is an alternative to doxycycline and is also useful for the treatment of rheumatoid arthritis, especially in the early stages of the disease. Resistance prevents these drugs from being particularly useful in the treatment of infections caused by staphylococcus, pseudomonas, and other nosocomial infections. Demeclocycline (Declomycin®), another tetracycline, is rarely used for infection because of its effect on the kidneys. It is, however, used to treat cases of hyponatremia (low blood levels of sodium) that are associated with excessive action of antidiuretic hormone, because demeclocycline blocks the action of antidiuretic hormone to cause the formation of very dilute urine, and removal of excess water.

hyponatremia Unusually low serum sodium levels.

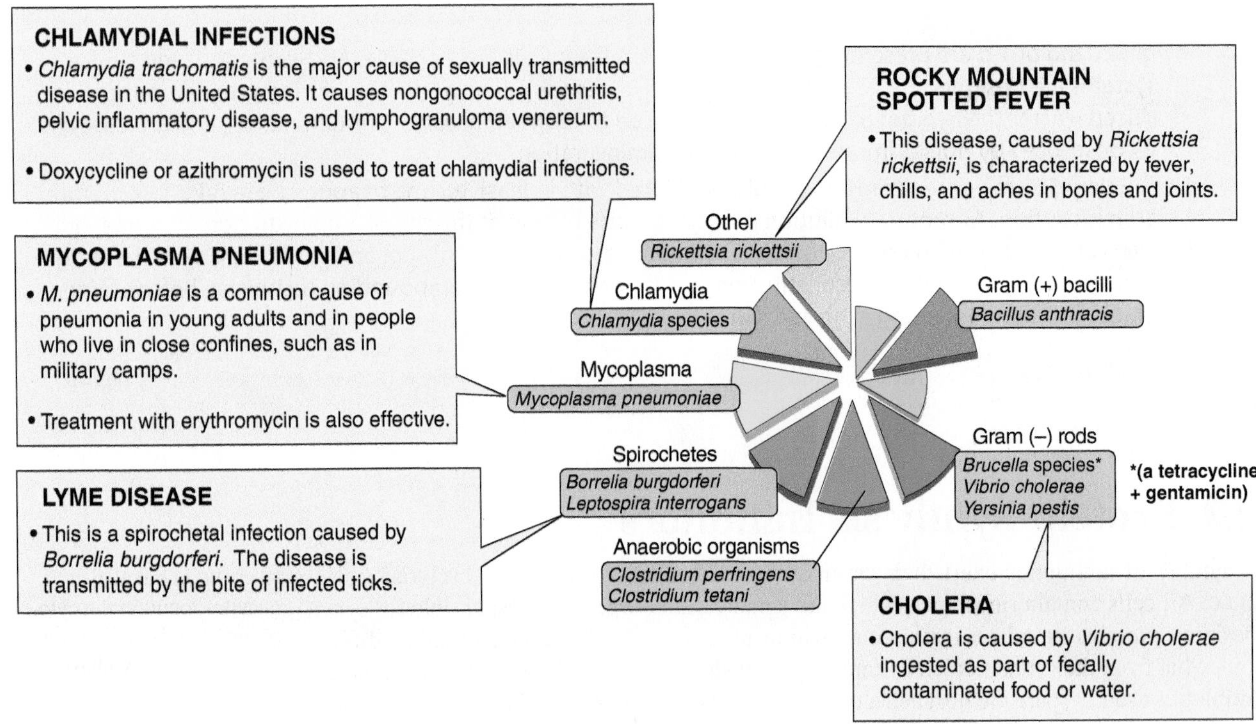

CHLAMYDIAL INFECTIONS
• Chlamydia trachomatis is the major cause of sexually transmitted disease in the United States. It causes nongonococcal urethritis, pelvic inflammatory disease, and lymphogranuloma venereum.
• Doxycycline or azithromycin is used to treat chlamydial infections.
ROCKY MOUNTAIN SPOTTED FEVER
• This disease, caused by Rickettsia rickettsii, is characterized by fever, chills, and aches in bones and joints.
MYCOPLASMA PNEUMONIA
• M. pneumoniae is a common cause of pneumonia in young adults and in people who live in close confines, such as in military camps.
• Treatment with erythromycin is also effective.
LYME DISEASE
• This is a spirochetal infection caused by Borrelia burgdorferi. The disease is transmitted by the bite of infected ticks.
Other
Rickettsia rickettsii
Chlamydia
Chlamydia species
Gram (+) bacilli
Bacillus anthracis
Mycoplasma
Mycoplasma pneumoniae
Gram (–) rods
Brucella species*
Vibrio cholerae
Yersinia pestis
*(a tetracycline + gentamicin)
Spirochetes
Borrelia burgdorferi
Leptospira interrogans
Anaerobic organisms
Clostridium perfringens
Clostridium tetani
CHOLERA
• Cholera is caused by Vibrio cholerae ingested as part of fecally contaminated food or water.


**Figure 29.6** Uses and antimicrobial activity of the tetracyclines. (Adapted with permission from Harvey RA, Champe PC, Howland RD, et al. *Lippincott's Illustrated Reviews: Pharmacology*, 3rd edition. Baltimore: Lippincott Williams & Wilkins, 2006.)

## Administration

All tetracyclines are adequately but incompletely absorbed after oral administration. However, taking tetracycline with dairy foods significantly decreases absorption because tetracycline combines with calcium to form nonabsorbable compounds called chelates. The same interaction occurs when the tetracyclines are taken with magnesium and aluminum antacids and iron preparations. Besides oral administration, doxycycline and minocycline are also available in formulations for intravenous administration (refer to **Table 29.2** for a listing of available products).

After administration the tetracyclines are widely distributed throughout the body, but they concentrate in the liver, kidney, and skin, and they bind to teeth and bones. All tetracyclines cross the placental barrier and concentrate in fetal bones and teeth. As a result, the tetracyclines are contraindicated for use during pregnancy. Because they stay in the body longer, doxycycline and minocycline can be given once or twice daily, while tetracycline is generally administered 4 times daily.

## Side Effects

The most common side effects seen with this class of drugs are mild and reversible. GI distress results from irritation of the gastric mucosa. If this is severe, the drugs can be taken with food as long as dairy products or antacids are avoided. Because of their broad antibacterial spectrum the tetracyclines disrupt normal flora, which can result in diarrhea, sometimes quite severe. For the same reason, yeast infections, including oral or vaginal candidiasis, are a common result of tetracycline treatment. Severe sunburn can occur when a patient taking these medications receives excessive sun exposure, as a result of tetracycline-induced photosensitivity.

While generally safe, the tetracyclines can be associated with serious side effects. Deposition in the bones and teeth occurs when tetracyclines are given to growing children. This causes permanent discoloration of the teeth and a temporary slowing of growth. These

**Table 29.2** Names, Indications, and Formulations of Antibiotics That Inhibit Protein Synthesis

| Generic | Brand Name | Available as | Indications | Notes |
|---|---|---|---|---|
| **Tetracyclines** | | | | |
| Demeclocycline | Declomycin® | Tablets | Infections due to gram (-) & atypical bacteria, SIADH | Avoid dairy products and antacids |
| Doxycycline | Vibramycin®, Vibra-Tabs® | Capsule, tablets, powder for oral susp, powder for injection, syrup | Infections due to gram (-) & atypical bacteria (plague, brucellosis, chlamydia, cholera, etc.), some STDs, amebiasis, malaria prevention | Store injection in refrigerator or freezer after mixing |
| Minocycline | Minocin® | Capsule, tablets, oral suspension, powder for injection | Same infections as doxycycline plus early RA, treatment of asymptomatic meningococcal carriers | |
| Tetracycline | Sumycin® | Capsules, oral suspension | Same infections as doxycycline, plus treatment of acne | Avoid dairy products and antacids |
| **Aminoglycosides** | | | | |
| Amikacin | Amikin® | Solution for injection | Serious infections due to organisms resistant to tobramycin & gentamicin | Amikin® looks & sounds like Amicar® |
| Gentamicin | Garamycin® | Solution for inj, ADD-vantage, IVPB premix, cream & ointment, ophthalmic soln. & ointment | Treatment of infection due to sensitive gram (-) & gram (+), bacteria including respiratory, skin, soft tissue, bone, abdominal | CAUTION—adult and pediatric soln for injection concentrations are different |
| Neomycin | Neo-Fradin® | Tablets, bladder irrigant, with other abx in ointment, cream, ophthalmic | PO – Bowel prep for surgery, GU—bladder irrigant, topical-minor infections, ophthalmic infections | |
| Streptomycin | | Powder for injection | Tuberculosis, other mycobacterial infections | |
| Tobramycin | Nebcin® | Solution for injection, ophthalmic oint, ophthalmic solution | Infection due to sensitive bacteria, often gram (-) & staph, including respiratory, skin, soft tissue, bone, abdominal | CAUTION—adult and pediatric soln for injection concentrations are different |

*(continues)*

**Table 29.2** Names, Indications, and Formulations of Antibiotics That Inhibit Protein Synthesis *(continued)*

| Generic | Brand Name | Available as | Indications | Notes |
|---|---|---|---|---|
| **Macrolides** | | | | |
| Azithromycin | Zithromax®, Z-Pak® | Powder for injection, powder for oral suspension, tablets | Infections of respiratory tract, OM, STDs, COPD exacerbations & strep throat due to sensitive bacteria including myco-plasma, chlamydia, and others. | Macrolides useful in PCN allergic patients |
| Clarithromycin | Biaxin® | Tablets, ER tabs, granules for oral suspension | Same as azithromycin + mycobacterium avium, mycobacterium intra-cellulare, tx of *H. pylori* ulcer disease. | Shake well, do not store reconstituted suspen-sion in refrigerator. |
| Erythromycin base, estolate, ethylsuccinate, stearate, others | Erythrocin®, Eryc.®, E.E.S.® | Powder for injection, ADD-Vantage, tablets, EC tablets, ER caps, chew tabs, granules for oral suspension & oral susp, topical gel, solution ointment, ophthalmic ointment | Infections due to sensitive organisms, including STDs, strep throat, respiratory infections (mycoplasma), amoebic dysentery, acne, bowel prep, eye infections | Different salts are not interchangeable |
| **Other Inhibitors of Protein Synthesis** | | | | |
| Chloramphenicol | Chloro-mycetin.® | Powder for injection | Serious infections not susceptible to other antibiotics | |
| Clindamycin | Cleocin.® | Solution for injection, IVPB premix, capsules, granules for oral solu-tion, topical foam, gel, lotion, solution, vaginal cream & suppository | Infections due to sus-ceptible aerobic & anaerobic bacteria, PID, vaginal infections, acne | Do not store reconstituted oral solution in refrigerator. |
| Linezolid | Zyvox.® | IVPB premix, tablets, powder for oral sus-pension | Serious infections due to VRE or MRSA | Suspension, shake well |
| Quinupristin/ Dalfopristin | Synercid.® | Powder for injection | Life-threatening or serious infections due to VRE or MRSA | Refrigerate before and after mixing |

COPD, chronic obstructive pulmonary disease; EC, enteric coated; ER, extended release; GU, genitourinary; MRSA, methicillin resistant staph aureus; OM, Otitis Media; PCN, penicillin; PID, pelvic inflammatory disease; RA, rheumatoid arthritis; tx, treatment; SIADH, syndrome of inappropriate ADH; STD, sexu-ally transmitted disease; VRE, Vancomycin resistant enterococcus.

drugs should never be administered to children under the age of 9, or to nursing or pregnant women. Besides crossing the placenta, fatal liver toxicity can occur in pregnant women who receive high doses of tetracyclines.

The tetracyclines can suppress the formation of white blood cells in the bone marrow and can cause elevations in intracranial pressure known as pseudotumor cerebri. This side effect is more commonly seen in people taking minocycline, and is associated with headache and vision changes that can be quite serious if the drug is not discontinued. Lastly, as tetracycline deteriorates it becomes toxic to the kidneys. For this reason, patients should be warned against using outdated tetracycline.

### Tips for the Technician

When dispensing new prescriptions to outpatients, it is appropriate for technicians to encourage cllients to speak to the pharmacist about possible side effects. Attach auxiliary labels that instruct patients to avoid dairy products and antacids, and to complete all the medication unless otherwise directed. They should be warned to avoid exposure to sunlight, and to discard any remaining drug after the expiration date. Technicians who compound tetracyclines for intravenous use can improve patient comfort by diluting these antibiotics appropriately. The tetracyclines can cause pain and irritation during infusion, especially if they are not adequately diluted.

## Aminoglycosides

Aminoglycosides are antibiotics derived from soil organisms called actinomycetes. Although aminoglycosides were once the antibiotics of choice for serious infections caused by gram-negative bacilli (Fig. 29.1), there are now safer antibiotics, such as the antipseudomonal penicillins, third-generation cephalosporins, and the carbapenems, that are in many cases equally effective in these circumstances. The aminoglycoside antibiotics are still important for treatment however, especially when there is resistance to the cephalosporins. In life-threatening infections caused by gram-negative organisms, aminoglycosides are almost always used, often in combination with another antibiotic, such as the antipseudomonal penicillins or cephalosporins.

### Actions and Indications

Aminoglycosides diffuse through pores in the cell walls of bacteria. The antibiotics work by altering bacterial protein synthesis. Aminoglycosides irreversibly bind to the ribosome where they block protein synthesis or cause the ribosome to misread the genetic code, producing abnormal proteins. The aminoglycosides act synergistically with β-lactam antibiotics, because cephalosporins enhance passage of the aminoglycosides into the bacteria. This means that when the antibiotics from both classes are used together, their effects are greater than the sum of the effect of treatment with each alone. Aminoglycosides are bacteriocidal and are effective against most gram-negative organisms and some gram-positive organisms. They are ineffective against anaerobic bacteria, viruses, or fungi.

synergistic effect An effect from the combination of two drugs that is greater than the sum of the effect of the two substances acting alone.

The aminoglycosides are usually reserved for serious infections, such as meningitis, postoperative infections, sepsis, or endocarditis, when other antibiotics are not likely to be effective. They are very often given along with one of the penicillins or cephalosporins to improve effectiveness, especially for use against difficult to treat organisms such as pseudomonas or staphylococcus. They can also be used alone for some infections with susceptible gram-negative organisms. Streptomycin is rarely used for systemic infections, other than mycobacterium infections. It is considered a first-line drug against mycobacterium tuberculosis, where it may be combined with other first-line antibiotics. However, it is less likely to be used than safer antitubercular drugs.

## Administration

Aminoglycoside antibiotics are not absorbed after oral administration, and are therefore given parenterally for system infections. They can be given by intravenous or intramuscular injection. For treatment of infections of the central nervous system, they must be injected into the space around the spinal cord (intrathecal injection) or into the ventricles of the brain. Gentamicin (Garamycin®), tobramycin (Nebcin®), and amikacin (Amikin®) are the aminoglycosides most frequently used for systemic infections and they are available in a variety of different preparations.

Aminoglycosides can be used for their local bacteriocidal effects. Neomycin (Neo-Fradin®) is never used for systemic infections, but it is given orally to reduce the bacterial count in preparation for bowel surgery. It is frequently combined with other antibiotics (Neosporin®, a combination of neomycin, bacitracin, and polymyxin) in preparations for superficial skin infections, ophthalmic infections or for infections of the ear canal. Gentamicin is available in a variety of topical preparations for treatment of superficial wounds or minor infections, and as ophthalmic ointment and solution for treatment of conjunctivitis or other infections of the outer surfaces of the eye or lids. Tobramycin is available for ophthalmic use, and in a preparation for inhalation.

When administered systemically, the aminoglycosides are dependant upon the kidney for removal from the body. Because they are concentrated in the kidneys, they can be quite useful for treating severe or resistant infections of the kidney and bladder. Aminoglycosides are not metabolized by the liver. Dosages of these drugs must be adjusted based on the kidney function of the patient and results of serum drug levels, to avoid toxicity. This is a function most often undertaken by hospital pharmacists.

## Side Effects

Toxicity from the aminoglycosides is related to high doses and prolonged therapy. These drugs concentrate in the inner ear and kidney after prolonged therapy, a fact that is likely related to their tendency to cause hearing loss and kidney failure (**Fig. 29.7**). Deafness can be irreversible when early signs of hearing loss are undetected and the drug is continued. Patients that receive another ototoxic drug simultaneously, such as the loop diuretics, are particularly at risk for hearing loss. Vertigo and loss of balance (especially in patients receiving streptomycin) may also occur because of the drug's effect on the inner ear. Kidney damage ranging from mild, reversible renal impairment to severe renal failure, which can be irreversible, can also occur with prolonged or high dose aminoglycoside therapy.

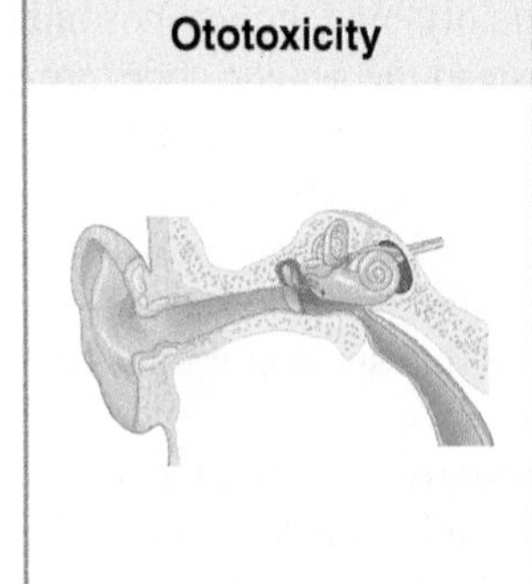


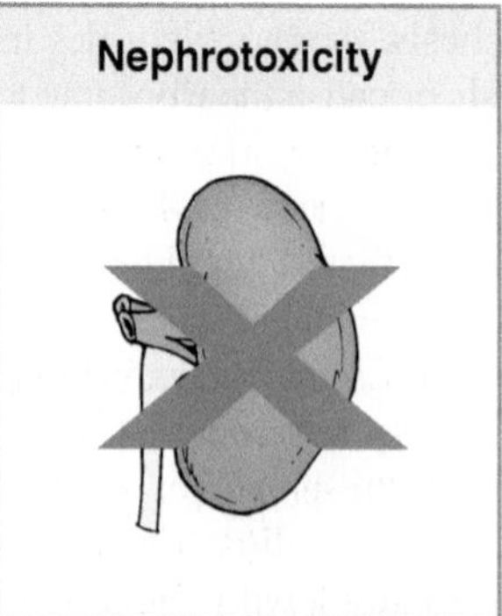


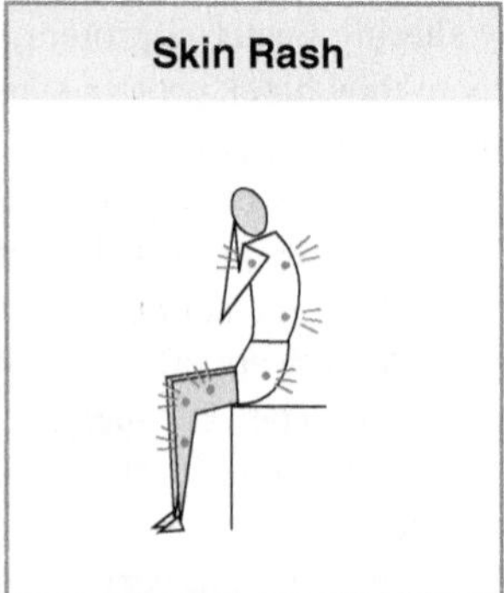


**Figure 29.7** Side effects commonly associated with aminoglycoside use. (Adapted with permission from Harvey RA, Champe PC, Howland RD, et al. *Lippincott's Illustrated Reviews: Pharmacology*, 3rd edition. Baltimore: Lippincott Williams & Wilkins, 2006.)

Advanced age, dehydration, and concurrent use of other nephrotoxic drugs are additional risk factors for developing renal failure.

Much less frequently, the aminoglycosides can cause temporary paralysis and they can prolong and increase the effects of the neuromuscular blocking agents. They can also suppress the ability of the bone marrow to produce white blood cells and platelets. Most experts regard tobramycin as the safest of the systemic aminoglycoside preparations.

Topical neomycin is a well-recognized cause of contact dermatitis. When ophthalmic preparations are used, contact inflammation reactions can be mistaken for symptoms of ongoing infection. True allergic reactions from systemic administration of an aminoglycoside can occur, but are uncommon. Patients who have such a reaction are considered to be allergic to all aminoglycosides.

### Tips for the Technician

Except for topical preparations, the aminoglycoside antibiotics are more likely to be handled by pharmacy technicians working in inpatient pharmacy settings. Technicians need to carefully calculate the volume of aminoglycoside to be withdrawn for preparation of intravenous admixtures. Have calculations double-checked by another technician before making the preparation, and note the volume for the final check by the pharmacist. Be careful not to confuse amikacin with Amicar® or tobramycin with Trobicin® (an antibiotic sometimes used to treat gonorrhea), two completely different drugs with sound-alike names.

It is appropriate for the pharmacist to advise patients who receive aminoglycoside ophthalmic preparations on techniques to maintain the sterility of the product. Patients should be advised to contact their physician if irritation and tearing continues beyond the first few days of treatment for eye infections. Suspensions, such as Cortisporin® Otic suspension, should be labelled with "shake well" instructions.

## Macrolide Antibiotics

Like the aminoglycosides, the first macrolide antibiotic, erythromycin, was derived from the soil microbe Streptomyces. Erythromycin (Erythrocin®, others) was the first antibiotic marketed as an alternative to penicillin for use in individuals who are penicillin allergic. The newer members of this family, clarithromycin (Biaxin®) and azithromycin, (Zithromax®) have some features in common with erythromycin, but also improve upon some of its less desirable characteristics.

### Actions and Indications

The macrolides bind irreversibly to the bacterial ribosome, where they inhibit certain steps of protein synthesis. Their actions are similar to those of clindamycin and chloramphenicol, two other antibiotics that block protein synthesis by bacteria. The macrolides are generally considered to be bacteriostatic, but they can be bacteriocidal at higher doses.

Erythromycin is effective against many of the same organisms as penicillin G, which justifies its use as a penicillin substitute in penicillin-allergic patients. Clarithromycin has a spectrum of antibacterial activity similar to that of erythromycin, but it is also effective against *Haemophilus influenzae* and *Moraxella catarrhalis*, common causes of upper respiratory infections. Its activity against some other pathogens, such as Chlamydia and *Helicobacter pylori*, is greater than that of erythromycin. Azithromycin has a spectrum of activity similar to clarithromycin. In spite of its higher cost, azithromycin is usually prescribed more often than clarithromycin, because it is less likely to cause some annoying side effects.

otitis media Infection and inflammation of the middle ear.

The macrolides are indicated for upper respiratory infections, such as bronchitis or sinus infections caused by susceptible organisms. They are often effective for otitis media (inner ear infections) in children and adults. The macrolides can be used for mild to moderate community acquired pneumonia caused by the most common bacteria and by mycoplasma. They are the drugs of choice for use when penicillins are indicated, but patients are allergic. Erythromycin may be used with neomycin for preparation of the bowel before surgery. Clarithromycin and azithromycin are used for eradication of *H. pylori* in the treatment of peptic ulcer disease, for treatment of Chlamydia, and other atypical bacterial infections.

## Administration

The macrolide antibiotics are absorbed to varying degrees after oral administration. Erythromycin base is acid labile, but use of enteric-coated preparations or erythromycin salts prevents this problem. The absorption of clarithromycin is the most consistent of the three macrolides, and unlike azithromycin, when taken with food there is no reduction in total drug absorbed. Azithromycin must be taken on an empty stomach. Erythromycin must be administered 4 times daily, clarithromycin (regular release) twice daily, and azithromycin can be given once each day, because of a longer half-life.

Azithromycin and erythromycin can also be administered intravenously. They are extremely irritating to tissues and cannot be given intramuscularly. When given IV, they must be adequately diluted and infused slowly to avoid irritation of the vein, known as phlebitis.

phlebitis Inflammation of a vein.

All of the macrolides are metabolized in the liver and can interact with other drugs that are detoxified by the same enzyme systems. When macrolide antibiotics are administered along with digoxin, theophylline, phenytoin, and carbamazepine, for example, increases in serum levels of these drugs can occur. The macrolides can also increase the effects of warfarin.

## Side Effects

While generally considered safe, the macrolide antibiotics cause annoying side effects that can reduce patient compliance. This is especially true of erythromycin. Epigastric distress is common and sometimes quite severe. Clarithromycin and azithromycin seem to be better tolerated by the patient, but gastrointestinal problems, including stomach pain and diarrhea, are the most common side effects reported. Clarithromycin causes an unpleasant, metallic taste in the mouth. The macrolides are less likely to cause more serious side effects, but they can occur. Both erythromycin and azithromycin have been reported to cause jaundice and liver damage. Azithromycin is sometimes associated with serious allergic skin reactions and angioedema.

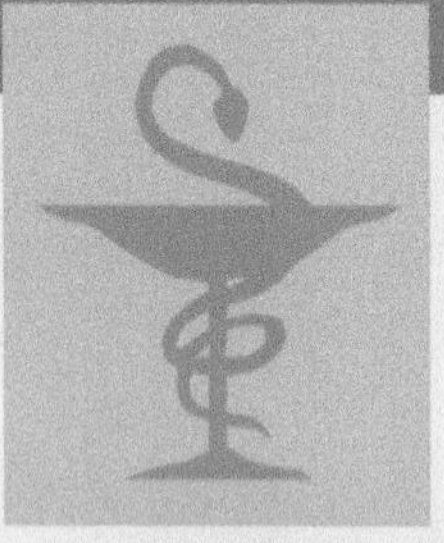

### Tips for the Technician

When dispensing prescriptions for erythromycin base and azithromycin suspension it is appropriate to attach auxiliary labels instructing patients to take these medications on an empty stomach. Enteric-coated erythromycin and erythromycin stearate can be taken without regard to food, as can clarithromycin tablets. Technicians should check the specific product inserts when unsure about auxiliary labelling. Attach a label instructing patients to "complete all of the medication unless otherwise directed by the physician" to all prescriptions for oral antibiotics.

Azithromycin may be prescribed as a Z-Pak®, a 5-day course frequently ordered for upper respiratory infections, such as sinus infections or bronchitis. Although handy for dispensing purposes, this packaging is inflexible because it limits patients to a 5-day initial course of antibiotic, which is often inadequate for complete treatment. Many physicians will include one refill with these prescriptions, and it is important that patients be aware that they should get a refill if symptoms return.

Hospital based technicians need to be aware that erythromycin is much less stable when mixed in 5% dextrose in water, and therefore it is usually diluted in normal saline for intravenous administration. When dextrose solutions are used, they must be buffered (pH controlled) with sodium bicarbonate. Both erythromycin and azithromycin piggybacks must be adequately diluted to prevent pain on injection.

buffer Compound(s) in solution that stabilizes the hydrogen-ion concentration by neutralizing both acids and bases.

## Other Inhibitors of Protein Synthesis

There are a number of other miscellaneous antibiotics that act by inhibiting protein synthesis, which are worthy of mention for different reasons. Clindamycin (Cleocin®) is unique for its action against anaerobic bacteria, quinupristin/dalfopristin (Synercid®) and linezolid (Zyvox®) for their ability to kill a few particularly resistant bacteria, and chloramphenicol (Chloromycetin®) for its very serious side effects.

### Actions and Indications

Clindamycin binds to bacterial ribosomes in the same location as the macrolides to inhibit bacterial protein synthesis. It is prescribed primarily for the treatment of infections caused by anaerobic bacteria, such as *Bacteroides fragilis*, which often cause abdominal infections as a result of trauma, perforated appendix, or abdominal surgery. In addition, it has significant activity against some gram-positive cocci.

Quinupristin/dalfopristin is a combination of two streptogramin antibiotics that bind to two separate sites on the bacterial ribosome. They synergistically interrupt protein synthesis. This combination drug is bactericidal and its effects continue for some time after the drug has disappeared from the blood stream. Linezolid binds to a site on the ribosome that causes it to block the translation of nucleic acids necessary for production of proteins. In some cases it is bactericidal, but against the organisms it is most often used to treat, it is bacteriostatic. Both Synercid® and linezolid are reserved for the treatment of MRSA and vancomycin resistant enterococci (VRE). Enterococci are gram-positive cocci that up until

### Case 29.1

Tom Jones is going to school to become a pharmacy technician. In class he was asked to read about MRSA skin infections on the CDC website and he learned that the infection can occur among athletes, military recruits, children, and prisoners, and that deaths have occurred as a result. Because resistance to antibiotics is rapidly spreading, he knows that the number of effective antibiotics available to treat serious MRSA infections is dwindling. He learned that linezolid, the only oral drug effective against MRSA, is extremely expensive. He is just finishing his homework when his son calls asking to be picked up from school because of a very sore throat. Tom arranges for his son to be seen by the physician's assistant, Misty Mark, one of Tom's acquaintances, at the doctor's office. Misty takes a look at the boy's throat, takes a throat culture, and tells Tom that it looks like strep throat. In an effort to save Tom some money, Misty rummages around for some antibiotic samples, and pulls out a box of Zyvox. "Here you go," she says, "this stuff will kill anything." Tom is stunned. He does not want to seem ungrateful, but feels that using this powerful antibiotic is not right. What should Tom do?

the 1980s were considered to be part of the genus Streptococcus. These two groups of organisms are difficult to distinguish from one another. Enterococcus lives in the intestine and rarely causes diseases, but in hospitals this organism can cause wound infections, urinary tract infections, or worse. In the past, Enterococci were susceptible to treatment with ampicillin or vancomycin, but more recently resistance has become a significant problem.

Like the other drugs in this section, chloramphenicol binds to the bacterial ribosome to inhibit protein synthesis. Because the binding site in bacteria is similar to the comparable mammalian ribosome, chloramphenicol can produce serious toxicity, especially at higher doses. Chloramphenicol is active against a wide range of gram-positive and gram-negative organisms. However, because of its toxicity, its use is restricted to life-threatening infections for which no alternatives exist. An example might include a life-threatening infection with *Salmonella typhi*. Veterinarians sometimes use chloramphenicol for treatment of infections in animals, where it causes less toxicity.

## Administration

Clindamycin is well absorbed by the oral route and it can be administered intravenously or topically (for treatment of acne), as well. It distributes into all body fluids, except the CSF and urine, and into bone. Linezolid is rapidly and completely absorbed when given orally. It is available for both oral and intravenous use, and no change in dose is required when switching from the intravenous to the oral route of administration. Synercid® is administered by intravenous piggyback. Penetration into tissues is good, except for poor penetration into the central nervous system. Chloramphenicol, though rarely used in humans, is administered intravenously or topically for eye infections. It is absorbed orally, but because of the risks of toxicity no oral preparations are available.

## Side Effects

Most side effects of clindamycin are related to overgrowth of nonsusceptible organisms. Clindamycin use can result in vaginitis due to yeast overgrowth. The most serious adverse effect is potentially fatal colitis caused by overgrowth of *C. difficile*, which produces toxins very damaging to the colon. Oral administration of either metronidazole (Flagyl®) or vancomycin is usually effective in controlling this serious problem. Skin rashes, nausea, and impaired liver function are other possible side effects.

Venous irritation commonly occurs in association with quinupristin/dalfopristin administration. Muscle and joint aches and pain, as well as headache have been reported, especially when higher doses of the drugs are used. This combination can also affect the liver, causing abnormal liver function tests in as many as 25% of patients, and rarely, jaundice. Concomitant administration with cyclosporine, calcium channel blockers, and a number of other drugs could result in elevated levels and effects from those drugs because Synercid® is metabolized by the same enzyme systems in the liver. A drug interaction with digoxin can also occur, causing increased digoxin levels.

Chloramphenicol is infamous for causing aplastic anemia, a rare but usually fatal condition that occurs when the bone marrow ceases to produce blood cells, usually in response to a toxin. Aplastic anemia from chloramphenicol is idiosyncratic, meaning that it is individual and unpredictable. This effect is independent of dose and may occur after therapy has ceased. Agranulocytosis and thrombocytopenia are other reported adverse effects of chloramphenicol. These forms of anemia are reversible, dose related, and occur during therapy. "Gray baby" syndrome occurs in neonates if the dosage regimen of chloramphenicol is not properly adjusted. Neonates have a low capacity to metabolise the antibiotic and they have underdeveloped kidney function. If the drug accumulates, it leads to poor feeding, depressed breathing, cardiovascular collapse, cyanosis (low levels of oxygen that result in a bluish tint to the lips and pallor, hence the term "gray baby"), and death.

idiosyncratic Of an unexpected nature; resulting from individual differences or peculiarities.

cyanosis Bluish discoloration of the skin or mucous membranes due to deficient oxygenation of the blood.

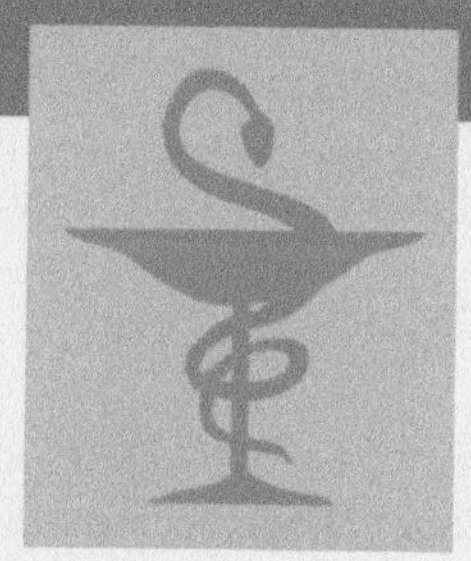

## Tips for the Technician

With the exception of clindamycin, hospital pharmacy technicians will encounter the drugs covered in this segment of the chapter more often than retail pharmacy technicians, because they are most often administered intravenously, for very serious infections. Clindamycin and linezolid are both available in premixed intravenous piggyback bags. Neither requires refrigeration, and both should be left in the protective outer wrapping until they are used. Clindamycin is also manufactured in vials. Technicians should be aware that this drug is viscous and prone to foaming. For these reasons, clindamycin can be more difficult to work with than other solutions for injection. Vials of quinupristin/dalfopristin powder must be refrigerated before use and reconstituted immediately before dilution. Quinupristin/dalfopristin must be diluted in 5% dextrose in water for intravenous administration because the drug is incompatible with normal saline.

Linezolid and clindamycin are both available for reconstitution as oral suspensions. These products do not require refrigeration, and in fact the manufacturer recommends clindamycin not be stored in the refrigerator because it becomes so thick it is difficult to pour. Clindamycin is stable for 14 days and linezolid is stable for 21 days at room temperature. Linezolid and quinupristin/dalfopristin are extremely expensive. Technicians should take great care to reconstitute these drugs exactly as recommended to avoid waste.

# Review Questions

## Multiple Choice

Choose the best answer for the following questions.

1. Circle the letter below that does not correspond to an antistaphylococcal penicillin.
   a. Amoxicillin
   b. Nafcillin
   c. Methicillin
   d. Oxacillin
   e. Dicloxacillin

2. Which of the following drugs is a second-generation cephalosporin that can be administered by mouth?
   a. Cephalexin
   b. Cefprozil
   c. Cefdinir
   d. Cefotetan
   e. None of the above can be administered by mouth.

3. Of the following side effects, which is likely to be associated with elevated serum levels of aminoglycoside antibiotics?
   a. Hearing loss
   b. Kidney damage
   c. Severe diarrhea
   d. a and b
   e. All of the above

4. Children younger than 9 years of age should not receive tetracyclines because these agents:
   a. Cause rupture of tendons
   b. Do not cross into the cerebrospinal fluid
   c. Are not bactericidal
   d. Deposit in teeth to cause discoloration of permanent teeth
   e. Can cause overgrowth of yeast

5. When administered together, the macrolide antibiotics can cause increased activity of which of the following medications?
   a. Theophylline
   b. Digoxin
   c. Carbamazepine
   d. Warfarin
   e. All of the above

## True/False

6. Vancomycin is never administered by the oral route except for the treatment of colitis caused by overgrowth of *C. difficile*.
   a. True
   b. False

7. Prescriptions for tetracycline should be labelled with auxiliary labels warning patients to avoid concomitant administration of antacids or consumption of dairy products while taking these medications.
   a. True
   b. False

8. Cephalosporin prescriptions should be labelled with a warning to patients to avoid excessive sun exposure.
   a. True
   b. False

9. A 1-gram dose of vancomycin should be diluted in at least 100 ml of appropriate fluid for piggyback administration.
   a. True
   b. False

10. Ceftriaxone is a third-generation cephalosporin often used in the treatment of meningitis because it reaches effective concentrations in the cerebrospinal fluid.
    a. True
    b. False

## Matching

For numbers 11–15, match the word or phrase with the correct lettered definition from the list below. Choices will not be used more than once and may not be used at all.

11. Antibiotic
12. Bacteriocidal
13. Bacteriostatic
14. Nosocomial
15. Antibacterial

a. An infection acquired while a patient is in a hospital
b. A drug that kills or inhibits the growth of microbes
c. Chemical substances produced by micro-organisms that inhibit the growth of other micro-organisms
d. Pain or irritation of the vein usually caused by infusion of an irritating drug
e. Inhibits the growth and reproduction of bacteria, but does not kill them
f. Any drug used to kill or suppress the growth of bacteria
g. Kills bacteria

## Short Answer

16. Why should highly effective antibiotics such as meropenem, imipenem, linezolid, and vancomycin be restricted to only the most seriously ill patients with difficult to treat infections?

17. Compare and contrast the use of a third-generation cephalosporin, such as ceftriaxone, versus the use of an aminoglycoside, such as tobramycin, for a serious infection caused by a susceptible gram-negative organism. Consider administration, side effects, and any other advantages or disadvantages.

18. For what kind of infections might tetracycline be prescribed? List any limitations for its, use, two common side effects, and auxiliary labels that are necessary to include with prescription labelling.

19. List the generic and brand names and route(s) of administration for one drug from each of the four "generations" of cephalosporins.

20. Pearl E. Gates is 81 years old and a regular client who lives independently across the street from the Pharm Aid Drug Store where you work. She brings in a prescription for Ceftin® tablets for a sinus infection. You notice she has a penicillin allergy listed on her patient profile. Should the prescription be filled? What other information is needed in order to make an informed decision about filling the prescription?

# FOR FURTHER INQUIRY

The Center for Disease Control and Prevention promotes the responsible use of antibiotics to both the public and health care professionals. The "Get Smart" campaign includes material that can be downloaded free of charge or ordered for use in a pharmacy. Read the material for the consumers and print items for family members or friends that might benefit from it.

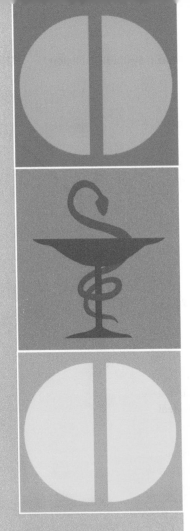

KEY TERMS

- crystalluria
- excoriation
- peripheral neuropathy

Chapter **30**

# Antibacterials: Sulfonamides, Quinolones, Urinary Antiseptics, and Antituberculars

## OBJECTIVES

After studying this chapter, the reader should be able to:

- Compare the mechanisms of action of the sulfonamides and the fluoroquinolones, describe an indication for use of each, and list an example of a drug from each class.
- List the appropriate auxiliary labelling that should be used with outpatient prescriptions for the sulfonamide antibacterial drugs.
- Name a common side effect and a rare side effect of the fluoroquinolones. Explain why there are restrictions on the use of these drugs in children.
- Describe a major side effect associated with prolonged use of nitrofurantoin, and explain how this side effect compares to adverse effects that may occur with short-term use.
- Describe three factors that contributed to the increase in tuberculosis cases seen in the early 1990s, list the five first line antitubercular drugs, and explain why multi-drug regimens are now standard treatment for tuberculosis.

## DRUGS COVERED IN THIS CHAPTER

### Antibacterial Agents

| Sulfonamides & Folic Acid Inhibitors | Fluoroquinolones | Urinary Tract Antiseptics | Antitubercular Drugs |
|---|---|---|---|
| Sulfacetamide | Ciprofloxacin | Methenamine | Ethambutol |
| Sulfadiazine | Gatifloxacin | Nitrofurantoin | Isoniazid |
| Sulfisoxazole | Levofloxacin | | Pyrazinamide |
| Sulfasalazine | Moxifloxacin | | Rifampin |
| Trimethoprim/Sulfamethox-azole (Cotrimoxazole) | Norfloxacin | | Rifabutin |
| | Ofloxacin | | Rifapentine |
| | Sparfloxacin | | Streptomycin |
| | Trovafloxacin | | |

A number of the drugs we commonly refer to as antibiotics are, strictly speaking, antibacterials. These drugs are neither derived from, nor related to, other compounds derived from living organisms. Although they were born in laboratories, the antibacterial compounds discussed here include some of our earliest, and some of today's most important anti-infective drugs.

# Sulfonamides and Other Folic Acid Inhibitors

In 1932, the German chemist Gerhard Domagk observed that the dye, Prontosil, had antibacterial properties in mice when they were infected with streptococcus. By 1935, a group of physicians discovered that sulfanilamide was the compound responsible for this antibacterial effect, and shortly thereafter it was made available to the public for treatment of infections. To the medical profession, the success of sulfanilamide in the treatment of infections seemed miraculous, and very soon other sulfa compounds were isolated and put to use. Although they did not cure all infections, for the first time in human history there was an effective treatment for scarlet fever, postpartum infections, pneumonia, and meningitis. The use of these drugs prompted pharmacologists and chemists to continue their search for better treatments, which eventually led to the discovery of penicillin. Together these drugs saved thousands of lives in World War II, not to mention the millions of lives saved since then.

## Actions and Indications

Folic acid is required by all living cells to synthesize precursors of RNA and DNA, and other compounds necessary for cell growth and replication. When folic acid is not available, cells cannot grow or divide. Humans depend on dietary intake of folic acid (also known as folate) because we cannot synthesize our own. In contrast, many bacteria must rely on their ability to synthesize folic acid because they cannot absorb it. The sulfonamides are a family of antibacterials that block some microbes' ability to synthesize folic acid. As a result of this action, bacteria survive but are unable to reproduce. The sulfonamides are considered bacteriostatic drugs because they only inhibit the growth and reproduction of bacteria, and leave the destruction of the organisms to the immune system.

A second type of folic acid antagonist, trimethoprim (Proloprim®), prevents the conversion of folic acid to the active form. Both trimethoprim and the sulfonamides interfere with the ability of an infecting bacterium to divide, but through slightly different mechanisms. The sulfonamide sulfamethoxazole, used together with trimethoprim, produce synergistic antibacterial activity. The generic name of this effective two-drug combination is cotrimoxazole

(Bactrim®, Septra®). Cotrimoxazole, sulfacetamide (Bleph-10®), sulfasalazine (Azulfidine®), and sulfadiazine are the most frequently used sulfa compounds today.

Cotrimoxazole is indicated for infections of the prostate, upper respiratory tract, ears, and urinary tract when they are caused by sensitive organisms. Is is the drug of choice for the treatment of Pneumocystis jiroveci (previously named Pneumocystis carinii), a common cause of opportunistic pneumonia in AIDS patients (**Fig. 30.1**). Sulfonamides combined with other agents are useful for certain other protozoal parasites as well. Silver sulfadiazine (Silvadene®) is an important topical antibacterial agent for treatment of wounds and burns. Sulfacetamide is frequently used as an ophthalmic antibacterial. Sulfasalazine is indicated for use in inflammatory bowel disease and other autoimmune conditions. Sulfadiazine, once widely used for infections, is now mainly used for toxoplasmosis, an opportunistic parasitic infection of the central nervous system associated with AIDS.

As with all antimicrobial drugs, resistance can adversely affect the usefulness of these drugs. Organisms that obtain folic acid without synthesizing it are naturally resistant to sulfa drugs. Bacterial resistance to the sulfa drugs can arise from plasmid transfers or random mutations, and organisms resistant to one member of this drug family are resistant to all.

## Administration

With the exception of sulfasalazine, the sulfonamides are well absorbed from the GI tract after oral administration. Although sulfasalazine is administered orally, it is minimally absorbed and is thought to exert most of its effect on the local organisms of the GI tract and through breakdown products created by the action of bacteria on the drug. Cotrimoxazole is the only sulfonamide antimicrobial available for parenteral administration. It is diluted and administered by intravenous piggyback for serious or complicated infections. Information on the brand names, formulations and routes of administration for the drugs covered in this chapter is available in **Table 30.1**.

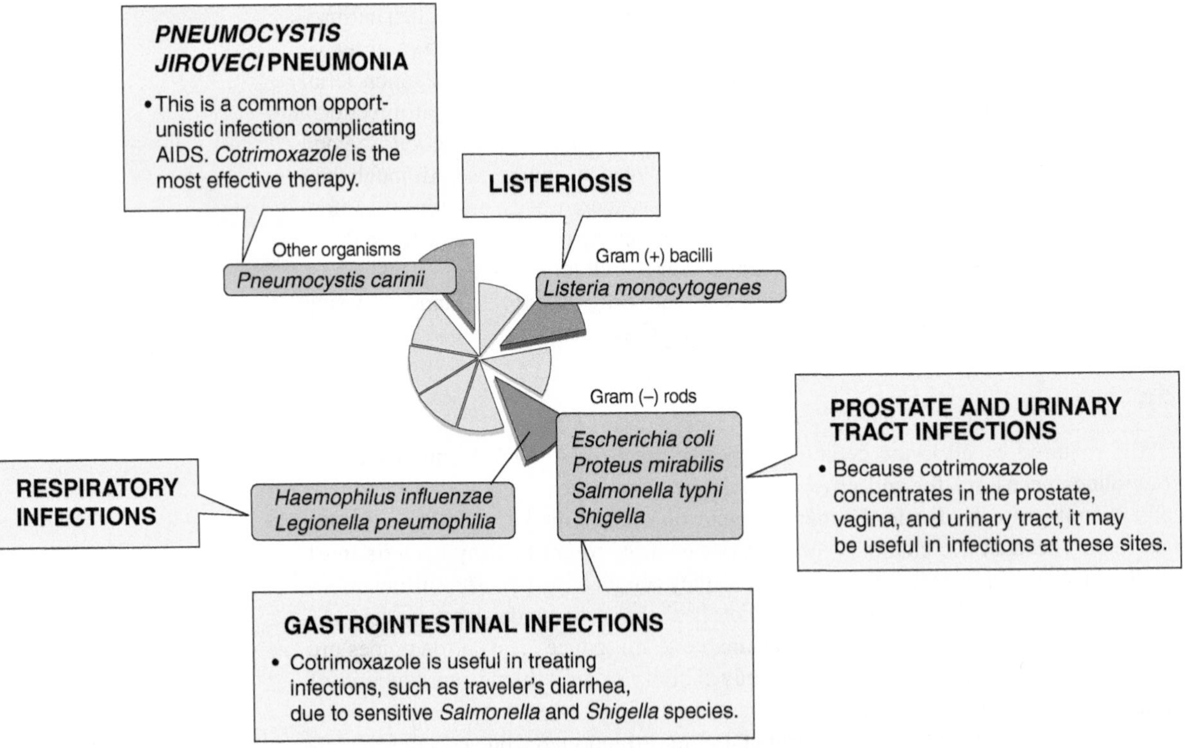


**Figure 30.1** Some important uses of trimethoprim plus sulfamethoxazole (cotrimoxazole). (Adapted with permission from Harvey RA, Champe PC, Howland RD, et al. *Lippincott's Illustrated Reviews: Pharmacology*, 3rd edition. Baltimore: Lippincott Williams & Wilkins, 2006.)

**Table 30.1** Generic and Brand Names, Indications, and Formulations of the Drugs Covered in This Chapter

| Generic | Brand Name | Available as | Indications | Notes |
|---|---|---|---|---|
| **Sulfonamides** | | | | |
| Sulfacetamide | Bleph-10®, AK-Sulf® | Ophthalmic solution & ointment | Superficial eye infections & adjunct in trachoma | Do not use in sulfa allergic pt. |
| Sulfadiazine | | Tablets | Toxoplasmosis | |
| Silver sulfadiazine | Silvadene®, SSD® | Cream | Infections related to burns | Do not use in sulfa allergic pt. |
| Sulfisoxazole | Gantrisin Ped® | Tablets, suspension | Toxoplasmosis, OM, trachoma | Also combined w/ erythromycin |
| Sulfasalazine | Azulfidine® | Tablets, EC tablets | Autoimmune disorders | |
| TMP/SMX (Co-trimoxazole) | Bactrim®, Septra® | Tablets, DS tablets, oral suspension, injection | UTI, Pneumocystis pneumonia, traveler's diarrhea, OM | |
| **Fluoroquinolones** | | | | |
| Ciprofloxacin | Cipro® | Tablets, ER tabs, injection, powder for suspension, premix IVPB | UTI, prostatitis, sinus infections, other infections due to sensitive organism | |
| Gatifloxacin | Tequin® | Tablets, injection, premix IVPB | Infections due to sensitive organism | Avoided in elderly or diabetics |
| Levofloxacin | Levaquin® | Tablets, injections premix IVPB | UTI, prostatitis, sinus infections, other infections due to sensitive organism | |
| Moxifloxacin | Avelox® | Tablets, premix IVPB | Sinusitis, bronchitis, pneumonia, skin infections | |
| Norfloxacin | Noroxin® | Tablets | UTI | |
| Ofloxacin | Floxin® | Tablets | UTI, prostatitis, STDs, pneumonia | |
| Sparfloxacin | Zagam® | Tablets | CAP, bronchitis | |
| Trovafloxacin | Trovan® | Injection | Life-threatening infection | Liver toxicity |

(continues)

**Table 30.1** Generic and Brand Names, Indications, and Formulations of the Drugs Covered in This Chapter *(continued)*

| Generic | Brand Name | Available as | Indications | Notes |
|---|---|---|---|---|
| **Urinary Tract Antiseptics** | | | | |
| Methenamine | Hiprex®, Mandelamine® | Tablets, suspension | Chronic UTI | Also combined w/ urine acidifiers |
| Nitrofurantoin | Macrodantin® Macrobid® | Capsules | UTI | |
| **Antituberculars** | | | | |
| Ethambutol | Myambutol® | Tablets | 1st-line treatment, TB | |
| Isoniazid | Nydrazid® | Tablets, syrup, injection | 1st-line treatment, TB | |
| Pyrazinamide | | Tablets | 1st-line treatment, TB | |
| Rifampin | Rifadin®, Rimactane® | Capsules, injection | 1st-line treatment, TB, leprosy, prevention of meningitis | |
| Rifabutin | Mycobutin® | Capsules | 2nd-line treatment, TB | |
| Rifapentine | Priftin® | Tablets | 2nd-line treatment, TB | |
| Streptomycin | | Lyophilized powder for injection | 2nd-line treatment, TB | |

CAP, community acquired pneumonia; DS, double strength; EC, enteric coated; ER, extended release; NPB, intravenous piggyback; OM, otitis media; SMX, sulfamethoxazole; STDs, sexually transmitted diseases; TB, tuberculosis; TMP, trimethoprim; UTI, urinary tract infection.

The sulfonamides are at least partly metabolized in the liver, and the kidneys excrete the metabolites and remaining drug. Sulfonamides penetrate into a variety of body tissues and fluids, such as the prostate, lung tissues, and the eye, a property that adds to their usefulness. They easily cross the placenta and are excreted in breast milk. They can increase the risk of jaundice in newborns, and are therefore avoided in pregnancy or in breast-feeding mothers. Topically applied sulfa can be absorbed in small amounts through the skin, especially when the product covers a large area, when burns or excoriation (scratched or scraped outer surface of the skin) exist, or when used on young children. Consequently, patients who are sulfa allergic cannot be treated with topical or ophthalmic products, and individuals who are not allergic can become sensitized through topical use of these drugs.

excoriation abraded or raw lesion of the skin.

## Side Effects

The sulfa drugs are well known for causing hypersensitivity reactions. Allergic reactions can be as straightforward as fever, itching, and rash, or as severe as angioedema, Stevens-Johnson syndrome, or other types of exfoliative dermatitis (inflammation and peeling of the skin). Cross sensitivity between the sulfa drugs occurs. Therefore, when a patient is sulfa allergic they should not receive any type of sulfonamide drug. Other typical side effects include photosensitivity and GI upset, such as nausea and vomiting or diarrhea (**Fig. 30.2**). Liver toxicity is rare, but can include a range of symptoms from elevated liver function tests to jaundice and hepatitis.

Crystalluria

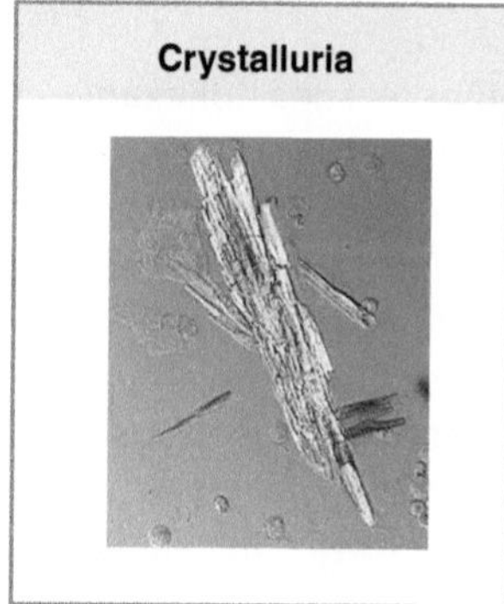

Allergic Reactions

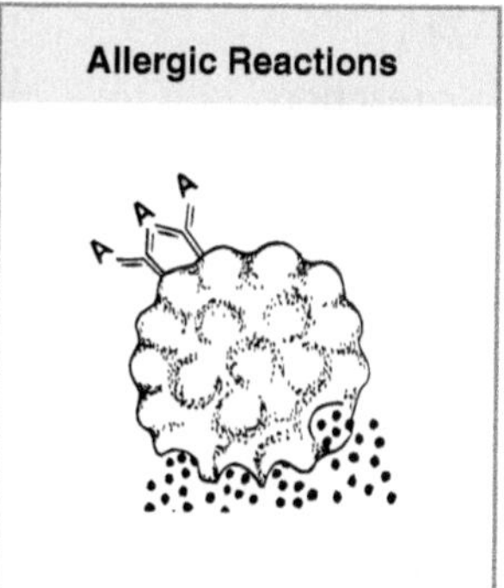

Hemolytic Anemia

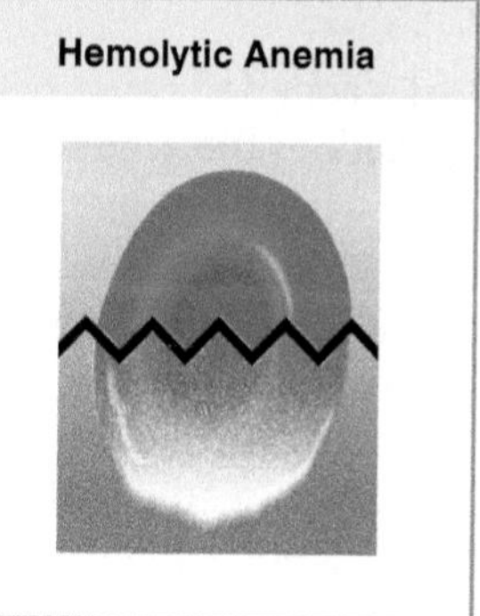

Nausea and Vomiting

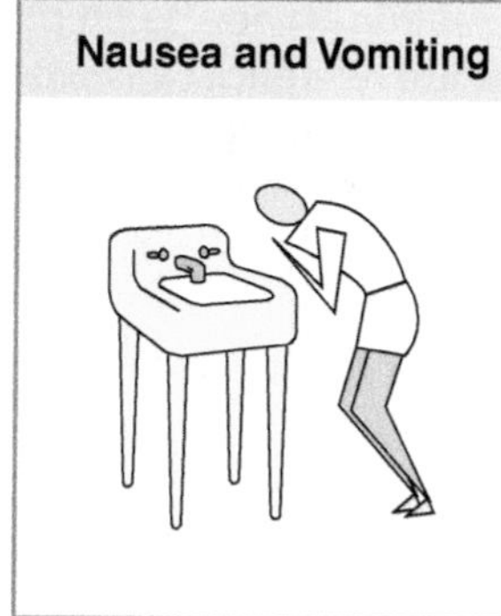

Jaundice

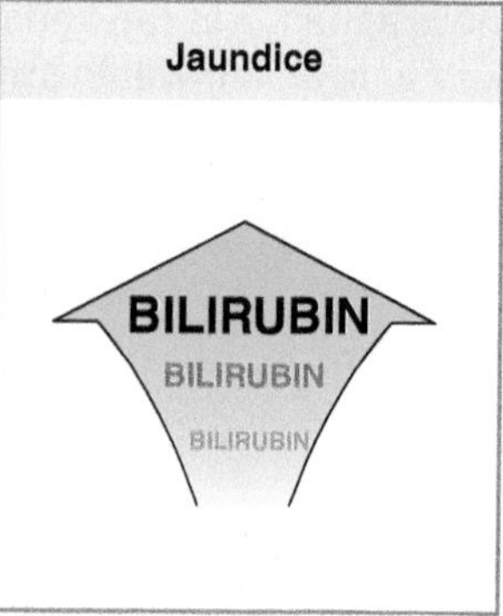


**Figure 30.2** Although generally safe, the sulfa antibacterials can cause some well-recognized side effects. (Adapted with permission from Harvey RA, Champe PC, Howland RD, et al. *Lippincott's Illustrated Reviews: Pharmacology*, 3rd edition. Baltimore: Lippincott Williams & Wilkins, 2006.)

When the sulfonamides were first introduced, nephrotoxicity sometimes occurred because the sulfa drugs, which are not particularly water soluble, crystallized in the urine as it was being formed (crystalluria). As the use of sulfadiazine declined, and the use of more water-soluble sulfonamides such as sulfamethoxazole increased, crystalluria became less of a problem. Prescriptions for sulfadiazine are on the upswing, however, because of the increase in the numbers of patients with immunosuppression due to AIDS or immunosuppressive drug therapy. Crystalluria and kidney damage can be prevented if patients drink an adequate volume of fluid so that the urine remains dilute.

crystalluria Excretion of crystals in the urine.

Blood disorders, including thrombocytopenia and leukopenia, can occur as a result of sulfonamide use. Hemolytic anemia is likely to occur in glucose-6-phosphate dehydrogenase (G6PD) deficient patients who receive sulfonamides. G6PD is an enzyme involved in carbohydrate metabolism, which in addition protects the red blood cells from oxidizing substances, such as metabolites of certain medications, including the sulfonamides. G6PD deficiency is the most common enzyme deficiency in humans.

## Tips for the Technician

Pharmacy technicians play an important role in preventing accidental exposure to drugs in patients who are allergic. Always check the patient profile for allergies first, before filling any prescription. Always clean the equipment before and after use when working with automated dispensing machines, packaging equipment, or other equipment that comes in contact with tablet dust. Counting trays should be wiped at intervals throughout the day, and after counting any medication that leaves dust, or is known as a common cause of allergic reactions, or is toxic for other reasons (for example, cytotoxic drugs). Medications that frequently cause allergies include the penicillins, the sulfonamides, and codeine.

Outpatient prescriptions for sulfonamide antibacterials require a number of auxiliary patient instructions. These include instructions to avoid excessive sun exposure, to complete all medications as ordered except on the advice of the physician, and directions to take with food if nausea is a problem. Prescriptions filled for women of childbearing age should include a warning against taking the drugs during pregnancy or while breast-feeding. All patients should be instructed to drink plenty of water when taking any sulfonamides, and a minimum of twelve 8-oz glasses of water every day while taking sulfadiazine.

Technicians compounding intravenous admixtures can find information on how to prepare co-trimoxazole solutions in the package insert or in an intravenous admixture reference. This product must be adequately diluted and infused over one hour or more depending on the dose. Co-trimoxazole cannot be refrigerated because of the risk of crystallization in the IV bag. Diluted solutions must be used within 6 hours of preparation.

# The Fluoroquinolones

Although we think of them as a relatively new family of antibacterial agents, in truth the fluoroquinolones in use today are second-generation quinolones. Nalidixic acid was the first quinolone, accidently discovered by a pharmaceutical scientist looking for a treatment for malaria in the early 1960s. Although it was available for many years as a urinary tract antibacterial, it was of limited usefulness. Norfloxacin (Noroxin®) was the first fluorinated quinolone. It, too, is of limited importance because it does not reach blood levels adequate to treat systemic infections. Later additions to the fluoroquinolone family include some of the most effective and widely used of all antimicrobials.

## Actions and Indications

The fluoroquinolones are bacteriocidal antimicrobials with a unique mechanism of action. They enter the bacterium by passive diffusion through pores in the outer membrane. Once inside, fluoroquinolones inhibit the action of two bacterial enzymes that are responsible for maintaining the conformation (the double-stranded structure, **Fig. 30.3**) of the bacterial DNA. If the DNA is not properly maintained, it cannot unwind. In order for bacteria to multiply, the DNA must unwind, separate and be replicated. The fluoroquinolones exert their effects by damaging the bacterial DNA, thereby preventing replication, and bacterial reproduction. Fortunately, the enzymes acted upon by the fluoroquinolones are specific for bacteria and not shared by humans. Because this mechanism of action is unique to the fluoroquinolones, resistance develops more slowly than with other antibiotics, but nevertheless, does occur.

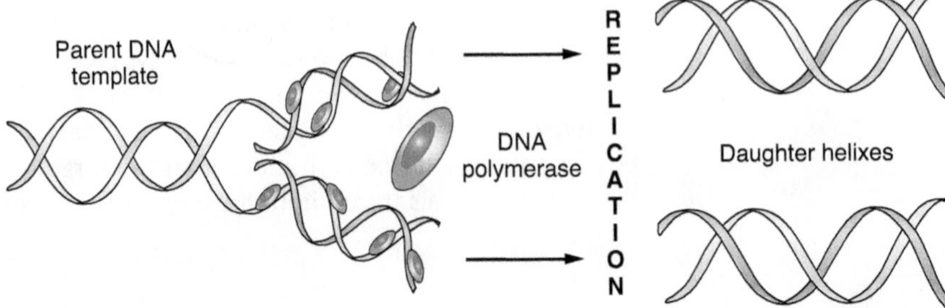


**Figure 30.3** In order for bacteria to replicate, the double-stranded structure of DNA (left) must be maintained so that it can unwind (right), separate, and be replicated.

Fluoroquinolones are broad spectrum, systemic antimicrobials that are most useful in the treatment of infections caused by gram-negative organisms such as the Enterobacteriaceae, *Pseudomonas species*, *Haemophilus influenzae*, *Moraxella catarrhalis*, and others. They are effective in the treatment of gonorrhea but not syphilis. The newer agents, such as levofloxacin (Levaquin®), gatifloxacin (Tequin®), and sparfloxacin (Zagam®) have improved activity against some gram-positive organisms, such as *Streptococcus pneumoniae*, but other drugs (cephalosporins and penicillins, for example) are more effective and have fewer side effects. The fluoroquinolones are now considered standard treatment for urinary tract infections and bacterial gastroenteritis caused by sensitive bacteria. They are used routinely (and many experts believe excessively) as empiric treatment for acute sinusitis, bacterial bronchitis, and other respiratory infections. The fluoroquinolones are also useful against a number of atypical bacteria.

Ciprofloxacin is the most prescribed of the fluoroquinolones and is one of the most prescribed drugs in the United States (**Fig. 30.4**). It is particularly useful in treating infections caused by many gram-negative bacilli, including for example, traveler's diarrhea caused by *E. coli*. Ciprofloxacin is the drug of choice for prophylaxis and treatment of anthrax infection. Of the fluoroquinolones, it is the most effective for treating *Pseudomonas aeruginosa* infections, and it is used in the treatment of pseudomonal infections associated with cystic fibrosis in children. Ciprofloxacin can be of benefit in treating resistant tuberculosis. Together with levofloxacin, these two drugs are the workhorse fluoroquinolones.

Levofloxacin is a close second behind ciprofloxacin as the most prescribed fluoroquinolone. Because of its increased activity against gram-positive organisms, levofloxacin is a treatment options for community-acquired pneumonia. Besides its use for respiratory infections and UTI, it is recommended for the treatment of sexually transmitted diseases, including chlamydia and gonorrhea.

## Administration

With the exception of norfloxacin, all of the fluoroquinolones are rapidly and nearly completely absorbed when taken orally. This characteristic eliminates the need for intravenous

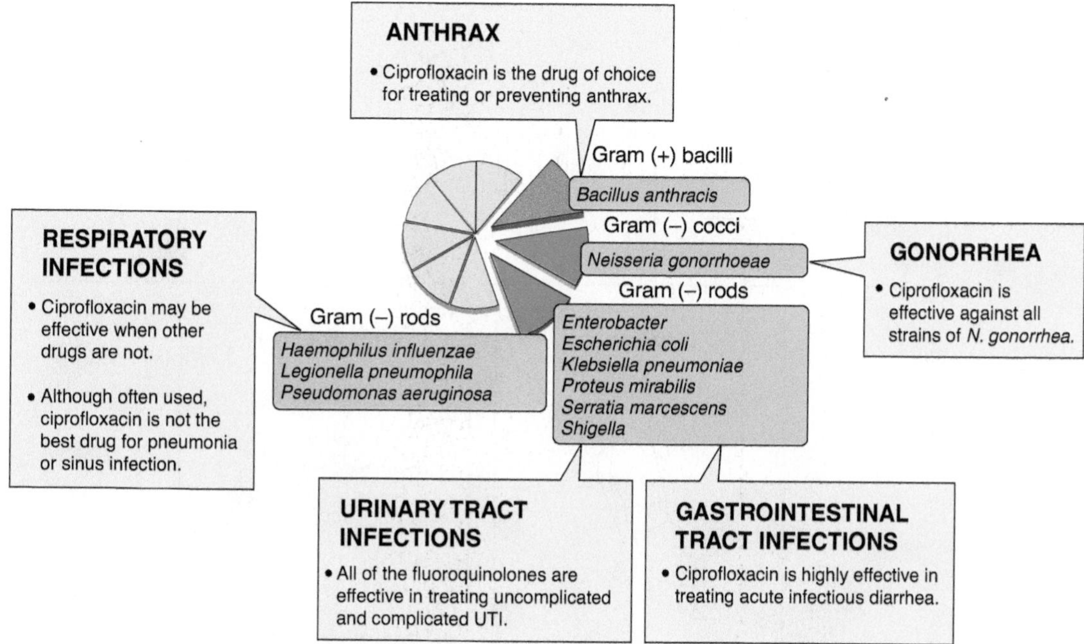


**Figure 30.4** Some important uses of ciprofloxacin. (Adapted with permission from Harvey RA, Champe PC, Howland RD, et al. *Lippincott's Illustrated Reviews: Pharmacology*, 3rd edition. Baltimore: Lippincott Williams & Wilkins, 2006.)

injection in many infections. For severe infections, intravenous preparations of ciprofloxacin, levofloxacin, and gatifloxacin are available. Trovafloxacin (Trovan®) is available only as an IV preparation.

When the fluoroquinolones are taken with sucralfate, antacids, or dietary supplements containing iron or zinc, absorption of the antibacterial is reduced. Because of their long half-lives, levofloxacin, moxifloxacin (Avelox®), sparfloxacin, and trovafloxacin can be given once daily. Ciprofloxacin requires twice-daily dosing. The fluoroquinolones penetrate all body tissues, except the CNS, quite well. Concentrations in the lung exceed those found in the blood stream for most of these drugs. These drugs are, for the most part, excreted unchanged in the urine, and their doses must be adjusted in people with severe renal failure.

## Side Effects

Although they are generally very well tolerated, the fluoroquinolones may cause side effects (**Fig. 30.5**). The most common adverse effects associated with the class are nausea, vomiting, and diarrhea. Headache, dizziness, or light-headedness occur somewhat less often, but are not considered unusual. Patients taking fluoroquinolones may develop sun sensitivity and should be advised to avoid excessive sunlight and to apply sunscreens. Fluoroquinolones are avoided in pregnancy, in nursing mothers, and in children (with the exception of treating infections in children with cystic fibrosis) because of potential damage to connective tissue in growing infants and children. Although rare, adults can experience tendonitis or tendon rupture, a related form of connective tissue damage observed with fluoroquinolone use. Serious allergic reactions are rare, but can occur.

Trovafloxacin is associated with serious liver injury, and therefore use of the drug is restricted to infections that are life threatening. Sparfloxacin and moxifloxacin cause abnormalities in the cardiac conduction system and should not be used in patients with arrhythmias. In early 2006, the manufacturer of Tequin® (gatifloxacin) warned health care providers of the risk of abnormal blood sugar levels related to use of gatifloxacin. This effect was especially marked in elderly patients, and the drug is no longer recommended for use in diabetics or the elderly.

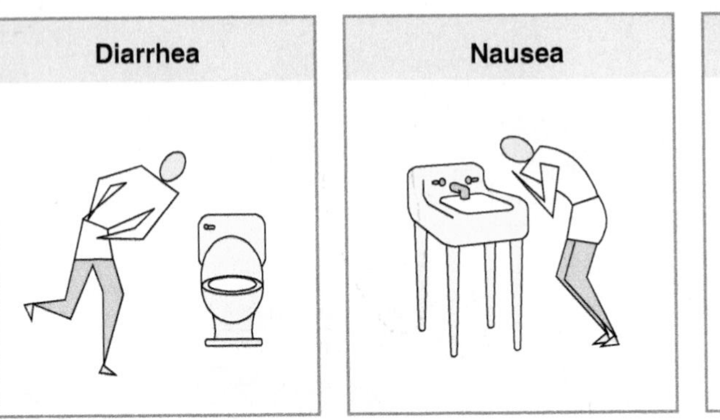


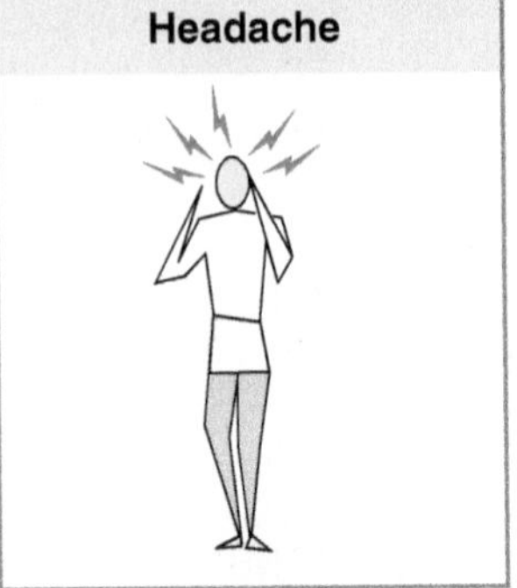


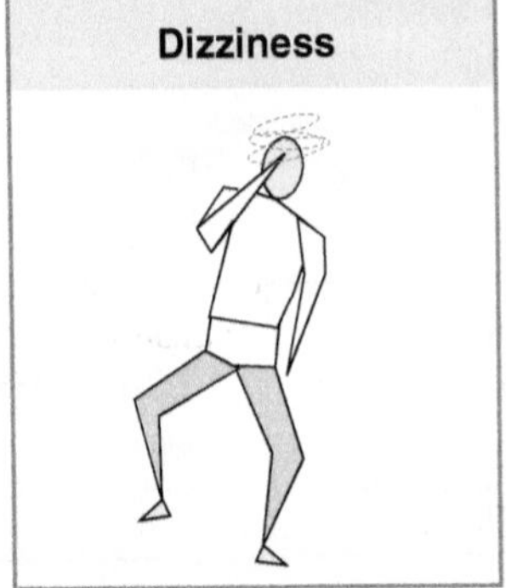


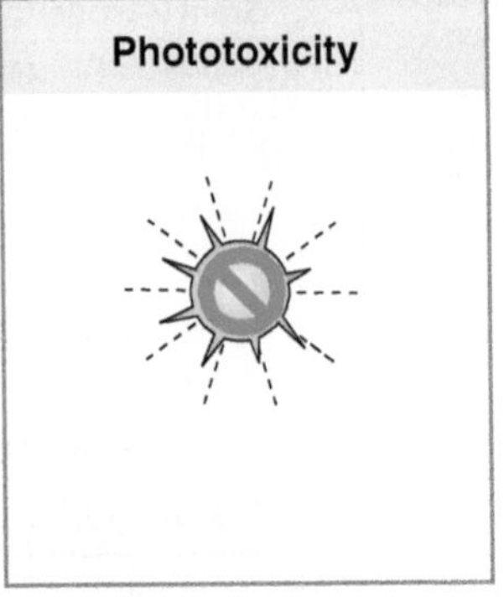


**Figure 30.5** Some typical side effects of fluoroquinolones. (Adapted with permission from Harvey RA, Champe PC, Howland RD, et al. *Lippincott's Illustrated Reviews: Pharmacology*, 3rd edition. Baltimore: Lippincott Williams & Wilkins, 2006.)

This class of antibacterials is involved with a number of drug interactions, including the effect of antacids on absorption previously mentioned. Ciprofloxacin and levofloxacin interfere with the metabolism of theophylline and can significantly raise theophylline levels, an effect that can result in toxicity if the theophylline dose is not adjusted.

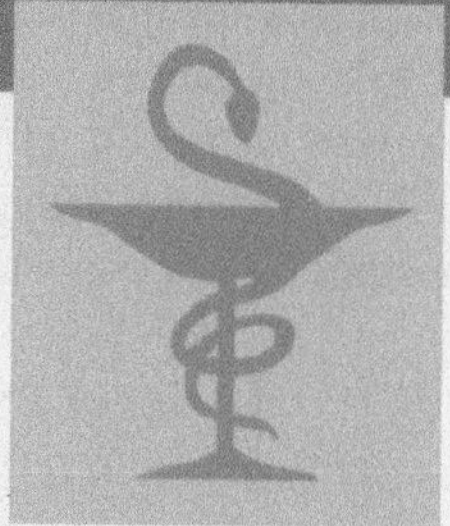

**Tips for the Technician**

The fluoroquinolones are among the most prescribed of all antibiotics. They cause some fairly unique side effects, and patients should be educated about these effects by the pharmacist. Like all antibiotics, it is important for patients to complete the prescribed course of therapy to avoid the development of resistant organisms. It is appropriate for technicians to affix an auxiliary label instructing patients to complete all of the medication unless otherwise directed by their physician. Other auxiliary labelling should include instructions to avoid the use of antacids, and a recommendation to restrict sun exposure and apply sunscreen when in the sun. Technicians should alert the pharmacist to any drug interaction warnings that appear during computerized order entry of the fluoroquinolones.

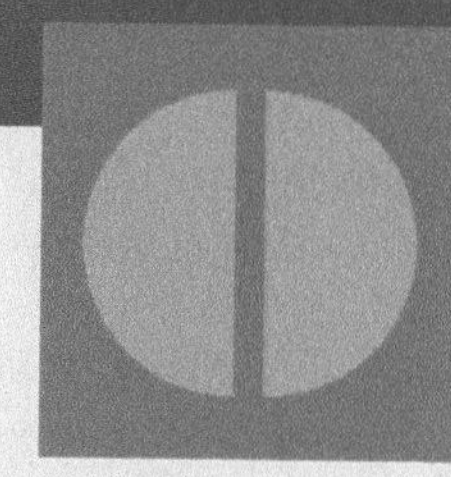

**Case 30.1**

It was a busy day at Bill's Pills Pharmacy, and Bill was up to his elbows in prescriptions that needed filling. As Bill was rushing to get the work done, his pharmacy technician, Annie Danow was feeling the pressure. To add to the stress, Mrs. Parson, a regular at Bill's Pills, was waiting for a prescription, and looked and sounded as though she was in misery. Mrs. Parson has asthma and chronic bronchitis, and she was there on that day to get a prescription for ciprofloxacin to treat a sinus infection and another bout of respiratory infection. Annie entered the prescription into the pharmacy computer system, and skipped through the flashing drug interaction warning, so that she could get poor Mrs. Parson on her way. Annie rationalized that these warnings went off all the time, and usually weren't important. The next week, the Reverend Mr. Parson called to inform the pharmacy staff that Mrs. Parson was in the intensive care unit because she was having seizures. The ICU doctor told Mr. Parson that if her doctor and the pharmacy staff had done their jobs correctly, Mrs. Parson would not be in the hospital. What is the likely cause of Mrs. Parson's seizures? What could Annie have done differently that would have prevented the problem? Besides putting Mrs. Parson in the hospital, what other unfortunate outcome could result from this case?

##  Urinary Antiseptics

Urinary tract infections (UTI) are a common problem in women of childbearing age and in the elderly. *Escherichia coli* is the most common pathogen, causing about eighty percent of uncomplicated infections. Although the fluoroquinolones and cotrimoxazole are more commonly used for treatment, nitrofurantoin (Macrodantin®) and methenamine may be useful in some situations.

### Actions and Indications

These two drugs are chemically unrelated and have different mechanisms of action. Their use is limited to infections of the urinary tract. Methenamine is intended for long-term suppression or prevention of recurring bladder infections. It is available as two different salts, methenamine mandelate (Mandelamine®) and methenamine hippurate (Hiprex®). When exposed to acidic urine in the bladder, methenamine is broken down into ammonia and formaldehyde, which is bacteriocidal. The effectiveness of the drug is dependent upon acidic urine, and occasionally a second drug is given to acidify the urine.

Nitrofurantoin is indicated for treatment of UTI caused by susceptible organisms. Although it was used for prevention of UTI in the past, it is not indicated for this use because of potentially serious adverse effects when taken chronically. Like methenamine, this drug is also more active in acidic urine, but does not require acid urine for effect. Nitrofurantoin breaks down in the body to an active form that inhibits bacterial enzymes and interferes with bacterial metabolism. Nitrofurantoin is bacteriostatic in low concentration and bacteriocidal in high urine concentrations.

## Administration

Both methenamine and nitrofurantoin are only administered by mouth. These medications are given with food. Nitrofurantoin absorption is improved when administered with food, and GI upset is reduced when methenamine is given with meals. Methenamine hippurate is given twice daily and methenamine mandelate is administered four times daily. Nitrofurantoin is given four times daily unless the monohydrate form (Macrobid®) is used. The longer-acting nitrofurantoin monohydrate capsules can be given twice daily.

### Side Effects

Methenamine typically can cause GI upset, rash, and in high doses, crystallization of uric acid in the bladder. Bladder irritation and pain with urination, symptoms that are typical of bladder infections, can be made worse by this medication. Rarely, it can cause shortness of breath and edema.

Nitrofurantoin can cause serious side effects in the lungs. Pulmonary toxicity is well documented, and can either be acute or chronic. Acute pulmonary reactions occur early in therapy and include shortness of breath, cough, fever and chills. Although dangerous, these symptoms reverse quickly once the drug is discontinued. This is a hypersensitivity reaction, and patients who experience this type of reaction should be considered allergic to nitrofurantoin. A second type of pulmonary toxicity occurs with prolonged therapy of 1 to 6 months duration. This type of toxicity is associated with an insidious onset of shortness of breath, dry cough, and complaints of tiredness or weakness. In these cases, pneumonitis and pulmonary fibrosis can occur, which results in permanent damage to the lungs and sometimes death. Nitrofurantoin can also cause GI distress, including vomiting, headache, pain in the legs, rashes (sometimes severe), hemolytic anemia in people with glucose-6-phosphate dehydrogenase deficiency, and liver toxicity.

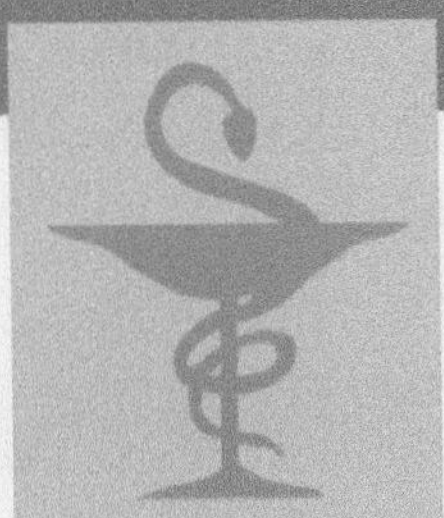

## Tips for the Technician

As with all antibacterial medications, patients should be encouraged to comply with the prescriber's instructions and complete their medication unless the doctor tells them to stop taking it. These medications should be taken with food, and methenamine should be taken with plenty of water. Some prescribers may encourage patients to take methenamine with cranberry juice or tablets to enhance the production of acid urine. Nitrofurantoin can cause brown discoloration of the urine, and prescriptions should be labelled with a "may discolor urine" warning. Technicians should affix the appropriate auxiliary labels (take with food, complete all the medication) to the prescription vials before dispensing these medications. Patients taking nitrofurantoin should be warned to immediately report any lung symptoms to the doctor or pharmacist.

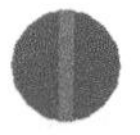

# Tuberculosis and Other Mycobacterial Infections

Tuberculosis (TB) is one of the two most deadly infectious diseases in the world today, killing more than 1.5 million people worldwide every year. Tuberculosis has a long and ferocious history with humanity. It was one of the most dreaded infectious diseases, causing prolonged suffering and inevitable death, for many centuries before the initiation of intense public health initiatives and the advent of antibiotics. During the 19th century, there was a tuberculosis epidemic in the westernized nations, as evidenced by the numerous accounts of death by TB in the fiction of the time. At the turn of the nineteenth century, death rates were nearly 200 per 100,000 persons. By the 1970s, this number was reduced to about 10 per 100,000 through intense public health efforts and extensive treatment with antibiotics. A sense of complacency accompanied the declining death rates in the late 20th century, and attention and funding for public health programs waned. At about the same time, increased immigration from nations where TB flourished and immunodeficiency from AIDS intersected to produce a resurgence of TB that has become increasingly difficult to treat.

An organism of the genus *Mycobacterium* causes tuberculosis. These bacteria are hardy and slow growing with a cell wall that is difficult to penetrate. Other members of this genus cause leprosy, and Mycobacterium avium-intracellular complex (MAC), a disease found in immunologically compromised patients. A subspecies of *Mycobacterium avium* causes disease in food animals and is being studied as a cause of the chronic inflammatory bowel diseases.

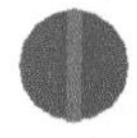

# Drugs for Treatment of Mycobacterial Infections

There are at least a dozen different drugs available for the treatment of tuberculosis, but only five of these are considered drugs of first choice. Streptomycin, an aminoglycoside antibiotic, was discussed in Chapter 29. In-depth discussion here will be limited to the first-line drugs used for treatment of TB. Isoniazid, rifampin, ethambutol, and pyrazinamide are considered the principal, or first-line drugs for TB because of their safety and efficacy.

Because of the increasingly high rate of resistance in tuberculosis, the Center for Disease Control now recommends initial treatment with four antituberculosis drugs for several weeks, followed by four or more month's additional treatment with at least two drugs (**Table 30.2**). These recommendations are likely to change, as multiple drug resistant organisms become more prevalent. The World Health Organization has discovered tuberculosis organisms that are resistant to both first- and second-line drugs. The organisms resistant to first and second line drugs are referred to as extensive drug resistant (XDR) tuberculosis.

## Action and Indications

Isoniazid (INH) is a synthetic relative of the B vitamin pyridoxine, and is a prodrug that is changed to the active form inside the bacteria. It is one of the most effective of the antitubercular drugs, and works by interfering with production of the bacterial cell wall. It is considered to be bacteriocidal when the bacteria are actively dividing. Resistance to this drug develops quickly if it is the only drug used. It is specifically indicated for treatment of *M. tuberculosis* infection, and it is used in combination with other anti-tubercular drugs.

Rifampin is a true antibiotic and a member of a class of drugs referred to as rifamycin antibiotics. Two related antibiotics, rifabutin and rifapentine, are second-line drugs in the treatment of TB. The rifamycin antibiotics work by inhibiting an enzyme that is necessary

**Table 30.2** CDC Recommendations for the Treatment of Tuberculosis

| Initial Phase | | | Continuation Phase | | |
|---|---|---|---|---|---|
| **Regimen** | **Drugs** | **Interval and doses (minimal duration)** | **Regimen** | **Drugs** | **Interval and doses (minimal duration)** |
| 1 | INH<br>RIF<br>PZA<br>EMB | Seven days per week for 56 doses (8 wk) or 5 d/wk for 40 doses (8 wk) | 1a | INH/RIF | Seven days per week for 126 doses (18 wk) or 5 d/wk for 90 doses (18 wk) |
| | | | 1b | INH/RIF | Twice weekly for 36 doses (18 wk) |
| | | | 1c | INH/RPT | Twice weekly for 18 doses (18 wk) |
| 2 | INH<br>RIF<br>PZA<br>EMB | Seven days per week for 14 doses (2 wk), then twice weekly for 12 doses (6 wk) or 5 d/wk for 10 doses (2 wk), then twice weekly for 12 doses (6wk) | 2a | INH/RIF | Twice weekly for 36 doses (18 wk) |
| | | | 2b | INH/RPT | Once weekly for 18 doses (18 wk) |
| 3 | INH<br>RIF<br>PZA<br>EMB | Three times weekly for 24 doses (8 wk) | 3a | INH/RIF | Three times weekly for 54 doses (18 wk) |
| 4 | INH<br>RIF<br>EMB | Seven days per week for 56 doses (8 wk) or 5 d/wk for 40 doses (8 wk) | 4a | INH/RIF | Seven days per week for 217 doses (31 wk) or 5 d/wk for 155 doses (31 wk) |
| | | | 4b | INH/RIF | Twice weekly for 62 doses (31 wk) |

EMB, Ethambutol; INH, isoniazid; PZA, pyrazinamide; RIF, rifampin; RTP, rifapentine.

Reprinted from Treatment of Tuberculosis: American Thoracic Society, CDC, and Infectious Diseases Society of America. *Morbidity and Mortality Weekly Report* 52(RR11);1–77. June 20, 2003 (published by the Centers for Disease Control and Prevention). Accessed from http://www.cdc.gov/mmwr July 25, 2007.

for bacterial RNA synthesis. Rifampin is bacteriocidal, and effective against not only species of mycobacterium, but also some gram-positive and gram-negative bacteria. Rifampin is indicated for treatment of tuberculosis, and for preventing meningitis in individuals exposed to *Neisseria meningitidis* or *Haemophilus influenzae* meningitis.

Rifampin is the most active anti-leprosy drug presently available, but to delay the emergence of resistant strains it is usually given in combination with other drugs. Leprosy, or Hansen disease, is rare in the United States, but a small number of cases are reported each year. Worldwide, it is a much larger problem. Rifampin, dapsone, and clofazimine are given for 6 to 24 months for the treatment of leprosy.

Pyrazinamide is a synthetic antitubercular agent used in combination with isoniazid and rifampin. It is bacteriocidal to actively dividing organisms, but the mechanism of its action is unknown. Pyrazinamide must be converted to the active form of the drug by a bacterial enzyme. Some resistant strains lack the enzyme required for conversion. Pyrazinamide is specifically active against tubercle bacilli, and is therefore only indicated for treatment of tuberculosis.

Ethambutol is bacteriostatic and works because it inhibits an enzyme that is important for the synthesis of the mycobacterial cell wall. It is specific for most strains of *M. tuberculosis*. Ethambutol resistance is not a serious problem if the drug is employed with other antitubercular agents. It is used in combination with pyrazinamide, isoniazid, and rifampin to treat tuberculosis.

The second-line treatments for tuberculosis are either no more effective and less well tolerated than the first-line agents, or they are particularly active against resistant and atypical strains of mycobacteria, and are therefore reserved. Second-line drugs include aminosalicylic acid, cycloserine, capreomycin, ethionamide, rifabutin, and rifapentine. The fluoroquinolones, discussed earlier in this chapter, play an important role in the treatment of multidrug-resistant tuberculosis. Macrolides (Chapter 29) are part of the regimen used for the treatment of MAC.

## Administration

With the exception of streptomycin, all of the first-line antituberculars are administered orally. They are readily absorbed after oral administration and distribute widely throughout the body. Isoniazid and rifampin can be given parenterally when needed. Isoniazid is given IM, and rifampin is given in cases where oral administration is not feasible. The drugs are administered once daily, often in a clinic setting where patients can be directly observed, to improve compliance.

## Side Effects

The incidence of adverse effects caused by isoniazid is fairly low. Most adverse effects are related to the dosage and duration of administration. Peripheral neuropathy (injury to the nerves that supply sensation to the arms and legs), which is the most common adverse effect, appears to be due to INH antagonism of the actions of pyridoxine. This and other effects on the nervous system can be corrected by pyridoxine (vitamin $B_6$) supplementation. Potentially fatal hepatitis is the most severe side effect associated with isoniazid, but seizures and drug related anemias also occur. The incidence of hepatitis increases in the elderly, among patients who take rifampin along with INH, or among those who drink alcohol daily.

peripheral neuropathy
Disease or injury to the nerves that supply sensation to the arms and legs.

Adverse effects are generally a minor problem with rifampin, but can include nausea and vomiting, and allergic reactions, sometimes presenting as rash and fever. The drug is used judiciously in patients with chronic liver disease, alcoholics, and the elderly, because rifampin can cause liver toxicity. High doses are associated with more severe side effects, such as renal failure and suppressed production of blood cells. When taken with birth control pills, anticoagulants, digoxin, phenytoin, and many other drugs, rifampin is likely to reduce the effects of the other drugs. Sometimes dose adjustments of the other drugs must be made, and women taking hormonal contraceptives are advised to use an additional form of contraception while on rifampin.

Pyrazinamide and ethambutol are quite well tolerated. They both can increase the risk of gouty attacks in people with gout, and can cause GI upset, rash, and a feeling of tiredness. Pyrazinamide causes minor muscle and joint aches and pains on a fairly frequent basis. The most serious side effects associated with pyrazinamide use are a possible reduction in the number of platelets, and an additive effect on the liver when combined with other liver toxic antitubercular drugs. The most important adverse effect caused by ethambutol is optic neuritis, which results in diminished vision and loss of ability to discriminate between red and green. When the drug is discontinued, vision usually returns to normal. Ethambutol can also cause reduced platelet counts, dizziness, and confusion.

## Tips for the Technician

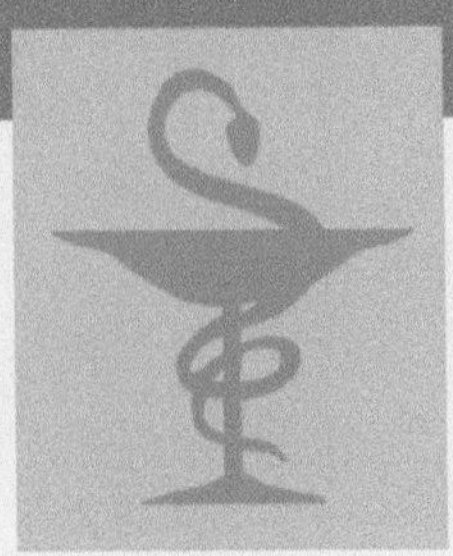

These drugs are often dispensed at outpatient clinics, and they are used in hospitals when tuberculosis is newly diagnosed, or when TB patients are admitted to the hospital for other reasons. The pharmacist should advise patients on the importance of adhering to the prescribed drug regimen and potential side effects. The technician will label all antitubercular medications with auxiliary labels encouraging patients to complete the medication unless otherwise directed. INH, rifampin, and pyrazinamide prescriptions must include a warning for the patient to avoid alcohol consumption while taking these medications. Technicians can warn patients that rifampin turns urine a red-orange color by attaching the appropriate auxiliary label.

# Review Questions

## Multiple Choice

Choose the best answer for the following questions:

1. Which of the following drugs is the sulfonamide-antibacterial combination frequently used for upper respiratory or ear infections and the opportunistic pneumonia sometimes seen in AIDS patients?
   a. Cotrimethobenzamide
   b. Piperacillin-Tazobactam
   c. Cotrimoxazole
   d. Erythromycin-sulfamethoxazole
   e. Cogentin®

2. Inhibition of bacterial folic acid metabolism is the mechanism of action for which of the following antibacterial agents?
   a. Sulfadiazine
   b. Sulfacetamide
   c. Trimethoprim
   d. Sulfamethoxazole
   e. All of the above

3. Of the following antibacterial drugs, circle the one that is not a quinolone derivative.
   a. Nalidixic acid
   b. Nitrofurantoin
   c. Norfloxacin
   d. Levofloxacin
   e. Gatifloxacin

4. Which of the following are side effects associated with the use of fluoroquinolones?
   a. Headache, dizziness, GI upset
   b. Connective tissue damage
   c. Hemolytic anemia

d. a and b
e. All of the above

5. Which of the following are first-line treatments for tuberculosis?
   a. Streptomycetes
   b. Isoniazid
   c. Rifabutin
   d. Ethionamide
   e. Cycloserine

## True/False

6. Bacteria of the genus Mycobacterium cause tuberculosis, leprosy, MAC, and may even be linked to inflammatory bowel diseases.
   a. True
   b. False

7. When given for extended periods of time, the urinary antibacterial nitrofurantoin can cause irreversible pulmonary toxicity.
   a. True
   b. False

8. Fluoroquinolones inhibit bacterial replication by elevating the pH within the cell, causing release of bacterial enzymes that result in lysis of the organism.
   a. True
   b. False

9. In acidic urine methenamine is broken down into formaldehyde and ammonia.
   a. True
   b. False

10. Sulfonamides are avoided in pregnant or nursing women because they easily cross the placenta and enter breast milk.
    a. True
    b. False

## Matching

For numbers 11 to 15, match the statement with the correct lettered choice from the list below. Choices will not be used more than once and may not be used at all.

11. Drinking plenty of water is essential while taking these drugs.
12. Drug class that works by inhibiting the enzymes responsible for maintaining bacterial DNA.
13. Can cause dysglycemia.
14. Bacterial genus responsible for tuberculosis.
15. Side effects include optic neuritis.

a. Dihydrogen oxide
b. Ethambutol
c. Mycobacterium
d. Fluoroquinolones
e. Gatifloxacin
g. Sulfonamides
h. Agrobacterium

## Short Answer

16. Explain why the folic acid antagonism caused by the sulfonamides is safe for humans but damaging to bacteria.

17. Which fluoroquinolones only need to be taken once a day? Why?
18. List the side effects of the urinary antiseptic methenamine.
19. What factors have contributed to the recent increase in tuberculosis infections?
20. Why are fluoroquinolone antibiotics not recommended for use in children? What related, rare side effect is seen in adults?

## FOR FURTHER INQUIRY

Investigate the use of the second-line drugs for tuberculosis on the Center for Disease Control website. See if you can determine why they are not considered drugs of first choice. How and when would these agents be used? Visit the World Health Organization web site to learn where XDR-TB occurs and why it appeared. Find out what, if any, treatment options are available for people with XDR-TB.

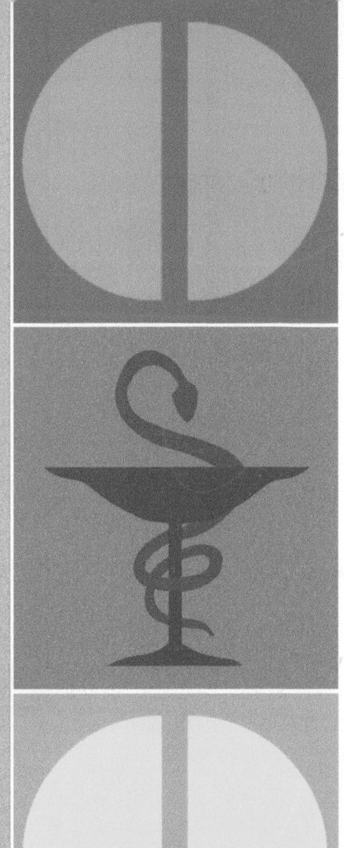

Chapter **31**

# Drug Treatment of Fungal and Parasitic Infections

*KEY TERMS*

- colloid
- endemic
- eukaryote
- helminth
- malaise
- mycosis
- nit
- onychomycoses
- opportunistic infection
- prokaryote
- thrush

## OBJECTIVES

After studying this chapter, the reader should be able to:

- Explain why fungal infections are more difficult to treat than bacterial infections, why antibiotics will not kill fungi, and why serious fungal infections are becoming more common.
- List four significant characteristics of amphotericin B products that pharmacy technicians must know in order to compound safe, stable, and effective intravenous preparations.
- Describe two advantages of azole antifungals over amphotericin, and list three azole antifungal drugs, their indications, available formulations, and most common side effects.
- List one protozoal and one helminth infection that are fairly common parasitic infections in the United States and state the drug of choice to treat each infection.
- Evaluate the characteristics of metronidazole and describe which characteristic of the drug you think is most unique, which side effect is most likely to reduce patient compliance, and which indication for its use is most important, and why.

## DRUGS COVERED IN THIS CHAPTER

| Antifungal Drugs | | | Drugs for Parasitic Infections | |
|---|---|---|---|---|
| **Antifungals for Systemic Mycoses** | **Azole Antifungals** | **Antifungals for Cutaneous Mycoses** | **Antiprotozoal Agents** | **Other Antiparasitic Drugs** |
| Amphotericin B | Fluconazole | Clotrimazole | Chloroquine | Mebendazole |
| Caspofungin | Itraconazole | Econazole | Mefloquine | Permethrin |
| Flucytosine | Ketoconazole | Griseofulvin | Metronidazole | Pyrantel Pamoate |
| | Voriconazole | Miconazole | Paromomycin | Pyrethrin |
| | | Nystatin | Primaquine | |
| | | Terbinafine | Quinine | |
| | | Tolnaftate | | |
| | | Undecylenic Acid | | |

Until recently, the risk of acquiring any fungal infection worse than athlete's foot, ringworm, or a vaginal yeast infection was small. Likewise, the parasitic infections likely to occur in developed countries were generally limited to pinworms, roundworms, lice, or scabies. The convergence of the increased use of immunosuppressant drugs, the spread of AIDS, and the increase in world travel and trade have changed the demographics of fungal, parasitic, and viral infections worldwide. This fact has given rise to a growing need for drugs to combat infection and a growing sense of alarm, especially regarding potential world-wide epidemics, within the developed countries of the world. This chapter will emphasize the most important, in terms of frequency and the risk to human life, fungal and parasitic infections.

Fungi are a large group of organisms (more than 100,000 species have been identified) that range from mushrooms to yeast. Organisms are placed into this taxonomic classification because they reproduce through spores and absorb nutrients in solution through their cell walls. Most fungi are beneficial to humans. They decompose organic material in the soil, provide us with antibiotics, and are essential for fermentation and as leavening for bread. Parasites are members of a variety of different kingdoms and phyla. Any organism that depends upon another organism for the requirements of life is considered a parasite. Parasites are as varied as mistletoe and orchids, to mites and lice, to parasitic worms. A few of these organisms live in humans, and cause a great deal of pain and suffering for the human race.

Fungi and parasites are far more complex organisms than bacteria, and therefore infections caused by these organisms are more difficult to treat. Fungi and parasites are considered eukaryotic organisms. Eukaryotic cells contain many more organelles and operate on metabolic processes that are more sophisticated than those of bacteria, which are prokaryotic organisms. In bacteria, genetic material consists of simple strands of DNA, while in the eukaryotes there is a nucleus that is separated from the rest of the cellular material by a membrane, and contains chromosomes that hold the organism's DNA. Although there are single celled fungi and parasites, most are multicellular organisms.

eukaryote Organisms composed of one or more cells that contain nuclei and organelles.

prokaryote Typically unicellular micro-organisms that lack a distinct nucleus and membrane-bound organelles; for example, bacteria.

The biological make-up and metabolic processes of fungi and parasites are important to pharmacologists because mammalian cells are also eukaryotes. Because of their greater similarity to mammalian cells, drugs that kill fungi and parasites are more likely to cause toxicity to human cells.

# Fungal Infections

Infectious diseases caused by fungi are called mycoses, and are often chronic in nature. Fungal infections are classified according to their location in body tissues. Infections of the skin surfaces or hair are considered superficial, while infections of deeper skin structures and nails are called cutaneous infections. Systemic infections pose a greater threat to the host and are more difficult to treat. Systemic fungal infections, those that overwhelm the host defenses and spread to the bloodstream or internal organs, are not likely to occur in people with normal immune systems. When they occur in people with impaired immune systems, they are referred to as opportunistic infections.

mycosis An infection or disease caused by a fungus.

opportunistic infection Infectious disease caused by an organism that is not usually a pathogen, because the patient's immune system is suppressed.

Nonopportunistic fungal infections follow a typical geographic pattern related to the presence of these organisms in the local soil or other areas of the environment. For example, Coccidioides immitis is native to the soil of the Southwestern United States (**Fig. 31.1**). Individuals who either live in this area or travel through it are the only otherwise healthy people likely to contract coccidioidomycoses. Overwhelming, systemic fungal infections are often life threatening, and although they can be suppressed, they are not typically cured.

People with ineffective or impaired immune system, such as those who take immunosuppressive drugs, individuals with AIDS, or patients in hospitals who develop nosocomial infections, are much more likely to contract systemic fungal infections than healthy individuals. Fungal infections that occur in people with poor immune defenses are increasing and are becoming a fairly common cause of sepsis, or infection of the bloodstream. Although there is some overlap of drug classes, on the whole drugs that are used to treat systemic fungal infection are different from those used to treat cutaneous or superficial infection.

The life cycles and metabolic processes of fungi are very different from those of bacteria. For this reason, antibacterial drugs are inherently ineffective against fungi and antifungal drugs are likewise ineffective treatment for bacterial infections. The composition of the fungal cell wall is a case in point. Bacterial and fungal cell walls are completely different, with the fungal cell wall depending upon complex lipids called sterols to control the passage of small molecules into and out of the cells. On the other hand, bacterial cell walls

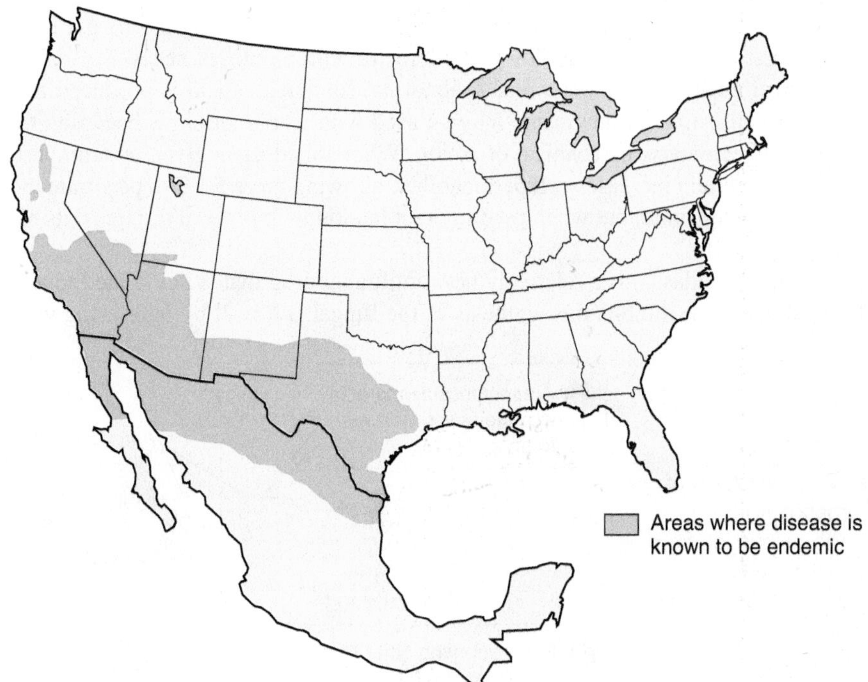


**Figure 31.1** Nonopportunistic fungal infections occur in a geographic pattern related to their presence in the local environment. This map shows where Coccidioides immitis lives, and where coccidioidomycoses is endemic. (Source: U.S. Geological Survey)

are made up mainly of sugars and amino acids. Antifungal agents must, therefore, be designed to take advantage of different targets in fungal cells, rendering them ineffective against other organisms.

# Antifungal Agents Used for Systemic Mycoses

In response to the increasing incidence of systemic fungal infections, ongoing development of new antifungal drugs has produced effective therapy for all but the most serious fungal infections. Unfortunately, some of the antifungals used for systemic infections are very toxic, and depending on the site of the infection, antifungal agents may only suppress it, not cure it. The treatments for systemic mycoses include the unrelated drugs amphotericin B, flucytosine, and caspofungin, and a few drugs from a group of newer, chemically related, antifungals. The newer agents are members of the azole antifungals class, some of which are used systemically and others that are used for superficial mycoses.

## Amphotericin B, Flucytosine, Caspofungin

Amphotericin B (1956) and flucytosine (1964) were the only systemic antifungal agents available until the introduction of the first systemic azole antifungal in the early 1980s. Amphotericin B (Fungizone®) remains the gold standard for treatment of life threatening systemic fungal infections. However, the azole antifungals are preferred for their safety.

### Actions and Indications

Amphotericin B molecules bind to molecules in the plasma membranes of sensitive fungal cells. When they bind, a channel is formed through the membrane that disrupts its ability to function. As a result, electrolytes and small molecules leak from the cell, which causes cell damage or death (**Fig. 31.2**). Amphotericin B is either fungicidal or fungistatic, depending on the organism being treated, its sensitivity, and the serum concentration of the drug that is attained with treatment. It is effective against a wide range of fungi, including *Candida albicans*, *Histoplasma capsulatum*, *Cryptococcus neoformans*, *Coccidioides immitis*, and many strains of aspergillus.

Flucytosine (often abbreviated 5-FC, Ancobon®) works by entering the fungal cells where it is converted to a toxic metabolite that competes with a nutrient necessary for the synthesis of fungal nucleic acids. As a result, abnormal ribonucleic acid is produced and protein synthesis is disrupted. Flucytosine may be used with amphotericin B because of a different, but complementary, mechanism of action. When this drug is given with amphotericin B, the amphotericin increases cell permeability, allowing more 5-FC to penetrate the cell. Flucytosine is fungistatic, but when used in combination with other antifungals, its effectiveness is improved.

Caspofungin (Cancidas®) is a relatively new antifungal drug that is not related to any other antifungal agents. It inhibits the synthesis of the fungal cell wall by interfering with

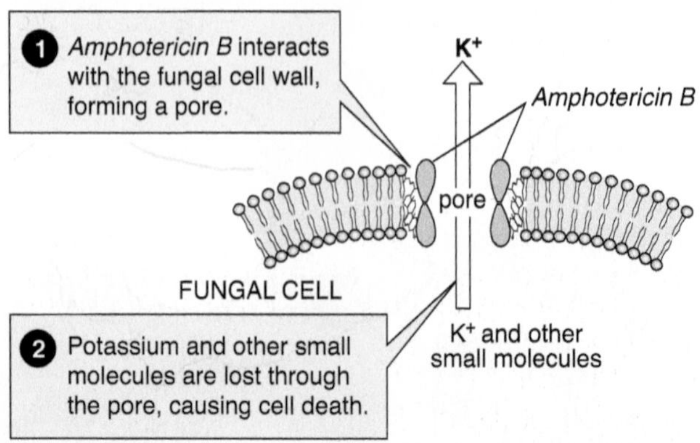


**Figure 31.2** Mechanism of action of amphotericin. (Adapted with permission from Harvey RA, Champe PC, Howland RD, et al. *Lippincott's Illustrated Reviews: Pharmacology*, 3rd edition. Baltimore: Lippincott Williams & Wilkins, 2006.)

the production of one integral component. Lack of a functional cell wall leads to cell death. Caspofungin is indicated only for the treatment of invasive aspergillus, a fungal infection that can develop in the lungs, especially in immunosuppressed patients. Its use is usually restricted to those patients who cannot tolerate amphotericin.

## Administration

Amphotericin B is highly insoluble in water, and therefore is manufactured as a colloid. Although it is clear on reconstitution, a colloid is actually a suspension of microscopic particles in liquid. Amphotericin B is administered by intravenous infusion over several hours, and must be reconstituted and diluted in accordance with the manufacturer's recommendation, only in 5% dextrose in water. Within the last 10 years, several new formulations of amphotericin, compounded with lipids, became available. These liposomal preparations (AmBisome®, Abelcet®, Amphotec®) have the primary advantage of reduced kidney and infusion related toxicity. However, because of their high cost, they are reserved mainly for those individuals with life-threatening fungal infections that cannot tolerate conventional amphotericin B.

colloid Microscopic particles, smaller than $1 \times 10^{-6}$, suspended in a liquid.

Besides intravenous administration, amphotericin B can be injected into the cerebrospinal fluid for the treatment of meningitis caused by fungi that are sensitive to the drug. It is also available as a cream, ointment or lotion for topical use, and as an oral suspension for local treatment of oropharyngeal yeast infections. It is sometimes used off-label for inhalation and for ophthalmic administration.

Flucytosine is well absorbed by the oral route, and is only available for oral administration. The presence of food reduces the absorption of the drug. Once absorbed, the drug distributes throughout the body and penetrates well into the organs, eyes, and cerebrospinal fluid. Most of the dose (75% to 90%) is excreted unchanged by the kidneys, and the dose must be adjusted in patients with compromised renal function.

Caspofungin is not active when given orally and must be administered by intravenous infusion. Unlike amphotericin B, this drug must be diluted only in normal saline, not dextrose. In order to avoid pain on infusion, the manufacturer recommends that all strengths of the drug be diluted in 250 mL of normal saline solution. Caspofungin remains in the body for a very long time, and undergoes slow metabolism in the liver. People with liver failure are usually given a reduced dose.

## Side Effects

If it were not for the grave threat to the patient posed by systemic fungal infections, and the few drug therapy options available, amphotericin B might have been removed from the market long ago. It has a very narrow therapeutic index, and the total daily dose of the original formulation should never exceed 1.5 mg amphotericin B/kg body weight. Some fungal infections require doses up to this maximum, even though higher doses have been reported to cause cardiovascular or respiratory collapse, or even death in some patients. A typical dose of conventional amphotericin B for an average weight adult is generally in the range of 50 to 70 mg. The dosing recommendations for the lipid based amphotericin products are very different from the conventional form and from each other, and can in some cases be as high as 5 mg drug/kg body weight. A typical dose of one of these products could be as high as 350 mg. Obviously, the name similarities and dosing differences create an opportunity for dangerous errors.

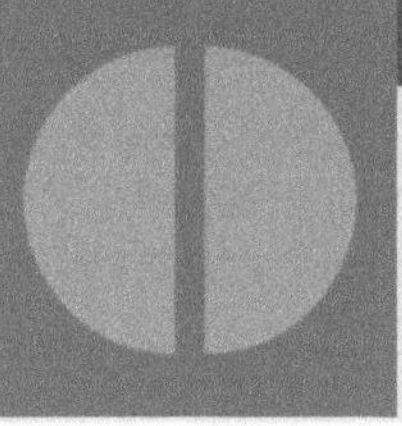

### Case 31.1

Marissa Hernandez is a very conscientious hospital-based technician who is making the IV admixtures for the day at Hospital of the Sequoias. She is preparing the drug that some pharmacists jokingly refer to as "amphoterrible" for a new patient with a serious case of coccidioidomycoses. Marissa knows amphotericin is a very toxic drug, so she reviews the order, which reads amphotericin B 200 mg IVPB daily. Marissa retrieves four vials of Fungizone® from the refrigerator and has the IVPB almost finished when Catherine Crabbe, the only pharmacist on at the time, sticks her head in to warn Marissa that she is going to the "code blue" that was just announced. Moments later, Nurse Ratchet calls to demand the amphotericin B for her patient. Marissa tells her that the IV is made, but that she cannot release it until it is checked. "Listen, sweetheart," Nurse Ratchet begins, "this woman is scared, she wants to get her treatment started, and she's too big for me to argue with, so bring me my IV."

"I really need for it to be checked," Marissa says.

"Fine. I'll be up to pick it up and I'll check it."

"That's very nice of you to offer . . . " Marissa says as she wonders what she should do.

Discuss this case in class and investigate name confusion for these drugs on the Institute for Safe Medication Practices web site. Afterwards, write a possible ending for this case.

malaise Generalized feeling of physical discomfort.

The most common side effects observed with the systemic use of amphotericin B include headache, malaise (a general feeling of physical discomfort), irritation at the site of injection, and fever and chills associated with infusion of the drug (**Fig. 31.3**). GI upset, anemia, bronchospasm, and cardiac arrhythmias can occur, and can sometimes be very serious. Impaired kidney function, often accompanied by loss of potassium, is quite common, and kidney damage can be permanent. It is this side effect that frequently limits the ability to continue with treatment. Because of the nephrotoxic effect of amphotericin, other drugs that cause nephrotoxicity are usually avoided while the patient is receiving amphotericin therapy.

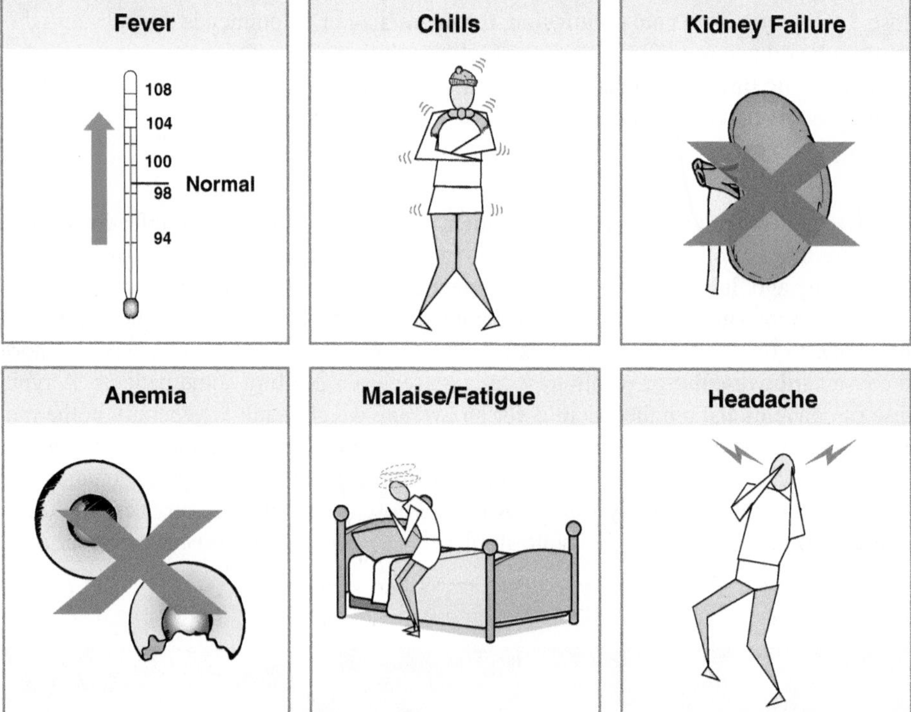


**Figure 31.3** Adverse effects most commonly experienced due to systemic use of amphotericin. (Adapted with permission from Harvey RA, Champe PC, Howland RD, et al. *Lippincott's Illustrated Reviews: Pharmacology*, 3rd edition. Baltimore: Lippincott Williams & Wilkins, 2006.)

Flucytosine can cause a number of serious side effects, but these are rare. Reversible neutropenia, thrombocytopenia, and occasional bone marrow depression can occur. Flucytosine is associated with myocardial toxicity, which can be life threatening, but is rare. When this drug is given along with amphotericin it can add to the already problematic kidney toxicity. Gastrointestinal disturbances, such as nausea, vomiting, and diarrhea, are common, and severe colitis can occur. Some of these adverse effects may be related to the formation of fluorouracil by intestinal organisms. Fluorouracil is the active, and highly toxic metabolite that results when fungal cells act upon the drug. When this same reaction occurs in the gut, some of the active metabolite, which is also used in cancer chemotherapy, may cause damage to human cells.

Caspofungin causes a number of unpleasant side effects but serious complications are rare. Typical side effects include tingling in the limbs, loss of appetite, and muscle pain. Infusion reactions, such as chills, fever, pain at the injection site, rash, itching, rapid respirations, and a feeling of warmth can all occur with some frequency. This drug should not be given with cyclosporine because of possible additive hepatotoxic effects.

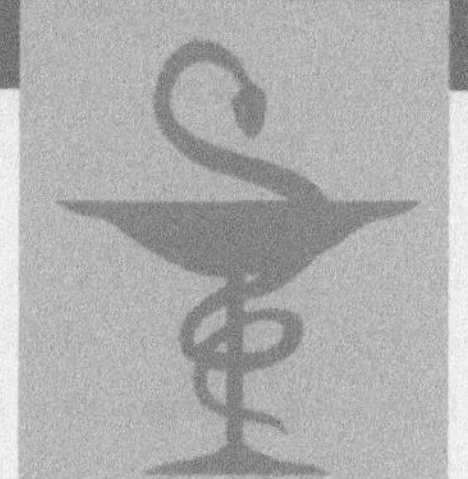

## Tips for the Technician

Colloids are inherently prone to separation, and amphotericin B is no exception. The lipid-complex forms of amphotericin are more stable than the original formulation, and by following manufacturer recommendations reconstitution separation can be avoided. All of the amphotericin B dry powder formulations should be reconstituted with preservative free sterile water only, to prevent precipitation of the drug. All formulations are further diluted with 5% dextrose in water. The original amphotericin B formulation should not be filtered because filters remove the microscopic drug particles. When the lipid-complex formulations are filtered, follow each manufacturer's specific instructions for filter pore size to avoid removing active ingredient. Amphotericin B should not be piggybacked with any other solutions or medications. The original amphotericin B preparation (Fungizone®) is unstable in the presence of light and, therefore, requires protection from light.

Technicians should be aware that different amphotericin B products are not interchangeable, not only because the formulations are not equivalent, but most importantly because the doses of the products vary. Drug errors can be prevented if the products are not located near each other on the shelf, and special policies relating to the use of these drugs are followed precisely.

# Azole Antifungals

The azole antifungals are a group of several related compounds, important in the treatment of systemic and cutaneous fungal infections. Ketoconazole (Nizoral®), the first orally active azole antifungal, set the stage for the development of many other azole antifungal agents, which are now the most frequently prescribed antifungal drugs. Ketoconazole, fluconazole (Diflucan®), itraconazole (Sporanox®), and voriconazole (Vfend®) are azole antifungal agents used for systemic mycoses.

## Actions and Indications

The azole antifungal drugs inhibit the synthesis of ergosterol, a sterol compound, which is a principal component of fungal cell membranes. Through this bacteriostatic drug action, the cell membrane structure is disrupted and function is impaired, resulting in inhibition of fungal cell growth and replication. Unfortunately, human cells also depend upon sterols (cholesterol, for example) for many functions, and the azole drugs vary in their specificity for ergosterol. Ketoconazole, which is less specific in its inhibition of sterols, is less likely to be selected for systemic use than the newer, more specific azole antifungals, such as fluconazole, itraconazole, or voriconazole.

Fluconazole is used to prevent fungal infections in people undergoing bone marrow transplantation, and is the drug of choice for some fungal infections, including candidemia, and some cases of systemic coccidioidomycosis. It is especially useful when patients are unable to receive amphotericin B, or where the infection is limited to the lungs. Fluconazole is effective against most forms of candidiasis, however resistance seems to be on the rise. Itraconazole is a recent addition to the azole family of antifungal agents, with a broad antifungal spectrum. Itraconazole is now the drug of choice for the treatment of a number of infections, including aspergillosis, and histoplasmosis. Voriconazole is the newest azole antifungal. It is approved for the treatment of invasive aspergillosis and a few other serious and difficult to treat fungal diseases.

## Administration

The azole antifungals are adequately absorbed when given by mouth. Ketoconazole and itraconazole tablet dissolution and absorption are increased in an acidic environment. Drugs such as antacids, $H_2$ receptor blockers, and proton-pump inhibitors can hamper the absorption of these drugs. When ketoconazole and itraconazole are taken with a full meal or acidifying beverages such as cola drinks, absorption is enhanced. Absorption of fluconazole and voriconazole is excellent and is not dependent on gastric acidity.

Fluconazole, itraconazole, and voriconazole are available in preparations for intravenous administration. Fluconazole is sold in premixed bags, but the other two must be compounded. Refer to **Table 31.1** for a summary of the brand names, indications, and formulations of antifungal drugs discussed in this chapter. The liver is responsible for removal of a large proportion of ketoconazole, itraconazole, and voriconazole through metabolism. Ethnicity (about 20% of Asians are slow metabolizers), increasing patient age, and liver disease can reduce the metabolism of voriconazole, and as a result, increase the risk of side effects. Fluconazole is excreted via the kidney, and doses are adjusted in patients with impaired kidney function.

**Table 31.1** Generic and Brand Names, Indications, and Available Formulations of the Antifungal Drugs

| Generic | Brand Name | Available as | Indications | Notes |
|---|---|---|---|---|
| **Drugs for Serious Systemic Mycoses** | | | | |
| Amphotericin B | Fungizone® | Powder for injection | Life-threatening systemic mycoses | Doses not equivalent to lipid based products |
| Amphotericin B Lipid Based | Abelcet®, AmBisome® | Susp. for injection<br>Powder for injection | Life-threatening mycoses if amphotericin B not tolerated | Doses not equivalent to each other or original product |
| Caspofungin | Cancidas® | Powder for injection | Invasive aspergillosis | |
| Flucytosine | Ancoban® | Capsules | Serious infections due to Cryptococcus or Candida | |

(continues)

| Generic | Brand Name | Available as | Indications | Notes |
|---|---|---|---|---|
| **Azole Antifungals** | | | | |
| Fluconazole | Diflucan® | Tablets, premix IVPB, powder for oral suspension | Systemic, cutaneous, and localized candidiasis, Cryptococcal meningitis | |
| Itraconazole | Sporanox® | Capsules, injection, powder for oral solution | Systemic mycoses. Oral or esophageal candida—solution only. Onychomycoses, prevent infection in immunosuppressed | Capsules—with food, solution—empty stomach |
| Ketoconazole | Nizoral® | Tablets, cream, shampoo | Systemic or cutaneous mycoses due to sensitive organisms | |
| Voriconazole | Vfend® | Tablets, powder for injection & oral suspension | Serious systemic mycoses, invasive aspergillosis, esophageal candidiasis | |
| **Drugs for Superficial and Cutaneous Mycoses** | | | | |
| Ciclopirox | Loprox®, Penlac® | Cream, gel, topical suspension, shampoo | Tinea infections of skin, hair, or nails | |
| Clotrimazole | Lotrimin®, Mycelex®, many others | Troche, cream, lotion, solution, vaginal suppository, cream | Superficial, oral, or vaginal candidiasis, tinea infections | Lotrimin® brand on several different antifungal agents |
| Econazole | Spectazole® | Cream | Tinea infections of skin | |
| Griseofulvin | Fulvicin®, Gris-PEG® | Tablets | Tinea infections of skin, hair, or nails | Doses not equivalent between brands |
| Miconazole | Monistat®, many others | Cream, ointment, powder, spray powder, vaginal cream, vaginal suppository | Superficial, or vaginal candidiasis, tinea infections | |
| Nystatin | Mycostatin® | Powder, troches, oral suspension, cream, ointment | Oral, vaginal, superficial candidiasis | |
| Terbinafine | Lamisil® | Tablets, cream, spray | Onychomycosis, cutaneous mycoses due to tinea species | |
| Tolnaftate | Tinactin®, Ting® | Cream, solution, gel, powder, spray liquid, spray powder | Infections of skin and scalp from tinea and others | |
| Undecylenic Acid | Cruex®, Caldesene® | Powder, cream, solution, soap | Prevention of diaper rash, tinea infections of skin (not scalp) | |

Susp, suspension.

### Side Effects

The risk of side effects caused by the use of azole antifungals varies from drug to drug. Because of less specific action on sterol synthesis, ketoconazole can affect synthesis of human hormones, and result in a reduction in libido or menstrual irregularities. It is more likely to cause GI upset, rash, or headache, a side effect profile comparable to that seen with the other azole drugs. Use of these drugs is associated with rare, but serious, hepatotoxicity. Itraconazole is a potent inhibitor of one class of drug metabolizing liver enzymes, the cytochrome P450 system, and is prone to numerous, very significant drug interactions (see **Table 31.2** for a display of important antifungal drug interactions). The other azole drugs are also involved with significant drug interactions, but in some cases to a lesser degree. For example, concomitant use of itraconazole with the lipid-lowering statin drugs is not advised, whereas a dose reduction is advised when these drugs are given with voriconazole. These drugs cause a significant increase in anticoagulation and bleeding risk when they are used with warfarin.

**Table 31.2** Potential Antifungal Drug Interactions

| Antifungal drug | Interacting Drugs | Possible Outcome |
|---|---|---|
| Amphotericin | Nephrotoxic drugs, including aminoglycosides, cyclosporine, others | ↑ Risk of nephrotoxicity |
| Fluconazole | Antacids, proton-pump inhibitors, $H_2$ receptor antagonists | Decreased fluconazole absorption |
| Fluconazole | Oral hypoglycemics (all classes) | Increased hypoglycemia possible |
| Itraconazole | Antacids, proton-pump inhibitors, $H_2$ receptor antagonists | Decreased itraconazole absorption |
| Itraconazole | HMG-CoA reductase inhibitors | Do not use together, increased risk rhabdomyolysis |
| Itraconazole | Oral hypoglycemics (all classes) | Increased hypoglycemia possible |
| Voriconazole | Ritonavir and other antiretroviral drugs | ↑ Metabolism of voriconazole |
| All systemic azole antifungals | Warfarin<br>Oral hypoglycemics<br>Cyclosporin<br>Tacrolimus<br>Phenytoin<br>Carbamazepine<br>Benzodiazepines<br>Isoniazid<br>Rifampin<br>Rifabutin<br>Antiarrhythmic Agents | ↑ Levels of interacting drugs,<br>↑ risk of adverse effects |
| All systemic azole antifungals | Isoniazid<br>Rifampin<br>Phenytoin<br>Carbamazepine<br>Phenobarbital | ↑ Metabolism of azole antifungal |

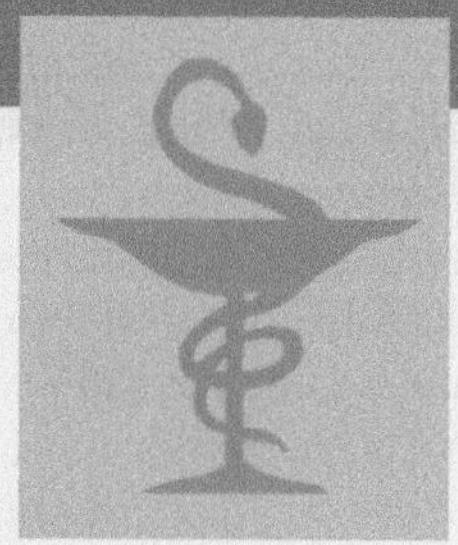

### Tips for the Technician

Pharmacy technicians who work in hospitals or home infusion centers will be called upon to compound IV antifungal medications. Be sure to check the package insert or a compounding reference before reconstituting these drugs. Always follow the manufacturer recommendations for reconstitution, dilution, and storage.

The antifungals used to treat systemic mycoses are implicated in numerous. significant drug interactions. When technicians participate in entering prescriptions into the pharmacy computer system, they must pay attention to drug interaction warnings and advise the pharmacist when warning messages appear. One important interaction occurs when antacids or acid suppressant drugs are taken with itraconazole or ketoconazole. These two drugs should carry an auxiliary warning that encourages patients to avoid antacids and take the medications after meals. On the other hand, voriconazole is taken on an empty stomach and should be appropriately labelled. As is true with all antimicrobial medications, it is advisable to add an auxiliary label that instructs patients to take all of the oral antifungal medication unless otherwise directed by the physician.

## Antifungal Agents for Superficial or Cutaneous Mycoses

Not all fungal infections are life threatening or even particularly serious. Superficial infections of the skin and vagina are common and are frequently self-diagnosed and treated with over the counter medications. Other infections, including fungal nail infections, and sometimes Candida infections of the mouth (thrush) require oral prescription medications. Fungi that cause superficial skin infections, such as athlete's foot or ringworm, are called dermatophytes. "Ringworm" is the common name for a fungal infection of the skin, which takes its name from the raised, red, and circular appearance of the infection (**Fig. 31.4**). Fungi that cause infections of the vagina, external genitalia, the diaper area in infants, and sometimes the oropharynx in people receiving potent antibiotics are yeast, usually Candida albicans. Terbinafine (Lamisil®) and griseofulvin (Grifulvin®) are oral antifungal agents that are used for nail infections. Fluconazole and itraconazole are also sometimes used for this type of infections. The other drugs discussed in this section, including clotrimazole, miconazole, nystatin, tolnaftate, and others, are used for their local effects.

thrush Superficial yeast infection of the oral cavity.

### Actions and Indications

There are a number of medications that are useful for onychomycoses, or nail infections, but treatment of this condition requires long-term therapy and may still not result in a complete cure. Terbinafine is the drug of choice for treating onychomycoses, although itracona-

onychomycoses Fungal infection of the nails.

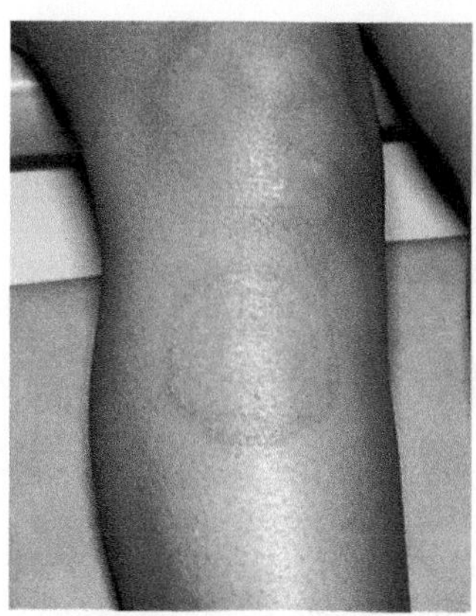

**Figure 31.4** Photograph of a typical dermatophyte infection commonly referred to as ringworm. (Reprinted with permission from Goodheart HP. *Goodheart's Photoguide of Common Skin Disorders*, 2nd edition. Philadelphia: Lippincott Williams & Wilkins, 2003.)

zole and griseofulvin are also indicated for this use. Terbinafine requires a shorter duration of therapy (usually 3 months), and is more effective than either itraconazole or griseofulvin. Terbinafine indirectly inhibits the synthesis of ergosterol and causes accumulation of toxic amounts of a precursor, which results in the death of the fungal cell. The antifungal activity of terbinafine is limited to dermatophytes and *Candida albicans*.

Griseofulvin is much less likely to be used than in the past for infections of the nails, since better, safer treatments are now available. Griseofulvin requires treatment of 6 to 12 months in duration, and it is only fungistatic. Griseofulvin accumulates in new keratin-containing tissue, such as skin and nails, where it causes inhibition of fungal reproduction.

Ciclopirox (Loprox®) is the only topical preparation approved for treatment of fungal nail infections. Its cure rate is quite low compared with that of terbinafine, but it is a useful alternative for people who cannot take the oral antifungal agents because of liver disease or for other reasons. Ciclopirox is thought to work by binding metal ions that are required by fungal enzymes in order to perform certain metabolic processes. It is active against Tinea, the most common dermatophytes, and against some yeast, including Candida. Ciclopirox penetrates skin better than other topical products.

Nystatin (Mycostatin®) is related to amphotericin B, with a similar mechanism and spectrum of activity. Because of its toxicity when used systemically, it is administered topically only. Other topical antifungals include members of the azole antifungal family, miconazole (Monistat®, others), clotrimazole (Lotrimin®, Mycelex®), econazole (Spectazole®), and others, which have mechanisms of action and antifungal spectrums that are the same as ketoconazole. The azole antifungals and nystatin are effective against Candida and are useful for skin and vaginal yeast infections. In addition, the topical azole drugs and the older antifungal agents, tolnaftate (Tinactin®) and undecylenic acid, are indicated for the treatment of tinea infections such as athlete's foot, ringworm, or jock itch.

## Administration

Terbinafine is well absorbed and effective when administered orally. It is deposited in the skin, nails, and fat and releases slowly from these tissues. Terbinafine accumulates in breast milk and is not prescribed for nursing mothers. It is extensively metabolized in the liver, and is not recommended for people with serious liver disease. Some systemic absorption occurs when this drug is used topically, but it is not enough to cause problems. Griseofulvin is taken by mouth and the newer preparations containing ultrafine crystals are absorbed adequately from the gastrointestinal tract. Taking the medication with a high-fat meal enhances absorption. Griseofulvin stimulates the activity of cytochrome P450 drug metabolizing enzymes, and as a result increases the rate of metabolism of a number of drugs, including anticoagulants.

Nystatin is negligibly absorbed from the gastrointestinal tract. It is administered as an oral suspension ("swish and swallow"), or as a lozenge for the treatment of oral candidiasis. Oral doses are nearly completely recovered in the feces. Nystatin is also available as a topical powder, and as a cream or ointment, for yeast infections of the skin. Vaginal tablets and cream are used for treatment of vaginal yeast infections. Clotrimazole, miconazole, and the other azole antifungals appropriate for topical use are available in an extensive assortment of drug formulations (see Table 31.1), and most of them can be purchased without a prescription. Products vary by drug, but miconazole and clotrimazole are available in vaginal preparations, powders, creams, and lotions, among others. Clotrimazole is available as a lozenge for oral *Candida albicans* infections. Ketoconazole can be applied topically and is available as a shampoo and cream. Tolnaftate, ciclopirox, and undecylenic acid are used for topical treatment only and are available in a number of formulations.

## Side Effects

The most common adverse effects due to terbinafine are headache, GI disturbances, and rash. Taste and visual disturbances, and transient changes in liver function tests can occur. Rarely terbinafine can cause hepatotoxicity and neutropenia. Griseofulvin is not as well tolerated as terbinafine by most patients. CNS symptoms, including headache, dizziness, and confusion can occur. Rash and hives occur in a significant percentage of patients. Griseofulvin can cause leukopenia and other abnormal blood findings, and may exacerbate intermittent porphyria, an inherited metabolic disease. Patients should not drink alcoholic beverages during therapy, because of potential for liver toxicity and because griseofulvin potentiates the intoxicating effects of alcohol.

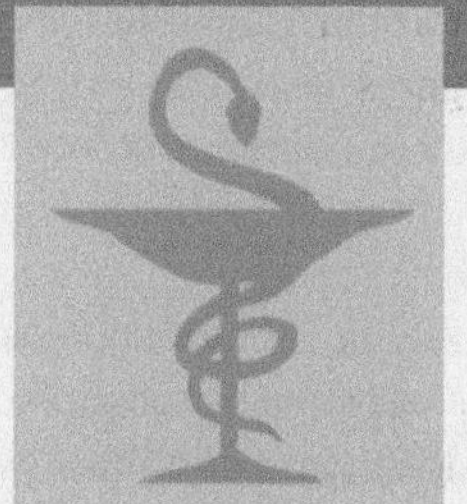

### Tips for the Technician

Technicians should be aware of the terbinafine sound-alike terbutaline. Lamisil®, the brand name of terbinafine, can be confused with Lamictal®, the brand name of lamotrigine. An auxiliary label, advising patients to complete all of their medication unless otherwise instructed, is appropriate labelling for all oral antifungal medications. Patients receiving prescriptions for griseofulvin should be warned to report side effects to the prescriber immediately and to avoid alcohol. Technicians must include auxiliary labels warning against alcohol consumption and cautioning patients that their ability to drive may be impaired on griseofulvin prescription vials. Technicians should be aware that different griseofulvin formulations are not equivalent.

Oral products intended for the treatment of oropharyngeal yeast infections work by being in contact with infected areas. Nystatin suspension should be swished around the mouth and held for several minutes before swallowing. Label prescriptions with a "shake well" auxiliary label. When antifungal lozenges are prescribed, inform the patient that lozenges should be allowed to dissolve slowly, not chewed, and label the prescription appropriately. When topical medications are dispensed, they should be labelled "for external use only," and the appropriate site of application spelled out on the prescription label. For instance, vaginal products should be labelled "for vaginal use only." Products formulated for use on one area of the body are not usually interchangeable with other products. As a case in point, cream designed for skin surfaces should not be applied to the external genitalia or used in the vagina.

## Parasitic Infections

Parasites are single- or multiple-celled organisms that live on or inside the body, and obtain food from the body of the host organism. Although North Americans are spared the worst parasitic infections, travelers to areas where, for example, malaria or schistosomiasis are endemic (consistently present in a geographic area), may contract these diseases and require treatment at home. In the United States, medication to treat parasitic infections not commonly found in North America is obtained directly from the manufacturer or the Center for Disease Control and Prevention (CDC).

endemic Present or occurring in a particular geographic area or population.

Discussion of drugs prescribed to combat parasitic diseases will be limited to the parasites found in North America and the drugs used to treat them, and treatment and prevention of malaria. Enterobius vermicularis and Ascaris lumbricoides, two helminths (parasitic worms that live in the intestines), are endemic multicellular parasites. Although they may not seem to qualify, lice and scabies are considered parasites because they must live on a host. The recommended treatments for lice (parasitic insects) and scabies (parasitic mites) will also be discussed.

helminth Parasitic worm, usually a parasite that lives in the intestine of a vertebrate.

## Life Cycle of Parasites and Spread of Disease

The life cycle of parasites varies between organisms and can be quite complex. Some parasites grow and reproduce in only one type of host, and spend most of their life cycle in one place. Head lice represent an example of this type of life cycle. More often than not, parasites live in more than one type of host, and they must survive in the environment in order to become established in a new host. The primary host is the site where adult parasites live and reproduce. In most parasitic life cycles, the ova (or cysts) leave the primary host, and may be present temporarily in soil or water. An intermediate host is infected through contact with the immature form of the parasite, which undergoes maturation inside the intermediate host to an infectious, or larval, stage. Transmission from the intermediate host back to a primary host animal can occur through a variety of processes, including ingestion of the intermediate host. Tapeworms, including those found in fish or pork, are representative of this type of life cycle. **Figure 31.5** shows the simplified life cycle of Plasmodium falciparum, which causes malaria.

Prevention of parasitic infections is as important as treatment, and is safer and easier. Many of the antiparasitic drugs required for serious parasitic diseases, such as schistosomiasis or leishmaniasis, are highly toxic. By understanding the basic stages of the life cycle of parasites, the vectors that carry them, and the factors that contribute to their spread, people traveling to foreign countries can avoid infections altogether. As a general rule, travelers to foreign countries should avoid drinking tap water or using ice made from tap water, wear shoes at all times, avoid eating raw vegetables, fruit (unless it is peeled by the consumer), or undercooked or raw fish or meat, and avoid swimming in fresh water. Effective prevention of parasitic disease requires that people become informed of the diseases endemic in the area where they live or plan to travel.

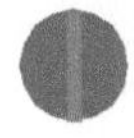

# Drugs Used to Treat or Prevent Protozoal Infections

Protozoa are single-celled, motile parasites that typically spend most of their life cycle within their primary host, often humans. Examples of protozoal parasites include the amoeba-like *Giardia intestinalis* (also known as *G. lamblia*) and *Cryptosporidium parvum*,

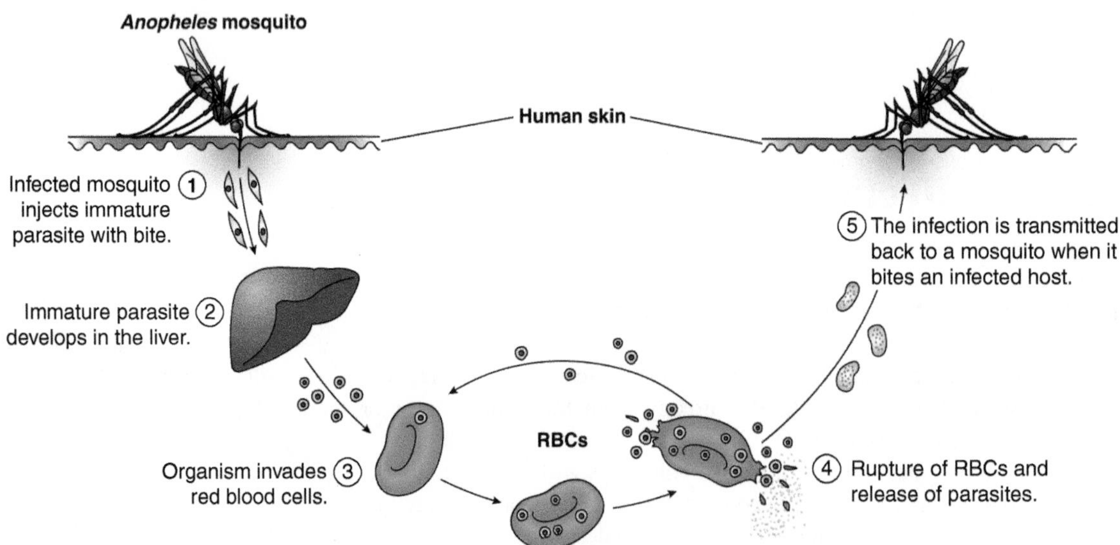


**Figure 31.5** The simplified life cycles of *Plasmodium falciparum*, the organism that causes malaria. (Adapted with permission from Rubin E and Farber JL. *Pathology*, 3rd edition. Philadelphia: Lippincott Williams & Wilkins, 1999.)

two parasites that occur fairly commonly in the United States. The protozoal genus Plasmodium causes malaria, one of the leading causes of death worldwide.

## Actions and Indications

Metronidazole (Flagyl®) is the drug of choice for treating *Giardia intestinalis* infections, amebic dysentery, and the sexually transmitted vaginal protozoa *Trichomonas vaginalis*. It is also very effective for treating infections caused by anaerobic bacteria, and can be used as part of the antibiotic regimen when abdominal infections occur after GI surgery or a perforated appendix. Metronidazole is indicated for the treatment of colitis caused by the anaerobic, gram-positive bacillus *Clostridium difficile*, which can invade the intestines when normal flora is reduced after use of broad-spectrum antibiotics. The chemical structure of metronidazole is altered inside the infecting organism, and the resulting compound disrupts the structure of the organism's DNA and inhibits the ability of the organism to synthesize nucleic acids.

Paromomycin (Humatin®), an aminoglycoside antibiotic, is only effective against the life stages of amoeba that reside in the intestine, because it is not significantly absorbed from the gastrointestinal tract. It is an alternative agent for treatment of cryptosporidiosis, protozoa that cause diarrhea in children where the water sources are contaminated, in people working with infected food animals, and in immunocompromised patients. In a normal healthy adult who contracts a cryptosporidium infection, treatment is usually supportive and the infection resolves on its own. However, immunocompromised patients and children can be treated with paromomycin, azithromycin, or nitazoxanide, a drug not readily available through normal channels. Paromomycin exerts direct amebicidal action, probably due to an effect on the infecting organism's cell membranes, where it causes leakage of electrolytes and small molecules.

Chloroquine (Aralen®) is a synthetic quinine derivative that remains the mainstay of antimalarial therapy when the local organisms are not resistant. It is the drug of choice in the treatment of some stages of the malaria life cycle. Chloroquine is less effective against malaria caused by some species of Plasmodium. The mechanisms of action by which chloroquine kills plasmodial parasites is still incompletely understood, however the following processes are known to be involved in the drug's lethal action. In certain stages of its life cycle, the malaria parasite invades red blood cells and feeds on the host's hemoglobin to obtain essential amino acids. During consumption of the hemoglobin, large amounts of a byproduct that is toxic to the parasite are produced. Normally, the parasite converts this byproduct to a nontoxic pigment. Chloroquine works by moving into red blood cells and concentrating inside the parasite, where it binds to the toxic breakdown product, and prevents its conversion to the nontoxic pigment. The accumulation of the toxic breakdown products results in damage to the parasite cell membranes, leading to destruction of both the parasite and the red blood cell. All quinine derivatives are thought to act in a similar way.

Malaria is spread through the bite of an infected *Anopheles* mosquito, and preventative measures include avoidance of mosquito bites when visiting countries where malaria is endemic. However important, preventive measures are inadequate for complete protection, and the CDC recommends several prescription medications to prevent malaria infections. Many of these drugs are also quinine derivatives. Refer to **Table 31.3** for a listing of these drugs.

## Administration

All of the medications discussed here for protozoal infections or for malaria prevention can be administered orally. In addition, metronidazole is available for intravenous use in premixed IVPB bags. Metronidazole is completely and rapidly absorbed after oral administration and distributes well throughout body tissues and fluids. Therapeutic levels can be found in vaginal and seminal fluids, saliva, breast milk, and cerebrospinal fluid. The drug accumulates in patients with severe hepatic disease. See **Table 31.4** for a summary of the antiparasitic drugs covered in this chapter.

**Table 31.3** Recommended Malaria Prophylaxis Regimens for Travellers

| Drug Name | Use | Adult Dose | Notes |
|---|---|---|---|
| Atovaquone/ proguanil (Malarone™) | Prophylaxis in areas with chloroquine-resistant or mefloquine-resistant *Plasmodium falciparum* | Adult tablets contain 250 mg atovaquone and 100 mg proguanil hydrochloride.<br><br>1 tablet orally, daily | Begin 1–2 days before travel & continue x 7 days after leaving malaria infested area.<br><br>Take daily at the same time each day. Malarone® should be taken with food or a thick drink. Not recommended for children <11 kg or pregnant women. |
| Chloroquine phosphate (Aralen™ and generic) | Prophylaxis only in areas with chloroquine-sensitive *P. falciparum* | Tablets contain 500 mg<br><br>1 tablet orally, once/week | Begin 1–2 weeks before travel & continue for 4 weeks after leaving malaria-infested area.<br><br>Take weekly on the same day of the week. May exacerbate psoriasis. |
| Doxycycline (Vibramycin® and generic) | Prophylaxis in areas with chloroquine-resistant or mefloquine-resistant *P. falciparum* | Tablets or capsules contain 50 or 100 mg<br><br>100 mg orally, daily | Begin 1–2 days before travel & for 4 weeks after leaving malaria-infested areas.<br><br>Take daily at the same time each day. Contraindicated in children <8 years of age and pregnant women. |
| Hydroxychloroquine sulfate (Plaquenil™) | Alternative to chloroquine for primary prophylaxis only in areas with chloroquine-sensitive *P. falciparum* | Tablets contain 200 mg<br><br>400 mg orally, once/week | Begin 1–2 weeks before travel & continue for 4 weeks after leaving malaria-infested area.<br><br>Take weekly on the same day of the week. May exacerbate psoriasis. |
| Mefloquine (Lariam™ and generic) | Prophylaxis in areas with chloroquine-resistant *P. falciparum* | 250 mg orally, once/week | Begin 1–2 weeks before travel & continue for 4 weeks after leaving malaria-infested area.<br><br>Take weekly on the same day of the week. Contraindicated in people with depression, other psychiatric disorders, or seizures. Not recommended for people with cardiac conduction abnormalities. |

Very little of an oral dose of paromomycin is absorbed, but the drug that is absorbed is excreted in the urine. Quinine and its derivatives chloroquine, primaquine, and mefloquine (Lariam®) are all well absorbed orally. Taking these medications with meals may improve tolerance, and in the case of mefloquine, is recommended to improve absorption. Although the majority of a chloroquine dose is excreted unchanged in the urine, the other quinine derivatives and quinine itself are mainly metabolized.

**Table 31.4** Drugs for Parasitic Diseases

| Generic | Brand Name | Available as | Indications | Notes |
|---|---|---|---|---|
| **Antimalarials and Amebicides** | | | | |
| Chloroquine | Aralen® | Tablets | Treatment and prevention of malaria | |
| Mefloquine | Lariam® | Tablets | Acute malaria infections, malaria prevention | |
| Metronidazole | Flagyl® | Tablets, capsules, IVPB Premix | Giardia intestinalis, amebiasis, trichomonas vaginalis, anaerobic bacterial infections | Do not refrigerate IVPB |
| Paromomycin | Humatin® | Capsules | Intestinal amebiasis | |
| Primaquine | | Tablets | Treatment of *P. vivax* malaria | |
| Quinine | | Capsules | Treatment of chloroquine resistant malaria | |
| **Other Antiparasitic Agents** | | | | |
| Mebendazole | Vermox® | Chewable tablets | Helminth infections—pinworm and others | |
| Permethrin | Elimite®, Nix® | Lotion, cream rinse for head lice | Head lice, scabies | External use only |
| Pyrantel Pamoate | Antiminth®, Pin-X® | Capsules, oral suspension, liquid | Roundworms and pinworms | |
| Pyrethrin | A-200®, RID® | Lotion, shampoo, gel, mousse | Head lice, body lice, and pubic lice | External use only |

Susp, suspension.

## Side Effects

Metronidazole is used extensively for a variety of bacterial infections, as well as parasitic infections, and is well tolerated. The most common adverse effects take place in the gastrointestinal tract, including nausea, vomiting, and epigastric distress. An unpleasant, metallic taste can occur. Rarely, toxicity in the nervous system, such as dizziness, vertigo, and numbness, and very rarely, seizures, can result from metronidazole therapy. When metronidazole is taken with alcohol, severe nausea and vomiting can result from the combination.

Because of its insignificant absorption, side effects from paromomycin are limited to the local effects in the GI tract. They are due mainly to the effects of the drug on the local flora, and include diarrhea, nausea and vomiting, and abdominal cramps.

Most quinine derivatives, including chloroquine and primaquine, can cause hemolysis of red blood cells in people with glucose-6-phosphate dehydrogenase deficiency, but mefloquine does not cause the same response. The quinine derivatives should be administered very cautiously to people with cardiac rhythm disorders. As previously discussed in the chapter on antiarrhythmic drugs, quinidine, an isomer of quinine, is a potent inhibitor of cardiac conduction, and all of the quinine derivatives have some of the same effects. Side effects observed with low doses are usually limited to mild GI upset, and transient headache. At higher doses, diarrhea, headache, tinnitus, vision disturbances, and seizures can occur. Reduced white blood cell count and other blood abnormalities can occur.

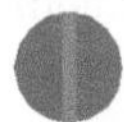

### Tips for the Technician

The importance of compliance with the drug regimen should be emphasized to all patients, whether they are being treated for protozoal infections, or are receiving malaria prophylaxis medications. Although this is a responsibility of the pharmacist, technicians can reinforce the instructions by affixing an auxiliary label that instructs the patient to complete the medication unless instructed to do otherwise by the physician. Prescriptions for metronidazole must be labelled with instructions to avoid alcohol while taking the medication. Patients should be warned about possible nervous system symptoms and report them to their physician if they occur.

Patients taking any of the quinine-related drugs should also report nervous system symptoms, such as numbness, vision changes, or persistent headache, to their physician. If a patient has a known allergy to quinine or quinidine, prescriptions for other quinine derivatives should be brought to the attention of the pharmacist.

## Other Antiparasitic Drugs

Helminths are parasitic worms that can infect humans (**Fig. 31.6**). Although there are three major groups of helminths, the nematodes are the most commonly encountered in North America. Examples include roundworms, pinworms, and hookworms. These organisms are usually spread by accidental ingestion of eggs or some other infectious stage of the parasite, or by penetration of the skin. Mebendazole (Vermox®) and pyrantel pamoate (Pin-X®, others) are used for these parasitic infections.

Lice (insects) and mites (related to spiders) are parasites that are quite common in institutional settings, such as preschools, elementary schools, and nursing homes (see **Fig. 31.7**). Lice live on the head or body, and both organisms are transmitted during close physical contact, or in the case of lice, through contact with hats, pillows, hairbrushes, or other items shared by an infected host. The female *Sarcoptes scabei* mite, the cause of scabies, burrows under the skin of the host to lay eggs, and their presence causes an intensely itchy allergic reaction and classic scabies rash. Neither lice nor mites can survive off of the human host for more than 2 days. These infestations are treated with mild insecticides.

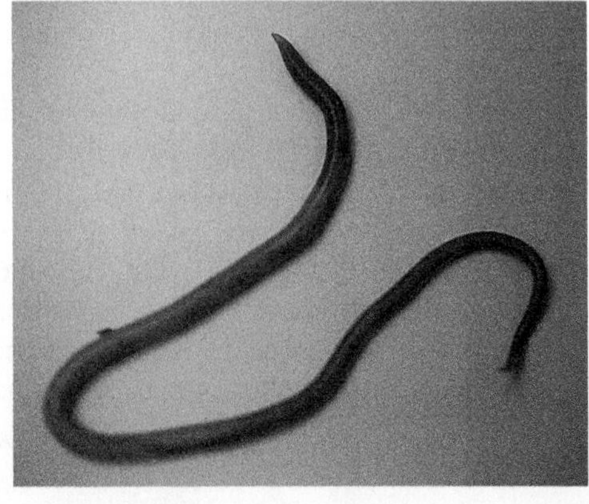

**Figure 31.6** A photograph of a roundworm, one of the more likely helminths to occur in North America. (Reprinted with permission from Fleisher GR, Ludwig W, Baskin MN. *Atlas of Pediatric Emergency Medicine.* Philadelphia: Lippincott Williams & Wilkins, 2004.)

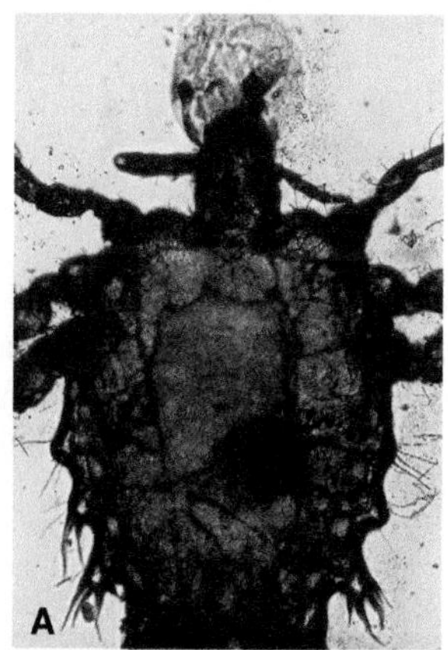


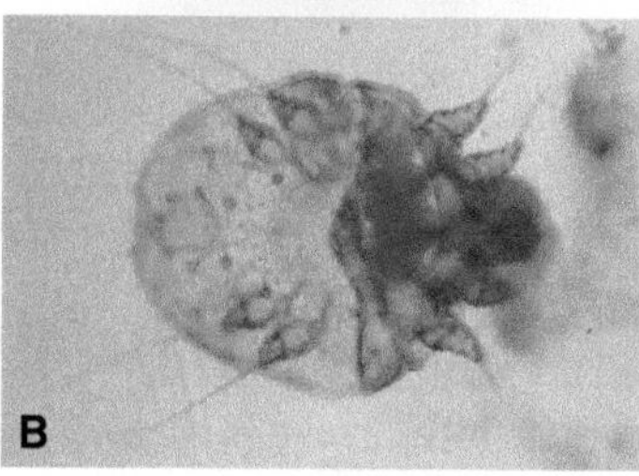


**Figure 31.7** Photomicrograph **A** is *Pediculus capitis*, human head lice (3 to 4 mm in length), and **B** is *Sarcoptes scabei*, scabies mite (0.3 to 0.4 mm in length). (A: reprinted with permission from Fleisher GR, Ludwig W, Baskin MN. *Atlas of Pediatric Emergency Medicine*. Philadelphia: Lippincott Williams & Wilkins, 2004; B: Goodheart HP. *Goodheart's Photoguide of Common Skin Disorders*, 2nd edition. Philadelphia: Lippincott Williams & Wilkins, 2003.)

## Actions and Indications

Mebendazole is effective against a wide spectrum of intestine-dwelling nematodes. It is a drug of choice in the treatment of infections by whipworm, pinworm (Enterobius vermicularis), hookworms, and roundworm (Ascaris lumbricoides). Mebendazole inhibits the ability of sensitive organisms to take up small molecules that are needed for nutrition, such as glucose. As nutrients are depleted, the organisms die and are expelled in the feces.

Pyrantel pamoate is effective in the treatment of infections caused by roundworms, pinworms, and hookworms. It exerts its effects in the intestinal tract, where it acts as a depolarizing, neuromuscular-blocking agent, causing paralysis in the parasite. The paralyzed worm is then expelled from the host's intestinal tract.

Drug treatment of scabies and lice are similar and consist of mild insecticides applied topically. Permethrin (Elimite®, Nix®) is the drug of choice for the treatment of both scabies and lice. Pyrethrin (A-200® Maximum Strength, others) can also be used. Lindane (Kwell®) is no longer recommended as a drug of first choice because of the risk of toxicity, especially in infants and small children. Permethrin, pyrethrin, and lindane work by paralyzing the nervous systems of the infecting organisms, resulting in their death.

## Administration

Mebendazole and pyrantel pamoate are administered orally and work on the parasites in the intestine. They are not intended to be systemically absorbed. Little of an oral dose of mebendazole is absorbed by the body, unless it is taken with a high-fat meal. The small amount that is absorbed undergoes first pass metabolism to inactive compounds. Pyrantel pamoate is also poorly absorbed.

Permethrin is applied topically, according to the infection being treated. For example, to treat head lice the lotion is applied to the shampooed hair like crème rinse, left on for 10 minutes, and then rinsed off. A second application 7 to 10 days later is recommended to kill any emerging insects because the drug is not completely effective at killing lice nits (eggs). In the treatment of scabies, permethrin is applied after a shower, from the chin and hairline on the neck to the toes, and left on for 10 to 12 hours, then washed off. The itching rash may take weeks to resolve after the treatment, because the antigenic material (dead mites and eggs) remains under the skin until the immune system clears it. Pyrethrin and lindane products are also applied topically, and then removed.

nit The egg of a louse.

## Side Effects

Because mebendazole and pyrantel pamoate are not extensively absorbed, systemic side effects are rare. Patients may complain of abdominal pain and diarrhea from either drug. Nervous system symptoms, such as dizziness, headache, and restlessness have been reported rarely with both drugs.

Permethrin and pyrethrin rarely cause systemic effects when used appropriately. Skin irritation, rashes, redness, and burning are typical side effects. Lindane, on the other hand, is known to be more extensively absorbed. There have been several reported deaths after the improper use of this drug, which is absorbed when left on the skin and causes toxicity to the nervous system, including refractory seizures. This medication should not be used on infants or small children, or people with seizure disorders.

### Tips for the Technician

Pyrantel pamoate is sold as tablets or suspension, and a "shake well" label should be applied to bottles of the suspension when filled as a prescription. However, this product is available without prescription. Because pinworms are easily passed between family members, the entire family is usually treated when this diagnosis is made. Family members should be informed that a repeat dose after 2 weeks is recommended. Mebendazole is a prescription only product that is provided as a chewable tablet. When this drug is used for pinworms or other organisms that live exclusively in the GI tract, the drug should not be taken with food because meals increase systemic absorption.

Many products sold for the treatment of lice are available without prescription. Make sure that clients read the instructions carefully, especially when treating small children. When dispensing products for scabies and lice as a prescription, apply a "for external use" label to the container. Be sure that the pharmacist advises patients on the proper use of lindane, and that the written patient instructions are included with the prescription. The CDC advises that patients not bathe immediately before applying lindane because warm, moist skin will absorb more of the active ingredient.

Along with drug treatment of both scabies and lice, patients should be advised to thoroughly launder all potentially contaminated linens and clothing, and dry them with high heat to destroy any organisms. In the case of head lice, the patient or family member should use a nit comb to remove eggs from the hair. Other family members should be checked for infestation and treated when necessary.

# Review Questions

## Multiple Choice

Choose the best answer for the following questions:

1. Systemic fungal infections are most apt to occur when
   a. People spend a lot of time in gymnasiums
   b. People take too many antibiotics
   c. Nutrition is poor
   d. The immune system is suppressed or weakened
   e. People travel to Alaska

2. Why do drugs to treat fungal infections often cause more side effects than drugs to treat bacterial infections?
   a. Drugs to treat bacterial infections have been improved over time.
   b. Fungal cells and human cells are both eukaryotic and share some similarities.
   c. Fungal infections require more intensive treatment.
   d. Bacterial cells and human cells are prokaryotic.
   e. None of the above is correct.

3. Why can Flucytosine and Amphotericin be used effectively together?
   a. They should never be given together because they both cause kidney toxicity.
   b. Flucytosine can be used with any other antifungal drug because it is so safe.
   c. Their mechanisms of action are complementary.
   d. Because amphotericin and flucytosine are compatible mixed in the same IV.
   e. Because they have very different side effects.

4. People with liver disease should use Ciclopirox rather than other onychomycoses treatments because?
   a. Ciclopirox is taken in a low dose for a shorter period than other treatments.
   b. Ciclopirox is used topically and is not systemically absorbed.
   c. The cure rate with ciclopirox treatment is higher than that with terbinafine treatment.
   d. Ciclopirox reverses the symptoms of cirrhosis.
   e. Ciclopirox is excreted by the kidneys.

5. The drug of choice for *Giardia intestinalis* (or *G. lamblia*) infection is which of the following drugs?
   a. Metronidazole
   b. Chloroquine
   c. Mebendazole
   d. Amphotericin B
   e. All of the above

## True/False

6. Cryptosporidiosis is a protozoal infection, contracted from contaminated water sources, that causes serious diarrhea for which otherwise healthy adults almost always require treatment.
   a. True
   b. False

7. Dermatophytes usually cause uncomplicated fungal infections of the skin that can be treated with OTC antifungal products.
   a. True
   b. False

8. Malaria infection, which is spread through the bite of the Anopheles mosquito, can be prevented during travel where malaria is endemic by taking a quinine derivative or other medication recommended by the CDC.
   a. True
   b. False

9. It does not matter if clotrimazole antifungal lozenges are chewed or allowed to dissolve because it will all end up in the stomach anyway.
   a. True
   b. False

10. Mebendazole is a good choice for the treatment of pinworm or roundworm infection.
    a. True
    b. False

## Matching

For numbers 11 to 15, complete the statement with the correct lettered choice from the list below. Choices will not be used more than once and may not be used at all.

11. Quinine derivatives taken by G6PD deficient patients can cause ______
12. Most common antiprotozoal medications are administered ______
13. Azole antifungal agents work by inhibiting ______
14. Amphotericin B should be reconstituted with ______
15. Ketoconazole may cause ______

a. Orally
b. Reduction of libido or menstrual irregularities
c. Intramuscularly
d. Temporary blindness and darkening of the gums
e. 5% dextrose
f. Sterile water
g. Sterols in the cell membrane
h. Hemolysis of red blood cells

## Short Answer

16. List four important facts that technicians need to know in order to safely compound amphotericin B IV admixtures.

17. List three azole antifungals, their indications, and their formulations. Include one that can be used in systemic mycoses as an alternative to amphotericin B and one that is used for superficial fungal infections.

18. Metronidazole is used for a number of very different infections, from *C. difficile* to Giardia infections, to *Trichomonas vaginalis*. Describe potential side effects to the drug, especially any that you think might prevent clients from completing the course of therapy as directed.

19. How is the proverb "an ounce of prevention is worth a pound of cure" relevant to people who travel to countries where parasitic diseases are endemic?

20. Compare and contrast scabies and lice infestations and describe one treatment useful for both and how it is used.

## FOR FURTHER INQUIRY

Nosocomial fungal infections are increasing, especially in the elderly or people taking immunosuppressive medications. The most common pathogens are Candida, Aspergillus, and Malassezia species. Use the Internet to identify additional risk factors for hospitalized patients, find out how these infections are acquired, and what drugs are used to treat nosocomial fungal infections.

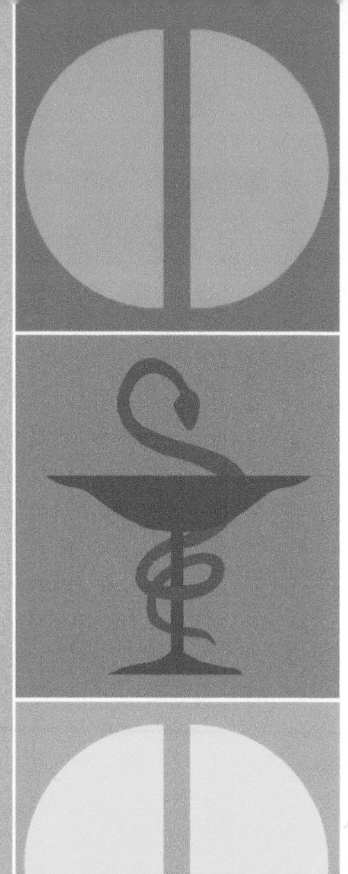

Chapter **32**

# Antiviral Drugs and Vaccines

## *KEY TERMS*

- active immunity
- alopecia
- antigen
- epidemic
- immunization
- pandemic
- passive immunity
- vaccination
- vaccine

## OBJECTIVES

After studying this chapter, the reader should be able to:

- Explain how the simple structure and the changeable nature of some viruses make them very difficult to target with either drugs or immunizations.
- List names of one drug each from the neuraminidase inhibitors and the adamantine derivatives, the indications for their use, typical side effects, and available formulations.
- List three common diseases caused by the members of the herpesvirus family, and explain how these viruses protect themselves from the immune system defenses.
- Compare and contrast lamivudine, or another nucleoside reverse transcriptase inhibitor of your choice, with ritonavir, or another protease inhibitor of your choice, including mechanism of action, administration, and side effects.
- Define the following terms: epidemic, pandemic, immunization, antigen, and passive immunity.

## DRUGS COVERED IN THIS CHAPTER

| Antiviral Drugs | | | Vaccines | |
|---|---|---|---|---|
| **Antiviral Agents for Influenza and RSV** | **Antiviral Agents for Herpes and CMV** | **Antiretroviral Agents (for HIV infection)** | **Viral Vaccines** | **Bacterial Vaccines** |
| Amantadine<br>Oseltamivir<br>Ribavirin<br>Rimantadine<br>Zanamivir | Acyclovir<br>Cidofovir<br>Famciclovir<br>Foscarnet<br>Ganciclovir<br>Trifluridine<br>Valacyclovir<br>Valganciclovir | **Nonnucleoside Reverse Transcriptase Inhibitors (NNRTI)**<br>Delavirdine<br>Efavirenz<br>Nevirapine<br>**Nucleoside Reverse Transcriptase Inhibitors (NRTI)**<br>Abacavir<br>Didanosine<br>Emtricitabine<br>Lamivudine<br>Stavudine<br>Tenofovir<br>Zalcitabine<br>Zidovudine<br>**Protease Inhibitors**<br>Amprenavir<br>Atazanavir<br>Indinavir<br>Lopinavir<br>Nelfinavir<br>Ritonavir<br>Saquinavir<br>Tipranavir | Hepatitis A & B<br>Herpes Zoster<br>Human Papilloma Virus<br>Measles<br>Mumps<br>Polio<br>Rabies<br>Rubella<br>Smallpox | HIB<br>Meningitis<br>Pneumonia<br>Diphtheria<br>Tetanus |

epidemic A sudden occurrence that affects an unexpectedly large percentage of a given population at the same time.

pandemic An epidemic that affects an unusually large geographic area and percent of the population.

immunization A process that exposes an individual to antigens from an organism in order to create immunity to that organism.

Viral infections are the most common form of infectious diseases in humans. It is not unusual for infants to contract a viral infection within months of their birth, and viruses continue to plague us throughout life. Viral infections that occur in otherwise healthy individuals usually resolve without treatment. Common self-limiting infections include rhinovirus infections, which are the cause of the common cold, and rotavirus infections, which are responsible for most cases of "stomach flu." However, viral epidemics (outbreaks of infectious disease that exceed the expected number of cases) pose a tremendous threat to humankind. The deadliest pandemic (an epidemic that spreads over a large part of the world) of all time was not the plague, or AIDS, but the influenza outbreak of 1918, which may have killed as many as 100 million people in only 2 years time. Prevention of viral infection through immunization , a process used to increase the body's ability to react to a specific infectious agent and thereby resist illness, or cautious behavior is the most effective strategy available to combat the spread of serious viral infections. Even this strategy has limitations if viruses are highly contagious and change rapidly. Highly contagious viruses are often spread to other people before the infected individual shows any symptoms of illness. In this chapter, the discussion of antiviral drug treatment is grouped according to the viruses affected and the diseases they cause. A review of immunization follows the discussion of drug therapy.

Viruses are infectious agents that inhabit the gray area between living organisms and nonliving biochemical complexes. They are much smaller than bacteria and can only be seen through an electron microscope. They operate as biological minimalists, requiring only a single strand of either DNA or RNA (never both) encased in a protein capsule (**Fig. 32.1**). While some viruses may have greater variation in the envelope that surrounds them, or have more pieces of nucleic acid, they are all very simple structures. Viruses undergo some of the processes that identify an organism as living, but they lack many others. They possess no cell walls or membranes, no organelles, and do not carry out any sort of metabolic processes. Although viruses can reproduce, they only accomplish this process when they insinuate themselves into the nucleus of host cells. Once a virus enters the nucleus, it commandeers the cellular nucleic acid replication machinery for its own replication. When the replicated viruses are released, the cell dies. Because they must be inside host cells when they reproduce, viruses are considered intracellular parasites.

Viruses are grouped according to a number of characteristics, including the type of genetic material they contain, their shape, size, the nature of their protein coat, and the species of host they infect. Only a few virus groups respond to available antiviral drugs. Drug development is extremely difficult, because there are few viral processes to target. It is difficult to kill intracellular parasites without damaging host cells, and few available antiviral drugs are selective enough to prevent viral replication without injury to the host's cells. Therapy for viral diseases is further complicated by the fact that the clinical symptoms of viral infections appear late in the course of the disease, at a time when most of the virus particles have been copied. At this late, symptomatic stage of the viral infection, administration of antiviral drugs has limited usefulness. Immunization is very successful against viruses whose antigens, the parts of foreign cells or organisms to which the immune system reacts, undergo very little change. However, developing vaccines to viruses with antigens that change regularly is either only partly successful (influenza) or a total failure (AIDS, to date). Nevertheless, research to find new antiviral drugs or vaccines that might treat or prevent AIDS, influenza, or some unknown future epidemic, continues.

antigen Any substance foreign to the body that evokes an immune response.

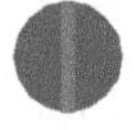

## Antiviral Agents for Influenza and Respiratory Syncytial Virus

Viral infections of the respiratory tract are among the most common of the viral infections. No treatments or immunizations exist for most of them. Consider, for example, the common cold. Because there are so many different virus types that undergo constant change,

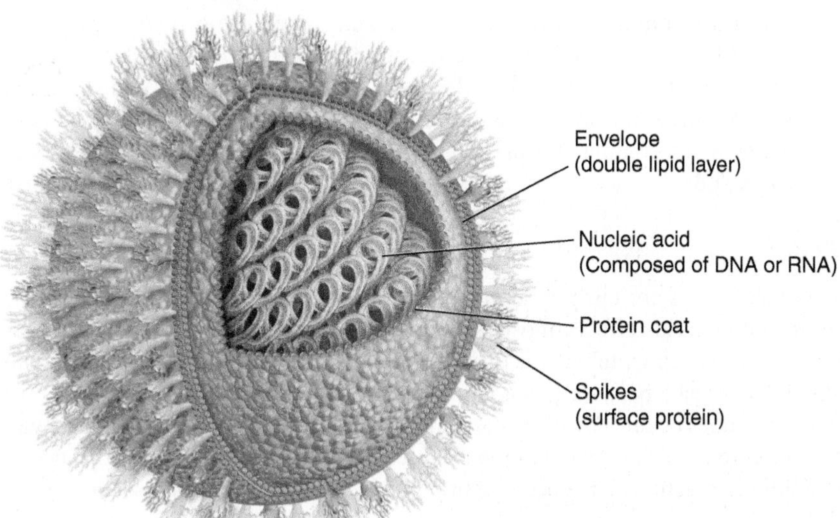


**Figure 32.1** A cross-sectional view of a virus. (Image provided by Anatomical Chart Co.)

developing products for immunization is impractical. People with normal immune systems recover easily from colds, so consequently there is no real need for drug therapy. There are other respiratory viruses, however, that can cause serious harm, especially to the elderly and very young. Two of these, influenza and respiratory syncytial virus (RSV), are common causes of pneumonia and hospitalization in the elderly and infants under 1 year of age, respectively. Fortunately, effective drug treatments and immunizations exist for both.

## Neuraminidase Inhibitors

A classic case of influenza comes on quickly, with a fever, congestion, cough, muscle aches and pains, and a general sense of feeling unwell. In debilitated people, this illness can progress to pneumonia and death. Influenza is caused by the orthomyxoviruses, which can be classified into types A, B, and C. Influenza types A and B cause the greatest risk of disease because their antigenic material changes from season to season. As a result individuals who contract the disease develop long-lasting immunity, but to last year's virus. The antigenic material contained in influenza type C does not change with time.

### Actions and Indications

Orthomyxoviruses contain the enzyme neuraminidase, which is essential to the replication and life cycle of the virus. Neuraminidase is involved with viral replication and dispersal, and is inhibited by oseltamivir (Tamiflu®) and zanamivir (Relenza®). These drugs prevent the release of new virus particles and their spread from cell to cell. Unlike some anti-influenza drugs, oseltamivir and zanamivir are effective against both type A and type B influenza viruses.

These drugs are indicated for the prevention and early treatment of influenza in at-risk patients who cannot or have not received immunization against influenza. Neuraminidase inhibitors prevent infection when they are administered prior to influenza exposure. When administered within the first 24 to 48 hours of the onset of infection, they cause a modest reduction in the intensity and duration of symptoms.

### Administration

Oseltamivir is an orally active prodrug that is rapidly hydrolyzed by the liver to its active form. Zanamivir, on the other hand, is not active orally, and is administered intranasally. Refer to **Table 32.1** for a listing of the antiviral drugs (other than those used for HIV), their indications, and formulations. The active forms of these drugs are eliminated by the kidneys. Because of the pharmacokinetics of oseltamivir, the usual dose must be reduced in people with serious renal failure.

When used for prevention of influenza, the drugs are administered as soon as possible after exposure, with a recommended maximum time since exposure of two days. When these drugs are used for treatment of an active infection, they must be started within two days of symptom onset, or they will not be effective. Oseltamivir can be used in children as young as 1 year of age, and zanamivir is approved for children aged 7 years and older. Preventative treatment can continue for up to 6 weeks, while treatment of an active infection is continued for 5 days.

### Side Effects

Side effects to these drugs are fairly mild and are much easier to tolerate than the disease itself. The most common side effects of oseltamivir are gastrointestinal discomfort and nausea, which can be alleviated by taking the drug with food. Zanamivir is not associated with gastrointestinal disturbance because it is administered directly to the airways. Irritation of the respiratory tract does occur, however. Zanamivir should be avoided in individuals with severe asthma or chronic obstructive pulmonary disease because bronchospasm can occur. No important drug interactions have been reported.

**Table 32.1** Generic and Brand names, Indications, and Formulations for the Antiviral Drugs for Respiratory Tract and Herpesvirus Infections

| Generic | Brand Name | Available as | Indications | Notes |
|---|---|---|---|---|
| **Drugs for Viral Respiratory Infection** | | | | |
| Amantadine | Symmetrel® | Capsules, tablets, syrup | Influenza A prevention and treatment, if sensitive | |
| Oseltamivir | Tamiflu® | Capsules, powder for oral suspension | Treatment and prevention of influenza | May refrigerate suspension |
| Ribavirin | Virazole®, Rebetol® | Powder for aerosol, capsules, tablets | Serious respiratory syncytial virus infection (inhalation), hepatitis C | Reconstitute in a biological safety cabinet |
| Rimantadine | Flumadine® | Tablets, syrup | Treatment and prevention of influenza A, if sensitive | |
| Zanamivir | Relenza® | Powder for Inhalation | Influenza A & B treatment | |
| **Drugs for Herpesvirus** | | | | |
| Acyclovir | Zovirax® | Tablets, capsules, oral suspension, injection, ointment | HSV infections, children & adults, shingles, genital herpes, HSV encephalitis | |
| Famciclovir | Famvir® | Tablets | HSV in AIDS, shingles, genital herpes | |
| Foscarnet | Foscavir® | Injection | CMV retinitis in AIDS patients, acyclovir resistant HSV | |
| Ganciclovir | Cytovene® | Capsules, injection | CMV retinitis, prevention of CMV disease in AIDS and transplant patients | |
| Trifluridine | Viroptic® | Ophthalmic solution | Herpes keratoconjunctivitis | |
| Valacyclovir | Valtrex® | Tablets | Shingles, genital herpes, cold sores | |
| Valganciclovir | Valcyte® | Tablets | CMV retinitis, Prevention of CMV disease | AIDS & organ transplant patients |

CMV, Cytomegalovirus; HSV, Herpes simplex virus.

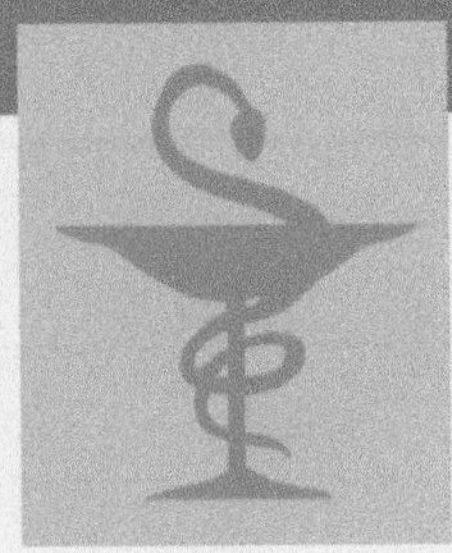

## Tips for the Technician

Oseltamivir suspension is reconstituted in the pharmacy and should be labelled, as always, with a "shake well" label. This suspension does not require refrigeration and is good for ten days. Patients who purchase zanamivir may need a demonstration to understand how the inhaler is used. The pharmacist is responsible for making sure patients feel comfortable with using this medication. Be sure that the manufacturer-provided patient instructions are included with the prescription. Asthmatics who receive zanamivir are usually instructed to use a short-acting bronchodilator, such as albuterol, before administering the zanamivir. Patients should be reminded to take the full 5 days of therapy, even if they begin to fell better before that time. Technicians can reinforce this point by labelling prescriptions with instructions to complete the full course of medication unless otherwise directed by the physician.

## Adamantine Derivatives

The adamantine derivatives, amantadine and rimantadine, are two older antiviral agents that can be useful for the treatment and prevention of Influenza type A. Amantadine was first developed as a drug for Parkinson's disease. One alert observer noticed that elderly people in nursing homes were less likely to contract influenza if they were taking amantadine, and in 1976 the FDA approved its use for prevention of influenza.

### Actions and Indications

Amantadine (Symmetrel®) and rimantadine (Flumadine®) are closely related compounds that are thought to prevent sensitive viruses from fusing with the host cell. When the virus cannot fuse with the cell, its entrance and shedding of the protein coat is blocked. These two steps are required in order for the virus to invade the host nucleus to replicate.

The antiviral activity of these agents is limited to influenza A infections, for which the drugs have been shown to be equally effective in both treatment and prevention. In the past the adamantine derivatives were 70% to 90% effective at preventing influenza if treatment was begun at the time of, or prior to, exposure to the virus. Both drugs reduced the duration and severity of systemic symptoms if started within the first 48 hours after exposure to the virus. Unfortunately, the influenza type A virus is capable of dramatic changes in its protein coat, and can develop resistance to these drugs. Influenza type A that circulated during the 2005 to 2006 influenza season was resistant to these drugs.

### Administration

Both amantadine and rimantadine drugs are well absorbed orally, and are available as solid oral dosing forms and as liquids. The dose is either administered once or twice a day. Amantadine distributes throughout the body and readily penetrates into the central nervous system, whereas rimantadine does not enter the brain to the same extent. Amantadine is excreted unchanged in the urine and may accumulate in patients with renal failure. On the other hand, rimantadine undergoes metabolism in the liver.

### Side Effects

Both amantadine and rimantadine cause a similar array of side effects, but they occur with different frequencies. Side effects are mainly associated with the central nervous system and the gastrointestinal tract, and are generally minor. Neurologic symptoms include insomnia, dizziness, and irritability. Because amantadine penetrates the central nervous system to a greater degree, CNS side effects are more likely with its use. More serious side effects, such as hallucinations, can occur with amantadine use but are rare. Both drugs can cause nausea.

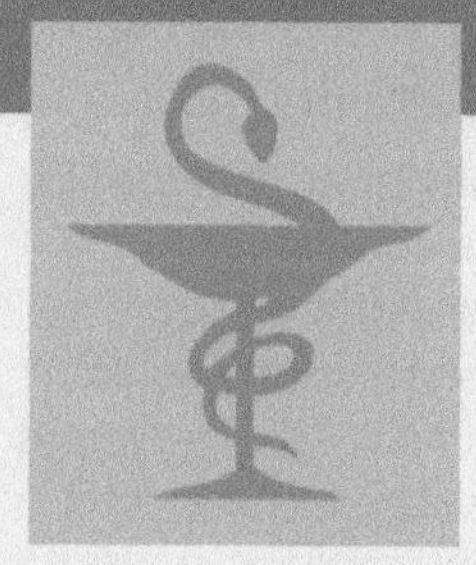

## Tips for the Technician

The adamantine derivative suspensions have no special storage requirements, but prescription bottles should be labelled "shake well." Patients should be advised to take all of the medication as directed. The central nervous system side effects can impair an adult patient's ability to drive. Warn patients to avoid driving until they are certain of how the medication will affect them by placing the appropriate warning label on prescription containers. Individuals should also avoid consumption of alcoholic beverages because of their potential for making CNS effects worse. These drugs can cause insomnia. Parents of children taking the medication should be advised to give the dose well before bedtime. This is especially important when the drug is taken twice daily.

# Ribavirin

Ribavirin (Virazole®) is an antiviral agent with activity against a broad spectrum of RNA and DNA viruses. For instance, ribavirin can be used to treat infants and young children infected with respiratory syncytial virus (RSV), and as part of combined therapy for hepatitis C. Although RSV infection is generally not serious in older children and adults, it can cause pneumonia in newborns, elderly, and other at-risk people.

## Actions and Indications

The mechanism of action of ribavirin is not completely understood. Ribavirin is thought to interfere with RNA and DNA synthesis, possibly by inhibiting RNA polymerase, the enzyme responsible for making RNA from the host cell's DNA template. It also may inhibit protein synthesis, needed for completion of the protein coating for replicated viruses. Ribavirin is indicated for the treatment of hospitalized infants and young children infected by RSV. It is also used in combination with interferon for the treatment of chronic hepatitis C. It has been used investigationally for the treatment of influenza.

## Administration

Ribavirin is effective orally and by inhalation. Oral absorption is fairly low, and is increased if the drug is taken with a meal. The manufacturers recommend this medication be taken consistently, either with food or without, so that serum levels remain consistent. When the drug is taken with other antiviral medications, recommendations for administration vary, but since taking the medication with food is always either recommended or an option, it is more common to recommend that this medication be given with food. Ribavirin is available in capsules or tablets, and is given twice daily in combination with other antiviral medication for the treatment of hepatitis C.

The aerosol form is used only in pneumonia caused by RSV. The drug is absorbed from lung tissue to a minor degree. Administration by the respiratory route requires the use of special respiratory equipment and a ventilated room because of the toxicity of the drug to health care staff. Female respiratory care practitioners who are pregnant should not administer this medication.

## Side Effects

Ribavirin was toxic to fetuses in every type of animal tested before the drug was approved, at doses less than those recommended for human use. It is designated as a pregnancy risk category X and should not be administered to women who are pregnant or plan to become pregnant in the near future, or to male partners of women who are pregnant. This also has implications for pharmacy employees and health care workers who handle these medications (see Tips for the Technician).

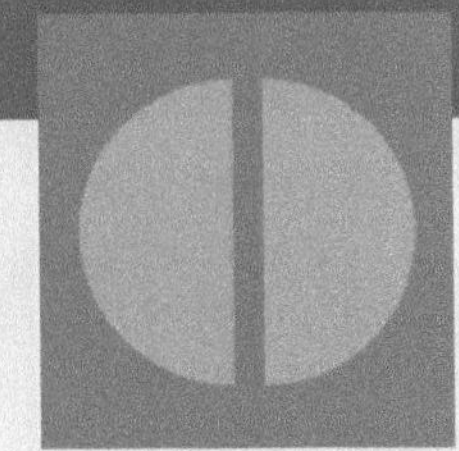

## Case 32.1

Pharmacy technician Hope Nobrythinsky is asked to deliver ribavirin to the floor for a patient with severe RSV. As she arrives at the nursing unit she notifies the nurse that his respiratory medication has been delivered. The nurse asks if it is the albuterol and the tech says she isn't sure. The medication is appropriately labelled, but is now in the medication room. The respiratory care practitioner (RCP) arrives at the unit. The nurse informs the RCP that the medication is available, so he picks it up and enters the patient's room. The RCP thinks he has the albuterol and pours it into a nebulizer, a device that converts the medication to a mist breathed in by the patient. Nebulizers are not closed systems, and the excess ribavirin mist floats into the room, exposing the patient, the nurse, the parents, and the respiratory care practitioner to the ribavirin. What should the pharmacy technician have done differently, to minimize the risk to all involved?

alopecia Baldness or loss of hair from skin areas where it is normally present.

Side effects reported for oral use of ribavirin include nausea, loss of appetite, dizziness, headache, fatigue, insomnia and irritability, hair loss (alopecia), rash, itching, muscle and joint pain, and transient anemia, including reduced levels of nearly any blood component. These occur at rates of anywhere from 10% to 60%, but amazingly, the drug is still employed because of the serious nature of hepatitis. The aerosol is somewhat safer, although respiratory function in infants can deteriorate because of bronchospasm after initiation of aerosol treatment.

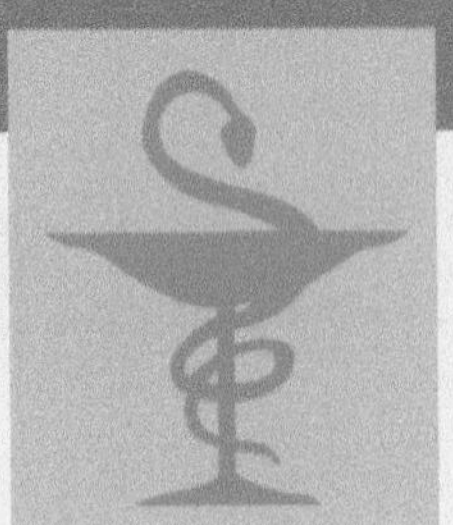

## Tips for the Technician

Pharmacy technicians who handle ribavirin should be aware of the dangerous nature of this drug and take every precaution to avoid contact with it. Hospital pharmacies have policies to direct employees who handle high-risk drugs, but not all retail pharmacies will have written policies. Automated counting machines or repackaging equipment should not be used with drugs such as ribavirin, where exposure to the dust is dangerous and cross-contamination with other products can occur. Counting trays should be cleaned after they are used to count ribavirin capsules or tablets. The product for inhalation comes to the pharmacy as a sterile dry powder, and requires reconstitution. Reconstitution should always take place in a biological safety cabinet (vertical flow hood).

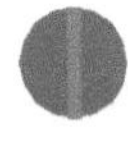

# Antiviral Agents for Herpes and Cytomegalovirus Infections

Herpesviruses are associated with a number of familiar and some less familiar infections. Herpes related diseases include chicken pox and shingles (varicella-zoster virus), cold sores and genital infections, as well as herpes encephalitis (brain infection), and herpes keratitis (eye infection). Cytomegalovirus, a member of the same family, causes infectious mononucleosis. Other viruses of the same group have been implicated as the underlying cause of certain cancers. These viruses are problematic because they can protect themselves from the human immune system. After an acute infection, they hide in nerve cells in a latent form, undetected by immune system cells, or they can prevent host cell death (a self defense mechanism used by the host) so that cells can continue to turn out viral proteins, and they can shield their own antigens so that the host immune system is less able to respond. Clearly, this is a well-adapted DNA virus family, able to penetrate host defenses with ominous results.

## Actions and Indications

The drugs that are effective against the herpes virus family exert their actions during the acute phase of viral infections and are without effect during the latent phase. Except for foscarnet (Foscavir®) and fomivirsen (Vitravene®), the antiherpes drugs inhibit viral DNA synthesis. The antiviral drugs related to acyclovir are analogs of the purines and pyrimidines, the building blocks of DNA. They work by inhibiting the action of the enzyme DNA polymerase, which is required to build the new viral DNA, and by being substituted into the DNA in place of the real purine or pyrimidine, producing faulty viral DNA. Most of the purine and pyrimidine analogs are inactive until they are converted to the active drug inside cells contaminated with the virus. A viral enzyme important in preparing genetic material for replication starts the activation process. As a result, uninfected cells are less likely to be damaged by the drug.

Acyclovir (Zovirax®) is the prototype of the purine and pyrimidine analogs. It is effective against herpes simplex virus types 1 and 2 (HSV-1 and -2), varicella-zoster virus (VZV), and some Epstein-Barr virus infections. It is the treatment of choice in disseminated herpes infections, such as herpes encephalitis. Acyclovir is the drug most frequently prescribed for cold sores (HSV-1) and genital herpes (HSV-2), two common herpesvirus infections. It is also the drug of choice for shingles, but is not effective against cytomegalovirus (CMV). Valacyclovir (Valtrex®) is an acyclovir prodrug that is converted immediately after absorption to acyclovir. It is indicated for the treatment of genital herpes and shingles.

Cidofovir (Vistide®) is another nucleotide analog, but with much more limited usefulness than acyclovir. It is approved for treatment of CMV-induced retinitis in patients with AIDS. It can also be used to treat herpesviruses that are resistant to acyclovir. Cidofovir is not dependent on viral enzymes for conversion to the active form, and it is therefore more toxic to host cells. Ganciclovir (Cytovene®) is another relative of acyclovir that has activity against CMV, the only viral infection for which it is approved. Famciclovir (Famvir®) is a prodrug that is metabolized to the active drug penciclovir. It is presently approved only for treatment of acute herpes zoster, although it is also effective against CMV. Trifluridine (Viroptic®) is a highly active thymidine analog with activity similar to acyclovir.

Unlike most of the antiviral agents, foscarnet is not a purine or pyrimidine analog. Foscarnet works by reversibly inhibiting viral DNA and RNA polymerases, thereby inhibiting the formation of the nucleic acids. Because it inhibits both RNA and DNA synthesis, foscarnet has a broad spectrum of antiviral activity. It is approved for CMV retinitis in patients with impaired immune function and for acyclovir-resistant HSV and herpes zoster infections. Fomivirsen is an antiviral of minor importance used for CMV retinitis in people with HIV. Its use is limited to those who cannot tolerate, or have failed, other therapies.

## Administration

Many of the purine and pyrimidine analogs are effective when taken by mouth. Acyclovir, ganciclovir, famciclovir, valacyclovir, and valganciclovir (Valcyte®) are available in preparations for oral use. Acyclovir can also be given by the intravenous route and can be applied to the skin. After oral or intravenous administration, it distributes well throughout the body and enters the cerebrospinal fluid (CSF), a fact that makes it useful for herpes encephalitis. Acyclovir is only partially metabolized to an inactive product, and can accumulate in patients with renal failure. Valacyclovir, the acyclovir prodrug, is better absorbed after an oral dose than acyclovir, and attains serum drug levels comparable to those from intravenous acyclovir.

Cidofovir and ganciclovir are both available for use in the eye. Cidofovir must be injected into the eye's fluid between the lens and the retina, while ganciclovir is available as an implant that is inserted into the vitreous humor. Like cidofovir, fomivirsen is injected into the vitreous fluid of the eye. Cidofovir and ganciclovir, however, are also provided as preparations for intravenous injection. While ganciclovir can be taken by mouth, cidofovir cannot. Valganciclovir, the ganciclovir prodrug, is only manufactured as tablets for oral administration. Famciclovir is effective when given orally. Trifluridine, the last of the purine and pyrimidine analogs discussed here, is only available as an ophthalmic solution.

Foscarnet is poorly absorbed orally and must be injected intravenously. While this drug can be administered to nonhospitalized patients, it must be given every 8 to 12 hours for 2 to 3 weeks to avoid relapse, a dosing schedule that can cause hardship for patients. The drug is dispersed throughout the body, and more than ten percent of a dose enters the bone, from which it slowly leeches back into the bloodstream.

## Side Effects

The purine and pyrimidine analogs might be expected to cause a similar array of side effects, because their mechanisms of drug action are similar. This is true, to a degree, for the purine and pyrimadine analogs used systemically (ie, by mouth or IV). The rates of the side effects differ, based on whether or not the drug is selectively changed to the active form only in cells infected by viruses, as in the case of acyclovir. **Figure 32.2** summarizes these side effects.

These drugs can affect the central nervous system, causing varying degrees of malaise, headache, confusion or a feeling of fatigue referred to as lethargy. Some people experience seizures. Most of these drugs have been reported to suppress the ability of the bone marrow to make the cellular components of the blood. This is especially true of ganciclovir and valganciclovir, which carry "black box" warnings required by the FDA to caution health care professionals about this risk. The purine and pyrimidine analogs can cause toxicity to the kidneys. This side effect is more likely if patients are dehydrated. The risk of kidney damage is greatest with cidofovir, which carries an FDA required warning regarding the

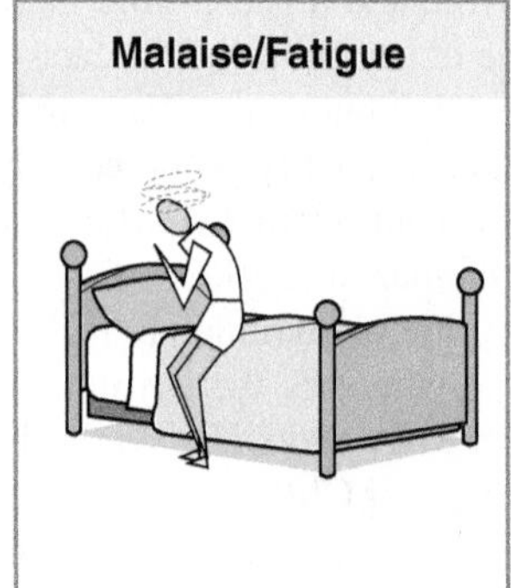


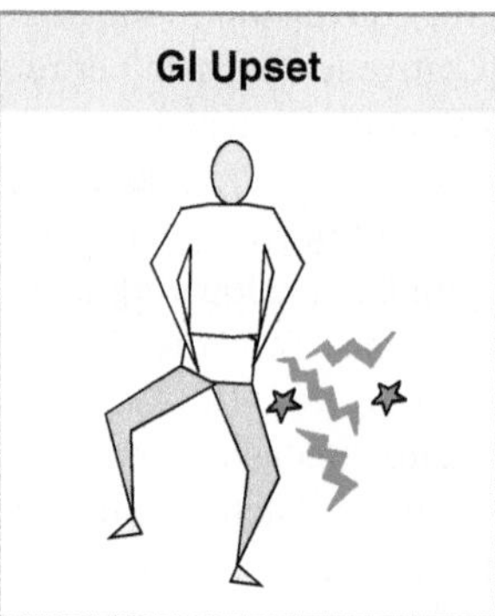


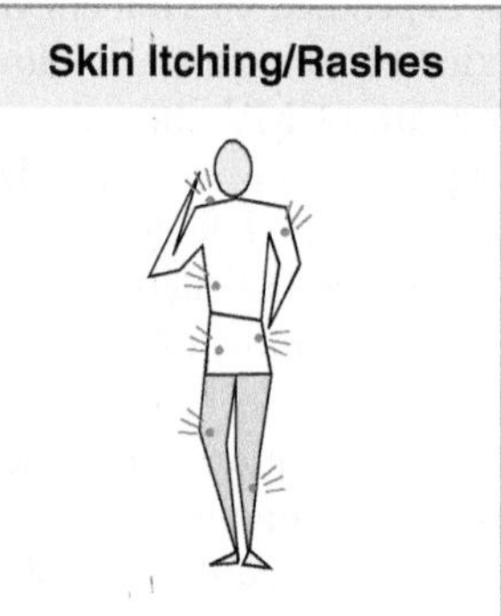


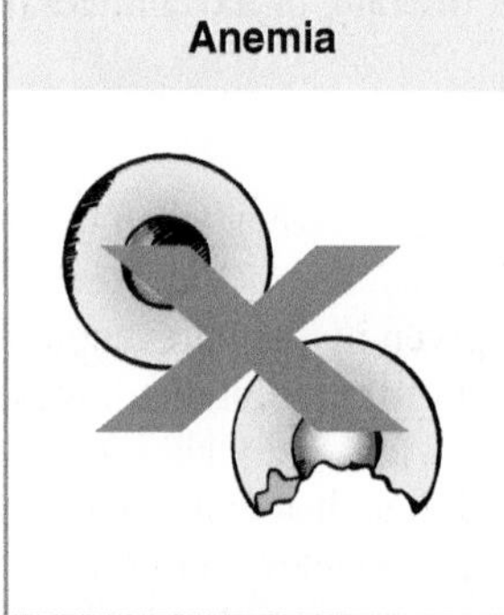


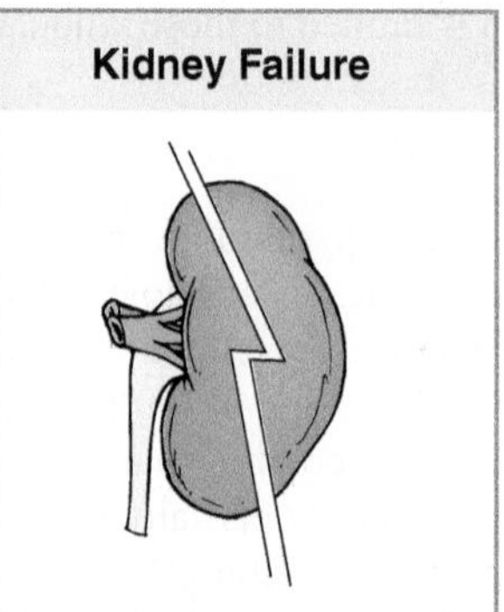


**Figure 32.2** Typical side effects of the purine and pyrimidine analogs. (Adapted with permission from Harvey RA, Champe PC, Howland RD, et al. *Lippincott's Illustrated Reviews: Pharmacology*, 3rd edition. Baltimore: Lippincott Williams & Wilkins, 2006.)

risk of serious kidney damage. Ganciclovir, valganciclovir, and cidofovir were toxic to embryos in animal studies. These drugs should not be given to pregnant women or to men who wish to conceive a child. Use of these drugs may cause infertility, and because they are mutagenic, they are treated as potentially carcinogenic. Patients taking these medications, especially cidofovir and ganciclovir, who also receive zidovudine or didanosine, are at greater risk for adverse effects from the latter drugs.

More frequent and less serious side effects seen across the board with these drugs include GI upset, diarrhea, rashes, and itching. Topical treatments are often associated with burning and irritation. Intravenous administration is associated with burning at the site of the infusion.

The risk of side effects from the use of foscarnet could be characterized as monumental. This may be partly due to the poorer state of health in people who are likely to receive this drug. Nevertheless, the risk of side effects ranges from 10% (seizures) to 65% (fevers). The rate of occurrence of nausea, vomiting, diarrhea, kidney toxicity, and headache ranges from about 25% to 50%.

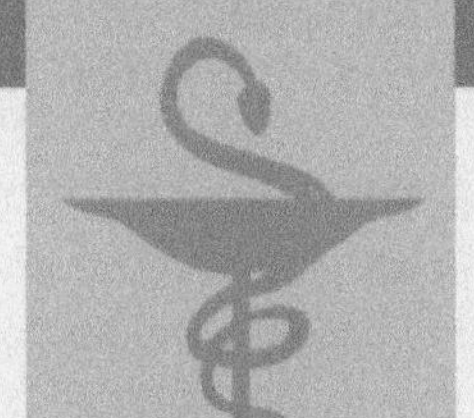

### Tips for the Technician

When dispensing oral purine or pyrimidine analogs, it is appropriate for pharmacy technicians to attach auxiliary labels that instruct patients to complete the course of medication unless advised otherwise by the physician. These drugs can cause lethargy and dizziness, therefore include labelling to caution patients about driving, or consuming alcoholic beverages. Label prescription vials with directions to take these medications with a full glass of water.

The pharmacist should be involved with counselling all patients with new prescriptions for these medications, but especially those with ganciclovir or valganciclovir. Prescription labels for these two medications should include warnings regarding the risk of use by pregnant women. Pharmacy technicians can protect themselves and others by not using automated packaging or dispensing equipment when handling ganciclovir or valganciclovir capsules or tablets. Clean counting trays after using them to count these drugs. A biological safety cabinet is used to reconstitute and compound IV admixtures containing ganciclovir and cidofovir. Follow the manufacturers recommendation for dilution of these drugs and foscarnet.

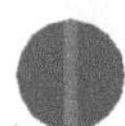

## Human Immunodeficiency Virus

Human immunodeficiency virus (HIV) is a member of the family of viruses called retroviruses. HIV attacks the human immune system, destroying T cell lymphocytes in the process, and makes its victims susceptible to opportunistic infections, many of which are life threatening. HIV causes AIDS, acquired immunodeficiency syndrome. Patients who are not treated lose weight, develop organ dysfunction, and eventually succumb to infections or cancer. HIV is transmitted by contact between mucous membranes and infected body fluids, such as blood or semen. Transmission is much more likely if the mucous membranes are not intact. The virus can pass during sexual contact, sharing of needles, the birth of an infant to an infected mother, or in health care workers, through accidental sticks with contaminated needles.

The first cases of AIDS may have appeared as early as the middle of the twentieth century, although it was not yet recognized as a distinct disease entity. AIDS did not draw attention until the late 1970s when clusters of individuals with unusual opportunistic infections and cancers began to appear in medical centers of large European and American cities. Although the epidemic was described and publicized by the CDC beginning in 1981, the causative virus was not isolated until 1983.

The infection came from Africa, where a related virus occurs in apes, and was possibly transferred to man when hunters in Africa killed infected animals. The disease took hold in the United States and Europe in earnest in the mid 1970s in the gay community, and by 1981 when the syndrome was recognized, it had spread to epidemic proportions. Since 1981, the AIDS pandemic has killed more than 25 million people of all ages, nationalities, and sexual orientation. Although there is no cure, and the virus readily mutates, antiretroviral therapy is now quite effective at controlling the virus and prolonging lives.

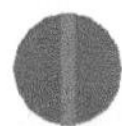

## Antiretroviral Therapy

When AIDS was first discovered there were no antiretroviral drugs and treatment was aimed at controlling opportunistic infections. Now there are three classes of antiretroviral drugs, and recommended treatments include a combination of these drugs. Drug classes include nucleoside reverse transcriptase inhibitors (NRTI), nonnucleoside reverse transcriptase inhibitors (NNRTI) and protease inhibitors (PI). The current recommendation for treatment of newly diagnosed HIV infections is to administer two NRTI drugs along with either a PI or an NNRTI agent. These combinations are sometimes referred to as HAART, or highly active antiretroviral therapy (**Fig. 32.3**).

At present there are two subtypes of HIV viruses, referred to as HIV-1 and HIV-2. The most prevalent virus in North America and Europe is HIV-1. Not all antiretroviral drugs are effective against both viral types. Drug resistance occurs, and is becoming more common. Selection of the appropriate drug regimen is based on the genetic characteristics of the virus, the patient's ability to comply with the various drug regimens, and current recommendations from CDC or National Institute of Health experts.

### Nucleoside Reverse Transcriptase Inhibitors

The nucleoside reverse transcriptase inhibitors (NRTI) are similar to the precursors of RNA. They and the nonnucleoside reverse transcriptase inhibitors target one of the early steps in viral replication, the reproduction of the viral genetic material.

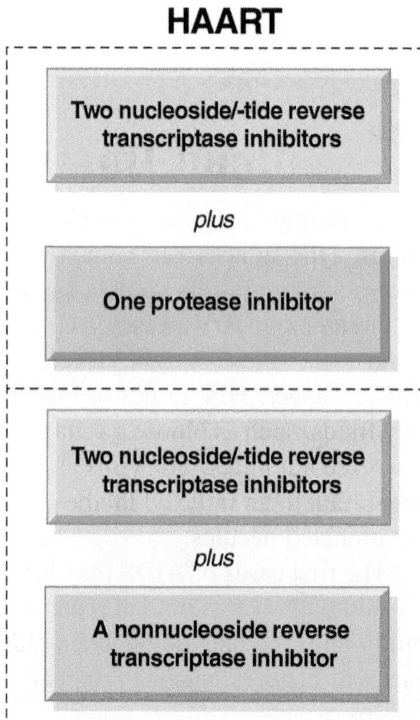


**Figure 32.3** Highly active antiretroviral therapy (HAART) for HIV/AIDS. (Adapted with permission from Harvey RA, Champe PC, Howland RD, et al. *Lippincott's Illustrated Reviews: Pharmacology*, 3rd edition. Baltimore: Lippincott Williams & Wilkins, 2006.)

## Actions and Indications

NRTI drugs are analogs of the precursors of ribonucleic acid. Normally these precursors are used by retroviruses inside the host cells to replicate viral RNA. When the drug is substituted into the growing chain of nucleic acid, the chain becomes faulty, and viral replication cannot proceed. **Figure 32.4** is a representation of the life cycle of the HIV virus that also illustrates the points at which the antiretroviral drugs work. As with the purine and pyrimidine analogs used to treat herpesviruses, these drugs must be converted to an active form inside the cells. When the uninfected human cell is better able to distinguish between the drug and the normal precursors of nucleic acid than the infected cell, the drug is likely to be less toxic. This is because the uninfected cells will be more selective and less likely to convert the drug to the active form.

Zidovudine (Retrovir®, sometimes referred to as AZT) is the prototype of the NRTI agents, and was approved by the FDA in 1987 for the treatment of HIV/AIDS. It is one of the cornerstones of the treatment of AIDS and is approved for use in both children and

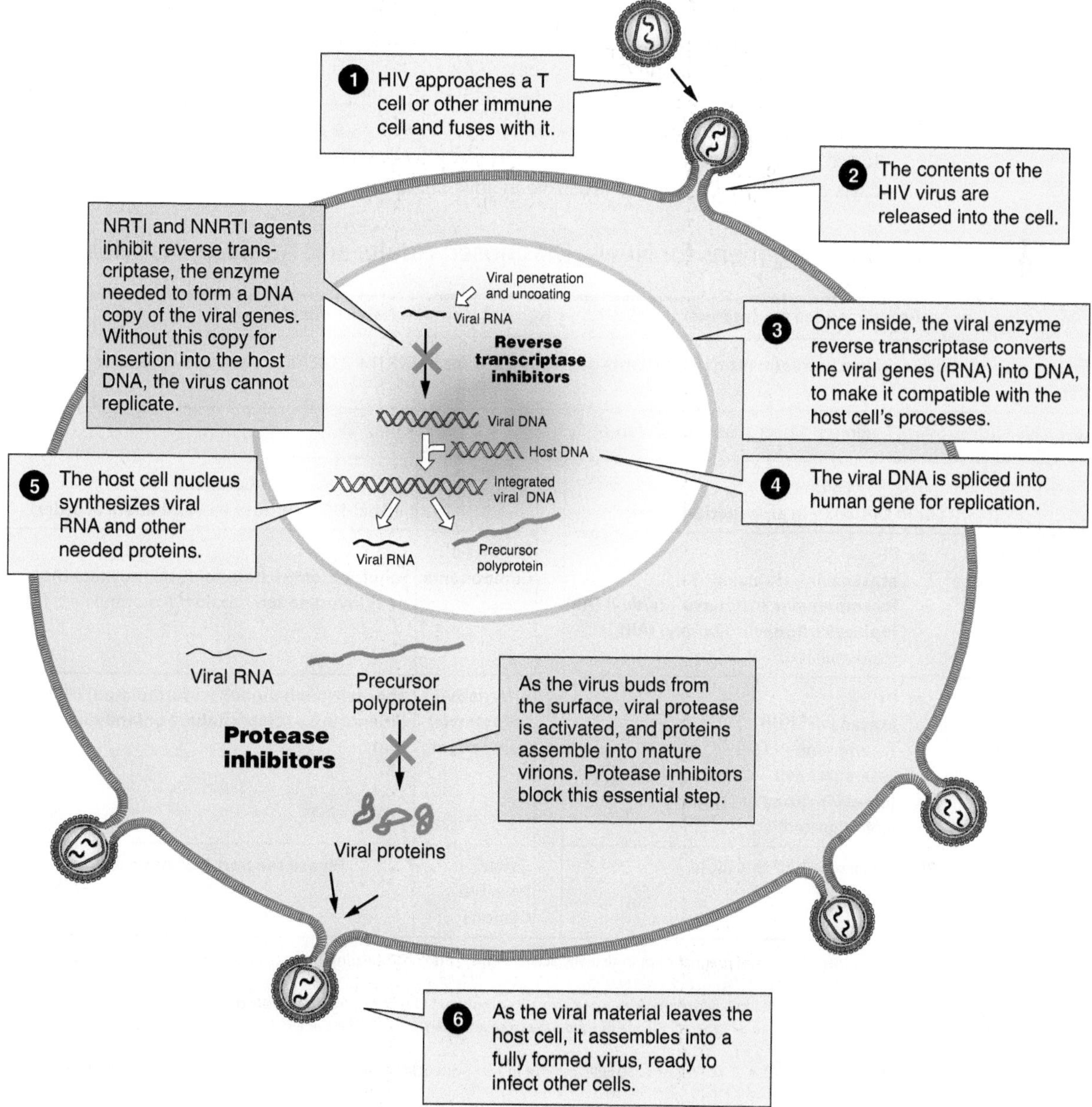


**Figure 32.4** The life cycle of the HIV virus and action of antiretroviral drugs. (Adapted with permission from Harvey RA, Champe PC, Howland RD, et al. *Lippincott's Illustrated Reviews: Pharmacology*, 3rd edition. Baltimore: Lippincott Williams & Wilkins, 2006.)

adults. Zidovudine is also used as part of the prevention strategies in individuals who have been exposed to the virus, and in addition is used to prevent prenatal HIV infection in pregnant, HIV positive mothers. When it is combined with other drugs, zidovudine reduces the viral load and increases the number of T cells. In 2006, the preferred HIV treatment included zidovudine (or tenofovir, Viread®) plus two other drugs. **Table 32.2** shows examples of preferred HIV regimens in newly diagnosed patients. Because of changing viral sensitivity patterns, treatment recommendations change fairly frequently.

The second drug approved to treat HIV infection was didanosine (Videx®, sometimes abbreviated ddI). Like zidovudine, didanosine is administered along with other antiretroviral drugs and is effective in adults and children, but it is only effective against HIV-1. Zalcitabine (Hivid®, sometimes called dideoxycytidine or ddC) can be used with zidovudine. Like other drugs in this group, it is converted to the active form and then inhibits reverse transcriptase and causes formation of abnormal viral DNA. Stavudine (Zerit®) and lamivudine (Epivir®) are other members of this class with similar mechanisms of action. Along with zidovudine, lamivudine is also a routine part of most preferred or alternate regimens because it is better tolerated than many other agents. Besides being effective treatment for HIV, lamivudine can also be used to treat hepatitis B virus. Emtricitabine (Emtriva®), a derivative of lamivudine, is as effective as lamivudine in the treatment of HIV, and is used as an alternative to lamivudine. Abacavir (Ziagen®), which plays a role in some alternative HIV drug regimens, is used in children and adults with AIDS who cannot tolerate or who are failing current regimens. Tenofovir can be used as a zidovudine substitute in the preferred NNRTI based regimen. Although cross-resistance with other members of this drug class can occur, tenofovir is effective against some zidovudine-resistant strains.

## Table 32.2a Preferred Drug Regimens for Newly Diagnosed Adults and Adolescents With HIV

**Antiretroviral Components Recommended for Treatment of HIV-1 Infection in Treatment Naïve Patients**

**A combination antiretroviral regimen in treatment-naïve patients generally contains 1 NNRTI + 2 NRTIs or a single or ritonavir-boosted PI + 2 NRTI.**

**To Construct an Antiretroviral Regimen, Select 1 Component from Column A + 1 from Column B**

| | Column A (NNRTI or PI Options – in alphabetical order) | | | Column B (Dual-NRTI Options – in alphabetical order) |
|---|---|---|---|---|
| **Preferred Components** | **NNRTI- efavirenz[1] (AII)** or **PI- atazanavir + ritonavir (AIII)<br>fosamprenavir + ritonavir (2x/day) (AII)<br>lopinavir/ritonavir[2] (2x/day) (AII)** (coformulated) | | **Preferred Components** | **tenofovir/emtricitabine[3]** (coformulated) **(AII); or zidovudine/lamivudine[3]** (coformulated) **(AII)** |
| **Alternative to Preferred Components** | **NNRTI – nevirapine[4] (BII)** or **PI atazanavir[5] (BII)<br>fosamprenavir (BII)<br>fosamprenavir + ritonavir (1x/day) (BII)<br>lopinavir/ritonavir (1x/day) (BII)** (coformulated) | + | **Alternative to Preferred Components** | **abacavir/lamivudine3 (coformulated) (BII)<br>didanosine + (emtricitabine or lamivudine) (BII)** |
| **Other Possible Options** | **Please see part b of this table** | | **Other Possible Options** | **Please see part b of this table** |

[1]Efavirenz is not recommended for use in the 1st trimester of pregnancy or in sexually active women with child-bearing potential who are not using effective contraception.

[2]The pivotal study that led to the recommendation of lopinavir/ritonavir as a preferred PI component was based on twice-daily dosing. A smaller study has shown similar efficacy with once-daily dosing but also showed a higher incidence of moderate to severe diarrhea with the once-daily regimen (16% vs. 5%).

[3]Emtricitabine may be used in place of lamivudine and vice versa.

[4]Nevirapine should not be initiated in women with CD4$^+$ T cell count >250 cells/mm$^3$ or in men with CD4$^+$ T cell count >400 cells/mm$^3$ because of increased risk of symptomatic hepatic events in these patients.

[5]Atazanavir must be boosted with ritonavir if used in combination with tenofovir.

*(continues)*

**Table 32.2b** Preferred Drug Regimens for Newly Diagnosed Adults and Adolescents With HIV *(continued)*

| Antiretroviral Components That Are Acceptable as Initial Antiretroviral Components but Are Inferior to Preferred or Alternative Components | | |
|---|---|---|
| **Antiretroviral Drugs or Regimens (in Alphabetical Order)** | **Reasons for Generally Not Recommending the Drugs or Regimens as Initial Therapy** | **Special Circumstances in Which the Drugs or Regimens May Be Used** |
| Abacavir/lamivudine/ zidovudine (coformulated) as triple-NRTI combination regimen **(CII)** | • Inferior virologic efficacy | • When PI or NNRTI-based regimens cannot be used based on toxicities or concerns of significant drug-drug interactions |
| Nelfinavir **(CII)** | • Inferior virologic efficacy | • Most experience with pregnant patients with good tolerability and adequate pharmacokinetic data |
| Saquinavir (ritonavir-boosted) **(CII)** | • Inferior to lopinavir/ritonavir<br>• Minimal efficacy data in treatmentnaïve patients | • When preferred or alternative PI components cannot be used based on toxicities or concerns of significant drug-drug interactions |
| Stavudine + lamivudine **(CII)** | • Significant toxicities including lipoatrophy, peripheral neuropathy, hyperlactatemia including symptomatic and life-threatening lactic acidosis, hepatic steatosis, and pancreatitis | • When preferred or alternative dual-NRTI combination cannot be used |

(Adapted from *Guidelines for the Use of Antiretroviral Agents in HIV-1-Infected Adults and Adolescents*, October 10, 2006. Developed by the DHHS Panel on Antiretroviral Guidelines for Adults and Adolescents – A Working Group of the Office of AIDS Research Advisory Council (OARAC). Accessed July 30, 2007 from http://aidsinfo.nih.gov.)

## Administration

All of the nucleoside reverse transcriptase inhibitors are taken orally, but some are better absorbed than others. Zidovudine is well absorbed after oral administration. When taken with food, peak levels can be lower, but the total amount of drug absorbed is unchanged. Zidovudine is taken every 8 hours. This drug is available for intravenous use. **Table 32.3** lists pertinent information about zidovudine and the other drugs presently used to treat HIV.

Lamivudine, stavudine, and abacavir are well absorbed orally. These drugs are usually taken twice daily. Emtricitabine and tenofovir, unlike many antiretroviral medications, are given once a day as a single capsule or tablet. Due to its instability in the presence of stomach acid, didanosine is administered as either a chewable, buffered tablet, extended release capsule, or in a buffered solution. Absorption is acceptable if taken on an empty stomach, but food causes decreased absorption. Zalcitabine is very well absorbed orally, but the presence of magnesium/aluminum-containing antacids reduces absorption.

## Side Effects

The nucleoside reverse transcriptase inhibitors are associated with a few class-wide side effects. The most common of these effects is GI upset, including nausea, vomiting, and diarrhea. Serious liver toxicity can also occur with these medications. In rare instances, fat is deposited in the liver, and severe metabolic changes can occur that result in death.

In addition to the class side effects, these drugs can cause other, sometimes serious side effects specific to one or more drugs. Stavudine, didanosine, and zalcitabine are known to cause pancreatitis, which is inflammation of the pancreas, and peripheral neuropathy. These drugs are not used in combination because their toxicities are additive when combined. Tenofovir and zidovudine can cause headache and weakness. In addition zidovudine can suppress the production of blood cells in the bone marrow, and tenofovir can damage the

**Table 32.3** Generic and Brand names, Indications, and Formulations for Drugs Used in the Treatment of HIV/AIDS

| Generic Name | Brand Name | Available as | Indications | Notes/Combinations |
|---|---|---|---|---|
| **Nucleoside Reverse Transcriptase Inhibitors** | | | | |
| Abacavir | Ziagen® | Tablets, oral solution | With other agents to treat HIV/AIDS | Also Trizivir® tablets w/ 3TC, Epzicom® tablets w/ AZT+3TC |
| Didanosine | Videx® | EC tabs, buffered chew tabs, buffered powder for oral soln | With other agents to treat HIV/AIDS | Take on an empty stomach |
| Emtricitabine | Emtriva® | Capsules, oral solution | With other agents to treat HIV/AIDS | Also Truvada® w/TDF |
| Lamivudine | Epivir® | Tablets, oral solution | With other agents to treat HIV/AIDS | Also Combivir® w/ AZT, Epzicom®, Trizivir® |
| Stavudine | Zerit® | Capsules, oral solution | HIV, after long-term AZT use | |
| Tenofovir | Viread® | Tablets | With other agents to treat HIV/AIDS | Also Truvada® |
| Zalcitabine | Hivid® | Tablets | Late stages of HIV | |
| Zidovudine | Retrovir® | Capsules, tablets, IV solution, oral solution | With other agents to treat HIV/AIDS | Also Combivir®, Trizivir® |
| **Nonnucleoside Reverse Transcriptase Inhibitors** | | | | |
| Delavirdine | Rescriptor® | Tablets | With other agents to treat HIV/AIDS | |
| Efavirenz | Sustiva® | Capsules | With other agents to treat HIV/AIDS | Take on empty stomach, food causes some ↑ in absorption |
| Nevirapine | Viramune® | Tablets, oral solution | With other agents to treat HIV/AIDS | Also used as single dose to prevent mother to child transmission |
| **Protease Inhibitors** | | | | |
| Amprenavir or Fosamprenavir | Agenerase® or Lexiva® | Capsules, oral solution | With other agents to treat HIV/AIDS | Do not use together, same active drug. Avoid high-fat meals with Agenerase® |
| Atazanavir | Reyataz® | Capsules | With other agents to treat HIV/AIDS | Take with food, avoid antacids |
| Indinavir | Crixivan® | Capsules | With other agents to treat HIV/AIDS | Encourage fluid intake |
| Lopinavir + Ritonavir | Kaletra® | Tablet, oral solution | With other agents to treat HIV/AIDS | Take solution with food, refrigerate |
| Nelfinavir | Viracept® | Tablets, powder for oral solution | With other agents to treat HIV/AIDS | Take with food |
| Ritonavir | Norvir® | Capsules, oral solution | With other agents to treat HIV/AIDS | Refrigerate capsules, not solution |
| Saquinavir | Invirase® | Capsules, tablets | With other agents to treat HIV/AIDS | |
| Tipranavir | Aptivus® | Capsules | With other agents to treat HIV/AIDS | Refrigerate capsules |

AZT, Zidovudine; 3TC, Lamivudine; EC, enteric coated; TDF, Tenofovir.

kidneys. Abacavir can cause serious allergic reactions that are sometimes fatal. Symptoms of hypersensitivity reactions include fever, rash, and cough or shortness of breath. Lamivudine and emtricitabine are the least toxic members of this class.

## Tips for the Technician

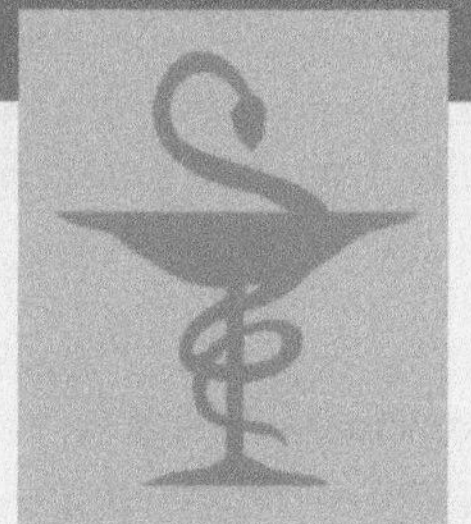

Patient compliance is an important issue in the treatment of HIV/AIDS. The number of tablets patients must take, the frequency of administration, and side effects play an important role in determining compliance. For this reason, many antiretroviral drugs are available as combination products. When combination products are dispensed, make sure that applicable auxiliary labelling for both drug components are included.

It is important that patients with HIV understand that none of these drugs can cure an HIV infection, but results are improved when the medications are taken correctly. The risk of resistance increases when the medications are not taken exactly as prescribed. Patients are better able to tolerate side effects when they are educated about them in advance, and pharmacists can help to ensure clients are informed about the antiretroviral drugs they take.

Technicians can help improve compliance by labelling all antiretroviral medications with auxiliary labels to advise clients to take the medication exactly as ordered, and not to stop unless specifically instructed to do so by the physician. Prescription vials containing didanosine should include instructions to take the drug on an empty stomach (30 minutes before or 2 hours after a meal). The manufacturer of zidovudine recommends that it be taken on an empty stomach, so it too should be labelled with the appropriate auxiliary label.

## Nonnucleoside Reverse Transcriptase Inhibitors

Nonnucleoside reverse transcriptase inhibitors (NNRTI) are highly selective, noncompetitive inhibitors of HIV reverse transcriptase. There are only three of these drugs, but they play an important role in combination therapies.

### Actions and Indications

Efavirenz (Sustiva®), delavirdine (Rescriptor®), and nevirapine (Viramune®) are the three NNRTI agents used in combination with other antiretroviral agents in the treatment of HIV infection or AIDS. They act by binding to the HIV reverse transcriptase to prevent it from working. Because this mechanism of action is different from the mechanism of the NRTI agents, they have an additive effect when used in combinations. The NNRTI agents can increase T cell counts, decrease viral load, and reduce the rate of transmission of the virus to the fetus in pregnancy.

### Administration

All of the NNRTI are manufactured in solid formulations (tablets or capsules) for oral administration. Only one, nevirapine, is available in a liquid formulation. Absorption after an oral dose of delavirdine and nevirapine is excellent. These products can be taken without regard to meals. Efavirenz absorption is affected by the presence of food in the stomach. High fat or high calorie meals can increase absorption by about forty to nearly eighty percent. To avoid wide variations in serum levels, these products should be taken on an empty stomach.

The three NNRTI drugs have varying half-lives and are, therefore, administered with different frequencies. Delavirdine is rapidly removed from the bloodstream and must be taken three times a day. Nevirapine is longer acting and is taken twice a day, while efavirenz has the longest half-life and is taken once a day.

### Side Effects

As a class, the NNRTI agents are known for causing allergic skin reactions. Rashes occur in as many as 40% or more of patients receiving an NNRTI agent in combination with other antiretroviral drugs. These can include life-threatening reactions, such as Stevens-Johnson syndrome. Other side effects include abnormal elevations in liver enzymes sometimes seen with use of delavirdine and efavirenz. Liver toxicity, that although uncommon can be fatal, is associated with nevirapine use. Resistance develops easily in this class of drugs, and when a virus is resistant to one member of the class, it is resistant to all.

Of the NNRTI agents, efavirenz is the best tolerated. The most common adverse effects associated with its use originate in the CNS, and include dizziness, headache, vivid dreams, and loss of concentration. Nearly half of the patients experience these complaints, which usually resolve within a few weeks. This drug was teratogenic in primates, so it should not be given to pregnant women.

Delavirdine can cause CNS effects similar to those caused by efavirenz. Delavirdine inhibits the metabolism of some drugs, including the protease inhibitors. Ritonavir levels are not altered significantly by the presence of delavirdine, but the levels of saquinavir and indinavir are significantly increased. Nevirapine increases the metabolism of a number of drugs, such as oral contraceptives, ketoconazole, methadone, metronidazole, quinidine, theophylline, and warfarin. It is also the most likely to cause rash and liver injury.

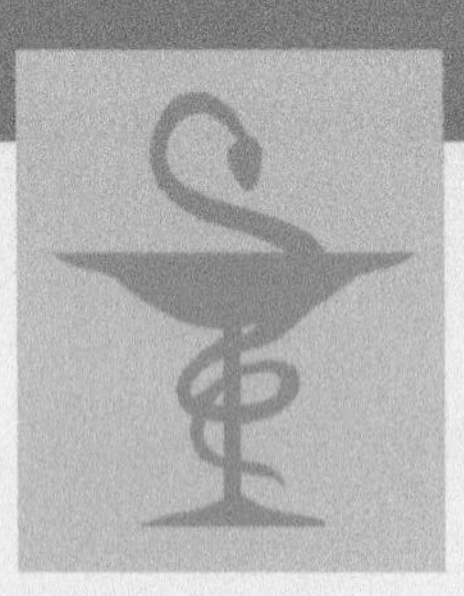

### Tips for the Technician

As with other antiretroviral agents, the importance of patient compliance cannot be overstated. It is important that patients with HIV understand that none of these drugs can cure an HIV infection, but results are improved when the medications are taken correctly. The risk of resistance increases when the medications are not taken exactly as prescribed. Label all prescription vials with an auxiliary label that underscores the importance of compliance with dosing instructions. Efavirenz should be labelled "take on an empty stomach." Be sure to alert the pharmacist to any drug interaction alerts when entering NNRTI orders on the pharmacy computer system. Many antiviral medications begin with vir-, including Viramune®, Viracept®, Viread®, and Virazole®. Be careful to clarify any potentially confusing prescriptions so that look-alike, sound-alike errors are avoided.

## Protease Inhibitors

The first protease inhibitors (PI) were introduced in 1995. Within a year of their introduction, the number of deaths in the United States due to AIDS declined dramatically. Although there are eight different drugs in this class, only two are presently included in the preferred regimens for HIV treatment.

### Actions and Indications

All the drugs in this group are reversible inhibitors of HIV protease. Protease is the viral enzyme responsible for converting newly synthesized viral proteins into the enzymes and structures required for maturation of the virus. The action of these drugs results in the production of non-infectious viruses. The protease inhibitors exhibit a much greater affinity for HIV enzymes than for comparable human proteases. As a result of this selectivity, they are less toxic than would otherwise be expected. Treatment with a protease inhibitor and two

NRTI agents, in patients who have never had HIV therapy, results in a decrease in the plasma viral load to undetectable levels in 60% to 95% of patients. Treatment failures are most likely due to a lack of patient adherence to the prescribed drug regimen. The protease inhibitors are indicated for the treatment of HIV/AIDS when combined with other agents.

## Administration

The protease inhibitors are administered orally, but most have poor absorption. High-fat meals substantially improve the absorption of some, such as atazanavir (Reyataz®), nelfinavir (Viracept®), saquinavir (Invirase®), and ritonavir (Norvir®). The bioavailability of indinavir (Crixivan®) is decreased in the presence of high-fat meals, and it should be taken on an empty stomach. High fat meals should be avoided with amprenavir (Agenerase®) administration, but it can be taken with or without food. The other PI agents are essentially unaffected by meals.

Saquinavir, which is available as tablets, capsules, and soft gelatin capsules, is the poorest absorbed of all the protease inhibitors. To maximize bioavailability, the soft gelatin capsules should be used and the drug given along with a low dose of ritonavir. Ritonavir also increases the plasma levels of amprenavir and thereby lowers the total daily dose needed. This is a distinct advantage, because when amprenavir is taken alone, patients must take 16 large tablets. Ritonavir tastes bad, however, and can be taken with chocolate milk or nutritional supplements to improve palatability.

## Side Effects

Protease inhibitors frequently cause nausea, vomiting, and diarrhea. Disturbances in glucose and lipid metabolism also occur, including diabetes, hypertriglyceridemia, and hypercholesterolemia (**Fig. 32.5**). Chronic use can result in fat redistribution from the arms and legs to the abdomen, the base of the neck, and the breasts. Fat distribution to the base of

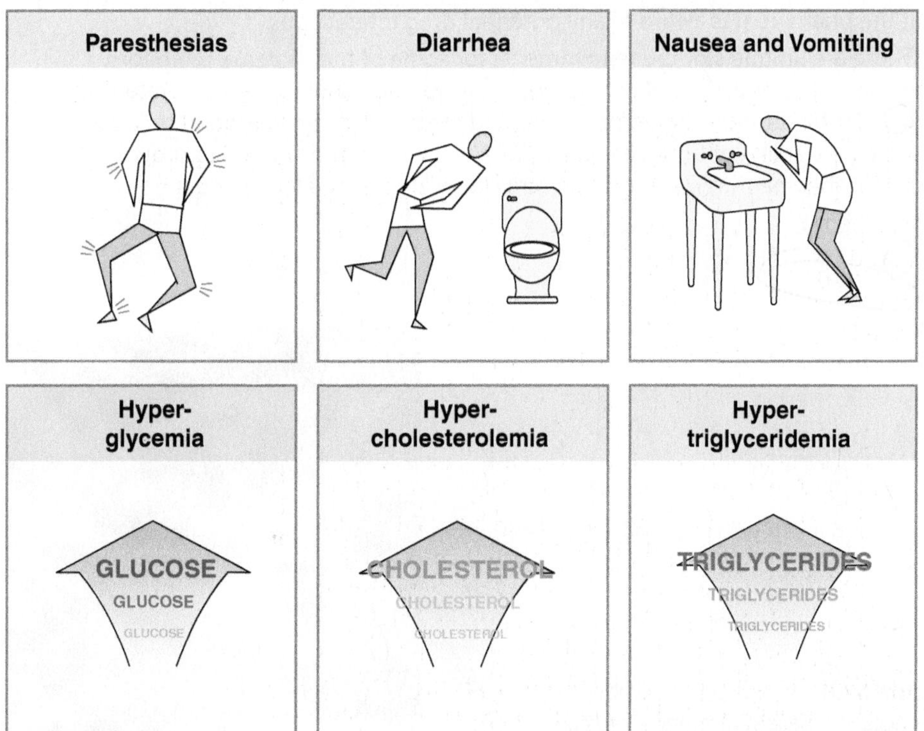


**Figure 32.5** Well-known adverse effects associated with the protease inhibitors. (Adapted with permission from Harvey RA, Champe PC, Howland RD, et al. *Lippincott's Illustrated Reviews: Pharmacology*, 3rd edition. Baltimore: Lippincott Williams & Wilkins, 2006.)

the neck (sometimes referred to as a buffalo hump) is unsightly and distressing to patients (**Fig. 32.6**). A number of these agents are associated with central nervous system side effects, such as headache, dizziness, and tingling in the limbs. They can cause an abnormal taste in the mouth.

Drug interactions are a common problem for all protease inhibitors, because they are potent inhibitors of the cytochrome P drug metabolizing enzymes. Ritonavir is the most potent inhibitor, and saquinavir, the least potent inhibitor of the class. Drugs that rely on metabolism by these enzymes can, in some cases, accumulate to toxic levels. Examples of potentially dangerous interactions include excessive sedation from midazolam or triazolam, bleeding from warfarin, respiratory depression from fentanyl, and low blood pressure from sildenafil (see **Fig. 32.7**). Other drugs that induce these enzymes can cause low concentrations of the protease inhibitor, resulting in treatment failures. Drugs such as rifampin, barbiturates, and carbamazepine should be avoided for this reason.

Amprenavir oral solution is made with propylene glycol and should not be used in pregnant women or children less than 4 years of age because of a high risk of toxicity. Kidney stone formation is a common problem seen with indinavir and other protease inhibitors. Adequate hydration is important to reduce this risk, and patients should drink at least six to eight full glasses of water daily.

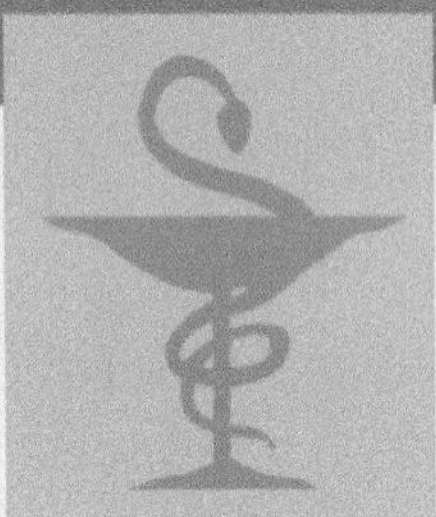

## Tips for the Technician

As is the case with all antiretroviral agents, compliance with administration instructions is of the utmost importance. When dispensing these medications, the technician is expected to include auxiliary instructions that reinforce the importance of compliance with dosing instructions. It is important that atazanavir, nelfinavir, ritonavir, saquinavir, and tipranavir (Aptivus®) be labelled "take with food," while indinavir prescription vials should be labelled "take on an empty stomach." Be sure that the pharmacist is aware of any potential drug interactions.

There are unique storage requirements for some of the protease inhibitors. Ritonavir capsules and ritonavir plus lopinavir solution should be refrigerated. Ritonavir oral solution should not be kept in the refrigerator. Refrigeration also improves the stability of tipranavir capsules. Make sure that drugs are appropriately stored in the pharmacy, and that prescription vials are labelled "refrigerate" when appropriate.

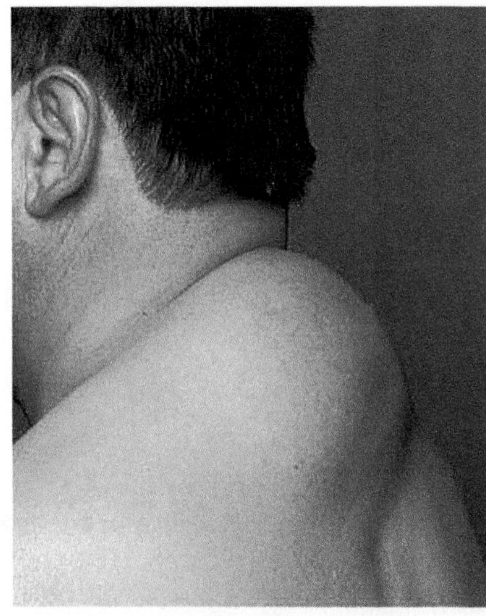

**Figure 32.6** Redistribution of fat to the base of the neck in a patient receiving a protease inhibitor. (Reprinted with permission from Harvey RA, Champe PC, Howland RD, et al. *Lippincott's Illustrated Reviews: Pharmacology*, 3rd edition. Baltimore: Lippincott Williams & Wilkins, 2006.)

**Protease Inhibitors**

| DRUG CLASS | EXAMPLE |
|---|---|
| ANTIARRHYTHMICS | Quinidine |
| ERGOT DERIVATIVES | Ergotamine |
| ANTIMYCOBACTERIAL DRUGS | RIfampin |
| BENZODIAZEPINES | Midazolam |
| BARBITURATES | Phenobarbital |
| ANTICOAGULANTS | Warfarin |
| HERBAL SUPPLEMENTS | St. John's wort |
| PHOSPHODIESTERASE TYPE 5 INHIBITORS | Sildenafil |

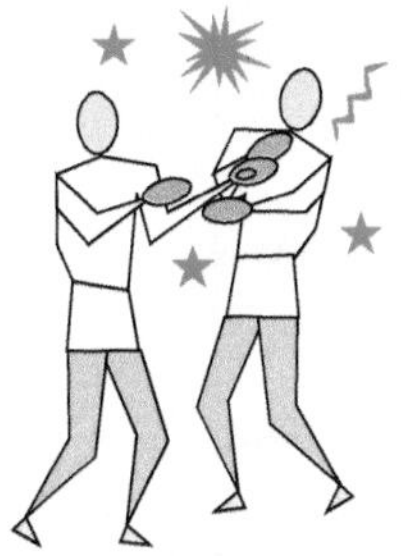

**Contraindicated**

**Figure 32.7** These drugs should not be given to patients taking protease inhibitors because the combinations can cause significant drug interactions. (Adapted with permission from Harvey RA, Champe PC, Howland RD, et al. *Lippincott's Illustrated Reviews: Pharmacology*, 3rd edition. Baltimore: Lippincott Williams & Wilkins, 2006.)

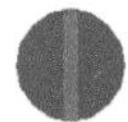

# Vaccines

Long before the development of antiviral medications, people protected themselves against viral infections through vaccination. Edward Jenner is credited with developing the first vaccine in the late 1790's, but in fact he took the idea for vaccination from milkmaids, who believed that if they were infected by cowpox (a virus that we now know is similar to smallpox) they could not contract smallpox. He tested this theory on an 8-year-old boy, by exposing a small wound on his arm to secretions from a cowpox on a milkmaid's hand. The boy was later exposed to smallpox, but did not contract the disease. Jenner coined the word "vaccine" from the Latin "vacca" for cow, and named the process of conferring active immunity in this manor, vaccination.

vaccine A preparation of killed or attenuated microorganisms administered in order to produce immunity to a specific infectious disease.

vaccination The administration of a vaccine to a person or animal in order to produce immunity.

## Actions and Indications

Modern vaccines are some of the most important advances in medicine. When a large majority of children are immunized, epidemics of childhood viral infections are prevented. Worldwide, this amounts to millions of lives saved and the aftermath of diseases, such as crippling from polio, prevented.

Vaccination is the process of administering weakened or inactivated viruses or bacteria to a patient in order to establish an immune response against that specific organism, and therefore prevent the disease. Immunization is done in advance of actual exposure to an infection. This process induces artificial active immunity, which is as effective, but not as long lasting as natural active immunity. In contrast, administration of a product that con-

active immunity Resistance to infection that is acquired because white blood cells are exposed to antigens and produce antibody to the infectious agent.

passive immunity
Immunity acquired by transfer of antibodies from another individual.

tains antibodies confers passive immunity, immunity that is acquired through the transfer of antibodies from one individual to another individual. Passive immunity is used after a patient is exposed or potentially exposed to an illness. Passive immunity lasts only as long as the antibodies stay in the body.

Vaccinees are administered to children and adolescents according to the schedule illustrated in **Figure 32.8**. While the majority of immunizations are administered in childhood or adolescence, some are administered to other high-risk populations. For example, college students living in dormitories, military recruits, and microbiologists are immunized for bacterial meningitis, the elderly living in long-term care facilities are immunized against pneumococcal pneumonia, and travelers to foreign countries may wish to be immunized against hepatitis A virus. Health care workers are a high-risk group routinely immunized against hepatitis B virus and influenza.

DEPARTMENT OF HEALTH AND HUMAN SERVICES • CENTERS FOR DISEASE CONTROL AND PREVENTION

**Recommended Immunization Schedule for Persons Aged 0–6 Years—UNITED STATES • 2007**

| Vaccine ▼ Age ▶ | Birth | 1 month | 2 months | 4 months | 6 months | 12 months | 15 months | 18 months | 19–23 months | 2–3 years | 4–6 years |
|---|---|---|---|---|---|---|---|---|---|---|---|
| Hepatitis B[1] | HepB | HepB | | *see footnote 1* | HepB | | | | HepB Series | | |
| Rotavirus[2] | | | Rota | Rota | Rota | | | | | | |
| Diphtheria, Tetanus, Pertussis[3] | | | DTaP | DTaP | DTaP | | DTaP | | | | DTaP |
| *Haemophilus influenzae* type b[4] | | | Hib | Hib | *Hib*[4] | Hib | | Hib | | | |
| Pneumococcal[5] | | | PCV | PCV | PCV | PCV | | | | PCV<br>PPV | |
| Inactivated Poliovirus | | | IPV | IPV | IPV | | | | | | IPV |
| Influenza[6] | | | | | Influenza (Yearly) | | | | | | |
| Measles, Mumps, Rubella[7] | | | | | | MMR | | | | | MMR |
| Varicella[8] | | | | | | Varicella | | | | | Varicella |
| Hepatitis A[9] | | | | | | HepA (2 doses) | | | | HepA Series | |
| Meningococcal[10] | | | | | | | | | | MPSV4 | |

Range of recommended ages

Catch-up immunization

Certain high-risk groups

DEPARTMENT OF HEALTH AND HUMAN SERVICES • CENTERS FOR DISEASE CONTROL AND PREVENTION

**Recommended Immunization Schedule for Persons Aged 7–18 Years—UNITED STATES • 2007**

| Vaccine ▼ Age ▶ | 7–10 years | 11–12 YEARS | 13–14 years | 15 years | 16–18 years |
|---|---|---|---|---|---|
| Tetanus, Diphtheria, Pertussis[1] | *see footnote 1* | Tdap | Tdap | | |
| Human Papillomavirus[2] | *see footnote 2* | HPV (3 doses) | HPV Series | | |
| Meningococcal[3] | MPSV4 | MCV4 | MCV4[3]<br>MCV4 | | |
| Pneumococcal[4] | PPV | | | | |
| Influenza[5] | Influenza (Yearly) | | | | |
| Hepatitis A[6] | HepA Series | | | | |
| Hepatitis B[7] | HepB Series | | | | |
| Inactivated Poliovirus[8] | IPV Series | | | | |
| Measles, Mumps, Rubella[9] | MMR Series | | | | |
| Varicella[10] | Varicella Series | | | | |

Range of recommended ages

Catch-up immunization

Certain high-risk groups

**Figure 32.8** Childhood and adolescent immunization recommendations from the Department of Health and Human Services, Centers for Disease Control and Prevention. (Accessed from http://www.cdc.gov/vaccines/recs/schedules/child-schedule.htm July 24, 2007)

## Administration

Most vaccines are administered by intramuscular injection. Exceptions include the oral poliovirus vaccine used in some countries, a version of influenza vaccine that is administered intranasally, and a few vaccines that are given subcutaneously, including measles, mumps, and rubella vaccine, and varicella (chickenpox) vaccine. Polio (IPV) vaccine for injection is either given subcutaneously or by intramuscular injection.

These products are biologicals, and as such, require special storage conditions. While most vaccines are stored refrigerated (Measles-Mumps-Rubella or MMR, pneumococcal, polio, influenza, hepatitis B, rabies, and others) and cannot be frozen, the rare product requires freezing (Varicella vaccine, yellow fever vaccine, and oral polio vaccine, which is no longer used in the United States).

## Side Effects

Immunization has allowed the worldwide eradication of smallpox, and elimination of polio from the western hemisphere and most of the rest of the world. Although a number of vaccines can cause mild febrile illness or pain at the site of injection, more serious reactions are rare. Some vaccines can cause allergic reactions because of the way the viruses or bacteria are cultured. For example, some influenza viruses are cultured in eggs, so patients with egg allergies should not receive the vaccine.

Public awareness of the risks of vaccination and controversy over their use has increased, however. This is largely due to the fact that the more people that are vaccinated, the more likely rare but serious side effects will occur. These side effects may be highly publicized, in some cases. When investigating vaccine side effects as a student or parent, it is important to keep in perspective how devastating the diseases can be that are being prevented. Nevertheless, it is public pressure and concern about side effects from vaccines that push pharmaceutical companies to improve their products. A case in point is the pertussis vaccine, given along with diphtheria and tetanus vaccines in a combination commonly know as DPT. In years past, the pertussis component caused high fevers in some children and, rarely, seizures or even coma. Studies that connected the two, lawsuits, and the increasing numbers of parents who refused to immunize their children eventually led to the development of diphtheria, acellular pertussis, and tetanus vaccine, a product that is not associated with the same safety concerns.

### Tips for the Technician

These products are nearly always provided to patients by clinics, doctor's offices, or hospitals. Although pharmacies may purchase them, they do not supply them directly to patients. These products are expensive, and the most important role the technician plays is to ensure they are properly stored in the pharmacy, and safely transported to the clinics or offices where they are administered.

# Review Questions

## Multiple Choice

Choose the best answer for the following questions:

1. The deadliest pandemic of all time was caused by which of the below?
   a. Influenza
   b. Bubonic plague
   c. Tuberculosis
   d. HIV
   e. Cholera

2. Of the following statements, which is not an adaptation by the herpesvirus to avoid the host's immune response?
   a. They change into a new viral coat, unrecognizable to the immune system.
   b. They hide in nerve cells in a latent form.
   c. They prevent the host cell from dying, forcing it to continue to churn out viruses.
   d. They can shield their own antigens so that the host immune system is less able to respond.
   e. All of the above are adaptations.

3. Which of the following can be causes of noncompliance with antiretroviral medications in HIV/AIDS patients?
   a. Number of tablets to take
   b. Side effects
   c. Frequency of administration
   d. a and b
   e. All of the above

4. Circle the letter that corresponds to the NNRTI agent below
   a. Lamivudine
   c. Acyclovir
   c. Efavirenz
   d. Indinavir
   e. Ribavirin

5. Of the following choices, the side effects most likely to be experienced by a child after being immunized are?
   a. Autism
   b. Guillain Barré syndrome
   c. Seizures and coma
   d. Pain at the injection site
   e. None is likely to occur

## True/False

6. Zanamivir, a drug used to treat influenza, is not active orally and is administered intranasally.
   a. True
   b. False

7. Parents of children taking the adamantine derivatives should be advised to give the dose immediately before bedtime because they cause drowsiness.
   a. True
   b. False

8. The purine and pyrimidine derivatives can cause lethargy and dizziness. Therefore, technicians should include a caution label to advise patients to avoid driving or consuming alcoholic beverages while taking these medications.
   a. True
   b. False

9. Stavudine, didanosine, and zalcitabine are not used together because they can each cause pancreatitis, and the risk is higher when they are used together.
   a. True
   b. False

10. All of the NNRTI are manufactured in liquid formulations for oral administration.
   a. True
   b. False

## Matching

For numbers 11 to 15, match the word or phrase with the correct lettered definition from the list below. Choices will not be used more than once and may not be used at all.

11. Epidemic
12. Pandemic
13. Passive Immunity
14. Immunization
15. Antigen

a. A process used to increase the body's ability to react to a specific infectious agent and thereby resist illness
b. An outbreak of infectious disease that exceeds the expected number of cases
c. A feeling of fatigue
d. Substances that increase the risk of cancer
e. An epidemic that spreads over a large part of the world
f. A formulation of attenuated or killed microorganisms administered to prevent disease
g. The parts of foreign cells or organisms to which the immune system reacts
h. Immunity that is acquired through the transfer of antibodies from one individual to another

## Short Answer

16. Identify the role of ribavirin in viral infections, the potential risks to health care workers who handle the medication, and measures that should be employed to prevent toxicity.

17. Explain why it is more difficult for pharmacologists to develop antiviral agents that are safe and effective than it is to develop safe and effective antibiotics.

18. List an NRTI drug that is considered a good first choice for treatment of HIV, and provide a description of its mechanism of action, administration, and side effects.

19. List one of the protease inhibitors considered a good first choice for treatment of HIV, and provide a description of its mechanism of action, administration, and side effects.

20. List a vaccine that must be frozen, a vaccine that is administered subcutaneously, and the most common side effects observed with vaccination.

## FOR FURTHER INQUIRY

The lay press and some Internet sites have recently promoted the idea that MMR® vaccine is the cause of the increase in cases of autism over the past few years. Some parents are even refusing to get their children immunized for these childhood illnesses because of this fear. Investigate this or another claim about diseases linked with immunizations (Anthrax vaccine and Gulf War syndrome, for example) either in the library or on the Internet. Does the association appear to be valid?

UNIT VII

# Chemotherapy and Other Drug Therapies

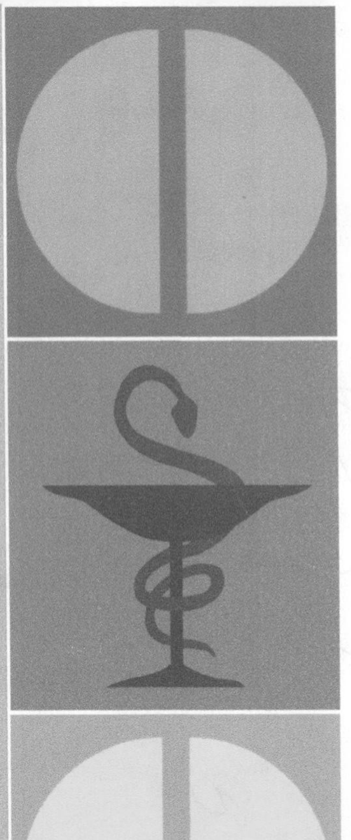

Chapter **33**

# Cancer Chemotherapy

## KEY TERMS

- actinic keratosis
- apoptosis
- benign
- cell cycle specific
- contact inhibition
- cytotoxic
- extravasate
- immunosuppression
- lymphoma
- malignant
- metastases
- metastasize
- monoclonal antibody
- mutagenic
- nucleotides
- oncology
- palliative therapy
- phagocytosis
- tumor lysis syndrome

## OBJECTIVES

After studying this chapter, the reader should be able to:

- Describe two differences between normal and cancerous cells, explain how these changes promote development of cancer, and list two of the most common forms of cancer in adults.
- Describe three measures that are used to either protect patients or health practitioners from improper use of, or exposure to, cytotoxic drugs.
- Identify one drug from each of the following chemotherapeutic drug classes, describe a problem encountered when dispensing the drug, and how technicians could prevent problems associated with the drug or class: antimetabolites, cytotoxic antibiotics, alkylating agents, and microtubule inhibitors.
- Explain the idea behind the use of biological response modifiers in cancer therapy, name one drug currently in use, and describe, in general terms, its mechanism of action.
- Define the following terms: oncology, malignant, metastasize, cytotoxic, carcinogenic, intrathecal, palliative therapy.

## DRUGS COVERED IN THIS CHAPTER

### Cytotoxic Drugs

**Antimetabolites**

5-Fluoruracil
Gemcitabine
5-Mercaptopurine
Methotrexate
6-Thioguanine

**Antibiotics**

Bleomycin
Daunorubicin
Doxorubicin (Adriamycin)
Mitomycin

**Alkylating Agents**

Carmustine
Cyclophosphamide
Dacarbazine
Melphalan

**Microtubule Inhibitors**

Paclitaxel
Vinblastine
Vincristine

**Other Cytotoxic Drugs**

Asparaginase
Cisplatin
Carboplatin
Etoposide

### Biologic Response Modifiers

Interferons
Bevacizumab
Cetuximab
Gemtuzumab
Rituximab
Trastuzumab

### Endocrine Therapies

Anastrozole
Leuprolide
Megestrol Acetate
Prednisone
Tamoxifen

It is estimated that one in three Americans will be diagnosed with some form of cancer in their lifetimes. Cancer is actually a group of different diseases, with differing prospects for recovery, and different treatments. Although there is no single known cause of these diseases, there are many well-known environmental, occupational, and lifestyle risk factors associated with developing cancer. These include exposure to radiation (leukemia, breast, thyroid, lung cancers), ultraviolet rays from the sun (skin cancer), some viral infections (leukemia, lymphoma, and cervical cancer), asbestos exposure (lung cancer), tobacco use (oropharynx and lung cancers), and dietary factors, including high-fat and low-fiber diets (colon, breast cancers). Other risk factors for nearly all cancers (except most pediatric cancers) include hereditary risks and advancing age. The most common forms of cancer in adults are skin, breast, lung, colorectal, uterine, including cervical, and prostate cancers, and in children, leukemia.

Drug treatment for cancer is almost always administered in hospitals or hospital-managed outpatient clinics. Hospital pharmacies have established procedures for storing, compounding, and disposing of chemotherapeutic agents to protect both the patient from errors, and pharmacy staff members from unnecessary exposure. USP 797, regulations developed by the United States Pharmacopeia, include specific clean air requirements, physical layout, protective garb, and compounding practices, and equipment for pharmacy clean rooms, to assure the lowest possible risk of IV contamination. This is especially important in patients who receive chemotherapy, because they are much less able to fight infection.

Managing cancer chemotherapy requires highly specialized and current knowledge because the drugs used in treatment are very dangerous, and new treatments are continuously being introduced. In many facilities, pharmacists and technicians become experts in oncology pharmacy (treatment of cancer). Once trained, these specialists are used as dedicated staff members, assigned only to oncology units. In some cases, when very high-risk drugs

oncology The study of cancers or tumors.

are used, pharmacists will compound and deliver the drug directly to the physician for administration to the patient. Regulating bodies recommend, and hospital polices increasingly require that physicians, pharmacists, and nurses take time for what is referred to as a "time out" to concentrate while verifying the medication before administering it. Other measures used to ensure patient safety are mentioned throughout this chapter.

Because this area of pharmacy practice is so specialized, and the number of drugs and regimens for their use so extensive, this chapter will briefly cover the most commonly encountered chemotherapeutic agents used for the most common forms of cancer only. The main focus of the chapter will be on potential pitfalls in handling these very dangerous, and sometimes very expensive medications.

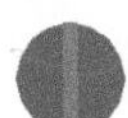

## Cancer Basics

The body is made up of many different kinds of cells or tissues. Normally, these cells grow, reproduce, and die at a rate that is specific for each cell type. Blood cells, for example, are constantly being produced and have a short lifespan within the body, whereas nervous system tissue is very long-lived, and is rarely replaced. Reproduction rate is controlled by factors within and outside of the cell. For example, the presence of other cells surrounding a cell inhibits its growth of normals cells (contact inhibition) and helps to prevent cells from reproducing at will. For most tissues types, self-destruction is programmed within the nucleus. If the nucleus receives signals that indicate that the cell is aging, or in ill health (for example, the presence of a virus in the cell), the nucleus will cause the cell to die. The process of programmed cell death is called apoptosis.

contact inhibition Inhibition of growth and replication of a cell or cells due to physical contact with other cells.

apoptosis Normal, programmed cell death, initiated by signals from the cell nuclei, when cell age or health dictates.

malignant Tumors likely to invade nearby tissues and metastasize.

benign In relationship to tumors, not cancerous, does not metastasize.

metastasize To spread to another part of the body through the blood or lymphatic system.

lymphoma A malignant tumor of lymphoid tissue.

Some initial event must cause a change in a normal cell's DNA in order for it to multiply outside of normal parameters. When a cell becomes altered, or mutates, it loses the ability to respond to contact inhibition, and even the normal apoptosis-driven cell death. If these altered cells are not recognized and destroyed by the body's immune system, uncontrolled replication can occur and cause a tumor. Tumors may either be malignant (cancerous) or benign (not cancerous). The seriousness of a cancerous lesion is characterized by the degree of difference from normal cells and the propensity to invade other layers or types of tissues, or metastasize (break off and move via the blood stream to other parts of the body).

Cancerous tissue does not function normally and cannot carry on the normal processes of the particular cell type. When solid tumors are formed, such as in lung or colon cancer, they put pressure on adjacent cells and disrupt the ability of normal tissue to function, adding stress to an already weakened organ system. Diffuse tumors, such as leukemias or lymphomas (a malignancy of the precursors of the white blood cells called lymphoblasts), undermine the production of normal white and red blood cells by using up the resources of the bone marrow for the production of abnormal cells. This results in anemia and a compromised immune system. Patients with compromised immunity are at risk for life-threatening infections.

Cancerous tumors cause the proliferation of blood vessels in their vicinity in order to direct the delivery of nutrients to the rapidly reproducing malignant cells. The growth of new vessels provides the tumor with oxygen and nutrients, and consequently deprives the rest of the body of needed nutrients. In addition, the chaotic network of blood vessels around the malignancy can carry cancerous cells to other parts of the body. When tumors metastasize to other areas, such as the lungs, liver, or brain, they disrupt normal tissue function there as well. At the same time that proliferating tumor cells are diverting needed nutrients, cancer patients may have a poor appetite and altered sense of taste due to drug therapy.

Of all the diseases that afflict the human race, the diagnosis of cancer is probably the most dreaded. Cancer patients can suffer from pain, malfunctioning organ systems, cancer-related symptoms, and weakness and malnutrition. When the disease is untreatable, and the cancer is rapidly growing, patients experience a rapid decline in health; they become weak and quickly succumb to the disease. People with treatable disease may have to undergo treatments that seem worse than the disease itself. However, the effective treatment of cancer is advancing, and as it does, life expectancy after diagnosis is lengthened. Early detection is much more likely now than even 20 years ago, and cures are far more common with early detection.

## Goals of Cancer Treatment

There are generally four goals of cancer therapy. The first goal is to completely remove the tumor and achieve a cure. This is more likely to be possible with some forms of cancers than others, and with early stages of cancer rather than late stages. Treatment options include surgical removal of solid tumors, radiation therapy, chemotherapy, and targeted therapy with biological response modifiers and other specific treatments. The second goal is to prevent a recurrence, or growth of a new tumor of the same type in the same or a different place. Patients may change their lifestyle (quit smoking, eat healthier foods), or use hormones or hormone suppressants, when indicated, to help prevent cancer recurrences. Even if the cancer is not completely removed or does grow back, the third goal, to prolong life, may be achievable. Whether any of the above goals can be realized, the last goal, to make the patient's life better through pain relief, treatments that reduce unwanted effects of the tumor, or therapies that ameliorate side effects of treatment, is always attainable (**Table 33.1**).

Cancer-related symptom relief does nothing to alter the growth of the cancer, but is simply designed to improve the quality of the cancer patient's life. This is called palliative therapy, and can be used alongside treatments directed at the tumor. Pharmacists and technicians in retail settings may play an important role in supporting palliative care by cooperating with pain-management programs, providing nutrition supplements and other products, such as skin or wound care treatments, for outpatients.

palliative therapy
Procedures or drug therapy used to improve patient comfort, not to cure disease.

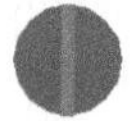

# Chemotherapy

Cancer chemotherapy strives to deliver a lethal blow to cancer cells in order to arrest a tumor's progression. The attack is mainly directed against metabolic processes essential to cell replication. Ideally, the anticancer drugs would affect only malignant cells. Unfortunately, most currently available anticancer drugs do not specifically recognize neoplastic cells, but rather, affect all reproducing cells, whether normal or cancerous. Therefore, almost all antitumor agents have a narrow therapeutic index. More often than not, adverse effects are related to damage to rapidly replicating cells, such as the epithelial

**Table 33.1** Goals and Treatment Options for Patients with Cancer

| Goal | Treatment Options | Limitations |
|---|---|---|
| Tumor removal and cure | Surgery, radiation, chemotherapy, targeted therapies | Late stages, and some forms of cancer are not amenable to cure |
| Prevent recurrence | Lifestyle changes, hormones, or hormone suppressants | As yet undiscovered metastases may already be present at diagnosis |
| Prolong life | Surgery, radiation, chemotherapy, targeted therapies may reduce tumor size, hormones and hormone suppressants may slow growth | Advanced stage of tumor at diagnosis, poor health of the patient at diagnosis |
| Improve quality of life (palliative care) | Analgesics, nutritional supplements, antiemetics, drugs for specific tumor-related symptoms | Side effects of drugs |

cells that line the gastrointestinal tract, the bone marrow that produces our blood cells, and hair follicles. As a result, the classic side effects of vomiting, sores in the mouth, hair loss, and bone marrow suppression occur to a greater or lesser degree with nearly all of the antineoplastic agents.

metastases Cancer cells from a primary tumor that moved via metastasis to a secondary site.

Chemotherapy is used as a supplemental treatment of the primary tumor after surgery or radiation, and to attack undetectable metastases, clusters of cancer cells that have broken off from the main tumor and have begun to replicate elsewhere in the body. It is used alone when tumors are disseminated and are not amenable to surgery or other treatments. Chemotherapy protocols combine agents with different mechanisms of action to provide the best results. **Table 33.2** displays some well-known chemotherapy protocols for breast cancer.

When drugs with a narrow therapeutic index are used, mistakes in the drug regimen are dangerous or even life threatening to the patient. Certain measures have become a routine part of cancer management as a way of protecting patients from errors. Cancers are treated according to well-defined drug protocols. By using protocols, treatment is standardized and health professionals become very familiar with recommended doses, routes of administration, and procedures for use. Although the use of protocols helps, it is important to understand that protocols are constantly changing and improving. In order for pharmacy staff members to stay current, they must keep up with changes through continuing education.

Chemotherapy experts continually try to devise methods that will limit the toxicity or maximize the effects of these drugs. Use of combination chemotherapy drug protocols is one example of these strategies. Using unique methods of drug administration is another example. In some cases, chemotherapy will be delivered to the site of the tumor through a vein that directly feeds the tumor. For ovarian cancer, chemotherapeutic agents are delivered directly into the abdomen through an intraperitoneal catheter.

Another method employed to ensure safe drug administration is the use of a uniform system for calculating doses. Doses of chemotherapeutic agents are not calculated based on body weight, but rather on body surface area. Body surface area is determined from the height and weight of the patient, using a mathematical formula. Dosage calculations that

**Table 33.2** A Sample of the Possible Chemotherapy Protocols Used in Some Patients With Breast Cancer

| Without Trastuzumab | With Trastuzumab |
|---|---|
| FAC CHEMOTHERAPY<br>5-Fluorouracil 500 mg/m IV days 1 & 8 or days 1 & 4<br>Doxorubicin 50 mg/m IV day 1 (or by 72 h continuous infusion)<br>Cyclophosphamide 500 mg/m IV day 1<br>Cycled every 21 days for 6 cycles. | AC FOLLOWED BY PACLITAXEL CHEMOTHERAPY WITH TRASTUZUMAB<br>Doxorubicin 60 mg/m IV day 1<br>Cyclophosphamide 600 mg/m IV day 1<br>Cycled every 21 days for 4 cycles.<br>Followed by:<br>Paclitaxel 80 mg/m by 1 h IV weekly for 12 weeks with Trastuzumab 4 mg/kg IV with first dose of paclitaxel<br><br>Followed by:<br>Trastuzumab 2 mg/kg IV weekly to complete 1 year of treatment. |
| AC CHEMOTHERAPY<br>Doxorubicin 60 mg/m IV day 1<br>Cyclophosphamide 600 mg/m IV day 1<br>Cycled every 21 days for 4 cycles. | |
| AC FOLLOWED BY PACLITAXEL CHEMOTHERAPY<br>Doxorubicin 60 mg/m IV day 1<br>Cyclophosphamide 600 mg/m IV day 1<br>Cycled every 21 days for 4 cycles.<br>Followed by:<br>Paclitaxel 175-225 mg/m by 3 h IV infusion day 1<br>Cycled every 21 days for 4 cycles. | |

Adapted from NCCN.org breast cancer protocols.

use body surface area are more accurate than those calculated based on weight alone, because they take the patient's build and proportions into consideration. When both height and weight are considered, variables such as frame size and muscle mass are minimized. All of the safety measures discussed in this chapter help pharmacy personnel to attain the ultimate goal in caring for cancer patients: to deliver the appropriate drug to the patient in the safest way possible.

## Antimetabolites

Both normal cells and tumor cells go through growth cycles. The growth cycle is made up of stages where the cell is involved in specific metabolic tasks (**Fig. 33.1**). In a slowly growing tumor, more cells will be resting than growing. In a rapidly growing tumor, many or most cells are in some stage of active growth. Some chemotherapeutic agents are effective only against replicating cells, or in other words, cells that are in the growth phases of the cell cycle. These are said to be cell-cycle specific. The antimetabolites are all cell-cycle specific drugs.

cell cycle specific Refers to chemotherapeutic agents that are only effective when the cancerous cells are replicating (within the cell replication cycle).

### Actions and Indications

The antimetabolites are similar to compounds found in cells that are used for cell growth and reproduction. Most of these drugs work by interfering with the production of precursor components, called nucleotides, used by the cell to make new DNA or RNA. The antimetabolites either inhibit the synthesis of precursors, or in some cases, because of their

nucleotides Basic building blocks of nucleic acids, made up of amino acids (cytosine, thymine, uracil, adenine, or guanine) joined with a sugar.

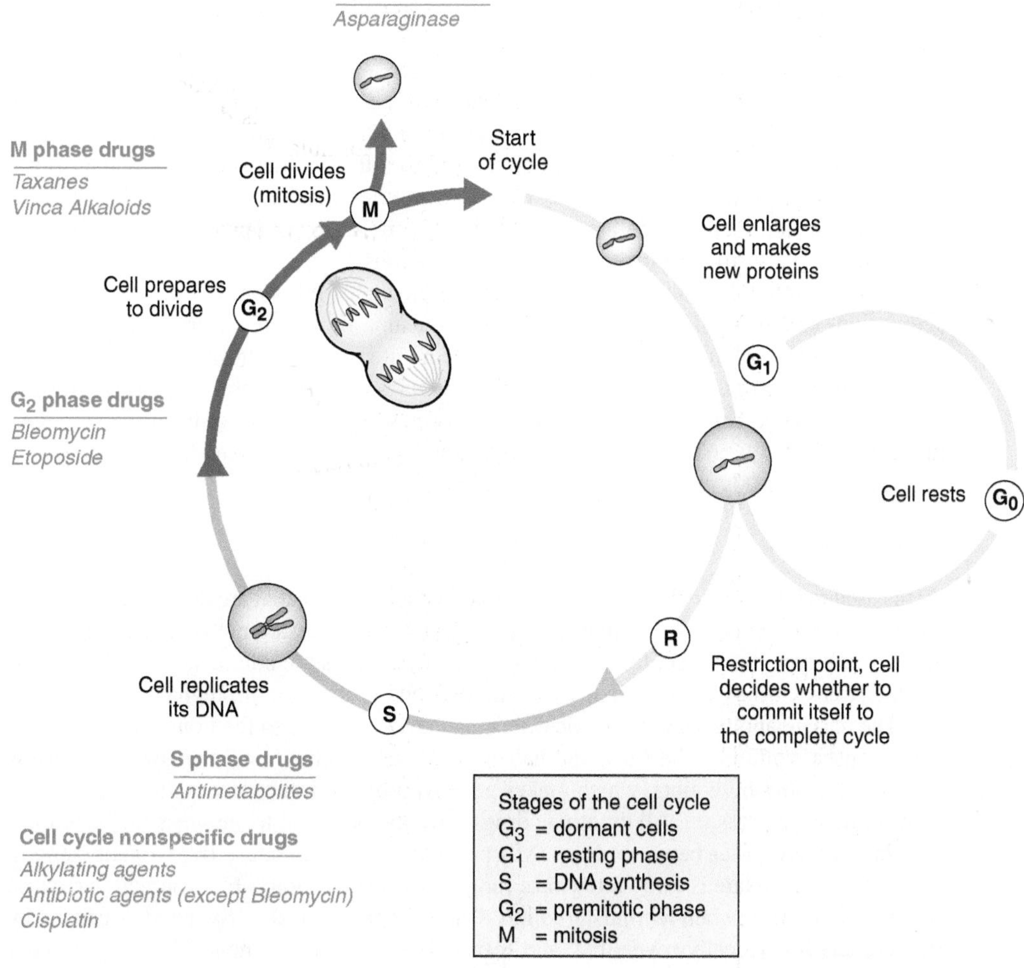


**Figure 33.1** The stages of the cell-cycle and the cell-cycle specific chemotherapeutic agents that work in each stage.

chemical similarity, they are substituted into the precursors, resulting in the production of nonfunctional DNA or RNA. As a result of this interference, cells go on to die instead of replicating. Methotrexate (Trexall®) is unique among the antimetabolites in that it antagonizes the vitamin folic acid. Folates are required for a number of metabolic processes in cells, including DNA synthesis.

The antimetabolites likely to be encountered by pharmacy technicians include methotrexate, fluorouracil (Adrucil®), thioguanine (Tabloid®), gemcitabine (Gemzar®), and mercaptopurine (Purinethol®). Methotrexate and fluorouracil are part of one breast cancer protocol that was widely used in the past and is still seen. Fluorouracil is combined with leucovorin for colorectal cancer, and methotrexate or thioguanine is combined with other drugs for different stages of treatment for certain lymphomas. Fluorouracil can be used to treat skin cancers or precancerous skin lesions. Methotrexate and mercaptopurine are used in different stages of therapy, along with agents from other classes, for acute lymphocytic leukemia, the leukemia most often encountered in childhood. Gemcitabine is used with other drugs for the treatment of some types of lung cancer. **Table 33.3** displays the most important medications for the antimetabolites and other drugs used in cancer chemotherapy.

## Administration

Cancer drug regimens are given cyclically in order to take maximum advantage of tumor growth patterns and to allow healthy tissues to recover. For example, in the cyclophosphamide, methotrexate, and fluorouracil (CMF) regimen for breast cancer, cyclophosphamide is given by mouth on days 1 through 14, and the methotrexate and fluorouracil are given by injection on days 1 and 8. The entire cycle is repeated every 28 days. Although the drugs, the routes of administration, and the cycles may change, this same principle is used in all drug protocols.

Methotrexate is available in products that can be administered by mouth or by injection, however it is generally given by intravenous infusion for cancer chemotherapy. Some cancer chemotherapy protocols for leukemias require intrathecal injection (injected into the cerebrospinal fluid, or CSF). This method is used to kill cells that sequester in the central nervous system of leukemia patients, where chemotherapeutic agents cannot penetrate. Oral methotrexate preparations are more likely to be prescribed to patients taking the drug for rheumatoid arthritis or other autoimmune conditions.

actinic keratosis A disease of the skin marked by overgrowth of keratin and caused by excessive sun exposure.

In most protocols, fluorouracil is given by intravenous infusion. For the precancerous skin lesions called actinic keratosis, and for certain superficial skin cancers, fluorouracil is applied topically. Mercaptopurine and thioguanine are available from the manufacturers only as tablets for oral use. However, some pharmacies compound oral suspensions for use in the very young. Thioguanine is available as an investigational drug, from the manufacturer, in a powder to be reconstituted for injection. Like other cytotoxic drugs, gemcitabine is given intravenously, as part of a cyclic regimen.

## Side Effects

cytotoxic Toxic to cells; often used in reference to drugs or chemicals.

Drugs used to kill tumor cells are dangerous to other cells. Drugs that are designed to kill cells are called cytotoxic agents, meaning cell toxic. Cytotoxic drugs are not cancer-cell specific, and any cell type that is rapidly replicating when these drugs are administered will be damaged. Cytotoxic drugs are also toxic to sperm, ova, and in the case of pregnancy, the fetus.

immunosuppression Suppression of normal immune response to infectious agents or other antigens, often a result of medication use.

The antimetabolites are cytotoxic drugs, and cause damage to the bone marrow, stomatitis, nausea, vomiting, diarrhea, and hair loss. Damage to the bone marrow often results in reduced neutrophil counts, which makes patients prone to infections, a situation referred to as immunosuppression. All cytotoxic drugs have the potential to suppress the bone marrow, but the risk varies between drugs. Most of these drugs can cause liver toxicity, and in addition, methotrexate is known to cause lung and kidney toxicity. Fluorouracil can cause skin reactions, both when administered intravenously and topically. Skin rashes caused by fluorouracil are typically reversible, and responsive to local treatment. Skin is especially sensitive to sun during topical treatment with fluorouracil.

When methotrexate is administered into the CSF, it can cause seizures or other neurotoxicity, especially if excessive doses are injected in error. Bone cancer (osteosarcoma) and

**Table 33.3** Generic and Brand names, Formulations, and Indications of the Most Commonly Used Chemotherapeutic Agents

| Generic | Brand Name | Available as | Indications | Notes |
|---|---|---|---|---|
| **Antimetabolites** | | | | |
| Fluorouracil | Adrucil®, Efudex® | Injection, topical cream and solution | CA of colon & others, CA & precancerous lesions of skin | Avoid excessive sun exposure |
| Gemcitabine | Gemzar® | Powder for injection | Lung and breast CA | Take before meals |
| Mercaptopurine | Purinethol® | Tablets | Acute lymphocytic leukemia | |
| Methotrexate | Trexall® | Powder & solution for injection, tablets | Breast, lung & other CA, hematologic CA, arthritis | Caution: high-risk medication. Verify dosage & route |
| Thioguanine | | Tablet | Lymphoblastic & myelogenous leukemias | |
| **Antibiotics** | | | | |
| Bleomycin | Blenoxane® | Injection | Testicular CA, lymphoma | |
| Daunorubicin | Cerubidine® | Injection | Acute lymphocytic & non-lymphocytic leukemias | Look-alike, sound-alike: doxorubicin |
| Doxorubicin | Adriamycin®, Rubex® | Injection | Breast, gastric, pancreatic, bladder CA, lymphomas, multiple myeloma | Look-alike, sound-alike: daunorubicin |
| Mitomycin | Mutamycin® | Powder for injection | Gastric cancer | |
| **Alkylating Agents** | | | | |
| Carmustine | BiCNU®, Gliadel® | Powder for injection, implant | Lymphoma, brain tumors, multiple myeloma | |
| Cyclophosphamide | Cytoxan® | Tablets, powder for injection | Lymphomas, leukemias, breast, testicular, lung, other CA | Look-alike, sound-alike: cyclosporine |
| Dacarbazine | DTIC® | Powder for Injection | Hodgkin's lymphoma, malignant melanoma | Refrigerate, protect from light |
| Melphalan | Alkeran® | Powder for injection, tablet | Multiple myeloma, some ovarian & breast CA | Look-alike, sound-alike: Myleran® |
| **Microtubule Inhibitors** | | | | |
| Paclitaxel | Taxol® | Injection | Breast, lung, ovarian CA | Look-alike, sound-alike: Paxil®, Taxotere® |
| Vinblastine | | Powder, solution for injections | Lymphomas, testicular, lung, head & neck, breast CA & others | Look-alike, sound-alike: vincristine<br>Refrigerate. Do not give IT |
| Vincristine | Vincasar PFS® | Injection | Leukemias, lymphomas, others | Look-alike, sound-alike: vinblastine<br>Refrigerate. Do not give IT |

*(continues)*

**Table 33.3** Generic and Brand names, Formulations, and Indications of the Most Commonly Used Chemotherapeutic Agents *(continued)*

| Generic | Brand Name | Available as | Indications | Notes |
|---|---|---|---|---|
| **Other Cytotoxic Agents** | | | | |
| Asparaginase | Elspar® | Powder for injection | Acute lymphocytic, leukemia, lymphoma | Refrigerate, may filter with 5 micron filter |
| Carboplatin | Paraplatin® | Powder & solution for injection | Ovarian CA | Look-alike, sound-alike: Platinol®, cisplatin. Avoid Al needles |
| Cisplatin | Platinol® | Solution for injection | Ovarian, testicular, breast CA, lymphomas, head & neck CA | Look-alike, sound-alike: Paraplatin®, carboplatin |
| Etoposide | Toposar®, VePesid® | Capsules, solution for injection | Lymphomas, some leukemias lung, testicular, prostate CA | |
| **Biological Response Modifiers** | | | | |
| Interferon alpha 2A | Roferon-A® | Solutions for injection | Some leukemias, Kaposi sarcoma | Look-alike, sound-alike: interferon alpha 2B. Refrigerate, do not shake |
| Interferon alpha 2B | Intron® | Powder & solution for injection | Some leukemias, lymphomas, Kaposi sarcoma | Look-alike, sound-alike: interferon alpha 2B. Refrigerate |
| Bevacizumab | Avastin® | Injection | Colorectal carcinoma, others | Refrigerate |
| Rituximab | Rituxan® | Injection | Non-Hodgkin's lymphoma | Refrigerate |
| Trastuzumab | Herceptin® | Powder for injection | Some breast CA | Refrigerate |
| **Endocrine Treatments** | | | | |
| Anastrozole | Arimidex® | Tablets | Some breast CA | |
| Leuprolide | Lupron®, Eligard® | Injection, depot injection, implant | Prostate CA, advanced | Injection – cool room temp or refrigerate. Implant – room temp. |
| Tamoxifen | Nolvadex® | Tablets | Breast CA, palliative and prevention | Look-alike, sound-alike: raloxifene |

AL, aluminum; CA, cancer; IT, intrathecal.

lymphoma can be intentionally treated with highly toxic doses of methotrexate. When methotrexate is administered systemically in high doses, either intentionally or unintentionally, folinic acid, also known as leucovorin, is administered to counteract toxicity. This is referred to as leucovorin "rescue." Leucovorin does not reverse neurotoxicity caused by intrathecal methotrexate.

The antimetabolites are involved in a few important drug interactions. Mercaptopurine should not be used with allopurinol because of increased risk of toxicity from the mercaptopurine. Hepatotoxic compounds (alcohol, acetaminophen) will increase the risk of liver toxicity when used with the antimetabolites. While folinic or folic acid antagonizes the effects of methotrexate, it increases the effects of systemically administered fluorouracil. Fluorouracil and leucovorin used together in the treatment of colorectal cancer takes advantage of this interaction.

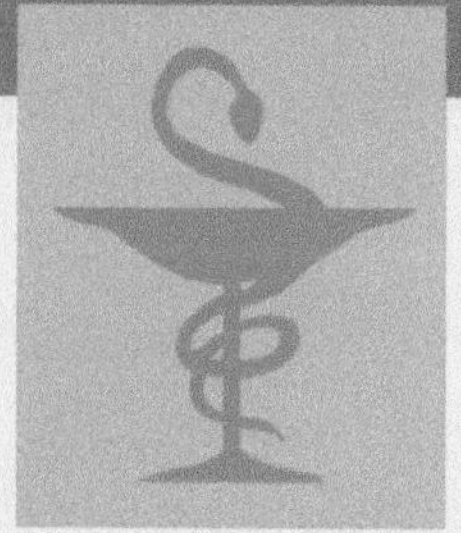

## Tips for the Technician

The English poet Alexander Pope wrote "to err is human, to forgive divine," meaning it is only human to make mistakes, and godly to forgive them. Chemotherapy is one area where mistakes are not easily forgiven, either by the recipient, their family, or the health care team. This is because most chemotherapy errors are devastating to the patient. Sterile compounding of cancer chemotherapy drugs is a job generally reserved for people who are highly trained and experienced. Individuals who are exceptionally meticulous, focused, and never make avoidable mistakes are well suited to this role. Handling chemotherapeutic agents requires familiarity with the drugs and protocols, applicable policies and procedures, and the use of biological safety cabinets or barrier isolator hoods, and other personal protective equipment (refer to **Fig. 33.2**).

Specifically, technicians who handle antimetabolites should follow all recommended precautions because frequent or prolonged exposure to these drugs is associated with long-term toxicities. With prolonged exposure these drugs are mutagenic (cause an increased rate of mutations to cells), carcinogenic, and teratogenic, causing an increased risk of malformations in a fetus.

mutagenic Inducing genetic mutations.

The doses of drugs that are injected into the CSF are very different than those used systemically. In addition, only preservative-free drugs can be administered intrathecally. When reconstitution is necessary, only diluents without preservatives can be used. Obviously, this increases the risk of bacterial contamination in patients who are already immunosuppressed, and therefore requires compounding personnel to use excellent sterile technique.

Technicians who handle oral formulations of antimetabolites should not use automated packaging or counting equipment for these drugs. Clean all surfaces, such as counting trays, used in the dispensing of these medications. Patients who take these medications by mouth must be warned to avoid alcohol consumption. Place the appropriate "avoid alcohol" auxiliary label on prescription vials. Men and women on methotrexate therapy should be warned not to plan a pregnancy while taking this drug. Technicians can help by applying the appropriate warning label. The pharmacist should instruct patients to use contraceptives for at least 3 months after discontinuing methotrexate. Topical fluorouracil requires a "for external use only" label. Methotrexate and fluorouracil (especially topical) can cause photosensitivity, and require a warning to patients to avoid sun exposure.

# Cytotoxic Antibiotics

Bleomycin (Blenoxane®), dactinomycin (Cosmegen®), daunorubicin (Cerubidine®), doxorubicin (Adriamycin®), and mitomycin (Mutamycin®) are antibiotic substances, derived from living organisms, with cytotoxic properties. With the exception of bleomycin, these drugs are cell cycle nonspecific. Dactinomycin was the first to be used for treatment of cancer, but is not a drug used for commonly occurring tumors today.

## Actions and Indications

The cytotoxic antibiotics work by interacting with DNA and disrupting its functions. They may accomplish this by causing breaks in the strands, by causing the DNA to unwind, by converting oxygen to hydrogen peroxide, a compound that is toxic to tumors, or through other actions.

Doxorubicin, which is often referred to by the brand name of Adriamycin® to avoid name confusion with daunorubicin, is one of the most widely used chemotherapeutic drugs. Despite their structural similarity and their apparently similar mechanisms of action, indi-

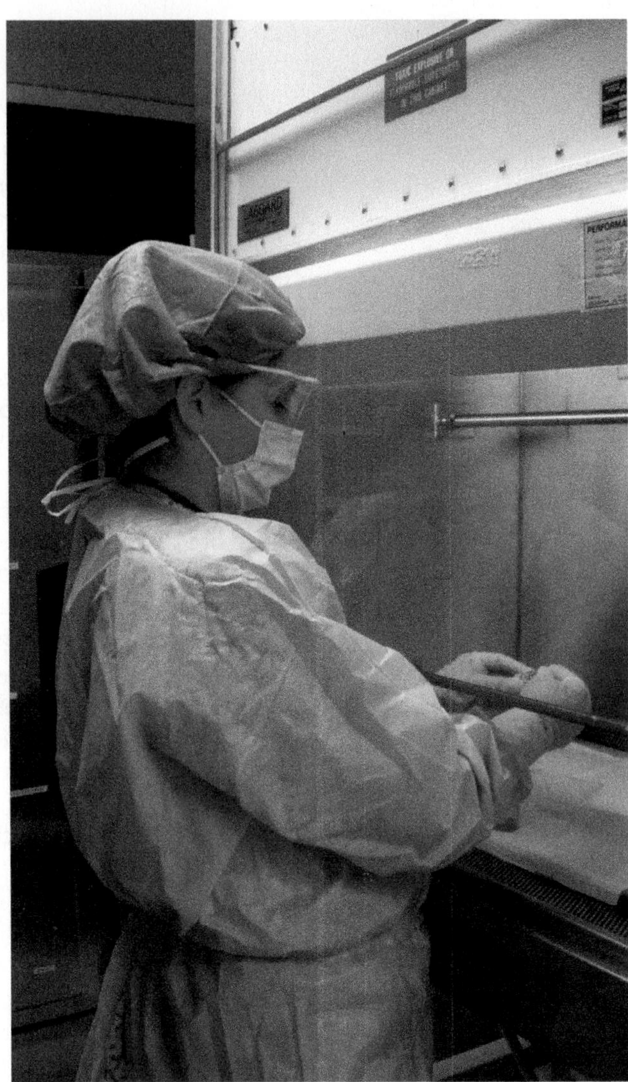

**Figure 33.2** Appropriate use of a biological safety cabinet and personal protective equipment is designed to protect pharmacists and technicians from exposure to cytotoxic agents.

cations for use of daunorubicin and doxorubicin are different. Doxorubicin is used in some breast cancer protocols, for bladder cancer, some lung cancers, and lymphomas. Daunorubicin is used in some cancers of the blood or lymphatic tissues such as leukemias or lymphomas. Bleomycin is indicated for testicular cancer and mitomycin is used for some less common tumors.

## Administration

extravasate To pass by infiltration from a blood vessel into surrounding tissue.

The antibiotic chemotherapeutic agents are administered as part of chemotherapy protocols that include use of other drugs. Daunorubicin and doxorubicin are given by intravenous infusion, or after appropriate dilution, by IV push. The health care providers who administer these drugs must monitor the infusion sites carefully. If extravasation (leakage from the vein into surrounding tissue) occurs, these drugs can cause serious tissue damage. Because bleomycin is much less irritating, it can be given IM or subcutaneously, as well as by intravenous injection.

## Side Effects

Like all cytotoxic agents, these drugs cause nausea, vomiting, stomatitis, and bone marrow suppression. Daunorubicin and doxorubicin are considered to be moderately to highly emetogenic (**Fig. 33.3**). These drugs cause very serious, drug-specific toxicity, in some cases. Doxorubicin and daunorubicin cause irreversible toxicity to the heart. This toxicity affects the myocardium and causes heart failure. It is directly related to the total dose of the drug

| High | High to Moderate | Moderate to Low | Low |
|---|---|---|---|
| Carmustine* | Carboplatin | Etoposide | Bleomycin |
| Cisplatin* | Cyclophosphamide PO | Fluorouracil | 6-Thioguanine |
| Cyclophosphamide* | Daunorubicin | Mitomycin | Vinblastine |
| Dacarbazine | Doxorubicin | Paclitaxel | Vincristine |
| * Lower doses result in moderation of emetogenicity | Methotrexate* | | |

**Figure 33.3** Emetogenic potential of some common chemotherapeutic agents. (Source: Koda-Kimble MA, et al. *Handbook of Applied Therapeutics*, 8th edition. Lippincott Williams & Wilkins, 2007)

the patient receives over time, and can be avoided by using lower doses, especially in people who already have cardiac disease. Bleomycin and mitomycin are associated with dose-related pulmonary toxicity, which usually resolves if the causative drug is discontinued soon enough. Pulmonary toxicity can, however, be progressive and fatal.

## Tips for the Technician

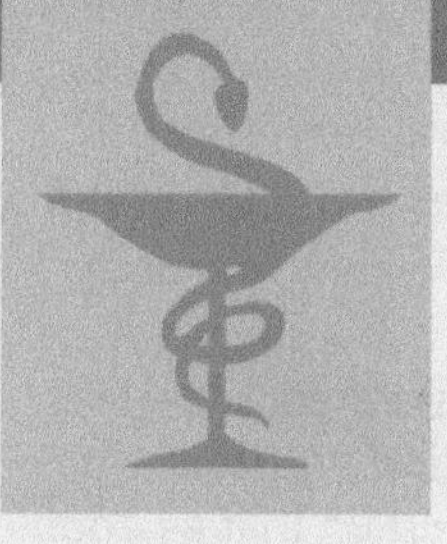

Doxorubicin and daunorubicin look alike after dilution (both solutions are red) and have sound-alike names. Hospital based technicians will need to assure compliance with the institution's safety procedures in order to avoid confusion between the two drugs. Hospital policies may require shelving the two drugs by brand names so they are not adjacent to one another, special checking procedures, or physician ordering by brand name. As with all cytotoxic drugs, these agents must be prepared by trained personnel, using a biological safety cabinet or barrier isolator hood, and personal protective equipment.

# Alkylating Agents

Alkylating agents are derivatives of nitrogen mustard (mustard gas) that was used as a chemical weapon in World War I. Drugs in this family include the original nitrogen mustard, mechlorethamine, and several related compounds. Cyclophosphamide (Cytoxan®) is a versatile drug used in a wide range of tumor types. Other drugs in this class include chlorambucil (Leukeran®), dacarbazine (DTIC-Dome®), and melphalan (Alkeran®). The alkylating agents are cell cycle nonspecific.

## Actions and Indications

The alkylating agents work through similar mechanisms of action. They bind to DNA, an action that prevents normal functions such as synthesis of RNA and proteins. Although these drugs are considered cell-cycle nonspecific, they work best in tumors that are rapidly growing.

The alkylating agents are used in combination with other agents to treat a variety of lymphatic and solid tumors. Cyclophosphamide, the most widely used, is a part of protocols for breast and ovarian cancers, and for a variety of lymphomas. Carmustine is one of the few agents that enter the central nervous system, making it suitable to treat some brain tumors. Dacarbazine and mechlorethamine are used for the treatment of Hodgkin's lymphoma.

## Administration

Although many of the alkylating agents are available in oral dosage forms, it is common for chemotherapy protocols to call for intravenous administration. Cyclophosphamide and melphalan are both available in tablets and injection. Melphalan injection, a highly unstable drug, must be reconstituted with the diluent provided by the manufacturer and infused right away. It begins to degrade significantly almost immediately, and the entire dose should be administered within an hour of reconstitution. Dacarbazine, carmustine, and mechlorethamine are administered intravenously. Chlorambucil, which is more often used in autoimmune conditions, is only available as tablets.

### Side Effects

The alkylating agents are some of the chemotherapeutic agents most likely to cause vomiting, and are considered highly emetogenic. They are well known for bone marrow suppression, an effect that in many situations delays therapy. Cyclophosphamide can cause bladder hemorrhage, which has the potential to result in permanent damage to the bladder. Cyclophosphamide, carmustine, and melphalan are associated with pulmonary fibrosis, a very serious form of lung damage. These drugs can impair fertility and are carcinogenic.

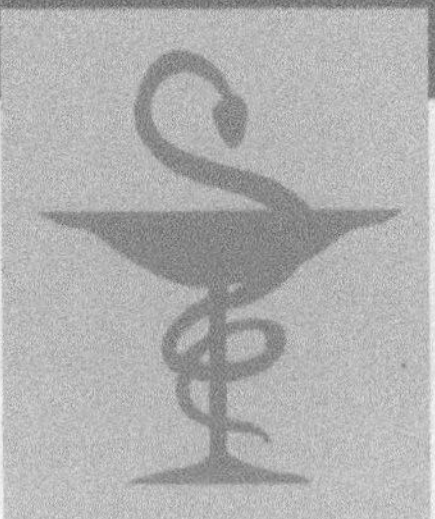

### Tips for the Technician

As is the case with all cytotoxic drugs, technicians and all persons who handle these medications should follow procedures to protect themselves from exposure. There is evidence collected from the years before personal protection was routine that indicates that personnel who handled chemotherapeutic agents without using protective equipment developed fertility impairment, among other long-term effects.

A number of these drugs are particularly unstable and require attention to the instructions for reconstitution and dilution before beginning the compounding process. The importance of double checks of the drug name, double checks of dosage calculations, and route of administration cannot be overstated. Especially when handling chemotherapeutic agents, these checks are critical for patient safety. To prevent wasting these unstable medications, make certain that all double checks of the dosage and compounding instructions are carried out before beginning the reconstitution process.

When melphalan and chlorambucil are dispensed in oral form, the pharmacist should be sure to consult with the patient about potential side effects. Because of the potential for bone marrow suppression, patients taking these medications are advised to stay away from people who are sick and report any unusual bruising or bleeding to the doctor. Patients need to continue to take these drugs in spite of nausea and vomiting and it is appropriate to place an auxiliary label instructing them to "continue this medications unless otherwise directed by your physician."

## Microtubule Inhibitors

The mitotic spindle, a cellular structure made of minute tubes called microtubules, is essential for the equal division of DNA between the two daughter cells that are formed when a cell divides. In mitosis, or cell division, the mitotic spindle segregates the chromosomes. Both the vinca alkaloids and the taxanes prevent the normal functioning of the mitotic spindle. The drugs in this class are cell-cycle specific, and act in the last phase of the cell cycle.

### Actions and Indications

The microtubule inhibitors, which include the vinca alkaloids, and paclitaxel and docetaxel, are plant derivatives. The vinca alkaloids, vincristine (Vincasar®), vinblastine, and vinorelbine (Navelbine®) are derived from the Madagascar periwinkle plant. Folk healers thought these plants were beneficial for the treatment of diabetes. During studies designed to verify this belief, scientists discovered that although of no use for diabetes they did suppress the growth of tumors. The vinca alkaloids act to prevent the formation of microtubules from the precursor substance, tubulin. A normal mitotic spindle cannot be formed without microtubules, and as a result cancer cells are prevented from dividing, and they eventually die. Although the vinca alkaloids are structurally very similar to each other, their therapeutic indications are different. Vincristine is used in the treatment of some forms of acute leukemia in children, some lymphomas, and a few other tumors. Vinblastine is used in Hodgkin's lymphoma and a few other cancers.

The taxanes, including the widely used paclitaxel (Taxol®), are derived from the Pacific yew tree. Paclitaxel, the original taxane derivative, was first discovered through the efforts of a joint National Cancer Institute and US Department of Agriculture program to find natural compounds with potential for treating cancer. Collection of the drug required harvesting of thousands of trees, a process that clearly would eventually cause extinction of the slow-growing yew tree. Paclitaxel may never have become an important anticancer drug, except for the efforts of organic chemists who eventually developed a means of synthesizing this complex molecule. Paclitaxel works by promoting the formation of microtubules, and prevents cells from disassembling them. As a result, cells fill with nonfunctional microtubules and cannot replicate, and the cells eventually die. **Figure 33.4** compares the mechanisms of action of the vinca alkaloids with that of paclitaxel. The taxanes are indicated for the treatment of breast, ovarian, and some forms of lung cancer, among others.

## Administration

The microtubule inhibitors are administered with other agents as part of chemotherapy protocols. Vincristine and vinblastine are administered only by intravenous injection. They are irritating to the tissues, so they are injected fairly quickly into a running IV line to reduce the contact time with tissues. Vincristine and methotrexate are both part of drug protocols for certain lymphomas, and they are sometimes given on the same day. Methotrexate is administered intrathecally, in some cases, but vincristine is always given intravenously. Special labelling of vincristine syringes is required by law to prevent it from ever being injected by the intrathecal route.

### Case 33.1

In a few disastrous mix-ups, vincristine has been administered intrathecally, an error that is almost always fatal. Although the following case is not about a real patient, the errors made are taken from actual situations.

A.L., a 14-year-old boy, was being treated at ABC Children's Hospital in Albuquerque, New Mexico, for lymphoma, a cancer of immature lymphocytes. On the first day of his maintenance cycle, his doctor was to inject methotrexate into the cerebrospinal fluid, and on the same day, he would receive vincristine 2 mg by IV push. Luke La Blanc, the oncology pharmacy technician, was making the chemotherapy products in the second floor satellite the day A.L. was admitted. Luke was a stickler for following protocol and carefully double-checked that the over wrap for the vincristine syringe, stating "FOR INTRAVENOUS USE ONLY" was present. Luke also made a methotrexate syringe for the same boy, and labelled it for intrathecal use. He noticed that both syringes were the same size, and asked Lucy, the pharmacist, if that was okay. She explained to him that because vincristine can cause severe irritation to the veins, the pharmacy chooses not to make it too dilute, so it can be given quickly into a rapidly running IV. She checked the product and reassured Luke that with the labelling, no errors would be made.

Lucy carried the syringes to the floor and handed them to A. L.'s nurse, Christine Van. Lucy wanted to hand them directly to the physician, but he was conferring with A. L.'s parents in another room. It was busy and Christine was behind, so she prepared the room for the oncologist, removed the outer wrapping on the vincristine syringe, and went next door to continue her work. The oncologist hurried to the area, found the only available nurse, who happened to be a recent graduate, and began the procedure. He was ready for the drug; he grabbed the closest syringe, and injected it. Christine arrived a moment later and the oncologist told her A.L. was now ready for his vincristine. As she looked at the syringe labels, she was horrified; the vincristine syringe was empty. In spite of a herculean effort to lavage the drug out of the spinal fluid, A.L. began to feel pain, then lost function of his lower limbs. Two days later he died.

After reading this "case," see if you can pinpoint places where opportunities for error occurred. Research preventative measures on the Internet, and decide how the errors could have been prevented.

Paclitaxel and the related docetaxel (Taxotere®) are also administered by intravenous injection, but these drugs are diluted and administered slowly. Both of the taxanes interact with some types of plastic. As a result, glass bottles or IV bags that do not contain polyvinyl chloride, a compound found in some plastics, are recommended for intravenous admixtures made with these drugs.

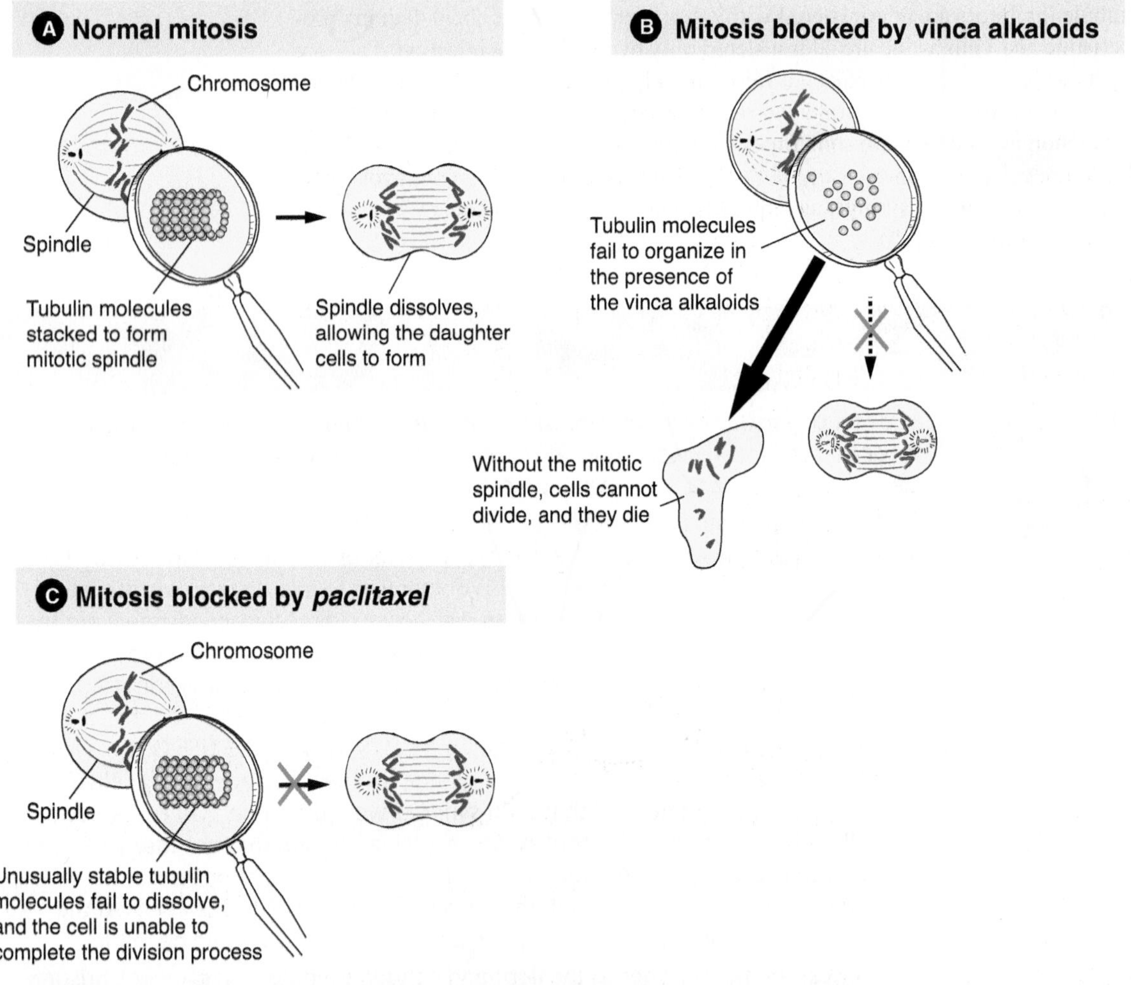
A Normal mitosis
Chromosome
Spindle
Tubulin molecules stacked to form mitotic spindle
Spindle dissolves, allowing the daughter cells to form
B Mitosis blocked by vinca alkaloids
Tubulin molecules fail to organize in the presence of the vinca alkaloids
Without the mitotic spindle, cells cannot divide, and they die
C Mitosis blocked by paclitaxel
Chromosome
Spindle
Unusually stable tubulin molecules fail to dissolve, and the cell is unable to complete the division process

**Figure 33.4** A comparison of the mechanisms of action of the vinca alkaloids and the taxanes. (Adapted with permission from Harvey RA, Champe PC, Howland RD, et al. *Lippincott's Illustrated Reviews: Pharmacology*, 3rd edition. Baltimore: Lippincott Williams & Wilkins, 2006.)

### Side Effects

The side effects observed with the vincristine, vinblastine, and vinorelbine share similarities, but they are not identical. Besides nausea, vomiting, diarrhea, and hair loss, these drugs are highly irritating to tissues, and can cause tissue damage if they extravasate. The vinca alkaloids can cause damage to peripheral nerves (peripheral neuropathy), with symptoms of tingling in the feet and hands and loss of reflexes. They can cause autonomic nerve damage that results in constipation. Allergic reactions, including bronchospasm, can occur with the vinca alkaloids.

As byproducts of natural substances, hypersensitivity reactions are common with the taxanes. Because allergic reactions can be quite serious, it is standard practice to pretreat patients with antihistamines before they receive paclitaxel. Peripheral neuropathy can develop with the taxanes. Hair loss and GI symptoms occur, but vomiting and diarrhea are less common than with some other agents. The most serious and limiting side effect observed with paclitaxel is bone marrow suppression. Patients are especially likely to experience neutropenia, which makes it more difficult for them to fight off infection. This reaction can be so severe as to postpone the use of the drug. The biologic response modifiers filgrastim, and sargramostim stimulate the production of granulocytes in the bone marrow, and can be used to help prevent infection and restore production of neutrophils and other granulocytes (refer back to Chapter 14 for a review of blood cell types and function) so that chemotherapy can continue.

#### Tips for the Technician

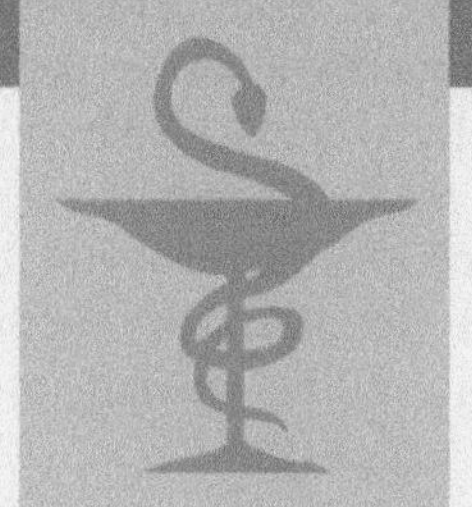

Both the vinca alkaloids and the taxanes present opportunities to the technician, who may be caught unaware to make serious drug errors. Name confusion is a very well documented pitfall and results in many drug administration errors. The generic names of the vinca alkaloids, vincristine, vinblastine, and vinorelbine, are obvious look-alike, sound-alike traps. The brand names of the two taxanes, Taxol® and Taxotere®, are also prone to name confusion. The doses of these drugs are different, and the use of one at doses prescribed for the other can have very serious or sometimes lethal consequences. The disastrous results previously mentioned, of the use of vincristine by the wrong route are worth repeating. Hospitals and clinics have policies in place to prevent these errors, including separation of the products on the shelf, use of warning labels, and procedures for professionals who write drug orders. Technicians can avoid possible pitfalls by meticulously following error prevention policies, and by having a basic understanding of the pharmacology, and a thorough understanding of the risks associated with every drug they touch.

## Other Cytotoxic drugs

Other commonly used chemotherapeutic agents include the platinum derivatives, cisplatin (Platinol®) and carboplatin (Paraplatin®), asparaginase (Elspar®), and etoposide (Toposar®). Asparaginase is a cell-cycle specific enzyme derived from bacteria, and etoposide is a cell-cycle specific derivative of the alkaloid podophyllotoxin, found in the May apple plant.

### Actions and Indications

Cisplatin and carboplatin work by binding to DNA to inhibit its replication, and to a lesser degree, they inhibit the synthesis of other proteins. Their mechanism of action is similar to that of the alkylating agents. The platinum derivatives are used with other drugs in the treatment of lung cancer, ovarian and testicular cancers, other solid tumors, and some lymphomas.

Asparaginase works by inactivating the amino acid asparagine, a necessary precursor for protein synthesis. Because cancer cells cannot synthesize their own asparagine, asparaginase stops protein formation, and eventually stops DNA synthesis and replication. It is indicated as part of the protocol for the treatment of the most common childhood leukemia, acute lymphocytic leukemia.

Etoposide and other members of this class work by inhibiting an enzyme (topoisomerase) that allows DNA bonds to be broken. If the bonds cannot be broken, DNA cannot be copied, and it cannot be repaired when damaged. Etoposide is used for the treatment of lung cancer and testicular cancer. Irinotecan (Camptosar®), and topotecan (Hycamtin®) are two newer drugs, which also inhibit DNA topoisomerase.

## Administration

Of the chemotherapeutic agents discussed in this section, only etoposide is available in a formulation for oral administration. Both of the platinum derivatives are typically administered by IV infusion, but they can also be administered directly into the peritoneal cavity for ovarian cancer or intra-arterially for more direct perfusion of a specific organ. Asparaginase is destroyed by stomach acid and is administered by intramuscular or intravenous injection.

## Side Effects

The platinum derivatives are well known for causing severe nausea and vomiting. Because these symptoms can be so severe with cisplatin, patients are usually pretreated with antinauseant drugs. Cisplatin causes dose-related kidney toxicity, which can result in discontinuation of treatment. Carboplatin can impair renal function, but to a lesser degree. Physicians ameliorate this toxicity by ensuring that patients are fully hydrated, and by treating them with diuretics. Damage to hearing and the peripheral nerves can occur as a result of treatment with these drugs, but it is much less severe with carboplatin than cisplatin. Use of other drugs that cause hearing loss or kidney failure add to the risk of toxicity. Both of the platinum derivatives cause bone marrow suppression, which can limit therapy, especially with carboplatin.

The side effect profile of asparaginase is quite different from that of most chemotherapeutic agents. Because it is a foreign protein, allergic reactions to asparaginase are fairly common, and are more likely to occur with each exposure. This drug can cause kidney damage, and it reduces the production of blood clotting factors, which can result in bleeding complications. The most important side effect seen with etoposide is bone marrow suppression, which can limit treatment. Nausea, vomiting, and hair loss also occur.

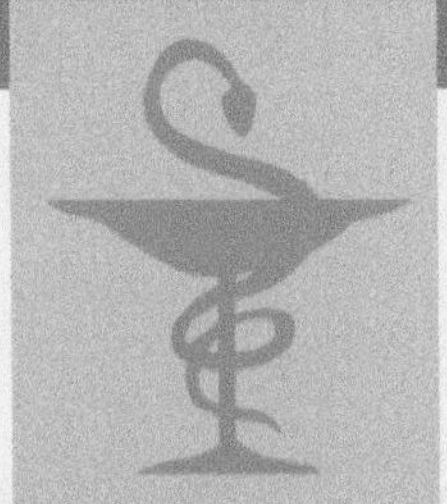

### Tips for the Technician

As is the case with all cytotoxic drugs, these chemotherapy agents are reconstituted in a biological safety cabinet or barrier isolator hood. The platinum derivatives interact with aluminum to form precipitates. Therefore, only stainless steel needles can be used for reconstitution and compounding of these products. In addition, cisplatin can only be diluted in normal saline. Solutions of cisplatin cannot be refrigerated because precipitation can occur.

Pharmacy technicians are advised to wear gloves whenever handling etoposide, and should wash the hands thoroughly if contact with the drug occurs to avoid contact skin reactions. Etoposide capsules are stored in the refrigerator and should be labelled with auxiliary instructions to keep the drug in the refrigerator. Vials of injectable etoposide do not require refrigeration.

Asparaginase is stored in the refrigerator before reconstitution. Vigorous shaking of the vials during reconstitution can result in decreased drug potency, and is avoided. When reconstituted, the solution may appear cloudy. It can be filtered to remove particulate matter, but only with larger sized filters (do not use 0.2 micron filter) to avoid potency loss. Asparaginase IV solution must be used within 8 hours of reconstitution.

## Biological Response Modifiers and Targeted Therapy

It was known for many years that although malignant cells regularly appear in the body, they do not often develop into cancer. The question was, why not? Researchers discovered that human cells produce chemicals and antibodies to defend against the abnormal cells. By isolating these chemical substances, and developing an understanding of the processes the body uses for self-defense, pharmacologists, immunologists, and oncologists were able to synthesize or create new biological products that reinforce or stimulate our natural defenses against malignancy. Interferon, isolated in 1957, was the first of these substances to find application in the treatment of malignant diseases.

Recall from the discussion in Chapter 28, that once B-lymphocytes are sensitized to foreign proteins, they produce specific antibody to those proteins when they are encountered again. In the late 1970s, as recombinant DNA technology developed, researchers were able to combine the genetic material from antibody producing, healthy human lymphocytes with mouse myeloma cells (cancerous mouse lymphocytes) to create an "immortal" cell line that would produce large quantities of a specific antibody, called monoclonal antibody (MAb). Initially, these monoclonal antibodies were created to use against bacteria, for the treatment of overwhelming infectious disease, but the results were disheartening.

monoclonal antibody An antibody that can be synthesized in the laboratory with one population of cells.

A major therapeutic breakthrough came in 1979, when a cancer researcher in Boston created an antibody to a cancer associated antigen. Unfortunately, the early monoclonal antibodies, made mostly of mouse protein, caused too many allergic reactions in patients. A new cell line was developed to produce antibodies to the same antigen that were "humanized" to contain much less mouse protein. The positive response to this form of treatment ushered in a new era in cancer treatment, with numerous monoclonal antibody products, interferon, and interleukin-2 now available to treat specific cancers. The natural ability of the body to defend against malignancies continues to be the subject of intensive study and great promise in the struggle to heal people with cancer.

### Actions and Indication

Drugs that stimulate or reinforce the actions of the body's own natural defense mechanisms to fight disease are called biologic response modifiers. When these drugs are used in cancer chemotherapy they are referred to as targeted therapies. Products available to date include three major types of interferon (alpha, beta, and gamma), interleukin-2, the monoclonal antibodies, and others. Interferon alpha-2a (Roferon®), and alpha-2b (Intron A®) are used in the treatment of certain malignancies of blood components. Interleukin-2 (Proleukin®) is used in a specific type of lung cancer.

Interferon and interleukin-2 are cytokines, chemicals that activate systems in the body, including the immune system. The cytokines are small protein molecules secreted when biological factors trigger their synthesis by specific cells. The precise mechanism of interferon action is not completely understood. However, when interferon binds to surface receptors on other cells, a number of intracellular responses occur. Suppression of cell proliferation, increased phagocytosis (the engulfing and digestion of other cells) by macrophages, and increased ability of lymphocytes to kill cells are among the responses that contribute to the anticancer activity.

phagocytosis The process of engulfing and destroying foreign material, an essential part of the immune response.

Monoclonal antibodies are used against tumor-associated antigens. The monoclonal antibody rituximab (Rituxan®) is used for certain lymphomas, and trastuzumab (Herceptin®) is indicated for some patients with breast carcinoma. Bevacizumab (Avastin®) is approved for use as a first-line drug against metastatic colorectal cancer. Other monoclonal antibodies, such as cetuximab (Erbitux®), and gemtuzumab (Mylotarg®) are available for less commonly occurring neoplasms.

Although the key role of monoclonal antibodies (binding to antigens), is similar to all specific effects of monoclonal antibodies differ because they each bind to unique antigens. Rituximab binds to a specific antigen on B lymphocytes to stimulate immune functions, including cytotoxicity of the B cells, and apoptosis. Rituximab is used with other combinations of anticancer agents to maximize effective tumor cell killing.

The details of the action of trastuzumab are less well delineated. About one third of breast tumors overproduce a growth factor receptor, called human epidermal growth factor receptor-2 (HER-2), which, when activated, encourages tumor cell growth. Trastuzumab binds to the HER-2 receptor sites on the tumor, prevents its activation, and thereby inhibits the proliferation of cells.

The monoclonal antibody bevacizumab is the first in a new class of anticancer drugs that prevents the formation of new blood vessels triggered by a tumor. It attaches to, and neutralizes the action of, the chemical responsible for stimulating the formation of new blood vessels. As part of this drug's effect, blood vessels already formed in the vicinity of the tumor are normalized. This allows for delivery of chemotherapy drugs to the existing tumor while preventing formation of new vessels needed for growth and proliferation of new cancer cells. Bevacizumab is approved for use against metastatic colorectal cancer, and is given along with other drugs.

## Administration

The interferons and the monoclonal antibodies are proteins, and because the GI tract contains enzymes that destroy proteins, administration by the oral route is impossible. The interferons are given by intravenous infusion, or by intramuscular or subcutaneous injection. The monoclonal antibodies are infused intravenously.

## Side Effects

Although all of the biologic response modifiers are at least partly "humanized" proteins, they are to varying degrees recognized by the body as foreign. As such, these drugs are often involved in hypersensitivity reactions, including infusion reactions with fever, chills, rashes, and a general sense of feeling unwell. In addition, each drug is associated with specific side effects.

The interferons can cause psychiatric symptoms that are sometimes quite severe. They are used with caution in patients with a history of psychiatric problems. Depression, with suicidal behavior, mania, and psychoses are all possible side effects of the interferon compounds.

The most common adverse effects of treatment with bevacizumab are infusion reactions, diarrhea, and other GI symptoms, loss of protein through the urine, and hypertension. Less common are bleeding in the GI tract and potential for bowel perforation. This drug has an adverse effect on wound healing, and can cause old surgical wounds to reopen. People who have had recent surgery must wait to begin treatment with bevacizumab. Rituximab most frequently causes infusion and hypersensitivity reactions. Cardiac arrhythmias, and a low platelet count can also occur.

tumor lysis syndrome
Syndrome that occurs as a result of cytotoxic therapy, and the large scale death of tumor cells; hyperuricemia, hyperkalemia, and hypocalcemia are common.

Tumor lysis syndrome, a syndrome associated with the rapid destruction of tumor cells, can occur with these and many combinations of cytotoxic drugs. The kidneys must remove a great deal of waste during chemotherapy because tumor cells are being killed quickly. When the kidneys are deluged with waste products, such as uric acid and electrolytes, they may not be able to adequately process the waste. As a result, acute renal failure, abnormal electrolyte levels, and hyperuricemia can occur.

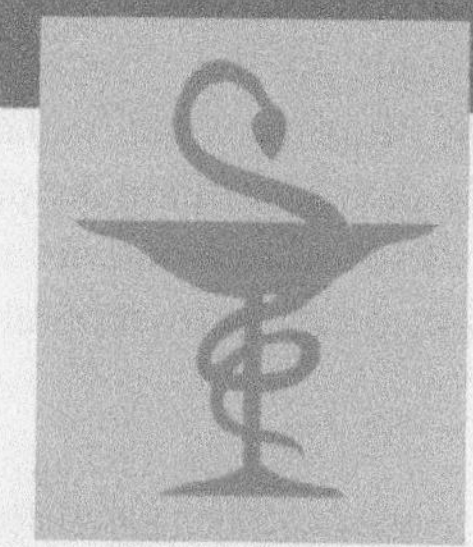

## Tips for the Technician

All of the biological response modifiers discussed must be stored in the refrigerator, and used as soon as possible after reconstitution. Interferon alfa-2B can be given intravenously, but only the powder for reconstitution is appropriate for this route. Technicians should be cautious when ordering and mixing this drug. There are many interferon products with confusing names; be sure to double-check before mixing these expensive products.

Bevacizumab is stable for 8 hours after dilution and rituximab for 24 hours after dilution. Bevacizumab cannot be mixed with dextrose solution. These products should not be shaken because of the potential, to damage the proteins with vigorous shaking. Monoclonal antibody products tend to froth when agitated, which makes withdrawal from the vial difficult. All of the biological response modifiers are very expensive. It is important for technicians to be aware of the storage and dilution requirements to prevent unintentional waste.

# Hormone Therapy

Some tumors are sensitive to the sex hormones and corticosteroids. In some cases the hormones cause tumors to regress, and in others, hormones cause tumors to grow. Tumors that may be hormone sensitive include breast cancer, prostate cancer, and lymphomas or leukemias. The sex hormones and corticosteroids, several of which are used as part of chemotherapy protocols, were covered in Chapter 27. However, a brief introduction of two additional drugs and a review of one already mentioned are appropriate.

## Actions and Indications

Tamoxifen (Nolvadex®) and leuprolide (Lupron®) are hormone antagonists used for breast cancer and prostatic cancer, respectively. Tamoxifen is related to raloxifene, the antiestrogen used for treatment of postmenopausal osteoporosis. Tamoxifen is used for first-line therapy in the treatment of estrogen receptor–positive breast cancer. It attaches to the estrogen receptors on the tumor, but it has no significant estrogenic activity. As a result, the growth-promoting effects of the natural hormone are suppressed. Leuprolide antagonizes the effects of gonadotropin-releasing hormone in the pituitary. Gonadotropin-releasing hormone is responsible for the secretion of testosterone by the testes. In prostatic cancer that is testosterone sensitive, the reduction in testosterone levels caused by leuprolide results in regression of the tumor.

Anastrozole (Arimidex®) is a member of a class of drugs called aromatase inhibitors. Aromatase is the enzyme responsible for the conversion of estrogen precursors in liver, fat, muscle, skin, and breast tissue, including cancerous breast tissue, to active estrogen. Conversion of estrogen precursors is an especially important source of estrogen in postmenopausal women. Estrogen sensitive tumors of the breast grow when exposed to estrogen. By inhibiting aromatase, the production of estrogen is reduced, and tumor growth is inhibited.

## Administration

Most of the hormone antagonists are active when administered by the oral route. Leuprolide, and the related goserelin (Zoladex®) are the exception. Leuprolide is given subcutaneously, or if the long-acting form is used, by intramuscular injection. Anastrazole and other aromatase inhibitors, tamoxifen, megestrol acetate (Megace®), and many other useful hormones and hormone antagonists can be given orally.

### Side Effects

Tamoxifen and the aromatase inhibitors cause side effects similar to the effects of menopause. These effects can be pronounced, and include headache, dizziness, hot flashes, tiredness, and mood disturbances. Both tamoxifen and anastrozole cause musculoskeletal and joint pain. Leuprolide, goserelin, and megestrol are associated with nausea and vomiting, testicular atrophy, mood disturbances, and worsening angina or other heart problems in men.

## Tips for the Technician

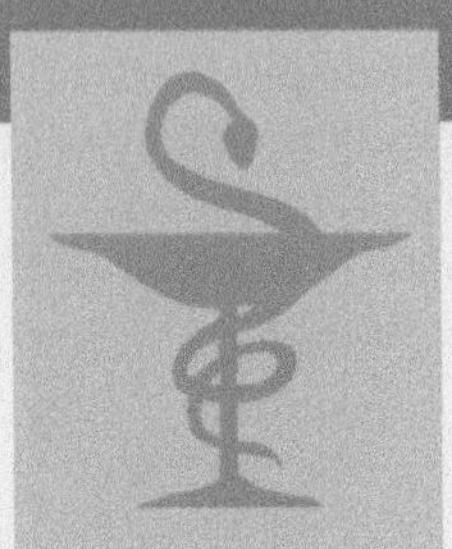

All of the drugs mentioned in this section can be dispensed and used by people outside of a hospital setting. Patients or their family members will likely be responsible for injecting leuprolide subcutaneously, but if the long-acting injection is used it will probably be administered in the doctor's office. The pharmacist is responsible for assuring that the patient who self-injects is comfortable with that process. The manufacturer states that Lupron® injection should be stored below room temperature, which, for practical purposes, means refrigerate. Lupron Depot® powder for reconstitution can be stored at room temperature.

Since central nervous system side effects, such as dizziness or a sensation of weakness or tiredness, can occur with anastrazole and leuprolide, an auxiliary label warning patients to use caution if operating an automobile or other dangerous machinery is appropriate. It is important that pharmacy staff members encourage patients to continue hormonal anti-cancer prescriptions as ordered, except on the advice of the physician, and prescription vials should be labelled accordingly.

## Analogy

Roadmaps are error prevention tools used in cancer chemotherapy. As the name implies, a roadmap is analogous to a map that you would use when you travel. Much like the packet you pick up from a travel agent before you leave on a long trip, the roadmap is a step-by-step itinerary for cancer treatment, based on protocols, that helps assure that the correct drugs, doses, and monitoring is completed while patients are on the road from point A, cancer, to point B, a hoped-for remission or cure. The roadmap, which is usually several pages long, includes important patient data, a schedule of when drugs are to be given, and laboratory and other therapeutic or diagnostic procedures are to be completed. The roadmap stays with the patient chart and is updated constantly so that team members will know where they are at all times. A copy of the protocol or plan for future treatment is a part of the permanent record. Chemotherapy dosing is based on body surface area (BSA), a measurement derived from height and weight. This and other crucial patient information is updated on the roadmap each time a patient comes in for treatment.

# Review Questions

## Multiple Choice

Choose the best answer for the following questions:

1. Which of the following cancers is not one of the most common forms of cancer in adults?
   a. Lung cancer
   b. Bladder cancer
   c. Breast Cancer
   d. Skin Cancer
   e. Prostate Cancer

2. Which of the following are goals of cancer treatment?
   a. Complete removal or destruction of the tumor, resulting in a cure
   b. Prevent a recurrence of the same type of tumor
   c. Prolong the life of the patient
   d. Improve the quality of the patient's life by treating pain and reducing tumor effects
   e. All of the above are goals

3. Measures used to protect patients or pharmacy employees from risks associated with cytotoxic agents include which of the following?
   a. Use of a biological safety cabinet when compounding sterile cytotoxic preparations
   b. Use of protocols
   c. Enforced "time out" for employees caught not following policies
   d. a and b
   e. a, b, and c

4. Circle the letter that corresponds to the best description of the antimetabolite drugs.
   a. Antimetabolites are antibodies to tumor-associated antigens.
   b. Antimetabolites are compounds derived from living organisms, which kill cancer cells by interacting with DNA and disrupting its functions.
   c. Antimetabolites are similar to natural compounds essential for growth and reproduction and work by interfering with the action of the naturally occurring compound.
   d. Antimetabolites are hormone antagonists that work by blocking hormone receptors on tumor cells that would normally to stimulated to grow by the presence of the hormones.
   e. None of the above describes the antimetabolite drugs.

5. Which of the following environmental, occupational, or lifestyle conditions are risk factors for the development of leukemia?
   a. Caffeine consumption
   b. Exposure to ultraviolet radiation
   c. Exposure to radiation
   d. Infections with certain viruses
   e. c and d

## True/False

6. Besides contributing to heart disease and high blood pressure, smoking is a risk factor for lung cancer and cancers if the oropharynx.
   a. True
   b. False

7. There is no known risk of using automated counting machines to dispense thioguanine or methotrexate tablets.
   a. True
   b. False

8. Although the names sound alike, technicians need not worry about confusing daunorubicin and doxorubicin because when reconstituted daunorubicin is green and doxorubicin is red.
   a. True
   b. False

9. Intrathecal administration of vincristine nearly always results in the death of the patient, and therefore this route of administration should never be used.
   a. True
   b. False

10. Since folinic acid (leucovorin) is an antidote for methotrexate toxicity, technicians should take responsibility to make certain there is always adequate product on the shelf.
    a. True
    b. False

## Matching

For numbers 11 to 15, match the word or phrase with the correct lettered definition from the list below. Choices will not be used more than once and may not be used at all.

11. Cytotoxic
12. Carcinogenic
13. Intrathecal
14. Palliative therapy
15. Metastasize

a. Therapy used for treatment of tumor lysis syndrome
b. The propensity of a tumor to spread to a distant location by "seeding" of tumor cells through the blood stream
c. Injection into a joint
d. Therapy that improves a patient's life through pain relief, treatments that reduce unwanted effects of the tumor, or therapies that ameliorate side effects of treatment
e. Toxic to cells
f. Injected into the cerebrospinal fluid
g. Causes an increased risk of fetal abnormalities
h. Causes an increased risk of cancer

## Short Answer

16. Many forms of cancer are associated with well-documented risk factors. List three of the most common forms of cancer and at least one associated risk factor.

17. Describe three measures used by hospitals where cancer chemotherapy is administered that are designed to protect patients from improper administration of a cancer chemotherapy agent.

18. Explain the idea behind the use of biological response modifiers in cancer treatment. Specifically, how does rituximab work and when is it used?

19. What information does a technician need before compounding an IV containing one of the alkylating agents?

20. What is a common cause of error when compounding and dispensing daunorubicin and doxorubicin, and how might these errors be prevented?

## FOR FURTHER INQUIRY

Visit the United States Pharmacopeia web site to learn more about USP chapter 797. This document contains guidelines for state of the art clean room use. USP 797 is frequently updated based on new information and technology, and the web site provides insight into the complexity of the use of clean rooms to provide product integrity and patient and personnel safety.

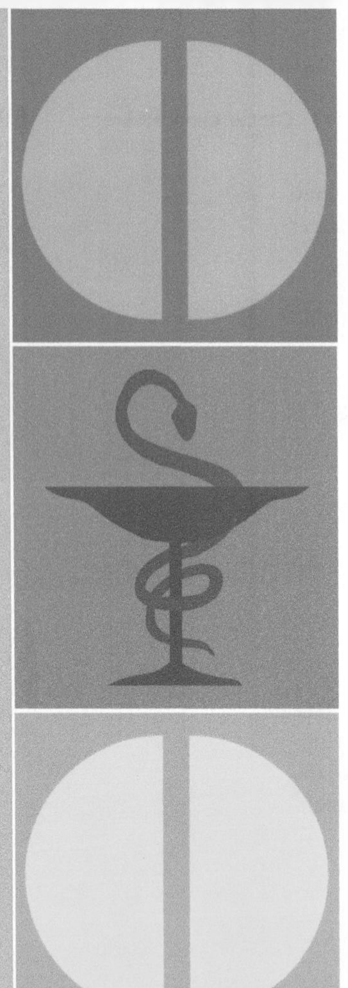

Chapter **34**

# Fluids, Nutrients, and Electrolytes

*KEY TERMS*

- cofactor
- dehydration
- dextrose
- electrolytes
- embolism
- free radical
- hypernatremia
- nasogastric tube
- osmolality
- provitamin
- recommended dietary allowance
- total parenteral nutrition

## OBJECTIVES

After studying this chapter, the reader should be able to:

- Describe three causes of dehydration, and explain why infants or the elderly may be more prone to develop this condition.
- Explain why potassium and magnesium are considered high-risk medications, and describe how a hospital might control access to these drugs.
- List three fat-soluble vitamins and three water-soluble vitamins important sources of these vitamins, and describe their roles in the human body.
- Describe the role of the following minerals and a formulation available for treatment of deficiency states: iron, zinc, copper, and chromium.
- Compare and contrast the indications for use, administration, and risks associated with complete enteral nutrition and total parenteral nutrition.

## FLUID AND NUTRIENTS COVERED IN THIS CHAPTER

| Fluids and Electrolytes | Vitamins | Minerals | Complete Diets |
|---|---|---|---|
| IV solutions<br>Oral fluid and electrolyte replacement products<br>Calcium<br>Magnesium<br>Potassium<br>Sodium | **Water-Soluble Vitamins**<br>B Vitamins<br>Vitamin C<br>**Fat-Soluble Vitamins**<br>Vitamin A<br>Vitamin D<br>Vitamin E<br>Vitamin K | Chromium<br>Cobalt<br>Copper<br>Fluoride<br>Iodine<br>Iron<br>Manganese<br>Molybdenum<br>Selenium<br>Zinc | Total Parenteral Nutrition<br>Enteral Feedings |

High school chemistry teachers used to love to tell students that the human body was composed of two dollars (or with inflation maybe twenty dollars) worth of chemicals. While it is impossible to create a complete human being from these basic ingredients without the amazing biochemical processes that make up our genetic inheritance, the fact is that we are made of water and the same organic compounds found in all other living things. Of the material that comprises our bodies, 96% is made of only four main elements: oxygen, carbon, hydrogen, and nitrogen. The rest of the human body is composed of more than twenty salts and minerals that play a crucial role in bone structure, the function of nerves and muscles, and many other functions. Included in this list are calcium, sodium, phosphorus, potassium, sulfur, iron, and iodine. Because the human body undergoes constant maintenance and repair, the substances of which we are made must constantly be replaced through our diets.

If "you are what you eat," then it should be no surprise that people who eat a healthy diet of grains, fresh fruits and vegetables, and adequate proteins enjoy better health. People who consistently consume food that is unhealthful or for medical or other reasons cannot eat adequately become malnourished, and suffer an inability to respond to physical insults or injury the way a healthy person can. This chapter focuses on the nutritional supplements, fluids, and electrolyte replacement therapy that may be prescribed for those individuals who have temporary or chronic nutritional needs that are not met by their diets. Because most of the compounds discussed in this chapter are considered nutritional supplements, a slightly different chapter format is used that will include the role of the nutrient in the body and indications for replacement, some of the available products, risks associated with their use, and tips for the technician.

# Fluids and Electrolytes

The human body is largely water; an average adult body is about 55% to 60% water while an infant's body contains about 70% water, a value that gradually approaches the adult percentage with increasing age. An average-sized adult loses almost 2.5 liters of water each day, through evaporation, urination, and defecation. This is water that we must replace every day in order to avoid dehydration, which can lead to serious disruption of body function.

## The Role of Fluid and Electrolytes and Indications for Replacement

Water keeps us cool through evaporation, keeps our skin intact, our blood flowing, and our kidneys working. Water dissolves the impurities that our kidneys remove and carries them out in the urine. Our metabolic processes depend on water, and without water our lungs would not function. Water provides the solvent for electrolytes, without which our nervous systems and heart cannot work. Fortunately for most of us, with a reasonable intake of water, our healthy kidneys are able to maintain the needed balance of fluid and electrolytes upon which so many functions depend.

dehydration Condition that results from either excessive loss or inadequate intake of water.

Without adequate water replacement, the body becomes dehydrated, a condition caused by a loss of body fluids. An individual who is dehydrated will feel thirsty first, and will experience a very dry mouth. Later, the dehydrated person will feel listless, will produce small amounts of dark urine, and eventually will become feverish because of the loss of evaporative cooling. The heartbeat may become irregular and the kidneys will quit functioning if fluids are not replaced. Dehydration will kill an individual far more quickly than starvation.

electrolytes A substance that dissociates into ions when in solution and as a result is capable of conducting electrical current; in the body electrolytes contribute to nerve conduction, muscle contraction, and many other processes.

Wherever there is water in the human body, there are also electrolytes. Electrolytes are the charged, or ionized components of molecules that dissolve in water. For example, when table salt, also known as sodium chloride, is dissolved in water it disassociates into $Na^+$ and $Cl^-$ ions. These charged particles can conduct electricity, thus the name "electrolyte." Electrolytes regulate important physiological functions, such as nerve conduction, muscle contraction, and normal cardiac rhythm, to name just a few. For each electrolyte, there is a concentration range in the serum that is considered normal. Refer to **Table 34.1** for the role and normal ranges of a few important electrolytes. Because electrolytes are dissolved in body fluids, dehydration is often accompanied by electrolyte imbalances.

Fluid replacement therapy is indicated in a number of conditions. Fluids and electrolytes are administered intravenously to hospitalized patients who cannot adequately replace, through oral intake, the fluids and electrolytes required to maintain the status quo. Individuals of all ages who are temporarily unable to eat or drink for a variety of reasons may require rehydration. Examples include people who undergo surgery or pregnant women who experience prolonged childbirth. Some forms of kidney failure are treated with fluid replacement, followed by diuretics.

Dehydration, or the prevention of dehydration, is the most important indication for replacement of fluids. Infants and the elderly are the most likely to become dehydrated in ordinary circumstances. Infants cannot convey to parents or caretakers that they are thirsty, and they cannot get their own water. Because babies' bodies contain more water per pound than adults, they require a greater volume per pound of replacement fluids. The elderly have a blunted sense of thirst, and because of disability, may not be able to get drinks as easily as a younger adult. Young, healthy adults can become dehydrated during extreme conditions, such as vigorous exercise in the heat. Extreme heat even without excessive

**Table 34.1** The Roles of Some Important Electrolytes and Their Normal Serum Concentration

| Electrolyte | Functions in the body | Normal Serum Levels |
|---|---|---|
| Calcium | Necessary for muscle contraction, nerve function, blood clotting, cell division | 4.5 to 5.5 mEq/L |
| Chloride | Major anion (- charge) in extracellular fluid; helps maintain fluid balance in the body | 97 to 107 mEq/L |
| Potassium | Major intracellular cation (+ charge); role in nerve and muscle contraction, especially heart rhythm regulation, helps maintain fluid balance | 3.5 to 5.3 mEq/L |
| Magnesium | Necessary for muscle contraction, nerve function, heart rhythm, bone strength | 1.5 to 2.5 mEq/L |
| Sodium | Major cation in extracellular fluid; maintains fluid balance and necessary for muscle contraction and nerve function | 136 to 145 mEq/L |

exercise can cause dehydration in infants or the elderly. Dehydration can also occur as a result of prolonged fever, diarrhea, or vomiting.

Electrolytes are administered to meet daily requirements, correct deficiencies, and in some cases for their therapeutic effects. For example, magnesium is used for treatment of eclampsia or pre-eclampsia syndrome of pregnancy. Pre-eclampsia is a disease associated with hypertension, and in eclampsia, seizures can develop. Magnesium sulfate is the best agent available for the treatment and prevention of the seizures associated with this illness. Oral magnesium salts are administered as laxatives.

Another example is the use of calcium for the treatment of osteoporosis. Calcium replacement is usually combined with other treatment modalities to prevent further bone loss in this disease. Calcium chloride or gluconate is used during cardiac emergencies to stabilize the myocardium when potassium levels are elevated. Calcium and phosphate levels are dependent upon each other. When calcium levels are elevated, phosphate levels fall, and vice versa. Calcium is used to treat elevated phosphate levels.

## Fluid and Electrolyte Replacement Products

The variety of available fluid and electrolyte replacement products is extensive and includes everything from sports drinks, such as Gatorade® or Powerade®, to intravenous solutions, such as normal saline (contains the normal concentration of sodium chloride, 0.9%, found in the blood), 5% dextrose in water, or lactated Ringer's solution, among others. **Table 34.2** shows some of the available combination fluid and electrolyte replacement

**Table 34.2** A Few of the Oral and Injectable Solutions Used for Fluid and Electrolyte Replacement

| Name | Electrolytes (mEq/L) | | | | Other Additives | Use | Provided as |
|---|---|---|---|---|---|---|---|
| **Oral Fluid and Electrolyte Replacement Products** | | | | | | | |
| | $Na^+$ | $K^-$ | $Cl^-$ | Other | | | |
| Pedialyte® | 45 | 20 | 35 | 30 citrate | 25 g/L dextrose | Maintain or replace fluid & electrolytes lost from diarrhea, vomiting | Ready-to-use solution or popsicles |
| Rehydralyte® | 75 | 20 | 65 | 30 citrate | 25 g/L dextrose | Same as Pedialyte® | Ready-to-use solution |
| Temp Tab® | 180 | 15 | 287 | | | Minimize effects of high temperature | Tablets |
| **Intravenous Fluids** | | | | | | | |
| Normal Saline | 154 | - | 154 | - | | Maintain or replace fluids | 1L, 0.5L, 0.25L & IVPB* bags |
| 5% D/Water | - | - | - | - | 50 g/L dextrose | Maintain or replace fluids | 1L, 0.5L, 0.25L, & IVPB bags |
| 5%D/0.45% NaCl | 77 | - | 77 | - | 50 g/L dextrose | Maintain or replace fluids | 1L, 0.5L, 0.25L |
| Lactated Ringer's Soln. | 130 | 4 | 109 | 28 lactate | 3 mEq/L $Ca^{++}$ | Maintain or replace fluids | 1L, 0.5L, 0.25L |
| Normosol-R® | 140 | 5 | 98 | 27 acetate | 23 gluconate, 3 mEq/L $Mg^{++}$ | Maintain or replace fluids | 1L, 0.5L |

IVPB, intravenous piggy-back; L, liter.

solutions sold for therapeutic purposes. Although combination products are available for oral use at home, fluids and electrolytes are usually prescribed as separate entities for hospitalized patients and compounded in the hospital pharmacy. This allows for individualized therapy based on a specific patient's needs. Electrolytes are available in concentrated solutions that are added to base solutions for intravenous infusion. Electrolyte solutions must be diluted before intravenous administration.

Many electrolytes are available as products for oral administration. For example, potassium may be depleted during treatment with diuretics. The lost potassium, usually as the chloride salt, can be replaced using a wide variety of oral liquids, tablets, or capsules. Sodium, calcium, phosphate, and magnesium are other examples of electrolytes that can be replaced with oral or intravenous products. Most electrolytes are available in many different salt forms. For example, calcium is available as calcium carbonate, calcium chloride, calcium gluconate, calcium lactate, and others. Different salts are chosen for their absorption characteristics, the amount of the elemental form of the electrolyte or mineral available in the product, and their side effect profiles, among other reasons. Some examples of electrolyte replacement products are shown in **Table 34.3**.

## Risks of Fluid and Electrolyte Therapy

Even though it might seem that there could be nothing dangerous about water and salts, there are serious risks associated with fluid and electrolyte therapy when replacement is inappropriate. Some people may be surprised to learn that even water, consumed in excess, can cause intoxication. Too much water, administered or consumed rapidly, without the ap-

**Table 34.3** Some Examples of Products Used for Either Oral or Injectable Electrolyte Replacement

| **For IV Use** | | | |
|---|---|---|---|
| **Name** | **Strength** | **Use** | **Provided as** |
| Sodium Chloride for injection | 23.4% (4 mEq/ml), 14.6% (2.5 mEq/ml) | Source of sodium for IV compounding | 30–250 ml vials 20–250 ml vials |
| Sodium Acetate for injection | 2 mEq, 4 mEq/ml | IV compounding | 20–250 (2 mEq) vials 50–100 (4 mEq) vials |
| Potassium Chloride | 2 mEq/ml Injection | IV compounding | 5–250 mL vials |
| Potassium Phosphate | 4.4 mEq $K^+$, 3 mmol phosphate/ml | IV compounding | 5–50 mL vials |
| Calcium gluconate | 10% (0.46 mEq/ml) | IV compounding | 10–200 mL vials |
| Magnesium sulfate | 50% (500mg/ml) | IV compounding | 2–50 mL vials |
| **For Oral Use** | | | |
| Sodium Chloride | 1 gram, 650 mg | Salt replacement | Tablets |
| Potassium Chloride (Klor-Con®, Kay Ciel®, K-Lyte®, others) | 8 mEq, 10 mEq, 15 mEq, 20 mEq (ER tablets), 25 & 50 mEq (effervescent) tabs, 10%, 15%, 20% liquid | Potassium replacement | ER Tablets, effervescent tablets, solution |
| Potassium & sodium phosphates (K-Phos®, Neutra-Phos®) | Many | Phosphate replacement, to lower calcium levels | Powder, tablets |

propriate electrolytes, causes water to move from outside to inside the cells. Cells can actually rupture if the imbalance is not corrected. Symptoms of water intoxication begin with light-headedness and can proceed to swelling of the brain and seizures. Fortunately, in the normal individual who is drinking water, the kidneys are able to form dilute urine and conserve electrolytes to keep water toxicity from occurring. Plain water is never infused intravenously because of the risk of causing cell rupture and hyponatremia.

When electrolytes become elevated in the blood of a normal person, the kidneys begin to conserve water and will naturally correct the imbalance, as long as the individual is drinking fluids. Risks of electrolyte excess are more likely to occur when replacement therapy is prescribed or administered incorrectly, in people with abnormal kidney function, or when an individual becomes dehydrated.

Some electrolytes are extremely dangerous in the undiluted, injectable form and can only be dispensed by the pharmacist. For example, potassium chloride, if administered rapidly in the undiluted form, can cause extreme pain at the site of injection, and more ominously, arrhythmias that can result in death. Twenty years ago, undiluted potassium was routinely available to nurses as floor stock. After a number of people were killed by inadvertent injection, this high-risk medication was taken off of nursing units.

High-risk, or high-alert medications are drugs that are likely to cause serious harm if given incorrectly. Hospitals regulate the use of potassium chloride and other high-risk medications through policies and procedures. In the case of electrolyte concentrates, policies may restrict access to the drugs in undiluted form, and control the maximum concentration or infusion rate that can be prescribed. Because of the importance of potassium in cardiac conduction, extremely high or low potassium levels are always considered a medical emergency. Very low levels of potassium are fairly easy to correct with potassium replacement. Excessive potassium levels are more difficult to manage and may require treatment with sodium polystyrene sulfonate (Kayexalate®), an exchange resin that binds potassium in the GI tract.

Along with potassium, injectable magnesium is considered a high-risk medication if used inappropriately. A fall in blood pressure or cardiac arrest can occur if IV magnesium is administered too rapidly. Elevated serum magnesium levels result in CNS depression, heart block, and if levels are high enough, death.

Although excessive sodium levels, or hypernatremia, usually occur as a result of inadequate water intake, they can be caused by inappropriate administration of sodium chloride. When sodium levels are elevated, the nervous system is the first to be affected. Most sodium stays outside of cells, and when levels are elevated, water moves out of cells to normalize sodium levels. As a result cells begin to shrink and malfunction. The initial symptom of hypernatremia (besides thirst) is likely to be mental confusion. Hypernatremia can result in death if not corrected.

hypernatremia
Abnormally elevated serum sodium level.

Too rapid administration of injectable calcium can cause slowed heart rate or other arrhythmia, and if IV calcium extravasates, it can cause tissue damage and necrosis. Oral calcium replacement products can cause constipation. Phosphate depletion is unusual, and technicians are most likely to encounter phosphate replacement as part of intravenous nutritional support.

## Tips for the Technician

Calcium and phosphate salts chemically interact when concentrations of either or both are too high. The result of this interaction is formation of a precipitate. When chemicals precipitate they are reacting to form a new compound that is insoluble in the solution. Technicians who manufacture sterile products for intravenous use need to be aware that the order in which these two electrolytes are added to the solution is important, especially when the final concentrations are higher than usual. If the two are added one after the other without dispersing them through the solution, the risk of precipitation increases.

Retail and hospital technicians should be aware that all forms of potassium chloride are highly irritating if administered undiluted. Oral potassium chloride liquid (Kaon-Cl®, others) must be diluted before administration according to manufacturers recommendations. Potassium chloride is highly unpalatable to most people. It is salty, but does not have the pleasant saltiness we associate with table salt. Diluting it in vegetable or tomato juice makes it easier for some patients to swallow. Potassium chloride delayed-release tablets (Klor-Con®, others), or the granules in delayed-release capsules (Micro-K®) should not be crushed. Many delayed-release oral potassium chloride formulation are microencapsulated (K-Dur®, others), so that they can be mixed in water or juice without tasting bad.

# Vitamins

The word vitamin was coined from the combination of the words "vital" and "amine" because they were initially thought to be amines, and were considered to be essential for life. While it is true that they are essential for life, they are not all amines. Except for vitamin K, the vitamins were assigned letters in order of their discovery. Vitamin K was named for the German spelling of coagulation, because it is required for the formation of several clotting factors. The vitamins can be subdivided according to whether they are fat or water soluble. The B vitamins and vitamin C are water soluble, and vitamins A, D, E, and K are fat soluble.

## The Role of the Vitamins and Indications for Replacement

recommended dietary allowance Amount of a nutrient that is recommended for daily consumption.

provitamin A vitamin precursor that is converted to the active form in the body.

Vitamins are not synthesized by the body and must be consumed in the diet. They are an essential factor in many important biochemical reactions in the body. There is a recommended dietary allowance (RDA) for each vitamin, which is the suggested amount that should be consumed each day. The recommended intake varies based on factors that correlate with need, such as age, sex, or pregnancy. Healthy, well-balanced diets generally provide adequate vitamin intake. However, although the quantities needed are small, vitamins in foods break down during processing, when food is cooked, or over time. Some of the best food sources of vitamins, along with the adult RDA for each, are listed in **Table 34.4**.

Most people know of vitamin A (Aquasol A®) for its important role in good vision. However, it also stimulates the production and activity of white blood cells and promotes healthy epithelial tissue, which lines the gastrointestinal tract, the urinary tract, the respiratory tract, and the eyes. Vitamin A is essential for healthy skin as well. Vitamin A is actually a group of related compounds with differing potency. Carotenoids, including beta-carotene, are provitamins (precursors to the vitamin) that the body converts to vitamin A.

There are eight B vitamins: vitamin $B_1$ or thiamine, vitamin $B_2$ or riboflavin (Ribo-100®), vitamin $B_3$ or niacin, vitamin $B_6$ or pyridoxine (Aminoxin®), folic acid ($B_9$), cyanocobalamin (Nascobal®, $B_{12}$), pantothenic acid ($B_5$), and biotin. These vitamins often occur together in the same foods. The B vitamins play an important role in the health and maintenance of the nervous system, in the metabolism of carbohydrates and fats, and the maintenance of smooth muscle. They may also play a role in heart health. Riboflavin and thiamine deficiency can both result in damage to nerves. Niacin is essential for healthy skin and nerve function and is used therapeutically to reduce triglyceride levels in atherosclerotic vessel disease.

Folic acid is especially important for proper development of the nervous system in the fetus. Pregnant women who do not get enough folic acid run a higher risk of giving birth to babies with birth defects, especially neural tube defects, including spina bifida. The CDC recommends all women take folic acid supplementation every day. Vitamins $B_{12}$ and folic

**Table 34.4** Common Food Sources and Recommended Daily Allowance (For Adults 19 to 24 Years Old) of Vitamins

| Vitamin Name | Food Source | RDA | |
|---|---|---|---|
| **Fat-Soluble Vitamins** | | **Men** | **Women** |
| Vitamin A | Whole milk, eggs, carrots, yellow squash, sweet potatoes | 3300 units | 2664 units |
| Vitamin D | Fortified dairy products, egg yolk | 400 units | 400 units |
| Vitamin E | Vegetable oil, margarine, wheat germ, nuts, sunflower seed, leafy green vegetables | 15 units | 12 units |
| Vitamin K | Leafy green vegetables, broccoli, cabbage | 70mcg | 60mcg |
| **Water-Soluble Vitamins** | | | |
| Vitamin C | Citrus fruit, leafy green vegetables, broccoli, tomatoes, berries, green and red peppers | 60 mg | 60 mg |
| Thiamine | Enriched or whole grain products, brewer's yeast, organ meats, pork, legumes (peas, beans) | 1.5 mg | 1.1 mg |
| Riboflavin | Enriched or whole grain products, organ meats, dairy products | 1.7 mg | 1.3 mg |
| Niacin | Enriched or whole grain products, beef, fish, chicken, pork, eggs | 19 mg | 15 mg |
| Pyridoxine | Beef, fish, chicken, pork, starchy vegetables, non-citrus fruits | 2 mg | 1.6 mg |
| Folic Acid | Leafy green vegetables, broccoli, legumes, enriched or whole grain products, orange juice | 200 mcg | 180 mcg* |
| Vitamine $B_{12}$ | Meat and dairy products, shellfish, liver | 2 mg | 2 mg |
| Biotin | Organ meats, dairy products, egg yolk, fresh vegetables | † | † |
| Pantothenic Acid | Beef, chicken, pork, fish, whole grain products, legumes | † | † |

*Folic Acid RDA in pregnancy=400mcg, † RDA not established

acid are essential for the formation of normal red blood cells (refer back to Chapter 18 to review pernicious anemia).

Vitamin C (Cecon®, many others), also known as ascorbic acid, is essential for normal connective tissue, and healthy gums, blood vessels, teeth, and bones. It is a powerful antioxidant, and most experts agree that adequate vitamin C intake helps the body's immune system fight off infection and may reduce the risk of developing cancer. Vitamin C is essential for synthesis of collagen and other substances and its deficiency causes scurvy. In the mid 18th century, a British physician hypothesized that something was missing from the diet of British sailors that caused them to fall ill with scurvy. Through an on-board experiment, he determined that citrus fruit reversed this condition. From then on British sailors received citrus fruit or juice on board, most often limes, which earned them the epithet "limeys."

Vitamin D (ergocalciferol, Calciferol®) regulates the absorption and utilization of calcium and phosphorus, both essential for the growth and maintenance of healthy bones. Experiments have demonstrated that vitamin D also affects the growth and differentiation of many types of cells. Vitamin D occurs in a number of forms and must be converted to the active form in the body. Ergocalciferol is the most active form available for replacement. Further activation of this and other vitamin D precursors takes place in the liver and kidneys. Vitamin D is unique because one form is produced in the skin. In order for this to occur, the skin must be exposed to a certain amount of sunshine. Because it is an antioxidant, a healthy intake of vitamin D may reduce the risk of cancer.

Like vitamins A and D, vitamin E (Aquasol-E®) is actually a group of related chemicals. Alpha tocopherol is the active form of the vitamin. The role of vitamin E is not completely understood. Studies indicate it may reduce platelet aggregation and influence smooth muscle functioning. Alpha tocopherol acts as an antioxidant as well. Cell membranes in the body are vulnerable to oxidation, which leads to cell death. Vitamin E protects the membranes of cells from oxidation. Although vitamin E supplementation was once thought to be helpful to reduce the risk of heart disease, this has not proven to be the case in controlled studies.

Vitamin K (phytonadione, Mephyton®) is another fat-soluble vitamin. It is the coenzyme that is required for the synthesis of 6 of the 13 clotting factors. While this is the most thoroughly understood role of vitamin K, it also is necessary for bone health. Although vitamin K is found in leafy green vegetables, synthesis by enteric bacteria provides a significant source of the vitamin.

Young, healthy adults who have normal absorption through the gastrointestinal tract and eat nutritious, balanced diets generally do not need vitamin supplementation. However, there are situations where vitamin replacement therapy is recommended. Pregnant women should always take prenatal vitamins (Natalins®, StuartNatal®) with additional folic acid, since lack of folic acid is well documented to be associated with birth defects. Infants, toddlers, and young children, who can be notoriously poor eaters, are usually given multivitamins with minerals and fluoride to meet the needs of their rapidly developing bodies. Individuals whose diets or GI absorption provide lower levels of vitamins than necessary are candidates for vitamin replacement. Included in this group are people with gastric bypass surgery, malabsorption syndromes, alcoholics, people with pernicious anemia, and the elderly. An ongoing deficiency of a particular vitamin from the diet results in a deficiency syndrome, such as scurvy. Obviously, patients with vitamin deficiency syndromes are candidates for replacement therapy.

Some vitamins are used therapeutically in certain circumstances. Vitamin D is generally given with calcium supplements in the treatment of osteoporosis. Vitamin K is used to reverse the effects of warfarin, when anticoagulation is excessive. Folic acid is used to reverse the effects of methotrexate, and pyridoxine is used to reverse isoniazid or other drug-induced peripheral neuropathy.

## Vitamin Products

Vitamins are available in nearly every form imaginable. Most of the water-soluble vitamins are available singly, in combinations such as B Complex (a combination of all the B vitamins), B complex with vitamin C (Albee with C®), and in a variety of multivitamin combinations (One-A-Day®, Flintstones®, others) that include the fat-soluble vitamins. Riboflavin is sold as a single agent in tablets or capsules. Pyridoxine is manufactured in tablet and capsule form, and in solution for injection. Thiamine and folic acid can be purchased as tablets or injection. Cyanocobalamin is most often administered by injection because poor oral absorption is the usual cause of $B_{12}$ deficiency states. Patients who adequately absorb the drug through the GI tract rarely need supplementation. Nevertheless, vitamin $B_{12}$ also comes in tablets and extended-release tablets. In addition, it is manufactured as an intranasal gel, sublingual tablet, and lozenge. The only B vitamins that are not available as single agents are biotin and pantothenic acid. Vitamin C is sold for use as an injection, an oral liquid, regular and chewable tablets, capsules, extended-release capsules, and powder for oral solution. The oral formulations of most of the water-soluble vitamins and most multiple vitamins are available without a prescription. The exceptions are products that contain more than 0.4 mg of folic acid, which are prescription medications.

The fat-soluble vitamins are available singly and in combination with water-soluble vitamins as daily multivitamin preparations. Although the oral route is preferred for the administration of vitamins A and D, both products are available for IM injection. Vitamin A derivatives are often applied topically for skin conditions, such as acne and prevention of skin aging. Vitamins A and D are routinely added to protectant skin preparations. Vitamin E is available only for oral or topical use, in capsules, oral solution, and in creams and oils. Vitamin K is available in tablets and injectable formulations. All vitamin K products are prescription only, while vitamin E products are available without prescription. Depending on dosage strength, some vitamin A and some vitamin D products are available by prescription only. **Table 34.5** lists a few of the prescription and nonprescription vitamin and mineral products available.

## Risks of Vitamin Therapy

When a person takes more of a water-soluble vitamin than the body can use, the excess is excreted in the urine. As a result of this characteristic, it should be no surprise that toxicity from excessive doses of the water soluble vitamins is rare and side effects from normal doses are extremely unusual. The most common side effects from water-soluble vitamins taken appropriately are GI upset, loss of appetite, or rarely, allergic reactions. Chronic use of large doses of vitamin C, which were touted in the past as an effective preventative against colds, may contribute to the formation of kidney stones in some individuals. High doses of niacin cause vasodilation and flushing, and can, in rare cases, cause liver impairment. Large doses of thiamine or pyridoxine may cause reversible neurological symptoms. In comparison, the fat-soluble vitamins, which are stored in the liver, other organs, and the fat, are much more likely to cause problems when taken inappropriately.

Excessive doses of most of the fat-soluble vitamins can cause serious toxicity. Toxicity can occur as a result of chronic use of higher than usual doses (the more common problem) or acute ingestion. Hypervitaminosis A is characterized by muscle and bone pain, insomnia, and loss of appetite. Other symptoms include hair loss, elevated cholesterol levels, liver damage, vision problems, fatigue, and nausea. Hypervitaminosis D causes elevated levels of calcium in the blood stream. Early signs of hypercalcemia may include weakness, fatigue, headache, loss of appetite, taste perversion, GI upset, and dizziness. Problems occurring later in the syndrome can be more serious, and include deposition of calcium in kidneys, blood vessels, and other tissues. Excessive doses of vitamin E are associated with relatively minor toxicity, including fatigue, weakness, and diarrhea. People taking aspirin or warfarin will have an increased risk of bleeding when taking these drugs with higher than usual doses of vitamin E.

### Tips for the Technician

Pharmaceutical companies design and advertise vitamin products for specific customer groups. Multivitamin products, for instance, are sold in colorful character-shaped chewable vitamins marketed to children, and different combinations and marketing are directed to the needs of women, or geriatric adults. Heavy advertising forces up costs, increases the appeal of the product, and increases the customer's interest in it. Because there are such a variety of products available, consumers may ask your advice on which vitamin product to choose. Suggest that they compare the ingredients on the labels. Many less expensive products contain similar vitamins, in similar doses as expensive, heavily advertised alternatives. There is no advantage to spending more money on high-profile vitamin products, when nearly identical generic drugs are available. In addition, it is important for technicians to understand that vitamin products are drugs, and carry risks. Remind parents that all drugs, and especially those that children may find appealing, should be kept out of the reach of childrden.

## Table 34.5 Examples of Vitamin and Mineral Preparations for Both Oral and Intravenous Use

| Name | Strength | Use | Provided as |
|---|---|---|---|
| **Oral and Injectable Vitamins** | | | |
| Individual vitamins A, D, E, K, C, $B_{1, 2, 3, 5, 6, 12}$ Folic acid | Varies | Deficiency or therapeutic indications | Tablets, chewable tabs (Vit C), Injection (Vit $B_{1, 6, 12}$, Vit C, folic acid, Vit A, D, K), lozenges ($B_{12}$, Vit C) |
| Multivitamins (One-A-Day®, Centrum®, Flintstones®, others) | Varies, contain all or most vitamins, may include minerals | Daily supplement | Tablets, chewable tabs, liquids, drops |
| Multivitamins (MVI-12, Berocca, Infuvite®) | Vitamins A, D, E, vitamin B complex + folic acid, vitamin C (+ Vit K – Peds) | IV, TPN vitamin replacement | 2-, 5-, 10-ml vials or ampules |
| Vitamin B complex (B-Ject-100®) | Contains $B_{1,2,3,5,6}$ | Vitamin B replacement | 30-ml vials |
| B Complex with C (Albee with C®, Vicam® injection) | Contains $B_{1,2,3,5,6\ \&\ 12}$ plus vitamin C | Vitamin B & C replacement | capsules, tablets, 10-ml vials |
| **Oral Minerals** | | | |
| Calcium carbonate (Tums®, Os-Cal 500, others) | 500 mg, 750 mg, 1,000 mg, 1,200 mg, 1,500 mg | Calcium replacement, osteoporosis | Tablets, chew tabs, suspension, some combined with vitamin D |
| Calcium acetate (PhosLo®) | 667 mg, 333.3 mg | Calcium replacement in renal failure, used to lower phosphate levels | Tablets, capsules, gelcaps |
| Magnesium oxide (Mag-Ox 400®) | 400 mg | Magnesium replacement | Tablets |
| Magnesium chloride (Slow-Mag®) | 535 mg | Magnesium replacement | ER Tablets* |
| Ferrous Sulfate (Feosol®, Fer-In-Sol, Slow FE®, others) | 160 mg, 200 mg, 325 mg 220 mg/5ml | Iron deficiency, iron supplement | Tablets, ER tablets, liquid |
| Ferrous Gluconate (Fergon®, others) | 240 mg, 325 mg | Iron deficiency, iron supplement | Tablets |
| **Minerals for Injection** | | | |
| M.T.E.-4®, MulTE-PAK-4® | Chromium 4 mcg/ml, copper 0.4 mg/ml, manganese 0.1 mg/ml, zinc 1 mg/ml | IV compounding | 3-, 10-, 30-ml vials |
| M.T.E.-6®† | Chromium 4mcg/ml, copper 0.4 mg/ml, iodine 25 mcg/ml, manganese 0.1 mg/ml, selenium 20 mcg/ml, zinc 1 mg/ml | IV compounding | 10-ml vial |
| Iron Dextran (InFeD®) | 50 mg/ml | Iron deficiency | Injection |
| Calcium gluconate, Calcium chloride | 10% (1g/10ml) | TPN, cardiac emergencies | chloride—10-ml vials, syringes gluconate:—10-ml amps, vials 50-ml vials |

*ER, extended release.

†Trace metals are available singly in vials for injection.

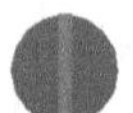

# Minerals

The body requires minerals in significant to minute amounts for building healthy bones, carrying oxygen to cells, normal healing, and other functions. Calcium, the mineral present in highest quantities, serves as both an electrolyte, where it is important for the normal contraction of muscles, and as a mineral, where it is deposited in bones and teeth as hydroxyapatite. Other important minerals are found in small to trace amounts and include iodine, iron, zinc, fluoride, copper, chromium, manganese, molybdenum, and selenium.

## The Role of Minerals in the Body and Indications for Replacement

The two most abundant minerals in the body, calcium and iron, play key roles in normal body function. The majority of the calcium we consume is used for formation and maintenance of the skeleton. Iron is essential for carrying oxygen from lungs to the tissues via hemoglobin, the iron-protein component of red blood cells that gives them their color. Zinc is essential for a healthy immune system and growth and repair of tissues. After zinc, fluoride is the next most abundant mineral in the body. In recommended quantities, fluoride helps teeth to resist decay, and hardens bones. Iodine is necessary for the thyroid gland to function normally. People with less than adequate iodine intake can develop goiter and hypothyroidism.

The rest of the trace minerals help in a variety of important events in the cell, such as interacting with enzymes to catalyze chemical reactions or moving electrons during energy production. For example, copper is an enzyme cofactor (a necessary complement of an enzyme reaction) involved in the production of connective tissue, generation of cellular energy, and neutralization of free radicals (highly reactive molecules that cause tissue damage). Although the actions of manganese are not as clearly defined, it is also involved in protecting cells from free radicals and is found in some enzymes. Manganese deficiency results in skeletal abnormalities and impaired fertility in a number of animal species. Chromium plays an important role in the action of insulin and metabolism of carbohydrates.

cofactor A substance that is required by an enzyme for catalysis to take place; in humans, cofactors are often essential minerals or vitamins.

free radical A highly reactive atom or atoms with one or more unpaired electrons that seeks or releases electrons to other compounds in order to achieve stability, and in the process can damage cells or biological processes.

With the exception of iron deficiency, mineral deficiencies are not common. Iron deficiency occurs fairly frequently in growing adolescents and women who menstruate. The demand for iron is high in this population due to high rates of growth and metabolism, or loss of iron that occurs every month with the menstrual flow (refer back to Chapter 18 for more details on iron deficiency anemia). Poor calcium intake can contribute to early deterioration of bones in osteoporosis. Iodine deficiency and resulting goiter can occur when there is no seafood in the diet and noniodized salt is used. The only other time mineral deficiencies are likely to occur is when the oral diet or absorption is completely inadequate, such as in eating disorders or malabsorption syndromes. Iron or other mineral replacement is indicated whenever a deficiency state occurs. When patients require intravenous feeding, trace metals are added as standard components of most intravenous nutrition protocols.

Short-term zinc replacement therapy is used in some instances in patients with wounds who might be zinc deficient, such as chronically ill or elderly patients with pressure ulcers, in the hope of improving healing. In fact, this type of short-term zinc therapy and zinc replacement for patients who receive their nutritional requirements intravenously are the most important and best-researched uses of zinc. Although zinc is touted in the lay press as effective for everything from curing colds to promoting growth, scientific studies supporting these claims are unavailable in some cases, or provide mixed results in others.

## Mineral Replacement Products

Of the calcium salts available, calcium carbonate (Tums®, Os-Cal®) is the supplement most often chosen for the treatment or prevention of osteoporosis. As previously mentioned, calcium is also available in other salts, for oral or injectable administration. Iron supplements, like calcium, are available in a variety of formulations and for administration by both oral and parenteral routes (Table 34.5). Ferrous sulfate (Feratab®, many others) is probably the most frequently administered iron salt, but ferrous gluconate (Fergon®) and ferrous fumarate (Femiron®, others) are also available without prescription for oral administration. The elemental iron content of each salt differs slightly. Recommendations for iron intake are based on elemental iron. Iron dextran (INFeD® for IM or IV use) and iron sucrose (Venofer® for intravenous administration) are used when oral iron replacement is not possible or more rapid replacement of stores is desirable.

Iodine is available in prescription supplements, as discussed in Chapter 25, but is also found in iodized salt and sea salt. Zinc, as the sulfate (Orazinc®), is sold as tablets, capsules, and nasal spray. The trace minerals are available as single agents for injection, and in a variety of set combination formulations, mainly used for compounding intravenous nutrition solutions. Although calcium, iron, fluoride, and manganese are sold as single drugs, other minerals are combined with vitamins in multivitamin supplements for oral use.

### Risks of Mineral Replacement Therapy

Minerals, when given in the usual amounts contained in a multivitamin plus mineral formulation or as part of intravenous nutrition solutions, are very unlikely to cause any adverse effects. However, some mineral preparations are associated with specific adverse effects. Intramuscular iron must be given very cautiously because the risk of infusion and allergic reactions from these products is significant. Intramuscular iron can cause similar allergic reactions and requires a special administration technique, called z-track administration, to avoid staining of the skin. Oral iron is not associated with allergic reactions, but frequently causes GI upset in the form of nausea, constipation, or less commonly, diarrhea. GI upset is the most common complaint associated with oral zinc. If it is used in excess, it can impair the absorption of copper, which can result in copper deficiency and symptoms of easy bruising or bleeding, tiredness, and anemia. Intranasal zinc can temporarily impair the sense of smell. Excess iodine is associated with dysfunction of the thyroid gland.

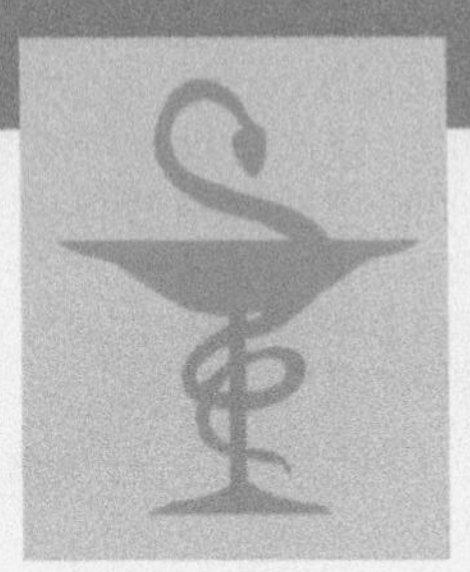

#### Tips for the Technician

Technicians need to be aware of the difference between the elemental form of the mineral replaced versus the strength of the tablet or capsule. For example, a 220-mg zinc sulfate capsule provides 50 mg of elemental zinc. Different mineral salts deliver different quantities of the mineral in its elemental form. For instance, 325 mg of ferrous gluconate provides 36 mg elemental iron, whereas 325 mg of ferrous sulfate provides 65 mg elemental iron. Check with the pharmacist if you are unsure of how to interpret a drug order or prescription to avoid inadvertently over or underdosing a patient.

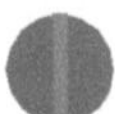

## Complete Diet Replacement

total parenteral nutrition
Intravenous feedings that provide patients with all their nutritional requirements when they are unable to take nutrients in via the enteral route.

People who are permanently or temporarily unable to chew or swallow or are unable to absorb adequate nutrition through the intestinal tract must receive all or part of their nutrition another way. Other than the traditional way of eating, two different options for nutrient intake exist. These include enteral nutrition, complete feedings administered into the GI tract through a tube, or total parenteral nutrition (TPN), complete nutrition administered through an intravenous catheter.

## Role and Indications for Enteral or Total Parenteral Nutrition.

When an individual is unable (or sometimes unwilling) to chew or swallow, but food is adequately absorbed through the GI tract, feedings can be given into the stomach or the intestines through a tube. Feedings that are administered in this manner are called enteral feedings, or sometimes tube feedings. Examples of the type of patients who might require enteral feedings include people who require long-term nutritional support because they are in a coma, or who have had damage to the part of the brain that coordinates swallowing, or simply have such high metabolic needs they cannot meet them through a normal diet alone.

A nasogastric tube, a small, flexible tube fed through the nose into the stomach, can be used for short-term conditions where enteral feeding is possible. In instances where a more permanent feeding method is needed, a tube can be surgically placed directly into the stomach using a procedure called percutaneous endoscopic gastrostomy (PEG). Gastric tubes (commonly referred to as PEG tubes or G-tubes) are fairly permanent and are suitable for long-term use. This type of feeding tube is far more frequently used than a tube into the jejunum (J-tube), which provides another site for tube placement. Feedings can be run continuously, with the assistance of a special pump, or can be administered in divided "meals" or bolus feedings administered by a caretaker.

nasogastric tube A flexible tube that is passed through the nostril and nasopharynx in order to access the stomach.

When an individual is not expected to require long-term feedings, or cannot absorb food through the GI tract, total feedings can be given parenterally, through an intravenous catheter surgically placed in a large, central vein, usually the subclavian. Patients recovering from extensive GI surgery, burn victims, cancer patients, or patients with unusual fluid and electrolyte abnormalities may require TPN. Some people who refuse to eat, as in the case of minors with anorexia, can be fed with TPN. TPN requires administration with an IV pump for accuracy and safety.

## Complete Diet Replacement Products

Many premixed or powdered enteral feedings are commercially available (**Table 34.6** displays a few examples) Enteral feedings include the recommended daily allowances of fats,

**Table 34.6** A Few Examples of Commercially Available Enteral Feedings

| Name | Provided as | Protein/L | Carbohydrates/L | Fats/L | Other Ingredients/Notes |
|---|---|---|---|---|---|
| Glucerna® | Liquid 1 cal/lmL | 41 g | 93 g | 55 | Electrolytes, vitamins, minerals. Specialty formula for patients with diabetes. |
| Jevity 1.5® | Liquid 1.5 cal/mL | 63.4 | 214.2 | 29.6 | Electrolytes, vitamins, minerals |
| Sustacal® | Liquid 1cal/ml | 60.4 | 138 | 23 | Electrolytes, vitamins, minerals |
| Ensure® | Liquid & powder 1.06 cal/mL | 37 | 143 | 37 | Electrolytes, vitamins, minerals |
| Ensure w/ fiber® | Liquid 1.1 cal/l | 39 | 160 | 37 | Electrolytes, vitamins, minerals + fiber |
| Vivonex T.E.N.® | Powder 1 cal/mL | 38.2 | 205 | 2.77 | Electrolytes, vitamins, minerals. Protein from crystalline amino acids. |
| Pulmocare® | Liquid 1.5 cal/mL | 62 | 104 | 92 | Electrolytes, vitamins, minerals. Specialty formula for lung disease. |

carbohydrates, protein, vitamins, and minerals. Some formulas are designed specifically for patients with certain disease states. For example, Glucerna® derives more of its calories from unsaturated fats and less from carbohydrates, which makes it better suited for patients with diabetes. Formulas designed for patients with liver disease include less protein, to reduce the buildup of ammonia. Formulas are available with higher fiber content to reduce constipation, without lactose for lactose intolerant patients, and with amino acids instead of whey or soy proteins for people who have trouble digesting and absorbing protein. As a subset of complete diet formulas, baby formulas are designed to suit the nutritional demands of growing infants.

While there are a few commercially available, premixed TPN preparations, most institutions compound their own preparations. There are advantages and disadvantages to compounding TPN solutions. By compounding the complete TPN, the pharmacy has greater flexibility and is better able to precisely meet the patient's nutritional requirements. It is also less expensive to purchase dextrose in a variety of concentrations and amino acids in different strengths and then mix the desired combination. Advantages of the ready to use combination products include fewer manipulations, and therefore less risk of contamination.

Hospitals usually have TPN protocols, or guidelines, to inform prescribers of available dextrose and amino acid concentrations. **Table 34.7** is an example of typical ingredients contained in a total parenteral nutrition regimen. Concentrations of electrolytes, dextrose (carbohydrate), and amino acids (for protein synthesis) are adjusted as needed based on laboratory findings and clinical results.

dextrose Dextrorotatory isomer of glucose.

Dextrose, which is the same sugar as glucose, is the ingredient used in TPN solutions to provide calories from carbohydrates. Dextrose is available in large volume IV bags in many concentrations, but the ones typically used for TPN include 20%, 30%, 40%, and 50%, in 500 ml bags. When 500 ml of dextrose is mixed with 500 ml of one of the amino acids, the final concentration of dextrose is half the original concentration, or 10%, 15%, 20%, or 25% dextrose. TPN solutions with a final concentration of 10% dextrose or less can be given through a smaller, peripheral vein, but usually cannot provide enough calories to completely replace an oral diet.

**Table 34.7** A Typical TPN Formula for an Adult, With Additives Listed per Liter of Finished Product

| Nutrient Name | Concentration or mEq/L | Typical Daily Intake |
|---|---|---|
| Dextrose | 20% | 400–500 g |
| Amino acids | 4.25% | 100 g |
| Sodium | 44 mEq/l | 110 mEq |
| Potassium | 13 mEq/l | 32.5 mEq |
| Magnesium | 3 mEq/l | 7.5 mEq |
| Chloride | 37 mEq/l | 92.5 mEq |
| Acetate | 31 mEq/l | 77.5 mEq |
| Phosphorus | 3.5 mmol/l | 10 mmol/l |
| Multivitamins | | 1 vial |
| Trace minerals | | 1–3 mL |

Amino acids (Aminosyn®, others) are added to the TPN so that the body can synthesize proteins. Products include essential amino acids in soluble form, in a variety of formulations suitable for different disease states. For instance, there are formulations for patients with renal failure (Aminosyn-RF®, NephrAmine®) and for people with liver failure (HepatAmine®). Injectable vitamins, and trace metals are included in TPN solutions according to the hospital protocol, and are usually added to one TPN bag each day.

Lipids, which are an important source of calories and essential nutrients, are also included in TPN regimens. Most of the time, emulsions of essential fatty acids (Intralipid®, Liposyn®) are delivered into the same IV line, but are not mixed into the dextrose, amino acid, and electrolyte solution. Solutions containing only the dextrose, amino acids, electrolytes, and vitamins are sometimes referred to as two-in-one admixtures. When lipids are included in the same container, the product is referred to as a three-in-one preparation. Although three-in-one mixtures are more easily administered, they are more difficult to check for incompatibility or contamination. Lipids are available as 10% or 20% fat emulsions.

## Risks of Complete Diet Replacements

Whether total feedings are given enterally or parenterally there are risks involved. Risks are more closely related to the condition of the patient and the route of administration than the content of these products. An older man who drinks a can of Ensure® to supplement his diet because he feels he needs more protein runs very little risk of any ill effects. If the same person were unable to swallow and required feeding through a PEG tube, risks increase significantly. There are dangers associated with surgical placement of the feeding tube, including risks from the surgery itself, infection, and irritation at the site of the tube. The patient who receives tube feedings faces the possibility of regurgitating his feeding and aspirating the contents of his stomach. A person who cannot swallow usually cannot communicate either, and he cannot tell caregivers when he is hungry or when he is full. As a result, people on enteral nutrition are often overfed and gain weight, which can contribute to ill health. Electrolyte imbalances and hyperglycemia can occur, and are more likely in people who have diabetes or kidney failure to begin with.

Because these diets are highly concentrated sources of calories, patients may not tolerate them well. The high osmolality (the concentration of osmotically active particles) of enteral products causes GI side effects. A high concentration of sugars and other particles draws fluid into the GI tract, resulting in diarrhea, nausea, and if sugars are not rapidly absorbed, flatulence. If diets are not carefully selected for patients who are allergic to certain proteins, intolerance will result.

osmolality Concentration of osmotically active particles in solution measured in osmols or milliosmoles per kg of solvent.

When nutrition is given intravenously the greatest risks are related to the presence of a central venous catheter. These catheters can become infected, and as a result cause serious systemic infections in patients. TPN solutions are designed to feed people, but when sloppy sterile technique is used they serve as an excellent growth medium for bacteria and fungi, too. Although contamination of TPN fluid is a less common cause of infection in a patient than an infected catheter, it certainly can happen. Infections that occur as a result of parenteral nutrition are all the more serious because patients receiving TPN are already very ill. Catheter tips can create a site for formation of blood clots, and air embolism (obstructs blood flow) although rare, is a catastrophic consequence of central venous catheter placement or removal.

embolism Sudden obstruction of vessel by a blood clot or foreign material.

Other risks of TPN are metabolic in nature and are related to the composition of the fluids themselves. These can include electrolyte abnormalities, elevated ammonia levels, and hyperglycemia. Treatment with lipids can result in elevated serum lipid levels, liver, or lung toxicity. Patients receiving TPN who are appropriately monitored by the pharmacist, dietitian, or physician usually have little risk of serious metabolic abnormalities.

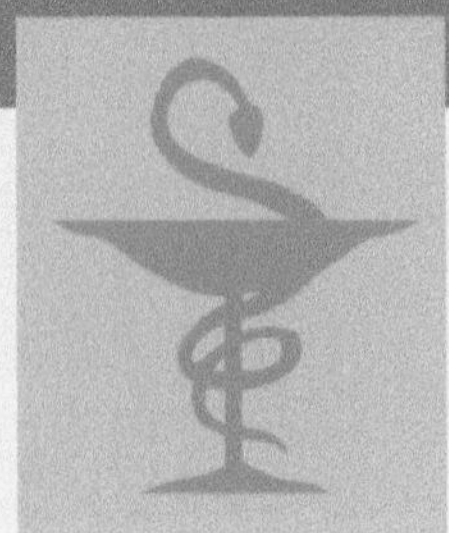

## Tips for the Technician

Except for baby formula and Ensure® supplements, the retail pharmacy based technician is unlikely to deal with many complete diet formulations. However, technicians based in hospitals and pharmacies that provide services to long-term care facilities will find that they are frequently handling parenteral nutrition products, and sometimes, enteral nutrition products.

Most pharmacies that make TPN will require technicians to prove their competency before being permitted to compound TPN solutions. Because TPN solutions have many additives, they are considered moderate risk solutions under the American Society of Health-System Pharmacists sterile compounding guidelines. They must be compounded, using sterile technique, in a clean room or barrier isolator IV hood, and sterile technique. Some hospital pharmacies have mechanical TPN compounders to improve efficiency and to reduce risk of contamination. This equipment is very expensive, and requires time to set up and calibrate on a daily basis, but dramatically reduces the number of manipulations required during the compounding process.

Besides expertise in sterile compounding, pharmacy technicians must understand the TPN additives, be familiar with the risks associated with electrolytes, and their potential physical and chemical interactions. Some additives can precipitate at higher concentrations, and the order in which they are added to a TPN is important. Information about additive stability and chemical incompatibilities can be found in a good reference text, such as *Trissel's Handbook of Injectable Drugs*.

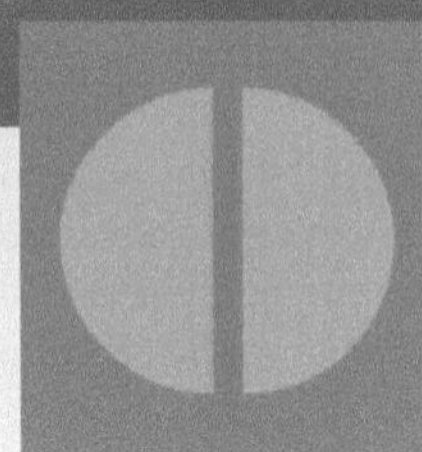

## Case 34.1

Abel Cooke was proud to have recently completed the TPN competencies required by Saint Joseph's Hospital Pharmacy. Saint Joe's Hospital was a very busy, 650-bed facility, with adult medicine, a cancer unit, pediatrics, and a burn unit, so making TPN solutions for the place consumed an entire day. Abel was spending his first full day assigned to making the TPN solutions. By the end of six hours, he was on a roll, his technique was very smooth, but he was aware that he was becoming mechanical.

Abel's last TPN of the day was for Dustin Rhodes, a 10-year-old boy who was in an accident while riding his ATV. Dusty's accident caused a small grass fire and he sustained burns and a broken tibia, which was pushing Dusty's calorie requirements way up. As Abel finished making the complicated bag of TPN for Dusty, he double-checked his work. "Let's see—500 mL D40%, 500 mL 10% amino acids, 9 mL sodium acetate (2mEq/mL), 6.2 mL potassium acetate (2mEq/ml), 4 mL potassium phosphate, 30 mL Calcium Gluconate, . . . MVI—check, trace metals—check. Looks good." As Abel cleared away his mess, he realized that instead of one partially used vial of potassium acetate, he was removing one empty 20-mL vial and one partially used vial. "Hmm," he thought to himself, "how did this get in here? I'm pretty sure I put in 6.2 mL, but I'm also pretty sure I only took one vial from the shelf." He noticed that the other electrolyte vials were all accounted for. "Man, I do not want to make this thing over, and I don't want to waste all this material" he thought. He wondered if perhaps a telephone call he received while he was making the TPN had distracted him. "What should I do?" Abel wondered out loud. What do you think Abel should do?

# Review Questions

## Multiple Choice

Choose the best answer for the following questions:

1. Which of the following conditions may result in dehydration?
   a. Blunted sense of thirst
   b. Vomiting or diarrhea
   c. Exposure to extreme heat
   d. Prolonged fever
   e. All of the above

2. Of the following, which is an indication for electrolyte administration?
   a. Daily replacement
   b. Correction of deficiency
   c. Therapeutic uses
   d. A and B
   e. A, B, and C

3. Which of the following statements about potassium chloride is correct?
   a. Potassium chloride for injection can be administered without regard to final concentration.
   b. Potassium chloride is relatively safe whether given by mouth or by injection.
   c. Potassium chloride for injection is considered a high-risk medication because when administered in undiluted form, it can cause severe irritation and cardiac arrhythmia.
   d. Potassium chloride is indicated for treatment of pre-eclampsia.
   e. None of the above is correct.

4. Of the following, which are considered fat-soluble vitamins?
   a. Vitamin C, folic acid, cyanocobalamin
   b. Vitamin K, vitamin A, vitamin D
   c. Vitamin E, vitamin C, vitamin $B_1$
   d. Pyridoxine, thiamine, folic acid
   e. Riboflavin, fat emulsion, vitamin B complex

5. Circle the letter that corresponds to the nonprescription fluid and electrolyte replacement product indicated for use in infants and young children.
   a. Gatorade®
   b. Normosol R®
   c. Lactated Ringer's solution
   d. Pedialyte®
   e. Ensure®

## True/False

6. Iron deficiency occurs fairly commonly in growing adolescents and women under fifty because the body's need for iron is higher in these populations.
   a. True
   b. False

7. Sucrose is the sugar used in TPN as the source of carbohydrate.
   a. True
   b. False

8. Blood clots or air embolism are potential side effects of enteral nutrition.
   a. True
   b. False

9. The most important roles for zinc therapy are to improve wound healing in patients known to be deficient and to prevent zinc deficiency in patients receiving TPN.
   a. True
   b. False

10. An average adult loses almost 2.5 liters of water each day, which must be replaced in order to avoid dehydration.
    a. True
    b. False

## Matching

For numbers 11 to 15, match the word or phrase with the correct lettered choice from the list below. Choices will not be used more than once and may not be used at all.

11. Carbohydrate used in TPN
12. Building blocks of protein
13. Trace metal associated with normal production of connective tissue
14. Mineral important for normal thyroid function
15. Key electrolyte for maintaining normal fluid balance

a. Lactose
b. Iodine
c. Copper
d. Sodium
e. Amino acids
f. Magnesium
g. Glucose

## Short Answer

16. How and why is enteral nutrition (tube feeding) administered to a patient? What are some of the risks associated with its use?

17. How and why is total parenteral nutrition administered to a patient? What are some of the risks associated with its use?

18. Why is undiluted magnesium considered a high-risk medication?

19. Name three water-soluble vitamins, an important food source of each, and describe the role of each in the body.

20. What measures do pharmacies use to prevent errors with high-risk electrolytes?

## FOR FURTHER INQUIRY

Although pediatricians agree that the best first food for a baby is breast milk, some women need or prefer to feed their infant baby formula. How would you imagine that baby formula and a complete enteral diet such as Ensure® differ? Investigate the source of protein, and compare the carbohydrates, fat, and vitamin content of Ensure® versus a typical baby formula. What assurance do parents have that formula will provide adequate nutrition for their infant?

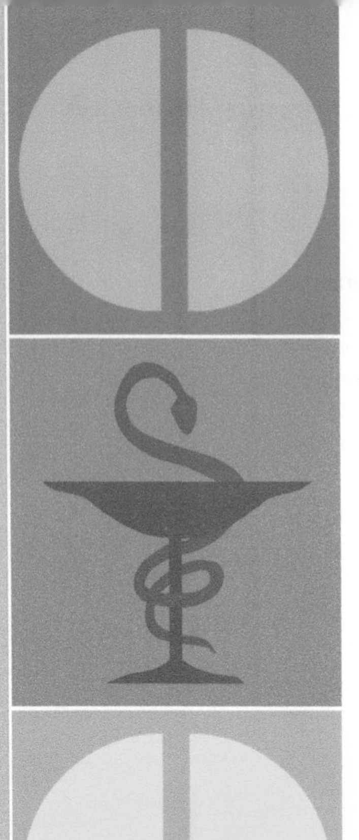

Chapter **35**

# Antidotes and Antivenins

## KEY TERMS

- antidote
- chelate
- decontaminate
- envenomation
- gastric lavage

## OBJECTIVES

After studying this chapter, the reader should be able to:

- Define poisoning, and describe the problem, risks, and general treatment of unintentional poisoning.
- Identify three measures that members of any household can take to reduce the risk of poisoning in children.
- List three antidotes, the poisons for which they are used, and their mechanisms of action.
- Explain when use of antivenin is indicated in black widow spider bites, rattlesnake bites, and coral snakebites.
- Describe the risks associated with the use of one antidote and one type of antivenin.

## DRUGS COVERED IN THIS CHAPTER

| Antidotes and Other Treatments | | Antivenins |
|---|---|---|
| Acetylcysteine | Flumazenil | Antivenin, crotalidae polyvalent |
| Activated charcoal | Glucagon | Antivenin, micrurus fulvius |
| Atropine | Ipecac syrup | Antivenin, lactrodectus mactans |
| Calcium disodium edetate | Methylene blue | |
| Calcium gluconate | Naloxone | |
| Cyanide antidote kit | Physostigmine | |
| Deferoxamine mesylate | Pralidoxime | |
| Diazepam | protamine | |
| Digoxin immune Fab | Sodium bicarbonate | |
| Dimercaprol | Vitamin K | |
| Diphenhydramine | | |

Poisoning is defined as an exposure to a poisonous or toxic substance that causes harm. Every year, tens of thousands of people die from intentional or unintentional poisoning. The most recent statistics from the Center for Disease Control and Prevention indicate that in 2003 almost 29,000 people died from poisonings, or ten deaths per 100,000 people per year in the United States. Unintentional poisoning is second only to automobile accidents as a cause of death from accidental injuries. Clearly, the risk of death or harm from poisoning and efforts aimed at prevention are an important concern for people working in pharmacy and other areas of health care.

This chapter will focus on poison prevention, common poisons, general treatment, and specific antidotes, which are drugs that counteract the effects of a poison. Antidotes can work either directly or indirectly, and include such drugs as naloxone, atropine, and physostigmine. This chapter also includes a brief discussion of poisonous bites, called envenomations, caused by spiders or snakes, and the use of antivenin. Because of the unique nature of this topic, the format of this chapter varies slightly from earlier chapters, and will include indications and administration of antidotes and antivenins, and risks of their use.

antidote A drug used to counteract the effects of a poison.

envenomation Injection of venom by a bite, sting, or spine.

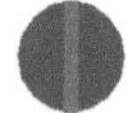

# Poison Prevention

As Benjamin Franklin so aptly wrote, "an ounce of prevention is worth a pound of cure." This is especially true of poison prevention; the treatments for poisoning can be very unpleasant and are not always successful. Several important poison prevention measures, enacted during and since the 1970's, have dramatically reduced the number of deaths due to poisoning in children. The Poison Prevention Packaging Act of 1970, which required that medication be packaged in childproof containers, is credited with reducing the death rate of children under four by about 45% in the first 20 years after its enactment.

Other important legislated prevention measures include education programs, such as National Poison Prevention Week, and the establishment and accessibility of poison control centers. During Poison Prevention Week, families with young children are taught basic steps to take in case of accidental poisoning, as well as the importance of keeping toxic substances in cupboards that are safe from children or pets. Parents are encouraged to teach children that putting things into their mouths without Mom or Dad's permission is dangerous to them. Some programs encourage parents to show their youngsters the substances around the home that are dangerous, and provide stickers that children can place on toxins to remind them of the danger (**Fig. 35.1**) One of the most important measures families can take is to have the telephone number of the poison control center on or near every telephone.

**Figure 35.1** Mr. Yuk is an example of a sticker that parents can place on toxic substances to remind children not to touch them. (Used with permission of Pittsburgh Poison Center at the University of Pittsburgh Medical Center.)

Poison control centers are established around the country to provide information regarding acute poison exposures to the public and health care professionals. In 2004, poison control centers in this country received almost 2.5 million calls. A large majority of these calls were for unintentional poisonings, nearly all of which occur in the home. More than 500,000 people visited the emergency room because of unintentional poisonings in 2004. Although people of any age can be victims of unintentional poisonings, more than half of the calls to poison centers are concerning poison exposure in children under the age of six. Fortunately, because of poison prevention efforts across the nation and improvements in the treatment of poisonings, deaths due to poisoning in young children are much less common now than 30 years ago.

# Common Poisons and Their General Treatment

In young children, exposure to cleaning products, pain relievers (especially acetaminophen Tylenol®), cough and cold products, cosmetics, and plants are among the most common poison exposures. In adults, exposure to pain relievers, sedatives, and cleaning substances are common. Industrial exposures may include skin, eye, or inhalation exposure with pesticides, lead or other metals, organic solvents, and petroleum products.

The first step in treatment and care of people with poison exposure is learning with what, when, and how the person was exposed. When pharmacy staff members receive calls regarding poisonings, the best advice is to encourage parents or victims to call the poison control center immediately, and to have the name of the potential poison readily available. Poison control center staff members are experts in toxicology and can advise both professionals and patients on the correct course to take in any potential exposure.

When a visit to the emergency room is necessary, efforts will be made to remove the poison from the system. Once a patient is stabilized (given fluids, oxygen, or treatment for seizures, for example) decontamination of the patient, or in other words, removal of the poison is attempted. If the skin is exposed to a toxin, clothes are removed and the patient showers or is washed, and after exposure to the eyes, the eyes are flushed with copious amounts of water.

decontaminate To rid of contamination, as in toxic exposures or drug overdoses.

After swallowing a poison, decontamination is accomplished by emptying the stomach. Either gastric lavage (a procedure used to wash out the contents of the stomach), or administration of syrup of ipecac is standard practice for removing toxins that are swallowed. Syrup of ipecac induces vomiting, and is only useful when used early, ideally within an hour of the poisoning. It is not used if the victim has swallowed caustic material or pe-

gastric lavage A procedure used to empty the stomach of its contents, especially in the treatment of ingestions of toxins or drugs.

troleum distillates. In the past, parents of young children were encouraged to keep syrup of ipecac in the home in case of overdose. The more current thinking is that gastric lavage is preferable because ongoing vomiting can delay the use of activated charcoal.

Use of activated charcoal (Actidose®) is a very important method of decontaminating the GI tract. It can be used alone or after gastric lavage. Activated charcoal works by binding the poison, but has no pharmacologic activity of its own to complicate the care of the patient. Activated charcoal is mixed with water to form a charcoal slurry, which is then swallowed. Charcoal slurries are gritty and unpleasant looking and tasting. Quite often the slurry is administered through a nasogastric tube to avoid the challenge of trying to get a child to swallow the mixture in the necessary quantities. Other therapies used to remove a toxin from the GI tract include use of cathartics, such as polyethylene glycol or magnesium citrate. If the patient cannot be adequately treated with decontamination and supportive therapy alone, specific antidotes to the poison may be used.

## Antidotes

The majority of poison exposures can be effectively treated by removing as much of the toxin as possible and preventing further absorption through the use of activated charcoal. When a patient is exposed to a large dose of toxin, or there is considerable delay in the time to treatment, the use of an antidote may be necessary. Some poisons require immediate reversal or treatment with antidotes, either because they are extremely toxic, work very quickly, or because reversing agents are readily available and safe to use. According to the American Association of Poison Control Centers, the most commonly used antidotes are acetylcysteine (Mucomyst®), naloxone (Narcan®), atropine, deferoxamine (Desferal®), and antivenins. **Table 35.1** lists the antidotes, the toxins for which they are given, and how quickly they need to be administered.

### Indications and Administration

Some antidotes are direct antagonists of the drug or compound that caused the poisoning. They work by preferentially attaching to the target receptors to prevent stimulation by the toxin or overdosed drug. The direct antagonists include atropine, naloxone, and flumazenil (Romazicon®). Other antidotes work less directly, for example by binding to the toxin in question to neutralize it, by causing an opposing pharmacologic effect, or by affecting metabolism of the toxin. Pralidoxime (Protopam®), physostigmine (Antilirium®), and calcium gluconate are examples of drugs that work indirectly.

Atropine is indicated for overdoses with drugs or toxic substances that elevate acetylcholine levels, including the cholinesterase inhibitors, and organophosphates. Some insecticides, such as ethyl parathion and malathion, are organophosphates. A few, highly toxic mushroom species are stimulants of muscarinic cholinergic receptors, and atropine is used to treat ingestion of these mushrooms, as well. Atropine binds to acetylcholine receptors in the peripheral nervous system (muscarinic receptors) to prevent the effects of excessive receptor stimulation from acetylcholine or cholinergic substances. Atropine is preferably administered intravenously, early in the treatment of the toxicity. Pralidoxime has anticholinergic effects through an indirect mechanism. It is given IV to treat organophosphate poisoning because it can reactivate cholinesterase following inactivation by these insecticides. By rejuvenating the enzyme, breakdown of excess accumulated acetylcholine can proceed. Pralidoxime is always used with atropine in organophosphate poisoning. Pralidoxime is also indicated for anticholinesterase overdoses.

Physostigmine is used to reverse atropine or other anticholinergic poisoning. Physostigmine blocks the action of cholinesterase, thereby increasing the levels of acetylcholine in the synapse. It is administered by IM or IV injection. Additional information about physostigmine and atropine is available in Chapter 5.

The flow of calcium through channels in cardiac tissue is important to the electrical activity of the heart. Calcium channel blockers work by partially blocking this flow in order to reduce the excitability of this tissue. In overdose situations, these drugs dramatically re-

**Table 35.1** The Most Commonly Used Antidotes, Their Indications, and Routes of Administration

| Antidote Name | For reversal of | Administration/Notes |
|---|---|---|
| Acetylcysteine (Mucomyst®) | Acetaminophen | Orally, within 2 hours of poisoning if possible, but no more than 8 hours after. Give for next 72 hours. Keep adequate supplies. |
| Activated charcoal (Actidose®, others) | All orally ingested poisons | Given as slurry mixed with sorbitol or water. Pharmacy must keep adequate supply. Used first, not a true antidote. |
| Atropine | Cholinesterase inhibitors, organophosphates, some poisonous mushrooms | IV boluses, within 2 hours of exposure, if possible. IV infusion until stable, if necessary. |
| Calcium EDTA (Calcium disodium Versenate®) | Lead | IV or IM, dose based on blood lead levels, given over several days. Drug depletes iron and zinc. |
| Calcium gluconate | Calcium channel blockers | IV, if cardiovascular symptoms occur. |
| Cyanide antidote kit: amyl nitrite, sodium nitrite, & sodium thiosulfate | Cyanide | Immediate—Amyl nitrite, inhaled; then sodium nitrite IV; then sodium thiosulfate IV. |
| Deferoxamine mesylate (Desferal®) | Iron intoxication | Acute toxicity, IM preferred but may be given slow IV. SC or IM for chronic iron overload. |
| Digoxin Fab (Digibind®) | Digoxin | IV infusion; dose based on nature of overdose, degree of toxicity |
| Dimercaprol (BAL in oil®) | Arsenic, gold, mercury, lead | Deep IM injection, begin as early as possible after basic support initiated. |
| Flumazenil (Romazicon®) | Benzodiazepines | IV, after patient stabilized. May require repeated doses. |
| Glucagon | Insulin, hypoglycemia | SC, IM, IV, as soon as possible. Emergency kits available for home use. |
| Ipecac syrup | Oral ingestions—induces vomiting | Not a true antidote. Orally, within 30 minutes of ingestion. May cause excessive vomiting & treatment delay. Use no longer encouraged. |
| Methylene Blue | Methemoglobinemia due to nitrites, other toxins | IV in low doses, converts methemoglobin back to Hgb to increase ability to carry oxygen. |
| Naloxone (Narcan®) | Opioids | Immediate, IV. Used routinely in respiratory depression if poison is unknown. |
| Physostigmine (Antilirium®) | Anticholinergic agents | IM or IV, used early in treatment |
| Pralidoxime (Protopam®) | Cholinesterase inhibitors, organophosphates | IV injection, within 2 hours if possible |
| Protamine | Heparin | IV, as soon as possible |
| Sodium Bicarbonate | Aid to removal of some toxins | IV infusion, if need determined. Not a true antidote. |
| Vitamin K (AquaMEPHYTON®) | Warfarin | Oral or IV, depends on overdose, lab work |

duce electrical activity, resulting in a slow heart rate and hypotension that is especially dangerous to children. Calcium gluconate, in high doses, can be used to overcome the effects of the calcium channel blocking drugs. It works indirectly, to create a concentration gradient that forces calcium ion into cells. When administered in adequate doses, calcium improves cardiac and blood pressure status in patients who have overdosed on calcium channel blockers.

Naloxone and flumazenil are indicated for narcotic overdoses and benzodiazepine overdoses, respectively. Because naloxone has no intrinsic pharmacologic activity, it is routinely administered to patients who have respiratory depression due to an unknown cause. Naloxone has a short half-life, and must be repeated until the causative substance is cleared from the body. Flumazenil is also safe, but is used less frequently because benzodiazepines are less likely to be the cause of serious toxicity or respiratory depression.

Other antidotes work by binding or chelating the substance in question. Toxic metals, such as lead, mercury, arsenic, gold, or excessive iron are removed by chelating agents. Dimercaprol (BAL in Oil®) is given by IM injection, and acts by forming complexes with arsenic, mercury, and gold. It is the drug of choice in these poisonings and for lead poisoning. In lead poisoning, it is used along with calcium disodium edetate (Calcium EDTA®, or calcium disodium Versenate®), which is administered intravenously. Deferoxamine, given IV or IM, is used for acute iron toxicity or chronic iron overload.

chelate To form a complex chemical compound in which a metallic ion is bound into a stable ring structure; chelates are not absorbable through the GI tract.

Protamine and digoxin immune Fab (DigiFab®, Digibind®) likewise bind to their target drugs to neutralize them. Protamine, which is strongly basic, binds to the acidic anticoagulant heparin, to reverse heparin related bleeding. Digoxin immune Fab is fragments of antibody to digoxin, and it is used to treat both acute and chronic overdoses. The antibody binds to the digoxin, which prevents it from binding to receptors, and allows for elimination through the kidneys. The dose of the antidote differs for acute or chronic overdoses.

Some antidotes prevent the production or block the action of toxic metabolites. Acetaminophen, which is one of the top causes of poisoning in the United States, produces toxic metabolites that can destroy the liver and acetylcysteine reduces the extent of the damage done by these toxins. Acetylcysteine can be diluted in diet cola and given orally or be injected intravenously, but it must be given as soon as possible after the ingestion. The dose and duration of treatment is based on acetaminophen blood levels, but an average sized adult who is poisoned can easily require treatment with forty 10 mL vials of 20% acetylcysteine. Having an adequate supply of this medication, either on hand or readily accessible, is vitally important for any hospital with an emergency department.

Methylene blue, in low doses, converts methemoglobin, which cannot carry oxygen, back to hemoglobin in the red blood cells. Methemoglobinemia can occur as a result of nitrite therapy used in the treatment of cyanide toxicity. Methylene blue is given IV for treatment of acute methemoglobinemia. Although cyanide exposure is uncommon, it is very toxic and acts quickly. Hospitals with emergency rooms should carry cyanide kits, which contain sodium nitrite and sodium thiosulfate as antidotes to this substance.

Lastly, some drugs are used to treat symptoms of poisonings or to increase the rate of removal of the toxins. Included in this category are the benzodiazepines, which are used to treat seizures if they occur, oxygen, which may be used in respiratory depression or carbon monoxide poisoning, or sodium bicarbonate, which aids in the removal of some substances through the kidneys and can reverse abnormal metabolic states caused by acidic drugs.

## Risks of Antidote Use

Although all antidotes are lifesaving when used appropriately, many are inherently dangerous. For this reason, health professionals are advised to contact a poison control center before using any antidotes. Cyanide kits for example, although lifesaving, can cause methemoglobinemia, which will itself require treatment.

Use of naloxone and flumazenil is very safe in acute overdoes in nonaddicted patients. Neither drug has significant intrinsic activity. However, use of either drug can precipitate withdrawal when given to patients addicted to benzodiazepines (flumazenil) or narcotics (naloxone). Withdrawal syndromes occur because these reversal agents are so effective at blocking their respective receptors that they cause a state akin to complete (although temporary) removal of the addictive drug. Atropine, pralidoxime, and physostigmine are intrinsically active and will cause symptoms of either cholinergic deficit (atropine and pralidoxime) or cholinergic excess (physostigmine).

Use of the chelating agents may be associated with significant toxicity. Dimercaprol consistently causes an increase in blood pressure and tachycardia that are dose related. If the urine is not alkalinized, the dimercaprol-metal complexes, which are toxic, can break down in the kidneys and cause kidney failure. Other chelating agents may likewise cause a fall in blood pressure, cardiac arrhythmias, and very serious kidney damage. Nausea, vomiting, headache, and neurological changes may occur as a result of treatment with these drugs.

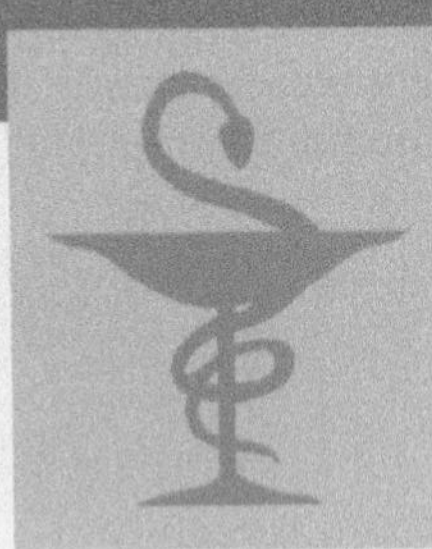

## Tips for the Technician

The use of antidotes and drugs for acute poisonings is most likely to occur in large hospitals with busy emergency rooms. It is the job of the technician in these facilities to be sure that the antidotes are stocked in adequate quantities, are fresh, and readily available for emergencies when they occur. The pharmacy and therapeutics committee in the hospital determines which antidotes to carry. Many small hospitals carry less than needed amounts of antidotes, and rely on arrangements with other area hospitals to borrow the rest of the drug to complete therapy. The thinking is that while the initial dose is administered, the rest of the drug needed can be borrowed. Although this may reduce waste, it is an unreliable system and is discouraged.

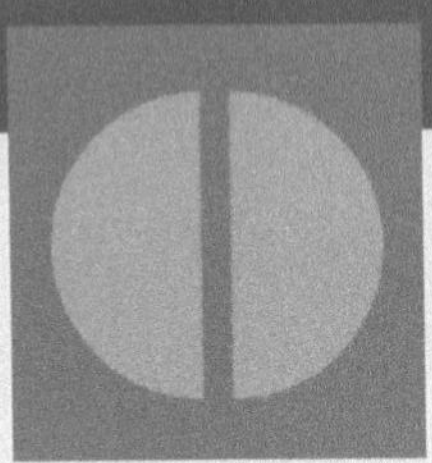

## Case 35.1

Florissa Pham was excited about her third month of work as a pharmacy technician at Sleepy Hollow Children's Hospital. Things were going very well, and her boss liked the fact that she had learned and was following pharmacy policies. She was in the process of pulling the medication for the refill of the automated drug dispensing cabinet when she received a call from the emergency room. The ER nurse, Tom Gunn, said they were out of flumazenil and requested that Florissa deliver some right away. "Not a problem," she said, "just fax over a floor stock requisition and I'll get some to you as soon as I can."

"A floor stock requisition, you've got to be kidding!" snapped Tom.

"No," replied Florissa, "I'm not—that is pharmacy policy."

"This is a fine time to start enforcing policies," Nurse Gunn fired back at her as he slammed down the telephone.

Moments later Florissa's boss flew out of her office. "Florissa, take four vials of Romazicon® down to the ER right now, then report back to my office."

"Yes, ma'am." As Florissa ran down to the emergency room, she realized she was in trouble and wondered what she had done wrong. Where was Florissa's mistake, and how could she have avoided it?

# Common Envenomations and Their General Treatment

Envenomation is the act of injecting venom by a bite or sting. In North America, there are about 20 species of poisonous snakes, out of more than 170 snake species. The two groups of spiders most likely to cause envenomations in the United States are Latrodectus (the widow spiders) and Loxosceles genus (which includes the brown recluse spider), although other spiders can cause painful bites. Although frightening and possibly painful, the vast majority of envenomations that occur in the United Sates, whether from snakes or spiders, are treated successfully and resolve without significant damage.

All but one (the coral snake) of the poisonous snakes found in the United States are members of the subfamily Crotalidae, also known as the pit vipers. This group includes the rattlesnakes, cottonmouth, and copperhead. The venom of the Crotalidae is comprised mainly of enzymes. When a member of the Crotalidae family bites an adult, the major risk is local tissue destruction. The coral snake (Micrurus fulvius) is a member of the family Elapidae. Coral snake venom contains neurotoxins, and a coral snake bite is more dangerous than that of the pit vipers. Before the advent of coral snake antivenin, only about twenty percent of coral snakebites were fatal. Now, with improving methods of treatment and the availability of antivenom, death from the bite of any native snake species in the United States is exceedingly rare. Estimates are that there are about 5 to 10 deaths due to snakebite annually, as compared with about 16 deaths due to dog bites each year. The four types of poisonous snakes found in the United States are pictured in **Fig. 35.2**.

Death from spider bite is also rare. In fact no deaths from spider bites were reported from 1989 to 1993. It is likely that fewer than 3 people die in the United States every year from spider bites, as compared with the more than 80 people who die each year from lightening strikes. Spider bites are of greatest concern in the very young or the elderly. Black widow spider venom contains neurotoxins, and brown recluse spider venom, for which there is no antivenin, causes tissue necrosis. Although widow spiders can be found all over the United States, the brown recluse is only found from Iowa south, and east to Georgia.

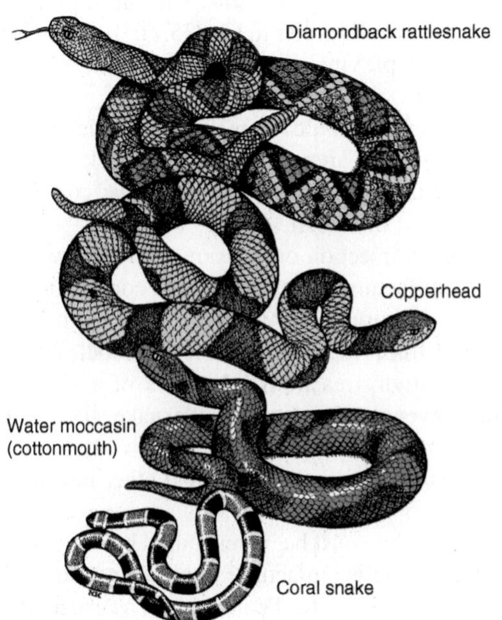


**Figure 35.2** The four types of poisonous snakes found in the United States. (Courtesy of Neil O. Hardy, Westpoint, CT.)

## Antivenins

Antivenins are biological products used to treat envenomations. When a small amount of the desired venom is injected into a horse or other large animal, the animal will mount an immune response and produce antibodies to the venom. The antibodies are harvested from the bloodstream of the animal and purified. The resulting antivenin preparation must meet international standards of purity and potency.

### Indication and Administration

The scientists of the Pasteur Institute developed the first antivenin in the 1890s, to be used against the bite of the Indian Cobra. The concept upon which antivenin is based is the same as that of passive immunity. The person who receives the antibodies never personally develops antibodies to the toxin or venom, but rather borrows temporary immunity from the host animal. Antivenin antibodies exert their effect by binding to the venom, thereby neutralizing and preparing it for removal from the body. Antivenins are either monovalent, containing antibodies to only one species, or polyvalent, containing antibodies to several species. Crotalidae antivenin is polyvalent, and contains antibodies to any of the rattlesnakes of North America, while coral snake antivenin is monovalent.

A large majority of snake or spider bites are made by nonvenomous species, and these bites obviously should not be treated with antivenin. Therefore, it is very important for patients to identify what bit them, whenever they can. Victims should try to remember color patterns, or when possible, take a digital snapshot from a safe distance of the animal in question.

Identification of snakes can be difficult, because the coloring of many harmless snake species resembles that of poisonous snakes. Gopher snakes, for example, have coloration very similar to rattlesnakes, and can coil and strike in a way similar to that of rattlesnakes. These animals are not only harmless, but also quite beneficial. The pit vipers, or rattlesnakes, are widely distributed across North America and are identified by the diamond shape of the head, pits on either side of the head where the heat-sensing organs are located, and the narrowed neck. Rattles on the snake are also proof that the snake is poisonous, but rattles are not always present. If a bite is known to be from a pit viper the decision to use antivenin, and the dose used, is based on an assessment of the degree of envenomation. Up to 20% of documented snakebites from rattlesnakes deliver no venom whatsoever.

Coral snakes are limited in their range, and occur naturally only in the South and the Southwest of the United States. The king snake and the milk snake can look very similar to coral snakes, however coral snakes always have red stripes against whitish to yellow stripes in a banding pattern of red-yellow-black-yellow-red (refer to Fig. 35.2). Because the bite of the coral snake is more toxic than that of the pit vipers, antivenin is routinely used after a coral snakebite.

Black widow spider antivenin is rarely indicated for adults. Some experts believe that all infants or small children should receive the antivenin after a documented black widow spider bite. Others believe that the risk incurred from the use of a product that contains horse serum is significantly more dangerous than the bite itself.

Antivenin is administered by slow intravenous injection or infusion after determination of prior exposure to antivenin products. Manufacturers of products that contain horse serum recommend that patients be tested for sensitivity before the product is used. The newer Crotalidae antivenin (CroFab®) is derived from fragments of sheep antibodies, and is consequently less likely to cause serious sensitivity reactions. The dose of antivenin needed for snakebite varies, but for a moderate envenomation from a rattlesnake, six to ten vials are typically used. Coral snakebites are routinely treated with three to six vials, but up to ten vials may be needed. The available antivenins, their indications, and other information is presented in **Table 35.2**.

Antivenins are provided as lyophilized powder that must be reconstituted before injection with the diluent included or recommended by the manufacturer. Antivenins must be refrigerated. After reconstitution, antivenin is further diluted for IV infusion. The exception is black widow spider antivenin, which may be administered intramuscularly or intravenously, because the total dose is usually limited to one vial.

**Table 35.2** The Available Antivenins, Their Indications, and Methods of Administration

| Generic Name | For Treatment of | Administration/Notes |
|---|---|---|
| Antivenin, lactrodectus mactans, equine origin | Black widow spider bites in few patients | Refrigerate. May give IM or IV after test dose. |
| Antivenin, crotalidae, equine origin | Rattlesnake, copperhead or cotton-mouth bites. Use based on degree of envenomation. | Refrigerate. Give test dose, then by IV infusion. |
| Antivenin, crotalidae immune fab, ovine origin (CroFab®) | Rattlesnake, copperhead, or cotton-mouth bites. Use based on degree of envenomation. | Refrigerate. Give by IV infusion. |
| Antivenin, micrurus fulvius, equine origin | Confirmed coral snake bite | Refrigerate. Give test dose, then IV injection or infusion. |

## Risks of Antivenin Use

The only adverse reaction attributable to use of antivenin is hypersensitivity, but these reactions can be life threatening. Immediate reactions of flu-like syndrome, including nausea, headache, and chills, can be minimized by slowing the antivenin infusion. Very serious allergic reactions, including anaphylaxis, can occur. Hospital personnel monitor these patients very closely as they receive antivenin, and antihistamines such as diphenhydramine, and epinephrine must be kept readily available to treat serious allergic reactions.

Serum sickness is a late allergic reaction that occurs as a result of treatment with animal serum proteins. This late form of allergic reaction can occur from a few days to 3 weeks after administration of horse or sheep serum. Symptoms of serum sickness include fever, hives, joint pain, swollen lymph nodes, nausea and vomiting, and malaise. Serum sickness is treated with antihistamines, antipyretics, and sometimes corticosteroids.

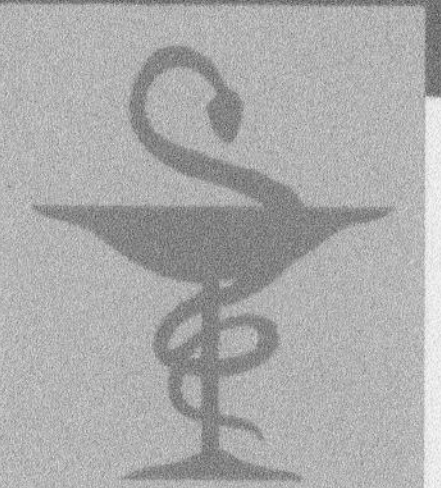

### Tips for the Technician

The challenge for technicians who deal with antivenin is to keep an adequate supply of fresh antivenin in stock, without breaking the pharmacy budget. Antivenin is expensive, and does not have a particularly long shelf life. It is not unusual for these products to be unavailable from the manufacturer, sometimes for long periods of time. These factors make the appropriate storage and reconstitution of antivenin all the more important. All antivenins are stored in the refrigerator before use. Because these products are made of antibody proteins, they should not be vigorously shaken during reconstitution. They can be rolled between the palms or swirled to aid in dissolution. Once reconstituted, antivenin should be used fairly quickly. Stability after reconstitution varies by the product and can be confirmed by checking in the package insert.

# Review Questions

## Multiple Choice

Choose the best answer for the following questions:

1. Which of the following is not a measure that will make a home more poison proof?
   a. Keep the telephone number of the local poison center on each telephone.
   b. Use child proof latches on cupboards that contain toxins.
   c. Show young children how to open their own multivitamin bottles.
   d. Teach children that only parents can handle medications or other dangerous substances.
   e. Properly store cleaning agents, chemicals, or pesticides out of reach of children.

2. Which of the following are general measures used in the treatment of oral poison ingestions?
   a. Identify the poison
   b. Remove the poison with gastric lavage
   c. Administer activated charcoal
   d. b and c
   e. a, b, and c

3. Circle the letter that corresponds to the antidote that works by chelation
   a. Deferoxamine
   b. Atropine
   c. Digibind®
   d. Activated charcoal
   e. Methylene blue

4. Of the following, which is a risk associated with naloxone administration?
   a. Inherent narcotic agonist activity of naloxone may further depress respiration
   b. Naloxone administration can induce withdrawals in addicts
   c. Excess CNS stimulation is associated with naloxone use
   d. Naloxone can cause nausea and constipation
   e. All of the above

5. When is coral snake antivenin administration indicated?
   a. Whenever a coral snake envenomation is verified
   b. Only in children weighing less than 100 pounds
   c. Only when elderly people or children are bitten
   d. In patients with documented snakebite who have not received antivenin before
   e. None of the above

## True/False

6. Every year, poison centers across the United States receive hundreds of thousands of calls and more than half of them are regarding poison exposures in children under six.
   a. True
   b. False

7. In up to 20% of documented rattlesnake bites, there is no envenomation.
   a. True
   b. False

8. Brown recluse spider venom is available as powder for reconstitution and can be given IM or IV.
   a. True
   b. False

9. Because Tylenol® overdose is common and requires large quantities of acetylcysteine for treatment, it is important to keep adequate supplies of the antidote on hand, especially in a large hospital with a busy emergency room.
   a. True
   b. False

10. The most important identifying characteristic of rattlesnakes and coral snakes is their unique coloration, which cannot be confused with any other snakes.
   a. True
   b. False

## Matching

For numbers 11 to 15, match the toxin with the correct lettered antidote from the list below. Choices will not be used more than once and may not be used at all.

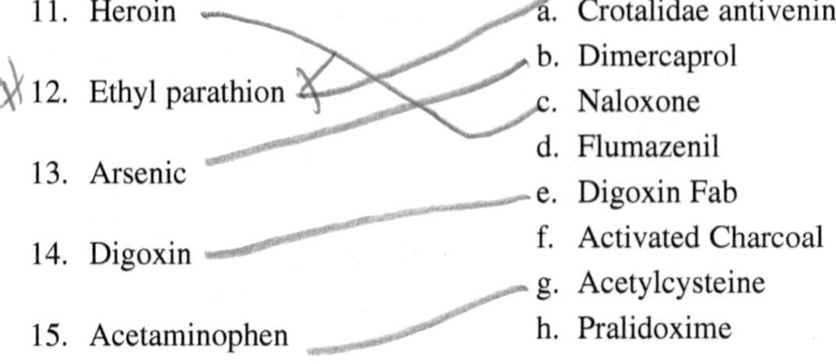

| | |
|---|---|
| 11. Heroin | a. Crotalidae antivenin |
| | b. Dimercaprol |
| 12. Ethyl parathion | c. Naloxone |
| | d. Flumazenil |
| 13. Arsenic | e. Digoxin Fab |
| | f. Activated Charcoal |
| 14. Digoxin | g. Acetylcysteine |
| 15. Acetaminophen | h. Pralidoxime |

## Short Answer

16. Besides the necessary quantities of antivenin, what other drugs must be kept in readiness when antivenin is used to treat snakebite, and why?

17. What two products are used for decontamination of the gut in oral ingestions of poisons but are not specific antidotes? Briefly describe how each is used, and list a drawback to the use of each product.

18. What legislation, enacted in the 1970s, dramatically reduced the rate of death from accidental poisonings in toddlers?

19. Define the term poisoning and describe the extent of the problem of poisoning in the United States.

20. What nonpoisonous species might be confused with rattlesnakes and coral snakes, and how might a snakebite victim know the difference?

## FOR FURTHER INQUIRY

Some poison control centers hire pharmacy technicians as staff members. Find out where the closest poison center in your area is located and how they staff the center. If pharmacy technicians are on staff there, find out in what capacity they are employed. If the center is reasonably close by and they allow visitors, plan a visit to the site to see how it operates.

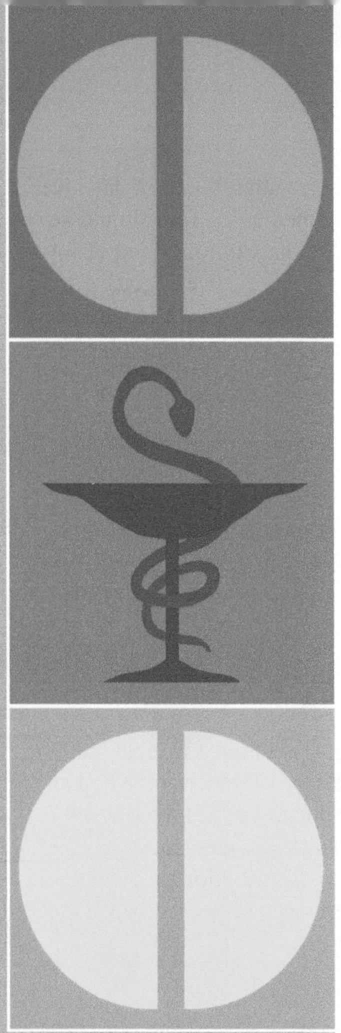

# Appendix A • Answers to Case Studies

## Case 1.1

It is important for pharmacy technicians to ask the pharmacist if they are unsure of what medication to select to fill a prescription. In this case, since the technician knows from the prescription that the prescribed medication is used for blood pressure control, he or she can check one of the reference books in the pharmacy for clarification. Another important source of information is the patient profile. Perhaps the patient has taken the prescription before. Lastly, if no one in the pharmacy can decipher the prescription, the physician should be called.

## Case 2.1

There are a number of facts to consider in making a decision. Some of these factors include the willingness of the child to take the liquid medication and the ability of the parents to manage the frequent dosing, the pain and expense of an IM injection, and the risk to the child if the required treatment is not completed.

## Case 3.1

Because alcoholics often eat poorly, they are frequently malnourished. In this case, the pharmacist was wise to bring up this likelihood, because phenytoin is highly protein bound and must be used in lower doses when albumin levels are low to prevent toxicity. The drug serum levels required for therapeutic effect are also lower than normal in patients with low albumin levels. This is an example of the way pharmacists and physicians can work together to improve the outcomes of drug treatment.

## Cases 4.1 and 4.2

No answers necessary.

## Case 5.1

Alden was aware that pancuronium was not used outside of the OR, ICU, or ER in his hospital, and he did not believe that it was usually used for agitation. He decided not to give the nurse the medications. To expedite Mrs. Windham's pain relief, he checked to see if there was morphine in floor stock and paged the pharmacist to return to the pharmacy. Pancuronium may be used in people who are on mechanical ventilators and are fighting the actions of the ventilator, but never for typical agitation in unventilated patients. The original order was poorly written, and should have more clearly described the indication for use. It is no longer considered acceptable to write orders to "continue same medications" when transferring patients to other units, because often the orders have not been reexamined by the physician. Preprinted orders and policies requiring medication review and rewriting of all orders on transfer will prevent these problems. In this case, continuing the pancuronium when the patient is off of the mechanical ventilator would likely result in her death.

## Case 6.1

Tom was in quite a pickle, but needed to give some advice or support quickly because allergic reactions have rapid and dire consequences. Hopefully, Tom advised the mother to immediately give the injection, even if it was slightly out of date. He should ask the mother to have someone at the picnic call 911 immediately. Tom should get a telephone number for the mother, so the pharmacist can call her back to follow-up. A follow-up telephone call could prevent any undesirable liability consequences because the pharmacist can verify information given by the technician and answer any additional questions. Following this course of action puts the best interest of the patient first and improves the odds that the only fireworks are at the picnic!

## Case 7.1

Local anesthetics appropriate for injection into the area around the spinal cord must be preservative free, and therefore can be used only once. Try to diffuse the issue by assuring the surgical technician that you will bring the lidocaine just as soon as it is checked, and then page the pharmacist and explain the situation. You are not allowed to dispense any medication without the pharmacist's check.

## Case 8.1

Any time there is an adverse result of drug therapy, there is a potential for legal action against care providers by the patient involved. For this reason, it is very important that pharmacy personnel fulfill all legal and ethical responsibilities, and document that these responsibilities have been fulfilled. Even though the pharmacist bears the ultimate legal and clinical responsibility to inform the patient about the risks of taking prescription medications, it is the ethical responsibility of technicians to support that effort so that patients receive the best pharmaceutical care at all times.

## Case 9.1

It is important for all technicians to know which medications might be used in emergencies. In this situation, Nurse Poppy was involved in treating a patient who was overdosed. Remember, the effects of naloxone last for a shorter period of time than most narcotics. Waiting to refill the automated dispensing machines might result in the recurrence of overdose symptoms before the needed medication arrives. Although Nurse Poppy shares responsibility for poor communication, the informed technician is aware that naloxone is often used in emergencies. By asking the nurse more about her need ("Is this an emergency?" or "Do you have a patient you need this drug for now?") the technician will serve the patient better and stay out of trouble!

## Case 10.1

In a situation like this, honesty, an apology, and the quick correction of the error work wonders. Fortunately, it sounds as if no medication has been given yet. First, Dee needs to get back on the telephone and confirm that Betty gave no medication to her son. Then Dee should ask Mrs. Bohm to kindly hold on for one more moment while Dee gets the pharmacist. The pharmacist will apologize for the error, thank Mrs. Bohm for her call, and make arrangements to replace the prescription with the correct medication right away. Dee can prevent this kind of look-alike, sound-alike medication error from occurring by knowing more about the medication she is dispensing. Inderal is for high blood pressure. If she paid closer attention to the patient profile she would have known that Adam Bohm is an 8-year-old boy, not a likely candidate for an antihypertensive medication. Although the ultimate responsibility for the error belongs to the pharmacist, Dee needs to acquire the knowledge and follow the processes that help prevent medication errors.

## Case 11.1

A quick look at the label will reveal that the Tylenol® cold product contains a decongestant, pseudoephedrine. Pseudoephedrine is an adrenergic agonist and should not be taken with MAOI antidepressants. The Robitussin DM® contains dextromethorphan, which also interacts. Although you may be well aware of the drug interactions, as a technician you do not have the authority to advise Mrs. Blue. The appropriate response would be to explain that there may well be a problem, and she was correct to check before purchasing either product. Then get the pharmacist, who will advise Mrs. Blue that she can safely take plain Robitussin®, but neither of the products she selected would be safe for her to take with her present medication.

## Case 12.1

While you cannot give her advice regarding her grandmother, there is nothing unethical or illegal about guiding your friend to information sources she and her family can use to learn more about the recent concerns. Recommend that she speak to a respected pharmacist or physician, or suggest that she check the FDA web site. You can also help her find journal articles from your local library, or help her do an Internet search.

## Case 13.1

It is possible that the medication is not being shaken adequately. As the medication settles, the drug concentrates at the bottom. This would explain the higher degree of side effects at the bottom of the bottle. Phenytoin suspensions are especially prone to this problem. This problem can be corrected by vigorous agitation of the phenytoin before each dose is poured.

## Case 14.1

Assuming he has visited his physician about the new onset of chest pain, you can best assist your father by encouraging him to learn about cardiac risk factors at one of the web sites listed, or any number of other sites with information on cardiac risk factors. Consider which lifestyle changes would be the easiest for him to accomplish and which would reap the most benefit. Write up a prioritized approach and discuss your plan in class. Consider examining your own risk factors and lifestyle. If you are over 20 and know your cholesterol levels and blood pressure, you can find risk-assessment calculators for yourself on the Internet. It is never too early to get healthy! www.americanheart.org or www.ynhh.org/cardiac/risk/

## Case 15.1

Cora should reassure Mr. Harte that while it is not within her scope of practice to answer questions about drug side effects, she will make sure that the pharmacist speaks to him about his problem. Amiodarone is known to cause thyroid dysfunction and could be the cause of Mr. Harte's problem. Since his arrhythmia was only noted during surgery, it is possible that the amiodarone is no longer needed. The pharmacist should contact the MD regarding the potential adverse reaction and suggest that the physician consider discontinuing the amiodarone. Before Cora takes Mr. Harte's question to the pharmacist, she should determine whether the prescribing physician for the levothyroxine is the same doctor who prescribed Mr. Harte's other medicines. It will also be important to know if Mr. Harte still takes his medications as prescribed.

## Case 16.1

Mrs. Valentine is trying to stay on top of her nitroglycerin needs, which is good, but she is going about it in the wrong way. Nitroglycerin is not a very stable product, and should never be kept in the glove compartment of a car, because cars get hot. Obviously, she does not use the drug very often at her daughter's house, so there is some question about whether it would be effective when she needed it. In order to preserve stability, patients should be advised to open only one bottle of nitroglycerin at a time. If they keep it with them, tightly closed in a pocket or purse, it will be fresh and available wherever they go. If Mrs.

Valentine is using her nitroglycerin fairly regularly, it makes sense to have an *unopened* vial, stored in a cool, dry place, such as a hall closet or other cupboard, at her home.

## Case 17.1

The best way to make sure employees enter the correct instruction into the computer is to have preprogrammed order sets for them to choose from. If this isn't an option where you work, the next best way to prevent errors is through a double check system. You can improve the chances of accurate administration of the medication by filling three separately labelled prescription vials that are appropriately dated. The first prescription label will read "Take one (1) capsule every night at bedtime for four (4) nights, from (date) to (date)." The second label will read "Take two (2) capsules every night at bedtime for five days from (date) to (date)," and so on.

## Case 18.1

This is a good example of a missed opportunity for communication. Mrs. Sanger is aware that she should not take OTC medications without getting advice. But although Rosie knows Mrs. Sanger is a customer with prescription medication, she misinterprets Mrs. Sanger's query about whether the medications she wishes to purchase are okay (to use with her warfarin, we can assume). Warfarin is unique among prescription drugs for the number of potentially significant drug interactions that are possible, including in this case vitamin K, acetaminophen, ibuprofen, and possibly some component of the cough and cold preparation.

Technicians need to be aware of signals from patients indicating that they may have questions. If reading people is not your strength, routinely incorporate some simple questions into your customer interactions. When you know that a patient receives prescription medications from the pharmacy, you can ask, "Would you like me to check with the pharmacist to see if these products are okay for you to take with your prescriptions?" Otherwise ask, "Are there any questions about your medicines the pharmacist can answer for you?"

## Case 19.1

Minnie's mistake was in assuming that general fitness would take the place of training for the specific type of exercise she was about to undertake. Backpacking is very strenuous, especially for the calves and thighs, and it is done at an altitude where there is a noticeable drop in oxygen pressure in the air, while carrying excess weight. Minnie had lactic acid buildup in her legs, and as her friends suggested, moving increases blood flow to the legs and will facilitate removal of lactic acid.

## Case 20.1

There are a number of things you can do for Mrs. Burroughs. You can be a good listener, and you should offer her encouragement in her quest to quit smoking. Direct her to the variety of smoking cessation products you have available. Suggest some helpful sources of information to her, such as "stop smoking" help lines. If you know where to look, the Internet has some great information sources. In this case, the CDC, Foundation for a Smoke Free America, the American Cancer Association, and the American Academy of Family Physicians have helpful and informative web sites dedicated to quitting. Most importantly, put her in touch with the pharmacist, who can answer her questions in more detail.

## Case 21.1

The presence of the young girlfriend and her mother undoubtedly inhibited the flow of conversation in this situation. Rules regarding confidentiality are designed to protect confidentiality of records, but have the added benefit of making the health care worker think about how culture and environment affect conversations with patients. Clearly, this conversation should have occurred in private.

## Case 22.1

Maalox® Total Stomach Relief is not an antacid, but bismuth subsalicylate. The practice of using a well-known, popular brand name on a product that contains something completely different from the original drug is known as "brand name extension," and is becoming common. For example, the brand name Kaopectate® used to contain kaolin-pectin suspension used for diarrhea. Now Kaopectate® is bismuth subsalicylate suspension, and Kaopectate® capsules contain docusate, a stool softener! Technicians and customers need to be aware of this practice and read the label to be sure of what is inside. Ivana should direct Perry to the antacid section and explain which medications are antacids.

## Case 23.1

Acetaminophen is the antipyretic and analgesic most often given to children. Unfortunately, many parents are unaware that acetaminophen is found in many OTC products meant for children, that acetaminophen products contain different concentrations of the drug, or even that Tylenol® and acetaminophen are the same drug. Parents are unlikely to know about the serious nature of acetaminophen overdose. This lack of information has resulted in unintentional overdoses and liver toxicity in infants and children. The best course for Henry is to give her this information and then hand her questions regarding dose over to the pharmacist.

## Case 24.1

Until the recent epidemic of childhood obesity, type II diabetes was never seen in children. Type II diabetes occurs when the pancreas cannot produce enough insulin to keep up with the demand, either because too much sugar is consumed or the tissues become resistant to insulin. Diabetes can cause kidney failure, neuropathy, and blindness. Type II diabetes is almost always preventable when children and adults lead a healthy lifestyle. It is a parent's responsibility to assure that children eat a balanced, nutritious diet, and stay physically fit through regular exercise.

## Case 25.1

If you were Brian, you could inform your friend that a pediatric endocrinologist would be able to determine if her son is normal and short, or has growth hormone deficiency. It is appropriate to let her know that growth hormone is available to use in children who meet certain stature criteria, but that it is given by injection, and is very expensive. Find two reliable, science-based Internet sources of information that you might refer someone to in this case. Examples of reputable sites include eMedicine, American Academy of Family Physicians, and the Food and Drug Administration. These Internet sites are professional and consistently reliable sources of information. Web sites with lots of advertising or that encourage the viewer to buy drugs or remedies off of the website are likely to be less reliable or unreliable.

## Case 26.1

This case is very similar to one that really happened. It cannot be overemphasized to parents purchasing a glucagon kit that they read the directions in advance and practice giving their child injections. Glucagon is much more viscous than insulin, but practice drawing any liquid from a vial into a syringe will help family members be prepared in an emergency.

## Case 27.1

No answer necessary.

## Case 28.1

No answer necessary.

## Case 29.1

Tom could suggest that Misty save this drug for someone who really needs it for a serious infection. He could point out to Misty that a full course of penicillin VK is under $15 at most pharmacies, and less than that in some cases.

## Case 30.1

Because Mrs. Parson has bronchitis and developed seizures after taking ciprofloxacin, we can deduce that she was probably also taking theophylline. Ciprofloxacin significantly increases theophylline levels. We also know that Annie skipped through the drug interaction warnings. Although it is true that some drug interactions flagged by computer systems are deemed to be insignificant, this is a decision the pharmacist must make. If Annie had notified the pharmacist of the warning, she might have kept Mrs. Parson out of the hospital and would certainly have relieved herself of any legal liability. Unfortunately, Annie could be held liable for her actions.

## Case 31.1

When confusion between lipid-based and conventional amphotericin B occurs, results can be disastrous. In this situation, even if the woman in question weighed 220 pounds, the dose would be too high for conventional amphotericin. It is likely that one of the lipid-based drugs was intended, but the physician wrote an unclear order. The Institute for Safe Medication Practices recommends that prescribers order lipid-based amphotericin products by the brand names to prevent confusion. To prevent errors, experts recommend that hospitals avoid storing conventional and lipid-based products in close proximity. As a rule of thumb, technicians should be concerned any time they compound an IV with multiple vials of any one drug, but especially with amphotericin B. Undoubtedly, Marissa will stand her ground and have the IV checked before she releases it.

## Case 32.1

Hope made at least two errors in this case. Most importantly, she did not know the medication she was delivering and did not make an effort to check. This case exemplifies the importance of a basic understanding of pharmacology for the person who works with medication. Hope's ignorance of the dangers of this medication directly resulted in the exposure of others to a high-risk product. The ideal technician knows high-risk drugs, and special policies designed for their handling. The model technician takes steps to answer questions posed by their customers (in this case, the nurse), and if that is not possible, refers the question to the pharmacist. Of course the RCP shares a great deal of responsibility for this error, because he did not read the label.

## Case 33.1

Because the potential for mistaking one syringe for another always exists, many experts recommend compounding vincristine in a small volume IV bag, which everyone would recognize as not to be used for intrathecal injection. The overwrap should never be removed before the procedure, and the syringe for IV use should not be placed in the area where the lumbar puncture will occur. Many hospital procedures require the pharmacist to hand the drug directly to the physician, and the physician to take a "time out" to verify contents.

## Case 34.1

"When in doubt, throw it out" is the rule in pharmacy compounding. If Abel is at all uncertain about his compounding, he should put aside concerns about his time, or the costs of ingredients, and start over. The Golden Rule, with a pharmacy twist, also applies. "Do not do unto others, what you would not have others do unto yourself." In other words, if you make a product that you would not be willing to use on yourself if you were the patient, then do not send it out to be used on anyone else. The patient's safety should always be your first concern.

## Case 35.1

Florissa fell into a common trap. First of all, she probably didn't learn the names and uses of drugs that are considered antidotes or are used in emergency situations. If she had, she would have realized that the ER nurse might be involved with the treatment of a drug overdose. Although the nurse did not communicate his need succinctly, Florissa should have asked him if his request was for a patient or for floor stock. Remember, in emergency situations, paperwork is always secondary to patient care.

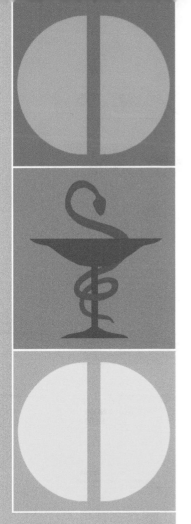

# Appendix B • **Auxiliary Prescription Labels**

Auxiliary prescription labels are affixed to the prescription container in the pharmacy. These labels are usually brightly colored to draw the patient's attention to the additional instructions contained there. Auxiliary labels may contain storage, administration, or side effect information, and are important tools to assure safe use of prescription medication. The labels contained here are some of the more commonly used auxiliary labels and include all of the labels referred to within the text.

Pharmex Original Copyrighted Warning Label information was printed with authorization by TimeMed Labeling Systems, Inc. for Medi-Dose®, Inc./EPS®, Inc.

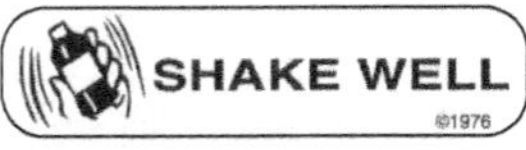


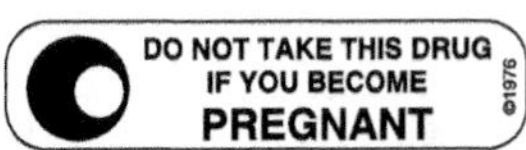


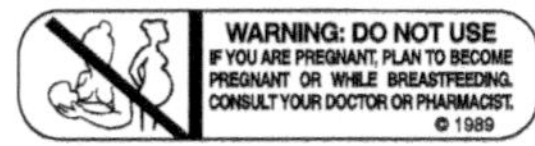


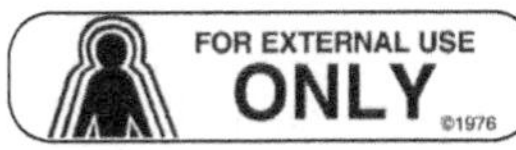


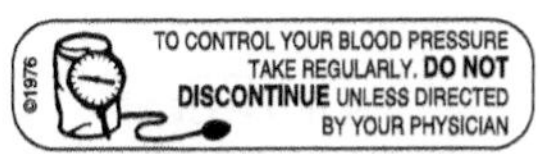


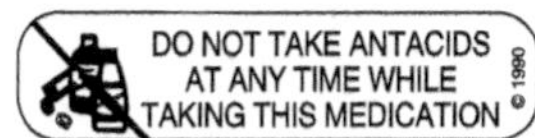


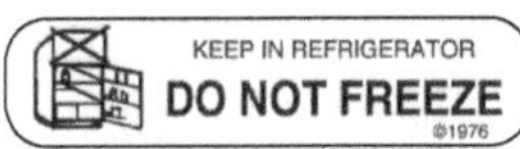


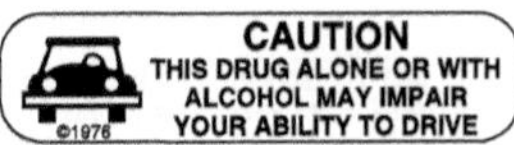


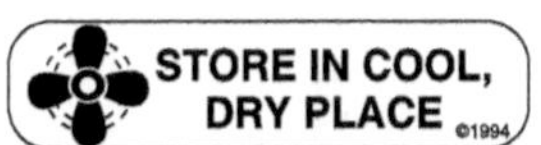


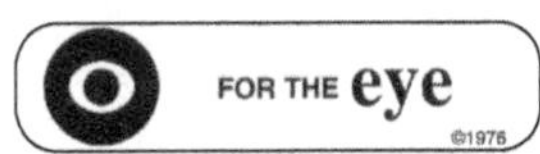


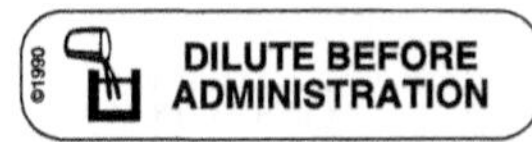


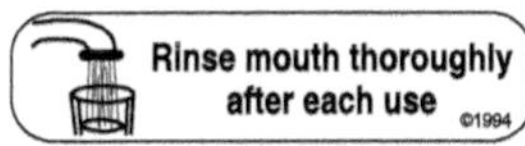


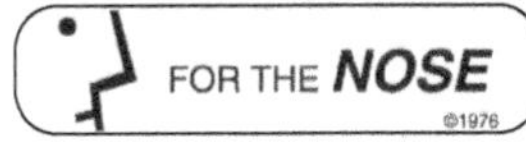


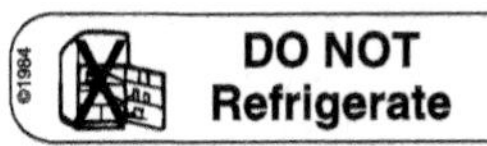


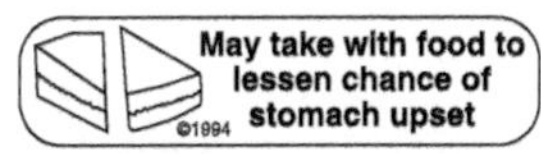


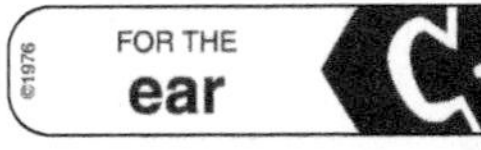


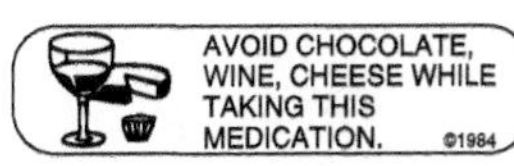


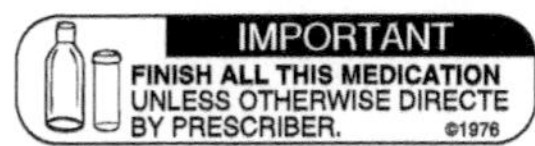


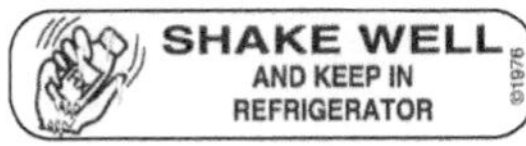


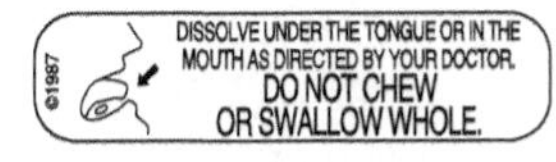


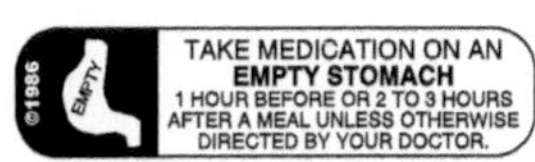


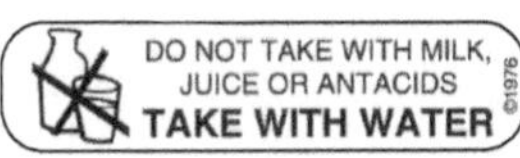


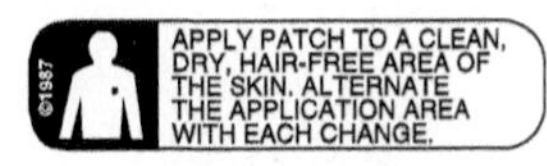


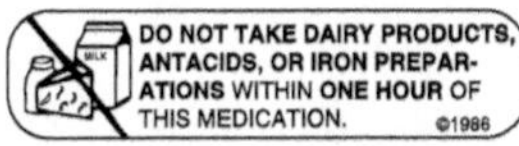


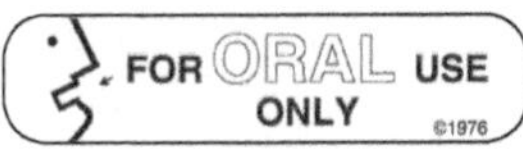


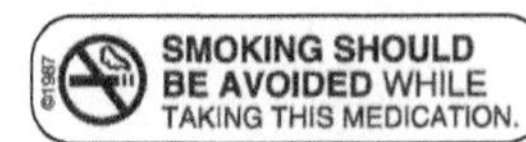


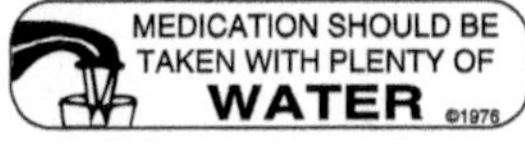


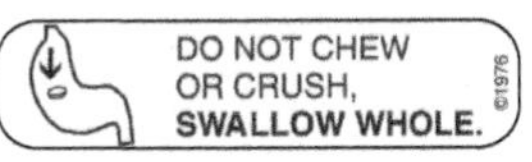


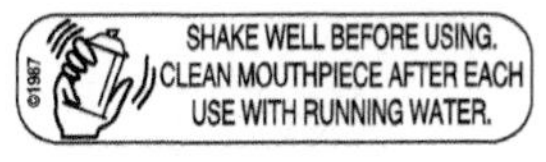


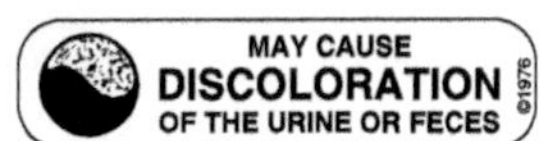

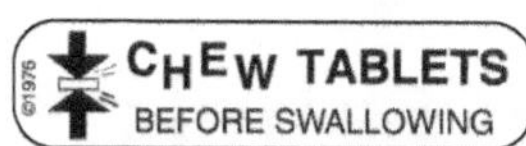
CHEW TABLETS
BEFORE SWALLOWING
©1976

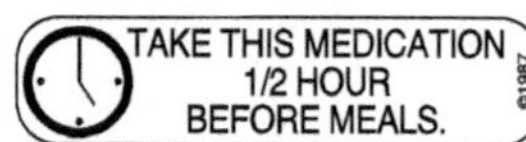
TAKE THIS MEDICATION
1/2 HOUR
BEFORE MEALS.
©1987

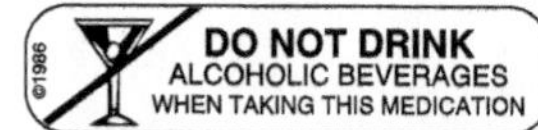
DO NOT DRINK
ALCOHOLIC BEVERAGES
WHEN TAKING THIS MEDICATION
©1986

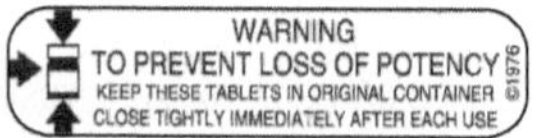
WARNING
TO PREVENT LOSS OF POTENCY
KEEP THESE TABLETS IN ORIGINAL CONTAINER
CLOSE TIGHTLY IMMEDIATELY AFTER EACH USE
©1976

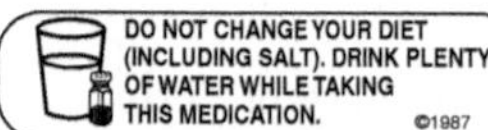
DO NOT CHANGE YOUR DIET
(INCLUDING SALT). DRINK PLENTY
OF WATER WHILE TAKING
THIS MEDICATION.
©1987

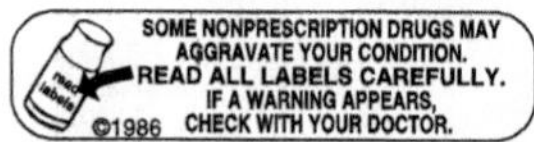
SOME NONPRESCRIPTION DRUGS MAY
AGGRAVATE YOUR CONDITION.
READ ALL LABELS CAREFULLY.
IF A WARNING APPEARS,
CHECK WITH YOUR DOCTOR.
©1986

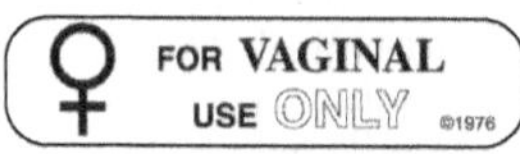
FOR VAGINAL
USE ONLY
©1976

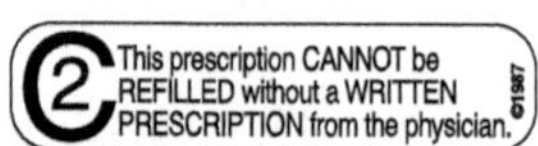
This prescription CANNOT be
REFILLED without a WRITTEN
PRESCRIPTION from the physician.
©1987

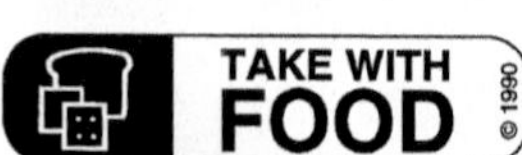
TAKE WITH
FOOD
©1990

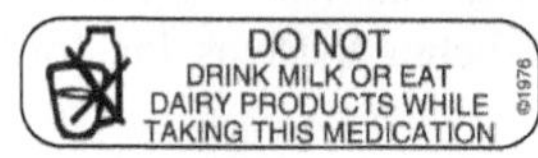
DO NOT
DRINK MILK OR EAT
DAIRY PRODUCTS WHILE
TAKING THIS MEDICATION
©1976

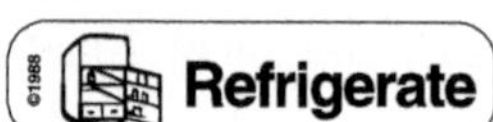
©1988
Refrigerate

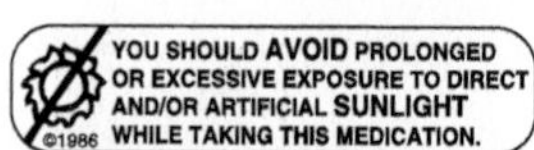
YOU SHOULD AVOID PROLONGED
OR EXCESSIVE EXPOSURE TO DIRECT
AND/OR ARTIFICIAL SUNLIGHT
WHILE TAKING THIS MEDICATION.
©1986

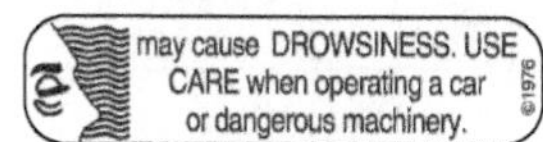
may cause DROWSINESS. USE
CARE when operating a car
or dangerous machinery.
©1976

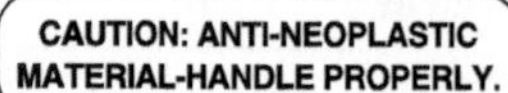
CAUTION: ANTI-NEOPLASTIC
MATERIAL-HANDLE PROPERLY.

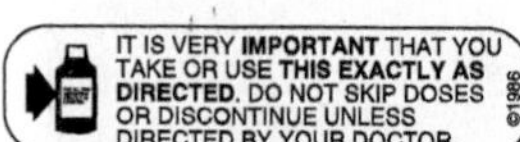
IT IS VERY IMPORTANT THAT YOU
TAKE OR USE THIS EXACTLY AS
DIRECTED. DO NOT SKIP DOSES
OR DISCONTINUE UNLESS
DIRECTED BY YOUR DOCTOR.
©1986

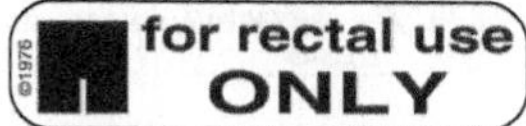
©1976
for rectal use
ONLY

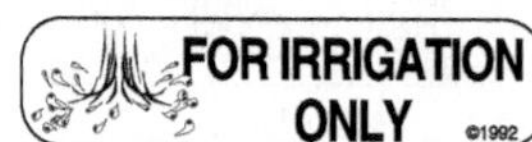
FOR IRRIGATION
ONLY
©1992

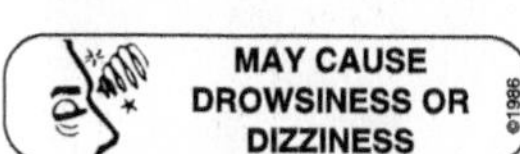
MAY CAUSE
DROWSINESS OR
DIZZINESS
©1986

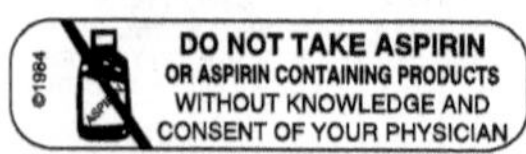
©1984
DO NOT TAKE ASPIRIN
OR ASPIRIN CONTAINING PRODUCTS
WITHOUT KNOWLEDGE AND
CONSENT OF YOUR PHYSICIAN

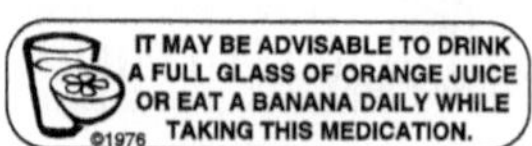
IT MAY BE ADVISABLE TO DRINK
A FULL GLASS OF ORANGE JUICE
OR EAT A BANANA DAILY WHILE
©1976
TAKING THIS MEDICATION.

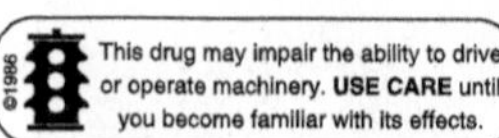
©1986
This drug may impair the ability to drive
or operate machinery. USE CARE until
you become familiar with its effects.

TAKE WITH
FOOD OR MILK
©1987

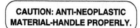

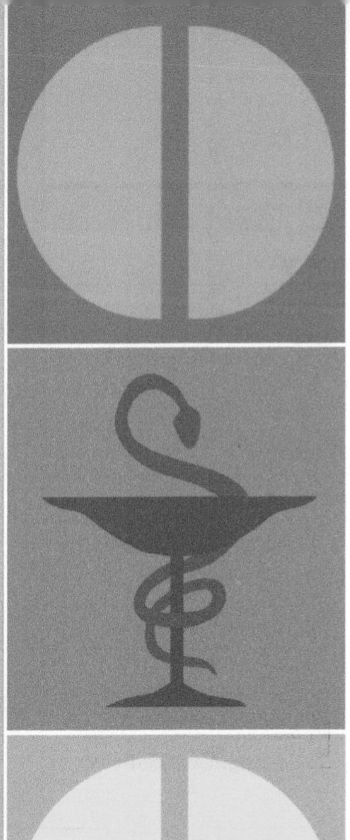
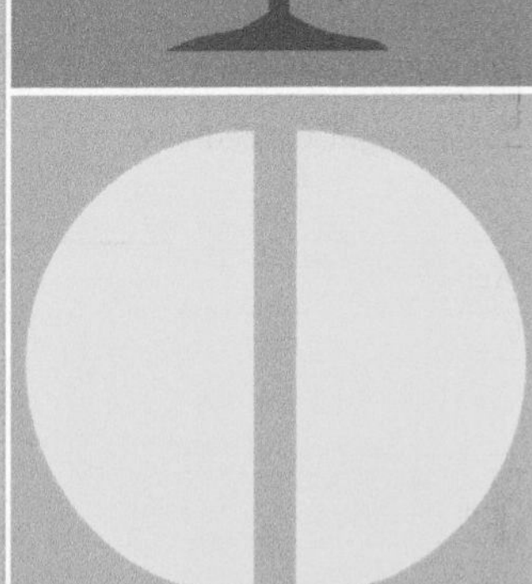

# Appendix C • **Error-Prone Drug Names and Abbreviations**

## ISMP's List of *Error-Prone Abbreviations, Symbols,* and *Dose Designations*

The abbreviations, symbols, and dose designations found in this table have been reported to ISMP through the USP-ISMP Medication Error Reporting Program as being frequently misinterpreted and involved in harmful medication errors. They should never be used when communicating medical information. This includes internal communications, telephone/verbal prescriptions, computer-generated labels, labels for drug storage bins, medication administration records, as well as pharmacy and prescriber computer order entry screens.

The Joint Commission on Accreditation of Healthcare Organizations (JCAHO) has established a National Patient Safety Goal that specifies that certain abbreviations must appear on an accredited organization's do-not-use list; we have highlighted these items with a double asterisk (**). However, we hope that you will consider others beyond the minimum JCAHO requirements. By using and promoting safe practices and by educating one another about hazards, we can better protect our patients.

| Abbreviations | Intended Meaning | Misinterpretation | Correction |
|---|---|---|---|
| µg | Microgram | Mistaken as "mg" | Use "mcg" |
| AD, AS, AU | Right ear, left ear, each ear | Mistaken as OD, OS, OU (right eye, left eye, each eye) | Use "right ear," "left ear," or "each ear" |
| OD, OS, OU | Right eye, left eye, each eye | Mistaken as AD, AS, AU (right ear, left ear, each ear) | Use "right eye," "left eye," or "each eye" |
| BT | Bedtime | Mistaken as "BID" (twice daily) | Use "bedtime" |
| cc | Cubic Centimeters | Mistaken as "u" (units) | Use "mL" |
| D/C | Discharge or discontinue | Premature discontinuation of medications if D/C (intended to mean "discharge") has beenmisinterpreted as "discontinued" when followed by a list of discharge medications | Use "discharge" and "discontinue" |
| IJ | Injection | Mistaken as "IV" or "intrajugular" | Use "injection" |
| IN | Intranasal | Mistaken as "IM" or "IV" | Use "intranasal" or "NAS" |
| HS<br>hs | Half-strength<br>At bedtime, hours of sleep | Mistaken as bedtime<br>Mistaken as half-strength | Use "half strength" or "bedtime" |
| IU** | International unit | Mistaken as IV (intravenous) or 10 (ten) | use "units" |
| o.d. or OD | Once daily | mistaken as "right eye" (OD-oculus dexter), leading to oral liquid medications administered in the eye | Use "daily" |
| OJ | Orange juice | Mistaken as OD or OS (right or left eye); drugs meant to be diluted in orange juice may be given in the eye | Use "orange juice" |
| Per os | By mouth, orally | the "os" can be mistaken as "left eye" (OS-oculus sinister) | Use "PO," "by mouth," or "orally" |
| q.d. or QD** | Every day | Mistaken as q.i.d., especially if the period after the "q" or the tail of the "q" is misunderstood as an "i" | Use "daily" |
| qhs | Nightly at bedtime | Mistaken as "qhr" or every hour | Use "nightly" |
| qn | Nightly or at bedtime | Mistaken as "qh" (every hour) | Use "nightly" or "at bedtime" |
| q.o.d. or QOD** | Every other day | Mistaken as "q.d." (daily) or "q.i.d." (four times daily) if the "o" is poorly written | Use "every other day" |
| q1d | Daily | Mistaken as q.i.d. (four times daily) | Use "daily" |
| q6PM, etc. | Every evening at 6 PM | Mistaken as every 6 hours | Use "6 PM nightly" or "6 PM daily" |
| SC, SQ, sub q | Subcutaneous | SC mistaken as SL (sublingual); SQ mistaken as "5 every;" the "q" in "sub q" has been mistaken as "every" (e.g., a heparin dose ordered "sub q 2 hours before surgery" misunderstood as every 2 hours before surgery) | Use "subcut" or "subcutaneously" |
| ss | Sliding scale (insulin) or ½ (apothecary) | Mistaken as "55" | Spell out "sliding scale;" use "one-half" or "1/2" |
| SSRI inhibitor | Sliding scale regular insulin | Mistaken as selective-serotonin reuptake | Spell out "sliding scale (insulin)" |
| SSI | Sliding scale insulin | Mistaken as Strong Solution of Iodine (Lugol's) | |
| i/d | One daily | Mistaken as "tid" | Use "1 daily" |
| TIW or tiw | 3 times a week | Mistaken as "3 times a day" or "twice in a week" | Use "3 times weekly" |
| U or u** | Unit | Mistaken as the number 0 or 4, causing a 10-fold overdose or greater (e.g., 4U seen as "40" or 4u seen as "44"); mistaken as "cc" so dose given in volume instead of units (e.g., 4u seen as 4cc) | Use "unit" |

(continues)

*(continued)*

| Dose Designations and Other Information | Intended Meaning | Misinterpretation | Correction |
|---|---|---|---|
| Trailing zero after decimal point (e.g., 1.0 mg)** | 1 mg | Mistaken as 10 mg if the decimal point is not seen | Do not use trailing zeros for doses expressed in whole numbers |
| "Naked" decimal point (e.g., .5 mg) | 0.5 mg | Mistaken as 5 mg if the decimal point is not seen | Use zero before a decimal point when the dose is less than a whole unit |
| Drug name and dose run together (especially problematic for drug names that end in "l" such as Inderal40 mg; Tegretol300 mg) | Inderal 40 mg<br>Tegretol 300 mg | Mistaken as Inderal 140 mg<br>Mistaken as Tegretol 1,300 mg | Place adequate space between the drug name, dose, and unit of measure |
| Numerical dose and unit of measure run together (e.g., 10mg, 100mL) | 10 mg<br>100 mL | The "m" is sometimes mistaken as a zero or two zeros, risking a 10- to 100-fold overdose | Place adequate space between the dose and unit of measure |
| Abbreviations such as mg. or mL. with a period following the abbreviation | mg<br>mL | The period is unnecessary and could be mistaken as the number 1 if written poorly | Use mg, mL, etc., without a terminal period |
| Large doses without properly placed commas (e.g., 100000 units; 1000000 units) | 100,000 units<br>1,000,000 units | 100000 has been mistaken as 10,000 or 1,000,000; 1000000 has been mistaken as 100,000 | Use commas for dosing units at or above 1,000, or use words such as one hundred thousand |

| Drug Name Abbrevations | Intended Meaning | Misinterpretation | Correction |
|---|---|---|---|
| ARA A | Vidarabine | Mistaken as cytarabine (ARA C) | Use complete drug name |
| AZT | Zidovudine (Retrovir) | Mistaken as azathioprine or aztreonam | Use complete drug name |
| CPZ | Compazine (prochlorperazine) | Mistaken as chlorpromazine | Use complete drug name |
| DPT | Demerol-phenergan-thorazine | Mistaken as diphtheria-pertussis-tetanus (vaccine) | Use complete drug name |
| DTO | Diluted tincture of opium or deodorized tincture of opium (Paregoric) | Mistaken as tincture of opium | Use complete drug name |
| HCl | Hydrochloric acid or hydrochloride | Mistaken as potassium chloride (The "H" is misinterpreted as "K") | Use complete drug name unless expressed as a salt of a drug |
| HCT | Hydrocortisone | Mistaken as hydrochlorothiazide | Use complete drug name |
| HCTZ | Hydrochlorothiazide | Mistaken as hydrocortisone (seen as HCT250 mg) | Use complete drug name |
| MgSO4** | Magnesium sulfate | Mistaken as morphine sulfate | Use complete drug name |
| MS, MS04** | Morphine sulfate | Mistaken as magnesium sulfate | Use complete drug name |
| MTX | Methotrexate | Mistaken as mitoxantrone | Use complete drug name |
| PCA | Procainamide | Mistaken as patient controlled analgesia | Use complete drug name |
| PTU | Propylthiouracil | Mistaken as mercaptopurine | Use complete drug name |
| T3 | Tylenol with codeine No. 3 | Mistaken as liothyronine | Use complete drug name |

*(continues)*

*(continued)*

| Drug Name Abbrevations | Intended Meaning | Misinterpretation | Correction |
|---|---|---|---|
| TAC | Triamcinolone | Mistaken as tetracaine, Adrenalin, cocaine | Use complete drug name |
| TNK | TNKase | Mistaken as "TPA" | Use complete drug name |
| ZnSO4 | Zinc sulfate | Mistaken as morphine sulfate | Use complete drug name |

| Stemmed Drug Names | Intended Meaning | Misinterpretation | Correction |
|---|---|---|---|
| "Nitro" drip | Nitroglycerin infusion | Mistaken as sodium nitroprusside infusion | Use complete drug name |
| "Norflox" | Norfloxacin | Mistaken as Norflex | Use complete drug name |
| "IV Vanc" | Intravenous vancomycin | Mistaken as Invanz | Use complete drug name |

| Symbols | Intended Meaning | Misinterpretation | Correction |
|---|---|---|---|
| ʒ | Dram | Symbol for dram mistaken as "3" | Use the metric system |
| ♍ | Minim | Symbol for minim mistaken as "mL" | |
| x3d | For three days | Mistaken as "3 doses" | Use "for three days" |
| > and < | Greater than and less than | Mistaken as opposite of intended; mistakenly use incorrect symbol; "< 10" mistaken as "40" | Use "greater than" or "less than" |
| / (slash mark) | Separates two doses or indicates "per" | Mistaken as the number 1 (e.g., "25 units/10 units" misread as "25 units and 110" units) | Use "per" rather than a slash mark to separate doses |
| @ | At | Mistaken as "2" | Use "at" |
| & | And | Mistaken as "2" | Use "and" |
| + | Plus or and | Mistaken as "4" | Use "and" |
| ° | Hour | Mistaken as a zero (e.g., q2$^{0}$ seen as q20) | Use "hr," "h," or "hour" |

** These abbreviations are included on the JCAHO's "minimum list" of dangerous abbreviations, acronyms, and symbols that must be included on an organization's "Do Not Use" list, effective January 1, 2004. Visit www.jcaho.org for more information about this JCAHO requirement.

# ISMP's List of *Confused Drug Names*

This list of confused drug names, which includes look-alike and sound-alike name pairs, consists ***only*** of those name pairs that have been involved in medication errors published in the *ISMP Medication Safety Alert!*® The errors involving these medications were reported to ISMP through the USP-ISMP Medication Errors Reporting Program (MERP).

The Joint Commission on Accreditation of Healthcare Organizations (JCAHO) established a National Patient Safety Goal that requires each accredited organization to identify a list of look-alike or sound-alike drugs used in the organization. Those names that appear on the JCAHO's list of look-alike or sound-alike names have been noted with a double asterisk (**) below.

| Drug Name | Confused Drug Name | *ISMP Medication Safety Alert!*® Acute Care Edition |
|---|---|---|
| ABELCET** | amphotericin B** | Vol. 8, Issue 13, 6/26/03 |
| ACCUPRIL | ACIPHEX | Vol. 5, Issue 9, 5/3/00 |
| acetazolamide** | acetohexamide** | Vol. 5, Issue 12, 6/14/00 |
| acetohexamide** | acetazolamide** | Vol. 5, Issue 12, 6/14/00 |
| ACIPHEX | ARICEPT | Vol. 5, Issue 24, 11/29/00 |
| ACIPHEX | ACCUPRIL | Vol. 5, Issue 9, 5/3/00 |
| ACTIVASE | TNKase | Vol. 8, Issue 11, 5/29/03 |
| ACTONEL | ACTOS | Vol. 9, Issue 13, 7/1/04 |
| ACTOS | ACTONEL | Vol. 9, Issue 13, 7/1/04 |
| ADDERALL | INDERAL | Vol. 1, Issue 4, 2/28/96 |
| ADVICOR | ALTOCOR | Vol. 7, Issue 9, 5/1/02 |
| AGGRASTAT | argatroban | Vol. 6, Issue 15, 7/25/01 |
| ALDARA | ALORA | Vol. 2, Issue 14, 7/16/97 |
| ALKERAN | LEUKERAN | Vol. 5, Issue 1, 1/12/00 |
| ALLEGRA | VIAGRA | Vol. 3, Issue 12, 6/17/98 |
| ALORA | ALDARA | Vol. 2, Issue 14, 7/16/97 |
| ALTOCOR | ADVICOR | Vol. 7, Issue 9, 5/1/02 |
| AMARYL** | REMINYL** | Vol. 9, Issue 18, 9/9/04 |
| AMBISOME** | amphotericin B** | Vol. 8, Issue 13, 6/26/03 |
| AMIKIN | KINERET | Vol. 7, Issue 13, 6/26/02 |
| amphotericin B** | ABELCET** | Vol. 8, Issue 13, 6/26/03 |
| amphotericin B** | AMBISOME** | Vol. 8, Issue 13, 6/26/03 |
| antacid | ATACAND | Vol. 4, Issue 25, 12/15/99 |
| ANTIVERT | AXERT | Vol. 7, Issue 21, 10/16/02 |
| ANZEMET | AVANDAMET | Vol. 7, Issue 22, 10/30/02 |
| APRESOLINE | PRISCOLINE | Vol. 6, Issue 22, 10/31/01 |
| argatroban | AGGRASTAT | Vol. 6, Issue 15, 7/25/01 |
| argatroban | ORGARAN | Vol. 7, Issue 4, 2/20/02 |
| ARICEPT | ACIPHEX | Vol. 5, Issue 24, 11/29/00 |
| aripiprazole | proton pump inhibitors | Vol. 8, Issue 5, 6/26/03 |
| aripiprazole | rabeprazole | Vol. 8, Issue 8, 4/17/03 |
| ASACOL | OS-CAL | Vol. 2, Issue 5, 3/12/97 |

*(continues)*

*(continued)*

| Drug Name | Confused Drug Name | *ISMP Medication Safety Alert!*® Acute Care Edition |
|---|---|---|
| ATACAND | antacid | Vol. 4, Issue 25, 12/15/99 |
| ATROVENT | NATRU-VENT | Vol. 4, Issue 22, 11/3/99 |
| AVANDAMET | ANZEMET | Vol. 7, Issue 22, 10/30/02 |
| AVANDIA | PRANDIN | Vol. 4, Issue 18, 9/8/99 |
| AVANDIA** | COUMADIN** | Vol. 5, Issue 15, 7/26/00 |
| AVINZA | INVANZ | Vol. 7, Issue 10, 5/15/02 |
| AVINZA** | EVISTA** | Vol. 9, Issue 5, 3/11/04 |
| AXERT | ANTIVERT | Vol. 7, Issue 21, 10/16/02 |
| BabyBIG | HBIG | Vol. 10, Issue 6, 3/24/05 |
| BAYHEP-B | BAYRAB | Vol. 2, Issue 4, 2/26/97 |
| BAYRAB | BAYRHO-D | Vol. 2, Issue 4, 2/26/97 |
| BAYRHO-D | BAYHEP-B | Vol. 2, Issue 4, 2/26/97 |
| BICILLIN C-R | BICILLIN L-A | Vol. 9, Issue 6, 3/25/04 |
| BICILLIN L-A | BICILLIN C-R | Vol. 9, Issue 6, 3/25/04 |
| BRETHINE | METHERGINE | Vol. 9, Issue 21, 10/21/04 |
| camphorated tincture of opium (paregoric) | opium tincture | Vol. 7, Issue 4, 2/20/02 |
| carboplatin** | cisplatin** | Vol. 1 Issue 22, 11/06/96 |
| CEDAX | CIDEX | Vol. 2, Issue 2, 1/29/97 |
| CELEBREX** | CELEXA** | Vol. 4, Issue 9, 5/5/99 |
| CELEXA | ZYPREXA | Vol. 3, Issue 18, 9/9/98 |
| CELEXA** | CELEBREX** | Vol. 4, Issue 9, 5/5/99 |
| CEREBYX | CELEXA | Vol. 4, Issue 3, 2/10/99 |
| CIDEX | CEDAX | Vol. 2, Issue 2, 1/29/97 |
| cisplatin** | carboplatin** | Vol. 1 Issue 22, 11/06/96 |
| CLARITIN-D | CLARITIN-D 24 | Vol. 1, Issue 25, 12/18/96 |
| CLARITIN-D 24 | CLARITIN-D | Vol. 1, Issue 25, 12/18/96 |
| CLOZARIL | COLAZAL | Vol. 6, Issue 9, 5/2/01 |
| COLACE | COZAAR | Vol. 1, Issue 23, 11/20/96 |
| COLAZAL | CLOZARIL | Vol. 6, Issue 9, 5/2/01 |
| colchicine | CORTROSYN | Vol. 5, Issue 2, 2/9/00 |
| COMVAX | RECOMBIVAX HB | Vol.8 , Issue 6, 3/20/03 |
| CORTROSYN | colchicine | Vol. 5, Issue 2, 2/9/00 |
| COUMADIN** | AVANDIA** | Vol. 5, Issue 15, 7/26/00 |
| COZAAR | COLACE | Vol. 1, Issue 23, 11/20/96 |
| COZAAR | ZOCOR | Vol. 1, Issue 1, 1/15/96 |
| dactinomycin | daptomycin | Vol. 8, Issue 22, 10/30/03 |
| daptomycin | dactinomycin | Vol. 8, Issue 22, 10/30/03 |

*(continues)*

*(continued)*

| Drug Name | Confused Drug Name | *ISMP Medication Safety Alert!*® Acute Care Edition |
|---|---|---|
| DARVON | DIOVAN | Vol. 2, Issue 19, 9/24/97 |
| daunorubicin** | idarubicin** | Vol. 6, Issue 22, 10/31/01 |
| daunorubicin** | daunorubicin citrate liposomal** | Special Alert, 8/18/98 |
| DENAVIR | indinavir | Vol. 2, Issue 13, 7/2/97 |
| DEPAKOTE | DEPAKOTE ER | Vol. 6, Issue 3, 2/7/01 |
| DEPAKOTE ER | DEPAKOTE | Vol. 6, Issue 3, 2/7/01 |
| DEPO-MEDROL | SOLU-MEDROL | Vol. 8, Issue 11, 5/29/03 |
| DIABINESE | DIAMOX | Vol. 5, Issue 14, 7/14/00 |
| DIABETA** | ZEBETA** | Vol. 5, Issue 18, 9/6/00 |
| DIAMOX | DIABINESE | Vol. 5, Issue 14, 7/14/00 |
| DIATEX (diazepam in Mexico) | DIATX | Vol. 7, Issue 16, 8/7/02 |
| DIATX | DIATEX (diazepam in Mexico) | Vol. 7, Issue 16, 8/7/02 |
| DILACOR XR | PILOCAR | Vol. 2, Issue 15, 7/30/97 |
| DILAUDID | DILAUDID-5 | Vol. 1, Issue 13, 7/3/96 |
| DILAUDID-5 | DILAUDID | Vol. 1, Issue 13, 7/3/96 |
| DIOVAL | DIOVAN | Vol. 2, Issue 19, 9/24/97 |
| DIOVAN | DIOVAL | Vol. 2, Issue 19, 9/24/97 |
| DIOVAN | ZYBAN | Vol. 2, Issue 19, 9/24/97 |
| DIOVAN | DARVON | Vol. 2, Issue 19, 9/24/97 |
| DIPRIVAN | DITROPAN | Vol. 7, Issue 6, 3/20/02 |
| DITROPAN | DIPRIVAN | Vol. 7, Issue 6, 3/20/02 |
| dobutamine | dopamine | Vol. 1, Issue 15, 7/31/96 |
| dopamine | dobutamine | Vol. 1, Issue 15, 7/31/96 |
| doxorubicin hydrochloride** | doxorubicin liposomal** | Vol. 9, Issue 14, 7/15/04 |
| DURICEF | ULTRACET | Vol. 7, Issue 6, 3/20/02 |
| ENBREL | LEVBID | Vol. 7, Issue 19, 9/18/02 |
| ENDOCET | INDOCID | Vol. 8, Issue 22, 10/30/03 |
| ENGERIX-B adult | ENGERIX-B pediatric/adolescent | Vol. 7, Issue 1, 1/5/02 |
| ENGERIX-B pediatric/adolescent | ENGERIX-B adult | Vol. 7, Issue 1, 1/5/02 |
| ephedrine** | epinephrine** | Vol. 8, Issue 8, 4/17/03 |
| epinephrine** | ephedrine** | Vol. 8, Issue 8, 4/17/03 |
| ESTRATEST | ESTRATEST HS | Vol. 1, Issue 19, 9/25/96 |
| ESTRATEST HS | ESTRATEST | Vol. 1, Issue 19, 9/25/96 |
| ethambutol | ETHMOZINE | Vol. 4, Issue 20, 10/6/99 |
| ETHMOZINE | ethambutol | Vol. 4, Issue 20, 10/6/99 |
| EVIST** | AVINZA** | Vol. 9, Issue 5, 3/11/04 |
| FEMARA | FEMHRT | Vol. 7, Issue 7, 4/3/02 |
| FEMHRT | FEMARA | Vol. 7, Issue 7, 4/3/02 |

*(continues)*

*(continued)*

| Drug Name | Confused Drug Name | *ISMP Medication Safety Alert!*® Acute Care Edition |
|---|---|---|
| fentanyl** | sufentanil** | Vol. 6, Issue 3, 2/7/01 |
| flavoxate | fluvoxamine | Vol. 10, Issue 4, 2/24/05 |
| fluvoxamine | flavoxate | Vol. 10, Issue 4, 2/24/05 |
| FOLEX | FOLTX | Vol. 10, Issue 2, 1/27/05 |
| FOLTX | FOLEX | Vol.10, Issue 2, 1/27/05 |
| folic acid** | folinic acid (leucovorin calcium)** | Vol. 8, Issue 20, 10/2/03 |
| folinic acid (leucovorin calcium)** | folic acid** | Vol. 8, Issue 20, 10/2/03 |
| FORADIL | TORADOL | Vol. 7, Issue 12, 6/12/02 |
| gentamicin | gentian violet | Vol. 3, Issue 21, 10/21/98 |
| gentian violet | gentamicin | Vol. 3, Issue 21, 10/21/98 |
| GRANULEX | REGRANEX | Vol. 3, Issue 9, 5/6/98 |
| HBIG | Baby BIG | Vol. 10, Issue 6, 3/24/05 |
| HEALON | HYALGAN | Vol. 9, Issue 9, 5/6/04 |
| heparin** | HESPAN** | Vol. 4, Issue 18, 9/8/99 |
| HESPAN** | heparin** | Vol. 4, Issue 18, 9/8/99 |
| HUMALOG** | HUMULIN** | Vol. 7, Issue 8, 4/17/02 |
| HUMALOG MIX 75/25** | HUMULIN 70/30** | Vol. 7, Issue 24, 11/27/02 |
| HUMULIN** | HUMALOG** | Vol. 7, Issue 8, 4/17/02 |
| HUMULIN 70/30** | HUMALOG 75/25** | Vol. 7, Issue 24, 11/27/02 |
| HYALGAN | HEALON | Vol. 9, Issue 9, 5/6/04 |
| HYDROGESIC | hydroxyzine | Vol. 7, Issue 4, 2/20/02 |
| hydromorphone** | morphine** | Vol. 9, Issue 12, 7/01/04 |
| hydroxyzine | HYDROGESIC | Vol. 7, Issue 4, 2/20/02 |
| idarubicin** | daunorubicin** | Vol. 6, Issue 22, 10/31/01 |
| INDERAL | ADDERALL | Vol. 1, Issue 4, 2/28/96 |
| indinavir | DENAVIR | Vol. 2, Issue 13, 7/2/97 |
| INDOCID | ENDOCET | Vol. 8, Issue 22, 10/30/03 |
| infliximab | rituximab | Vol. 9, Issue 3, 2/12/04 |
| influenza virus vaccine | tuberculin purified protein derivative (PPD) | Vol. 9, Issue 22, 11/4/04 |
| INSPRA | SPIRIVA | Vol. 10, Issue 4, 2/24/05 |
| INVANZ | AVINZA | Vol. 7, Issue 10, 5/15/02 |
| iodine | LODINE | Vol. 7, Issue 14, 7/10/02 |
| ISORDIL | PLENDIL | Vol. 4, Issue 22, 11/3/99 |
| isotretinoin | tretinoin | Vol. 1, Issue 22, 11/6/96 |
| K-PHOS NEUTRAL | NEUTRA-PHOS-K | Vol. 7, Issue 4, 2/20/02 |
| KALETRA | KEPPRA | Vol. 8, Issue 22, 10/30/03 |
| KEPPRA | KALETRA | Vol. 8, Issue 22, 10/30/03 |

*(continues)*

*(continued)*

| Drug Name | Confused Drug Name | *ISMP Medication Safety Alert!®* Acute Care Edition |
|---|---|---|
| KETALAR | ketorolac | Vol. 3, Issue 24, 12/2/98 |
| ketorolac | KETALAR | Vol. 3, Issue 24, 12/2/98 |
| KINERET | AMIKIN | Vol. 7, Issue 13, 6/26/02 |
| LAMICTAL** | LAMISIL** | Vol. 3, Issue 12, 6/17/98 |
| LAMISIL** | LAMICTAL** | Vol. 3, Issue 12, 6/17/98 |
| lamivudine | lamotrigine | Vol. 1, Issue 18, 9/11/96 |
| lamotrigine | lamivudine | Vol. 1, Issue 18, 9/11/96 |
| LANOXIN | levothyroxine | Vol. 5, Issue 18, 9/6/00 |
| LANTUS** | LENTE** | Vol. 6, Issue 16, 8/8/01 |
| LASIX | LUVOX | Vol. 1, Issue 3, 2/14/96 |
| LENTE** | LANTUS** | Vol. 6, Issue 16, 8/8/01 |
| leucovorin calcium** | LEUKERAN** | Vol. 8, Issue 20, 10/2/03 |
| LEUKERAN | MYLERAN | Vol. 5, Issue 1, 1/12/00 |
| LEVBID | ENBREL | Vol. 7, Issue 19, 9/18/02 |
| levothyroxine | LANOXIN | Vol. 5, Issue 18, 9/6/00 |
| LEXAPRO | LOXITANE | Vol. 8, Issue 25, 12/18/03 |
| LIPITOR | ZYRTEC | Vol. 8, Issue 7, 4/4/03 |
| liposomal doxorubicin (DOXIL) | doxorubicin hydrochloride | Vol. 9, Issue 14, 7/15/04 |
| LODINE | iodine | Vol. 7, Issue 14, 7/10/02 |
| LOTRONEX | PROTONIX | Vol. 5, Issue 24, 11/29/00 |
| LOXITANE | LEXAPRO | Vol. 8, Issue 25, 12/18/03 |
| LUPRON DEPOT-3 MONTH | LUPRON DEPOT-PED | Vol. 7, Issue 18, 9/4/02 |
| LUPRON DEPOT-PED | LUPRON DEPOT-3 MONTH | Vol. 7, Issue 18, 9/4/02 |
| LUVOX | LASIX | Vol. 1, Issue 3, 2/14/96 |
| MAXZIDE | MICROZIDE | Vol. 2, Issue 9, 5/7/97 |
| METADATE | methadone | Vol.8 , Issue 13, 6/26/03 |
| METADATE CD | METADATE ER | Vol. 6, Issue 24, 11/28/01 |
| METADATE ER | METADATE CD | Vol. 6, Issue 24, 11/28/01 |
| METADATE ER | methadone | Vol. 6, Issue 4, 2/21/01 |
| METFORMIN | metronidazole | Vol. 9, Issue 20, 10/7/04 |
| methadone | METADATE ER | Vol. 6, Issue 4, 2/21/01 |
| methadone | METADATE | Vol.8 , Issue 13, 6/26/03 |
| METHERGINE | BRETHINE | Vol. 9, Issue 21, 10/21/04 |
| methimazole | metolazone | Vol. 9, Issue 22, 11/4/04 |
| metolazone | methimazole | Vol. 9, Issue 22, 11/4/04 |
| metronidazole | METFORMIN | Vol. 9, Issue 20, 10/7/04 |
| MICRONASE | MICROZIDE | Vol. 2, Issue 9, 5/7/97 |
| MICROZIDE | MICRONASE | Vol. 2, Issue 9, 5/7/97 |

*(continues)*

*(continued)*

| Drug Name | Confused Drug Name | *ISMP Medication Safety Alert!*® Acute Care Edition |
|---|---|---|
| mifepristone | misoprostol | Vol. 7, Issue 15, 7/24/02 |
| MIRALAX | MIRAPEX | Vol. 7, Issue 20, 10/3/02 |
| MIRAPEX | MIRALAX | Vol. 7, Issue 20, 10/3/02 |
| misoprostol | mifepristone | Vol. 7, Issue 15, 7/24/02 |
| morphine** | hydromorphone** | Vol. 9, Issue 12, 7/01/04 |
| morphine—oral liquid concentrate** | morphine—nonconcentrated oral liquid** | Vol. 1, Issue 25, 12/18/96 |
| MS CONTIN | OXYCONTIN | Vol. 6, Issue 17, 8/22/01 |
| MUCINEX | MUCOMYST | Vol. 9, Issue 13, 7/1/04 |
| MUCOMYST | MUCINEX | Vol. 9, Issue 13, 7/1/04 |
| MYLERAN | ALKERAN | Vol. 5, Issue 1, 1/12/00 |
| NARCAN | NORCURON | Vol. 3, Issue 20, 10/7/98 |
| NUTRA-VENT | ATROVENT | Vol. 4, Issue 22, 11/3/99 |
| NAVANE | NORVASC | Vol. 9, Issue 7, 4/8/04 |
| NEULASTA | NEUMEGA | Vol. 9, Issue 8, 4/22/04 |
| NEUMEGA | NEUPOGEN | Vol. 4, Issue 5, 3/10/99 |
| NEUMEGA | NEULASTA | Vol. 9, Issue 8, 4/22/04 |
| NEUPOGEN | NEUMEGA | Vol. 4, Issue 5, 3/10/99 |
| NEURONTIN | NOROXIN | Vol. 7, Issue 3, 2/06/02 |
| NEUTRA-PHOS-K | K-PHOS NEUTRAL | Vol. 7, Issue 4, 2/20/02 |
| NORCURON | NARCAN | Vol. 3, Issue 20, 10/7/98 |
| NOROXIN | NEURONTIN | Vol. 7, Issue 3, 2/06/02 |
| NORVASC | NAVANE | Vol. 9, Issue 7, 4/8/04 |
| NOVOLIN 70/30** | NOVOLOG MIX 70/30** | Vol. 9, Issue 14, 7/15/04 |
| NOVOLOG MIX 70/30** | NOVOLIN 70/30** | Vol. 9, Issue 14, 7/15/04 |
| OCCLUSAL-HP | OCUFLOX | Vol. 6, Issue 11, 5/30/01 |
| OCUFLOX | OCCLUSAL-HP | Vol. 6, Issue 11, 5/30/01 |
| opium tincture | camphorate tincture of opium (paregoric) | Vol. 7, Issue 4, 2/20/02 |
| ORGARAN | argatroban | Vol. 7, Issue 4, 2/20/02 |
| OS-CAL | ASACOL | Vol. 2, Issue 5, 3/12/97 |
| oxycodone | OXYCONTIN | Vol. 6, Issue 17, 8/22/01 |
| OXYCONTIN | MS CONTIN | Vol. 6, Issue 17, 8/22/01 |
| OXYCONTIN | oxycodone | Vol. 6, Issue 17, 8/22/01 |
| paclitaxel | paclitaxel protein-bound particles for injectable suspension | Vol. 10, Issue 5, 3/10/05 |
| paclitaxel protein-bound particles for injectable suspension | paclitaxel | Vol. 10, Issue 5, 3/10/05 |
| PAMELOR | PANLOR DC | Vol. 6, Issue 18, 9/5/01 |

*(continues)*

*(continued)*

| Drug Name | Confused Drug Name | *ISMP Medication Safety Alert!*® Acute Care Edition |
|---|---|---|
| PANLOR DC | PAMELOR | Vol. 6, Issue 18, 9/5/01 |
| PATANOL | PLATINOL | Vol. 2, Issue 1, 1/15/97 |
| PAVULON | PEPTAVLON | Vol. 2, Issue 7, 4/9/97 |
| PAXIL | TAXOL | Vol. 2, Issue 1, 1/15/97 |
| PAXIL | PLAVIX | Vol. 7, Issue 12, 6/12/02 |
| PEPTAVLON | PAVULON | Vol. 2, Issue 7, 4/9/97 |
| PERCOCET | PROCET | ol. 6, Issue 18, 9/5/01 |
| PILOCAR | DILACOR XR | Vol. 2, Issue 15, 7/30/97 |
| PLATINOL | PANTANOL | Vol. 2, Issue 1, 1/15/97 |
| PLAVIX | PAXIL | Vol. 7, Issue 12, 6/12/02 |
| PLENDIL | ISORDIL | Vol. 4, Issue 22, 11/3/99 |
| pneumococcal 7-valent vaccine | pneumococcal polyvalent vaccine | Vol. 7, Issue 10, 5/15/02 |
| pneumococcal polyvalent vaccine | pneumococcal 7-valent vaccine | Vol. 7, Issue 10, 5/15/02 |
| PRANDIN | AVANDIA | Vol. 4, Issue 18, 9/8/99 |
| PRECARE | PRECOSE | Vol. 1, Issue 19, 9/25/96 |
| PRECOSE | PRECARE | Vol. 1, Issue 19, 9/25/96 |
| PRILOSEC | PROZAC | Vol. 1, Issue 17, 8/28/96 |
| PRISCOLINE | APRESOLINE | Vol. 6, Issue 22, 10/31/01 |
| probenecid | PROCANBID | Vol. 5, Issue 5, 3/8/00 |
| PROCANBID | probenecid | Vol. 5, Issue 5, 3/8/00 |
| PROCARDIA XL | PROTAIN XL | Vol. 5, Issue 20, 10/4/00 |
| PROCET | PERCOCET | Vol. 6, Issue 18, 9/5/01 |
| propylthiouracil | PURINETHOL | Vol. 8, Issue 17, 8/21/03 |
| PROTAIN XL | PROCARDIA XL | Vol. 5, Issue 20, 10/4/00 |
| protamine | PROTONIX | Vol. 9, Issue 6, 3/25/04 |
| Proton Pump Inhibitors | aripiprazole | Vol. 8, Issue 5, 6/26/03 |
| PROTONIX | LOTRONEX | Vol. 5, Issue 24, 11/29/00 |
| PROTONIX | protamine | Vol. 9, Issue 6, 3/25/04 |
| PROZAC | PRILOSEC | Vol. 1, Issue 17, 8/28/96 |
| PURINETHOL | propylthiouracil | Vol. 8, Issue 17, 8/21/03 |
| quinine | quinidine | Vol. 2, Issue 20, 10/8/97 |
| quinidine | quinine | Vol. 2, Issue 20, 10/8/97 |
| rabeprazole | apripiprazole | Vol. 8, Issue 8, 4/17/03 |
| RECOMBIVAX HB | COMVAX | Vol.8 , Issue 6, 3/20/03 |
| REGRANEX | GRANULEX | Vol. 3, Issue 9, 5/6/98 |
| REMINYL | ROBINUL | Vol. 7, Issue 4, 2/20/02 |
| REMINYL** | AMARYL** | Vol. 9, Issue 18, 9/9/04 |
| RETROVIR** | ritonavir** | Vol. 5, Issue 20, 10/4/00 |

*(continues)*

*(continued)*

| Drug Name | Confused Drug Name | *ISMP Medication Safety Alert!*® Acute Care Edition |
|---|---|---|
| RIFATER | RIFADIN | Vol. 6, Issue 24, 11/28/01 |
| RIFADIN | RIFATER | Vol. 6, Issue 24, 11/28/01 |
| RITALIN | ritodrine | Vol. 2, Issue 10, 5/21/97 |
| RITALIN LA | RITALIN SR | Vol. 6, Issue 24, 11/28/01 |
| RITALIN SR | RITALIN LA | Vol. 6, Issue 24, 11/28/01 |
| ritodrine | RITALIN | Vol. 2, Issue 10, 5/21/97 |
| ritonavir** | RETROVIR** | Vol. 5, Issue 20, 10/4/00 |
| rituximab | infliximab | Vol. 9, Issue 3, 2/12/04 |
| ROBINUL | REMINYL | Vol. 7, Issue 4, 2/20/02 |
| ROXANOL | ROXICODONE INTENSOL | Vol. 1, Issue 25, 12/18/96 |
| ROXANOL | ROXICET | Vol. 1, Issue 25, 12/18/96 |
| ROXICET | ROXANOL | Vol. 1, Issue 25, 12/18/96 |
| ROXICODONE INTENSOL | ROXANOL | Vol. 1, Issue 25, 12/18/96 |
| saquinavir (free base) | saquinavir mesylate | Vol. 3, Issue 13, 7/1/98 |
| saquinavir mesylate | saquinavir (free base) | Vol. 3, Issue 13, 7/1/98 |
| saquinavir | SINEQUAN | Special Alert, 4/11/96 |
| SARAFEM | SEROPHENE | Vol. 6, Issue 18, 9/5/01 |
| SEROPHENE | SARAFEM | Vol. 6, Issue 18, 9/5/01 |
| SEROQUEL** | SERZONE** | Vol. 7, Issue 11, 5/29/02 |
| sertraline | SORIATANE | Vol. 8, Issue 16, 8/7/03 |
| SERZONE** | SEROQUEL** | Vol. 7, Issue 11, 5/29/02 |
| SINEQUAN | saquinavir | Special Alert, 4/11/96 |
| SOLU-MEDROL | DEPO-MEDROL | Vol. 8, Issue 11, 5/29/03 |
| SORIATANE | sertraline | Vol. 8, Issue 16, 8/7/03 |
| SPIRIVA | INSPRA | Vol. 10, Issue 4, 2/24/05 |
| sufentanil** | fentanyl** | Vol. 5, Issue 7, 4/5/00 |
| sumatriptan | zolmitriptan | Vol. 3, Issue 4, 2/25/98 |
| TAXOL** | TAXOTERE** | Vol. 6, Issue 3, 2/7/01 |
| TAXOL | PAXIL | Vol. 2, Issue 1, 1/15/97 |
| TAXOTERE** | TAXOL** | Vol. 6, Issue 3, 2/7/01 |
| TEGRETOL | TEQUIN | Vol. 5, Issue 15, 7/26/00 |
| TEGRETOL | TEGRETOL XR | Vol. 1, Issue 21, 10/23/96 |
| TEGRETOL XR | TEGRETOL | Vol. 1, Issue 21, 10/23/96 |
| TEQUIN | TEGRETOL | Vol. 5, Issue 15, 7/26/00 |
| TEQUIN | TICLID | Vol. 7, Issue 4, 2/20/02 |
| TESTODERM | TESTODERM W/ ADHESIVE | Vol. 3, Issue 14, 4/8/98 |
| TESTODERM TTS | TESTODERM | Vol. 3, Issue 14, 4/8/98 |
| TESTODERM W/ ADHESIVE | TESTODERM TTS | Vol. 3, Issue 14, 4/8/98 |

*(continues)*

*(continued)*

| Drug Name | Confused Drug Name | *ISMP Medication Safety Alert!*® Acute Care Edition |
|---|---|---|
| tetanus diphtheria toxoid (Td) | tuberculin purified protein derivative (PPD) | Vol. 9, Issue 16, 8/12/04 |
| tiagabine** | tizanidine** | Vol.8 , Issue 3, 2/6/03 |
| TIAZAC | ZIAC | Vol. 1, Issue 6, 3/27/96 |
| TICLID | TEQUIN | Vol. 7, Issue 4, 2/20/02 |
| tizanidine** | tiagabine** | Vol.8 , Issue 3, 2/6/03 |
| TNKase | ACTIVASE | Vol. 8, Issue 11, 5/29/03 |
| TNKase | t-PA | Vol. 8, Issue 11, 5/29/03 |
| TOBRADEX | TOBREX | Vol. 4, Issue 13, 6/30/99 |
| TOBREX | TOBRADEX | Vol. 4, Issue 13, 6/30/99 |
| TOPAMAX | TOPROL XL | Vol. 7, Issue 16, 8/7/02 |
| TOPROL XL | TOPAMAX | Vol. 7, Issue 16, 8/7/02 |
| TORADOL | FORADIL | Vol. 7, Issue 12, 6/12/02 |
| t-PA | TNKase | Vol. 8, Issue 11, 5/29/03 |
| TRACLEER | TRICOR | Vol. 8, Issue 13, 6/26/03 |
| tramadol hydrochloride | trazodone hydrochloride | Vol. 7, Issue 19, 9/18/02 |
| trazodone hydrochloride | tramadol hydrochloride | Vol. 7, Issue 19, 9/18/02 |
| tretinoin | isotretinoin | Vol. 1, Issue 22, 11/6/96 |
| TRICOR | TRACLEER | Vol. 8, Issue 13, 6/26/03 |
| tuberculin purified derivative | influenza virus vaccine (PPD) | Vol. 9, Issue 22, 11/4/04 |
| tuberculin purified derivative | tetanus diphtheria toxoid (Td) (PPD) | Vol. 9, Issue 16, 8/12/04 |
| TYLENOL | TYLENOL PM | Vol. 8, Issue 8, 4/17/03 |
| TYLENOL PM | TYLENOL | Vol. 8, Issue 8, 4/17/03 |
| ULTRACET | DURICEF | Vol. 7, Issue 6, 3/20/02 |
| valacyclovir | valganciclovir | Vol. 7, Issue 13, 6/26/02 |
| VALCYTE | VALTREX | Vol. 7, Issue 13, 6/26/02 |
| valganciclovir | valacyclovir | Vol. 7, Issue 13, 6/26/02 |
| VALTREX | VALCYTE | Vol. 7, Issue 13, 6/26/02 |
| VARIVAX | VZIG | Vol.8 , Issue 2, 1/23/03 |
| VEXOL | VOSOL | Vol. 1, Issue 11, 6/5/96 |
| VIAGRA | ALLEGRA | Vol. 3, Issue 12, 6/17/98 |
| vinblastine** | vincristine** | Vol. 5, Issue 10, 5/17/00 |
| vincristine** | vinblastine** | Vol. 5, Issue 10, 5/17/00 |
| VIOKASE | VIOKASE 8 | Vol. 7, Issue 6, 3/20/02 |
| VIOKASE 8 | VIOKASE | Vol. 7, Issue 6, 3/20/02 |
| VIOXX | ZYVOX | Vol. 7, Issue 17, 8/21/02 |
| VIRACEPT | VIRAMUNE | Vol. 7, Issue 17, 8/21/02 |
| VIRAMUNE | VIRACEPT | Vol. 7, Issue 17, 8/21/02 |

*(continues)*

*(continued)*

| Drug Name | Confused Drug Name | *ISMP Medication Safety Alert!®* Acute Care Edition |
|---|---|---|
| VOSOL | VEXOL | Vol. 1, Issue 11, 6/5/96 |
| VZIG | VARIVAX | Vol.8 , Issue 2, 1/23/03 |
| WELLBUTRIN SR** | WELLBUTRIN XL** | Vol. 9, Issue 1, 1/15/04 |
| WELLBUTRIN XL** | WELLBUTRIN SR** | Vol. 9, Issue 1, 1/15/04 |
| XELODA | XENICAL | Vol. 4, Issue 18, 9/8/99 |
| XENICAL | XELODA | Vol. 4, Issue 18, 9/8/99 |
| ZANTAC** | ZYRTEC** | Vol. 5, Issue 22, 11/1/00 |
| ZEBETA | DIABETA | Vol. 5, Issue 18, 9/6/00 |
| ZEBETA | ZETIA | Vol. 8, Issue 11, 5/29/03 |
| ZESTRIL | ZETIA | Vol.8 , Issue 6, 3/20/03 |
| ZETIA | ZEBETA | Vol. 8, Issue 11, 5/29/03 |
| ZETIA | ZESTRIL | Vol.8 , Issue 6, 3/20/03 |
| ZIAC | TIAZAC | Vol. 1, Issue 6, 3/27/96 |
| ZOCOR | COZAAR | Vol. 1, Issue 1, 1/15/96 |
| zolmitriptan | sumatriptan | Vol. 3, Issue 4, 2/25/98 |
| ZOSTRIX | ZOVIRAX | Vol. 8, Issue 21, 10/16/03 |
| ZOVIRAX | ZYVOX | Vol. 7, Issue 17, 8/21/02 |
| ZOVIRAX | ZOSTRIX | Vol. 8, Issue 21, 10/16/03 |
| ZYBAN | DIOVAN | Vol. 2, Issue 19, 9/24/97 |
| ZYPREXA** | ZYRTEC** | Vol. 6, Issue 22, 10/31/01 |
| ZYPREXA | CELEXA | Vol. 3, Issue 18, 9/9/98 |
| ZYRTEC** | ZYPREXA** | Vol. 6, Issue 22, 10/31/01 |
| ZYRTEC** | ZANTAC** | Vol. 5, Issue 22, 11/1/00 |
| ZYRTEC | LIPITOR | Vol. 8, Issue 7, 4/4/03 |
| ZYVOX | VIOXX | Vol. 7, Issue 17, 8/21/02 |
| ZYVOX | ZOVIRAX | Vol. 7, Issue 17, 8/21/02 |

** These drugs are included on the JCAHO's list of look-alike or sound-alike drug names from which an accredited organization creates its own list to satisfy the requirements of the National Patient Safety Goals. Visit www.jcaho.org for more information about this JCAHO requirement.

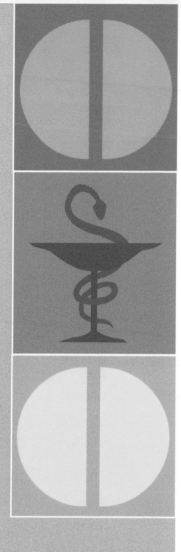

# Glossary

**absence** A generalized seizure that is marked by the transient loss of consciousness, usually with a blank stare, that begins and ends abruptly; also known as petit mal.

**absorption** The movement and uptake of substances into cells or across tissues, as with the absorption of nutrients or drugs in the small intestine.

**acetylcholinesterase** An enzyme that breaks down unused acetylcholine in the synaptic cleft.

**achlorhydria** The absence of hydrochloric acid from the gastric juices.

**acid labile** Chemically unstable in the presence of acid.

**acromegaly** A disorder that is caused by chronic overproduction of growth hormone by the pituitary gland, similar to gigantism.

**actinic keratosis** A disease of the skin marked by overgrowth of keratin and caused by excessive sun exposure.

**action potential** The sequential polarization and depolarization that travels across membranes of excitable tissue (such as nerve or muscle cells), in response to stimulation.

**active immunity** Resistance to infection that is acquired because white blood cells are exposed to antigens and produce antibody to the infectious agent.

**acute coronary syndrome** A set of signs and symptoms suggestive of sudden cardiac ischemia and including unstable angina and possibly heart attack.

**addiction** Compulsive use of a habit-forming substance known by the user to be physically, psychologically, or socially harmful.

**adipose** Fat- or tissue-containing fat cells.

**adrenergic** Neurons that are activated by, or secrete, norepinephrine, or another chemically similar catecholamine.

**adverse drug event** Any unexpected or unwanted effect caused by the administration of a drug.

**adverse effect** An unwanted or dangerous reaction to a drug.

**afferent** Moving or conducting inwardly. Refers to vessels, nerves, etc.

**aggregate** To collect or gather into a mass, as when platelets aggregate to form a thrombus.

**agonist** A drug capable of combining with a receptor on a cell and initiating the same reaction produced by an endogenous substance.

**agranulocytosis** An acute condition, often caused by drug therapy, characterized by a marked decrease in the number of granulocytes and associated with signs of infection.

**akathisia** A condition of motor restlessness or an urge to move about that is a common extrapyramidal effect due to antipsychotic medication.

**albumin** Any of a number of water-soluble proteins that occur in blood plasma or serum, and other animal substances.

**aldosterone** A steroid hormone produced by the adrenal glands that acts in the kidneys to contribute to the control of salt and water balance.

**alimentary** Concerned with or relating to nourishment, or the organs of digestion.

**alkaloid** Any one of the many pharmacologically active, complex, nitrogenous compounds found in plants.

**alopecia** Baldness or loss of hair from skin areas where it is normally present.

**alveoli** The small thin-walled compartments of the lung that are typically arranged in saclike clusters and are the site of air exchange.

**amenorrhea** The abnormal absence of menstruation.

**amnesia** Loss of memory; in some cases related to the use of anesthesia or other medications.

**anabolic** The aspect of metabolism concerned with molecular synthesis and tissue building.

**anal sphincter** The musculature surrounding and able to close the anus.

**analeptic** A drug that acts as a restorative or stimulant in the central nervous system, for example, caffeine.

**analgesic** An agent that relieves pain without causing loss of consciousness.

**anaphylaxis** An acute, life-threatening allergic reaction caused by release of histamine that can result in bronchoconstriction and hypotension.

**androgen** A general term referring to male sex hormones.

**anemia** A condition that results from a lack of red blood cells, hemoglobin, or total blood volume.

**angina pectoris** Irregular attacks of crushing chest pain, symptomatic of a lack of oxygen to the myocardium and usually precipitated by effort or emotion.

**angioedema** An often serious allergic skin reaction characterized by wheals and edema of the skin and the mucous membranes.

**angioplasty** Surgical reopening of a clogged blood vessel.

**anorexia** Loss of appetite for food; sometimes a symptom of drug therapy.

**antagonist** A drug that acts within the body to oppose the action of another drug or a substance occurring naturally in the body, by blocking its receptor.

**anterior** Located or situated toward the front of the body.

**antianxiety** Intended to prevent or relieve anxiety.

**antibacterial** Intended to kill or prevent the growth or reproduction of bacteria.

**antibiotic** A drug produced by or derived from a micro-organism, and able to kill or inhibit the growth and reproduction of another micro-organism.

**antibody** A protein that is produced by B lymphocytes, after sensitization by an antigen, to act specifically against the antigen in an immune response; also called immunoglobulin.

**anticholinergic** Opposing or blocking the physiological action of acetylcholine.

**antidote** A drug used to counteract the effects of a poison.

**antiemetic** A drug used to prevent or alleviate nausea or vomiting.

**antigen** Any substance foreign to the body that evokes an immune response.

**antimicrobial** A drug used to kill or suppress the growth of micro-organisms.

**antipsychotic** A drug that is indicated for, and effective in the treatment of psychosis.

**antipyretic** An agent that relieves or reduces fever.

**antitussive** A drug that relieves or suppresses cough.

**anxiety** An abnormal sense of apprehension and fear, often including physical signs such as sweating or racing pulse, which is a disproportionate response to an event.

**anxiolytic** A medication used to treat or relieve anxiety.

**aorta** The largest artery in the body; originates in the heart and branches to carry the blood through the body.

**aplastic anemia** A form of anemia, often caused by toxic agents or drugs, that occurs when the bone marrow ceases to produce sufficient red and white blood cells.

**apnea** Temporary cessation of breathing.

**apoptosis** Normal, programmed cell death, initiated by signals from the cell nuclei when cell age or health dictates.

**appendicular skeleton** The bones that make up the shoulder girdle, the pelvis, and the upper and lower extremities.

**aqueous** Made from or with water.

**arrhythmia** Any variation from the normal rhythm of the heartbeat.

**arthritis** Inflammation of the joints caused by infection, trauma, and metabolic or other causes.

**aseptic technique** Methods used by pharmacists and technicians to maintain the sterility of sterile products during compounding.

**aspirate** To draw in by breathing; inhale.

**asthma** A lung disorder of recurring episodes of airway constriction, with symptoms of labored breathing accompanied by wheezing and coughing.

**ataxia** Inability to coordinate voluntary muscle movements that can be an adverse drug effect or a symptom of some neurologic disorders.

**atherosclerosis** The progressive narrowing of the arteries caused by fatty deposits and fibrosis of the vessels.

**atopic dermatitis** An inflammatory skin condition characterized by dry skin, itchy, scaly rash, and often associated with allergies.

**atrial arrhythmia** Abnormal heart rhythm caused by conduction disturbances in the atria.

**atrial flutter** A rapid, organized atrial arrhythmia, with atrial rate of $>200$, but a slower ventricular rate.

**atrioventricular node** Tissue in the conduction system of the heart that passes impulses received from the sinoatrial node (atria) to the ventricles.

**aura** A subjective sensation that precedes an attack of a neurological disorder, such as epilepsy or migraine headache.

**autocrine** Of or related to self-signalling; secretion of a substance by cells that affects only members of the same cell type.

**autoimmune** Relating to conditions caused by antibodies or cells that react to tissues of the individual that produces them.

**automaticity** The ability of a cell, organ, or system to initiate its own activity.

**autonomic** Acting or occurring involuntarily; self-controlling.

**axial skeleton** The articulated bones of the head and trunk.

**axon** A long projection of the nerve cell that conducts efferent impulses from the cell body toward target cells.

**bacteriocidal** Capable of killing bacteria.

**bacteriostatic** Capable of inhibiting the growth and replication of bacteria.

**baroreceptors** Specialized tissue in the walls of the large arteries and the atria that senses changes in blood pressure.

**benign** Amenable to treatment; in relationship to tumors, not cancerous; does not metastasize.

**benign prostatic hypertrophy** Benign enlargement of the prostate gland usually seen in older men.

**bioavailability** Rate at which a drug is absorbed and becomes available to the target tissue.

**bioequivalent** Two different drug formulations with identical active ingredients that possess similar bioavailability and produce the same effect at the site of action.

**biologicals** Antibodies, vaccines, cultures, or other products usually derived from the serum of living organisms, and used to treat or prevent disease.

**biotransformation** Chemical alterations of a compound that occur within the body, as in drug metabolism.

**bipolar disorder** A mood disorder characterized by alternating episodes of excitement and depression.

**black box warning** The strongest type of side effect warning, required by the Food and Drug Administration to appear on some drugs that cause significant risk of serious or life-threatening side effects.

**blood dyscrasia** A general term used to describe any abnormality in the blood or bone marrow's cellular components.

**blood-brain barrier** An anatomical barrier that prevents many substance from entering the brain, which is created as a result of the relative impermeability of capillaries in the brain.

**bradycardia** A slowness of the heartbeat, as evidenced by slowing of the pulse rate to less than 60 beats per minute.

**broad spectrum** A term used to describe an antibiotic that is effective against a wide range of micro-organisms.

**bronchi (plural of bronchus)** The main airways that lead from the trachea to the lungs.

**bronchiole** One of many small, thin-walled branches off of the bronchus.

**bronchitis** Acute or chronic inflammation of the bronchi, often due to infection.

**bronchoconstriction** Narrowing of bronchioles.

**buffer** Compound(s) in solution that stabilizes the hydrogen-ion concentration by neutralizing both acids and bases.

**bursa** Singular of bursae; a small sack between tendon and bone that contains synovial fluid and facilitates smooth movement of joints.

**cancellous bone** Bone that has a lattice-like structure.

**capillary permeability** Property of capillary walls that allows for exchange of specific, fat-soluble molecules.

**carcinogenic** Substance that may produce or promote cancer.

**cardiac decompensation** Failure of the heart to maintain adequate blood circulation; symptoms include shortness of breath and edema.

**cardiac glycoside** Drugs derived from the foxglove plant that increase the contractility of the heart muscle.

**cardiac output** Measurement of the volume of blood ejected by the heart to the systemic circulation, expressed as liters per minute.

**cardioversion** Application of an electric shock, usually to the chest, in order to restore normal heartbeat.

**carrier-mediated transport** Movement of a chemical substance, using a carrier protein and with the expenditure of energy, against a concentration gradient.

**cartilaginous joint** A joint in which the bony surfaces of the two juxtaposed bones are united with cartilage, for example, the vertebral joints.

**catabolism** Destructive metabolism whereby complex materials are broken down into waste products and energy.

**catalyze** To accelerate, or bring about an increase in, the rate of a chemical reaction.

**catecholamine** A biogenic amine derived from the amino acid tyrosine that functions as a neurotransmitter or hormone.

**cathartic** A medication used to stimulate the clearing of the intestinal contents.

**cation** Positively charged ion.

**cecum** Pouch-like section of the intestine (off of which the appendix extends) that connects the ileum to the colon.

**cell-cycle specific** Refers to chemotherapeutic agents that are only effective when the cancerous cells are replicating (within the cell replication cycle).

**central nervous system** Part of the nervous system consisting of the brain, cranial nerves, and spinal cord, which supervises and coordinates the activity of the nervous system.

**cerebellum** Part of the posterior division of the brain. Concerned primarily with motor functions, coordination, and balance.

**cerebral cortex** The outer portion of the brain that is the part of the brain in which thought processes take place.

**cerebrospinal fluid** The fluid that fills the ventricles of the brain and the central canal of the spinal cord; serves to maintain uniform pressure within the CNS and cushion the brain and spinal cord.

**cerebrovascular accident** General term used to describe an acute loss of oxygen to some part of the brain due to an embolus or rupture of a blood vessel.

**cerumen** The waxy, acidic secretion found in the external ear canal; earwax.

**chelate** To form a complex chemical compound in which a metallic ion is bound into a stable ring structure; chelates are not absorbable through the GI tract.

**chemical name** The proper scientific name, based on the chemical structure, for a drug.

**cholinergic** Resembling acetylcholine in pharmacological action, stimulated by or releasing acetylcholine or a related compound.

**chronic obstructive pulmonary disease** Progressive, irreversible pulmonary diseases (emphysema or chronic bronchitis) related to smoking and characterized by difficulty breathing and a chronic cough.

**clotting cascade** The series of reactions among blood clotting factors that cause clotting or coagulation.

**cofactor** A substance that is required by an enzyme for catalysis to take place; in humans, cofactors are often essential minerals or vitamins.

**collagen** A fibrous protein of vertebrates, that is a major constituent of connective tissues, such as tendon, ligament, and skin.

**colloid** Microscopic particles, smaller than $1 \times 10^{-6}$, suspended in a liquid.

**colon** Also known as the large intestine, the colon extends from the cecum to the rectum.

**communicable** Capable of being transmitted from person to person or between animals of other species; especially disease.

**compact bone** Noncancellous; made up of layers of bone formed around a central canal.

**complement** A group of about 20 serum proteins which, working in tandem with other parts of the immune system, activate pathways that cause the destruction of specific antigens.

**complementary and alternative medicine** Nontraditional or unconventional forms of treatment that are used in addition to (complementary) or instead of (alternative) standard treatments.

**compliance** The process of following a prescribed regimen of treatment.

**concentration gradient** A variation in the concentration of a solute with regard to position; in pharmacology, especially in relationship to a semipermeable membrane.

**conduction system** The system in the heart responsible for moving electrical impulses from the atria to the ventricles; responsible for cardiac muscle contraction.

**congenital** Existing at birth; usually referring to conditions acquired during development of the fetus, regardless of their cause; i.e., congenital herpes.

**congestive heart failure** Inability of the heart to effectively pump returned venous blood, leading to accumulation of fluid in the lungs and lower extremities.

**conjunctiva** Clear, thin membrane that lines the inner surface of the eyelids and the outer surface of the eyeball.

**contact inhibition** Inhibition of growth and replication of a cell or cells due to physical contact with other cells.

**contraindication** A condition that makes a particular drug or procedure inadvisable.

**cornea** Multilayered, transparent structure on the anterior surface of the eye; its outer epithelial layer is continuous with the conjunctiva.

**crystalluria** Excretion of crystals in the urine.

**culture** To grow in a laboratory; especially bacteria in infectious diseases.

**cyanosis** Bluish discoloration of the skin or mucous membranes due to deficient oxygenation of the blood.

**cystitis** Inflammation of the urinary bladder (often caused by infection).

**cytokine** Small proteins secreted by cells that are involved with cell to cell communication and regulation, especially of the immune system.

**cytotoxic** Toxic to cells; used in reference to drugs or chemicals.

**decontaminate** To rid of contamination, as in toxic exposures or drug overdoses.

**dehydration** Condition that results from either excessive loss or inadequate intake of water.

**delirium** An acute, reversible mental disorder often due to illness or medications with symptoms of confusion, incoherent speech, and hallucinations.

**dendrite** Threadlike extensions of the cytoplasm of a neuron that conduct impulses toward the body of a nerve cell.

**dependence** In pharmacology, refers to habituation to the use of a drug that will result in withdrawal symptoms if the drug is discontinued.

**depolarization** The loss of the difference in charge between the inside and outside of a cell, due to a change in permeability and migration of sodium ions to the interior.

**depot injection** Formulation that uses a vehicle designed to remain in "storage" at the site of injection so that absorption and drug action occurs over a prolonged period .

**depression** A mood disorder; typical symptoms range from sadness, inactivity, and changes in sleep and eating patterns to anger, guilt, and suicidal thoughts.

**dermatitis** Inflammation of the skin.

**dextrose** Dextrorotatory isomer of glucose.

**diabetes, type 1** Form of diabetes that usually develops during childhood or adolescence and is characterized by a lack of insulin secretion requiring replacement.

**diabetes, type 2** Diabetes often seen in obese adults, characterized by impaired insulin utilization and inadequate compensation of insulin production; initially diet, exercise, and oral antidiabetic agents are used for treatment.

**dialysis** Medical procedure that uses a machine to filter waste products from the blood and adjust fluid and electrolyte imbalances in people with renal failure.

**diastole** Time between contractions when the heart chambers fill with blood.

**diencephalon** Posterior portion of the forebrain that houses the thalamus and hypothalamus.

**dissolution** Process of dissolving or separating into component parts.

**distal convoluted tubule** Winding portion of the nephron between the loop of Henle and the nonsecretory part of the nephron; important in the concentration of urine.

**distribution** The process by which a drug is carried to sites of action throughout the body by the bloodstream.

**diuretic** A drug that promotes the excretion of urine.

**diurnal** Having a daily cycle or occurring during the daytime.

**dose-response curve** A graph that shows the relationship between the dose of a drug and the degree of response it causes.

**drug** Any compound taken with the intent to alter some form or function of the body or treat a disease.

**duodenum** The first and shortest part of the small intestine that extends from the pylorus to the jejunum.

**dyskinesia** Impairment of normal voluntary muscle movement that results in halting or jerky movement.

**dysmenorrhea** Painful menstruation.

**dyspepsia** Stomach discomfort following meals; indigestion.

**dysphoria** A state of feeling disquiet, agitated, or unwell; opposite of euphoria.

**dyspnea** Shortness of breath; difficulty breathing.

**dystonia** Abnormal tone of muscles.

**eczema** A chronic inflammatory condition of the skin, which usually appears as itchy, red lesions that may ooze serous fluid and become scaly, crusted, or hardened over time.

**edema** Abnormal accumulation of fluid in the spaces between cells, especially subcutaneous tissue.

**effective dose range** Range of drug doses that cause an increase in the desired pharmacologic effect with increasing dose.

**effector** A molecule that activates, controls, or inactivates a process or action.

**efferent** Moving or carrying outward or away from a central part. Refers to vessels, nerves, etc.

**efficacy** The ability of a drug to treat or cure a disease.

**electroencephalogram** A diagnostic test that measures and records electrical activity of the brain.

**electrolytes** A substance that dissociates into ions when in solution and as a result is capable of conducting electrical current; in the body electrolytes contribute to nerve conduction, muscle contraction, and many other processes.

**elixir** A drug preparation in which the active ingredients are dissolved in an alcohol-based, sweetened liquid.

**embolism** Sudden obstruction of vessel by a blood clot or foreign material.

**emesis** Vomiting.

**emetogenic** Causes vomiting; usually in reference to a drug side effect.

**emphysema** A lung disease usually due to smoking, in which distention and reduced elasticity of alveoli causes air accumulation and impaired air exchange.

**emulsify** To disperse in an emulsion or convert immiscible liquids into an emulsion.

**emulsion** Pharmaceutical preparation of one liquid dispersed in small globules through a second, immiscible liquid.

**enantiomer** Either of a pair of chemical compounds whose molecular structures have a mirror-image relationship to each other.

**endemic** Present or occurring in a particular geographic area or population.

**endocrine** Pertaining to glands or their secretions that are distributed in the body by way of the bloodstream.

**endogenous** Developing or growing within or arising from internal causes.

**endometriosis** Presence and growth of endometrial tissue outside the uterus that can result in severe pain with the menses, and infertility.

**endorphins** A group of endogenous opioid-type peptides found in the CNS that bind to opiate receptors and produce effects similar to the opioids.

**endothelium** Type of epithelial cells that line blood vessels and the cavities of the heart.

**enkephalins** Endogenous pentapeptides that bind to and activate opiate receptors in the CNS.

**enteral** A route of nutrient or drug delivery where delivery is made directly into the gastrointestinal tract.

**enteric coating** Coating used on drugs to prevent their dissolution until they leave the stomach and enter the small intestine.

**enuresis** Involuntary urination that occurs after the age where bladder control should have developed.

**envenomation** Injection of venom by a bite, sting, or spine.

**enzymes** A type of protein produced by a living organism that catalyzes biochemical reactions without itself being destroyed or altered.

**epidemic** A sudden occurrence that affects an unexpectedly large percentage of a given population at the same time.

**epidermis** The outer epithelial layer of the skin.

**epiglottis** A cartilaginous flap that covers the glottis while swallowing food or liquids.

**epiphysis** The part of the long bone where growth occurs; growth plate.

**epithelium** Membranous cellular tissue that lines internal and external body surfaces and is classified in types according to cell shapes and layers.

**equilibrium** A state of balance where no significant change occurs.

**erectile dysfunction** Routine inability to maintain an erection sufficient for sexual intercourse.

**erythrocytes** Red blood cells.

**essential hypertension** High blood pressure that occurs without an identifiable cause.

**eukaryote** Organisms composed of one or more cells that contain nuclei and organelles.

**euphoria** A feeling of well-being or elation; in pharmacology, the "high" associated with drugs of abuse.

**excoriation** Abraded or raw lesion of the skin.

**excretion** The act or process of excreting; one form of elimination from the body.

**exfoliative dermatitis** Generalized shedding of the skin in layers; often a drug reaction.

**exocrine** Secreting outwardly, usually via a duct, for example salivary glands.

**exophthalmos** Abnormal protrusion of the eyeball.

**expectorant** Drug that encourages the removal of mucus from the respiratory tract, usually by thinning secretions.

**extracellular** Outside of the cell or cells.

**extrapyramidal symptoms** Motor or movement abnormalities usually related to medication use.

**extravasate** To pass by infiltration from a blood vessel into surrounding tissue.

**febrile seizure** A seizure, usually seen in infants, caused by a rapid rise in body temperature.

**fibrillation** Twitching or contraction of individual muscle fibers; in cardiology an arrhythmia characterized by contraction of individual fibers in a disorganized fashion.

**fibrin** Insoluble fibrous protein formed from fibrinogen and essential to the blood clotting process.

**fibrinogen** Soluble plasma protein essential to normal clotting and the precursor to fibrin.

**fibrous joint** Union of two bones with fibrous tissue resulting in a joint that is nearly immobile; examples include joints between the bones of the skull.

**first-pass effect** Biotransformation of a drug before it reaches the systemic circulation.

**flatulence** The presence of gas or air in the GI tract to the degree that distention and discomfort occur.

**free radical** A highly reactive atom or atoms with one or more unpaired electrons that seeks or releases electrons to other compounds in order to achieve stability, and in the process can damage cells or biological processes.

**ganglia** A group of nerve cell bodies located outside of the central nervous system.

**gastric lavage** A procedure used to empty the stomach of its contents, especially in the treatment of ingestions of toxins or drugs.

**gastrin** A peptide hormone that is secreted by the gastric mucosa; contributes to the secretion of gastric acid.

**gastritis** Inflammation of the mucous membrane of the stomach.

**generic name** Nonproprietary name assigned to a drug or chemical and recommended or recognized by an official body.

**gingival hyperplasia** Proliferation of gum tissue, sometimes related to drug therapy.

**glial cells** Specialized cells that surround neurons and provide insulation, mechanical, and physical support.

**glomerular filtration** Filtration of the blood through the tuft of capillaries at the origin of the nephron in the kidney.

**glomerulonephritis** Inflammation of the capillary tuft in the nephron of the kidneys.

**glomerulus** An intertwined mass of capillaries that is situated at the origin of each nephron, and through which the blood is filtered.

**glottis** The vocal apparatus of the larynx, including both the vocal cord tissue and the opening between the vocal cord and surrounding cartilage.

**glucocorticoids** A group of corticosteroids that affect carbohydrate metabolism, especially by increasing blood sugar, and that have pronounced anti-inflammatory activity.

**glucose** The sugar that is the end product of carbohydrate metabolism and the main source of energy for living things.

**goiter** Enlargement of the thyroid gland that can result from insufficient iodine intake.

**gout** Metabolic disease marked by painful inflammation, deposits of uric acid crystals in the joints, and an excessive level of uric acid in the blood.

**granulocyte** White blood cells that contain granules in the cytoplasm.

**gynecomastia** Excessive development of the male mammary gland.

**heart block** Disturbance of cardiac impulse conduction that delays or completely prevents movement of the electrical impulse from the atria to the ventricles.

**heart failure** Condition where inefficient contraction of the heart muscle results in reduced blood circulation; compensatory mechanisms lead to fluid retention and further deterioration.

**helminth** Parasitic worm, usually a parasite that lives in the intestine of a vertebrate.

**hematoma** Localise, semisolid mass of blood that collects in a tissue or space due to a break in a vessel wall.

**hematopoietic** Relating to, or involved in, the formation of blood cells.

**hematopoietic stem cell** Cell that gives rise to distinct daughter cells, including a cell that will reproduce and differentiate into mature blood cells.

**hemodynamics** Forces and mechanisms involved with blood circulation.

**hemolysis** Rupture of red blood cells with resultant release of hemoglobin.

**hemolytic anemia** Anemia caused by rupture of red blood cells.

**hemostasis** Physiologic processes that arrest bleeding.

**hepatotoxicity** Liver toxicity or damage.

**hirsutism** Excessive hair growth, especially male patterned hair distribution in women.

**homeostasis** Relatively stable internal physiological conditions (as body temperature or the pH of blood) under fluctuating environmental conditions.

**hormone** An endogenous substance secreted into the bloodstream, which causes a specific response in target cells, usually located at a distant site.

**hydrophilic** Having an affinity for, readily absorbing, or mixing with water.

**hydrophobic** Resistant to absorption of water or lack of affinity for water.

**hyperalgesia** Increased sensitivity to pain.

**hyperglycemia** Abnormally elevated serum glucose level.

**hyperkalemia** Abnormally elevated serum potassium level.

**hyperkinesia** Abnormally increased and sometimes uncontrollable motor activity.

**hyperlipidemia** Abnormally high fat or lipid levels in the blood.

**hypernatremia** Abnormally elevated serum sodium level.

**hypersensitivity** A state of exaggerated immune system reactivity to foreign substances.

**hypertension** Persistently elevated blood pressure.

**hypertensive crisis** Sudden onset of dangerously high blood pressure requiring immediate treatment to prevent organ damage.

**hyperthyroidism** Excessive activity of the thyroid gland that results in signs of increased metabolic rate, an enlarged thyroid gland, and other symptoms.

**hypertrichosis** Excessive hair growth.

**hyperuricemia** Abnormally elevated serum uric acid level.

**hypnotic** Drug used to induce sleep.

**hypoglycemic agent** Drug used to reduce blood glucose levels.

**hypokalemia** Unusually low serum potassium levels.

**hyponatremia** Unusually low serum sodium levels.

**hypothyroidism** Deficient activity of the thyroid gland that results in a lowered metabolic rate and associated symptoms.

**hypovolemia** Abnormally low volume of the circulating blood.

**hypoxia** Inadequate oxygen supply to tissues due to low oxygen levels in the blood.

**idiopathic** Arising spontaneously with no known cause.

**idiosyncratic** Of an unexpected nature; resulting from individual differences or peculiarities.

**ileum** The last segment of the small intestine.

**ileus** Obstruction of the bowel or intestine usually due to failure of peristalsis.

**immediate-release** Drug formulation with normal dissolution characteristics; not delayed release.

**immunity** Ability of the body to resist an infectious disease; classified as active, passive, natural, or acquired.

**immunization** A process that exposes an individual to antigens from an organism in order to create immunity to that organism.

**immunosuppression** Suppression of normal immune response to infectious agents or other antigens, often a result of medication use.

**incontinent** Unable to voluntarily retain urine or feces.

**indication** A disease or symptom that suggests the use of a specific drug treatment or procedure.

**infectious disease** Disease caused by the presence and growth of pathogenic microorganisms.

**innervate** To supply with nerves; to stimulate an organ to activity.

**inotropic** Increasing or affecting the force of muscular contractions.

**insomnia** Recurring inability to fall asleep or stay asleep.

**insulin** Peptide hormone secreted by the pancreas that regulates blood sugar levels.

**integrative medicine** An approach to medical care that combines use of conventional medical treatments and unconventional treatments (for example, homeopathy).

**interstitial nephritis** Inflammation of the renal tubules and glomerulus; often a reaction to a medication.

**interstitial** Situated within or between parts of a particular organ or tissue.

**intracellular** Existing or functioning inside a cell or cells.

**intramuscular** A route of drug administration that utilizes injection into the muscle.

**intrathecal** Within or introduced into the space between the organs of the CNS and the sheath that surrounds them.

**intravenous** Drug administration that utilizes injection into a vein.

**intravenous bolus** A dose of a substance given by intravenous injection; includes large initial doses used to rapidly achieve the needed therapeutic blood levels.

**intravenous piggyback** A small-volume, single-dose, sterile preparation used to administer medications into an IV line at specific times.

**intrinsic activity** Inherent ability of a drug to bind to and activate a receptor, especially as compared to the endogenous compound that activates it; i.e., agonists have greater intrinsic activity than partial agonists.

**ion** An atom or group of atoms that carries a positive or negative electric charge as a result of having lost or gained one or more electrons.

**ischemia** Inadequate supply of oxygen to a part of the body, such as the heart or brain, due to obstruction of arterial blood flow.

**isotonic** Denoting solutions possessing the same osmotic pressure, especially as related to the osmotic pressure of the blood.

**jejunum** The section of the small intestine that connects the duodenum to the ileum.

**larynx** The part of the respiratory tract that is below the glottis and connected with the trachea; contains the vocal cords.

**lethargy** Abnormal drowsiness or sluggishness.

**leukemia** A malignancy of the blood forming tissues that occurs in people and other mammals, and is characterized by excessive production of white blood cells.

**leukocytes** General term for any type of white blood cells.

**ligament** Tough band of fibrous tissue that connects and supports the bones in a joint or supports or maintains the position of some organs.

**limbic system** The parts of the brain that are concerned especially with emotion and motivation.

**lipids** Water-insoluble, biologically active substances that are important components of, and sources of energy for living cells; includes fats, steroids, and related compounds.

**lipodystrophy** Abnormality of fat metabolism especially involving loss of fat from, or deposition of fat in, tissue.

**lipophilic** Having an affinity for, or ability to absorb or dissolve in, fats.

**lithotripsy** A procedure that uses sound waves to break up kidney stones into pieces small enough to be easily eliminated.

**loading dose** Large initial dose or doses of a drug given at the start of therapy in order to rapidly achieve a therapeutic level.

**locomotion** Movement, or the ability to move from place to place.

**Loop of Henle** The U-shaped portion of the renal tubule in vertebrates; begins at the proximal convoluted tubule and ends in the distal convoluted tubule.

**lozenge** Small, flavored, solid, medication formulation designed to be held in the mouth for slow dissolution; also known as a troche.

**lymph** Clear fluid similar to plasma that passes from the blood, to intercellular spaces of body tissue, into the lymphatic vessels and contains lymphocytes.

**lymphocyte** White blood cells, differentiated in the lymphatic tissue; B and T lymphocytes are responsible for the production of antibody and other aspects of immunity.

**lymphoma** A malignant tumor of lymphoid tissue.

**macrophage** A phagocytic cell that arises from the bone marrow and moves out to tissues where it functions in the destruction of foreign antigens and stimulates other immune system cells.

**malaise** Generalized feeling of physical discomfort.

**malignant** Tending to deteriorate and respond unfavorably to treatment; tumors likely to invade nearby tissues and metastasize.

**malignant hyperthermia** Rapidly rising fever and hypermetabolic state that occurs as a reaction to some neuromuscular blocking agents and anesthetic agents, and that is often fatal.

**mania** Excitement and mood elevation of excessive proportions, marked by mental hyperactivity and irrational behavior.

**mastication** Chewing with the teeth.

**materia medica** Materials used in the composition of remedies, also a general term for all the substances used as curative agents in medicine.

**mediastinum** The space in the chest behind the sternum and between the lungs.

**megaloblastic anemia** Anemia characterized by the presence of megaloblasts in the bloodstream; vitamin B12 and folic acid deficiencies cause this type of anemia.

**meninges** The membranes that surround the brain and spinal cord: the dura mater (outer layer), arachnoid membrane (middle layer), and the pia mater (inner layer).

**metabolism** The total of all processes used by organisms to produce and maintain all cells and systems; also all processes used to handle consumed substances, whether nutrients, drugs, or toxins.

**metabolite** A product or byproduct of metabolism.

**metastases** Cancer cells from a primary tumor that move via metastasis to a secondary site.

**metastasize** To spread to another part of the body through the blood or lymphatic system.

**metered-dose inhaler** A device for delivering measured doses of aerosolized medication to the airways.

**micro-organism** A microscopic organism.

**micturition** Urination.

**mineralocorticoid** Any of a group of corticosteroids that primarily regulate fluid and electrolyte balance.

**mitochondria** Cellular organelles, found in eukaryotic cells, responsible for energy production and cellular respiration.

**monoamine** An organic compound containing only one amino group; examples include the neurotransmitters epinephrine, norepinephrine, dopamine, and others.

**monoclonal antibody** An antibody that can be synthesized in the laboratory with one population of cells.

**motility** Spontaneous movement, as in the movement of the gastrointestinal tract.

**mucosa** A mucous membrane.

**muscarinic receptor** One of two types of cholinergic receptor, muscarinic receptors are found in the smooth muscle.

**muscular dystrophy** One of a group of hereditary diseases characterized by progressive degeneration of muscles.

**mutagenic** Inducing genetic mutations.

**mycosis** An infection or disease caused by a fungus.

**mydriasis** Excessive or prolonged dilation of the pupil.

**myelin** A soft, somewhat fatty material that forms a thick protective sheath around nerve axons.

**myocardial infarction** An area of tissue death in the myocardium resulting from obstruction of the local circulation due to a blood clot; heart attack.

**myocarditis** Inflammation of the muscular walls of the heart.

**myocardium** The muscular walls of the heart.

**myoclonic** Related to, or describing, uncontrollable muscle twitching; i.e., a myoclonic seizure.

**myopathy** A muscle disease.

**myopic** Suffering from nearsightedness.

**narcolepsy** A sleep disorder that includes involuntary sleep episodes in the daytime and disturbed sleep patterns at night.

**narcotic** A drug that in moderate doses reduces the sensation of pain and other senses and causes sedation, usually applied to opioids.

**nares** Nostrils.

**nasogastric tube** A flexible tube that is passed through the nostril and nasopharynx in order to access the stomach.

**nebulizer** A device used to convert a sterile medication solution into an extremely fine spray for inhalation into the lungs.

**necrosis** Death of living tissue in a structure or organ.

**nephron** Single excretory unit of the kidney, where blood is filtered and urine formed.

**neurogenic** Arising from, or caused by, the nervous system.

**neuroleptic** Antipsychotic.

**neuroleptic malignant syndrome** A reaction to the use of antipsychotic drugs that includes rigidity, stupor, fever, and unstable blood pressure, among other symptoms.

**neuromuscular junction** The junction of an efferent nerve fiber and a muscle fiber.

**neurons** Any of the cells of the nervous system that have the property of transmitting and receiving nervous impulses.

**neuropathic** Of or relating to pathology of the nervous system.

**neuropathy** An abnormal state or condition of the nervous system.

**neurotransmission** Passage of signals from one nerve cell to another via chemical substances and electrical signals.

**neurotransmitter** An endogenous substance that carries a nerve impulse across a synapse.

**neutropenia** An abnormally low white blood cell count chiefly due to a shortage of neutrophils.

**nicotinic receptor** One type of cholinergic receptor, found in the skeletal muscle, adrenal glands, and ganglia.

**nit** The egg of a louse.

**noncompliance** Failure or refusal to comply with instructions for taking prescribed medication.

**normal flora** Micro-organisms expected to be present on body surfaces or in the intestines and that under normal circumstances do not cause disease.

**normal sinus rhythm** The normal and regular heart rhythm, generated by the sinoatrial node.

**nucleotides** Basic building blocks of nucleic acids, made up of amino acids (cytosine, thymine, uracil, adenine, or guanine) joined with a sugar.

**nystagmus** Involuntary, rapid side to side or up and down eye movement; may be an adverse drug effect.

**off-label** Use of a drug for an indication or use other than those approved by the FDA.

**oncology** The study of cancers or tumors.

**onychomycoses** Fungal infection of the nails.

**opiate** Drug derived from the opium poppy.

**opioids** Originally used to describe synthetic drugs resembling opiates; now more commonly used to include both natural opiates and synthetic relatives.

**opportunistic infection** Infectious disease caused by an organism that is not usually a pathogen; occurs because the patient's immune system is suppressed.

**oral** Pertaining to the mouth; route of administration of medication given or taken by mouth.

**orbit** The bony cavity or socket in the skull where the eye is situated.

**osmolality** Concentration of osmotically active particles in solution measured in osmols or milliosmoles per kg of solvent.

**osteoarthritis** Degenerative arthritis that usually begins during middle or old age, marked by pain, swelling, and stiffness.

**osteoblast** Cell that gives rise to bone.

**osteoclast** A cell associated with bone resorption or breakdown.

**osteomalacia** Softening of the bones in adults that is analogous to rickets in the young.

**osteomyelitis** Inflammation of the bone, usually caused by infection of bacterial origin.

**osteoporosis** Bone disease, mainly of older women, which causes a decrease in bone mass and more porous and brittle bones that can lead to fracture.

**otic** Relating to the ear.

**otitis media** Infection and inflammation of the middle ear.

**ototoxic** Toxic to the nerves and other anatomical structures involved in hearing.

**over-the-counter** Sold without a prescription.

**oxidation** Removal of one or more electrons from a compound through interaction with oxygen.

**palliative therapy** Procedures or drug therapy used to improve patient comfort, not to cure disease.

**palpitations** Unpleasant sensation of irregular or abnormal heartbeat, which may or may not be symptomatic of heart disease.

**pandemic** An epidemic that affects an unusually large geographic area and percent of the population.

**paracrine** Substance secreted by a cell that acts on nearby cells.

**parasite** An organism that must get nutrition and shelter from another organism in order to survive.

**parasympathetic** Referring to the parasympathetic division of the autonomic nervous system.

**parenteral** Introduced into the body other than by way of the intestines; usually relates to drug administration by injection.

**paroxysmal** Episodic recurrences or attacks of a disease.

**passive diffusion** The process whereby particles become evenly spread solely as a result of spontaneous movement caused by their random thermal motion.

**passive immunity** Immunity acquired by transfer of antibodies from another individual.

**pathogenic** Capable of causing disease.

**pathology** The study of diseases and the structural and functional changes produced by them.

**patient package insert** A drug insert sometimes required by the FDA and designed specifically to inform patients about risks associated with specific medications.

**pepsin** An enzyme that in an acid medium digests most proteins.

**peptic ulcer** An ulcer in the mucous membrane of the wall of the stomach or duodenum.

**peptide** A compound made up of two or more amino acids; many biologically active compounds are peptides.

**perfuse** To force a fluid through tissue, especially by way of the blood vessels.

**pericardium** The membranous sac that encloses the heart and the roots of the great blood vessels.

**periosteum** Tough, fibrous connective tissue that surrounds bones except the joint surfaces.

**peripheral nervous system** The part of the nervous system that is outside the central nervous system.

**peripheral neuropathy** Disease or injury to the nerves that supply sensation to the arms and legs.

**peripheral resistance** Resistance to the flow of blood in peripheral arterial vessels.

**peristalsis** Waves of involuntary contraction passing along the walls of the GI tract responsible for the movement of food to the intestines and waste through the intestines.

**peritoneum** The smooth serous membrane that lines the cavity of the abdomen.

**pernicious anemia** Anemia marked by a decrease in number and increase in size of the red blood cell and caused by vitamin B12 deficiency.

**phagocyte** A cell capable of engulfing and destroying foreign material, such as bacteria.

**phagocytosis** The process of engulfing and destroying foreign material, an essential part of the immune response.

**pharmaceutical care** Direct involvement of the pharmacist in the design, implementation, and monitoring of a therapeutic drug plan intended to relieve symptoms or treat disease.

**pharmacodynamics** A branch of pharmacology dealing with the reactions between drugs and living systems, including the correlation of effects of drugs with their chemical structure.

**pharmacokinetics** The study of the characteristic interactions of a drug and the body, including its absorption, distribution, metabolism, and excretion.

**pharmacology** The study of drugs, including their origin, composition, actions, uses, and side effects.

**pharmacopoeia** A book describing the drugs and preparations used in medicine, usually issued by an officially recognized authority and serving as a standard.

**pharynx** The anatomical area situated between and connecting the cavity of the mouth and the esophagus.

**phlebitis** Inflammation of a vein.

**placebo** A pharmacologically inert substance used in controlled trials to test the efficacy of a drug.

**plasma proteins** Dissolved proteins of blood plasma, including albumin and antibodies.

**platelets** A tiny, disk-shaped, nonnucleated body found in the bloodstream that plays a key role in blood clotting.

**pneumonitis** Inflammation of the lung.

**polycythemia** An excessive number of red blood cells and concentration of hemoglobin.

**polydipsia** Excessive or abnormal thirst.

**polyphagia** Excessive or abnormal hunger.

**polyuria** Excessive secretion of urine.

**posterior** Situated at or toward the back part of the body.

**postprandial** Occurring after a meal.

**postsynaptic** Pertaining to or occurring after the synapse.

**postural hypotension** Low blood pressure that occurs upon arising from a bed or chair.

**potency** Refers to the relative amount of drug required to produce the desired response; related to strength of a drug, not efficacy.

**precipitate** An insoluble solid that settles out of a solution; also the formation of such a solid.

**precocious puberty** Unexpectedly early onset of puberty that can be due to a disease process in the glands that secrete sex hormones.

**premature ventricular contractions** Early contractions of the ventricles that occur because of abnormal electrical activity.

**pressor** Tending to raise blood pressure or producing vasoconstriction.

**presynaptic** Pertaining to or occurring before the synapse.

**priapism** A persistent, often painful erection that is a result of injury, disease, or an unwanted effect of medication.

**proarrhythmic** A compound that causes or creates an environment that encourages arrhythmias.

**prodrug** An inactive drug precursor that is converted in the body to the active drug form.

**prokaryote** Typically unicellular micro-organisms that lack a distinct nucleus and membrane-bound organelles; for example, bacteria.

**prototype** The first example of a drug class to which subsequent members of the class bear significant chemical and pharmacologic similarities.

**provitamin** A vitamin precursor that is converted to the active form in the body.

**proximal convoluted tubule** The portion of the vertebrate nephron that lies between the glomerulus and the loop of Henle.

**pruritus** Itching.

**psychomotor** Pertaining to motor effects of cerebral or psychic activity.

**psychomotor seizure** Seizure type marked by complex sensory, motor, and psychic components.

**psychotomimetic** Inducing psychoses or psychotic behavior.

**pyrogen** A substance that, when in the bloodstream, causes fever.

**recommended dietary allowance** Amount of a nutrient that is recommended for daily consumption.

**rectal** Pertaining to the rectum; as in rectal suppository.

**rectum** The last portion of the colon that connects the colon to the anus.

**reflex arc** The pathway followed by a nerve impulse that produces a reflex.

**reflux** A backward flow.

**refractory period** The interval after the passage of an action potential in an excitable cell and before the cell recovers the capacity to respond to another.

**renal cortex** The outer part of the kidney, which contains the glomerulus and parts of the tubules.

**renal medulla** The center portion of the kidneys where the urine collecting system is located.

**resistance** The failure of an infection or other disease to respond to treatment.

**resorption** The loss of substance, for example bone mass, through normal or disease processes.

**resting membrane potential** The tiny electrical charge that exists in excitable membranes at rest.

**reuptake** Reabsorption of a neurotransmitter following the movement of a nerve impulse across a synapse.

**rhabdomyolysis** Destruction of skeletal muscle cells, which is associated with the release of muscle cell contents into the circulation and causes serious metabolic disturbances.

**rheumatoid arthritis** Chronic, inflammatory, autoimmune disease marked by pain and inflammation of the joints leading to eventual joint destruction.

**rhinitis** Inflammation of the mucous membrane of the nose.

**ribosome** Granular organelles found in the cytoplasm of cells and responsible for protein synthesis.

**saturable process** A process with a limited capacity; i.e., in drug metabolism there is a limited supply of drug metabolizing enzymes that must be free in order to proceed.

**schizophrenia** Major psychotic disorder characterized by disturbances in thought and mood.

**sebaceous glands** Oil producing glands that open into hair follicles.

**seborrhea** Abnormal secretion of oils on the skin, often accompanied by yellowish scales on scalp, eyebrows, and some areas of the skin.

**secretagogue** Substance that stimulates secretion.

**seizure** Abnormal electrical discharge in the brain.

**sepsis** An infection of the bloodstream and the systemic response it causes.

**shock** Profound disruption of hemodynamic and metabolic processes characterized by pallor, rapid but weak pulse, rapid but shallow respirations, and low blood pressure.

**sinoatrial node** Tissue that is the site of origin of the impulses that stimulate the heartbeat.

**somatic** Of, relating to, supplying, or involving skeletal muscles.

**spermatogenesis** The process of male gamete formation.

**standardized** To compare with, or bring into conformity with, a standard.

**stasis** Slowing or stoppage of the normal flow of a substance, as in blood circulation.

**status epilepticus** A prolonged series of seizures without complete recovery of consciousness between them.

**steady state** A state of equilibrium; especially related to drug serum levels.

**stereoisomer** Molecules with the same formula in which atoms are linked in the same order, but differ in their spatial arrangement.

**steroid** A group of compounds that contain a 17-carbon ring system; includes some hormones and sterols.

**Stevens-Johnson syndrome** A severe and often life-threatening allergic drug reaction that causes inflammation and sometimes sloughing of the skin and mucous membranes.

**stomatitis** Inflammation of the mucous membranes of the oral cavity.

**stratum corneum** The outer layer of the skin consisting of several layers of keratinized cells.

**striated** Marked by parallel lines or grooves; as in striated muscle.

**structure-activity relationships** Relationship between the chemical structure or make-up of a compound and its pharmacologic activity.

**stye** An infected sebaceous gland at the margin of an eyelid.

**subcutaneous** Beneath the skin.

**sublingual** Under the tongue.

**substantia nigra** Layer of pigmented gray matter in the midbrain that contains dopamine-producing nerve cells.

**substrate** A substance acted upon by an enzyme.

**supraventricular** Originating or occurring above the ventricles.

**surfactant** Surface-active agent; increases the emulsifying and wetting properties of a product.

**suspension** A drug formulation of fine, insoluble particles dispersed evenly throughout a suitable vehicle.

**sustained-release** A drug formulation designed to slowly release the active ingredient over an extended period of time; also known as delayed or extended release.

**sympathetic** Referring to the sympathetic division of the autonomic nervous system.

**sympatholytic** Agents that oppose the actions of the sympathetic nervous system or sympathomimetic drugs.

**sympathomimetic** Drug that mimics, or an effect similar to, the actions of the sympathetic nervous action.

**synapse** The connection between two neurons at which a nervous impulse passes from one to the other.

**synaptic cleft** The narrow space between neurons at a nerve synapse.

**syncope** Temporary loss of consciousness due to lack of oxygen to the brain; faint.

**synergistic effect** An effect from the combination of two drugs that is greater than the sum of the effect of the two substances acting alone.

**synovial joint** Mobile joint that is lined with synovial membrane and contains synovial fluid.

**syrup** Concentrated solution of sugar and water; in pharmacy, flavored and used as a vehicle for a medicinal substance.

**systemic** Affecting the entire body.

**systole** Stage of cardiac cycle where ventricular contraction and blood ejection occurs.

**tachycardia** Rapid heart rate; usually applied to rates >100 beats/minute.

**tardive dyskinesia** Neurological disorder with involuntary movements of the mouth, tongue, and limbs; often as a side effect of chronic use of antipsychotic drugs.

**tendon** Strong, fibrous connective tissue that joins muscle to bone so that muscle can initiate movement at joints.

**teratogenic** Causing or tending to cause fetal malformations.

**thalassemia** Inherited anemias that occur due to an anomaly in hemoglobin; they tend to occur especially in people of Mediterranean, African, or Asian descent.

**therapeutic effect** The positive, or desirable, effect expected to occur when a drug is administered.

**therapeutic index** The ratio of the dose expected to cause toxicity in half the population (LD50) to the lowest effective dose in half the population (ED50), important in comparing drug safety.

**thoracic cavity** Division of the body cavity that lies above the diaphragm; the chest, which contains the heart and lungs.

**thrombin** An enzyme important in the clotting process; converts fibrinogen to fibrin.

**thrombocytopenia** An abnormally low platelet count with an increased risk of bleeding.

**thrombosis** Development or presence of a thrombus.

**thrombus** Immature blood clot (mainly platelets) formed within a blood vessel and remaining at the site of origin.

**thrush** Superficial yeast infection of the oral cavity.

**tincture** A formulation of a drug in an alcoholic solution.

**tinnitus** The sensation of noise, such as ringing or buzzing, in the ear.

**tolerance** A need for increasing doses of a drug to achieve the same response.

**tonic-clonic** A generalized seizure (also known as grand mal seizure) with muscle rigidity, followed by shaking, ending with confusion and drowsiness.

**tonicity** The osmotic pressure or tension of a solution, usually in relation to the blood.

**tophi** Uric acid crystals deposited in tissues characteristic of gout.

**topical** Drug formulation designed for, or involving, application to and action on the surface of a body part, especially the skin, eyes, and ears.

**torticollis** Abnormal contraction of the muscles of the neck that results in abnormal carriage of the head; sometimes a reaction to the phenothiazine antipsychotics.

**total parenteral nutrition** Intravenous feedings that provide patients with all their nutritional requirements when they are unable to take nutrients via the enteral route.

**tourette syndrome** A neuropsychiatric disorder that is characterized by involuntary motor and vocal tics.

**toxicity** Relative degree of being poisonous.

**trachea** The trunk of the airway that connects the larynx to the bronchi.

**transdermal** Absorption through the skin into the bloodstream or a drug formulation that supplies active ingredient for absorption through the skin.

**transient ischemic attack** Temporary ischemia in a part of the brain caused by a brief loss of blood flow to that area and accompanied by a reversible loss of neurological function.

**trigeminal neuralgia** Excruciating, intermittent pain in the areas of the face enervated by the trigeminal nerve.

**troche** Lozenge.

**tumor lysis syndrome** Syndrome that occurs as a result of cytotoxic therapy and the large scale death of tumor cells; hyperuricemia, hyperkalemia, and hypocalcemia are common.

**tympanic membrane** The eardrum.

**uricosuric** An agent that promotes, or relates to, the excretion of uric acid.

**vaccination** The administration of a vaccine to a person or animal in order to produce immunity.

**vaccine** A preparation of killed or attenuated micro-organisms administered in order to produce immunity to a specific infectious disease.

**vascular** Relating to blood vessels or indicating an area is well suppled with vessels.

**vasculature** The arrangement of blood vessels in an organ or area.

**vasoconstriction** Constriction of vascular smooth muscle, which causes the inside of a vessel to narrow.

**vasodilation** Relaxation of vascular smooth muscle, which causes the inside of a vessel to widen.

**vasopressor** A drug that causes a rise in blood pressure by exerting a vasoconstrictor effect.

**vector** An organism, such as an insect, that transmits a pathogen from one source to another.

**ventricular arrhythmia** An abnormal rhythm of the heart beat that arises in the ventricles.

**vestibular system** The vestibule of the inner ear with the end organs and nerve fibers that function in mediating the sense of balance.

**virulent** A markedly pathogenic organism able to rapidly overcome the body's defense mechanisms.

**visceral** Of, relating to, or located in, the organs of the abdominal cavity.

**viscosity** A physical property of fluids that describes their resistance to flow.

**vital signs** The signs of life, specifically the pulse rate, respiratory rate, body temperature, and blood pressure.

**volatile** Readily changes state from liquid to vapor at relatively low temperatures.

**volume of distribution** The hypothetical volume required if the amount of drug in the body was distributed throughout the body at the same concentration measured in the blood.

**zoonosis** An infectious disease that can pass from animals to humans under natural conditions.

**zygote** A single cell formed from the union of the male and female germ cells at fertilization and capable of developing into an embryo.

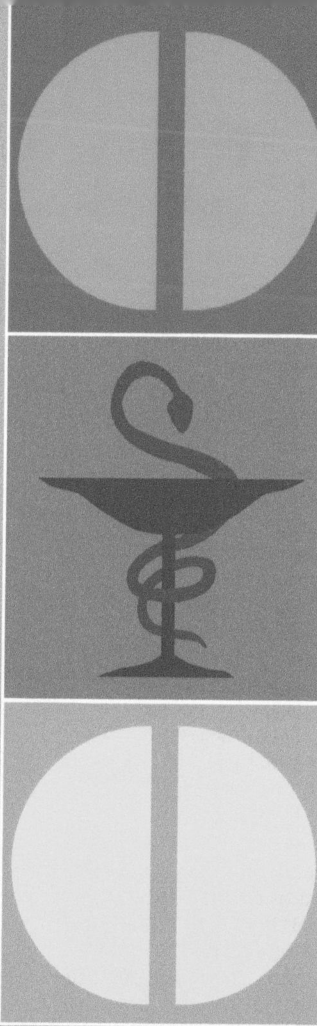

# Index

Page numbers in italics denote figures; those followed by a *t* denote tables.

## B

## C

## E

## Q



## R